Omega-3 and Omega-6 Polyunsaturated Fatty Acids in Food Systems

Advances and Opportunities in Product Formulation, Technology, and Delivery

Omega-3 and Omega-6 Polyunsaturated Fatty Acids in Food Systems

Advances and Opportunities in Product Formulation, Technology, and Delivery

Edited by

Pothiyappan Karthik
Department of Food Technology, Faculty of Engineering, Karpagam Academy of Higher Education, Coimbatore, Tamil Nadu, India

Bharathipriya Rajasekaran
Institute of Food Science and Technology, National Taiwan University, Taipei, Taiwan

Sajid Maqsood
Department of Food Science, College of Agriculture and Veterinary Medicine, United Arab Emirates University, Al Ain, United Arab Emirates

Tanmay Sarkar
Department of Food Processing Technology, Malda Polytechnic, West Bengal State Council of Technical Education, Government of West Bengal, Malda, West Bengal, India

ELSEVIER

ACADEMIC PRESS
An imprint of Elsevier

Academic Press is an imprint of Elsevier
125 London Wall, London EC2Y 5AS, United Kingdom
50 Hampshire Street, 5th Floor, Cambridge, MA 02139, United States

ISBN: 978-0-443-43810-3

For Information on all Academic Press publications
visit our website at https://www.elsevier.com/books-and-journals

Publisher: Mara Conner
Acquisitions Editor: Nicole Denis
Editorial Project Manager: Kritika Sharma
Production Project Manager: Jenela Priscy
Cover Designer: Gopalakrishnan Venkatraman

Typeset by MPS Limited, Chennai, India

Dedication

To my beloved mother, Jothi, father, Pothiyappan, and my loved ones, Sivasankari and Laksika, for their unconditional support and constant encouragement, which have been invaluable in molding my career. Finally, thank God for all.

—Dr. Pothiyappan Karthik

To my beloved husband, Pandiyarajan, my father and mother, Rajasekaran and Sumathi, and my brother, Balamanikandan, whose enduring love, guidance, and encouragement have shaped my path and strengthened my resolve.

With gratitude to God the Almighty for his boundless grace and presence in every step of my journey.

—Dr. Bharathipriya Rajasekaran

To my beloved mother, Arati Sarkar, father, Bholanath Sarkar, and sister, Tanusree Sarkar, whose unwavering love, support, and encouragement have shaped my journey.

And to God, for the strength and guidance throughout every step of the way.

—Dr. Tanmay Sarkar

To my students and researchers who have been an important part of my academic and research journey.

—Sajid Maqsood

Contents

8. High-pressure processing for retaining polyunsaturated fatty acids nutritional integrity

Sangeetha Karunanithi

Section III
Health and nutritional benefits

11. Docosahexaenoic acid and eicosapentaenoic acid in cardiovascular health: implications for functional food development

Monisha Prasad, Kalaiselvi Krishnamoorthy, Manoj Kumar Srinivasan and Muthu Thiruvengadam

12. Docosahexaenoic acid and eicosapentaenoic acid in inflammation regulation: opportunities in functional and nutraceutical foods

M.J. Rekha, K.L. Madhukala and Bharathi Suresh

Section VI
Advances in technology

Section VII
Case studies

31. Commercialization strategies for polyunsaturated fatty acid products with case study analysis: From concept to market

Sunayan Sharma and Soumi Chakraborty

32. Polyunsaturated fatty acids-based nutraceuticals and supplements: case studies and application in modern healthcare

Laureana de Quevedo Barcelos, Sergio Roberto Mortari, Elisângela Colpo and Carina Rodrigues Boeck

33. Polyunsaturated fatty acid utilization in emerging food sectors: case studies on technological advancement

Sureshkumar Sujithra, Ravi Sanjana, Kalaiselvi Krishnamoorthy, Safreena Kabeer, Kumar P. Kiran, Karthikeyan Velayutham and Pothiyappan Karthik

34. Polyunsaturated fatty acid-enriched foods in the market: case studies and strategies

Kalaivanan Rajalakshmi, Amit Ranjan, Govindharaj Sathishkumar and Munusamy Ajithkumar

Section VIII
Future opportunities

List of contributors

Billu Abraham Centre for Food Nanotechnology, Karpagam Academy of Higher Education, Coimbatore, Tamil Nadu, India; Department of Chemistry, Faculty of Arts, Science, Commerce, and Management, Karpagam Academy of Higher Education, Coimbatore, Tamil Nadu, India

Munusamy Ajithkumar Department of Genetics, Benchmark Genetics, Bergen, Norway

Sarra Akermi Laboratory of Microbial Biotechnology, Enzymatic and Biomolecules, Centre of Biotechnology of Sfax, Sfax, Tunisia

Plachikkattu Parambil Akhila Centre for Food Nanotechnology, Karpagam Academy of Higher Education, Coimbatore, Tamil Nadu, India; Department of Biotechnology, Faculty of Arts, Science, Commerce, and Management, Karpagam Academy of Higher Education, Coimbatore, Tamil Nadu, India

Sarojini Andiappan Paraprofessional Institute of Fisheries Technology, Tamil Nadu Dr. J. Jayalalithaa Fisheries University, Madhavaram Campus, Chennai, Tamil Nadu, India

Arfa Department of Nutrition & Dietetics, JSS Academy of Higher Education and Research, Mysuru, Karnataka, India

Kitipong Assatarakul Department of Food Technology, Faculty of Science, Chulalongkorn University, Bangkok, Thailand

Balakumaran Palanisamy Athiyaman Chemical Sciences and Technology Division, CSIR-National Institute for Interdisciplinary Science and Technology (CSIR-NIIST), Thiruvananthapuram, Kerala, India; Academy of Scientific and Innovative Research (AcSIR), Ghaziabad, Uttar Pradesh, India

Aria Babakhani Fisheries Department, Faculty of Natural Resources, University of Guilan, Sowmeh Sara, Guilan, Iran

Yuganthra Balaji Department of Biotechnology, Vel Tech Rangarajan Dr Sagunthala R&D Institute of Science and Technology, Chennai, Tamil Nadu, India

Tarun Kanti Bandyopadhyay Department of Chemical Engineering, National Institute of Technology Agartala, Jirania, Tripura, India

Ritesh Banerjee School of Biological and Environmental Sciences, Shoolini University, Solan, Himachal Pradesh, India

Laureana de Quevedo Barcelos Universidade Franciscana, Programa de Pós-graduação em Nanociências, Mestrado em Ciências da Saúde e da Vida, Santa Maria, Rio Grande do Sul, Brazil

Fakhreddine Ben Amara Laboratory of Microbial Biotechnology, Enzymatic and Biomolecules, Centre of Biotechnology of Sfax, Sfax, Tunisia

Bouthaina Ben Hadj Hmida Laboratory of Biochemistry and Enzymatic Engineering of Lipases, National Engineering School of Sfax, University of Sfax, Sfax, Tunisia

Carina Rodrigues Boeck Universidade Franciscana, Programa de Pós-graduação em Nanociências, Mestrado em Ciências da Saúde e da Vida, Santa Maria, Rio Grande do Sul, Brazil

Gokul C.S. Chemical Sciences and Technology Division, CSIR-National Institute for Interdisciplinary Science and Technology (CSIR-NIIST), Thiruvananthapuram, Kerala, India

Moufida Chaari Laboratory of Microbial Biotechnology, Enzymatic and Biomolecules, Centre of Biotechnology of Sfax, Sfax, Tunisia

Soumi Chakraborty Amity Institute of Food Technology, Amity University, Noida, Uttar Pradesh, India

Sook Chin Chew China-ASEAN College of Marine Sciences, Xiamen University Malaysia, Sepang, Selangor, Malaysia; Centre of Excellence for Sustainable Technologies for Agricultural Advancement and a Zero-Waste Economy (STARGAZE), Xiamen University Malaysia, Sepang, Selangor, Malaysia

Ahlem Chira Laboratory of Biomathematics Lr22es01, Faculty of Sciences of Sfax, Sfax, Tunisia

Elisângela Colpo Universidade Franciscana, Programa de Pós-graduação em Nanociências, Mestrado em Ciências da Saúde e da Vida, Santa Maria, Rio Grande do Sul, Brazil

Abhiramy D. S. Chemical Sciences and Technology Division, CSIR-National Institute for Interdisciplinary Science and Technology (CSIR-NIIST), Thiruvananthapuram, Kerala, India

Femil Selta Daniel Department of Biochemistry, Sri Ramakrishna College of Arts and Science for Women, Coimbatore, Tamil Nadu, India

Deeplina Das Department of Bio Engineering, National Institute of Technology Agartala, Jirania, Tripura, India

Vignaesh Dhanabalan Paraprofessional Institute of Fisheries Technology, Tamil Nadu Dr. J. Jayalalithaa Fisheries University, Madhavaram Campus, Chennai, Tamil Nadu, India

Mahdi Ebrahimi Department of Vet erinary Preclinical Sciences, Faculty of Veterinary Medicine, University Putra Malaysia, Serdang, Selangor, Malaysia

James Elegbeleye University of Pretoria, Pretoria, South Africa

Khaoula Elhadef Laboratory of Microbial Biotechnology, Enzymatic and Biomolecules, Centre of Biotechnology of Sfax, University of Sfax, Sfax, Tunisia

Olaniyi Amos Fawole Department of Botany and Plant Biotechnology, South African Chair in Sustainable Postharvest and Agroprocessing Research, University of Johannesburg, Johannesburg, South Africa; Postharvest and Agroprocessing Research Centre, Department of Botany and Plant Biotechnology, University of Johannesburg, Johannesburg, South Africa

Maryam Gharachorloo Department of Food Science and Technology, Science and Research Branch, Islamic Azad University, Tehran, Iran

Mehrdad Ghavami Department of Food Science and Technology, Science and Research Branch, Islamic Azad University, Tehran, Iran

Rakesh Kumar Gupta Agricultural and Food Engineering Department, Indian Institute of Technology, Kharagpur, West Bengal, India

Mayssa Hachem Department of Chemistry, College of Engineering and Physical Sciences, Khalifa University of Science and Technology, Abu Dhabi, United Arab Emirates; Food Security and Technology Center, Khalifa University of Science and Technology, Abu Dhabi, United Arab Emirates

Netravati Hiremath Department of Nutrition & Dietetics, JSS Academy of Higher Education and Research, Mysuru, Karnataka, India

Saeid Jafari Department of Food Science, Purdue University, West Lafayette, IN, United States; Department of Food Technology, Faculty of Science, Chulalongkorn University, Bangkok, Thailand

Vinay Jain Department of Pharmacognosy, ShriRam College of Pharmacy, Morena, Madhya Pradesh, India

Prajwal Jakhmola Applied Phycology and Food Technology Laboratory, Dietetics and Nutrition Technology Division, CSIR-Institute of Himalayan Bioresource Technology, Palampur, Himachal Pradesh, India

Mohammed Akram Javith Directorate of Extension Education, Tamil Nadu Dr. J. Jayalalithaa Fisheries University, Nagappattinam, Tamil Nadu, India

Sonia Jemli Centre of Biotechnology of Sfax, Tunisia; University of Sfax, Sfax, Tunisia

Safreena Kabeer Department of Food Technology, Faculty of Engineering, Karpagam Academy of Higher Education, Coimbatore, Tamil Nadu, India

Pothiyappan Karthik Department of Food Technology, Faculty of Engineering, Karpagam Academy of Higher Education, Coimbatore, Tamil Nadu, India

Masilan Karunanithi Department of Fish Processing Technology, TNJFU – Fisheries College and Research Institute, Tamil Nadu Dr. J. Jayalalithaa Fisheries University, Ponneri, Tamil Nadu, India

Sangeetha Karunanithi Food Technology, Vignan's Foundation for Science, Technology and Research (Deemed to be University), Guntur, Andhra Pradesh, India

Tafadzwa Kaseke Department of Botany and Plant Biotechnology, South African Chair in Sustainable Postharvest and Agroprocessing Research, University of Johannesburg, Johannesburg, South Africa; Postharvest and Agroprocessing Research Centre, Department of Botany and Plant Biotechnology, University of Johannesburg, Johannesburg, South Africa

Munazza Aslam Khan Department of Food Processing and Technology, Gautam Buddha University, Greater Noida, Uttar Pradesh, India

Kumar P. Kiran Department of Chemistry, Seshadripuram Institute of Technology, Mysuru, Karnataka, India

Prashanth Kotthapalli Department of Microbiology, JSS Academy of Higher Education and Research, Mysuru, Karnataka, India

Kalaiselvi Krishnamoorthy Centre for Herbal Pharmacology and Environmental Sustainability, Chettinad Hospital and Research Institute, Chettinad Academy of Research and Education, Chennai, Tamil Nadu, India

Srinivasan Krishnamoorthy National Institute of Food Technology Entrepreneurship and Management - Thanjavur, Thanjavur, Tamil Nadu, India

K.S. Krithiga Department of Food Technology, Faculty of Engineering, Karpagam Academy of Higher Education, Coimbatore, Tamil Nadu, India

Sumana Kumar Department of Microbiology, JSS Academy of Higher Education and Research, Mysuru, Karnataka, India

Rama Prabha M. Vellore Institute of Technology, Vellore, Tamil Nadu, India

Sameh Ben Mabrouk Laboratory of Biochemistry and Enzymatic Engineering of Lipases, National Engineering School of Sfax, University of Sfax, Sfax, Tunisia; Laboratory of Microbial Biotechnology, Enzymatic and Biomolecules, Centre of Biotechnology of Sfax, University of Sfax, Sfax, Tunisia; Faculty of Chemical & Metallurgical Engineering, Istanbul Technical University, Dr, Department of Food Engineering, Istanbul, Turkey

Aditya Madan Department of Food Technology, Parul Institute of Applied Sciences, Parul University, Vadodara, Gujarat, India

K.L. Madhukala Department of Life Sciences, Acharya Bangalore B-School, Lingadheeranahalli, Andrahalli, Bengaluru, Karnataka, India

Tendai Abgirl Makore University of Zimbabwe, Harare, Zimbabwe

Shreelekha Manthiri ICAR-Central Institute of Brackishwater Aquaculture, Chennai, Tamil Nadu, India

Mintu Martin Department of Food Technology, School of Engineering and Technology, D. Y. Patil Agriculture and Technical University, Talsande, Maharashtra, India

Tonderayi Mathew Matsungo University of Zimbabwe, Harare, Zimbabwe

Fatemehsadat Mirmohammadmakki Department of Food Science and Technology, Science and Research Branch, Islamic Azad University, Tehran, Iran; Medical Ethics and Law Research Center, Shahid Beheshti University of Medical Sciences, Tehran, Iran

Dharmendra Mishra Department of Food Science, Purdue University, West Lafayette, IN, United States

Shivani Mohan Department of Biotechnology, Vel Tech Rangarajan Dr Sagunthala R&D Institute of Science and Technology, Chennai, Tamil Nadu, India

Asma Moideen CMS College of Science and Commerce, Coimbatore, Tamil Nadu, India

Sergio Roberto Mortari Universidade Franciscana, Programa de Pós-graduação em Nanociências, Mestrado em Ciências da Saúde e da Vida, Santa Maria, Rio Grande do Sul, Brazil

Gurunath Mote Department of Food Technology, School of Engineering and Technology, D. Y. Patil Agriculture and Technical University, Talsande, Maharashtra, India

Brighton Marimanzi Mvumi University of Zimbabwe, Harare, Zimbabwe

Mondher Mzoughi Faculty of Chemical & Metallurgical Engineering, Istanbul Technical University, Dr, Department of Food Engineering, Istanbul, Turkey

Venkatachalapathy Natarajan National Institute of Food Technology Entrepreneurship and Management-Thanjavur, Thanjavur, Tamil Nadu, India

Yograj Neha Applied Phycology and Food Technology Laboratory, Dietetics and Nutrition Technology Division, CSIR-Institute of Himalayan Bioresource Technology, Palampur, Himachal Pradesh, India; AcSIR-Academy of Scientific and Innovative Research, Ghaziabad, Uttar Pradesh, India

Amiya Ojha Department of Bio Engineering, National Institute of Technology Agartala, Jirania, Tripura, India

Karthikanath P. R. Chemical Sciences and Technology Division, CSIR-National Institute for Interdisciplinary Science and Technology (CSIR-NIIST), Thiruvananthapuram, Kerala, India; Academy of Scientific and Innovative Research (AcSIR), Ghaziabad, Uttar Pradesh, India

Pavithra Palanisamy ICAR-Central Institute of Brackishwater Aquaculture, Chennai, Tamil Nadu, India

Dhivya Pandiyan Department of Food Technology, Faculty of Engineering, Karpagam Academy of Higher Education, Coimbatore, Tamil Nadu, India

Apoorwa Pathak Department of Pharmaceutics, Shriram College of Pharmacy, Morena, Madhya Pradesh, India

Namita Patil Department of Food Technology, School of Engineering and Technology, D. Y. Patil Agriculture and Technical University, Talsande, Maharashtra, India

Trust Mukudzeyi Pfukwa Department of Botany and Plant Biotechnology, South African Chair in Sustainable Postharvest and Agroprocessing Research, University of Johannesburg, Johannesburg, South Africa; Postharvest and Agroprocessing Research Centre, Department of Botany and Plant Biotechnology, University of Johannesburg, Johannesburg, South Africa

Monisha Prasad Molecular Nutrition and Genomics Laboratory, Department of Community Medicine, Saveetha Medical College and Hospital, Saveetha Institute of Medical and Technical Sciences, Saveetha University, Chennai, Tamil Nadu, India

Balasasirekha R. Avinashilingam Institute for Home Science and Higher Education for Women, Coimbatore, Tamil Nadu, India

Alireza Rabiepour Fisheries Department, Faculty of Natural Resources, University of Guilan, Sowmeh Sara, Guilan, Iran

Vijaya Raghavan Department of Bioresource Engineering, Sainte-Anne-de-Bellevue, Montreal, McGill University Canada, Montreal, QC, Canada

Kalaivanan Rajalakshmi Erode Bhavanisagar centre for Sustainable Aquaculture (EBCeSA), Tamil Nadu Dr. J. Jayalalithaa Fisheries University (TNJFU), Erode, Tamil Nadu, India

R. Rajam Department of Food Technology, Faculty of Engineering, Karpagam Academy of Higher Education, Coimbatore, Tamil Nadu, India

Devanampriyan Rajan Department of Food Technology, Kongu Engineering College, Erode, Tamil Nadu, India

Sankari Rajan Department of Food Technology, Kongu Engineering College, Erode, Tamil Nadu, India

Bharathipriya Rajasekaran Institute of Food Science and Technology, National Taiwan University, Taipei, Taiwan

Amit Ranjan Department of Fish Nutrition and Feed Technology, Tamil Nadu Dr. J. Jayalalithaa FIsheries University, Chennai, Tamil Nadu, India

Abiram Karanam Rathankumar Department of Biotechnology (FoE), Karpagam Academy of Higher Education, Coimbatore, Tamil Nadu, India

Sai Nandhini Ravi Department of Biotechnology, Vel Tech Rangarajan Dr Sagunthala R&D Institute of Science and Technology, Chennai, Tamil Nadu, India

M.J. Rekha Department of Life Sciences, Acharya Bangalore B-School, Lingadheeranahalli, Andrahalli, Bengaluru, Karnataka, India

Sandhiya S. Vellore Institute of Technology, Vellore, Tamil Nadu, India

Kongkona Saikia Department of Biochemistry, FASCM, Karpagam Academy of Higher Education, Coimbatore, Tamil Nadu, India

Karan Saini Applied Phycology and Food Technology Laboratory, Dietetics and Nutrition Technology Division, CSIR-Institute of Himalayan Bioresource Technology, Palampur, Himachal Pradesh, India

Maria del Rayo Sanchez-Carbente Autonomous University of the State of Morelos, Cuernavaca, Mexico

Ravi Sanjana Department of Food Technology, Faculty of Engineering, Karpagam Academy of Higher Education, Coimbatore, Tamil Nadu, India

A. Sarojini Department of Fish Processing Technology, TNJFU – Paraprofessional Institute of Fisheries Technology, Tamil Nadu Dr. J. Jayalalithaa Fisheries University, Chennai, Tamil Nadu, India

Govindharaj Sathishkumar GKSM, Department of Fish Nutrition and Feed Technology, Research & Development Department, The Waterbase Limited, Nellore, Andhra Pradesh, India

Faith Seke Department of Botany and Plant Biotechnology, South African Chair in Sustainable Postharvest and Agroprocessing Research, University of Johannesburg, Johannesburg, South Africa; Postharvest and Agroprocessing Research Centre, Department of Botany and Plant Biotechnology, University of Johannesburg, Johannesburg, South Africa

Eng Keng Seow Department of Food Science and Technology, Faculty of Applied Sciences, Universiti Teknologi MARA, Shah Alam, Selangor, Malaysia

Harish Sharma Department of Pharmaceutics, Shriram College of Pharmacy, Morena, Madhya Pradesh, India

Pankaj Sharma Department of Pharmaceutics, Shriram College of Pharmacy, Morena, Madhya Pradesh, India

Sunayan Sharma Amity Institute of Food Technology, Amity University, Noida, Uttar Pradesh, India

Knawang Chhunji Sherpa Academy of Scientific and Innovative Research (AcSIR), Ghaziabad, Uttar Pradesh, India; Environmental Technology Division, CSIR-National Institute for Interdisciplinary Science and Technology (CSIR-NIIST), Thiruvananthapuram, Kerala, India

Shivanand Shirkole Department of Food Technology, School of Engineering and Technology, D. Y. Patil Agriculture and Technical University, Talsande, Maharashtra, India

K. Shobana Department of Food Technology, Faculty of Engineering, Karpagam Academy of Higher Education, Coimbatore, Tamil Nadu, India

H.E. Shweatha Department of Nutrition & Dietetics, JSS Academy of Higher Education and Research, Mysuru, Karnataka, India

Keerthana Sivakumar Department of Biotechnology, Vel Tech Rangarajan Dr Sagunthala R&D Institute of Science and Technology, Chennai, Tamil Nadu, India

Slim Smaoui Laboratory of Microbial Biotechnology, Enzymatic and Biomolecules, Centre of Biotechnology of Sfax, Sfax, Tunisia

Manoj Kumar Srinivasan Saveetha Medical College, Saveetha Institute of Medical and Technical Science (SIMATS), Chennai, Tamil Nadu, India

Vidyashankar Srivatsan Applied Phycology and Food Technology Laboratory, Dietetics and Nutrition Technology Division, CSIR-Institute of Himalayan Bioresource Technology, Palampur, Himachal Pradesh, India; AcSIR-Academy of Scientific and Innovative Research, Ghaziabad, Uttar Pradesh, India

Jagan Karthik Sugumar Department of Food Technology, Faculty of Engineering, Karpagam Academy of Higher Education, Coimbatore, Tamil Nadu, India

Sureshkumar Sujithra Department of Food Technology, Faculty of Engineering, Karpagam Academy of Higher Education, Coimbatore, Tamil Nadu, India

Kalaivani Sundaravadivelu Department of Food Technology, Kongu Engineering College, Erode, Tamil Nadu, India

Bharathi Suresh Graduate School of Biomedical Science and Engineering, Hanyang University, Seoul, South Korea

Ajay Kumar Swarnakar Department of Agricultural Engineering, Triguna Sen School of Technology, Assam University Silchar, Assam, India

Muthu Thiruvengadam Department of Crop Science, College of Sanghuh Life Science, Konkuk University, Seoul, Republic of Korea

Vinoth Kumar Vaidyanathan Integrated Bioprocessing Laboratory, School of Bioengineering, SRM Institute of Science and Technology, Kattankulathur, Tamil Nadu, India

Karthikeyan Velayutham Centre for Nanotechnology, Karpagam Academy of Higher Education, Coimbatore, Tamil Nadu, India; Department of Food Technology, Faculty of Engineering, Karpagam Academy of Higher Education, Coimbatore, Tamil Nadu, India

Saranya Venkatajalam Department of Food Technology, Faculty of Engineering, Karpagam Academy of Higher Education, Coimbatore, Tamil Nadu, India

Ruchi Verma Department of Food Processing and Technology, Gautam Buddha University, Greater Noida, Uttar Pradesh, India

Anjaneyulu Vinukonda Formulation and Process Development, Strides Pharma Inc, New York, NY, United States

Fatemeh Zahmatkesh Fisheries Department, Faculty of Natural Resources, University of Guilan, Sowmeh Sara, Guilan, Iran

About the editors

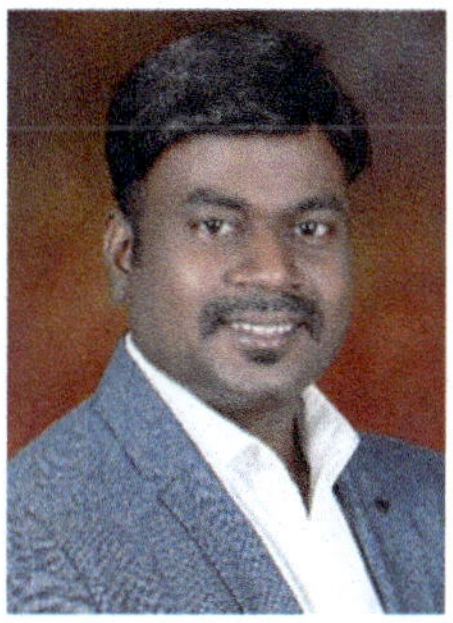

Dr. Pothiyappan Karthik is an associate professor and head of the Department of Food Technology, Faculty of Engineering, Karpagam Academy of Higher Education, Coimbatore, Tamil Nadu, India. He has done a PhD in engineering with a specialization in food technology at CSIR–Central Food Technological Research Institute (CFTRI), Mysore, Karnataka, India. He has experience as a postdoctoral fellow at Zhejiang Gongshang University, China. He has received a Senior Research Fellowship from CSIR for doctoral work, the Best Scientific Research Paper Award by CSIR–CFTRI, and the Young Scientist Award–2025 from the Academy of Sciences, Chennai. He is also a recipient of a funded major research project for sustainable utilization of millets from the Department of Science and Technology (DST), Government of India. His research interests include food nanotechnology, biopolymers, food colloids, nutraceuticals, and functional foods. His research is well documented with a total impact factor of 147 with 3193 citations, 18 book chapters, 2 granted international patents (Germany and China), and 1 Indian patent. He serves as an academic editor and editorial board member in the peer-reviewed international journals. He is the editor of two books to be published by Elsevier. He has been recognized as one of the Royal Society of Chemistry's outstanding reviewers lists for 2023 and 2024 (United Kingdom).

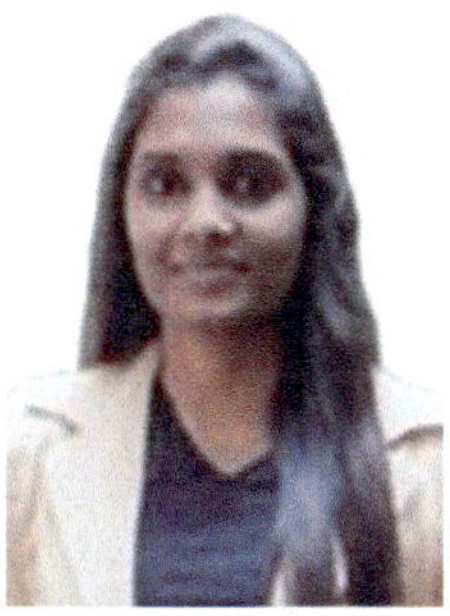

Dr. Bharathipriya Rajasekaran is a researcher at the Institute of Food Science and Technology, National Taiwan University, Taipei, Taiwan. She obtained her PhD in Food Science and Technology from Prince of Songkla University, Songkhla, Thailand, under the PSU President's Scholarship. Her research focuses on food nanotechnology, bioactive encapsulation, functional foods, and eco-friendly packaging. She has authored 21 peer-reviewed articles and 6 book chapters and served as editor for academic volumes published by Elsevier and CRC Press. She was honored with the Excellent Doctorate Thesis Award and has received multiple distinctions, including two scholarships, four research awards, one research grant, and two academic gold medals.

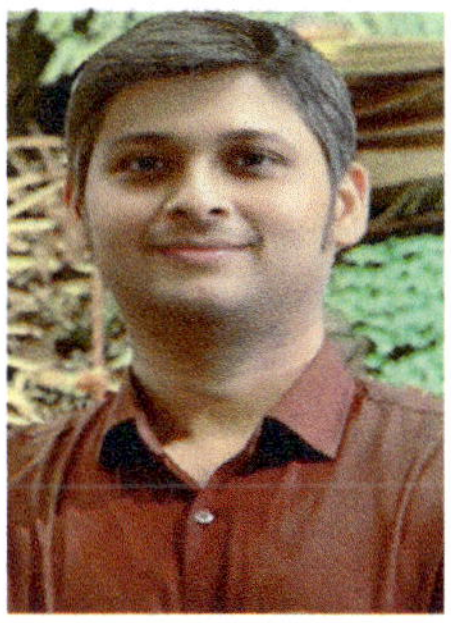

Dr. Tanmay Sarkar is currently working as a lecturer in the Government of West Bengal and as a visiting professor at the Center for Research and Development, Sri Eshwar College of Engineering, Coimbatore, Tamil Nadu, India. He has received his Bachelor of Technology, Master of Technology, and PhD in engineering from Jadavpur University, Kolkata, India. With 10 years of experience in both teaching and research, his areas of interest include bioactive components from natural sources, ethnic foods, mathematical modeling and AI, and phytochemicals. He is an editor for several SCI, SCIE, and Scopus-indexed journals and has edited 40 books with Elsevier, Springer, CRC Press, and Wiley. Dr. Sarkar has been recognized among the top 2% of globally highly cited researchers in the world rankings published by Stanford University, United States, for both 2024 and 2025.

https://orcid.org/0000-0003-3869-1604

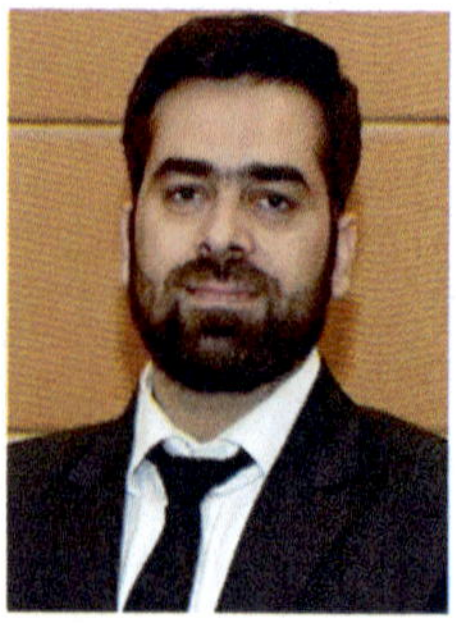

Sajid Maqsood is a professor at the Department of Food Science, College of Agriculture and Veterinary Medicine, United Arab Emirates University (UAEU), Al Ain, United Arab Emirates. His research is dedicated and aligned exclusively with the UAE's food and nutritional needs. He has established an innovative research program at the UAEU that focuses on bioactive molecules in camel milk and dates. Additionally, he is working on a circular economy of food waste and by-products generated during the UAE's agricultural practices and food processing phases. He has published more than 250 publications in highly reputed journals (mostly Q1-ranked) and was listed among the top 2% of highly cited scientists by a Stanford University-based study.

Preface

Polyunsaturated fatty acids (PUFAs), particularly omega-3 and omega-6 fatty acids, bridge nutrition, food technology, and health. Over the span of decades, eicosapentaenoic acid, docosahexaenoic acid, alpha-linolenic acid, and arachidonic acid have played a prominent role in shaping functional food innovation in a sustainable food system. Thus these lipids have carved their significance beyond basic nutrition.

This volume, *Omega-3 and Omega-6 Polyunsaturated Fatty Acids in Food Systems: Advances and Opportunities in Product Formulation, Technology, and Delivery*, assimilates the research foundations related to integration of PUFAs within modern food systems. It intricately carves the role of PUFAs in intelligent food designing. It showcases the integration of biochemical understanding with advanced processing, delivery technologies, and market strategy, highlighting omega-3 and omega-6 fatty acids as foundational components of next-generation functional foods.

The initial chapters establish the biochemical foundation, metabolic processes, and the emerging sources, including algae, microbial systems, and genetically engineered crops. The subsequent section explores stabilization strategies, encapsulation technologies, high-pressure processing, and structured lipid design, addressing one of the most persistent challenges in PUFA application: oxidative instability. PUFAs play a crucial role in health and nutrition, which is highlighted in the following chapters. It pivots around cardiovascular protection, cognitive function, inflammation regulation, and the expanding role of personalized nutrition.

This book is also an excellent reflection of the translational journey from the basic science of fatty acids to the engineering of innovative applications, which culminates in product formulation, commercialization, and sustainability. It caters to packaging, quality control, regulatory frameworks, and techno-economic analysis as well. A glimpse of real-world insights is presented in the last section through case studies of successful product formulation and market integration.

Aiming for food scientists, nutrition researchers, product developers, regulatory professionals, and industry leaders, this book can serve as an innovation roadmap for harnessing the full potential of PUFAs in building healthier and more sustainable food systems.

Section I

Introduction to PUFAs

Chapter 1

Introduction to omega-3 and omega-6 polyunsaturated fatty acids: sources and natural occurrence

Fatemehsadat Mirmohammadmakki[1,2], Maryam Gharachorloo[1], Mehrdad Ghavami[1], and Ritesh Banerjee[3]
[1]*Department of Food Science and Technology, Science and Research Branch, Islamic Azad University, Tehran, Iran,* [2]*Medical Ethics and Law Research Center, Shahid Beheshti University of Medical Sciences, Tehran, Iran,* [3]*School of Biological and Environmental Sciences, Shoolini University, Solan, Himachal Pradesh, India*

1.1 Introduction

1.1.1 Overview of omega-3 and omega-6 polyunsaturated fatty acids

Omega-3 and omega-6 fatty acids (FAs) are among the most important polyunsaturated fatty acids (PUFAs) that play a fundamental role in cell structure, regulation of inflammatory reactions, and physiological function in the body. These two groups of FAs are biochemically essential, meaning that the human body isn't able to produce them; therefore, they must be received through the diet (Balić et al., 2020; Gammone et al., 2018). Omega-3 FAs include three main types: docosahexaenoic acid (DHA), eicosapentaenoic acid (EPA), and α-linolenic acid (ALA) (Krupa et al., 2025). ALA is found primarily in plant sources like flaxseed, chia, and walnuts, while EPA and DHA are found in marine sources, including fatty fish like salmon, sardines, as well as fish oil. Omega-3 FAs are well known for their anti-inflammatory effects and have a pivotal part in heart, brain, eye, and immune system health (Burns-Whitmore et al., 2019; Saidaiah et al., 2024). These kinds of FAs can decrease the risk of cardiovascular disease, Alzheimer's, depression, and certain types of cancers (Das, 2008; Thomas et al., 2015). Omega-6 FAs are primarily known as linoleic acid (LA) and arachidonic acid (AA). The essential sources of omega-6 FAs include vegetable oils like sunflower and safflower oil, as well as seeds and nuts. The major sources of PUFA are shown in Fig. 1.1 (Alberio et al., 2016, Djuricic & Calder, 2021; Mercola & D'Adamo, 2023). Omega-6 is effective in the formation of eicosanoids, which play a crucial part in inflammatory responses, blood clotting, and immune function. Although omega-6 is essential for health, excessive consumption, especially when it is out of balance with omega-3, can lead to an increase in the amount of inflammation and a higher risk of chronic disorders (Djuricic & Calder, 2021; Zivkovic et al., 2011). The important thing about these two groups of FAs is their dietary intake ratio. Therefore, modifying dietary patterns by increasing the consumption of sources rich in omega-3 FAs and reducing sources with excessive omega-6 FAs can have a significant preventive impact on public health (Balić et al., 2020; Patterson et al., 2012; Simopoulos, 2002a).

1.1.2 Importance of identifying natural sources

Understanding the sources of omega-3 and omega-6 FAs is crucial, as these important compounds are obtained solely through our diet (Jones & Rideout, 2014; Rahman et al., 2024). A balanced intake of omega-3 FAs is important for controlling chronic diseases. Natural sources of these kinds of FAs enhance their health benefits by providing additional nutrients, including vitamins and antioxidants (Jones & Rideout, 2014; Krupa et al., 2025). These kinds of compounds effectively reduce blood triglycerides, improve vascular flexibility, enhance brain function, and support infants neural development during pregnancy (Banaszak et al., 2024; Jones & Rideout, 2014). ALA, seen in plant sources like flaxseed, walnuts, chia seeds, and canola oil, can also be converted to EPA and DHA in the body to some extent (Burns-Whitmore et al., 2019; Rizzo et al., 2023). Omega-6 FAs natural sources are mainly some animal products, seeds, unrefined

Omega-3 and Omega-6 Polyunsaturated Fatty Acids in Food Systems. DOI: https://doi.org/10.1016/B978-0-443-43810-3.00002-6

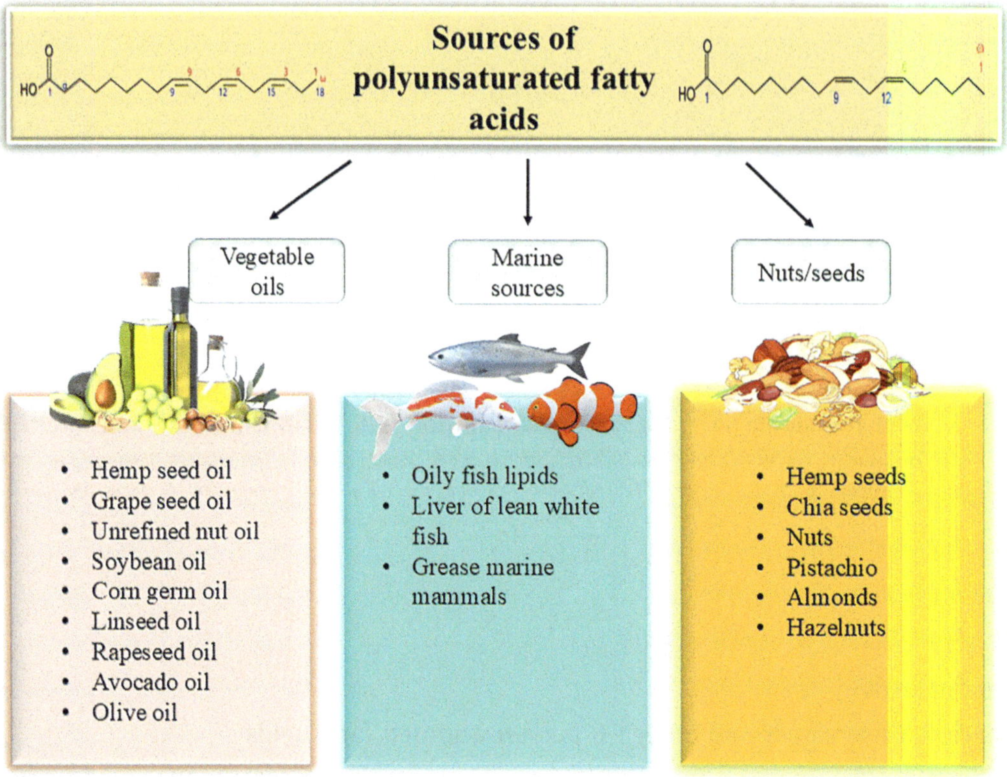

FIGURE 1.1 **Sources of polyunsaturated fatty acids (PUFAs).**

vegetable oils, and nuts. It is preferable to consume these sources in moderation, preferably in their unprocessed or minimally processed form, rather than industrial sources or processed foods containing omega-6-rich oils for general health. Excessive intake of omega-6 through a Western diet rich in industrial oils and processed foods can lead to increased systemic inflammation and metabolic imbalances (Haque et al., 2016; Kent, 2003; Rahim et al., 2023). Therefore, understanding the natural food sources of these two FAs groups and trying to contain them in the daily diet is one of the key strategies for promoting heart, brain, and immune health, as well as lowering the risk of inflammatory and chronic disorders (Liu et al., 2017; Tu et al., 2024; Velissaridou et al., 2024). It is also recommended that sources of omega-3 FAs in the diet be increased to maintain a favorable ratio of omega-6. A healthy, anti-inflammatory diet built on mindful, diversified, and natural intake is built on this equilibrium (DiNicolantonio & O'Keefe, 2021; Simopoulos, 2002a).

1.1.3 Factors influencing polyunsaturated fatty acid content in different sources

Several important and related subjects may be covered in order to understand the function and significance of PUFAs and to continue the preceding information. Each has a direct or indirect role in controlling overall health and creating efficient dietary plans (Mititelu et al., 2024). First, the biosynthesis and metabolism of PUFAs in the body should be addressed. LA and ALA, the key precursors of omega-3 and omega-6, are converted into more active shapes like AA, EPA, and DHA in the body with precise enzymes like delta-5-desaturases and delta-6-desaturases, as shown in Fig. 1.2 (Le et al., 2009). A major role in metabolic pathways is recreated by the competition for omega-3 and omega-6 for these enzymes. This rivalry can lower the conversion of ALA to DHA and EPA in food with extremely high amounts of omega-6 FAs, which eventually disrupts the metabolic equilibrium of FAs (Saini & Keum, 2018; Simopoulos, 2016).

The effects of PUFAs on inflammation and anti-inflammation are the next topic and are depicted in Fig. 1.2 Omega-3 FAs, particularly EPA and DHA, which are precursors of anti-inflammatory molecules that have a pivotal part in tissue regeneration, suppression of chronic inflammatory reactions, and prevention of autoimmune illness, asthma, and atherosclerosis (Simopoulos, 2002b; Zivkovic et al., 2011). Omega-6 FAs are crucial for immune responses but can

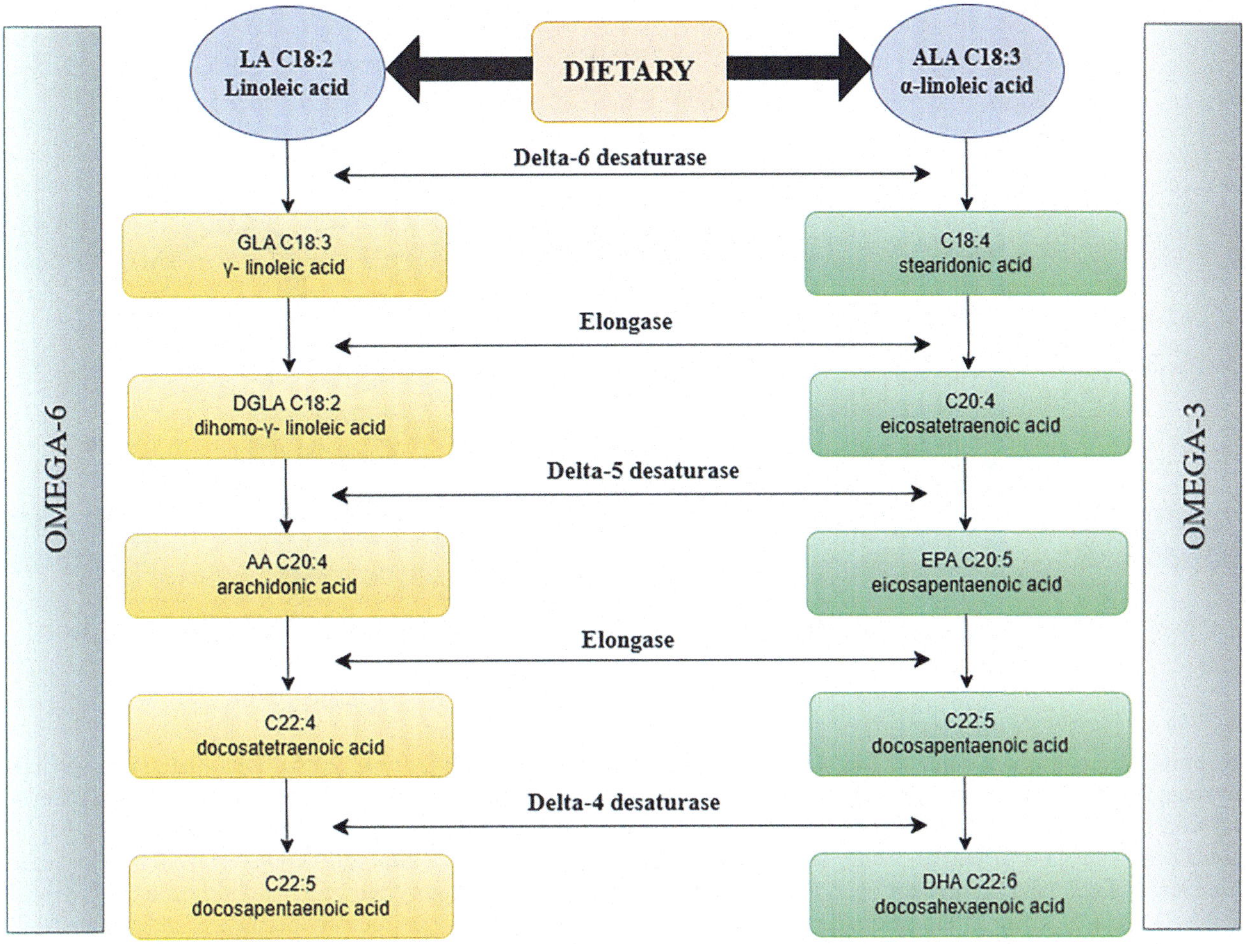

FIGURE 1.2 **Pathways of biosynthesis of unsaturated fatty acids omega-6 and omega-3 series (Simopoulos, 2016).**

promote inflammation if eaten excessively without adequate omega-3 FAs (Patterson et al., 2012). The stability and oxidation of PUFAs are important since their unsaturated structure makes them prone to oxidation from oxygen, light, and heat. This process creates free radicals and harmful compounds, decreasing the nutritional quality of food and potentially leading to cell destruction in the body and oxidative stress (Simopoulos, 2002a, 2016). The factors like PUFAs, proper storage of foods rich in avoiding excessive heating during cooking, and using suitable packaging are vital for obtaining their health benefits (Coniglio et al., 2023; Mititelu et al., 2025). Lastly, nutritional interventions and supplementation can also be examined. The use of supplements containing fish oil, DHA and EPA, can be advantageous for people who do not consume enough fish, especially in vulnerable groups such as heart patients, infants, pregnant women, and the elderly. Of course, choosing high-quality supplements with oxidation and heavy metal control certificates is necessary (Lange, 2020; Liao et al., 2022). All these parameters provide a clear picture of the medical, scientific, and nutritional significance of omega-3 and omega-6 FAs and highlight the demand for balance, quality, and awareness in consuming these compounds in the daily diet (Lange, 2020; Simopoulos, 2002b) (see Fig. 1.3.

eNOS: endothelial nitric oxide synthase, NO: nitric oxide, HSP90: heat shock protein 90, AMPK: AMP-activated protein kinase

1.2 Plant-based sources of omega-3 and omega-6 polyunsaturated fatty acids

1.2.1 Oilseeds and nuts

The diet's chemical solvents are the main source of FAs; therefore, edible oils significantly impact human health (National Research Council US, 1989a; Orsavova et al., 2015). The oil's composition of saturated, monounsaturated, and PUFAs

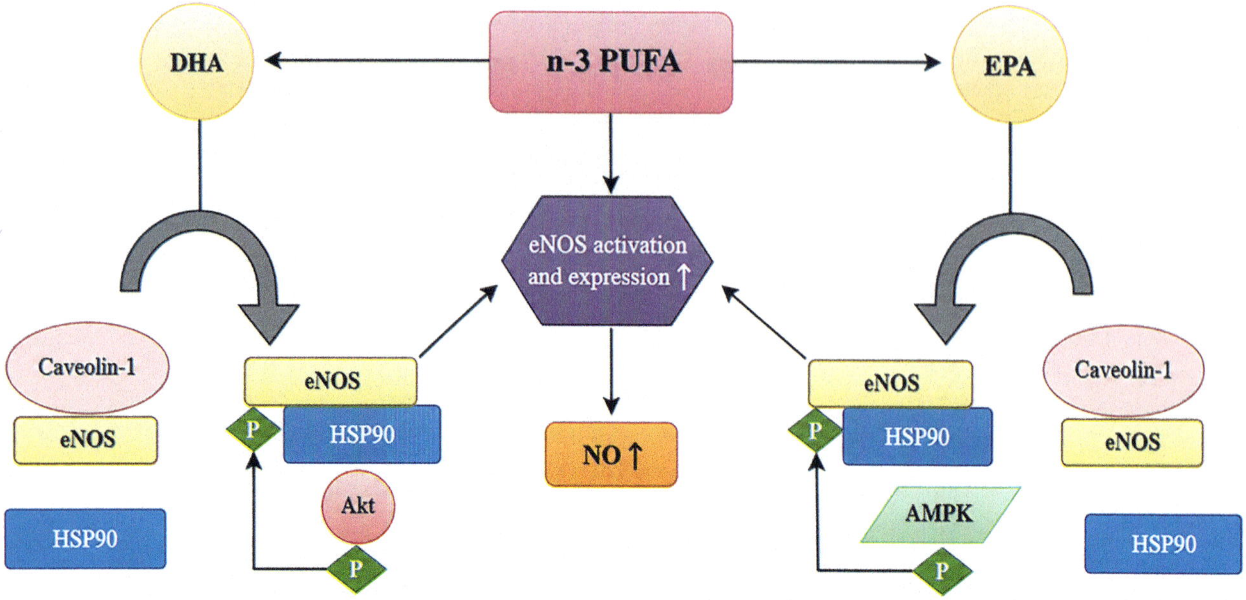

FIGURE 1.3 **n-3 polyunsaturated fatty acid (PUFA) mediated endothelial nitric oxide synthase modulation (Oppedisano et al., 2020).**

determines its nutritional value (DiNicolantonio & O'Keefe, 2022; Orsavova et al., 2015). Oils like sunflower, corn, soybean, and safflower are rich in LA (omega-6 FAs), the high consumption of which, without a balance with omega-3, can lead to increased inflammation. In contrast, oils like rapeseed and safflower contain ALA (omega-3 FAs) that help regulate the omega-6 to omega-3 ratio (Balić et al., 2020; Mariamenatu & Abdu, 2021). Olive oil, rich in oleic acid (monounsaturated) and polyphenols, is of interest because of its anti-inflammatory activities and improved cardiovascular health. In contrast, coconut and palm oils are more frequently utilized in the food industry because of their high stability and high content of saturated FAs (Isaakidis et al., 2023; Mehany et al., 2025).

Oil extraction and refining methods play a vital part in their quality. Mechanically extracted oils by cold-pressed retain their bioactive compounds better and are less susceptible to oxidation. In contrast, intensive refining with chemical solvents and high heat may diminish the loss of beneficial compounds and nutritional quality. Therefore choosing quality oils and paying attention to the ratio of FAs and extraction methods is crucial in ensuring nutritional health (Symoniuk et al., 2022; Wandhekar et al., 2022; Mungwari et al., 2025).

*1.2.1.1 Flaxseed (*Linum usitatissimum*): α-linolenic acid content and bioavailability*

Edible oils are crucial for lipid metabolism and overall body health as a significant source of dietary FAs (Zhu et al., 2025). The composition of saturated, monounsaturated, and PUFAs in each oil significantly determines its nutritional value. Oils like sunflower, corn, soybean, and safflower are great sources of LA (Ivanova et al., 2016; Orsavova et al., 2015; Ali et al., 2023; Zhu et al., 2025). High consumption of LA without adequate omega-3 intake can cause high inflammation. In contrast, rapeseed (canola) and flaxseed oils are high in ALA, which improves the omega-6 to omega-3 FAs ratio (Balić et al., 2020; Nguyen et al., 2018). Olive oil, which content high level of oleic acid (monounsaturated) and polyphenolic compounds, effectively decreases oxidative stress and enhances cardiovascular health because of its anti-inflammatory and vascular protective characteristics (Milena & Maurizio, 2025; Salvo & Tuttolomondo, 2025). Despite their good thermal stability, coconut and palm oils, high in saturated FAs, can enhance Low Density Lipoprotein (LDL) cholesterol when eaten in large amounts (Arias et al., 2023; Boateng et al., 2016).

Oil extraction methods affect oil quality; cold and mechanical extraction preserve bioactive compounds. On the other hand, harsh refining processes like high heat and chemical solvents can destroy sensitive FAs and decrease nutritional value (Li et al., 2023; Rahim et al., 2023). To preserve quality, proper storage of oils away from air, light, and heat is also crucial. Preventing chronic diseases, improving lipid metabolism, and advancing general health can all be greatly aided by selecting edible oils with knowledge of the omega-3 to omega-6 FAs ratio, variation in consumption, and appropriate processing (Calugar et al., 2024; Nagy et al., 2024; Mungwari et al., 2025).

1.2.1.2 Chia seeds (Salvia hispanica): nutritional composition and polyunsaturated fatty acid profile

Chia seeds (*Salvia hispanica*) are an important plant source of PUFAs, especially ALA, an omega-3 FAs. Almost 30% to 35% of chia's dry weight is fat, with a ratio of ALA to LA that is favorable, close to 3:1 (Khalid, Arshad, Ranjha, et al., 2022; Knez Hrnčič et al., 2019). This omega-3 to omega-6 FAs ratio has a vital role in lowering inflammation, supporting cardiovascular health, and balancing the metabolic balance of FAs in the body. Along with FAs, chia seeds have soluble and insoluble fiber, plant protein with a complete amino acid profile, minerals like calcium, magnesium, phosphorus, and iron, and B vitamins that help improve digestive function, decrease glucose and fat absorption, and enhance satiety (Djuricic & Calder, 2021; Simopoulos, 2002b).

Chia seeds form a gelatinous layer when mixed with water, which slows digestion and allows gradual nutrient release. Unlike flaxseeds, they can be consumed whole, but grinding them may increase the absorption of fats and micronutrients (Shydakova-Kameniuka et al., 2024; Waszkowiak et al., 2025). The presence of natural antioxidants in the seed structure also causes the high stability of ALA against oxidation. Frequent consumption of chia seeds as a "superfood" in plant-based and anti-inflammatory diets can help avoid metabolic illnesses and promote heart, brain, and digestive health (Jiang et al,. 2024; Agurla et al., 2024; Jeelani et al., 2023).

1.2.1.3 Walnuts (Juglans regia): polyunsaturated fatty acid contribution to diet

Walnuts (*Juglans regia*), one of the edible nuts with high nutritional value, are a rich source of PUFAs, especially ALA, a plant-based omega-3 FAs (Fan et al., 2023; Hayes et al., 2016; Thakur & Singh, 2013). Walnuts have almost 9% to 13% ALA by weight, which is a high quantity compared to other nuts. This makes walnuts the only common nut with a significant omega-3 content and helps improve the omega-6 to omega-3 FAs ratio in the diet (Ros, 2010; Zec et al., 2020). Walnuts also contain LA, an omega-6, but the ratio of ALA to LA is more balanced than in other plant sources. With their balanced PUFA content, walnuts may help reduce inflammation, protect the heart, and improve endothelial function (Djuricic & Calder, 2021; Zec et al., 2020). Although the ALA conversion rate to EPA and DHA is limited, ALA itself has beneficial effects on cardiovascular health.

Along with their unique fat composition, walnuts are enriched with natural antioxidants such as tocopherols, polyphenols, and melatonin, which contribute to walnuts anti-inflammatory and cardioprotective properties by inhibiting FA oxidation and reducing oxidative stress (Blondeau et al., 2015; Blondeau, 2016). Research has shown that regularly eating walnuts could lower LDL levels, lower the risk of cardiovascular disorders, and improve markers of inflammation. In addition to being tasty both raw and cooked, walnuts can lower the risk of chronic illness and support heart and brain health when included in a plant-based or Mediterranean diet (Banel and Hu, 2009; Kris-Etherton, 2014).

1.2.2 Edible oils and their fatty acid composition

Edible oils are an essential part of the diet, and their FA composition plays a fundamental part in metabolic health, regulation of inflammatory processes, and prevention of chronic illness. Each oil has a specific ratio of saturated, monounsaturated, and PUFAs that determine its nutritional quality (Chen, Ran, et al., 2023; Mititelu et al., 2025; Voon et al., 2024). Among these, PUFAs (especially omega-3 and omega-6 FAs) are particularly significant (Derbyshire et al., 2024). Oils such as sunflower, corn, and soybean are predominantly rich in omega-6, and their high consumption in the absence of adequate omega-3 intake can disrupt lipid balance and activate inflammatory pathways (Balić et al., 2020; Blasbalg et al., 2011). In contrast, canola oil and safflower oil, due to their ALA as an omega-3 FAs precursor, can improve the omega-6 to omega-3 FAs ratio in the diet and are therefore considered more suitable options for daily consumption (Balić et al., 2020; Lane et al., 2021; Simopoulos, 2016).

Olive oil is rich in polyphenols and oleic acid, which have important anti-inflammatory and antioxidant qualities despite having a lower PUFA content (Jimenez-Lopez et al., 2020; Tamburini et al., 2025). These properties, especially in extra virgin type of olive oil, help lower the risk of heart disorders and increase vascular health (Milena & Maurizio, 2025; Xia et al., 2022). On the other hand, oils like coconut and palm oil have high thermal stability due to the significant amount of saturated FAs, and prolonged usage of these oils may be linked to elevated LDL and compromised heart health (Boateng et al., 2016; Lordan et al., 2018). Also, the processing of oil as well as the method of its extraction significantly impacts its final quality; cold-pressed oils often retain their bioactive compounds, while industrial refining processes can reduce nutritional quality and increase oxidation potential. Therefore, informed choice of oil type and production methods has an important part in improving overall health (Mungwari et al., 2025; Durmaz & Gökmen, 2019; Lu et al., 2025; Momot et al., 2023).

1.2.2.1 Linseed oil versus canola oil: α-linolenic acid content and stability

Canola oil and linseed oil are vital plant sources of ALA, an omega-3 FAs. But, they differ significantly regarding ALA content, oxidative stability, and nutritional applications (Saini et al., 2021; Takić et al., 2024). One of the most abundant plant sources of omega-3 FAs is linseed oil, which contains 50%–60% ALA. However, because of its polyunsaturated composition, it is extremely vulnerable to oxidation under light, heat, and air. This suggests that safflower oil is mostly eaten raw and at low temperatures, and that it must be stored in dark containers at low temperatures to avoid the production of dangerous oxidative chemicals (Evans & Evans, 2009; Goyal et al., 2014; Rahim et al., 2023).

On the other hand, canola oil is renowned as a versatile oil for light cooking and raw ingestion because of its high oleic acid content, which makes it more resilient to heat and oxidation despite having less ALA (approximately 10%) (Falade et al., 2017; Moghadama & Moslehishad, 2020). This oil is mostly utilized in the food industry and home cooking. From the nutritional perspective, the combination of linseed and canola oil can effectively improve lipid balance, decrease inflammation, and enhance cardiovascular health in modern diets, where omega-6 to omega-3 FAs is often unequal (Abo Egila et al., 2023; Alagawany et al., 2019; Lin et al., 2013). Maintaining nutritional quality completely utilizing the functional qualities of omega-3 FAs requires careful, targeted, and selective consumption of these oils based on thermal conditions and the kind of application (Nagy et al., 2024; Usturoi et al., 2025).

1.2.2.2 Soybean and sunflower oils: high omega-6 concentration

Sunflower oil and soybean oils are globally consumed vegetable oils due to their wide accessibility, reasonable price, and relative stability at high temperatures. They are mostly used in the food industry and home cooking (Abrante-Pascual et al., 2024; Gharby et al., 2014; Mahmud et al., 2023). The balance of FAs in the diet has been seriously threatened by the lipid content of these oils, particularly the high concentration of LA, an omega-6 FAs. The omega-6 to omega-3 ratio might rise to a concerning degree due to the extensive use of soybean oil, which typically contains 50%–60% LA, in industrial products like margarine, sauces, and prepared dishes, as well as other sources of omega-6 FAs (Bilska & Krzywdzińska-Bartkowiak, 2025; Blasbalg et al., 2011; Mercola & D'Adamo, 2023). This imbalance causes enhanced activity of inflammatory pathways, formation of proinflammatory eicosanoids, and a high risk of cardiovascular, metabolic, and inflammatory disorders. Also, industrial processes such as hydrogenation can produce trans FA, which are known to compromise cardiovascular health by increasing LDL and decreasing High Density Lipoprotein (HDL) (Blasbalg et al., 2011; Iwata et al., 2011; Oteng & Kersten, 2020; Pipoyan et al., 2021; Raphael & Sordillo, 2013).

Sunflower oil is similarly high in omega-6 FAs (60%–70%), although, in recent years, modified varieties with high oleic acid have been developed to reduce the damage caused by unstable PUFAs. However, regular sunflower oil is still the most widely used type on the market and is prone to rapid oxidation at high temperatures, such as frying, producing harmful compounds (Akkaya, 2018; Chen, Zhao, et al., 2023; Ruiz-Domínguez et al., 2021). The optimum omega-6 to omega-3 ratio in the diet should be around 1:1 to 4:1, while in modern diets this ratio typically exceeds 15:1, increasing the risks of inflammation (DiNicolantonio & O'Keefe, 2021; Simopoulos, 2002a). Therefore, managing the consumption of the mentioned oils and gradually replacing them with the other oils that have a better balance between omega-3 and omega-6 FAs is an essential step in enhancing general health and decreasing the incidence of diseases like noncommunicable diseases associated with chronic inflammation (DiNicolantonio & O'Keefe, 2021; Simopoulos, 2002a, 2016).

1.2.2.3 Olive oil: balancing monounsaturated fatty acids and polyunsaturated fatty acids

Olive oil (extra virgin olive oil, particularly) is nutritionally superior due to its predominance of oleic acid (70%–80%), as an oxidation-stable monounsaturated fatty acid (Isaakidis et al., 2023; Majida et al., 2025; Milena & Maurizio, 2025; Mirrezaie Roodaki et al., 2016). This compound plays a significant part in regulating vascular health and preventing heart disease by lowering LDL, increasing HDL, and inhibiting inflammatory pathways. Olive oil also contains a balanced amount of PUFAs, including omega-6 and omega-3 FAs, with an average ratio of 10:1, but appears to be more balanced compared to other vegetable oils (Caffrey et al., 2023; Jump et al., 2012; Shramko et al., 2020). This feature and the presence of polyphenolic compounds, vitamin E, and squalene enhance antioxidant properties and reduce oxidative stress (Bucciantini et al., 2021; Cuffaro et al., 2024).

The relative stability of olive oil to moderate heat makes it appropriate for frying, light cooking, or using raw in foodstuffs like salads. In diets with a high omega-6 to omega-3 ratio, replacing olive oil with industrial oils such as soybean or sunflower can help restore lipid balance and reduce inflammation (Ambra et al., 2022; Nagy et al., 2024). Regular utilization of olive oil alongside marine sources of omega-3 FAs not only improves the dietary lipid profile but also has a crucial part in lowering the risk of chronic disorders and developing overall quality of life with its anti-inflammatory and heart-healthy properties (Banaszak et al., 2024; Bayram & Kızıltan, 2024; Gammone et al., 2018).

1.2.3 Legumes, leafy greens, and algal sources

Legumes, leafy greens, and algae are among the most effective plant sources of PUFAs, especially ALA, which are particularly important in vegetarian diets (Burns-Whitmore et al., 2019; Khalid, Arshad, Aziz, et al., 2022). Legumes like lentils, beans, and chickpeas provide fiber and protein, as well as adequate amounts of ALA, B vitamins, and minerals like magnesium and iron, which contribute to heart health and reduce inflammation (Burns-Whitmore et al., 2019; Guo et al., 2024; Khalid, Arshad, Aziz, et al., 2022; Polak et al., 2015). Although leafy greens such as spinach and kale contain lower amounts of ALA, they play an important role in improving vascular function, reducing oxidative stress, and reducing fat absorption with their high antioxidant, vitamin, and fiber content. Consuming these vegetables along with richer sources of omega-3 FAs, such as chia or flax seeds, is recommended (Ayaz et al., 2024; Crupi et al., 2023; Kalogerakou & Antoniadou, 2024).

Microscopic algae such as spirulina and chlorella are among the few plant sources that can directly produce DHA and EPA and, in the form of oil supplements, are a good alternative to fish oil in plant-based diets (Alagawany et al., 2021; Remize et al., 2021). These algae are rich in complete protein, beta-carotene, chlorophyll, and micronutrients such as iodine, in addition to omega-3 FAs, which are in plants effective in improving metabolic health and thyroid function (Podgórska-Kryszczuk, 2024; Wu et al., 2023). The bioavailability of plant-based sources is limited due to their fiber and antioxidant content. It is necessary to mention that consuming them with healthy fats and mild processing can improve absorption (Aydar et al., 2020; Nolden & Forde, 2023). Overall, including these food groups in plant-based diets is an effective way to provide omega-3 FAs and maintain an anti-inflammatory balance in the body (Banaszak et al., 2024; van Zonneveld et al., 2024).

1.2.3.1 Role of legumes in dietary polyunsaturated fatty acid intake

Legumes like beans, lentils, and chickpeas are well-known for their protein and fiber. This is especially important for vegetarian diets that lack marine sources. In addition, the presence of some bioactive compounds such as isoflavones in legumes with antioxidant and anti-inflammatory effects makes them an effective option for supporting cardiovascular health (Guo et al., 2024; Merdzhanova et al., 2021; Khalid, Arshad, Ranjha, et al., 2022). Leafy vegetables, despite their small contribution to the supply of ALA, also have a complementary part in enhancing lipid and oxidative stress reduction due to their richness in antioxidants such as polyphenols (Hassanpour & Doroudi, 2023; Michalak, 2022).

In addition to these sources, microalgae hold a special place in plant-based diets because, unlike most plant sources that only provide ALA, they directly produce DHA and EPA, long-chain FAs that are important for brain and heart health. Oils extracted from these algae are famous as plant-based omega-3 FAs supplements, especially among vegans, and are an effective alternative to fish oil. A balanced and diverse combination of these three food groups can help to efficiently provide PUFAs, lower inflammation, and promote overall health in plant-based diets (Merdzhanova et al., 2021; Barta et al., 2021; Jesionowska et al., 2023; Santigosa et al., 2021).

1.2.3.2 Marine algae: a sustainable source of eicosapentaenoic acid and docosahexaenoic acid

Seaweeds are a natural, sustainable, and beneficial source of long-chain omega-3 FAs like EPA and DHA because they are the main producers of these essential compounds in the marine food chain. This is especially true for vegetarian and vegan diets. Oil derived from algae is highly accessible, free of pollutants like mercury, and an excellent option for people who are sensitive to fish flavor, in contrast to animal sources like fatty fish. Growing algae is very environmentally sustainable, doesn't require freshwater or cropland, and helps reduce overfishing and store carbon dioxide from the ocean (Gladyshev & Sushchik, 2019; Oliver et al., 2020; Rocha et al., 2021). Along with essential FAs, algal oil also has natural antioxidants. Like carotenoids and chlorophyll, which make EPA and DHA more stable against oxidation, are significant antioxidants. Additionally, algae are rich in minerals (like magnesium and iron), making them a rich source of nutrients for promoting cardiac health, cognitive function, and lowering chronic inflammation (Kratzer & Murkovic, 2021; Michalak, Tiwari, et al., 2022; Sathasivam et al., 2019).

1.3 Animal-based sources of omega-3 and omega-6 polyunsaturated fatty acids

1.3.1 Marine sources: fish and seafood

Animal sources of PUFAs, especially omega-3 and omega-6 FAs, have an important role in providing the active forms of these FAs, like EPA and DHA, in the diet. Fatty fish are enriched with omega-3 FAs as they live in cold waters and feed on plankton (Alagawany et al., 2019; Saini & Keum, 2018). Regular consumption of fatty fish has been associated with improved vascular function, decreased blood triglycerides, and a lower risk of cardiac disorders. DHA-fortified eggs and grass-fed meat can also enhance the omega-3 to omega-6 ratio. On the other hand, processed animal sources or grain-fed usually are high in the amount of omega-6 (Hooper et al., 2004; McMullan et al., 2023). One of the most crucial points is that consuming large quantities of omega-3 FAs might raise the risk of chronic illness and inflammation (omega-3 FAs should be balanced with other nutrients). As a result, these sources must be used carefully, focusing on their natural origins, quality, and preserving a balance of vital fats (Rittenhouse et al., 2025; Simopoulos, 2002b).

Marine sources, like oily fish, are regarded as the most effective natural sources of EPA and DHA. Unlike plant sources, these don't need enzymatic conversion and have high bioavailability. Consuming food like oily fish (such as salmon, herring, and sardines) can play a vital part in lowering blood pressure, preventing atherosclerosis, and improving brain function (Alijani et al., 2025; Rodrigues et al., 2024). Seafood also has omega-3 FAs, but at reduced levels than oily fish. There are concerns about contamination of heavy metals in large marine species. Consuming seafood on a regular basis could enhance lipid profiles, prevent chronic diseases, and drastically decrease inflammation (Abera & Adimas, 2024; Zhuzzhassarova et al., 2024).

1.3.1.1 Cold-water fatty fish (salmon, mackerel, sardines) as rich sources of eicosapentaenoic acid and docosahexaenoic acid

Cold-water fatty fish (salmon, mackerel, and sardines) are one of the best sources of EPA and DHA, long-chain omega-3 FAs that have an essential part in heart health, brain function, reducing inflammation, and preventing diseases such as type 2 diabetes and Alzheimer's (Oliver et al., 2020; Rodrigues et al., 2024). Salmon (especially wild-caught salmon) is high in omega-3 FAs and rich in protein, vitamin D, and the antioxidant astaxanthin. Mackerel is also a great source of healthy fats, vitamin B12, and selenium, and its consumption could improve blood pressure and reduce triglycerides. Along with containing EPA and DHA, sardines are less contaminated and are a good source of calcium and vitamin B12 due to their short life cycle and low position in the food chain (Abera & Adimas, 2024; Awuchi et al., 2022; Hustad et al., 2022).

There are advantages to these kinds of oils. Fish offer a key advantage over plant sources of omega-3 FAs by providing direct DHA and EPA without requiring enzymatic conversion (which is beneficial for those with low metabolic capacity), like the elderly (Jerab et al., 2025; Krupa et al., 2024; Saini et al., 2021). To risk reduction of heavy metal contamination, it's best to choose smaller fish such as sardines or wild salmon. consuming excat amount of these kinds of fish per week, as recommended internationally, is an effective way to boost omega-3 FAs intake, support heart and brain health, and reduce inflammation (Abera & Adimas, 2024; Mititelu et al., 2025; Santos et al., 2023).

1.3.1.2 Shellfish and crustaceans: variability in polyunsaturated fatty acid content

Shellfish and crustaceans are important marine sources of PUFAs, especially omega-3 FAs like EPA and DHA, and their lipid composition is strongly influenced by species, habitat, and diet (Monteiro et al., 2024; Van Vliet et al., 2021). Crustaceans such as shrimp, crab, and lobster, although lower in PUFA, also contain high-quality protein and antioxidants such as astaxanthin, which protect lipids and reduce oxidative stress (Cholidis et al., 2024; Peng and Zhang, 2025; Šimat et al., 2022).

The lipid composition of crustaceans also varies depending on the culture environment; wild-caught fish typically have a more favorable ratio of omega-3 to omega-6, while farm-raised fish fed industrial feed may upset this balance (Alfio et al., 2021; Jensen et al., 2020; Roy et al., 2022). Despite the many nutritional benefits, eating wisely and selecting safe sources is crucial, as a few shellfish are susceptible to contamination with heavy metals. Finally, eating foods like crustaceans and shellfish along with other omega-3 FAs sources can support a number of bodily functions, including dietary fat balance, cardiac health, and brain function (Barchiesi et al., 2020; Demelash Abera & Alefe Adimas, 2024; Milanković et al., 2024).

1.3.1.3 Farmed versus wild fish: impact of diet on fatty acid profile

The composition of wild and farmed fish FAs differs significantly, largely due to their diets. Wild fish (like Alaskan salmon, sardines, and mackerel), which feed on plankton and algae in their natural habitat, contain high levels of EPA and

DHA and an optimal ratio of omega-3 to omega-6 FAs (Cahu et al., 2004; Fernandez-Jover et al., 2007; Taşbozan & Gökçe, 2017). This fat blend is linked to reduced inflammation, improved heart health, and cognitive function, while farmed fish (which are fed diets rich in grains and vegetable oils) tend to have a higher proportion of omega-6 FAs, lower omega-3 FAs, and a more unfavorable fat ratio. This situation can negatively impact the body's inflammatory balance (Banaszak et al., 2024; Daley et al., 2010; Rodrigues et al., 2024).

In addition to differences in FAs, wild fish tend to have higher levels of bioactive compounds such as astaxanthin, while farmed fish may have lower levels in this regard. Some advanced farms try to improve fat quality by adding algae oil or fish oil to the diet, but these approaches are expensive and less common (Alfio et al., 2021; Awuchi et al., 2022; Tsoupras et al., 2022). Lastly, based on nutritional quality, availability, sustainability of the catch, and environmental risks, an informed choice between farmed and wild fish should be made. A balanced intake of both types in the diet, along with consideration of the source and quality of production, can help to provide adequate omega-3 FAs and support overall health (Awuchi et al., 2022; Farmery et al., 2018; Pounds et al., 2022; Tsoupras et al., 2022).

1.3.2 Terrestrial animal sources

In modern diets, land-based animal sources like red meat, poultry, eggs, and dairy products provide most PUFAs, especially omega-6 FAs. However, the animal's diet strongly influences the composition of these FAs (Alagawany et al., 2019; Jeong et al., 2024; Mititelu et al., 2025). Grass-fed and herb-fed animals have meat and dairy products with a higher ratio of omega-3 to omega-6 FAs than grain-fed animals. Grass-fed and herb-fed animals also contain CLA (which has anti-inflammatory and anticancer effects) (Daley et al., 2010; Van Vliet et al., 2025). In contrast, corn- and soy-based diets increase omega-6 levels and disrupt the optimal lipid balance. Chickens fed omega-3 seeds like flaxseed produce eggs that are rich in DHA, which is beneficial for heart and brain health (Alagawany et al., 2019; Simopoulos, 2016; Usturoi et al., 2025).

Dairy products from pasture-raised animals also positively reduce inflammation and promote cardiovascular health due to their more favorable composition of FAs, especially omega-3 FAs and CLA. Diet in pigs also has a significant part in determining the ratio of PUFA; the use of ALA-rich sources can improve the fat quality of their meat (Fabjanowska et al., 2023; Jeong et al., 2024; Mollica et al., 2021). In summary, the conscious choice of livestock products of natural origin and proper nutrition (including pasture-raised dairy products, meat, and fortified eggs) is an effective strategy to improve the omega-3 to omega-6 ratio, decrease the risk of chronic diseases, and promote general health (Daley et al., 2010; Usturoi et al., 2025).

1.3.2.1 Ruminant meat and dairy: influence of grass-fed versus grain-fed diets

The diet strongly influences the fat composition of some products, like dairy and meat products from ruminants such as cattle, sheep, and goats. Grass-fed animals produce meat and dairy products with a higher ratio of omega-3 to omega-6 and higher amounts of conjugated linoleic acid (CLA) (Mollica et al., 2021; Ponnampalam et al., 2024). This fat compound is associated with anti-inflammatory, anticancer, and cardiovascular health protection. The natural diet of animals also increases the presence of antioxidants such as polyphenols in fat tissue, improving the nutritional quality of the products. In contrast, grain-fed diets increase omega-6 FAs, decrease the omega-3 FAs ratio, and are also associated with a high risk of chronic inflammation and heart disorders. These animals' meat and dairy products are often fattier, have lower nutritional value, and have fewer protective properties (Basak & Duttaroy, 2020; Cuchillo-Hilario et al., 2024; den Hartigh, 2019).

Grass-fed dairy products (like milk and butter) offer similar benefits and contain more CLA and omega-3 FAs, which help improve heart function and lower the risk of disorders like metabolic diseases. On the other hand, these products cost more; their higher nutritional value, better balance of FAs, and more sustainable farming methods make them a superior option for overall health (Alothman et al., 2019; Badawy et al., 2023; Grille et al., 2024; Pilar Gómez-Cortés et al., 2018). Making a conscious choice of pasture-raised meat and dairy can improve diet quality, maintain fat balance, and promote metabolic and immune health (Pânzaru et al., 2024; Vliet et al., 2021).

1.3.2.2 Poultry and eggs: omega-6 to omega-3 ratio in modern farming

Important sources of animal protein in the modern diet, like poultry and eggs, have a unique fat composition that industrial farming methods have heavily influenced. One of the most significant challenges in consuming these products is the unbalanced omega-6 to omega-3 ratio resulting from diets based on grains and oilseeds in industrial poultry farms (Alagawany et al., 2019; Cartoni Mancinelli et al., 2022; Usturoi et al., 2025).

In modern agriculture, poultry is typically fed with diets containing corn, soybeans, and other grains that are rich in LA, an omega-6 FAs. This dietary composition results in chicken meat and eggs with high levels of omega-6 FAs and much lower levels of omega-3 FAs (Alagawany et al., 2019; Attia et al., 2024). In contrast, free-range poultry farming methods or the use of omega-3-rich feeds such as flaxseed, algae, or fishmeal can help improve this ratio. Eggs produced in an omega-3-enriched manner can provide a better ratio of omega-3 to omega-6 by feeding the hens a diet rich in DHA or ALA. From a public health perspective, changes in poultry feeding practices can significantly impact the quality of fats found in meat and eggs (Ehr et al., 2017; Feng et al., 2020; Madacussengua et al., 2025).

There is an effective approach to improving the quality of poultry products to increase consumer awareness of the importance of FA balance and to prefer organic or fortified products. Also, using other food sources, such as fatty fish and omega-3-rich vegetable oils, can help compensate for the omega-3 FAs deficiency in diets high in industrially produced foodstuffs (Alagawany et al., 2019; Ali et al., 2022; Rodrigues et al., 2024). To protect public health and lower the risk of diseases linked to lipid imbalance, it is important to consume poultry products mindfully, particularly those from sources that prioritize natural farming practices. Improving community health and helping reduce cardiovascular issues can be significantly implemented by sustainable agricultural policies that enhance the quality of poultry nutrition (Connolly & Campbell, 2023; Grace et al., 2024; Marangoni et al., 2015).

1.3.2.3 Omega-3-enriched animal products: nutritional and functional benefits

Animal products that are enriched with omega-3, such as eggs, meat, and dairy, are produced by purposefully feeding livestock with sources like flaxseed, fish oil, or algae, and are designed to increase EPA and DHA content. These products effectively reduce blood triglycerides, improve lipid profiles, and reduce inflammation by improving fat composition, especially increasing DHA, and can be a suitable alternative for people whose fish intake is limited in their diet (Alagawany et al., 2019; Bourre, 2005; Konieczka et al., 2017). Enriched eggs are among the most successful examples in this area, and dairy products from animals fed with ALA-rich sources also contain more CLA and omega-3 and have higher nutritional value. From a physiological perspective, omega-3 FAs play a key role in heart disease prevention, type 2 diabetes, and cognitive disorders by improving cell membrane flexibility and vascular function and reducing inflammation (Nguyen et al., 2019; Patel et al., 2022; Usturoi et al., 2025). Despite challenges such as the high cost of production and difficulty in maintaining the stability of fats in processing, increasing public awareness has led to the growth of the market for these products. Ultimately, conscious and regular consumption of animal products enriched with omega-3 FAs is an effective strategy for promoting general health and improving the balance of dietary fat intake (Clemente-Suárez et al., 2023; Usturoi et al., 2025).

1.4 Environmental and agricultural factors affecting polyunsaturated fatty acid composition

1.4.1 Influence of soil and climate on polyunsaturated fatty acid content in plants

Plants are directly influenced by the physicochemical properties of some options like the soil and climatic conditions. For instance, soils that are rich in organic matter and micronutrients such as magnesium, zinc, and iron, together with a suitable pH and high water-holding capacity, provide favorable conditions for the long-chain FAs synthesis (like ALA) (Gatiboni, 2022; Johnston, 1986; Thapa et al., 2021). Otherwise, climatic factors (such as low temperature, limited light, and sufficient moisture) increase the production of PUFAs, especially omega-3 FAs, while hot, dry, or water-stressed conditions shift the FA composition towards saturated fats or omega-6 FAs. Applying sustainable agricultural strategies and selecting varieties resistant to environmental stresses play a crucial role in obtaining the improving the quality of vegetable oils and the best ratio of PUFAs (Mititelu et al., 2025; Nagy et al., 2024; Saini et al., 2021).

1.4.2 Feed composition and its impact on animal-based polyunsaturated fatty acid profiles

The composition of animal diets plays a decisive role in livestock products' PUFA profile. Feeding fresh forage and pasture plants to ruminants increases ALA, CLA, and the favorable omega-3 to omega-6 ratio in meat and dairy products. In contrast, the use of industrial diets rich in cereals and vegetable oils increases omega-6 FAs levels and shifts the ratio of PUFAs in favor of omega-6 FAs (Alfaia et al., 2009; Rueda García et al., 2024). In poultry and aquaculture, the addition of sources such as flaxseed, algae, or fish oil to the diet can also improve DHA and EPA levels. The particular use of omega-3-rich food sources can boost the nutritional content of products and play a crucial role in improving overall health and lowering inflammatory and cardiovascular illnesses, regardless of financial difficulties (Alagawany et al., 2019; Glencross et al., 2024; Rodrigues et al., 2024).

1.4.3 Seasonal and geographical variability in polyunsaturated fatty acid content in marine sources

The omega-3 FAs levels in marine sources are strongly influenced by seasonal and geographical factors. In fatty fish like sardines and salmon, PUFA storage increases during the cold seasons (winter and spring) to maintain cell membrane fluidity; as a result, fish caught during these seasons and in cold waters have a higher omega-3 FAs content. In contrast, in warmer seasons, the need for PUFA decreases, and the overall fat content of the fish also decreases (Gladyshev et al., 2018; Hossain, 2011).

Geographically, fish from polar regions and cold waters have a huge rate of EPA and DHA due to their feeding on plankton and algae rich in omega-3. Also, marine algae from cold and dimly lit areas, especially macroalgae, also produce a high content of DHA. Seasonal changes in the availability of marine food sources (such as phytoplankton) also indirectly affect the fat composition of fish. Choosing cold-water fish during the colder seasons can be very beneficial for optimizing omega-3 FAs intake in the diet (Dave & Routray, 2018; Gladyshev et al., 2018; Lordan et al., 2011; Schmidt et al., 2024).

1.4.4 Processing, storage, and oxidation: effects on polyunsaturated fatty acid stability

The stability of PUFAs, especially omega-3 and omega-6 FAs, is significantly affected by storage conditions, industrial processes, and oxidation, as their special bond (double-bonded structure) is naturally susceptible to oxidative degradation (Ayala et al., 2014; Saini et al., 2021). Processes such as high heating, deodorization of oils, and hydrogenation can destroy natural antioxidants such as vitamin E and produce trans FAs, which threaten heart health. In addition, environmental factors like heat, light, and oxygen are among the most important drivers of oxidation. They can form harmful compounds (like peroxides and aldehydes), which lower nutritional value and enhance oxidative stress in the body (Fadda et al., 2022; Ng et al., 2014).

To stop this process, it is advised to keep oils and items high in PUFAs in oxygen-controlled, low-temperature, dark containers. Important methods for preserving quality include the utilization of natural antioxidants, quick freezing for seafood, and protective packaging such as gelatin capsules in supplements (Saini et al., 2021; Sharma et al., 2019). Finally, the choice of gentle processing methods, such as cold pressing, and awareness of storage principles have an essential role in regulating the health benefits of PUFAs and producing products with high nutritional value (Ali et al., 2022; Mititelu et al., 2024; Mititelu et al., 2025).

1.5 Comparative analysis of omega-3 and omega-6 sources

1.5.1 Bioavailability and conversion efficiency of α-linolenic acid to eicosapentaenoic acid/docosahexaenoic acid in plant versus animal sources

The bioavailability and efficiency of conversion of ALA to DHA and EPA depend on the dietary source. Plant sources like flaxseed, chia, walnuts, and canola oil provide only ALA, which must be converted to EPA and then to DHA in the body for biological activity (Burns-Whitmore et al., 2019; Lane et al., 2021; Takic et al., 2022). This conversion is accomplished by enzymes such as delta-6-desaturases, but its efficiency is low; only about 5%–10% of ALA is converted to EPA and less than 1%–5% to DHA (Shi et al., 2015; Shi et al., 2016). Age, gender, hormonal status, and LA (omega-6 FAs) competition can reduce this rate. For example, women of childbearing age have a more efficient conversion, which is attributed to the effect of estrogen (Ko & Kim, 2020; National Research Council US, 1989b).

In contrast, animal sources such as fatty fish and fish oil supplements or algae contain EPA and DHA directly, which the body absorbs and uses without needing conversion. This makes the bioavailability of omega-3 FAs from these sources much higher and more effective (Li et al., 2023; Saini et al., 2021). Algal oil supplements containing DHA and EPA are recommended for people who follow a vegetarian diet or have low conversion rates. Industrial oils (containing omega-6 FAs) reduction can help increase the efficiency of ALA conversion (García-Maldonado et al., 2023; Li et al., 2023; Qin et al., 2023). These differences in understanding play a crucial role in designing a balanced diet (Liu et al., 2022; Qin et al., 2023).

1.5.2 Balancing omega-3 and omega-6 intake in different dietary patterns

Maintaining a balance between the intake of FAs is essential for metabolic and cardiovascular health (like omega-3 and omega-6 FAs). While omega-3 FAs have anti-inflammatory properties and support heart, brain, and vascular health, omega-6 FAs have a critical part in cell membrane structures and immune responses (Djuricic & Calder, 2021; Mititelu et al., 2025). However, excessive omega-6 FAs intake, especially in the absence of adequate omega-3 FAs, can activate inflammatory pathways and increase the risk of chronic disease (Djuricic & Calder, 2021; Redruello-Requejo et al., 2023; Simopoulos, 2016). In Western diets, high consumption of industrial oils from processed foods can result in an omega-6 to omega-3 ratio exceeding 20:1, far above the ideal ratio of 4:1 or less (Kousparou et al., 2023; Redruello-Requejo et al., 2023; Simopoulos, 2016).

In contrast, some traditional diets, such as the Mediterranean and Asian diets, which are rich in fish, algae, olive oil, and nuts, have a more favorable ratio of omega-3 to omega-6 FAs. In vegetarian diets, the imbalance is more likely due to the high reliance on plant sources of ALA and limited intake of DHA and EPA, but this can be improved by taking algae supplements and limiting industrial oils (Mititelu et al., 2025; Patel et al., 2022; Sebastiani et al., 2019). Choosing the right fats, like canola and olive oil, and consuming fatty fish or omega-3 FAs supplements regularly can regulate the balance and decrease chronic inflammation risk (Ali et al., 2024; Mititelu et al., 2025; Tomczyk, 2024).

1.5.3 Nutritional synergies and potential deficiencies

Nutrient interactions impact absorption and metabolism. A key example is the competition between omega-3 and omega-6 for shared enzymes. A high intake of FAs (omega-6 relative to omega-3) increases the production of inflammatory eicosanoids, while a proper balance of these two groups of fats leads to the synthesis of anti-inflammatory compounds that protect heart and brain health (Balić et al., 2020; Mititelu et al., 2025; Schulze et al., 2020). Due to this, consuming fatty fish, canola oil, and DHA supplements is an effective nutritional strategy along with reducing the intake of industrial omega-6 oils. Additionally, positive synergies between vitamins and minerals are also important (Alagawany et al., 2019; Kitessa et al., 2014; Mercola & D'Adamo, 2023). For example, vitamin D increases calcium absorption, and a deficiency can lead to bone problems. Vitamin C increases the absorption of nonvegetarian iron, while excessive intake of zinc can impair copper absorption. High fiber may also reduce the absorption of minerals, an issue that vegetarian diets need to manage (Institute of Medicine US et al., 2011; Kiani et al., 2022). Correct food combinations, like consuming plant-based iron with vitamin C or protein with complex carbohydrates, can enhance nutritional efficiency. Consuming antioxidants like vitamins E and C together can more effectively lower oxidative stress and enhance dietary planning (Jacobs et al., 2009; Kalogerakou & Antoniadou, 2024; Pruteanu et al., 2023; Wang et al., 2024).

1.6 Conclusion

The PUFAs omega-3 and omega-6 are important for vital functions of the body, such as heart, brain, and immune health, but maintaining a balance between them is a significant challenge in modern diets. Sources of omega-3 FAs include fatty fish and plant seeds, while omega-6 is mainly provided by industrial oils like soybean and sunflower. An imbalance caused by high omega-6 intake can increase the chance of chronic diseases and inflammation. The way livestock and poultry are fed also affects the composition of PUFAs in livestock products; meat and dairy products from pasture-raised animals are higher in omega-3 than industrial products. In addition, environmental factors such as the season of fishing and improper processing of oils also affect the stability of PUFAs. Future research should concentrate on optimizing the consumption of PUFAs and identifying sustainable sources for these nutrients. Genetic studies have shown that there are individual differences in the conversion rate of ALA to EPA and DHA, which could facilitate the design of individualized nutritional supplements. Also, raising fish with algae feed and producing vegetable oils with a more favorable omega-3 to omega-6 ratio would be effective in reducing environmental impacts. The development of advanced analytical technologies to accurately identify lipid composition and produce innovative products such as fortified supplements and modified oils will shape the future of research in this area. To achieve the optimal balance between omega-3 and omega-6 FAs, the consumption of industrial oils should be reduced, and oils with a more optimal profile, such as olive, canola, and safflower, should be used instead. In vegetarian diets, increasing the consumption of ALA sources such as flaxseed and walnuts and reducing omega-6 FAs can help improve the ratio. Choosing pasture-raised meat and dairy products and fortified eggs also plays an important role in providing omega-3 FAs. Proper storage of oils in the refrigerator and dark containers, using gentle processing methods, and avoiding prolonged frying are also effective in preserving the quality of PUFAs. These strategies, along with public education and modifying dietary patterns, can prevent chronic diseases and improve general health.

References

Abera, B. D., & Adimas, M. A. (2024). Health benefits and health risks of contaminated fish consumption: Current research outputs, research approaches, and perspectives. *Heliyon, 10*(13), e33905. https://doi.org/10.1016/j.heliyon.2024.e33905 ISSN 2405-8440.

Abo Egila, N. S. H., Dosoky, W. M., Khisheerah, N. S. M., Ahmed, M. H., Zahran, S. M., Almohmadi, N. H., Abusudah, W. F., Kamal, M., Moustafa, M., Tellez-Isaias, G., Al-Shehri, M., & Abd El-Hack, M. E. (2023). Does dietary linseed or canola oil affect lipid metabolism, immunity, and n-3 polyunsaturated fatty acids content in quail eggs? *Poultry Science, 102*(12), 103116. https://doi.org/10.1016/j.psj.2023.103116 Epub 2023 Sep 15. PMID: 37844526; PMCID: PMC10587527.

Abrante-Pascual, S., Nieva-Echevarría, B., & Goicoechea-Oses, E. (2024). Vegetable oils and their use for frying: A review of their compositional differences and degradation. *Foods, 13*(24), 4186. https://doi.org/10.3390/foods13244186.

Agurla, V., Sharma, M., Pawase, P. A., Shams, R., Ingale, O. S., & Dash, K. K. (2024). A review on extraction, functionality and application of chia seeds as a storehouse of bioactive components. *Measurement: Food, 15*, 100185. https://doi.org/10.1016/j.meafoo.2024.100185 ISSN 2772-2759.

Akkaya, M. R. (2018). Prediction of fatty acid composition of sunflower seeds by near-infrared reflectance spectroscopy. *Journal of Food Science and Technology, 55*(6), 2318–2325. https://doi.org/10.1007/s13197-018-3150-x Epub 2018 Apr 19. PMID: 29892132; PMCID: PMC5976617.

Alagawany, M., Elnesr, S. S., Farag, M. R., Abd El-Hack, M. E., Khafaga, A. F., Taha, A. E., Tiwari, R., Yatoo, M. I., Bhatt, P., Khurana, S. K., & Dhama, K. (2019). Omega-3 and omega-6 fatty acids in poultry nutrition: Effect on production performance and health. *Animals: An Open Access Journal from MDPI, 9*(8), 573. https://doi.org/10.3390/ani9080573 PMID: 31426600; PMCID: PMC6721126.

Alagawany, M., Taha, A. E., Noreldin, A., El-Tarabily, K. A., & Abd El-Hack, M. E. (2021). Nutritional applications of species of *Spirulina* and *Chlorella* in farmed fish: A review. *Aquaculture, 542*, 736841. https://doi.org/10.1016/j.aquaculture.2021.736841 ISSN 0044-8486.

Alfaia, C. P. M., Susana, P. A., Martins, S. I. V., Ana, S. H., Costa, A. S. H., Fontes, C. M. G. A., Lemos, J. P. C., Bessa, R. J. B., & Prates, J. A. M. (2009). Effect of the feeding system on intramuscular fatty acids and conjugated linoleic acid isomers of beef cattle, with emphasis on their nutritional value and discriminatory ability. *Food Chemistry, 114*(3), 939–946. https://doi.org/10.1016/j.foodchem.2008.10.041 ISSN 0308-8146.

Alfio, V. G., Manzo, C., & Micillo, R. (2021). From fish waste to value: An overview of the sustainable recovery of omega-3 for food supplements. *Molecules, 26*(4), 1002. https://doi.org/10.3390/molecules26041002.

Ali, A., Wei, S., Ali, A., Khan, I., Sun, Q., Xia, Q., Wang, Z., Han, Z., Liu, Y., & Liu, S. (2022). Research progress on nutritional value, preservation and processing of fish-a review. *Foods, 11*(22), 3669. https://doi.org/10.3390/foods11223669 PMID: 36429260; PMCID: PMC9689683.

Ali, Z., Al-Ghouti, M. A., Abou-Saleh, H., & Rahman, M. M. (2024). Unraveling the omega-3 puzzle: Navigating challenges and innovations for bone health and healthy aging. *Marine Drugs, 22*(10), 446. https://doi.org/10.3390/md22100446.

Alijani, S., Hahn, A., Harris, W. S., & Schuchardt, J. P. (2025). Bioavailability of EPA and DHA in humans – A comprehensive review. *Progress in Lipid Research, 97*, 101318. https://doi.org/10.1016/j.plipres.2024.101318 ISSN 0163-7827.

Alothman, M., Hogan, S. A., Hennessy, D., Dillon, P., Kilcawley, K. N., O'Donovan, M., Tobin, J., Fenelon, M. A., & O'Callaghan, T. F. (2019). The "grass-fed" milk story: Understanding the impact of pasture feeding on the composition and quality of bovine milk. *Foods, 8*(8), 350. https://doi.org/10.3390/foods8080350 PMID: 31426489; PMCID: PMC6723057.

Ambra, R., Lucchetti, S., & Pastore, G. (2022). A review of the effects of olive oil-cooking on phenolic compounds. *Molecules, 27*(3), 661. https://doi.org/10.3390/molecules27030661 PMID: 35163926; PMCID: PMC8838846.

Arias, A., Patron, A. R., Simmons, S., Bell, H., & Alvarez, V. (2023). Palm oil and coconut oil saturated fats: Properties, food applications, and health. *World Journal of Food Science and Technology, 7*(1), 9–19. https://doi.org/10.11648/j.wjfst.20230701.12.

Attia, Y., Hayat, Z., Alhotan, R. A., Abd El-Hamid, A. E. E., Khalil, H. M., El-Prollosy, A. A., Asiry, K. A., Tellez-Isaias, G., Hafez, H. M., Shehata, A. A., & Basiouni, S. (2024). Impact of omega-3/omega-6 fatty acid ratios and photoperiod on productivity, reproductive performance and immune response of dual-purpose hens. *European Poultry Science. 88*. https://doi.org/10.1399/eps.2024.402 ISSN 1612-9199, © Verlag Eugen Ulmer, Stuttgart.

Awuchi, C. G., Chukwu, C. N., Iyiola, A. O., Noreen, S., Morya, S., Adeleye, A. O., Twinomuhwezi, H., Leicht, K., Mitaki, N. B., & Okpala, C. O. R. (2022). Bioactive compounds and therapeutics from fish: Revisiting their suitability in functional foods to enhance human wellbeing. *BioMed Research International, 2022*, 3661866. https://doi.org/10.1155/2022/3661866 PMID: 36033572; PMCID: PMC9410824.

Ayala, A., Muñoz, M. F., & Argüelles, S. (2014). Lipid peroxidation: Production, metabolism, and signaling mechanisms of malondialdehyde and 4-hydroxy-2-nonenal. *Oxidative Medicine and Cellular Longevity, 2014*, 360438. https://doi.org/10.1155/2014/360438 Epub 2014 May 8. PMID: 24999379; PMCID: PMC4066722.

Ayaz, A., Zaman, W., Radák, Z., & Gu, Y. (2024). Harmony in motion: Unraveling the nexus of sports, plant-based nutrition, and antioxidants for peak performance. *Antioxidants (Basel), 13*(4), 437. https://doi.org/10.3390/antiox13040437 PMID: 38671884; PMCID: PMC11047508.

Aydar, E. F., Tutuncu, S., & Ozcelik, B. (2020). Plant-based milk substitutes: Bioactive compounds, conventional and novel processes, bioavailability studies, and health effects. *Journal of Functional Foods, 70*, 103975. https://doi.org/10.1016/j.jff.2020.103975 ISSN 1756-4646.

Badawy, S., Liu, Y., Guo, M., Liu, Z., Xie, C., Marawan, A., Marawan, M. A., Ares, I., Lopez-Torres, B., Martínez, M., Maximiliano, J. E., Martínez-Larrañaga, M. R., Wang, X., Anadón, A., & Martínez, M. A. (2023). Conjugated linoleic acid (CLA) as a functional food: Is it beneficial or not? *Food Research International, 172*, 113158. https://doi.org/10.1016/j.foodres.2023.113158 ISSN 0963-9969.

Balić, A., Vlašić, D., Žužul, K., Marinović, B., & Bukvić Mokos, Z. (2020). Omega-3 versus omega-6 polyunsaturated fatty acids in the prevention and treatment of inflammatory skin diseases. *International Journal of Molecular Sciences, 21*(3), 741. https://doi.org/10.3390/ijms21030741 PMID: 31979308; PMCID: PMC7037798.

Banaszak, M., Dobrzyńska, M., Kawka, A., Górna, I., Woźniak, D., Przysławski, J., & Drzymała-Czyż, S. (2024). Role of Omega-3 fatty acids eicosapentaenoic (EPA) and docosahexaenoic (DHA) as modulatory and anti-inflammatory agents in noncommunicable diet-related diseases – Reports from the last 10 years. *Clinical Nutrition ESPEN, 63*, 240–258. https://doi.org/10.1016/j.clnesp.2024.06.053 ISSN 2405-4577.

Banel, D. K., & Hu, F. B. (2009). Effects of walnut consumption on blood lipids and other cardiovascular risk factors: a meta-analysis and systematic review. *The American Journal of Clinical Nutrition, 90*(1), 56–63. https://doi.org/10.3945/ajcn.2009.27457 Epub 2009 May 20. PMID: 19458020; PMCID: PMC2696995.

Barchiesi, F., Branciari, R., Latini, M., Roila, R., Lediani, G., Filippini, G., Scortichini, G., Piersanti, A., Rocchegiani, E., & Ranucci, D. (2020). Heavy metals contamination in shellfish: Benefit-risk evaluation in central Italy. *Foods, 9*(11), 1720. https://doi.org/10.3390/foods9111720 PMID: 33238443; PMCID: PMC7700650.

Barta, D. G., Coman, V., & Vodnar, D. C. (2021). Microalgae as sources of omega-3 polyunsaturated fatty acids: Biotechnological aspects. *Algal Research, 58*, 102410. https://doi.org/10.1016/j.algal.2021.102410 ISSN 2211-9264.

Basak, S., & Duttaroy, A. K. (2020). Conjugated linoleic acid and its beneficial effects in obesity, cardiovascular disease, and cancer. *Nutrients, 12*(7), 1913. https://doi.org/10.3390/nu12071913 PMID: 32605287; PMCID: PMC7401241.

Bayram, S., & Kızıltan, G. (2024). The role of omega- 3 polyunsaturated fatty acids in diabetes mellitus management: A narrative review. *Current Nutrition Reports, 13*(3), 527–551. https://doi.org/10.1007/s13668-024-00561-9 Epub 2024 Jul 20. PMID: 39031306; PMCID: PMC11327211.

Bilska, A., & Krzywdzińska-Bartkowiak, M. (2025). The influence of vegetable oil addition levels on the fatty acid profile and oxidative transformation dynamics in liver sausage-type processed meats. *Foods, 14*(3), 380. https://doi.org/10.3390/foods14030380.

Blasbalg, T. L., Hibbeln, J. R., Ramsden, C. E., Majchrzak, S. F., & Rawlings, R. R. (2011). Changes in consumption of omega-3 and omega-6 fatty acids in the United States during the 20th century. *The American Journal of Clinical Nutrition, 93*(5), 950–962. https://doi.org/10.3945/ajcn.110.006643 ISSN 0002-9165.

Blondeau, N. (2016). The nutraceutical potential of omega-3 alpha-linolenic acid in reducing the consequences of stroke. *Biochimie, 120*, 49–55. https://doi.org/10.1016/j.biochi.2015.06.005 ISSN 0300-9084.

Blondeau, N., Lipsky, R. H., Bourourou, M., Duncan, M. W., Gorelick, P. B., & Marini, A. M. (2015). Alpha-linolenic acid: An omega-3 fatty acid with neuroprotective properties-ready for use in the stroke clinic? *BioMed Research International, 2015*, 519830. https://doi.org/10.1155/2015/519830 Epub 2015 Feb 19. PMID: 25789320; PMCID: PMC4350958.

Boateng, L., Ansong, R., Owusu, W. B., & Steiner-Asiedu, M. (2016). Coconut oil and palm oil's role in nutrition, health and national development: A review. *Ghana Medical Journal, 50*(3), 189–196 PMID: 27752194; PMCID: PMC5044790.

Bourre, J. M. (2005). Enrichissement de l'alimentation des animaux avec les acides gras omega-3: Impact sur la valeur nutritionnelle de leurs produits pour l'homme [Effect of increasing the omega-3 fatty acid in the diets of animals on the animal products consumed by humans]. *Medecine sciences: M/S, 21*(8-9), 773–779. https://doi.org/10.1051/medsci/2005218-9773 PMID: 16115466.

Bucciantini, M., Leri, M., Nardiello, P., Casamenti, F., & Stefani, M. (2021). Olive polyphenols: Antioxidant and anti-inflammatory properties. *Antioxidants (Basel), 10*(7), 1044. https://doi.org/10.3390/antiox10071044 PMID: 34209636; PMCID: PMC8300823.

Burns-Whitmore, B., Froyen, E., Heskey, C., Parker, T., & San Pablo, G. (2019). Alpha-linolenic and linoleic fatty acids in the vegan diet: Do they require dietary reference intake/adequate intake special consideration? *Nutrients, 11*(10), 2365. https://doi.org/10.3390/nu11102365.

Caffrey, C., Leamy, A., O'Sullivan, E., Zabetakis, I., Lordan, R., & Nasopoulou, C. (2023). Cardiovascular diseases and marine oils: A focus on omega-3 polyunsaturated fatty acids and polar lipids. *Marine drugs, 21*(11), 549. https://doi.org/10.3390/md21110549.

Cahu, C., Salen, P., & de Lorgeril, M. (2004). Farmed and wild fish in the prevention of cardiovascular diseases: Assessing possible differences in lipid nutritional values. *Nutrition, Metabolism, and Cardiovascular Diseases, 14*(1), 34–41. https://doi.org/10.1016/s0939-4753(04)80045-0 PMID: 15053162.

Calugar, L., Grozea, I., & Butnariu, M. (2024). Vegetable oils in maintaining health. *Journal of Medical and Clinical Nursing Studies*. https://doi.org/10.61440/JMCNS.2024.v2.53.

Cartoni Mancinelli, A., Mattioli, S., Twining, C., Dal Bosco, A., Donoghue, A. M., Arsi, K., Angelucci, E., Chiattelli, D., & Castellini, C. (2022). Poultry meat and eggs as an alternative source of n-3 long-chain polyunsaturated fatty acids for human nutrition. *Nutrients, 14*(9), 1969. https://doi.org/10.3390/nu14091969 PMID: 35565936; PMCID: PMC9099610.

Chen, J., Zhao, Y., Wu, R., Yin, T., You, J., Hu, B., Jia, C., Rong, J., Liu, R., Zhang, B., & Zhao, S. (2023). Changes in the quality of high-oleic sunflower oil during the frying of shrimp (*Litopenaeus vannamei*). *Foods, 12*(6), 1332. https://doi.org/10.3390/foods12061332.

Chen, X., Ran, J., Mazhar, M., Zhu, Y., Lin, Y., Qin, L., & Miao, S. (2023). The balanced unsaturated fatty acid supplement constituted by woody edible oils improved lipid metabolism and gut microbiota in high-fat diet mice. *Frontiers in Nutrition, 10*, 1203932. https://doi.org/10.3389/fnut.2023.1203932 PMID: 37545586; PMCID: PMC10399753.

Cholidis, P., Kranas, D., Chira, A., Galouni, E. A., Adamantidi, T., Anastasiadou, C., & Tsoupras, A. (2024). Shrimp lipid bioactives with anti-inflammatory, antithrombotic, and antioxidant health-promoting properties for cardio-protection. *Marine Drugs, 22*(12), 554. https://doi.org/10.3390/md22120554.

Clemente-Suárez, V. J., Beltrán-Velasco, A. I., Redondo-Flórez, L., Martín-Rodríguez, A., & Tornero-Aguilera, J. F. (2023). Global impacts of western diet and its effects on metabolism and health: A narrative review. *Nutrients, 15*(12), 2749. https://doi.org/10.3390/nu15122749 PMID: 37375654; PMCID: PMC10302286.

Coniglio, S., Shumskaya, M., & Vassiliou, E. (2023). Unsaturated fatty acids and their immunomodulatory properties. *Biology (Basel), 12*(2), 279. https://doi.org/10.3390/biology12020279 PMID: 36829556; PMCID: PMC9953405.

Connolly, G., & Campbell, W. W. (2023). Poultry consumption and human cardiometabolic health-related outcomes: A narrative review. *Nutrients, 15*(16), 3550. https://doi.org/10.3390/nu15163550 PMID: 37630747; PMCID: PMC10459134.

Crupi, P., Faienza, M. F., Naeem, M. Y., Corbo, F., Clodoveo, M. L., & Muraglia, M. (2023). Overview of the potential beneficial effects of carotenoids on consumer health and well-being. *Antioxidants (Basel), 12*(5), 1069. https://doi.org/10.3390/antiox12051069 PMID: 37237935; PMCID: PMC10215867.

Cuchillo-Hilario, M., Fournier-Ramírez, M.-I., Díaz Martínez, M., Montaño Benavides, S., Calvo-Carrillo, M.-C., Carrillo Domínguez, S., Carranco-Jáuregui, M.-E., Hernández-Rodríguez, E., Mora-Pérez, P., Cruz-Martínez, Y. R., & Delgadillo-Puga, C. (2024). Animal food products to support human nutrition and to boost human health: The potential of feedstuffs resources and their metabolites as health-promoters. *Metabolites, 14*(9), 496. https://doi.org/10.3390/metabo14090496.

Cuffaro, D., Bertolini, A., Silva, A. M., Rodrigues, F., Gabbia, D., De Martin, S., Saba, A., Bertini, S., Digiacomo, M., & Macchia, M. (2024). Comparative analysis on polyphenolic composition of different olive mill wastewater and related extra virgin olive oil extracts and evaluation of nutraceutical properties by cell-based studies. *Foods, 13*(20), 3312. https://doi.org/10.3390/foods13203312.

Daley, C. A., Abbott, A., Doyle, P. S., Nader, G. A., & Larson, S. (2010). A review of fatty acid profiles and antioxidant content in grass-fed and grain-fed beef. *Nutrition Journal, 10*(9), 10. https://doi.org/10.1186/1475-2891-9-10 PMID: 20219103; PMCID: PMC2846864.

Das, U. N. (2008). Can essential fatty acids reduce the burden of disease(s)? *Lipids in Health and Disease, 7*, 9. https://doi.org/10.1186/1476-511X-7-9 PMID: 18348729; PMCID: PMC2276500.

Dave, D., & Routray, W. (2018). Current Scenario of Canadian Fishery and Corresponding Underutilized Species and Fishery Byproducts: A Potential Source of Omega-3 Fatty Acids. *Journal of Cleaner Production, 180*, 617–641.

Derbyshire, E., Lane, K. E., & Djuricic, I. (2024). Editorial: Optimal omegas. *Front. Nutr. 11*, 1529722. https://doi.org/10.3389/fnut.2024.1529722.

Demelash Abera, B., & Alefe Adimas, M. (2024). Health benefits and health risks of contaminated fish consumption: Current research outputs, research approaches, and perspectives. *Heliyon, 10*(13), e33905. https://doi.org/10.1016/j.heliyon.2024.e33905 PMID: 39050454; PMCID: PMC11268356.

DiNicolantonio, J. J., & O'Keefe, J. (2021). The importance of maintaining a low omega-6/omega-3 ratio for reducing the risk of autoimmune diseases, asthma, and allergies. *Missouri Medicine, 118*(5), 453–459 PMID: 34658440; PMCID: PMC8504498.

DiNicolantonio, J. J., & O'Keefe, J. H. (2022). Monounsaturated fat vs saturated fat: Effects on cardio-metabolic health and obesity. *Missouri Medicine, 119*(1), 69–73 PMID: 36033137; PMCID: PMC9312452.

Djuricic, I., & Calder, P. C. (2021). Beneficial outcomes of omega-6 and omega-3 polyunsaturated fatty acids on human health: An update for 2021. *Nutrients, 13*(7), 2421. https://doi.org/10.3390/nu13072421 PMID: 34371930; PMCID: PMC8308533.

Durmaz, G., & Gökmen, V. (2019). Effect of refining on bioactive composition and oxidative stability of hazelnut oil. *Food Research International, 116*, 586–591. https://doi.org/10.1016/j.foodres.2018.08.077 ISSN 0963-9969.

Ehr, I. J., Persia, M. E., & Bobeck, E. A. (2017). Comparative omega-3 fatty acid enrichment of egg yolks from first-cycle laying hens fed flaxseed oil or ground flaxseed. *Poultry Science, 96*(6), 1791–1799. https://doi.org/10.3382/ps/pew462 PMID: 28108729; PMCID: PMC6280955.

Evans, W. C., & Evans, D. (2009). Chapter 19 - Hydrocarbons and derivatives, Editor(s): William Charles Evans, Daphne Evans. In *Trease and Evans' pharmacognosy (sixteenth edition)*. W.B. Saunders, 173–193. https://doi.org/10.1016/B978-0-7020-2933-2.00019-8 ISBN 9780702029332.

Fabjanowska, J., Kowalczuk-Vasilev, E., Klebaniuk, R., Milewski, S., & Gümüş, H. (2023). N-3 Polyunsaturated fatty acids as a nutritional support of the reproductive and immune system of cattle—A review. *Animals: An Open Access Journal from MDPI, 13*(22), 3589. https://doi.org/10.3390/ani13223589.

Fadda, A., Sanna, D., Sakar, E. H., Gharby, S., Mulas, M., Medda, S., Yesilcubuk, N. S., Karaca, A. C., Gozukirmizi, C. K., Lucarini, M., Lombardi-Boccia, G., Diaconeasa, Z., & Durazzo, A. (2022). Innovative and sustainable technologies to enhance the oxidative stability of vegetable oils. *Sustainability, 14*(2), 849. https://doi.org/10.3390/su14020849.

Falade, O., Oboh, G., & Okoh, I. (2017). A, potential health implications of the consumption of thermally-oxidized cooking oils – A review. *Ayodeji, Pol. J. Food Nutr. Sci. 67*(2), 95–105. https://doi.org/10.1515/pjfns-2016-0028.

Fan, N., Fusco, J. L., & Rosenberg, D. W. (2023). Antioxidant and anti-inflammatory properties of walnut constituents: Focus on personalized cancer prevention and the microbiome. *Antioxidants (Basel), 12*(5), 982. https://doi.org/10.3390/antiox12050982 PMID: 37237848; PMCID: PMC10215340.

Farmery, A. K., O'Kane, G., McManus, A., & Green, B. S. (2018). Consuming sustainable seafood: Guidelines, recommendations and realities. *Public Health Nutrition, 21*(8), 1503–1514. https://doi.org/10.1017/S1368980017003895 Epub 2018 Jan 21. PMID: 29352833; PMCID: PMC10284715.

Feng, J., Long, S., Zhang, H. J., Wu, S. G., Qi, G. H., & Wang, J. (2020). Comparative effects of dietary microalgae oil and fish oil on fatty acid composition and sensory quality of table eggs. *Poultry Science, 99*(3), 1734–1743. https://doi.org/10.1016/j.psj.2019.11.005 ISSN 0032-5791.

Fernandez-Jover, D., Lopez Jimenez, J. A., Sanchez-Jerez, P., Bayle-Sempere, J., Casalduero, F. G., Martinez Lopez, F. J., & Dempster, T. (2007). Changes in body condition and fatty acid composition of wild Mediterranean horse mackerel (Trachurus mediterraneus, Steindachner, 1868) associated to sea cage fish farms. *Marine Environmental Research, 63*(1), 1–18. https://doi.org/10.1016/j.marenvres.2006.05.002 ISSN 0141-1136.

Gammone, M. A., Riccioni, G., Parrinello, G., & D'Orazio, N. (2018). Omega-3 polyunsaturated fatty acids: Benefits and endpoints in sport. *Nutrients, 11*(1), 46. https://doi.org/10.3390/nu11010046 PMID: 30591639; PMCID: PMC6357022.

García-Maldonado, E., Alcorta, A., Zapatera, B., & Vaquero, M. P. (2023). Changes in fatty acid levels after consumption of a novel docosahexaenoic supplement from algae: A crossover randomized controlled trial in omnivorous, lacto-ovo vegetarians and vegans. *European Journal of Nutrition, 62*(4), 1691–1705. https://doi.org/10.1007/s00394-022-03050-3 Epub 2022 Nov 23. PMID: 36418565; PMCID: PMC9684969.

Gatiboni, L. (2022). Soils and plant nutrients, chapter 1. In K. A. Moore, & L. K. Bradley (Eds.). *North carolina extension gardener handbook*(2nd ed.). Raleigh, NC: NC State Extensionhttps://content.ces.ncsu.edu/extension-gardener-handbook/1-soils-and-plant-nutrients.

Gharby, S., Harhar, H., Boulbaroud, S., Bouzoubaâ, Z., Madani, N., Chafchaouni, I., & Charrouf, Z. (2014). The stability of vegetable oils (sunflower, rapeseed and palm) sold on the Moroccan market at high temperature. *IJCBS, 5*, 47–54.

Gladyshev, M. I., & Sushchik, N. N. (2019). Long-chain omega-3 polyunsaturated fatty acids in natural ecosystems and the human diet: Assumptions and challenges. *Biomolecules, 9*(9), 485. https://doi.org/10.3390/biom9090485 PMID: 31547473; PMCID: PMC6770104.

Gladyshev, M. I., Sushchik, N. N., Tolomeev, A. P., et al. (2018). Meta-analysis of factors associated with omega-3 fatty acid contents of wild fish. *Reviews in Fish Biology and Fisheries, 28*, 277–299. https://doi.org/10.1007/s11160-017-9511-0.

Glencross, B. D., Bachis, E., Betancor, M. B., Calder, P., Liland, N., Newton, R., & Ruyter, B. (2024). Omega-3 futures in aquaculture: Exploring the supply and demands for long-chain omega-3 essential fatty acids by aquaculture species. *Reviews in Fisheries Science & Aquaculture, 33*(2), 167–216. https://doi.org/10.1080/23308249.2024.2388563.

Goyal, A., Sharma, V., Upadhyay, N., Gill, S., & Sihag, M. (2014). Flax and flaxseed oil: An ancient medicine & modern functional food. *Journal of Food Science and Technology, 51*(9), 1633–1653. https://doi.org/10.1007/s13197-013-1247-9 Epub 2014 Jan 10. PMID: 25190822; PMCID: PMC4152533.

Grace, D., Knight-Jones, T. J. D., Melaku, A., Alders, R., & Jemberu, W. T. (2024). The public health importance and management of infectious poultry diseases in smallholder systems in Africa. *Foods, 13*(3), 411. https://doi.org/10.3390/foods13030411.

Grille, L., Vieitez, I., Garay, A., Romero, M., Jorcín, S., Krall, E., Méndez, M. N., Irigaray, B., Bejarano, E., & López-Pedemonte, T. (2024). Fat profiles of milk and butter obtained from different dairy systems (High and Low Pasture) and seasons (Spring and Fall): Focus on healthy fatty acids and technological properties of butter. *Dairy, 5*(3), 555–575. https://doi.org/10.3390/dairy5030042.

Guo, F., Danielski, R., Santhiravel, S., & Shahidi, F. (2024). Unlocking the nutraceutical potential of legumes and their by-products: Paving the way for the circular economy in the agri-food industry. *Antioxidants, 13*(6), 636. https://doi.org/10.3390/antiox13060636.

Haque, M. M., Rahman, M. N., Alam, M. J., & Akter, S. (2016). A possible approach for maintaining effective omega-6/ omega-3 fatty acid ratio from mixed vegetable oils. *Journal of Environmental Sciences & Natural Resources, 9*(2), 65–69.

den Hartigh, L. J. (2019). Conjugated linoleic acid effects on cancer, obesity, and atherosclerosis: A review of pre-clinical and human trials with current perspectives. *Nutrients, 11*(2), 370. https://doi.org/10.3390/nu11020370 PMID: 30754681; PMCID: PMC6413010.

Hassanpour, S. H., & Doroudi, A. (2023). Review of the antioxidant potential of flavonoids as a subgroup of polyphenols and partial substitute for synthetic antioxidants. *Avicenna Journal of Phytomedicine, 13*(4), 354–376. https://doi.org/10.22038/AJP.2023.21774 PMID: 37663389; PMCID: PMC10474916.

Hayes, D., Angove, M. J., Tucci, J., & Dennis, C. (2016). Walnuts (*Juglans regia*) chemical composition and research in human health. *Critical Reviews in Food Science and Nutrition, 56*(8), 1231–1241. https://doi.org/10.1080/10408398.2012.760516.

Hooper, L., Thompson, R. L., Harrison, R. A., Summerbell, C. D., Moore, H., Worthington, H. V., Durrington, P. N., Ness, A. R., Capps, N. E., Davey Smith, G., Riemersma, R. A., & Ebrahim, S. B. (2004). Omega 3 fatty acids for prevention and treatment of cardiovascular disease. *Cochrane Database System Reviews, 4*, CD003177. https://doi.org/10.1002/14651858.CD003177.pub2 Update in: Cochrane Database Syst Rev. 2018 Jul 18;7:CD003177. doi: 10.1002/14651858.CD003177.pub3. PMID: 15495044; PMCID: PMC4170890.

Hossain, M. A. (2011). Fish as source of n-3 polyunsaturated fatty acids (PUFAs), which one is better-farmed or wild? *Advance Journal of Food Science and Technology, 3*(6), 455–466. https://doi.org/10.1016/j.glohj.2020.01.004 ISSN: 2042-4876.

Hustad, K. S., Ottestad, I., Olsen, T., Sæther, T., Ulven, S. M., & Holven, K. B. (2022). Salmon fish protein supplement increases serum vitamin B12 and selenium concentrations: Secondary analysis of a randomised controlled trial. *European Journal of Nutrition, 61*(6), 3085–3093. https://doi.org/10.1007/s00394-022-02857-4 Epub 2022 Apr 1. PMID: 35362766; PMCID: PMC9363293.

Institute of Medicine (US) Committee to Review Dietary Reference Intakes for Vitamin D and Calcium. (2011). Overview of calcium. In A. C. Ross, C. L. Taylor, A. L. Yaktine, & H. B. Del Valle (Eds.), *Dietary reference intakes for calcium and vitamin D*. National Academies Press. https://www.ncbi.nlm.nih.gov/books/NBK56060/

Isaakidis, A., Maghariki, J. E., Carvalho-Barros, S., Gomes, A. M., & Correia, M. (2023). Is there more to olive oil than healthy lipids? *Nutrients, 15*(16), 3625. https://doi.org/10.3390/nu15163625 PMID: 37630815; PMCID: PMC10459315.

Ivanova, S., Marinova, G., & Batchvarov, V. (2016). Comparison of fatty acid composition of various types of edible oils, 2016. *Bulgarian Journal of Agricultural Science, 22*(5), 849–856.

Iwata, N. G., Pham, M., Rizzo, N. O., Cheng, A. M., Maloney, E., & Kim, F. (2011). Trans fatty acids induce vascular inflammation and reduce vascular nitric oxide production in endothelial cells. *PLoS ONE, 6*(12), e29600. https://doi.org/10.1371/journal.pone.0029600 Epub 2011 Dec 28. PMID: 22216328; PMCID: PMC3247279.

Jacobs, D. R., Jr, Gross, M. D., & Tapsell, L. C. (2009). Food synergy: An operational concept for understanding nutrition. *The American Journal of Clinical Nutrition, 89*(5), 1543S–1548S. https://doi.org/10.3945/ajcn.2009.26736B Epub 2009 Mar 11. PMID: 19279083; PMCID: PMC2731586.

Jeelani, P. G., Sinclair, B. J., Perinbarajan, G. K., et al. (2023). The therapeutic potential of chia seeds as medicinal food: A review. *Nutrire, 48*, 39. https://doi.org/10.1186/s41110-023-00224-9.

Jensen, I. J., Eilertsen, K. E., Otnæs, C. H. A., Mæhre, H. K., & Elvevoll, E. O. (2020). An update on the content of fatty acids, dioxins, PCBs and heavy metals in farmed, escaped and Wild Atlantic Salmon (*Salmo salar* L.) in Norway. *Foods, 9*(12), 1901. https://doi.org/10.3390/foods9121901 PMID: 33352671; PMCID: PMC7766777.

Jeong, H. Y., Moon, Y. S., & Cho, K. K. (2024). ω-6 and ω-3 polyunsaturated fatty acids: Inflammation, obesity and foods of animal resources. *Food Science of Animal Resources, 44*(5), 988–1010. https://doi.org/10.5851/kosfa.2024.e65 Epub 2024 Sep 1. PMID: 39246544; PMCID: PMC11377208.

Jerab, D., Blangero, F., da Costa, P. C. T., de Brito Alves, J. L., Kefi, R., Jamoussi, H., Morio, B., & Eljaafari, A. (2025). Beneficial effects of omega-3 fatty acids on obesity and related metabolic and chronic inflammatory diseases. *Nutrients, 17*(7), 1253. https://doi.org/10.3390/nu17071253.

Jesionowska, M., Ovadia, J., Hockemeyer, K., Clews, A. C., & Xu, Y. (2023). EPA and DHA in microalgae: Health benefits, biosynthesis, and metabolic engineering advances. *Journal of the American Oil Chemists' Society, 100*(11), 831–842. https://doi.org/10.1002/aocs.12718.

Jimenez-Lopez, C., Carpena, M., Lourenço-Lopes, C., Gallardo-Gomez, M., Lorenzo, J. M., Barba, F. J., Prieto, M. A., & Simal-Gandara, J. (2020). Bioactive compounds and quality of extra virgin olive oil. *Foods, 9*(8), 1014. https://doi.org/10.3390/foods9081014.

Johnston, A. E. (1986). Soil organic matter, effects on soils and crops. *Soil Use and Management, 2*(3), 97–105. https://doi.org/10.1111/j.1475-2743.1986.tb00690.x.

Jones, P. J. H., & Rideout, T. (2014). Lipids, sterols, and their metabolites. In A. C. Ross, B. Caballero, R. J. Cousins, K. L. Tucker, & T. R. Ziegler (Eds.). *Modern nutrition in health and disease*(11th ed.). Baltimore, MD: Lippincott Williams & Wilkins.

Jump, D. B., Depner, C. M., & Tripathy, S. (2012). Omega-3 fatty acid supplementation and cardiovascular disease. *Journal of Lipid Research, 53*(12), 2525–2545. https://doi.org/10.1194/jlr.R027904 Epub 2012 Aug 17. PMID: 22904344; PMCID: PMC3494243.

Kalogerakou, T., & Antoniadou, M. (2024). The role of dietary antioxidants, food supplements and functional foods for energy enhancement in healthcare professionals. *Antioxidants (Basel), 13*(12), 1508. https://doi.org/10.3390/antiox13121508 PMID: 39765836; PMCID: PMC11672929.

Kent, J. A. (2003). Animal and vegetable fats, oils, and waxes. In J. A. Kent (Ed.). *Riegel's handbook of industrial chemistry*Boston, MA: Springerhttps://doi.org/10.1007/0-387-23816-6_8.

Khalid, W., Arshad, M. S., Aziz, A., Rahim, M. A., Qaisrani, T. B., Afzal, F., Ali, A., Ranjha, M. M. A. N., Khalid, M. Z., & Anjum, F. M. (2022). Chia seeds (*Salvia hispanica* L.): A therapeutic weapon in metabolic disorders. *Food Science & Nutrition, 11*(1), 3–16. https://doi.org/10.1002/fsn3.3035 PMID: 36655089; PMCID: PMC9834868.

Khalid, W., Arshad, M. S., Ranjha, M. M. A. N., Różańska, M. B., Irfan, S., Shafique, B., Rahim, M. A., Khalid, M. Z., Abdi, G., & Kowalczewski, P. (2022). Functional constituents of plant-based foods boost immunity against acute and chronic disorders. *Open Life Sciences, 17*(1), 1075–1093. https://doi.org/10.1515/biol-2022-0104 PMID: 36133422; PMCID: PMC9462539.

Kiani, A. K., Dhuli, K., Donato, K., Aquilanti, B., Velluti, V., Matera, G., Iaconelli, A., Connelly, S. T., Bellinato, F., Gisondi, P., & Bertelli, M. (2022). Main nutritional deficiencies. *Journal of Preventive Medicine and Hygiene, 63*(2 Suppl 3), E93–E101. https://doi.org/10.15167/2421-4248/jpmh2022.63.2S3.2752 PMID: 36479498; PMCID: PMC9710417.

Kitessa, S. M., Abeywardena, M., Wijesundera, C., & Nichols, P. D. (2014). DHA-containing oilseed: A timely solution for the sustainability issues surrounding fish oil sources of the health-benefitting long-chain omega-3Oils. *Nutrients, 6*(5), 2035–2058. https://doi.org/10.3390/nu6052035.

Knez Hrnčič, M., Ivanovski, M., Cör, D., & Knez, Ž. (2019). Chia seeds (*Salvia hispanica* L.): An overview-phytochemical profile, isolation methods, and application. *Molecules, 25*(1), 11. https://doi.org/10.3390/molecules25010011 PMID: 31861466; PMCID: PMC6994964.

Ko, S. H., & Kim, H. S. (2020). Menopause-associated lipid metabolic disorders and foods beneficial for postmenopausal women. *Nutrients, 12*(1), 202. https://doi.org/10.3390/nu12010202 PMID: 31941004; PMCID: PMC7019719.

Konieczka, P., Czauderna, M., & Smulikowska, S. (2017). The enrichment of chicken meat with omega-3 fatty acids by dietary fish oil or its mixture with rapeseed or flaxseed—Effect of feeding duration: Dietary fish oil, flaxseed, and rapeseed and n-3 enriched broiler meat. *Animal Feed Science and Technology, 223*, 42–52. https://doi.org/10.1016/j.anifeedsci.2016.10.023 ISSN 0377-8401.

Kousparou, C., Fyrilla, M., Stephanou, A., & Patrikios, I. (2023). DHA/EPA (Omega-3) and LA/GLA (Omega-6) as bioactive molecules in neurodegenerative diseases. *International Journal of Molecular Sciences, 24*(13), 10717. https://doi.org/10.3390/ijms241310717.

Kratzer, R., & Murkovic, M. (2021). Food ingredients and nutraceuticals from microalgae: Main product classes and biotechnological production. *Foods, 10*(7), 1626. https://doi.org/10.3390/foods10071626.

Kris-Etherton, P. M. (2014). Walnuts decrease risk of cardiovascular disease: A summary of efficacy and biologic mechanisms. *The Journal of Nutrition, 144*(4 Suppl), 547S–554S. https://doi.org/10.3945/jn.113.182907 Epub 2014 Feb 5. PMID: 24500935.

Krupa, K. N., Fritz, K., & Parmar, M. (2025). Omega-3 fatty acids. In *StatPearls*. StatPearls Publishing. https://www.ncbi.nlm.nih.gov/books/NBK564314/

Krupa, K. N., Fritz, K., & Parmar, M. (2024). *Omega-3 Fatty Acids*. Treasure Island (FL): StatPearls Publishing Available from: nih.gov.

Lane, K. E., Wilson, M., Hellon, T. G., & Davies, I. G. (2021). Bioavailability and conversion of plant based sources of omega-3 fatty acids – A scoping review to update supplementation options for vegetarians and vegans. *Critical Reviews in Food Science and Nutrition, 62*(18), 4982–4997. https://doi.org/10.1080/10408398.2021.1880364.

Lange, K. W. (2020). Omega-3 fatty acids and mental health. *Global Health Journal, 4*(1), 18–30 ISSN 2414-6447.

Le, H. D., Meisel, J. A., de Meijer, V. E., Gura, K. M., & Puder, M. (2009). The essentiality of arachidonic acid and docosahexaenoic acid. *Prostaglandins, Leukotrienes, and Essential Fatty Acids, 81*(2-3), 165–170. https://doi.org/10.1016/j.plefa.2009.05.020 Epub 2009 Jun 18. PMID: 19540099; PMCID: PMC3361712.

Li, X., Guo, M., Xue, Y., & Duan, Z. (2023). Effect of extraction methods on the physicochemical properties, chemical composition, and antioxidant activities of samara oil. *Foods, 12*(17), 3163. https://doi.org/10.3390/foods12173163.

Liao, J., Xiong, Q., Yin, Y., Ling, Z., & Chen, S. (2022). The effects of fish oil on cardiovascular diseases: Systematical evaluation and recent advance. *Frontiers in Cardiovascular Medicine, 8*, 802306. https://doi.org/10.3389/fcvm.2021.802306 PMID: 35071366; PMCID: PMC8767101.

Lin, L., Allemekinders, H., Dansby, A., Campbell, L., Durance-Tod, S., Berger, A., & Jones, P. J. (2013). Evidence of health benefits of canola oil. *Nutrition Reviews, 71*(6), 370–385. https://doi.org/10.1111/nure.12033 Epub 2013 May 2. PMID: 23731447; PMCID: PMC3746113.

Liu, A. G., Ford, N. A., Hu, F. B., Zelman, K. M., Mozaffarian, D., & Kris-Etherton, P. M. (2017). A healthy approach to dietary fats: Understanding the science and taking action to reduce consumer confusion. *Nutrition Journal, 16*(1), 53. https://doi.org/10.1186/s12937-017-0271-4 PMID: 28854932; PMCID: PMC5577766.

Liu, Y., Ren, X., Fan, C., Wu, W., Zhang, W., & Wang, Y. (2022). Health benefits, food applications, and sustainability of microalgae-derived N-3 PUFA. *Foods, 11*(13), 1883. https://doi.org/10.3390/foods11131883.

Lordan, R., Tsoupras, A., Mitra, B., & Zabetakis, I. (2018). Dairy fats and cardiovascular disease: Do we really need to be concerned? *Foods, 7*(3), 29. https://doi.org/10.3390/foods7030029 PMID: 29494487; PMCID: PMC5867544.

Lordan, S., Ross, R. P., & Stanton, C. (2011). Marine bioactives as functional food ingredients: Potential to reduce the incidence of chronic diseases. *Marine Drugs, 9*(6), 1056–1100. https://doi.org/10.3390/md9061056 Epub 2011 Jun 14. PMID: 21747748; PMCID: PMC3131561.

Lu, C., Zhu, Y., Wang, Y., Zhang, L., Zhu, Y., & Wei, G. (2025). Effective Production of Branched-chain Biodiesel by the Hydrolysis-esterification of Castor Oil Using Porous Carbon-based Solid Acid. *Process Safety and Environmental Protection, 202*, 107658. https://doi.org/10.1016/j.psep.2025.107658 Accessed May 22, 2026.

Madacussengua, O., Mendes, A. R., Almeida, A. M., & Lordelo, M. (2025). Effects of using microalgae in poultry diets on the production and quality of meat and eggs: A review. *British Poultry Science*, 1–17. https://doi.org/10.1080/00071668.2024.2420330.

Mahmud, N., Islam, J., Oyom, W., Adrah, K., Adegoke, S. C., & Tahergorabi, R. (2023). A review of different frying oils and oleogels as alternative frying media for fat-uptake reduction in deep-fat fried foods. *Heliyon, 9*(11), e21500. https://doi.org/10.1016/j.heliyon.2023.e21500 PMID: 38027829; PMCID: PMC10660127.

Majida, A. W., Zeshan, A., Mohamed, A. A., Li, J., & Liu, Y. (2025). Enhancing extra virgin olive oil stability with chemically modified polysaccharides from *Lycium barbarum* L. leaves: Implications for heat resistance and shelf life. *Heliyon, 11*(4), e42504. https://doi.org/10.1016/j.heliyon.2025.e42504 PMID: 40040964; PMCID: PMC11876864.

Marangoni, F., Corsello, G., Cricelli, C., Ferrara, N., Ghiselli, A., Lucchin, L., & Poli, A. (2015). Role of poultry meat in a balanced diet aimed at maintaining health and wellbeing: An Italian consensus document. *Food & Nutrition Research, 59*, 27606. https://doi.org/10.3402/fnr.v59.27606 PMID: 26065493; PMCID: PMC4462824.

Mariamenatu, A. H., & Abdu, E. M. (2021). Overconsumption of omega-6 polyunsaturated fatty acids (PUFAs) versus deficiency of omega-3 PUFAs in modern-day diets: The disturbing factor for their "balanced antagonistic metabolic functions" in the human body. *Journal of Lipids, 2021*, 8848161. https://doi.org/10.1155/2021/8848161 PMID: 33815845; PMCID: PMC7990530.

Mititelu, M., Lupuliasa, D., Neacs,u, S. M., Olteanu, G., Busnatu, S. S., Mihai, A., Popovici, V., Măru, N., Boroghină, S. C., Mihai, S., et al. (2025). Polyunsaturated Fatty Acids and Human Health: A Key to Modern Nutritional Balance in Association with Polyphenolic Compounds from Food Sources. *Foods, 14*, 46. https://doi.org/10.3390/foods14010046.

Mungwari, C. P., Obadele, B. A., & King'ondu, C. K. (2025). Application of Response Surface Methodology (RSM) and Artificial Neural Network (ANN) for Bioactive Compounds Recovery from Mimosa Wattle Tree (Acacia Mearnsii) Bark Using Ultrasound-assisted Extraction. *Scientific African, 29*, e02934. https://doi.org/10.1016/j.sciaf.2025.e02934 Accessed May 22, 2026.

McMullan, J. E., Yeates, A. J., Allsopp, P. J., Mulhern, M. S., Strain, J. J., Wijngaarden, E. V., Myers, G. J., Shroff, E., Shamlaye, C. F., & McSorley, E. M. (2023). Fish consumption and its lipid modifying effects – A review of intervention studies. *Neurotoxicology, 99*, 82–96. https://doi.org/10.1016/j.neuro.2023.10.003 ISSN 0161-813X.

Mehany, T., González-Sáiz, J. M., & Pizarro, C. (2025). Improving the biostability of extra virgin olive oil with olive fruit extract during prolonged deep frying. *Foods, 14*(2), 260. https://doi.org/10.3390/foods14020260.

Mercola, J., & D'Adamo, C. R. (2023). Linoleic acid: A narrative review of the effects of increased intake in the standard american diet and associations with chronic disease. *Nutrients, 15*(14), 3129. https://doi.org/10.3390/nu15143129 PMID: 37513547; PMCID: PMC10386285.

Michalak, I., Tiwari, R., Dhawan, M., Alagawany, M., Farag, M. R., Sharun, K., Emran, T. B., & Dhama, K. (2022). Antioxidant effects of seaweeds and their active compounds on animal health and production - A review. *The Veterinary Quarterly, 42*(1), 48–67. https://doi.org/10.1080/01652176.2022.2061744 PMID: 35363108; PMCID: PMC9004519.

Michalak, M. (2022). Plant-derived antioxidants: Significance in skin health and the ageing process. *International Journal of Molecular Sciences, 23*(2), 585. https://doi.org/10.3390/ijms23020585.

Milanković, V., Tasić, T., Leskovac, A., Petrović, S., Mitić, M., Lazarević-Pašti, T., Novković, M., & Potkonjak, N. (2024). Metals on the menu—Analyzing the presence, importance, and consequences. *Foods, 13*(12), 1890. https://doi.org/10.3390/foods13121890.

Milena, E., & Maurizio, M. (2025). Exploring the cardiovascular benefits of extra virgin olive oil: Insights into mechanisms and therapeutic potential. *Biomolecules 2025, 15*(2), 284. https://doi.org/10.3390/biom15020284.

Mirrezaie, Roodaki, Sahari, M. S., Ghiassi, M. A., Tarzi, B., Barzegar, M., & Gharachorloo, M. (2016). Effect of refining and thermal processes on olive oil properties. *Journal of Agricultural Science and Technology. 18*, 629–641.

Mititelu, M., Lupuliasa, D., Neacşu, S. M., Olteanu, G., Busnatu, S., Mihai, A., Popovici, V., Măru, N., Boroghină, S. C., Mihai, S., Ioniță-Mîndrican, C. B., & Scafa-Udrişte, A. (2024). Polyunsaturated fatty acids and human health: A key to modern nutritional balance in association with polyphenolic compounds from food sources. *Foods, 14*(1), 46. https://doi.org/10.3390/foods14010046 PMID: 39796335; PMCID: PMC11719865.

Moghadama, K., & Moslehishad (2020). Advantages of thermal stability of virgin olive oil over canola and frying oil. *Journal of Food and Bioprocess Engineering, JFBE, 3*(1), 41–46.

Mollica, M. P., Trinchese, G., Cimmino, F., Penna, E., Cavaliere, G., Tudisco, R., Musco, N., Manca, C., Catapano, A., Monda, M., Bergamo, P., Banni, S., Infascelli, F., Lombardi, P., & Crispino, M. (2021). Milk fatty acid profiles in different animal species: Focus on the potential effect of selected pufas on metabolism and brain functions. *Nutrients, 13*(4), 1111. https://doi.org/10.3390/nu13041111 PMID: 33800688; PMCID: PMC8066999.

Momot, M., Stawicka, B., & Szydłowska-Czerniak, A. (2023). Physicochemical properties and sensory attributes of cold-pressed camelina oils from the polish retail market. *Applied Sciences, 13*(3), 1924. https://doi.org/10.3390/app13031924.

Monteiro, J. P., Domingues, M. R., & Calado, R. (2024). Marine animal co-products—How improving their use as rich sources of health-promoting lipids can foster sustainability. *Marine Drugs, 22*(2), 73. https://doi.org/10.3390/md22020073.

Nagy, K., Iacob, B. C., Bodoki, E., & Oprean, R. (2024). Investigating the thermal stability of omega fatty acid-enriched vegetable oils. *Foods, 13*(18), 2961. https://doi.org/10.3390/foods13182961.

National Research Council (US) Committee on Diet and Health. (1989). Fat-soluble vitamins. In *Diet and health: Implications for reducing chronic disease risk*. National Academies Press. https://www.ncbi.nlm.nih.gov/books/NBK218749/

National Research Council (US) Committee on Diet and Health. (1989). Fats and other lipids. In *Diet and health: Implications for reducing chronic disease risk*. National Academies Press. https://www.ncbi.nlm.nih.gov/books/NBK218759/

Ng, C., Leong, X., Masbah, N., Khadijah, A. S., Kamisah, Y., & Jaarin, K. (2014). Heated vegetable oils and cardiovascular disease risk factors. *Vascular Pharmacology, 61*(1), 1–9. https://doi.org/10.1016/j.vph.2014.02.004 ISSN 1537-1891.

Nguyen, D. V., Malau-Aduli, B. S., Cavalieri, J., Nichols, P. D., & Malau-Aduli, A. E. O. (2018). Supplementation with plant-derived oils rich in omega-3 polyunsaturated fatty acids for lamb production. *Veterinary and Animal Science, 6*, 29–40. https://doi.org/10.1016/j.vas.2018.08.001 ISSN 2451-943X.

Nguyen, Q. V., Malau-Aduli, B. S., Cavalieri, J., Malau-Aduli, A. E. O., & Nichols, P. D. (2019). Enhancing omega-3 long-chain polyunsaturated fatty acid content of dairy-derived foods for human consumption. *Nutrients, 11*(4), 743. https://doi.org/10.3390/nu11040743 PMID: 30934976; PMCID: PMC6520953.

Nolden, A. A., & Forde, C. G. (2023). The nutritional quality of plant-based foods. *Sustainability, 15*(4), 3324. https://doi.org/10.3390/su15043324.

Oliver, L., Dietrich, T., Marañón, I., Villarán, M. C., & Barrio, R. J. (2020). Producing omega-3 polyunsaturated fatty acids: A review of sustainable sources and future trends for the EPA and DHA market. *Resources, 9*(12), 148. https://doi.org/10.3390/resources9120148.

Oppedisano, F., Macrì, R., Gliozzi, M., Musolino, V., Carresi, C., Maiuolo, J., Bosco, F., Nucera, S., Caterina Zito, M., Guarnieri, L., & Scarano, F. (2020). The anti-inflammatory and antioxidant properties of n-3 PUFAs: Their role in cardiovascular protection. *Biomedicines, 8*(9), 306. https://doi.org/10.3390/biomedicines8090306.

Orsavova, J., Misurcova, L., Ambrozova, J. V., Vicha, R., & Mlcek, J. (2015). Fatty acids composition of vegetable oils and its contribution to dietary energy intake and dependence of cardiovascular mortality on dietary intake of fatty acids. *International Journal of Molecular Sciences, 16*(6), 12871–12890. https://doi.org/10.3390/ijms160612871 PMID: 26057750; PMCID: PMC4490476.

Oteng, A. B., & Kersten, S. (2020). Mechanisms of action of trans fatty acids. *Advances in Nutrition, 11*(3), 697–708. https://doi.org/10.1093/advances/nmz125 PMID: 31782488; PMCID: PMC7231579.

Pânzaru, C., Doliş, M. G., Radu-Rusu, R.-M., Pascal, C., Maciuc, V., & Davidescu, M.-A. (2024). Equine milk and meat: Nutritious and sustainable alternatives for global food security and environmental sustainability—A review. *Agriculture, 14*(12), 2290. https://doi.org/10.3390/agriculture14122290.

Patel, A., Sawant Desai, S., Kelkar Mane, V., Enman, J., Rova, U., Christakopoulos, P., & Matsakas, L. (2022). Futuristic food fortification with a balanced ratio of dietary ω-3/ω-6 omega fatty acids for the prevention of lifestyle diseases. *Trends in Food Science & Technology, 120*, 140–153. https://doi.org/10.1016/j.tifs.2022.01.006 ISSN 0924-2244.

Patterson, E., Wall, R., Fitzgerald, G. F., Ross, R. P., & Stanton, C. (2012). Health implications of high dietary omega-6 polyunsaturated fatty acids. *Journal of Nutrition and Metabolism, 2012*, 539426. https://doi.org/10.1155/2012/539426 Epub 2012 Apr 5. PMID: 22570770; PMCID: PMC3335257.

Peng, L., Zhang, Z., Li, Q., & Yang, H. (2025). Current challenges and issues in the application of astaxanthin. *Fishes, 10*(4), 159. https://doi.org/10.3390/fishes10040159.

Pilar Gómez-Cortés, P., Manuela Juárez, M., & de la Fuente, M. A. (2018). Milk fatty acids and potential health benefits: An updated vision. *Trends in Food Science & Technology, 81*, 1–9. https://doi.org/10.1016/j.tifs.2018.08.014 ISSN 0924-2244.

Pipoyan, D., Stepanyan, S., Stepanyan, S., Beglaryan, M., Costantini, L., Molinari, R., & Merendino, N. (2021). The effect of trans fatty acids on human health: Regulation and consumption patterns. *Foods, 10*(10), 2452. https://doi.org/10.3390/foods10102452.

Podgórska-Kryszczuk, I. (2024). Spirulina-an invaluable source of macro- and micronutrients with broad biological activity and application potential. *Molecules, 29*(22), 5387. https://doi.org/10.3390/molecules29225387 PMID: 39598773; PMCID: PMC11596570.

Polak, R., Phillips, E. M., & Campbell, A. (2015). Legumes: Health benefits and culinary approaches to increase intake. *Clinical Diabetes: A Publication of the American Diabetes Association, 33*(4), 198–205. https://doi.org/10.2337/diaclin.33.4.198 PMID: 26487796; PMCID: PMC4608274.

Ponnampalam, E. N., Priyashantha, H., Vidanarachchi, J. K., Kiani, A., & Holman, B. W. B. (2024). Effects of nutritional factors on fat content, fatty acid composition, and sensorial properties of meat and milk from domesticated ruminants: An overview. *Animals: An Open Access Journal from MDPI, 14*(6), 840. https://doi.org/10.3390/ani14060840.

Pounds, A., Kaminski, A. M., Budhathoki, M., Gudbrandsen, O., Kok, B., Horn, S., Malcorps, W., Mamun, A.-A., McGoohan, A., Newton, R., Ozretich, R., & Little, D. C. (2022). More than fish—framing aquatic animals within sustainable food systems. *Foods, 11*(10), 1413. https://doi.org/10.3390/foods11101413.

Prutcanu, L. L., Bailey, D. S., Grădinaru, A. C., & Jäntschi, L. (2023). The biochemistry and effectiveness of antioxidants in food, fruits, and marine algae. *Antioxidants, 12*(4), 860. https://doi.org/10.3390/antiox12040860.

Qin, J., Kurt, E., LBassi, T., Sa, L., & Xie, D. (2023). Biotechnological production of omega-3 fatty acids: Current status and future perspectives. *Frontiers in Microbiology, 14*, 1280296. https://doi.org/10.3389/fmicb.2023.1280296 PMID: 38029217; PMCID: PMC10662050.

Rahim, M. A., Ayub, H., Sehrish, A., Ambreen, S., Khan, F. A., Itrat, N., Nazir, A., Shoukat, A., Shoukat, A., Ejaz, A., Özogul, F., Bartkiene, E., & Rocha, J. M. (2023). Essential components from plant source oils: A review on extraction, detection, identification, and quantification. *Molecules, 28*(19), 6881. https://doi.org/10.3390/molecules28196881 PMID: 37836725; PMCID: PMC10574037.

Rahman, S. U., Weng, T. N., Qadeer, A., Nawaz, S., Ullah, H., & Chen, C. C. (2024). Omega-3 and omega-6 polyunsaturated fatty acids and their potential therapeutic role in protozoan infections. *Frontiers in Immunology, 15*, 1339470. https://doi.org/10.3389/fimmu.2024.1339470 PMID: 38633251; PMCID: PMC11022163.

Raphael, W., & Sordillo, L. M. (2013). Dietary polyunsaturated fatty acids and inflammation: The role of phospholipid biosynthesis. *International Journal of Molecular Sciences, 14*(10), 21167–21188. https://doi.org/10.3390/ijms141021167.

Redruello-Requejo, M., Samaniego-Vaesken, M.d L., Puga, A. M., Montero-Bravo, A., Ruperto, M., Rodríguez-Alonso, P., Partearroyo, T., & Varela-Moreiras, G. (2023). Omega-3 and omega-6 polyunsaturated fatty acid intakes, determinants and dietary sources in the spanish population: Findings from the ANIBES study. *Nutrients, 15*(3), 562. https://doi.org/10.3390/nu15030562.

Remize, M., Brunel, Y., Silva, J. L., Berthon, J. Y., & Filaire, E. (2021). Microalgae n-3 PUFAs production and use in food and feed industries. *Marine drugs, 19*(2), 113. https://doi.org/10.3390/md19020113 PMID: 33670628; PMCID: PMC7922858.

Rittenhouse, M., Khurana, S., Scholl, S., & Emerson, C. (2025). Examining the influence of omega-3 fatty acids on performance, recovery, and injury management for health optimization: A systematic review focused on military service members. *Nutrients, 17*(2), 307. https://doi.org/10.3390/nu17020307.

Rizzo, G., Baroni, L., & Lombardo, M. (2023). Promising sources of plant-derived polyunsaturated fatty acids: A narrative review. *International Journal of Environmental Research and Public Health, 20*(3), 1683. https://doi.org/10.3390/ijerph20031683.

Rocha, C. P., Pacheco, D., Cotas, J., Marques, J. C., Pereira, L., & Gonçalves, A. M. M. (2021). Seaweeds as valuable sources of essential fatty acids for human nutrition. *International Journal Of Environmental Research and Public Health, 18*(9), 4968. https://doi.org/10.3390/ijerph18094968 PMID: 34067088; PMCID: PMC8124752.

Rodrigues, M., Rosa, A., Almeida, A., Martins, R., Ribeiro, T., Pintado, M., Gonçalves, R. F. S., Pinheiro, A. C., Fonseca, A. J. M., Maia, M. R. G., Cabrita, A. R. J., Barros, L., & Caleja, C. (2024). Omega-3 fatty acids from fish by-products: Innovative extraction and application in food and feed. *Food and Bioproducts Processing, 145*, 32–41. https://doi.org/10.1016/j.fbp.2024.02.007 ISSN 0960-3085.

Ros, E. (2010). Health benefits of nut consumption. *Nutrients, 2*(7), 652–682. https://doi.org/10.3390/nu2070652 Epub 2010 Jun 24. PMID: 22254047; PMCID: PMC3257681.

Roy, V. C., Park, J.-S., Ho, T. C., & Chun, B.-S. (2022). Lipid indexes and quality evaluation of omega-3 rich oil from the waste of Japanese Spanish mackerel extracted by supercritical CO_2. *Marine drugs, 20*(1), 70. https://doi.org/10.3390/md20010070.

Ruiz-Domínguez, M. C., Toledo, C., Órdenes, D., Vílchez, C., Ardiles, P., Palma, J., & Cerezal, P. (2021). Variability of Omega-3/6 Fatty Acid Obtained Through Extraction-Transesterification Processes from Phaeodactylum tricornutum. *Acta Chim. Slov. 68*(3), 629–637.

Rueda García, A. M., Fracassi, P., Scherf, B. D., Hamon, M., & Iannotti, L. (2024). Unveiling the nutritional quality of terrestrial animal source foods by species and characteristics of livestock systems. *Nutrients, 16*(19), 3346. https://doi.org/10.3390/nu16193346.

Saidaiah, P., Banu, Z., Kha, A. A., Geetha, A., & Somraj, B. (2024). A comprehensive review of Omega-3 fatty acids: Sources, industrial applications, and health benefits. *Annals of Phytomedicine, 13*(1), 209–225. https://doi.org/10.54085/ap.2024.13.1.20.

Saini, R. K., & Keum, Y. S. (2018). Omega-3 and omega-6 polyunsaturated fatty acids: Dietary sources, metabolism, and significance - A review. *Life Sciences, 203*, 255–267. https://doi.org/10.1016/j.lfs.2018.04.049 Epub 2018 Apr 30. PMID: 29715470.

Saini, R. K., Prasad, P., Sreedhar, R. V., Akhilender Naidu, K., Shang, X., & Keum, Y. S. (2021). Omega-3 polyunsaturated fatty acids (PUFAs): Emerging plant and microbial sources, oxidative stability, bioavailability, and health benefits-a review. *Antioxidants (Basel), 10*(10), 1627. https://doi.org/10.3390/antiox10101627 PMID: 34679761; PMCID: PMC8533147.

Salvo, A., & Tuttolomondo, A. (2025). The role of olive oil in cardiometabolic risk. *Metabolites, 15*(3), 190. https://doi.org/10.3390/metabo15030190 PMID: 40137153; PMCID: PMC11943877.

Santigosa, E., Brambilla, F., & Milanese, L. (2021). Microalgae oil as an effective alternative source of EPA and DHA for gilthead seabream (*Sparus aurata*) aquaculture. *Animals: An Open Access Journal from MDPI, 11*(4), 971. https://doi.org/10.3390/ani11040971.

Santos, H. O., May, T. L., & Bueno, A. A. (2023). Eating more sardines instead of fish oil supplementation: Beyond omega-3 polyunsaturated fatty acids, a matrix of nutrients with cardiovascular benefits. *Frontiers in Nutrition, 10*, 1107475. https://doi.org/10.3389/fnut.2023.1107475 PMID: 37143475; PMCID: PMC10153001.

Sathasivam, R., Radhakrishnan, R., Hashem, A., & Abd_Allah, E. F. (2019). Microalgae metabolites: A rich source for food and medicine. *Saudi Journal of Biological Sciences, 26*(4), 709–722. https://doi.org/10.1016/j.sjbs.2017.11.003 ISSN 1319-562X.

Schmidt, K., Graeve, M., Hoppe, C. J. M., Torres-Valdes, S., Welteke, N., Whitmore, L. M., Anhaus, P., Atkinson, A., Belt, S. T., Brenneis, T., Campbell, R. G., Castellani, G., Copeman, L. A., Flores, H., Fong, A. A., Hildebrandt, N., Kohlbach, D., Nielsen, J. M., Parrish, C. C., ... Zhuang, Y. (2024). Essential omega-3 fatty acids are depleted in sea ice and pelagic algae of the Central Arctic Ocean. *Global Change Biology, 30*(1), e17090. https://doi.org/10.1111/gcb.17090 PMID: 38273483.

Schulze, M. B., Minihane, A. M., Saleh, R. N. M., & Risérus, U. (2020). Intake and metabolism of omega-3 and omega-6 polyunsaturated fatty acids: Nutritional implications for cardiometabolic diseases. *Lancet Diabetes Endocrinol, 8*(11), 915–930. https://doi.org/10.1016/S2213-8587(20)30148-0 Epub 2020 Sep 16. PMID: 32949497.

Sebastiani, G., Herranz Barbero, A., Borrás-Novell, C., Alsina Casanova, M., Aldecoa-Bilbao, V., Andreu-Fernández, V., Pascual Tutusaus, M., Ferrero Martínez, S., Gómez Roig, M. D., & García-Algar, O. (2019). The Effects of vegetarian and vegan diet during pregnancy on the health of mothers and offspring. *Nutrients, 11*(3), 557. https://doi.org/10.3390/nu11030557 PMID: 30845641; PMCID: PMC6470702.

Sharma, S., Cheng, S. F., Bhattacharya, B., & Chakkaravarthi, S. (2019). Efficacy of free and encapsulated natural antioxidants in oxidative stability of edible oil: Special emphasis on nanoemulsion-based encapsulation. *Trends in Food Science & Technology, 91*, 305–318. https://doi.org/10.1016/j.tifs.2019.07.030 ISSN 0924-2244.

Shi, H., Chen, H., Gu, Z., Song, Y., Zhang, H., Chen, W., & Chen, Y. Q. (2015). Molecular mechanism of substrate specificity for delta 6 desaturase from*Mortierella alpina* and *Micromonas pusilla*. *Journal of Lipid Research, 56*(12), 2309–2321. https://doi.org/10.1194/jlr.M062158 Epub 2015 Oct 20. PMID: 26486975; PMCID: PMC4655987.

Shi, H., Chen, H., Gu, Z., Zhang, H., Chen, W., & Chen, Y. Q. (2016). Application of a delta-6 desaturase with α-linolenic acid preference on eicosapentaenoic acid production in *Mortierella alpina*. *Microbial cell factories, 15*(1), 117. https://doi.org/10.1186/s12934-016-0516-5 PMID: 27364006; PMCID: PMC4929779.

Shramko, V. S., Polonskaya, Y. V., Kashtanova, E. V., Stakhneva, E. M., & Ragino, Y. I. (2020). The short overview on the relevance of fatty acids for human cardiovascular disorders. *Biomolecules, 10*(8), 1127. https://doi.org/10.3390/biom10081127 PMID: 32751513; PMCID: PMC7464661.

Shydakova-Kameniuka, O., Zagorulko, A., Kasabova, K., Mikhaylov, V., Shkliaiev, O., Rohova, A., Novik, A, & Lapytska, N. (2024). Applying chia seeds to improve the structural characteristics and nutrient composition of whipped candies. *Eastern-European Journal of Enterprise Technologies, 6*(11 (132), 73–83. https://doi.org/10.15587/1729-4061.2024.318530.

Šimat, V., Rathod, N. B., Čagalj, M., Hamed, I., & Generalić Mekinić, I. (2022). Astaxanthin from crustaceans and their byproducts: A bioactive metabolite candidate for therapeutic application. *Marine Drugs, 20*(3), 206. https://doi.org/10.3390/md20030206.

Simopoulos, A. P. (2002a). The importance of the ratio of omega-6/omega-3 essential fatty acids. *Biomedicine & Pharmacotherapy, 56*(8), 365–379. https://doi.org/10.1016/S0753-3322(02)00253-6 ISSN 0753-3322.

Simopoulos, A. P. (2002b). Omega-3 fatty acids in inflammation and autoimmune diseases. *Journal of the American College of Nutrition, 21*(6), 495–505. https://doi.org/10.1080/07315724.2002.10719248 PMID: 12480795.

Simopoulos, A. P. (2016). An increase in the omega-6/omega-3 fatty acid ratio increases the risk for obesity. *Nutrients, 8*(3), 128. https://doi.org/10.3390/nu8030128 PMID: 26950145; PMCID: PMC4808858.

Symoniuk, E., Wroniak, M., Napiórkowska, K., Brzezińska, R., & Ratusz, K. (2022). Oxidative stability and antioxidant activity of selected cold-pressed oils and oils mixtures. *Foods, 11*(11), 1597. https://doi.org/10.3390/foods11111597.

Takic, M., Pokimica, B., Petrovic-Oggiano, G., & Popovic, T. (2022). Effects of dietary α-linolenic acid treatment and the efficiency of its conversion to eicosapentaenoic and docosahexaenoic acids in obesity and related diseases. *Molecules, 27*(14), 4471. https://doi.org/10.3390/molecules27144471 PMID: 35889342; PMCID: PMC9317994.

Takić, M., Ranković, S., Girek, Z., Pavlović, S., Jovanović, P., Jovanović, V., & Šarac, I. (2024). Current insights into the effects of dietary α-linolenic acid focusing on alterations of polyunsaturated fatty acid profiles in metabolic syndrome. *International Journal of Molecular Sciences, 25*(9), 4909. https://doi.org/10.3390/ijms25094909.

Tamburini, B., Di Liberto, D., Pratelli, G., Rizzo, C., Barbera, L. L., Lauricella, M., Carlisi, D., Maggio, A., Palumbo Piccionello, A., D'Anneo, A., Caccamo, N., & Guggino, G. (2025). Extra virgin olive oil polyphenol-enriched extracts exert antioxidant and anti-inflammatory effects on peripheral blood mononuclear cells from rheumatoid arthritis patients. *Antioxidants, 14*(2), 171. https://doi.org/10.3390/antiox14020171.

Taşbozan, O., & Gökçe, M. A. (2017). *Fatty acids in fish*. InTech. 10.5772/68048.

Thakur, M., & Singh, K. (2013). Walnut (*Juglan regia* L.) a complete health and brain food. *Asian Journal of Bio Science, 8*(2), 276–288.

Thapa, S., Bhandari, A., Ghimire, R., Xue, Q., Kidwaro, F., Ghatrehsamani, S., Maharjan, B., & Goodwin, M. (2021). Managing micronutrients for improving soil fertility, health, and soybean yield. *Sustainability, 13*(21), 11766. https://doi.org/10.3390/su132111766.

Thomas, J., Thomas, C. J., Radcliffe, J., & Itsiopoulos, C. (2015). Omega-3 fatty acids in early prevention of inflammatory neurodegenerative disease: A focus on alzheimer's disease. *BioMed Research International, 2015*, 172801. https://doi.org/10.1155/2015/172801 Epub 2015 Aug 2. PMID: 26301243; PMCID: PMC4537710.

Tomczyk, M. (2024). Omega-3 fatty acids and muscle strength—Current state of knowledge and future perspectives. *Nutrients, 16*(23), 4075. https://doi.org/10.3390/nu16234075.

Tsoupras, A., Brummell, C., Kealy, C., Vitkaitis, K., Redfern, S., & Zabetakis, I. (2022). Cardio-protective properties and health benefits of fish lipid bioactives; The effects of thermal processing. *Marine drugs, 20*(3), 187. https://doi.org/10.3390/md20030187 PMID: 35323486; PMCID: PMC8955125.

Tu, Z., Yang, J., & Fan, C. (2024). The role of different nutrients in the prevention and treatment of cardiovascular diseases. *Frontiers in Immunology, 15*, 1393378. https://doi.org/10.3389/fimmu.2024.1393378 PMID: 38799425; PMCID: PMC11116626.

Usturoi, M. G., Rațu, R. N., Crivei, I. C., Veleșcu, I. D., Usturoi, A., Stoica, F., & Radu Rusu, R.-M. (2025). Unlocking the power of eggs: Nutritional insights, bioactive compounds, and the advantages of omega-3 and omega-6 enriched varieties. *Agriculture, 15*(3), 242. https://doi.org/10.3390/agriculture15030242.

Van Vliet, S., Provenza, F. D., & Kronberg, S. L. (2021). Health-promoting phytonutrients are higher in grass-fed meat and milk. *Frontiers in Sustainable Food Systems, 4*, 555426. https://doi.org/10.3389/fsufs.2020.555426.

Velissaridou, A., Panoutsopoulou, E., Prokopiou, V., & Tsoupras, A. (2024). Cardio-protective-promoting properties of functional foods inducing HDL-cholesterol levels and functionality. *Nutraceuticals, 4*(4), 469–502. https://doi.org/10.3390/nutraceuticals4040028.

Voon, P. T., Ng, C. M., Ng, Y. T., Wong, Y. J., Yap, S. Y., Leong, S. L., Yong, X. S., & Lee, S. W. H. (2024). Health effects of various edible vegetable oils: An umbrella review. *Advances in Nutrition, 15*(9), 100276. https://doi.org/10.1016/j.advnut.2024.100276 ISSN 2161-8313.

Wandhekar, S., Pawar, V. S., Shinde, S. T., & Gangakhedkar, P. S. (2022). Extraction of oil from oilseeds by cold pressing: A review Sangram Abstract College of Food Technology. *Indian Food Industry Mag, 4*(5), 63–69.

Wang, L., Meng, Q., & Su, C.-H. (2024). From food supplements to functional foods: Emerging perspectives on post-exercise recovery nutrition. *Nutrients, 16*(23), 4081. https://doi.org/10.3390/nu16234081.

Waszkowiak, K., Szymandera-Buszka, K., Kidoń, M., Kobus-Cisowska, J., Brzozowska, A., Kowiel, A., Jarzębski, M., & Radziejewska-Kubzdela, E. (2025). Application of chia and flaxseed meal as an ingredient of fermented vegetable-based spreads to design their nutritional composition and sensory quality. *Foods, 14*(3), 438. https://doi.org/10.3390/foods14030438.

Wu, J. Y., Tso, R., Teo, H. S., & Haldar, S. (2023). The utility of algae as sources of high value nutritional ingredients, particularly for alternative/complementary proteins to improve human health. *Frontiers in Nutrition, 10*, 1277343. https://doi.org/10.3389/fnut.2023.1277343 PMID: 37904788; PMCID: PMC10613476.

Xia, M., Zhong, Y., Peng, Y., & Qian, C. (2022). Olive oil consumption and risk of cardiovascular disease and all-cause mortality: A meta-analysis of prospective cohort studies. *Frontiers in Nutrition, 9*, 1041203. https://doi.org/10.3389/fnut.2022.1041203 PMID: 36330142; PMCID: PMC9623257.

Zec, M. M., Krga, I., Takić, M., Debeljak-Martačić, J., Koričanac, G., Ranković, S., Popović, T., Pantelić, M., & Glibetic, M. (2020). Walnut consumption induces tissue-specific omega-6/omega-3 decrease in high-fructose-fed wistar rats. *ACS Omega, 5*(43), 28136–28145. https://doi.org/10.1021/acsomega.0c03784.

Zhu, T., Kuai, Y., Guo, X., Bu, G., Yang, C., & Chen, F. (2025). Effect of dietary oils with different fatty acid compositions on serum lipid and gut microbiota of rats. *Foods, 14*(1), 61. https://doi.org/10.3390/foods14010061.

Zivkovic, A. M., Telis, N., German, J. B., & Hammock, B. D. (2011). Dietary omega-3 fatty acids aid in the modulation of inflammation and metabolic health. *Calif Agric (Berkeley), 65*(3), 106–111. https://doi.org/10.3733/ca.v065n03p106 PMID: 24860193; PMCID: PMC4030645.

van Zonneveld, S. M., van den Oever, E. J., Haarman, B. C. M., Grandjean, E. L., Nuninga, J. O., van de Rest, O., & Sommer, I. E. C. (2024). An anti-inflammatory diet and its potential benefit for individuals with mental disorders and neurodegenerative diseases—A narrative review. *Nutrients, 16*(16), 2646. https://doi.org/10.3390/nu16162646.

Zhuzzhassarova, G., Azarbayjani, F., & Zamaratskaia, G. (2024). Fish and Seafood Safety: Human Exposure to Toxic Metals from the Aquatic Environment and Fish in Central Asia. *Int J Mol Sci, 25*(3), 1590. https://doi.org/10.3390/ijms25031590 PMID: 38338869; PMCID: PMC10855114.

Further reading

Alberio, C., Izquierdo, N. G., Galella, T., Zuil, S., Reid, R., Zambelli, A., & Aguirrezábal, L. A. N. (2016). A new sunflower high oleic mutation confers stable oil grain fatty acid composition across environments. *European Journal of Agronomy, 73*, 25–33. https://doi.org/10.1016/j.eja.2015.10.003 ISSN 1161-0301.

Ali, S., Asif, N., Hayat, M., Bilal, R. M., Nauman, K., Nasir, J., Asghar, B., & Badar, I. (2023). Omega-3 fatty acids enriched flaxseed oil effects on meat quality and fatty acid profile of broiler chicks. *Kafkas Univ Vet Fak Derg, 29*(4), 327–334. https://doi.org/10.9775/kvfd.2022.27854.

Jiang, L., Wu, W., Wu, S., Wu, J., Zhang, Y., & Liao, L. (2024). Effect of different pretreatment techniques on quality characteristics, chemical composition, antioxidant capacity and flavor of cold-pressed rapeseed oil. *LWT, 201*, 116157. https://doi.org/10.1016/j.lwt.2024.116157 ISSN 0023-6438.

Merdzhanova, A., Panayotova, V., Dobreva, D. A., & Peycheva, K. (2021). Can fish and shellfish Species from the black sea supply health beneficial amounts of bioactive fatty acids? *Biomolecules, 11*(11), 1661. https://doi.org/10.3390/biom11111661 PMID: 34827659; PMCID: PMC8615860.

Mungwari, C. P., King'ondu, C. K., Sigauke, P., & Obadele, B. A. (2025). Conventional and modern techniques for bioactive compounds recovery from plants: Review. *Scientific African, 27*, e02509. https://doi.org/10.1016/j.sciaf.2024.e02509 ISSN 2468-2276.

Chapter 2

Nutritional importance and health benefits of n-3 and n-6 polyunsaturated fatty acids: essential fatty acids and dietary sources

Aria Babakhani, Fatemeh Zahmatkesh, and Alireza Rabiepour
Fisheries Department, Faculty of Natural Resources, University of Guilan, Sowmeh Sara, Guilan, Iran

2.1 Introduction

2.1.1 Definition and classification of lipids

Lipids and fats have played excessive roles in human societies from ancient times to the modern era. With the advancement of science, the sources of these bioactive compounds have changed and have been depicted in many usages. Polyunsaturated fatty acids (PUFAs) have been the matter of much preoccupation today owing to their single in-kind virtues in human health. In addition, producing high-value-added products based on fatty acids (FAs) is one of the things that industries are seeking to realize (Cerone & Smith, 2021). Lipids refer to a large set of molecules present in food products and living organisms. They are the main component of the food of humans and other organisms and play essential roles in providing energy, building and maintaining cell membranes, creating regulatory metabolites, and regulating gene expression. However, the use of some lipids, such as trans or saturated FAs, is harmful to humans and leads to disease. In addition to their impact on health, lipids have also been reported to have noteworthy traces in the chow industry in terms of texture, hardness, and savor of food (Domínguez et al., 2022). Miscellaneous classifications of lipids have been made. In the first type, fats include polar and neutral fats. The second kind is divided into two groups: saponifiable and unsaponifiable fats. Plain, blended, and derivative fats constitute the third lot. The fourth hilt contains triglycerides (TGs) and phospholipids (Zakipour Rahimabadi, 2021).

2.1.2 Fatty acids and their types

The maker fitments of lipids and crucial (cellular) membranes are designated FAs. Their estimable effects are very broad and can participate in cellular mechanisms (endocytosis and exocytosis), cell survival, modulation of ion channels and cell signaling potentials, and other functional activities (Iwabuchi et al., 2010; Simons & Toomre, 2000). FAs include three factions: saturated fatty acids (SFAs), monounsaturated fatty acids (MUFAs), and PUFAs. Eatable oils and lipids extracted from herb and animal reserves are among the reserves of fabrication of these FAs (Ahamad et al., 2024). Mankind can make FAs largely within their bodies. However, it cannot manufacture essential FAs. α-linoleic acid (ALA) and linoleic acid(LA) are conceived as essential FAs that must be fabricated from the foods we eat. SFAs, unlike unsaturated FAs, do not have binary grafts in their architecture. However, unsaturated FAs have from one to a large number of double bonds (Lunn & Theobald, 2006). MUFAs command purely one binary bond and subsume omega-7 and omega-9, while PUFAs hold two or further bipartite bonds.

2.1.3 Classification of polyunsaturated fatty acids

PUFAs include omega-3 and omega-6 FAs. These two FAs cannot be converted into each other, and balance amidst them is among the consistent factors in the operation of cell membranes and mankind health (Hulbert, 2021). In PUFAs, when

Omega-3 and Omega-6 Polyunsaturated Fatty Acids in Food Systems. DOI: https://doi.org/10.1016/B978-0-443-43810-3.00036-1

the first double bond occurs middle carbons 3 and 4, they are calculated as omega-3 FAs. Oppositely, the essence of the first double relationship between carbons 6 and 7 makes omega-6 PUFAs manifest (Rustan & Drevon, 2005). ALA (C18:3 n-3), eicosapentaenoic acid (EPA) (C20:5 n-3), docosahexaenoic acid (DHA) (C22:6 n-3), stearidonic acid (SDA) (C18:4 n-3), and docosapentanoic acid (DPA) (C22:5 n-3) are considered the most important omega-3 FAs. In contrast, LA (C18:2 n-6), γ-linolenic acid (GLA) (C18:3 n-6), dihomo-γ-linolenic acid (C20:3 n-6), arachidonic acid (AA) (C20:4 n-6), and adrenic acid (AdA) (C22:4 n-6) are nominated as the momentous omega-6 FAs (Ponnampalam et al., 2021).

2.1.4 Structural characteristics of omega-3 and omega-6 fatty acids

TGs are a kind of lipid subsisted in food and body fat. A glycerol is attached to three FAs to incorporate a TGs frame (Lunn & Theobald, 2006). The existence of a hydrocarbon armature with two carboxyl and methyl multitudes on contrary extremity establishes PUFAs. PUFAs contain two or more binary bonds versus other FAs. The chemical architecture of PUFAs is represented in Fig. 2.1. In omega-3 FAs, the presence of one more binary graft makes SDA distinct from ALA. The difference between EPA and DPA is in the number of carbon atoms. Versus the EPA, 22 carbon atoms are concentrated in the DPA structure, which is 2 carbons more than the EPA. DHA and DPA each have 22 carbon atoms; however, DPA has one less double bond than DHA (Guil-Guerrero, 2007; Zhan et al., 2021). In omega-6, the extra carbons in ADA make AA and ADA different. LA also differs from GLA in that LA has one less double bond.

2.2 Current scenario and literature review

2.2.1 Dietary reserves of n-3 and n-6 fatty acids

Chronic diseases have increased in human societies, which has led consumers to consume diets rich in PUFAs. It has been reported that camelina, chia, canola, flax, perilla, and watercress seed oils can provide high levels of ALA in mankind (Saini et al., 2021). Furthermore, *Vaccinium corymbosum*, *Vaccinum macrocarpon*, *Rubus occidentalis*, *Rubus ideaus*, *Ocimum spp.*, *Cannabis sativa*, *Hippophae rhamnoides*, *Lupinus albus L.*, *Juglans regia*, *Glycine max*, *Hevea brasiliensis*, Echium, and rose fruit seed oils are among the other sources of ALA in terricolous plants (Abedi & Sahari, 2014). Also, cow, lamb, pork, and chicken are nominated as terrestrial animals containing PUFAs, and meat, eggs, and milk are products originating from them (Abedi & Sahari, 2014). When organisms receive a diet rich in grains, we can observe an increased presence of omega-6 in their textures. While diets enriched with vegetables and plant seeds secure plentiful degrees of omega-3 FAs in the body (Bae et al., 2023). Omega-3 FAs come from fish (salmon, cod, mackerel, trout, sardines, tuna, herring, and halibut), walnuts, chia seed, and flaxseed; and omega-6 FAs come from plant oils (soybeans, sunflower, coconut, safflower, corn), almond, hazelnut, and walnut (Innis, 2008-; Ibrahim et al., 2018). Furthermore, sesame seed, pumpkin seed, and grape seed oil are omega-6 FA reserves (Froyen & Burns-Whitmore, 2020; Marangoni et al., 2020).

Aquatics and their derivatives are potential sources for the production of healthy foods and medicines. Bioactive substances produced from these aquatic organisms include PUFAs (Rabiepour & Babakhani, 2023). Algae and cyanobacteria are among the accessible reserves with superior potential to provide nutrients and generate food products for humans (Babakhani & ZahmatkeshInnis, 2024). Since algae are good producers of PUFAs, aquatic organisms can feed on them and pass PUFAs up the food chain (Chen and Li, 2023). In addition to fish oil (FO), which is a superlative reserve of PUFAs, DHASCO-B and life's DHA are among the algal nutritional supplements containing EPA and DHA (Saini et al., 2021). Diatoms, dinoflagellates, cryptophytes, cyanobacteria, green algae, and macrophytes can produce a significant portion of PUFAs in the bodies of fish, zooplankton, and invertebrates (Yan et al., 2024). Other aquatic

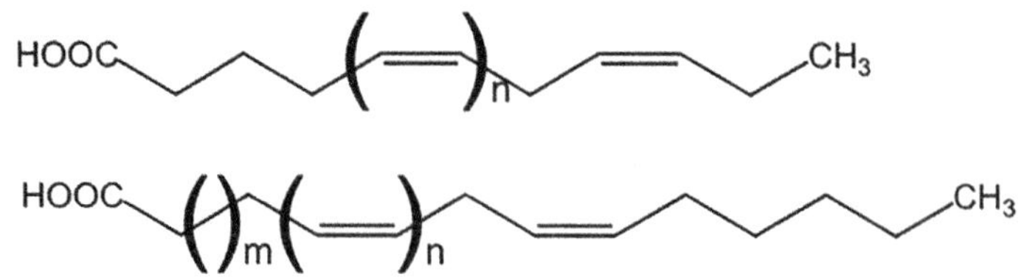

FIGURE 2.1 Chemical architecture of polyunsaturated fatty acids (omega-3 and omega-6 are indicated at the top and bottom, respectively) (Navalho and Ferrer-Ledo, 2025).

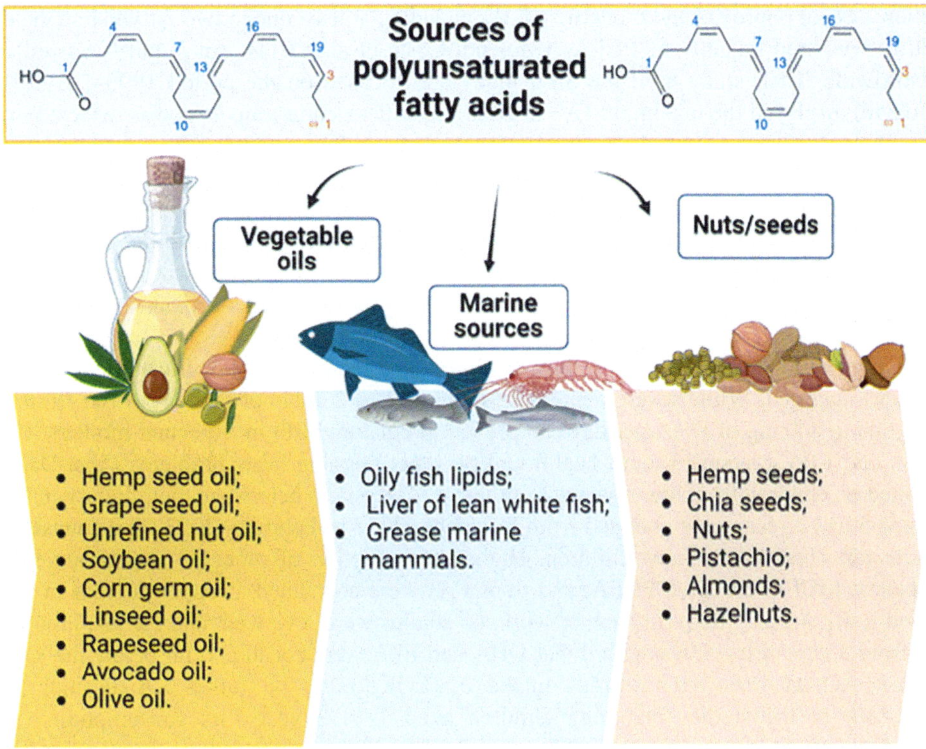

FIGURE 2.2 Food products containing polyunsaturated fatty acids. (Created with BioRender.com) (Mititelu et al., 2024).

organisms that are capable of producing PUFAs include bacteria, fungi, yeasts, and protozoa. Both aerobic and anaerobic pathways in these organisms lead to the biosynthesis of PUFAs (Tian et al., 2024). In addition to the reserves listed above, anchovies, *Thenus unimaculatus*, and *Solenocera hextii* are among the healthy food products that contain PUFAs. Cheek, age, genus, and hunting season are among the agents that affect the amount of fats and FAs in the body of these creatures (Chakraborty and Krishnan, 2021; Gil & Gil, 2015). The amount of PUFAs in fishery derivatives hinges on the processing strategies used (Nava et al., 2023). Besides, the kind of feed used also has a potential trace on the amount of PUFAs in the final processed product. One study argued that the use of a diet based on vegetable oils containing omega-6 was able to significantly enhance the levels of PUFAs in farmed salmon versus wild salmon (Strobel et al., 2012).

Krill is another aquatic animal with PUFA content. Research reported the presence of EPA and DHA in phospholipids and triacylglycerols of oil produced from krill powder (Xie et al., 2017). Fernandes et al. (2019) appraised the particulars of FAs of *Patella aspera* and *Patella candei*. The topmost degree of EPA was related to the *P. aspera*. In contrast, AA, oleic acid, and total PUFAs were found in *P. candei*. These two fishery products are considered healthy seafoods due to their estimable nutritional composition. In addition to the ones mentioned, other food options contain PUFAs. Breast milk is an appropriate reserve of PUFA, including DHA. This particular has led to its high ability to support brain and vision accretion and expansion. Therefore it leaves a profound mark on the supply of nutrients and the health of the infant (Kus-Yamashita et al., 2023). In addition, some well-known food products, including milk powder, dairy products, bread, biscuits, cookies, and other foods, have been fortified with DHA and EPA. These products have emerged as functional foods with health and nutritional benefits. Fig. 2.2 demonstrates food products containing PUFAs.

2.2.2 Global intake trends, recommendations, and deficiencies of polyunsaturated fatty acids

A slight consumption of PUFAs is connected with a variety of illnesses. Although some recommendations for PUFA intake or sources have been made by several organizations, few people follow these guidelines (Dicklin et al., 2024). The classes of omega-3 consumed in the West are down. Research demonstrates low intake of omega-3 in parturient and nursing mothers (Barrera et al., 2018). The advised amount of PUFAs by world organizations (FAO and WHO) and heart and dietary societies is being improved and modernized. By including at least one to two fatty fish in the diet per week, the body can provide the required quantity of PUFAs (Molendi-Coste et al., 2011). An inquiry showed that FA intake is highly uneven worldwide. Their study used the SEV index and focused on the period 1990–2019. The United States (Northern Hemisphere) displayed the maximal SEV. In addition, a diet rich in trans FAs was detected in this country (Hu et al., 2023). Forsyth et al. (2016) assessed universal DHA and arachidonic acid (ARA) consumption in 175 countries. ARA intakes below 150 mg/day and DHA intakes below 200 mg/day were found in 48% and 64% of 175 extended and extending states, respectively. Central and South Asia and Sub-Saharan Africa had the least consumption of ARA and DHA. Mao & Kong (2025) described that in 2021, little omega-6 consumption led to fatalities and disability-modified life years. The most affected groups were people over 75 years of age and men. Likewise, it was prognosticated that by 2030 and 2050, widespread troubles, including heart disease due to veritably low omega-6 intake, would occur in countries in Russia, Africa, and the Middle East.

The intake of PUFAs varies depending on the type of illness and its severity. For illustration, for depression, 200 to 300 mg/day has been suggested. While severe depression requires 1 to 2 g/day of omega-3 FAs. During pregnancy, it is recommended that 600 to 800 mg of DHA per day can prevent premature birth in expectant mothers. In addition, the use of 500 mg of DHA and EPA guarantees heart health and prevents possible heart problems (Van Dael, 2021). Another survey was conducted on children from low-revenue families in Malaysia to determine their dietary intake of FAs. A total of 182 children aged 5 to 12 years were assessed from December 2022 to February 2023. The counseled instructions for eating PUFAs were not observed by most children. Higher consumption of omega-3 was observed in children from Tawau. In discrepancy, MUFA, omega-6 PUFA, and trans FAs were consumed at upper degrees in children from Kota Kinabalu (Chen and Rafiz Azuan, 2024). In another work, 65 studies were reviewed, and the test group included children aged 1 to 7 years from 33 countries. It was found that DHA and EPA were consumed far below the levels recommended by the WHO and the FAO. ALA showed a very low intake (0.5%) in 50% of the studies. LA consumption was better than ALA. In fact, in 24% of the studies involving children aged 1 to 2 years, its consumption was not under the recommendations of the mentioned organizations (Monnard & Fleith, 2021). Despite the aforementioned studies revealing inadequate intake of PUFAs, it is expected that strict management approaches will be adopted by relevant organizations for the dietary intake of PUFAs by the population globally. Creating such regulations can be difficult, but it can provide health benefits for preventing and combating diseases.

2.2.3 Role of n-3 and n-6 in human health

The main hassle of human society is the developed diseases that require huge expenses. In addition, the use of inappropriate food diets that have artificial origins is also considered to be a factor causing diseases. To deal with these irresistible conditions, we must turn to the healthy food templates that are derived from natural means. The investment in these foods not only helps to obtain essential nutrients for the body, but also lays the foundation for permanent human health (Rabiepour et al., 2024). In this regard, much attention has been focused on PUFAs due to their health-promoting properties. PUFAs have amazing effects in reducing harmful lipids. EPA and DHA accomplish effective actions in reducing TGs and regulating cardiovascular activity, and controlling blood flow. They also act as antiinflammatory, antioxidant, and antithrombotic agents, and fight free radicals. Omega-6 has also been shown to help prevent the spread of other diseases by reducing LDL cholesterol (Djuricic & Calder, 2021). Brain development, improved psychological and behavioral traits (Noreen et al., 2024), treatment of depression, regulation of neural activity (Serefko et al., 2024), and anticancer effects against breast, prostate, and colon cancers (Akbar and Rahman, 2024) are just a few of the extraordinary potential applications of omega-3 FAs. PUFAs can also combat protozoa and the infections caused by them. They recognize and destroy disease-causing agents. Their effects are widespread and include increased phagocytosis and reduced inflammation. Given that parasitic infections pose a severe threat to the lives of organisms and humans, the consumption of PUFAs can reduce or eliminate the stresses created in this area (Rahman et al., 2024). Fig. 2.3 offers some of the bioactive effects of PUFAs (see Fig. 2.3).

Omega-3 FAs may have a profitable impress on sepsis patients by reducing oxidative stress and suppressing inflammation. This may subtract the duration of illness and the need for mechanical ventilation (Awasthi & Jerath, 2025). A study displayed that when a diet containing PUFAs and FO supplements was utilized in cancer patients, the prostate cancer progression index (Ki-67) subtracted in people addicted to this disease (Aronson and Grogan, 2025). A work was located that the combination of the cancer cure (5-fluorouracil) and FO led to greater inhibition of the colorectal cancer cell echelons (LS411N, LS513, HCT-8, and DLD-1) versus the therapy alone (Pettersen et al., 2023). Studies have shown the curative potential of ALA in viral diseases. For instance, ALA can control the Zika virus and forestall its propagation in the cells of the infected individual (Feng et al., 2023; Doaei and Gholami, 2021) concluded in an inquiry that omega-3-

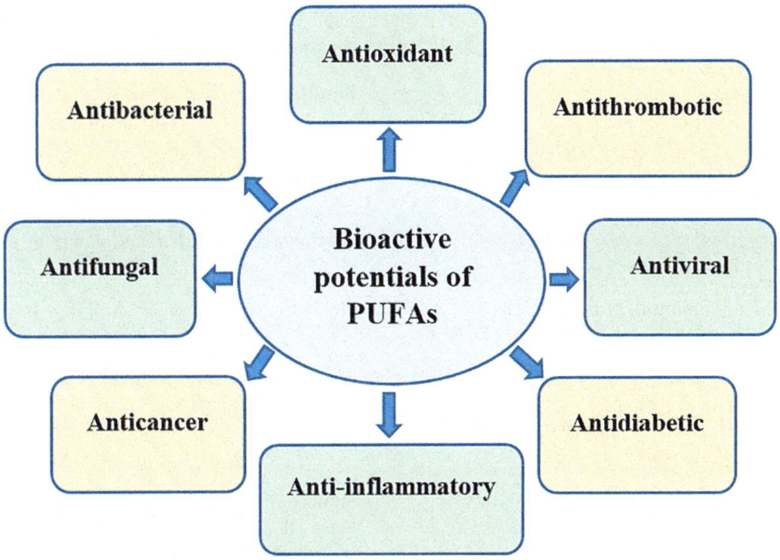

FIGURE 2.3 Bioactive effects of polyunsaturated fatty acids.

formulated supplements amended survival, respiratory, and renal status in COVID-19 sicks. Also, nanoencapsulated AA can provide a sizeable performance in the treatment of COVID-19 (Shoieb et al., 2021). MCI is a type of mild cognitive impairment. Omega-3-enriched diets establish a forceful operation in enhancing cognition in elderly individuals with this condition (Zhang et al., 2020).

Sharifi et al. (2017) worked on people infected with *Helicobacter pylori*. The first multitude received only specific drugs (Amoxicillin, Clarithromycin, and Omeprazole) against *H. pylori*, and the second multitude took PUFA supplements along with the mentioned drugs. Increased apoptosis in the second group and inhibition of bacterial growth were observed. This study proved that using PUFAs in the diet can eliminate antibiotic resistance in people infected with this bacterium and improve the treatment process. Adiponectin is a hormone whose low levels in the human body pose risks to humans in terms of its effect on the heart. In addition, attention should be paid to the level of this hormone in people with type 2 diabetes. A perusal by Müllner et al. (2014) was conducted on the effect of using food products containing PUFAs in patients with this type of diabetes. These people consumed 9 g of nuts and mixed oils per day. Adiponectin levels showed an increasing trend after 10 weeks. The results of another project investigating the utilization of FO supplementation in young adults (15–25 years) with symptoms of depression stated that taking 1.4 g of omega-3 per day improved cognitive function in persons with MDD (Rice et al., 2016). A study evaluated the use of chicken flesh fortified with omega-3 in healthy young men. The span of the investigation was 3 weeks, and the tentative groups included the first group (500 g of chicken meat) and the second group (1500 mg of meat containing omega-3). The second group showed an observable enhancement in antioxidant enzymes (Nađ et al., 2025).

Omega-3 and FO supplements may reduce the traces of the disorder in patients with multiple sclerosis (AlAmmar and Albeesh, 2021). Research examined the traces of FO supplementation on osteoarthritis (joint inflammation) in 40 to 65-year-old women. The duration of supplementation was 3 months, and the dosage was 100 mg of FO. The patients suffered from swelling and pain in the knee area. After the course of treatment with omega-3 FO, the severity of the disease and the resulting inflammation disclosed a remarkable reduction (Abd El-Fatah et al., 2016). The conclusions of a research study argued that curcumin-based nanoparticles loaded with ALA could be assigned as a novel option for the therapy of psoriasis. This method can eliminate the inflammation caused by this kind of skin sickness and prevent excessive proliferation of keratinocytes (Serini et al., 2025). A study explained that canola oils with an omega-6/omega-3 proportion (5.6:1) and FOs with a ratio of 2:1 can inhibit atherosclerosis and regulate immune system activity through their bioactive effects (Subash-Babu & Alshatwi, 2018). Table 2.1 declares the health actions of PUFAs on Mankind's life.

2.2.4 Imbalance of omega-6/omega-3 proportion and its health aftermaths

Mankind evolved with a omega-6/omega-3 proportion of about 1. In the Western diet, we see a shortage of omega-3 and a boost in omega-6. This upper proportion of omega-6 to omega-3 is connected with a comprehensive bound of

TABLE 2.1 The health actions of polyunsaturated fatty acids on mankind's life.

Type of disease/ disorder	Dosage	Results	References
Rheumatoid arthritis	Two capsules of omega-3 (each capsule contains 2.1 g DHA and 1.8 g EPA)	The syntax of antirheumatic cure (DMARDS) with omega-3 capsules for 12 weeks led to the elimination of inflammation and deduced agony in people.	(Rajaei et al., 2015)
Isolated systolic blood pressure (BP)	0.7 g (minimum) of EPA + DHA	Deducting in BP.	(Minihane et al., 2016)
Breast cancer	Three capsules (each capsule containing 50 mg of curcumin extract, 460 mg of EPA + DHA, and 125 mg of olive-extracted hydroxytyrosol)	Remedy for 30 days resulted in subtracted inflammation and muscle pain in subjects.	(Martínez et al., 2019)
Dry eye (DE)	Oral supplementation (300 mg DHA, 150 mg GLA, and 1200 mg EPA)	Subjects displayed a positive trend in letup DE and its symptoms after 3 months of oral supplementation.	(Ng and Woods, 2022)
Coronary artery disease	1200 mg of omega-3 daily	Taking omega-3 in patients (age 45 to 65 years) was able to subtract myostatin quantities and ultimately lead to improvement in patients with CAD.	(Sharifzadeh et al., 2024)
Epilepsy	0.3 to 1.7 g (EPA and DHA) per day	Eating omega-3 could be considered an effective treatment for people with epilepsy. This dietary supplement can reduce neurotic and seizure behaviors in patients.	(Wu et al., 2025)

indispositions, including autoimmune, cancer, cardiovascular, and inflammatory diseases (Simopoulos, 2002). About 100 years ago, this proportion was 4 to 1 or downer. Currently, in the West, the ratio is 20 to 1. This issue requires urgent attention. The solution in this regard is more utilization of reserves of omega-3, for instance, fish or fishery crops. In addition, a downward trend in the reception of full omega-6 means should be included in the Western diet (DiNicolantonio & O'Keefe, 2021). Jang et al. (2025) said that an upper omega-6/omega-3 proportion was a risk factor for AMD (macular degeneration) in Korean individuals. Fedacko et al. (2012) submitted that the cause of death in deceased Indian subjects was positively associated with their dietary intake and high and unbalanced omega-6/omega-3 proportion. Their inquiry was based on hospital records of the deceased as well as autopsy data from the World Health Organization. The obesity complication is because the phospholipids of the red blood cell (RBC) membrane contain a superior amount of omega-6 compared to omega-3 (Simopoulos, 2016). Also, very excessive levels of lipid agents generated from AA and LA can be manufactured with high omega-6/omega-3 proportions. This, in turn, causes inflammation, atheroma, thrombosis, and an overactive endocannabinoid system. To prevent these conditions from occurring, people should consume a balanced omega-6/omega-3 proportion (4–5/1) (Mariamenatu & Abdu, 2021).

It has been said that low DHA: AA ratios can increase preterm birth in African American pregnant women (Christian and Blair, 2016). Mood disorders are considered to be psychiatric disorders. Studies suggest that an unbalanced and high omega-6/omega-3 proportion creates a remarkable potential for the enlargement of this disorder in youths (Berger and Smesny, 2017). A superior omega-6 proportion is also associated with a superior platelet count and activity. Omega-3, on the other hand, can significantly reduce bleeding and has antithrombotic potential. Their moderate intake helps maintain heart health (DiNicolantonio & O'Keefe, 2019). The loss of the equilibrium of omega-3 and omega-6 also disrupts the principles of lipid accumulation. In addition, the liver is unable to eliminate fat. Ultimately, as the amount of fat in the liver increases, a person develops fatty liver (El-Badry et al., 2007). Explained that an upper omega-6/omega-3 proportion in older adults with knee osteoarthritis is associated with comorbidities such as pain, agitation derangements, and mobility limitations. An abnormal ratio of LA to ALA was sustained in epileptic infants versus healthy infants (Bahgat et al., 2019).

It has also been explained that ingesting plentiful quantities of omega-6 before or during pregnancy may have adverse effects on the fetus. These effects may be disseminated and may lead to health risks in later life (Shrestha et al., 2020).

2.3 Principles and methodology

2.3.1 Biosynthesis pathways of omega-3 and omega-6 fatty acids

Long-chain unsaturated FAs have a significant role in creating embedded within cell membranes and are precursors of bioactive combinations (Dyall and Balas, 2022; Uttaro, 2006). PUFA biosynthesis takes place via two main routes: the anaerobic route, which rely on polyketide synthesis enzymes, and the aerobic routes, which include elongases and desaturases (Uttaro, 2006). This anaerobic route was initially discovered in marine microorganisms and subsequently in terrestrial myxobacteria (Gemperlein et al., 2014). The aerobic route utilizes elongases and desaturases that are activated under oxygen-dependent situations (Uttaro, 2006).

A major enzyme contributing to the synthesis of unsaturated fats is FA desaturase. They are typically categorized into three primary groups: acyl lipid-dependent desaturases, acyl carrier protein-dependent desaturases, and acyl-CoA-dependent desaturases (Cerone & Smith, 2022). Δ9 desaturases, particularly stearoyl-CoA desaturase, function as a rate limiting enzymes in the manufacturing of unsaturated FAs. The enzyme is responsible for initiating the organization of a cis-type binary graft at the Δ9 position of the acyl-CoA molecule, an essential step in the desaturation pathway (Nagao et al., 2019).

Desaturases utilize a diiron active site to catalyze dehydrogenation processes that rely on molecular oxygen (O_2). Recent structural and functional investigations of castor oil desaturase have substantiated the concept of an ancestral oxidase enzyme that has contributed to the evolutionary functional variety of diiron enzymes (Shanklin et al., 2009). Recent examinations have greatly revised our learning of PUFA biosynthetic pathways, revealing that they are more complex than previously thought, involving 24-carbon intermediates and a partial beta-oxidation process in peroxisomes (Sprecher et al., 1995). This complex biosynthetic pathway requires intracellular transport between various organelles, including peroxisomes and the endoplasmic reticulum, which play important roles in completing the various steps of PUFA synthesis (Sprecher et al., 1995).

Among the model organisms that have been extensively employed to examine the molecular and genetic processes of PUFA biosynthesis is the nematode worm *Caenorhabditis elegans*. In this organism, one elongase and seven unique genes associated with desaturase activity have been identified by researchers, offering informative insights into the enzymatic regulation of this process (Napier & Michaelson, 2001). Significant advances in biotechnology, especially in areas such as industrial fermentation and enzyme engineering, have enabled the commercial and large-scale production of PUFAs for widespread functions in the food, pharmaceutical, and nutritional supplement industries (Ma et al., 2002).

2.3.2 Omega-3 and omega-6 analysis techniques

Determining the range of essential FAs in food, seafood products, and dietary supplements, particularly these omega-3 and omega-6 FAs, is of nutritional importance for quality control and determining their respective health benefits. Chromatography and spectroscopy methods are some of the most prevalent techniques for measuring and analyzing FAs. Gas and liquid chromatography with high-tech detectors are examples of chromatographic methods that are officially recognized and recommended for regular research because they are sensitive and specific (Curtis & Black, 2013; Rohman et al., 2023). Gas chromatography (GC)-multiple sclerosis (MS) has been effectively utilized to examine FOcapsules. The great susceptibility and specificity of GC-MS and LC-MS make them popular courses for FA analysis (Muriuki et al., 2012; Öztürk Er et al., 2020). These courses enable the precise amount of the presence of FAs within multiple biological systems. Among them, spectroscopic techniques such as infrared, Raman, and NMR, when combined with chemometric methods, are emerging as fast, reliable, and efficient options that can provide results comparable to conventional chromatographic methods (Irnawati et al., 2024; Rohman et al., 2023). On the other hand, they are helpful alternatives for performing accurate quantitative analyzes (Rohman et al., 2023). High-pressure liquid chromatography (HPLC) in blend with a charged aerosol detector provides consistent and reliable responses for nonvolatile analytes. It is, therefore an effective tool for analyzing and identifying lipid compounds (Acworth and Plante, 2011). To date, various analytical methods have demonstrated successful performance in identifying omega-3 and omega-6 PUFAs in diverse matrices, including food, seafood, dietary supplements, and human biological samples. Among these methods, reductive ozonolysis has been enlarged as a basic course for gauging the total omega-3 FAs in lipid mixtures (Ott & Meusel, 1990). Table 2.2 highlights the principal analytical procedures appropriate for the quantification of FAs. The selection of the appropriate tool for analysis is made according to the specific requirements of each application, including accuracy, selectivity, and the

TABLE 2.2 Comparison of analytical methods for the quantification of omega-3 and omega-6 fatty acids (*FAs*).

Method	Description of method and conditions	Sensitivity and accuracy	Advantages	Limitation	Application	References
HPLC-CAD	· C30 column · Mobile phase: water/ACN/THF · No derivatization required	· LOD: 1–10 ng · Linearity: $R^2 > 0.99$	· No derivatization needed · Simultaneous FA analysis	· Lower sensitivity compared to GC	· omega-3/omega-6 profiling in oils	(Acworth and Plante, 2011)
GC-MS	· Same as GC-FID · Detection in SIM mode (e.g., m/z 79 for EPA/DHA)	· LOD: 0.08 ng (EPA), 0.21 ng (DHA) · RSD < 1.1%	· High sensitivity · FA identity confirmed via mass spectra	· Expensive equipment · Time-consuming sample prep	· Confirmation of compounds in supplements · Complex matrices	Yi and Li, (2014), Wang et al. (2017)
LC-MS/MS	· C18 column · MRM transitions (e.g., EPA: m/z 301→257) · No derivatization	· LOD: pg/mg · Recovery: 90–110%	· Extremely high sensitivity · Suitable for bio-samples	· Matrix effects may require correction	· Blood/plasma samples · Pharmacokinetic studies	(Serafim et al., 2019)
NMR	· Detection of characteristic peaks (e.g., 2.39 ppm for DHA) · Internal std: dimethyl terephthalate	· Accuracy: ±5% · Recovery: 95–105%	· No derivatization · Structural information	· High cost · Lower sensitivity	· Absolute analysis in pure oils	(Lv et al., 2020)
GC-FID	· Polar capillary column (e.g., HP-88) · Programmed temp: 170–240°C · Internal std: methyl tricosanoate	· LOD: ~0.1 µg/g · RSD < 2% · Recovery: 95–105%	· High resolution · Low cost · USP compliant	· Requires derivatization to fatty acid methyl esters · High temp may degrade some FAs	· Fish oils and supplements · Quantification of EPA/DHA	(Muhammad Alinafiah et al., 2021); (Rohman et al., 2023)
FTIR + chemometrics	· Direct ATR-FTIR analysis · Spectral range: 1800–950 cm^{-1} · PLS modeling for prediction	· R^2 ~0.98 for EPA/DHA · RMSE ~1.6 mg/g	· Fast and nondestructive · Minimal sample prep	· Requires initial calibration	· Rapid screening of supplements	(Prado et al., 2022)

nature of the sample. Chromatographic techniques are seen to be the best choice for accurate analyzes because of their high precision and good resolution, whereas spectroscopy is more frequently employed as a quick and practical instrument for screening and exploratory research.

2.3.3 Modern techniques for extraction and purification

Researchers have been working on developing more effective methods for extracting and purifying omega-3 and omega-6 PUFAs in recent years. The main goals are to improve the quality, speed up the process, and make these compounds more stable. In this sense, microalgae have been identified as new and valuable biological producers of EPA and DHA acids, and scientists have looked into different ways to extract them (Karrar et al., 2024). Supercritical fluid extraction and supercritical fluid chromatography (SFC) as neoteric approaches, have shown significant potential in the manufacturing and purification of lipids from microalgae (Karrar et al., 2024). Among modern technologies, treatments, including urea adduction, low-temperature fractional crystallization, and distillation, have proven helpful for lipid purification (Senanayake, 2013). The application of HPLC and SFC offers advantages over conventional GC by avoiding thermal degradation associated with the high temperatures of GC analysis, thus enhancing the precision and quality of lipid analysis (Yves et al., 2016). These methods have helped optimize extraction yield while avoiding the degradation of sensitive components, including FAs and fat-soluble vitamins (Maqsood et al., 2012).

Improvements in synthetic biology and microbial fermentation are being investigated to generate n-3 PUFAs in a more sustainable and less costly manner. Among them, microorganisms such as bacteria, fungi, microalgae, and especially thraustochytrids are being studied because they could be a rich reservoir of omega-3 compounds (Hinzpeter et al., 2006). Thraustochytrids, which are macrocellular marine heterokonts, have high biological potential owing to their potency to fabricate significant quantities of DHA and EPA (Gupta et al., 2012). These microorganisms can synthesize elevated quantities of specific omega-3 PUFAs under heterotrophic conditions and also exhibit faster growth rates compared with other sources (Hinzpeter et al., 2006).

Microalgae can produce a significant amount of FAs, which is the reason for their extensive study. Recent research has focused on finding the best conditions for growth and using metabolic engineering to make production more efficient (Barta et al., 2021). In addition, microalgae, both in autotrophic and heterotrophic cultures, have been widely studied as emerging biofactories used in obtaining omega-3 PUFAs, especially for applications in aquatic feed and biofuels (Adarme-Vega and Lim, 2012). Extraction methods expanded for the recovery of these combinations include the use of solvents, mechanical processes, and solvent-free approaches (Verma et al., 2020). Meanwhile, enzymatic extraction using lipases has been proposed as a mild and environmentally friendly method that can preserve the structure and integrity of PUFAs (Wanasundara & Shahidi, 2020). However, challenges such as optimizing fermentation conditions, selecting efficient strains, and utilizing cheap carbon sources remain on the path to industrialization of these approaches (Gupta et al., 2012; Hinzpeter et al., 2006).

2.3.4 Challenges in analytical and nutritional research

PUFAs, including omega-3 and omega-6, face challenges in their analysis and application due to their vital roles in human health and their high sensitivity to oxidation. These FAs, particularly omega-3 and omega-6 types, must overcome obstacles related to oxidative stability to be effectively used in diets and supplements. Since their incorporation into food yields is accompanied by the risk of oxidative degradation, the use of efficient antioxidants and the application of new encapsulation technologies seem essential (Hernandez, 2014). Using natural antioxidants, particularly plant extracts, to safeguard omega-3-rich oils from oxidation has been suggested as a suitable and secure alternative to synthetic antioxidants. These natural components enhance the stability of FO against oxidative degradation and reduce concerns about the harmful consequences of artificial additives (Maqsood et al., 2012).

Due to the lack of established methods for analyzing these FAs, researchers have explored various testing methods. As Rohman et al. (2023) have pointed out, chromatographic and spectroscopic techniques, including GC and LC-MS, are generally used to perform sensitive and targeted analyzes. However, the existence of inferior grades of omega-3 FAs in supplements and fortified foods makes the extraction and analysis of samples a major challenge (Hernandez, 2014). For this reason, chromatographic techniques are considered the most effective options for continuous quality control due to their high accuracy and sensitivity (Rohman et al., 2023). Since PUFAs usually exist in minimal quantities in biological matrices, the profiling of lipid intermediates derived from these molecules requires the use of analytical techniques with high sensitivity and precision (Kasuga et al., 2015). In these studies, sample matrix effects and extraction efficiency are key factors that must be considered. However, sample matrix effects make Guo & Lankmayr (2011) claim that omega-3 and omega-6 research in biological matrices is highly challenging and complex. These matrix effects may increase or decrease the analyte response in LC-MS/MS-based biological analyzes.

Selected FAs such as omega-3 and omega-6 from RBC phospholipids can now be quantified utilizing a standardized and verified gas chromatography method with flame ionization detection, which is wellsuited for large-scale epidemiological examinations (Gupta and Dhatwalia, 2021). The standard procedure for analyzing omega-3 FAs includes lipid extraction, conversion of FAs to methyl esters, and ensuing assay utilizing several instrumental techniques (Curtis & Black, 2013). It is also recommended that consideration be given to the development of standardized spectroscopic techniques for future collaborative research and skill assessment (Irnawati et al., 2024).

Phospholipids, which are particularly abundant in biological samples, are a significant source of matrix effects that interfere with the washing and retention processes during normal-phase and reversed-phase chromatography (Guo & Lankmayr, 2011). Therefore accurately assessing matrix effects and preparing standard samples are crucial to overcoming these obstacles (Kasuga et al., 2015). Chromatographic techniques, particularly in conjunction with mass spectrometry in gas and liquid chromatography, yield sensitive and accurate data for continuous quality control (Rohman et al., 2023). The form of chemical bonding, matrix effects, and galenic structure are among the items that have an impact on the bioavailability of these omega-3 and omega-6 FAs (Schuchardt & Hahn, 2013). De Carvalho & Caramujo (2018) believe that FA profiles can elucidate interactions within food webs, identify organisms, and examine bacterial adaptations. The complexity of FA patterns in biological materials has been widely studied due to their diverse roles and potential as biomarkers. FAs are not only a reserve of energy storage but also establish a function in cell signaling processes and act as structural supports in cell membranes (De Carvalho & Caramujo, 2018).

Determining total fat intake and accounting for variables that influence FA deposition and mobilization, including genetic variation, disease status, and lifestyle changes, remains challenging (Tiuca et al., 2015). Cancer and cardiovascular illness are among the common health issues linked to a superior proportion of omega-6 to omega-3 in the Western nutritional regimen (Berquin et al., 2008). Yet, boosting the consumption of omega-3 FAs, primarily from sources like vegetable oils and seafood, has demonstrated potential for the effective deterrence and therapy of chronic disorders (Gazem & Chandrashekariah, 2014). Ensuring an appropriate equilibrium between omega-6 and omega-3 FA consumption is crucial for health preservation and the deterrence of inflammatory disorders (Gazem & Chandrashekariah, 2014).

Genetic variation mostly affects individual responses to both omega-3 and omega-6 FAs, hindering the formulation of uniform dietary regimens. Genes such as FADS1, FADS2, 5-lipoxygenase, and cyclooxygenase-2 have polymorphisms that affect FA metabolism and, consequently, health outcomes, including cancer risk, cardiovascular disease, and child development (Simopoulos, 2010). The connection between dietary FAs and genetic variation is a crucial element in the development of metabolic syndrome (O'Connor & Rudkowska, 2019). Recent dietary modifications and genetic variants affecting the production of an elongated chain of unsaturated FAs may lead to discrepancies in prevailing dietary patterns (Chilton and Dutta, 2017). Although a genotype-based diet is a promising strategy for reducing cardiovascular disease, there is still inadequate proof about the interactions between nutrients and genes.

Analysis of the part of omega-3 in depression has yielded mixed and sometimes contradictory results, with some studies failing to demonstrate apparent efficacy (Lange, 2021). These inconsistencies may arise from variations in experimental setup, omega-3 administration levels, and sample demographics (Sahye-Pudaruth & Ma, 2023). New and inconsistent evidence has challenged the role of omega-3 FAs in stopping various conditions and curing a range of illnesses, despite decades of preclinical study demonstrating their potential health advantages (Weylandt et al., 2015). Furthermore, complex interactions between PUFAs (omega-3 and omega-6), as well as other dietary ingredients, significantly influence their physiological effects. The superior proportion of omega-6 to omega-3 in Western diets, where omega-6 plays a proinflammatory role and omega-3 plays an inflammation-controlling role, leads to the exacerbation of chronic diseases (Simopoulos, 2008). The gut microbiota interacts with various dietary compounds, including phytochemicals, PUFAs, and prebiotics, and these interactions significantly impact their bioavailability and efficacy (Laparra & Sanz, 2010). Omega-3 FAs enhance the synthesis of the intestinal alkaline phosphatase enzyme, so decreasing inflammation and metabolic endotoxemia, underscoring the essential function of gut microbiota in facilitating these outcomes (Kaliannan et al., 2015).

2.4 Applications

2.4.1 Nutritional-therapeutic applications

A consideration by Aristotelous and Stefanakis, 2021 was conducted to estimate the trace of using the nutritional supplement Neuroaspis PLP10 on Cypriot women with multiple sclerosis (MS) who were taking the drug Interferon-β.

This supplement contained high levels of DHA, EPA, LA, and GLA, and amounts of antioxidant compounds. The intake period was 20 ml daily for 24 months. Gait parameters, sit-to-stand test, and 6-minute walk were improved in the multitude fed the dietary supplement versus the multitude that consumed only olive oil (20 ml). A study showed that AA supplementation of 4 g can increase platelet counts in the body. This, in turn, can suppress the detrimental effects of liver cirrhosis, which deduces platelet activity (Mitchell et al., 2018; Pantaleo et al., 2004) reported that 1.5 g of AA supplementation for 1 month may amplify muscle harmony for subsequent recovery in future days. Ribosome biogenesis was also augmented after 48 hours. AA can contribute to human health, but its use should not be excessive enough to cause human complications (Zhou et al., 2021). A project looked at the investment of PUFAs on fertility in men. An upward procedure in fertility rates was obtained with a higher intake of nuts and seeds, which are high in PUFAs (Schipper et al., 2025). Yamaguchi et al. (2022) assessed the effect of FO supplements (omega-3) and evening primrose oil (omega-6) in postmenopausal women. A sizable deduction in platelet secretion and aggregation was demonstrated in women. Therefore the risk of heart disease for postmenopausal women was reduced due to the neutralization of platelet reactivity.

Quispe-Fuentes et al. (2025) extracted oil from the hepatopancreas of the *Dosidicus gigas*. The resulting oil was rich in EPA, DHA, and antioxidants and indicated anticancer potential against colon cancer (Serini et al., 2018). In a study, made solid lipid nanoparticles with the help of resveratrol, which is a chemical derived from plants. Omega-3 PUFAs were able to easily approach the body and colorectal cancer cells using nanoencapsulation technology. Preventing the propagation of cancer cells and inhibiting their growth were among the traces of nanoparticles containing omega-3 and resveratrol. Furthermore, the magnitude of AA as a suitable curative option in the remedy of human coronavirus via nanoencapsulation has been emphasized by Shoieb et al. (2021). It has been shown that daily use of two Oravex capsules, which contain 40 mg DHA, 280 mg EPA, 20 mg green tea extract, 50 mg thyme extract, 7.5 mg zinc, 27.5 μg selenium, and 50 mg olive leaf extract, can together with the drug tacalcitol, treat psoriasis and its skin inflammation in patients (Balbás et al., 2011). An inquiry revealed that the supplementation of the isomer of LA, namely conjugated LA, can reduce the amount of OS in persons with COPD by having antioxidant properties. The supplementation period was 6 weeks, and at a dose of 3.2 g per day (Matin et al., 2018). An inquiry by Veselinovic et al. (2017) was conducted on the impressions of PUFA supplementation on rheumatoid arthritis. The treatment period was 12 weeks and included the use of five Omega-3 Cardio capsules (200 mg of EPA, 300 mg of DHA, 1 g of FO, and 100 mg of else unsaturated FAs) and a combination supplement consisting of two Omega-3 Cardio capsules and two Primrose Oil capsules (117 mg of GLA, 949 mg of LA, and 1300 mg of evening primrose oil) after meals. The results indicated a very good effect of the supplements in reducing disease symptoms and improving the performance of the subjects.

2.4.2 Functional foods (fortifying foods with polyunsaturated fatty acids)

Despite all the health benefits mentioned about PUFAs, we see low consumption of these FAs by people. Therefore food fortification with omega-3 FAs or encapsulation of bioactive FAs and their addition to food products can establish health benefits for humans besides enhancing the nutritional value of foods. Yogurt, milk, juices, cereals, fresh produce, oils, baby food, and other foods are some of the functional food products to which omega-3 FAs have been added (Yadav et al., 2020). Research invested in solid lipid micro- and nanoparticles to encapsulate FO containing EPA and DHA. They were then used to fortify milk. Omega-3 PUFAs encapsulated in micro- and nanoparticles created higher stability in milk (Rostamzad et al., 2022; Yan et al., 2024) inquired into the enrichment of tomato sauce with omega-3 FO microcapsules. Considering that the 6% omega-3 treatment achieved high efficiency in encapsulation, it was used to enrich tomato sauce. The results indicated that tomato sauce fortified with encapsulated omega-3 was acceptable in terms of sensory evaluations, and adding up to 1.5% encapsulated omega-3 could lead to the generation of a product with high nutritional value. Melilli et al. (2020) concluded in this study that adding 10% purslane to pasta resulted in a functional product with acceptable sensory properties owing to its upper levels of LA and ALA, as well as antioxidant and phenolic compounds. With these interpretations, some food products enriched with PUFAs are shown in Table 2.3.

2.4.3 Cosmetic-therapeutic applications

Research has shown that rich sources of PUFAs, including FO, can exhibit cosmeceutical-therapeutic skin protective effects. Skin protection from UV radiation, improvement of skin dryness, elimination of skin blemishes, and effective relief of itching and skin ulcers are among the benefits of taking supplements, creams, and medications containing omega-3 and omega-6 FAs (Huang and Wang, 2018). In a study, Lee et al. (2011) produced a shampoo containing omega-3. Then, the effect of this formulated shampoo on damaged and bleached hair was evaluated. Formulation of shampoo with 12% EPA/DHA was able to significantly strengthen and protect hair. Microneedling is a novel technique to enhance the

TABLE 2.3 Types of food products enriched with polyunsaturated fatty acids (*PUFAs*).

Food Products	Sources of PUFAs	Results	References
Fish cakes	Cod liver oil and microencapsulated fish oil (FO)	Microencapsulated FO maintained PUFAs, reduced PV index, and slowed the formation of secondary compounds in the refrigerated product.	(Dellarosa et al., 2015)
Ice cream	Microencapsulated flaxseed oil	Microencapsulation of flaxseed oil powder ensured its stability in the product. Fortification of ice cream with 4% encapsulated flaxseed oil powder terminated a functional crop with appropriate sensory properties.	(Gowda et al., 2018)
Yogurt	Flaxseed powder	Escalating in water holding valency, viscosity, acidity, pH, and also upper antioxidant properties of the fortified product compared to unfortified yogurt were seen.	(Marand et al., 2020)
Chocolate cookies, breadsticks, and whole-meal sliced bread	Flaxseed	High levels of PUFAs were observed after the product was cooked. The antiinflammatory and antithrombotic properties were greater in PUFA-enriched products than in nonenriched products.	(Karantonis et al., 2022)
Fruit smoothie drink	Microencapsulated chiaseed oil	Enhanced solubility, reduced moisture, low peroxide value, augmented encapsulated oil quality, and effective product enrichment with chia oil were among the factors identified in the powdered drink.	(Copado et al., 2024)

stimulation of collagen synthesis, wrinkle reduction, and skin rejuvenation with the goal of beautifying and improving skin. In a follow-up study in women, a novel formulation containing omega-3 FAs was used to reduce inflammation and improve skin over 4 weeks. The presence of omega-3 in this formulation resulted in faster wound healing and improved skin radiance after microneedling (Wong and Murphy, 2023).

2.4.4 Polyunsaturated fatty acids dietary supplements in livestock, poultry, and aquaculture industries

PUFAs can strengthen bones, increase growth, improve immune function, reduce disease, enhance fertility and sperm quality, and ultimately produce eggs with high nutritional value and quality meat in poultry (Alagawany and Elnesr, 2019). A perusal utilized FO, flaxseed, and rapeseed in the diet of 15-day-old chickens up to 36 days of age. EPA and DHA were augmented in the thighs and breasts of chickens. In addition, topper ALA and a less omega-6/omega-3 proportion were obtained in chickens nourished with flaxseed (Konieczka et al., 2017). The outcomes of a research by Zhang et al. (2023) confirmed that body TGs were reduced in ducks fed (for 4 weeks) with flaxseed oil supplementation.

Considering the benefits of PUFAs and their bioactive potential, their inclusion in livestock diets can lead to a boost in the accumulation of these FAs in meat and enhance animal health along with general activity (Alagawany and Elnesr, 2022). In a study, algal DHA supplementation was introduced into the diet of Holstein cows. Consumption of a diet based on 10% DHA improved reproductive performance, deduced gestation time, augmented protein content, enhanced daily milk production, and increased PUFAs in cow's milk (Sinedino et al., 2017). Mohammadabadi et al. (2025) worked on the omega-3 supplementation application for 1 month on lactating camels. The fat and PUFA content, protein, and antioxidant properties of milk, as well as its generation rate, declared an upward trend.

Zatti et al. (2023) focused on the exploitation of *Schizochytrium sp.* in *Salmo salar* nourishing. Feeding the fish with this algal complement terminated in augmented weight gain as well as higher quantities of DHA in the meat. A consideration centered on the exploitation of the herb *Lemna minor* in the nourishing of *Cyprinus carpio*. An upwelling procedure of omega-3 FAs in *C. carpio* was observed (Goswami and Sharma, 2022). Else project confirmed that the utilization of algal oil, owing to its plentiful measures of DHA and EPA, was able to promote development, functional activity, and nutritional worth in *Litopenaeus vannamei* (Santigosa et al., 2024).

2.5 Future perspectives

2.5.1 Innovations in omega-3 and omega-6 production

Biotechnological approaches have attracted widespread attention as promising alternatives for the generation of omega-3 PUFAs and provide a suitable response to the increasing demand for these nutrients (Hinzpeter et al., 2006). Recent progress in synthetic biology and the sketching of engineered microbial cell factories have provided new perspectives for the sustainable, economical, and high-yield production of FAs, which could greatly lower the limitations associated with traditional sources, such as FO (Qin et al., 2023).

"Precision nutrition" became more popular, and individuals began to focus on omega-3 supplements tailored to each individual's needs and genetics (Chilton and Dutta, 2017; Jauregibeitia et al., 2020). According to a new examination, unique helpers known as specialized pro-resolving mediators (SPMs) emanated from omega-3 FAs are momentous in managing and eliminating inflammation (Al-Shaer et al., 2021). Personalized antiinflammatory diets depend on insights into how polyunsaturated FAs affect SPM production, modulated by genetics and gender differences (Chilton and Dutta, 2017; Al-Shaer et al., 2021).

Recently, genomic data have shown that differences in genes, especially polymorphisms in genes involved in the metabolic pathways of PUFAs, like the FADS family genes, can affect how well the body can convert and use these FAs and, by extension, how well nutritional interventions work (Fernandez and Blomquist, 2021). In addition, other items such as overall nutritional profile, gut microbiota structure, diversity, and individual genetic and epigenetic differences are among the factors influencing the variability of responses to omega-3 supplementation in human intervention studies (Serini & Calviello, 2020). On the other hand, increasing evidence suggests that omega-3 FAs can regulate molecular pathways related to inflammation, reduce oxidative stress, and induce programmed cell demise (apoptosis) by interacting with specific genotypes, which may be effective in preventing various forms of cancer (Yurko-Mauro et al., 2020).

These chemicals have been documented to enhance metabolic parameters, including the optimization of blood lipid profiles, regulation of glycemia levels in someones with type 2 diabetes, and reduction of hepatic fat accumulation in individuals receiving medical care with nonalcoholic adipose liver disease (Djuricic & Calder, 2022). Recent research has found that the omega-3 Index and the percentage of omega-6 to omega-3 FAs are useful biomarkers for determining sufficient omega-3 intake and predicting individual variability in response to nutritional interventions, allowing for more individualized dietary approaches (Serini & Calviello, 2020).

2.5.2 Sustainable sources and environmental impacts

Microalgae and genetically engineered plants have garnered the attention of scientists and the food industry as new terrestrial sources to synthesize important PUFAs, mainly omega-3. These alternatives have been viewed as sustainable and effective substitutes for conventional marine sources like FO based on their potential for large-scale industrial production, excellent environmental sustainability, and economic feasibility (Zhou et al., 2023). Specifically, oilseed crops that have been genetically modified to alter their biological processes can be made to produce FAs that are similar in composition to FO and contain a high proportion of omega-3 to omega-6, thereby fulfilling the dietary requirements of both the aquaculture industry and human nutrition (Zhou et al., 2023). Additional alternatives, including krill and protozoan microalgae-like, have been suggested as reserves of PUFAs (Nichols et al., 2010). The other reference is to plants, particularly whole grains, nuts, and dried fruits, which are most important in supplying omega-6 FAs (Dhull & Punia, 2020). The application of biotechnology, including genetic modification and metabolic engineering of plants and microorganisms, has been intensively investigated to enhance the generation efficiency of vital FAs. The creation of these alternative sources has the potential to eliminate reliance on fossil fuels and finite fish stocks while contributing valuable environmental sustainability, cost-effectiveness, and promotion of public health simultaneously (Zhou et al., 2023).

2.6 Conclusion

In the modern epoch, the recognition and investment of bioactive ingredients fabricated from natural reserves have become a turning point in the nutrition-pharmaceutical (nutraceutical) knowledge-based industries and companies. PUFAs are a momentous and constituent component of lipids and are also among the worthwhile biological compounds manufactured from terrestrial and aquatic reserves. They have 2 or more dual grafts and contain omega-3 and omega-6 FAs. There are umpteen privileges of PUFAs that demonstrate their potential magnitude for utilization in sundry industries. Recent studies indicate that daily consumption of omega-3 supplements can support basic biological processes, particularly during development stages, inflammatory conditions, and pregnancy, when daily dietary requirements may be inadequate to sustain physiological needs. Given the superior prevalence of indispositions, diets comprising PUFAs can delay the progression of chronic illnesses and augment the operation of the immune system in terms of bioactive effects. This is while the consumption of omega-3 and omega-6 in the universe is negligible and does not comply with the recommendations delineated by global assemblies and organizations. In this regard, more robust enactments and management agendas should be executed to increase the consumption of PUFAs, especially omega-3. In making proper and scientifically backed recommendations for various population segments, additional studies must be conducted to establish the proper dosage and frequency of use. One efficacious solution is to enrich foods with PUFAs and extend functional foods. In addition to their nourishing worth, these foods have a vast confine of health-promoting benefits. These consequences comprise antiinflammatory, antioxidant, anticancer, antiviral, and antibacterial potentials. These beneficial effects can play many roles in the prophylaxis and treatment of chronic ailments, such as diabetes, obesity, cardiovascular illnesses, depression, cognitive impairment, and Alzheimer's. The balance and proportion of omega-3 and omega-6 are considered consequential precautions in disease interception. Because an imbalance and a high proportion of omega-6/omega-3 cause many human disorders and conditions. The deployment of dietary supplements containing PUFAs has been one of the accomplishments of mankind in combating illnesses and ameliorating human performance. Nanotechnology is one of the fields that has made significant progress in the background of drug delivery to patients. In the medical field, nanoparticles are nanostructures that can combat pathogenic cells. The syntax of this technology, with the exploitation of PUFA pharmaceutical supplements, can lead to the deduction and omission of disease and its resulting inflammation due to the faster delivery of encapsulated drugs to pathogenic cells. Furthermore, cosmetic health supplements based on omega-3 and -6 FAs, which have remedial virtues, can depict peculiar valences in rejuvenating the skin, strengthening hair, and also controlling skin conditions such as wounds, itching, and dry skin. PUFAs can display potential nutritional applications in the animal feed industry. Strengthening bones, enhancing reproductive activity, increasing weight and growth, escalating the body's defense function against diseases, generating meat and eggs containing PUFA with sublime quality, and increasing milk manufacturing with omnibus bioactive properties are just a few of their benefits in the livestock, poultry, and aquaculture industries. Despite all the benefits mentioned, more cultures should be created to consume the recommended amounts of PUFAs that the body needs. For this purpose, all relevant organizations should join hands and, under a collaborative attitude, decisions and principled plans should be made. Seaweeds, genetically modified plants, krill, and seafood by-products are novel and feasible sources that have provided alternative ways of procuring these acids without dependence on finite marine resources. Microbial sources, which construct heightened echelons of EPA and DHA, are acknowledged as sustainable and eco-friendly substitutes for conventional sources of FO. Complementing these advances requires sophisticated and precise analytical techniques to ensure the quality, safety, and dosing accuracy of FA supplements. Thus follow-up research must focus on the optimization of omega-3 intake, compare reserves of omega-3, and explore the long-term effects of supplement usage on inflammatory and chronic conditions, thereby creating evidence-based approaches to be integrated into nutritional policy frameworks.

References

Abd El-Fatah, N. K., Kheder, S. M. M., & El-Sayed, N. A. E. R. (2016). Effect of omega 3 polyunsaturated fatty acids supplementation on osteoarthritic knees among females. *International Journal of Health Sciences & Research, 6*(4), 362–369.

Abedi, E., & Sahari, M. A. (2014). Long-chain polyunsaturated fatty acid sources and evaluation of their nutritional and functional properties. *Food Science & Nutrition, 2*(5), 443–463.

Acworth, I. N., Plante, M., Crafts, C., & Bailey, B. (2011). Quantitation of underivatized omega-3 and omega-6 fatty acids in foods by HPLC and charged aerosol detection. *Planta Medica, 77*(12), 0032–0943. https://doi.org/10.1055/s-0031-1282608.

Adarme-Vega, T. C., Lim, D. K. Y., Timmins, M., Vernen, F., Li, Y., & Schenk, P. M. (2012). Microalgal biofactories: A promising approach towards sustainable omega-3 fatty acid production. *Microbial Cell Factories, 11*, 14752859. Available from: https://doi.org/10.1186/1475-2859-11-96Australia, http://www.microbialcellfactories.com/content/11/1/96.

Ahamad, J., Naquvi, K. J., Uthirapathy, S., Naim, M. J., & Majedi, S. (2024). Monounsaturated and polyunsaturated fatty acids. In *Bioactive compounds of edible oils and fats*. CRC Press, 71–87.

Akbar, S., Rahman, A., Ahmad, N., Imran, M., & Hafeez, Z. (2024). *191*, 57–93. Understanding the role of polyunsaturated fatty acids in the development and prevention of cancer191 http://doi.org/10.1007/978-3-031-55622-7_3 Springer Science and Business Media LLC .

Alagawany, M., Elnesr, S. S., Farag, M. R., Abd El-Hack, M. E., Khafaga, A. F., Taha, A. E., Tiwari, R., Yatoo, M. I., Bhatt, P., Khurana, S. K., & Dhama, K. (2019). Omega-3 and omega-6 fatty acids in poultry nutrition: Effect on production performance and health. *Animals, 9*(8), 20762615. Available from: https://doi.org/10.3390/ani9080573, https://www.mdpi.com/2076-2615/9/8/573/pdf.

Alagawany, M., Elnesr, S. S., Farag, M. R., El-Sabrout, K., Alqaisi, O., Dawood, M. A. O., Soomro, H., & Abdelnour, S. A. (2022). Nutritional significance and health benefits of omega-3, -6 and -9 fatty acids in animals. *Animal Biotechnology, 33*(7), 1678–1690. Available from: https://doi.org/10.1080/10495398.2020.1869562, www.tandf.co.uk/journals/titles/10495398.asp.

AlAmmar, W. A., Albeesh, F. H., Ibrahim, L. M., Algindan, Y. Y., Yamani, L. Z., & Khattab, R. Y. (2021). Effect of omega-3 fatty acids and fish oil supplementation on multiple sclerosis: A systematic review. *Nutritional Neuroscience, 24*(7), 569–579. Available from: https://doi.org/10.1080/1028415X.2019.1659560, http://www.tandfonline.com/loi/ynns20#.VvukQLdf1Hh.

Al-Shaer, A. E., Buddenbaum, N., & Shaikh, S. R. (2021). Polyunsaturated fatty acids, specialized pro-resolving mediators, and targeting inflammation resolution in the age of precision nutrition. *Biochimica et Biophysica Acta (BBA) - Molecular and Cell Biology of Lipids, 1866*(7), 158936.

Aristotelous, P., Stefanakis, M., Pantzaris, M., Pattichis, C. S., Calder, P. C., Patrikios, I. S., Sakkas, G. K., & Giannaki, C. D. (2021). The effects of specific omega-3 and omega-6 polyunsaturated fatty acids and antioxidant vitamins on gait and functional capacity parameters in patients with relapsing-remitting multiple sclerosis. *Nutrients, 13*(10), Available from: https://doi.org/10.3390/nu13103661, https://www.mdpi.com/2072-6643/13/10/3661/pdf.

Aronson, W. J., Grogan, T., Liang, P., Jardack, P., Liddell, A. R., Perez, C., Elashoff, D., Said, J., Cohen, P., Marks, L. S., & Henning, S. M. (2025). High omega-3, low omega-6 diet with fish oil for men with prostate cancer on active surveillance: The CAPFISH-3 randomized clinical trial. *of Clinical Oncology, 43*(7), 800–809. Available from: https://doi.org/10.1200/JCO.24.00608, https://ascopubs.org/loi/jco.

Awasthi, S. M., & Jerath, N. (2025). Omega-3 fatty acids as an adjunct therapy in sepsis: Insights and implications: A narrative review. *Journal of Clinical and Diagnostic research,* KE01–KE07. https://doi.org/10.7860/jcdr/2025/73918.20850.

Babakhani, A., & Zahmatkesh, F. (2024). Microalgae and cyanobacteria are potential sources of food in the future. In *Algae as a natural solution for challenges in water-food-energy nexus: Toward carbon neutrality*. Springer Nature Singapore, 771–786.

Bae, J. H., Lim, H., & Lim, S. (2023). The potential cardiometabolic effects of long-chain ω-3 polyunsaturated fatty acids: Recent updates and controversies. *Advances in Nutrition, 14*(4), 612–628.

Bahgat, K. A., Elhady, M., Abdel Aziz, A., Youness, E. R., & Zakzok, E. (2019). Omega-6/omega-3 ratio and cognition in children with epilepsy. *Anales de Pediatría (English Edition), 91*(2), 88–95. https://doi.org/10.1016/j.anpede.2018.07.005.

Balbás, G. M., Regaña, M. S., & Millet, P. U. (2011). Study on the use of omega-3 fatty acids as a therapeutic supplement in treatment of psoriasis. *Clinical, Cosmetic and Investigational Dermatology, 4*, 73–77.

Barrera, C., Valenzuela, R., Chamorro, R., Bascuñán, K., Sandoval, J., Sabag, N., Valenzuela, F., Valencia, M.-P., Puigrredon, C., & Valenzuela, A. (2018). The impact of maternal diet during pregnancy and lactation on the fatty acid composition of erythrocytes and breast milk of chilean women. *Nutrients, 10*(7), 839. https://doi.org/10.3390/nu10070839.

Barta, D. G., Coman, V., & Vodnar, D. C. (2021). Microalgae as sources of omega-3 polyunsaturated fatty acids: Biotechnological aspects. *Algal Research, 58*, 102410.

Berger, M. E., Smesny, S., Kim, S. W., Davey, C. G., Rice, S., Sarnyai, Z., Schlögelhofer, M., Schäfer, M. R., Berk, M., McGorry, P. D., & Amminger, G. P. (2017). Omega-6 to omega-3 polyunsaturated fatty acid ratio and subsequent mood disorders in young people with at-risk mental states: A 7-year longitudinal study. *Translational Psychiatry, 7*, 1–6. Available from: https://doi.org/10.1038/tp.2017.190, http://www.nature.com/tp/index.html.

Berquin, I. M., Edwards, I. J., & Chen, Y. Q. (2008). Multi-targeted therapy of cancer by omega-3 fatty acids. *Cancer Letters, 269*(2), 363–377.

Cerone, M., & Smith, T. K. (2021). A brief journey into the history of and future sources and uses of fatty acids. *Frontiers in Nutrition, 8*. Available from: https://doi.org/10.3389/fnut.2021.570401, journal.frontiersin.org/journal/nutrition.

Cerone, M., & Smith, T. K. (2022). Desaturases: Structural and mechanistic insights into the biosynthesis of unsaturated fatty acids. *IUBMB Life, 74*(11), 1036–1051. Available from: https://doi.org/10.1002/iub.2671, http://iubmb.onlinelibrary.wiley.com/hub/journal/10.1002/(ISSN)1521-6551/.

Chakraborty, K., Krishnan, S., Chakraborty, R. D., & Vijayagopal, P. (2021). Deep-sea mud shrimp and shovel-nosed lobster from the arabian sea as prospective sources of long-chain polyunsaturated fatty acids. *Indian Journal of Fisheries, 68*(3), 125–130. Available from: https://doi.org/10.21077/ijf.2021.68.3.111408-17, http://epubs.icar.org.in/ejournal/index.php/IJF/article/download/111408/45228.

Chen, A., Rafiz Azuan, N. B., Harun, N. M., Ooi, Y. B. H., & Khor, B. H. (2024). Nutritional status and dietary fatty acid intake among children from low-income households in Sabah: A cross-sectional study. *Human Nutrition and Metabolism, 36*. Available from: https://doi.org/10.1016/j.hnm.2024.200260, https://www.sciencedirect.com/science/journal/26661497.

Chen, W., Li, T., Du, S., Chen, H., & Wang, Q. (2023). Microalgal polyunsaturated fatty acids: Hotspots and production techniques. *Frontiers in Bioengineering and Biotechnology, 11*, 2296–4185. https://doi.org/10.3389/fbioe.2023.1146881.

Chilton, F. H., Dutta, R., Reynolds, L. M., Sergeant, S., Mathias, R. A., & Seeds, M. C. (2017). Precision nutrition and omega-3 polyunsaturated fatty acids: A case for personalized supplementation approaches for the prevention and management of human diseases. *Nutrients, 9*(11), 20726643. Available from: https://doi.org/10.3390/nu9111165, http://www.mdpi.com/2072-6643/9/11/1165/pdf.

Christian, L. M., Blair, L. M., Porter, K., Lower, M., Cole, R. M., & Belury, M. A. (2016). Polyunsaturated fatty acid (PUFA) status in pregnant women: Associations with sleep quality, inflammation, and length of gestation. *PLoS One, 11*(2), 19326203. Available from: https://doi.org/10.1371/journal.pone.0148752, http://www.plosone.org/article/fetchObject.action?uri=info:doi/10.1371/journal.pone.0148752&representation=PDF.

Copado, C. N., Ixtaina, V. Y., & Tomás, M. C. (2024). Enrichment of a fruit-based smoothie beverage with omega-3 fatty acids from microencapsulated chia seed oil. *Journal of the Science of Food and Agriculture, 104*(6), 3352–3360.

Curtis, J. M., & Black, B. A. (2013). Analysis of omega-3 fatty acids in foods and supplements. In *Food enrichment with omega-3 fatty acids*. Canada: Elsevier Inc, 226–254. http://doi.org/10.1533/9780857098863.2.226, http://www.sciencedirect.com/science/book/9780857094285.

De Carvalho, C., & Caramujo, M. (2018). The various roles of fatty acids. *Molecules (Basel, Switzerland), 23*(10), 2583. https://doi.org/10.3390/molecules23102583.

Dellarosa, N., Laghi, L., Martinsdóttir, E., Jónsdóttir, R., & Sveinsdóttir, K. (2015). Enrichment of convenience seafood with omega-3 and seaweed extracts: Effect on lipid oxidation. *LWT - Food Science and Technology, 62*(1), 746–752. https://doi.org/10.1016/j.lwt.2014.09.032.

Dhull, S. B., & Punia, S. (2020). Sources: Plants, animals and microbial. *In Essential Fatty Acids,* 19–56.

Dicklin, M. R., Anthony, J. C., Winters, B. L., & Maki, K. C. (2024). Omega-3 polyunsaturated fatty acid status testing in humans: A narrative review of commercially available options. *The Journal of Nutrition*.

DiNicolantonio, J. J., & O'Keefe, J. (2019). Importance of maintaining a low omega-6/omega-3 ratio for reducing platelet aggregation, coagulation and thrombosis. *Open Heart, 6*(1).

DiNicolantonio, J. J., & O'Keefe, J. (2021). The importance of maintaining a low omega-6/omega-3 ratio for reducing the risk of autoimmune diseases, asthma, and allergies. *Missouri Medicine, 118*(5), 453.

Djuricic, I., & Calder, P. C. (2022). Polyunsaturated fatty acids and metabolic health: Novel insights. *Current Opinion in Clinical Nutrition and Metabolic Care, 25*(6), 436–442. Available from: https://doi.org/10.1097/MCO.0000000000000865, http://journals.lww.com/co-clinicalnutrition/pages/default.aspx.

Djuricic, I., & Calder, P. C. (2021). Beneficial outcomes of omega-6 and omega-3 polyunsaturated fatty acids on human health: An update for 2021. *Nutrients, 13*(7), 2421. https://doi.org/10.3390/nu13072421.

Doaei, S., Gholami, S., Rastgoo, S., Gholamalizadeh, M., Bourbour, F., Bagheri, S. E., Samipoor, F., Akbari, M. E., Shadnoush, M., Ghorat, F., Mosavi Jarrahi, S. A., Ashouri Mirsadeghi, N., Hajipour, A., Joola, P., Moslem, A., & Goodarzi, M. O. (2021). The effect of omega-3 fatty acid supplementation on clinical and biochemical parameters of critically ill patients with COVID-19: Aa randomized clinical trial. *Journal of Translational Medicine, 19*(1), 14795876. Available from: https://doi.org/10.1186/s12967-021-02795-5, http://www.translational-medicine.com/home/.

Domínguez, R., Pateiro, M., Purriños, L., Munekata, P. E. S., Echegaray, N., & Lorenzo, J. M. (2022). Introduction and classification of lipids. In *Food Lipids: Sources, Health Implications, and Future Trends*. Elsevier Inc., Spain, 1–16. http://doi.org/10.1016/B978-0-12-823371-9.00018-6, https://www.sciencedirect.com/book/9780128233719.

Dyall, S. C., Balas, L., Bazan, N. G., Brenna, J. T., Chiang, N., da Costa Souza, F., Dalli, J., Durand, T., Galano, J. M., Lein, P. J., Serhan, C. N., & Taha, A. Y. (2022). Polyunsaturated fatty acids and fatty acid-derived lipid mediators: Recent advances in the understanding of their biosynthesis, structures, and functions. *Progress in Lipid Research, 86*. Available from: https://doi.org/10.1016/j.plipres.2022.101165, www.elsevier.com/locate/plipres.

El-Badry, A. M., Graf, R., & Clavien, P. A. (2007). Omega 3–Omega 6: What is right for the liver? *Journal of Hepatology, 47*(5), 718–725.

Fedacko, J., Vargova, V., Singh, R. B., Anjum, B., Takahashi, T., Tongnuka, M., Dharwadkar, S., Singh, S., Singh, V., Kulshresth, S. K., de Meester, F., & Wilson, D. W. (2012). Association of high w-6/w-3 fatty acid ratio diet with causes of death due to noncommunicable diseases among urban decedents in north India. *Open Nutraceuticals Journal, 5*(1), 113–123. https://doi.org/10.2174/1876396001205010113.

Feng, Y., Yang, Y., Zou, S., Qiu, S., Yang, H., Hu, Y., Lin, G., Yao, X., Liu, S., & Zou, M. (2023). Identification of alpha-linolenic acid as a broad-spectrum antiviral against zika, dengue, herpes simplex, influenza virus and SARS-CoV-2 infection. *Antiviral Research, 216*, 105666. https://doi.org/10.1016/j.antiviral.2023.105666.

Fernandes, I., Fernandes, T., & Cordeiro, N. (2019). Nutritional value and fatty acid profile of two wild edible limpets from the Madeira Archipelago. *European Food Research and Technology, 245*(4), 895–905.

Fernandez, M. L., Blomquist, S. A., Hallmark, B., & Chilton, F. H. (2021). Omega-3 supplementation and heart disease: A population-based diet by gene analysis of clinical trial outcomes. *Nutrients, 13*(7), Available from: https://doi.org/10.3390/nu13072154, https://www.mdpi.com/2072-6643/13/7/2154/pdf.

Forsyth, S., Gautier, S., & Salem Jr, N. (2016). Global estimates of dietary intake of docosahexaenoic acid and arachidonic acid in developing and developed countries. *Annals of Nutrition and Metabolism, 68*(4), 258–267.

Froyen, E., & Burns-Whitmore, B. (2020). The effects of linoleic acid consumption on lipid risk markers for cardiovascular disease in healthy individuals: A review of human intervention trials. *Nutrients, 12*(8), 2329.

Gazem, R. A. A., & Chandrashekariah, S. A. (2014). Omega fatty acids in health and disease: A review. *Journal of Pharmaceutical Research, 8*(8), 1027–1044.

Gemperlein, K., Rachid, S., Garcia, R. O., Wenzel, S. C., & Müller, R. (2014). Polyunsaturated fatty acid biosynthesis in myxobacteria: Different PUFA synthases and their product diversity. *Chemical Science, 5*(5), 1733–1741. https://doi.org/10.1039/c3sc53163e.

Gil, A., & Gil, F. (2015). Fish, a mediterranean source of n -3 PUFA: Benefits do not justify limiting consumption. *British Journal of Nutrition, 113*(S2), S58. https://doi.org/10.1017/s0007114514003742.

Goswami, R. K., Sharma, J. G., Shrivastav, A. K., Kumar, G., Glencross, B. D., Tocher, D. R., & Chakrabarti, R. (2022). Effect of *Lemna minor* supplemented diets on growth, digestive physiology and expression of fatty acids biosynthesis genes of *Cyprinus carpio*. *Scientific Reports, 12*(1), 20452322. Available from: https://doi.org/10.1038/s41598-022-07743-x, www.nature.com/srep/index.html.

Gowda, A., Sharma, V., Goyal, A., Singh, A. K., & Arora, S. (2018). Process optimization and oxidative stability of omega-3 ice cream fortified with flaxseed oil microcapsules. *Journal of Food Science and Technology, 55*(5), 1705–1715. https://doi.org/10.1007/s13197-018-3083-4.

Guil-Guerrero, J. L. (2007). Stearidonic acid (18:4 n -3): Metabolism, nutritional importance, medical uses and natural sources. *European Journal of Lipid Science and Technology, 109*(12), 1226–1236. https://doi.org/10.1002/ejlt.200700207.

Guo, X., & Lankmayr, E. (2011). Phospholipid-based matrix effects in LC–MS bioanalysis. *Bioanalysis, 3*(4), 349–352. https://doi.org/10.4155/bio.10.213.

Gupta, A., Barrow, C. J., & Puri, M. (2012). Omega-3 biotechnology: Thraustochytrids as a novel source of omega-3 oils. *Biotechnology Advances, 30*(6), 1733–1745.

Gupta, R., Dhatwalia, S., Chaudhry, M., Kondal, D., Stein, A. D., Prabhakaran, D., Tandon, N., Ramakrishnan, L., & Khandelwal, S. (2021). Standardization and validation of assay of selected omega-3 and omega-6 fatty acids from phospholipid fraction of red cell membrane using gas chromatography with flame ionization detector. *Journal of Analytical Science and Technology, 12*(1), 20933371. Available from: https://doi.org/10.1186/s40543-021-00287-1, jast-journal.springeropen.com/.

Hernandez, E. M. (2014). Issues in fortification and analysis of omega-3 fatty acids in foods. *Lipid Technology, 26*(5), 103–106. https://doi.org/10.1002/lite.201400004 Available from: http://www.interscience.wiley.com/jpages/0956-666X.

Hinzpeter, I., Shene, C., & Masson, L. (2006). Biotechnological alternatives for omega-3 polyunsaturated fatty acids production. *Grasas y Aceites, 57*(3), 336–342.

Hu, J. J., Dong, Y. M., Ding, R., Yang, J. C., Odkhuu, E., Zhang, L., & Ye, D. W. (2023). Health burden of unbalanced fatty acids intake from 1990 to 2019: A global analysis. *Cell Press, China Med, 4*(11), 778. Available from: https://doi.org/10.1016/j.medj.2023.08.002, www.cell.com/med.

Huang, T. H., Wang, P. W., Yang, S. C., Chou, W. L., & Fang, J. Y. (2018). Cosmetic and therapeutic applications of fish oil's fatty acids on the skin. *Marine Drugs, 16*(8), Available from: https://doi.org/10.3390/md16080256, http://www.mdpi.com/1660-3397/16/8/256/pdf.

Hulbert, A. J. (2021). The under-appreciated fats of life: The two types of polyunsaturated fats. *Journal of Experimental Biology, 224*(8). https://doi.org/10.1242/jeb.232538.

Ibrahim, D., El-Sayed, R., Khater, S. I., Said, E. N., & El-Mandrawy, S. A. (2018). Changing dietary n-6: n-3 ratio using different oil sources affects performance, behavior, cytokines mRNA expression and meat fatty acid profile of broiler chickens. *Animal Nutrition, 4*(1), 44–51.

Innis, S. M. (2008). Dietary omega 3 fatty acids and the developing brain. *Brain research, 1237*, 35–43.

Irnawati, I., Windarsih, A., Putri, A. R., Fadzillah, N. A., Azmi, A. A., Kusbandari, A., & Rohman, A. (2024). The use of spectroscopic methods in combination with multivariate data analysis for determination of omega fatty acids: A review. *Journal of Applied Pharmaceutical Science, 14*(1), 45–53. Available from: https://doi.org/10.7324/JAPS.2024.139258, www.japsonline.com/index.php.

Iwabuchi, K., Nakayama, H., Iwahara, C., & Takamori, K. (2010). Significance of glycosphingolipid fatty acid chain length on membrane microdomain-mediated signal transduction. *FEBS Letters, 584*(9), 1642–1652. https://doi.org/10.1016/j.febslet.2009.10.043.

Jang, W., Kim, Y., & Kim, H. (2025). Association between the dietary omega-6 to omega-3 fatty acid ratio and age-related macular degeneration in Korean adults. *Nutrition Journal, 24*(1), 29.

Jauregibeitia, I., Portune, K., Amezaga, J., Tueros, I., & Arranz, S. (2020). A Journey through ω-3 Supplements: Future perspectives for precision nutrition. *Journal of Food and Nutrition Research, 8*(10), 556–560. https://doi.org/10.12691/jfnr-8-10-3.

Kaliannan, K., Wang, B., Li, X. Y., Kim, K. J., & Kang, J. X. (2015). A host-microbiome interaction mediates the opposing effects of omega-6 and omega-3 fatty acids on metabolic endotoxemia. *Scientific Reports, 5*, 11276.

Karantonis, H. C., Nasopoulou, C., & Skalkos, D. (2022). Functional bakery snacks for the post-COVID-19 market, fortified with omega-3 fatty acids. *Sustainability, 14*(8), 4816.

Karrar, E., Albakry, Z., Mohamed Ahmed, I. A., Zhang, L., Chen, C., Wu, D., & Li, J. (2024). Docosahexaenoic acid and eicosapentaenoic acid from microalgae: Extraction, purification, separation, and analytical methods. *Algal Research, 77*, 103365. https://doi.org/10.1016/j.algal.2023.103365.

Kasuga, K., Suga, T., & Mano, N. (2015). Bioanalytical insights into mediator lipidomics. *Journal of Pharmaceutical and Biomedical Analysis, 113*, 151–162.

Konieczka, P., Czauderna, M., & Smulikowska, S. (2017). The enrichment of chicken meat with omega-3 fatty acids by dietary fish oil or its mixture with rapeseed or flaxseed—Effect of feeding duration: Dietary fish oil, flaxseed, and rapeseed and n-3 enriched broiler meat. *Animal Feed Science and Technology, 223*, 42–52.

Kus-Yamashita, M. M. M., Cano, C. B., Monteiro, V. C. B., & Catarino, R. M. (2023). Human milk: Fast determination of docosahexaenoic acid (DHA). *Analytica, 4*(1), 54–65. Available from: https://doi.org/10.3390/analytica4010006, www.mdpi.com/journal/analytica.

Lange, K. W. (2021). Lack of evidence for efficacy of omega-3 fatty acids in depression. *Acta Psychiatrica Scandinavica, 144*(4), 415–416. Available from: https://doi.org/10.1111/acps.13357, http://onlinelibrary.wiley.com/journal/10.1111/(ISSN)1600-0447.

Laparra, J. M., & Sanz, Y. (2010). Interactions of gut microbiota with functional food components and nutraceuticals. *Pharmacological Research, 61*(3), 219–225. https://doi.org/10.1016/j.phrs.2009.11.001.

Lee, B. R., Lee, O. S., Kang, T. J., & Lim, S. C. (2011). Development of shampoo formulated by EPA for the damaged hair. *Korean Journal of Clinical Pharmacy, 21*(3), 256–269.

Lunn, J., & Theobald, H. E. (2006). The health effects of dietary unsaturated fatty acids. *Nutrition Bulletin, 31*(3), 178–224. https://doi.org/10.1111/j.1467-3010.2006.00571.x.

Lv, J., Wang, C., Zhang, X., Lv, Z., & Yu, M. (2020). 1H NMR quantification of DHA and EPA in fish oil. *Journal of Ocean University of China, 19*(5), 1193–1197. https://doi.org/10.1007/s11802-020-4395-3.

Ma, Y. P., Li, D. H., & Wang, Z. P. (2002). *The Biosynthesis of Polyunsaturated Fatty Acids*.

Mao, Q., & Kong, Y. (2025). Effect of diet low in omega-6 polyunsaturated fatty acids on the global burden of cardiovascular diseases and future trends: Evidence from the Global Burden of Disease 2021. *Frontiers in Medicine, 11*. https://doi.org/10.3389/fmed.2024.1485695.

Maqsood, S., Benjakul, S., & Kamal-Eldin, A. (2012). Extraction, processing, and stabilization of health-promoting fish oils. *Recent Patents on Food, Nutrition & Agriculture, 4*(2), 141–147.

Marand, M. A., Amjadi, S., Marand, M. A., Roufegarinejad, L., & Jafari, S. M. (2020). Fortification of yogurt with flaxseed powder and evaluation of its fatty acid profile, physicochemical, antioxidant, and sensory properties. *Powder Technology, 359*, 76–84.

Marangoni, F., Agostoni, C., Borghi, C., Catapano, A. L., Cena, H., Ghiselli, A., La Vecchia, C., Lercker, G., Manzato, E., Pirillo, A., Riccardi, G., Risé, P., Visioli, F., & Poli, A. (2020). Dietary linoleic acid and human health: Focus on cardiovascular and cardiometabolic effects. *Atherosclerosis, 292*, 90–98. Available from: https://doi.org/10.1016/j.atherosclerosis.2019.11.018, www.elsevier.com/locate/atherosclerosis.

Mariamenatu, A. H., & Abdu, E. M. (2021). Overconsumption of omega-6 polyunsaturated fatty acids (PUFAs) versus deficiency of omega-3 PUFAs in modern-day diets: The disturbing factor for their "balanced antagonistic metabolic functions" in the human body. *Journal of Lipids, 2021*, 8848161.

Martínez, N., Herrera, M., Frías, L., Provencio, M., Pérez-Carrión, R., Díaz, V., Morse, M., & Crespo, M. C. (2019). A combination of hydroxytyrosol, omega-3 fatty acids and curcumin improves pain and inflammation among early stage breast cancer patients receiving adjuvant hormonal therapy: results of a pilot study. *Clinical and Translational Oncology, 21*(4), 489–498. https://doi.org/10.1007/s12094-018-1950-0.

Matin, S., Nemati, A., Ghobadi, H., Alipanah-Moghadam, R., & Rezagholizadeh, L. (2018). The effect of conjugated linoleic acid on oxidative stress and matrix metalloproteinases 2 and 9 in patients with COPD. *International Journal of Chronic Obstructive Pulmonary Disease, 13*, 1449–1454. https://doi.org/10.2147/copd.s155985.

Melilli, M. G., Pagliaro, A., Scandurra, S., Gentile, C., & Di Stefano, V. (2020). Omega-3 rich foods: Durum wheat spaghetti fortified with *Portulaca oleracea*. *Food Bioscience, 37*, 100730. https://doi.org/10.1016/j.fbio.2020.100730.

Minihane, A. M., Armah, C. K., Miles, E. A., Madden, J. M., Clark, A. B., Caslake, M. J., Packard, C. J., Kofler, B. M., Lietz, G., Curtis, P. J., Mathers, J. C., Williams, C. M., & Calder, P. C. (2016). Consumption of fish oil providing amounts of eicosapentaenoic acid and docosahexaenoic acid that can be obtained from the diet reduces blood pressure in adults with systolic hypertension: A retrospective analysis. *Journal of Nutrition, 146*(3), 516–523. Available from: https://doi.org/10.3945/jn.115.220475, http://jn.nutrition.org/content/146/3/516.full.pdf.

Mitchell, C. J., D'Souza, R. F., Figueiredo, V. C., Chan, A., Aasen, K., Durainayagam, B., Mitchell, S., Sinclair, A. J., Egner, I. M., Raastad, T., David, C. S., & Markworth, J. F. (2018). Effect of dietary arachidonic acid supplementation on acute muscle adaptive responses to resistance exercise in trained men: A randomized controlled trial. *Journal of Applied Physiology, 124*(4), 1080–1091. Available from: https://doi.org/10.1152/japplphysiol.01100.2017, https://www.physiology.org/doi/pdf/10.1152/japplphysiol.01100.2017.

Mititelu, M., Lupuliasa, D., Neacşu, S. M., Olteanu, G., Busnatu, Ş. S., Mihai, A., Popovici, V., Măru, N., Boroghină, S. C., Mihai, S., & Ioniţă-Mîndrican, C. B. (2024). Polyunsaturated fatty acids and human health: A key to modern nutritional balance in association with polyphenolic compounds from food sources. *Foods, 14*(1), 46.

Mohammadabadi, T., Chaji, M., Hoseini, S., & Davar, S. A. (2025). The use of protected fat supplement on milk production, quality and fatty acid profiles in dairy camels: Protected fat supplement of dairy camel. *Veterinary Medicine and Science, 11*(3), Available from: https://doi.org/10.1002/vms3.70351, tinyurl.com/y7omcl8y.

Molendi-Coste, O., Legry, V., & Leclercq, I. A. (2011). Why and how meet n-3 PUFA dietary recommendations? *Gastroenterology Research and Practice, 2011*, 364040.

Monnard, C., & Fleith, M. (2021). Total fat and fatty acid intake among 1–7-Year-old children from 33 Countries: Comparison with International recommendations. *Nutrients, 13*(10), 3547. https://doi.org/10.3390/nu13103547.

Muhammad Alinafiah, S., Azlan, A., Ismail, A., & Mahmud Ab Rashid, N.-K. (2021). Method development and validation for omega-3 fatty acids (DHA and EPA) in fish using gas chromatography with flame ionization detection (GC-FID). *Molecules (Basel, Switzerland), 26*(21), 6592. https://doi.org/10.3390/molecules26216592.

Muriuki, M., Purdie, N., & Dumancas, G. (2012). Quantification of the major ω-3, ω-6 PUFAs using the Purdie assay and their ratios in different cholesterol types and the effects of gender and cholesterol on PUFA levels. *Trends in Analytical Chemistry, 31*, 157–164.

Müllner, E., Plasser, E., Brath, H., Waldschütz, W., Forster, E., Kundi, M., & Wagner, K.-H. (2014). Impact of polyunsaturated vegetable oils on adiponectin levels, glycaemia and blood lipids in individuals with type 2 diabetes: A randomised, double-blind intervention study. *Journal of Human Nutrition and Dietetics, 27*(5), 468–478. https://doi.org/10.1111/jhn.12168.

Nagao, K., Murakami, A., & Umeda, M. (2019). Structure and function of Δ9-fatty acid desaturase. *Chemical and Pharmaceutical Bulletin, 67*(4), 327–332.

Napier, J. A., & Michaelson, L. V. (2001). Genomic and functional characterization of polyunsaturated fatty acid biosynthesis in caenorhabditis elegans. *Lipids, 36*(8), 761–766. Available from: https://doi.org/10.1007/s11745-001-0782-9, http://www.springerlink.com/content/0024-4201.

Nava, V., Turco, V. L., Licata, P., Panayotova, V., Peycheva, K., Fazio, F., Rando, R., Di Bella, G., & Potortì, A. G. (2023). Determination of fatty acid profile in processed fish and shellfish foods. *Foods, 12*(13), Available from: https://doi.org/10.3390/foods12132631, www.mdpi.com/journal/foods.

Navalho, S., Ferrer-Ledo, N., Barbosa, M. J., & Varela, J. (2025). Nannochloropsis lipids and polyunsaturated fatty acids: Potential applications and strain improvement. *Marine Drugs, 23*(3), 16603397. Available from: https://doi.org/10.3390/md23030128, http://www.mdpi.com/journal/marinedrugs.

Nađ, T., Kolobarić, N., Mihaljević, Z., Drenjančević, I., Šušnjara, P., Stupin, A., Kardum, D., Kralik, Z., Kralik, G., Košević, M., & Jukić, I. (2025). Effect of n-3 polyunsaturated fatty acids enriched chicken meat consumption in relation to oxidative stress marker levels in young healthy individuals: A randomized double-blind study. *Antioxidants, 14*(2), 204. https://doi.org/10.3390/antiox14020204.

Ng, A., Woods, J., Jahn, T., Jones, L. W., & Ritter, J. S. (2022). Effect of a novel omega-3 and omega-6 fatty acid supplement on dry eye disease: A 3-month randomized controlled trial. *Optometry and Vision Science, 99*(1), 67–75. Available from: https://doi.org/10.1097/OPX.0000000000001826, http://journals.lww.com/optvissci.

Nichols, P. D., Petrie, J., & Singh, S. (2010). Long-chain omega-3 oils–an update on sustainable sources. *Nutrients, 2*(6), 572–585.

Noreen, S., Anmol, S., Fatima, S., Sattar, R., Yameen, Z., Arshad, S., Khan, A. U., & Pane, Y. S. (2024). Emerging role of polyunsaturated fatty acids (PUFAs) on human brain development and neurological diseases: A systematic review. *Tropical Journal of Natural Product Research, 8*(12), 9363–9369. Available from: https://doi.org/10.26538/tjnpr/v8i12.3, https://tjnpr.org/index.php/home/article/download/5418/5119.

O'Connor, S., & Rudkowska, I. (2019). Dietary fatty acids and the metabolic syndrome: A personalized nutrition approach. *Advances in Food and Nutrition Research, 87*, 43–146.

Ott, K., & Meusel, D. (1990). A method for the quantitative determination of ω-3-polyunsaturated fatty acids by reductive ozonolysis. *Food / Nahrung, 34*(1), 93–94. https://doi.org/10.1002/food.19900340124.

Öztürk Er, E., Şahin, A., & Bakırdere, S. (2020). Accurate, sensitive determination of omega-6 and omega-3 polyunsaturated fatty acids in human plasma and urine samples. *Biomedical Chromatography, 34*(12), e4951.

Pantaleo, P., Marra, F., Vizzutti, F., Spadoni, S., Ciabattoni, G., Galli, C., Villa, G. L. A., Gentilini, P., & Laffi, G. (2004). Effects of dietary supplementation with arachidonic acid on platelet and renal function in patients with cirrhosis. *Clinical Science, 106*(1), 27–34. https://doi.org/10.1042/cs20030182.

Pettersen, C. H. H., Samdal, H., Sætrom, P., Wibe, A., Hermansen, E., & Schønberg, S. A. (2023). The Salmon Oil OmeGo reduces viability of colorectal cancer cells and potentiates the anti-cancer effect of 5-FU. *Marine Drugs, 21*(12), Available from: https://doi.org/10.3390/md21120636, http://www.mdpi.com/journal/marinedrugs.

Ponnampalam, E. N., Sinclair, A. J., & Holman, B. W. (2021). The sources, synthesis and biological actions of omega-3 and omega-6 fatty acids in red meat: An overview. *Foods, 10*(6), 1358.

Prado, E., Eklouh-Molinier, C., Enez, F., Causeur, D., Blay, C., Dupont-Nivet, M., Labbé, L., Petit, V., Moreac, A., Taupier, G., Haffray, P., Bugeon, J., Corraze, G., & Nazabal, V. (2022). Prediction of fatty acids composition in the rainbow trout *Oncorhynchus mykiss* by using Raman micro-spectroscopy. *Analytica Chimica Acta, 1191*, 339212. https://doi.org/10.1016/j.aca.2021.339212.

Qin, J., Kurt, E., LBassi, T., Sa, L., & Xie, D. (2023). Biotechnological production of omega-3 fatty acids: Current status and future perspectives. *Frontiers in Microbiology, 14*. https://doi.org/10.3389/fmicb.2023.1280296.

Quispe-Fuentes, I., Valenzuela, P., Roco, T., Pérez-Won, M., Espinoza, J., Bernal, G., Bernal, C., & Martínez, R. (2025). Isolation and characterization of polyunsaturated fatty acid-rich oil from jumbo squid (Dosidicus gigas) Viscera: Antioxidant potential and anticancer activity on colorectal cancer cells. *Waste and Biomass Valorization, 16*(7), 3507–3517. https://doi.org/10.1007/s12649-024-02862-0.

Rabiepour, A., & Babakhani, A. (2023). Functional and health properties of bioactive compounds from aquatics. *Aquaculture Sciences, 11*(2), 47–73.

Rabiepour, A., Zahmatkesh, F., & Babakhani, A. (2024). Preservation techniques to increase the shelf life of seafood products: An overview. *Journal of Food Engineering and Technology, 13*(1), 1–24.

Rahman, S. U., Weng, T. N., Qadeer, A., Nawaz, S., Ullah, H., & Chen, C. C. (2024). Omega-3 and omega-6 polyunsaturated fatty acids and their potential therapeutic role in protozoan infections. *Frontiers in Immunology, 15*. Available from: https://doi.org/10.3389/fimmu.2024.1339470, https://www.frontiersin.org/journals/immunology#.

Rajaei, E., Mowla, K., Ghorbani, A., Bahadoram, S., Bahadoram, M., & Dargahi-Malamir, M. (2015). The effect of omega-3 fatty acids in patients with active rheumatoid arthritis receiving DMARDs therapy: Double-blind randomized controlled trial. *Global Journal of Health Science, 8*(7), 18. https://doi.org/10.5539/gjhs.v8n7p18.

Rice, S. M., Hickie, I. B., Yung, A. R., Mackinnon, A., Berk, M., Davey, C., Hermens, D. F., Hetrick, S. E., Parker, A. G., Schäfer, M. R., McGorry, P. D., & Amminger, G. P. (2016). Youth depression alleviation: The fish oil youth depression study (YoDA-F): A randomized, double-blind, placebo-controlled treatment trial. Blackwell Publishing, Australia. *Early Intervention in Psychiatry, 10*(4), 290–299. Available from: https://doi.org/10.1111/eip.12166, http://onlinelibrary.wiley.com/journal/10.1111/(ISSN)1751-7893.

Rohman, A., Irnawati, Windarsih, A., Riswanto, F. D. O., Indrayanto, G., Fadzillah, N. A., Riyanto, S., & Bakar, N. K. A. (2023). Application of chromatographic and spectroscopic-based methods for analysis of omega-3 (ω-3 FAs) and omega-6 (ω-6 FAs) fatty acids in marine natural products. *Molecules (Basel, Switzerland), 28*(14), Available from: https://doi.org/10.3390/molecules28145524, http://www.mdpi.com/journal/molecules.

Rostamzad, H., Babakhani, A., Fakouri, Z., & Esmaeilzadeh, M. (2022). Production and evaluation of microcapsules containing omega-3 to enrich tomato sauce. *Aquaculture Sciences, 10*(2), 134–148.

Rustan, A.C., Drevon, C.A. (2005). Fatty acids: structures and properties Encyclopedia of life sciences. Wiley. 10.1038/npg.els.0003894.

Sahye-Pudaruth, S., & Ma, D. W. L. (2023). Assessing the highest level of evidence from randomized controlled trials in omega-3 research. *Nutrients, 15*(4), 1001. https://doi.org/10.3390/nu15041001.

Saini, R. K., Prasad, P., Sreedhar, R. V., Akhilender Naidu, K., Shang, X., & Keum, Y.-S. (2021). Omega−3 polyunsaturated fatty acids (PUFAs): Emerging plant and microbial sources, oxidative stability, bioavailability, and health benefits—A review. *Antioxidants, 10*(10), 1627. https://doi.org/10.3390/antiox10101627.

Santigosa, E., Lemos, D., Rafael, T. I., Coelho, I., & Carr, C. (2024). Bailey, omega-3 EPA and DHA from algal oil improve pacific white shrimp zootechnical performance and nutritional quality without changing sensory quality. *Aquaculture Research, 2024*(1). https://doi.org/10.1155/2024/7543478.

Schipper, M. C., Jaddoe, V. W., Bekkers, E. L., Mulders, A. G., & Gaillard, R. (2025). Dietary intake of poly-unsaturated fatty acids, their food sources and fertility in females and males: A preconception prospective population-based cohort study. *The American Journal of Clinical Nutrition.*

Schuchardt, J. P., & Hahn, A. (2013). Bioavailability of long-chain omega-3 fatty acids. *Prostaglandins, Leukotrienes, and Essential Fatty Acids, 89*(1), 1–8. https://doi.org/10.1016/j.plefa.2013.03.010.

Senanayake, S. N. (2013). Methods of concentration and purification of omega-3 fatty acids. In *In Separation, extraction and concentration processes in the food, beverage and nutraceutical industries*. Woodhead Publishing, 483–505.

Serafim, V., Tiugan, D. A., Andreescu, N., Mihailescu, A., Paul, C., Velea, I., Puiu, M., & Niculescu, M. D. (2019). Development and validation of a LC–MS/MS-based assay for quantification of free and total omega 3 and 6 fatty acids from human plasma. *Molecules (Basel, Switzerland), 24*(2), Available from: https://doi.org/10.3390/molecules24020360, https://www.mdpi.com/1420-3049/24/2/360/pdf.

Serefko, A., Jach, M. E., Pietraszuk, M., Świąder, M., Świąder, K., & Szopa, A. (2024). Omega-3 Polyunsaturated fatty acids in depression. *International Journal of Molecular Sciences, 25*(16), 8675. https://doi.org/10.3390/ijms25168675.

Serini, S., Cassano, R., Corsetto, P. A., Rizzo, A. M., Calviello, G., & Trombino, S. (2018). Omega-3 PUFA loaded in resveratrol-based solid lipid nanoparticles: Physicochemical properties and antineoplastic activities in human colorectal cancer cells in vitro. *International Journal of Molecular Sciences, 19*(2), Available from: https://doi.org/10.3390/ijms19020586, http://www.mdpi.com/1422-0067/19/2/586/pdf.

Serini, S., & Calviello, G. (2020). Omega-3 PUFA responders and non-responders and the prevention of lipid dysmetabolism and related diseases. *Nutrients, 12*(5), 2072–6643. https://doi.org/10.3390/nu12051363.

Serini, S., Trombino, S., Cassano, R., Marino, M., & Calviello, G. (2025). Anti-inflammatory effects of curcumin-based nanoparticles containing α-linolenic acid in a model of psoriasis in vitro. *Nutrients, 17*(4), 692. https://doi.org/10.3390/nu17040692.

Shanklin, J., Guy, J. E., Mishra, G., & Lindqvist, Y. (2009). Desaturases: Emerging models for understanding functional diversification of diiron-containing enzymes. *Journal of Biological Chemistry, 284*(28), 18559–18563. Available from: https://doi.org/10.1074/jbc.R900009200, http://www.jbc.org/cgi/reprint/284/28/18559.

Sharifi, R., Nouri, M., Eidi, A., Noormohammadi, Z., Dolatkhah, H., & Shirmohammadi, M. (2017). Dietary PUFA increase apoptosis in stomach of patients with dyspeptic symptoms and infected with H. pylori. *Lipids, 52*(6), 549–558. https://doi.org/10.1007/s11745-017-4257-y.

Sharifzadeh, M., setayesh, L., Emami, M. R., Salim, S. J., & Javanbakht, Mh. H. (2024). The effects of omega-3 fatty acid supplementation on serum myostatin, body composition, blood glucose, lipid profile and hs-CRP level in overweight men with coronary heart disease: A randomized double-blind placebo controlled clinical trial. *Human Nutrition and Metabolism, 36*. Available from: https://doi.org/10.1016/j.hnm.2024.200248, https://www.sciencedirect.com/science/journal/26661497.

Shoieb, S. M., El-Ghiaty, M. A., & El-Kadi, A. O. (2021). Targeting arachidonic acid–related metabolites in COVID-19 patients: Potential use of drug-loaded nanoparticles. *Emergent Materials, 4*(1), 265–277.

Shrestha, N., Sleep, S. L., Cuffe, J. S. M., Holland, O. J., Perkins, A. V., Yau, S. Y., McAinch, A. J., & Hryciw, D. H. (2020). Role of omega-6 and omega-3 fatty acids in fetal programming. *Clinical and Experimental Pharmacology and Physiology, 47*(5), 907–915. Available from: https://doi.org/10.1111/1440-1681.13244, http://onlinelibrary.wiley.com/journal/10.1111/(ISSN)1440-1681.

Simons, K., & Toomre, D. (2000). Lipid rafts and signal transduction. *Nature Reviews. Molecular Cell Biology, 1*(1), 31–39. https://doi.org/10.1038/35036052.

Simopoulos, A. P. (2002). The importance of the ratio of omega-6/omega-3 essential fatty acids. *Biomedicine & Pharmacotherapy, 56*(8), 365–379. https://doi.org/10.1016/s0753-3322(02)00253-6.

Simopoulos, A. P. (2008). The omega-6/omega-3 fatty acid ratio, genetic variation, and cardiovascular disease. *Asia Pacific Journal of Clinical Nutrition, 17*(1), 131–134. Available from: http://apjcn.nhri.org.tw/server/APJCN/Volume17/vol17suppl.1/131-134S6-6.pdf.

Simopoulos, A. P. (2010). Genetic variants in the metabolism of omega-6 and omega-3 fatty acids: Their role in the determination of nutritional requirements and chronic disease risk. *Experimental Biology and Medicine, 235*(7), 785–795. Available from: https://doi.org/10.1258/ebm.2010.009298, http://ebm.rsmjournals.com/cgi/reprint/235/7/785.

Simopoulos, A. P. (2016). An increase in the Omega-6/Omega-3 fatty acid ratio increases the risk for obesity. *Nutrients, 8*(3), Available from: https://doi.org/10.3390/nu8030128, http://www.mdpi.com/2072-6643/8/3/128/pdf.

Sinedino, L. D. P., Honda, P. M., Souza, L. R. L., Lock, A. L., Boland, M. P., Staples, C. R., Thatcher, W. W., & Santos, J. E. P. (2017). Effects of supplementation with docosahexaenoic acid on reproduction of dairy cows. *Reproduction (Cambridge, England), 153*(5), 707–723. Available from: https://doi.org/10.1530/REP-16-0642, http://www.reproduction-online.org/content/153/5/707.full.pdf+html.

Sprecher, H., Luthria, D. L., Mohammed, B. S., & Baykousheva, S. P. (1995). Reevaluation of the pathways for the biosynthesis of polyunsaturated fatty acids. *Journal of Lipid Research, 36*(12), 2471–2477. https://doi.org/10.1016/s0022-2275(20)41084-3.

Strobel, C., Jahreis, G., & Kuhnt, K. (2012). Survey of n-3 and n-6 polyunsaturated fatty acids in fish and fish products. *Lipids in Health and Disease, 11*, 1–10.

Subash-Babu, P., & Alshatwi, A. A. (2018). Effects of increasing ratios of dietary omega-6/omega-3 fatty acids on human monocyte immunomodulation linked with atherosclerosis. *Journal of Functional Foods, 41*, 258–267. Available from: https://doi.org/10.1016/j.jff.2017.12.020, http://www.elsevier.com/wps/find/journaldescription.cws_home/717426/description#description.

Tian, L., Chi, G., Lin, S., Ling, X., & He, N. (2024). Marine microorganisms: natural factories for polyunsaturated fatty acid production. *Blue Biotechnology, 1*(1). https://doi.org/10.1186/s44315-024-00012-8.

Tiuca, I., Nagy, K., & Oprean, R. (2015). Recent developments in fatty acids profile determination in biological samples—A review. *Revista Romana de Medicina de Laborator, 23*(4), 371–384.

Uttaro, A. D. (2006). Biosynthesis of polyunsaturated fatty acids in lower eukaryotes. *IUBMB Life, 58*(10), 563–571. https://doi.org/10.1080/15216540600920899.

Van Dael, P. (2021). Role of n-3 long-chain polyunsaturated fatty acids in human nutrition and health: Review of recent studies and recommendations. *Nutrition Research and Practice, 15*(2), 137–159. Available from: https://doi.org/10.4162/nrp.2021.15.2.137, https://www.ncbi.nlm.nih.gov/pmc/articles/PMC8007408/pdf/nrp-15-137.pdf.

Verma, M. L., Kishor, K., Sharma, D., Kumar, S., & Sharma, K. D. (2020). Microbial production of omega-3 polyunsaturated fatty acids. *In Biotechnological Production of Bioactive Compounds,* 293–326.

Veselinovic, M., Vasiljevic, D., Vucic, V., Arsic, A., Petrovic, S., Tomic-Lucic, A., Savic, M., Zivanovic, S., Stojic, V., & Jakovljevic, V. (2017). Clinical benefits of n-3 PUFA and γ-linolenic α-linolenic acid in patients with rheumatoid arthritis. *Nutrients, 9*(325), 2–11.

Wanasundara, U. N., & Shahidi, F. (2020). Biotechnological methods for concentrating omega-3 fatty acids from marine oils. In *Seafood safety, processing, and biotechnology*. CRC Press, 225–233.

Wang, P., Sun, M., Ren, J., Djuric, Z., Fisher, G. J., Wang, X., & Li, Y. (2017). Gas chromatography–mass spectrometry analysis of effects of dietary fish oil on total fatty acid composition in mouse skin. *Scientific Reports, 7*(1), 42641.

Weylandt, K. H., Serini, S., Chen, Y. Q., Su, H. M., Lim, K., Cittadini, A., & Calviello, G. (2015). Omega-3 polyunsaturated fatty acids: The way forward in times of mixed evidence. *BioMed Research International, 2015*, 143109.

Wong, R., Murphy, A., Lira, M., Sichmann, M. Gd. O., Kim, A. R., Saechee, V. D., Hermanson, K. D., & Hawkins, S. S. (2023). Microneedling with a novel, n-3-PUFA-rich formulation accelerates inflammation resolution to improve skin recovery outcomes in adults with healthy skin. *Dermatology and Therapy, 13*(12), 3057–3069. Available from: https://doi.org/10.1007/s13555-023-01049-0, https://www.springer.com/journal/13555.

Wu, W. C., Meng, X., & Zhou, K. (2025). Can omega-3 fatty acid supplementation support the clinical management of drug-resistant epilepsy? A meta-analysis of randomized controlled trials. *Seizure: European Journal of Epilepsy*.

D. Xie, J. Jin, J. Sun, L. Liang, X. Wang, W. Zhang, X. Wang, Q. Jin, Comparison of solvents for extraction of krill oil from krill meal: Lipid yield, phospholipids content, fatty acids composition and minor components. Food Chemistry. **233** (2017), 434–441, doi: 10.1016/j.foodchem.2017.04.138.

Yadav, P., Chauhan, A. K., & Al-Sebaeai, M. A. (2020). Omega-3 fatty acid from plant sources and its application in food technology. *In Innovations in Food Technology: Current Perspectives and Future Goals,* 41–52.

Yamaguchi, A., Stanger, L., Freedman, J. C., Prieur, A., Thav, R., Tena, J., Holman, T. R., & Holinstat, M. (2022). Supplementation with omega-3 or omega-6 fatty acids attenuates platelet reactivity in postmenopausal women. *Clinical and Translational Science, 15*(10), 2378–2391. Available from: https://doi.org/10.1111/cts.13366, http://onlinelibrary.wiley.com/journal/10.1111/(ISSN)1752-8062.

Yan, K., Guo, F., Kainz, M. J., Li, F., Gao, W., Bunn, S. E., & Zhang, Y. (2024). The importance of omega-3 polyunsaturated fatty acids as high-quality food in freshwater ecosystems with implications of global change. *Biological Reviews, 99*(1), 200–218. Available from: https://doi.org/10.1111/brv.13017, http://onlinelibrary.wiley.com/journal/10.1111/(ISSN)1469-185X.

Yi, T., Li, S. M., Fan, J. Y., Fan, L. L., Zhang, Z. F., Luo, P., Zhang, X. J., Wang, J. G., Zhu, L., Zhao, Z. Z., & Chen, H. B. (2014). Comparative analysis of EPA and DHA in fish oil nutritional capsules by GC-MS. *Lipids in Health and Disease, 13*(1), Available from: https://doi.org/10.1186/1476-511X-13-190, http://www.lipidworld.com/home/.

Yurko-Mauro, K., Van Elswyk, M., & Teo, L. (2020). A scoping review of interactions between omega-3 long-chain polyunsaturated fatty acids and genetic variation in relation to cancer risk. *Nutrients, 12*(6), 1647.

Yves, H., Korma, S. A., Ali, A. H., Tuyishime, M. A., Habinshuti, I., & Abed, S. M. (2016). Extraction, refining and purification of ω-3 PUFA through different techniques—A review. *American Journal of Food Science and Nutrition Research, 4*, 18–26.

Zakipour Rahimabadi, A. (2021). *Book of seafood products*. University of Guilan Press.

Zatti, K. M., Ceballos, M. J., Vega, V. V., & Denstadli, V. (2023). Full replacement of fish oil with algae oil in farmed Atlantic salmon (Salmo salar) – Debottlenecking omega 3. *Aquaculture (Amsterdam, Netherlands), 574*. Available from: https://doi.org/10.1016/j.aquaculture.2023.739653, http://www.journals.elsevier.com/aquaculture/.

Zhan, J., Tang, X., Wang, F., & Han, J. (2021). Association between daily dietary eicosatetraenoic acid intake and the lower risk of psoriasis in American adults. *Clinical, Cosmetic and Investigational Dermatology, 14*, 1541–1549. https://doi.org/10.2147/ccid.s333288.

Zhang, X., Han, H., Ge, X., Liu, L., Wang, T., & Yu, H. (2020). Effect of n-3 long-chain polyunsaturated fatty acids on mild cognitive impairment: A meta-analysis of randomized clinical trials. *European Journal of Clinical Nutrition, 74*(4), 548–554. https://doi.org/10.1038/s41430-019-0544-4.

Zhang, Y., Cao, Z., Wang, L., Dong, B., Qi, S., Xu, X., Bao, Q., Zhang, Y., Xu, Q., Chang, G., & Chen, G. (2023). Effects of linseed oil supplementation duration on fatty acid profile and fatty acid metabolism-related genes in the muscles of Chinese crested white ducks. *Poultry Science, 102*(10), 102896. https://doi.org/10.1016/j.psj.2023.102896.

Zhou, X. R., Yao, Z. J., Benedicto, K., Nichols, P. D., Green, A., & Singh, S. (2023). New sustainable oil seed sources of omega-3 long-chain polyunsaturated fatty acids: A journey from the ocean to the field. *Sustainability, 15*(14), 11327. https://doi.org/10.3390/su151411327.

Zhou, Y., Khan, H., Xiao, J., & Cheang, W. S. (2021). Effects of arachidonic acid metabolites on cardiovascular health and disease. *International Journal of Molecular Sciences, 22*(21), 12029. https://doi.org/10.3390/ijms222112029.

Chapter 3

Biological mechanisms of PUFAs: metabolism and health impacts of EPA, DHA, ALA, AA, and linoleic acid

Ruchi Verma[1], Munazza Aslam Khan[1], and Eng Keng Seow[2]

[1]*Department of Food Processing and Technology, Gautam Buddha University, Greater Noida, Uttar Pradesh, India,* [2]*Department of Food Science and Technology, Faculty of Applied Sciences, Universiti Teknologi MARA, Shah Alam, Selangor, Malaysia*

3.1 Introduction

Polyunsaturated fatty acids (PUFAs) are essential dietary lipids which characterized by the presence of multiple double bonds within their hydrocarbon chains, and these structural features confer unique biochemical properties that influence cellular membrane fluidity, gene expression, and the synthesis of bioactive lipid mediators (Calder, 2020). PUFAs are of two major categories based on the position of the first double bond from the methyl end: omega-3 (n-3) and omega-6 (n-6) fatty acids. They are both essential fatty acids that must be obtained from the diet. The omega-3 fatty acids include alpha-linolenic acid (ALA), eicosapentaenoic acid (EPA), and docosahexaenoic acid (DHA). ALA is derived from plant sources such as flaxseed, chia, and walnuts, while EPA and DHA are abundant in marine oils. The omega-6 family includes linoleic acid (LA) and arachidonic acid (AA), derived from vegetable oils and animal-derived products. Humans lack the desaturase enzymes required to introduce double bonds at the n-3 or n-6 positions, making LA and ALA essential fatty acids (Innes & Calder, 2020). PUFAs are no longer viewed solely as dietary nutrients but are increasingly recognized as bioactive compounds with therapeutic and preventive potential. Their role in functional foods, disease management, and biotechnology reflects a multidimensional value across health domains. Once ingested, these essential fatty acids undergo elongation and desaturation through shared enzymatic pathways. However, the conversion rate of ALA to EPA and DHA is generally low, influenced by genetic, dietary, and hormonal factors. The end products of PUFA metabolism serve as precursors to eicosanoids, resolvins, protectins, and lipid mediators that modulate inflammation, immune function, and cell signaling (Calder, 2020). The physiological relevance of PUFAs has attracted renewed interest due to their implications in chronic diseases neurodevelopmental processes, and the health implications of PUFAs are vast. Omega-3 fatty acids, particularly EPA and DHA, have been associated with reduced risks of cardiovascular disease (CVD), neurodegenerative disorders, and chronic inflammation. In contrast, excessive intake of omega-6 PUFAs relative to omega-3s has been linked to pro-inflammatory states and metabolic dysfunction. Thus achieving a balanced n-6/n-3 ratio is increasingly recognized as critical for disease prevention and optimal health outcomes. PUFAs are a subgroup of unsaturated fatty acids that possess two or more carbon–carbon double bonds in their aliphatic chain. These double bonds are typically in the cis configuration, introducing structural "kinks" that prevent the molecules from packing tightly together. Fatty acids are essential constituents of lipids, serving as energy sources, signaling molecules, and structural elements in cell membranes. They comprise a hydrocarbon chain and a terminal carboxyl group (-COOH). Fatty acids are generally classified by the presence and number of double bonds in their carbon chain into saturated fatty acids (SFAs), monounsaturated fatty acids, and PUFAs (Gunstone, 2009). PUFAs, which possess two or more double bonds, contribute to membrane fluidity and participate in a variety of metabolic processes and metabolic pathways; the functions of essential PUFAs are shown in Table 3.1. They are essential for the synthesis of eicosanoids, resolvins, and protectins, which regulate inflammation and immunity (Calder, 2020). Recent research has increasingly focused on the physiological importance of PUFAs, particularly their roles in chronic diseases and brain development.

Omega-3 and Omega-6 Polyunsaturated Fatty Acids in Food Systems. DOI: https://doi.org/10.1016/B978-0-443-43810-3.00001-4

TABLE 3.1 Metabolic pathways and physiological functions of essential polyunsaturated fatty acids (*PUFAs*).

PUFA	Chemical name	Metabolic pathway	Health impacts	References
Alpha-linolenic acid (ALA)	α-LA (18:3 n-3)	Plant-derived; Δ6/Δ5-desaturases convert to EPA/DHA (~5%–10% efficiency)	Cardiovascular protection; limited brain delivery	Liu et al. (2015)
Eicosapentaenoic acid (EPA)	EPA (20:5 n-3)	ALA conversion/fish sources; cyclooxygenase/ lipoxygenase competition with AA forms resolvins	Lowers triglycerides, antithrombotic	Calder (2020); Furse et al. (2022)
Docosahexaenoic acid (DHA)	DHA (22:6 n-3)	EPA → peroxisomal β-oxidation; brain phospholipid accumulation	Neuroprotection, retinal/ cognitive function	Liu et al. (2015); Gladine et al. (2014); Furse et al. (2022)
Linolenic acid (LA)*	LA (18:2 n-6)	Essential; Δ6-desaturase → AA precursor	Energy; excess competes with n-3 conversion	Marklund et al. (2019).
Arachidonic acid (AA)	AA (20:4 n-6)	LA → PLA2 release → prostaglandins	Immunity/cell growth; chronic inflammation risk	Calder (2020); Liu et al. (2015); Furse et al. (2022)

The current dietary pattern, which shows a high intake of omega-6 fatty acids compared to omega-3s, poses significant public health concerns, particularly regarding CVD, obesity, metabolic syndrome, and inflammatory disorders. Consequently, augmenting the consumption of long-chain omega-3 fatty acids, whether through dietary modifications or supplementation, is increasingly acknowledged as a financially viable strategy for mitigating disease prevalence and enhancing public health outcomes. Public health guidelines are consequently evolving to prioritize the optimization of the omega-6 to omega-3 fatty acid ratio. Furthermore, the promotion of sustainable EPA and DHA sources, including algae-based products and genetically engineered oilseeds, is being encouraged. Investigations into the metabolism and physiological functions of PUFAs underscore the significance of dietary recommendations and public health campaigns aimed at ensuring adequate omega-3 fatty acid intake. This discussion will examine the biological processes involved in how PUFAs are metabolized. The focus will be on the physiological functions and health effects of EPA, DHA, ALA, AA, and LA.

3.1.1 Saturated, monounsaturated, and polyunsaturated fatty acids

Animal fats and tropical oils contain SFAs that do not have any double bonds. This has been linked to high intake in terms of LDL cholesterol increases and cardiovascular risk generation, although more recent metaanalyzes indicate that this association might be contingent on replacement nutrients (Astrup et al., 2020). Oleic acid, which is monounsaturated, has a single cis-double bond and is present in olive oil, nuts, and avocados, and it has been demonstrated to reduce inflammation and lead to better lipid profiles. PUFAs, which are omega-3 and omega-6, vary in where the first double bond is located along the chain between the methyl (omega) end of the chain. These are liquid at room temperature and have a pro- and antiinflammatory effect, which depends on their structure and balance.

3.1.2 Polar structure and classification of polyunsaturated fatty acids

The unsaturated fatty acids are further divided into PUFAs, which contain two or more carbon–carbon double bonds in their aliphatic chain. These two bonds tend to be in a cis arrangement, and this arrangement creates structural kinks that hinder close molecular assembly. This molecular structure gives PUFAs unique physicochemical properties, such as lower melting points and high membrane fluidity; these are properties that are essential to maintaining the structural integrity and functional flexibility of biological membranes (Dyall, 2015). The chemical structure and classification of PUFAs are illustrated in Fig. 3.1. Moreover, PUFAs represent a form of fatty acids, that is, characterized by several double bonds in the carbon chain. These are commonly broken by a methylene group (–CH_2), forming a methylene-interrupted structure. PUFAs are categorized according to the location in the chain of fatty acids of the first double bond (relationship between

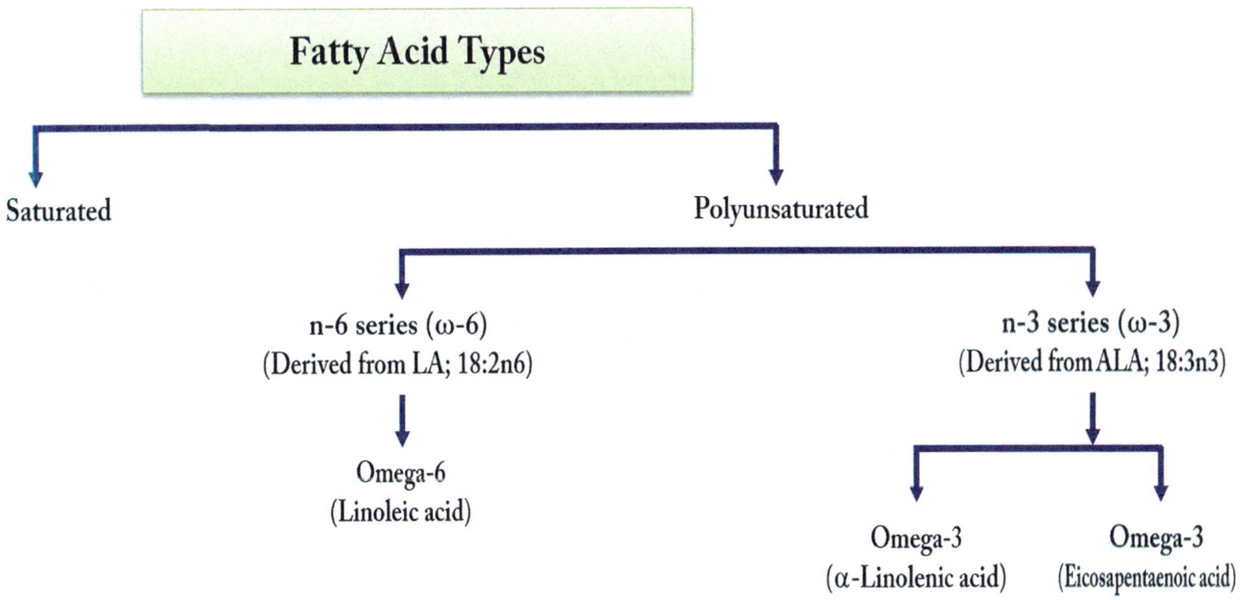

FIGURE 3.1 Types and classification of fatty acids.

the methyl [omega] end and the first double bond). The omega-3 (n-3) and omega-6 (n-6) fatty acids are considered the most important groups in this classification. To illustrate the example of the first double bond, ALA (18:3 n-3) has a first double bond on the third carbon from the methyl end, whereas LA (18:2 n-6) has the first double bond on the sixth carbon. The chemical structure of a PUFA has a direct influence on its physical and biological properties. The multiplicity of the number of carbon chain double bonds gives the structure of a kinked carbon chain that may not allow the molecules to fit tightly to each other, which is the reason why such molecules are in the liquid state at room temperature. This is contrary to the solid state of SFAs. There is typically a cis configuration of each of the two bonds, and this renders cell membranes more fluid. Ordinary omega-3 PUFAs are EPA (20:5 n-3) and DHA (22:6 n-3), and AA (20:4 n-6) is one of the omega-6 PUFAs. They can also be named as essential or nonessential PUFAs. Some of the essential PUFAs (ALA and LA) cannot be synthesized in the human body as the enzymes 12- and 15-desaturases, which add double bonds at the 12th and 15th carbon positions, are missing. Thus these should be acquired in the diet. On the contrary, essential fatty acids may be converted into nonessential PUFAs such as EPA, DHA, and AA, but the conversion efficacy is low in humans (Burdge and Wootton, 2002). Structurally, PUFAs typically occur in biological systems as constituents of complex lipids, including phospholipids and triglycerides. Long-chain PUFAs such as DHA are also found to contribute to the membrane curvature and fluidity in membrane phospholipids, particularly in neural and retinal tissues. In addition, the functional properties of PUFAs can be categorized. Antiinflammatory and cardiovascular effects are generally associated with omega-3 PUFAs; omega-6 PUFAs, on the contrary, although necessary, may even trigger pro-inflammatory reactions in case of over consumption in relation to omega-3s.

Therefore it follows that a broad understanding of the nature and structure of PUFAs is key to understanding the nature of metabolism, physiological roles, and general health impact of such fats. Lipidomics and molecular biology have achieved great advances, which have led to a more precise comprehension of PUFA isomers, their oxidation end-products, and their integration into diverse lipid classes. This increased knowledge, in its turn, has made it possible to develop more targeted nutritional and treatment strategies (Lemaitre et al., 2015).

3.1.3 Biosynthesis and metabolism of polyunsaturated fatty acids

3.1.3.1 Enzyme pathways: desaturases and elongases

PUFAs are processed metabolically through a series of enzymatic activities, and these are desaturases and elongases. Desaturases are involved in adding the double bonds into the carbon chain, and the elongases are involved in adding the carbon atoms into the chain, which extends the length of the chain. Δ6-desaturase (FADS2) and Δ5-desaturase (FADS1) are two important enzymes involved in the biosynthesis of polyunsaturated fatty acids (PUFAs). The rate-limiting step in the metabolism of ALA (18:3 n−3) and LA (18:2 n−6) into their longer-chain derivatives is catalyzed by Δ6-desaturase. Subsequently, ELOVL enzymes, particularly ELOVL5 and ELOVL2, elongate C18 and C20 polyunsaturated fatty acids (PUFAs). Subsequently, the intermediates generated are then desaturated by Δ5-desaturase to give EPA and AA. Substantial regulation of the functionality of these enzymes is provided by transcription factors, such as SREBP-1c and PPAR, and is also influenced by nutritional status, hormonal responses, and genetic differences (Martinelli et al., 2022). The metabolic pathway of omega-3 and omega-6 fatty acids is presented in Fig. 3.2.

3.1.3.2 Metabolic retransformation of alpha-linolenic acid to eicosapentaenoic acid and docosahexaenoic acid

The n-3 PUFAs biosynthetic pathway is initiated by a fatty acid, ALA (18:3 n-3), which is found in the flaxseed, chia, and walnut oils. ALA is also exposed to 86-desaturation, forming stearidonic acid (18:4 n-3), then elongated to form eicosatetraenoic acid (20:4 n-3), and finally 5-desaturated to form EPA (20:5 n-3). Conversion of EPA to DHA (22:6 n-3) requires further extension to docosapentaenoic acid (22:5 n-3) and an essential step, peroxisomal 2-oxidation, after extension to 24:5 n-3 and 24:6 n-3 in the endoplasmic reticulum. DHA is produced in the peroxisomes by shortening the chain of 24:6 n-3, which is a unique metabolic process to distinguish DHA synthesis and other PUFA conversions (Brenna et al., 2009). However, humans have poor conversion efficiency, and only about 5%–10% of ALA is converted to EPA, and a smaller percentage is converted to DHA.

3.1.3.3 Metabolic conversion of linoleic acid to arachidonic acid

LA (18:2 n-6), a vital n-6 fatty acid, is converted into gamma-linolenic acid ([GLA], 18:3 n-6) via Δ6-desaturase. Following this, GLA is elongated to produce dihomo-γ-linolenic acid ([DGLA], 20:3 n-6), which is then desaturated by Δ5-desaturase, yielding AA (20:4 n-6). AA is a key precursor for bioactive lipid mediators, such as prostaglandins,

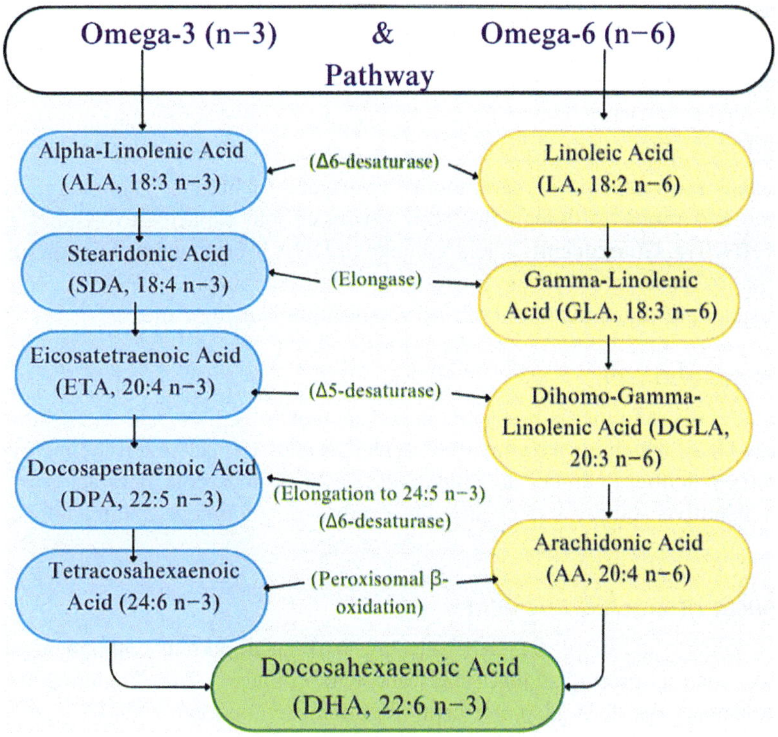

FIGURE 3.2 Metabolic pathway of omega-3 and omega-6 fatty acids (Borghi & Cicero, 2006).

thromboxanes, and leukotrienes, all of which are fundamental to inflammatory and immune responses. Analogous to EPA, AA can be esterified into membrane phospholipids and subsequently released by phospholipase A2 for signaling purposes. Although LA is abundant in Western diets, an overconsumption of n-6 PUFAs, combined with a low intake of n-3 PUFAs, can trigger a pro-inflammatory condition.

3.1.3.4 Alpha-linolenic acid metabolism

ALA, an important omega-3 fatty acid, is mainly found in plant-based foods such as flaxseed, chia seeds, and walnuts. After consumption, ALA is processed in the liver through desaturation and elongation. This process leads to the creation of EPA, which is then converted into DHA. The enzymatic steps involved in this transformation include Δ6-desaturase, elongase, and Δ5-desaturase (Brenna et al., 2009). Despite this, the conversion efficiency of ALA to EPA is comparatively low, approximated at 5%–10%, and the conversion to DHA is even less effective, with human values falling below 1% (Brenna, 2002; Burdge and Calder, 2005).

3.1.3.5 Eicosapentaenoic acid metabolism

EPA is synthesized from ALA or consumed directly from fatty fish such as salmon and mackerel. It plays an important role in antiinflammatory processes by serving as a precursor for eicosanoids, such as prostaglandins (PG3) and leukotrienes (LT5), which are less inflammatory than those derived from AA (Calder, 2020). EPA can also be further elongated and desaturated to form DHA through a series of complex enzymatic steps involving elongase and desaturase enzymes (Leonard et al., 2004). PUFAs serve as precursors for eicosanoids that are bioactive lipid mediators involved in inflammation, immunity, and hemostasis. The metabolic pathways include the following:

- Cyclooxygenase (COX) pathway: converts AA to prostaglandins and thromboxanes, which are generally pro-inflammatory.
- Lipoxygenase (LOX) pathway: converts AA to leukotrienes, also pro-inflammatory.
- Cytochrome P450 pathway: produces various hydroxyl-eicosatetraenoic acids (HETEs) and epoxy-eicosatrienoic acids (EETs).

In contrast, EPA and DHA give rise to resolvins, protectins, and maresins that are collectively termed specialized pro-resolving mediators, which actively resolve inflammation and promote tissue healing (Calder, 2017). The balance between pro-inflammatory and antiinflammatory eicosanoids is influenced by the dietary ratio of omega-6 to omega-3 fatty acids.

3.1.3.6 Docosahexaenoic acid metabolism

DHA, an essential omega-3 fatty acid, is of paramount importance to human physiology, especially concerning the development of the brain and retina. Although the body possesses the capacity to synthesize DHA from EPA, this conversion is not highly effective. Consequently, dietary intake of DHA is critical for maintaining its homeostasis. Fig. 3.2 presents the enzymatic pathways involved in the biosynthesis and metabolism of PUFAs. After being absorbed, DHA becomes part of the phospholipid membranes in both nerve and light-sensing cells.

3.1.3.7 Linoleic acid metabolism

LA is the essential omega-6 fatty acid that is easily found in vegetable oils, nuts, and seeds. Δ6-desaturase is involved in the metabolism of ALA to GLA, which is then converted to DGLA and AA. However, the incorporation of large amounts of dietary LA may have the potential to hinder the conversion of ALA since both fatty acids are competing for the same desaturase enzymes. Competitive activity can reduce the production of omega-3 fatty acids, as reported by Goyens et al. (2006).

3.1.3.8 The metabolism of arachidonic acid

AA may be of animal origin, or it can be derived from LA. It is an important component of the production of pro-inflammatory eicosanoids, such as prostaglandins (PG2) and leukotrienes (LT4) (Calder, 2008). Though AA has been considered a pro-inflammatory agent, it also performs significant functions regarding cell signaling and immune responses, thus a balance of the right amount is vital.

3.1.3.9 Synthesis and signaling pathways of eicosanoids

Eicosanoids are a general family of bioactive lipid mediators based on 20-carbon PUFAs, predominantly, AA (an omega-6 fatty acid) and EPA and DHA, which are omega-3 fatty acids. These metabolites play significant roles in the physiological and pathological processes of diverse physiological functions, especially related to inflammation, immunity, and hemostasis (Calder, 2020). Eicosanoids are synthesized mainly by three enzyme pathways, namely, the COX pathway, the LOX pathway, and the cytochrome P450 (CYP450) epoxygenase pathway. All these pathways produce different types of lipid mediators that have varied biological actions. The COX pathway transforms AA to prostaglandin H 2 (PGH 2), which is the precursor of the other prostanoids, such as prostaglandins (PGs), prostacyclins (PGIs), and thromboxanes (TXs). The effects of these lipid mediators are far-reaching since they modulate the vascular tone, platelet aggregation, and the production of fever. COX exhibits two isoforms, COX-1 and COX-2, which perform differing functions, with COX-1 always expressed in most tissues and performing homeostatic functions, and with COX-2 being inducible and mostly expressed in the case of inflammation. The LOX pathway entails the oxygenation of AA by various LOX isoenzymes (5-LOX, 12-LOX, 15-LOX) to form leukotrienes (LTs), lipoxins (LXs), and HETEs. As an illustration, the AA is converted to leukotriene A4 (LTA4) by the 5-LOX and could be further turned into LTB4 or LTC4, which are strong agents of leukocyte recruitment and bronchoconstriction (Back and Powell, 2016). Notably, the LOX pathway also oxidizes omega-3 fatty acids into resolvins, protectins, and maresins, which play a central role in the resolution of inflammation. Due to the work of the CYP450 pathway, the EETs and the omega-terminal hydroxylated products, such as 20-HETE, are produced. EETs, the derivatives of AA, mostly have a vasodilatory and antiinflammatory effect, whereas 20-HETE may be pro-hypertensive and pro-inflammatory (Imig, 2016). EPA and DHA are also metabolized by this pathway to similar epoxides and hydroxylated products, which can potentially produce positive cardiovascular effects. PUFA determines the bioactivity of the eicosanoids to a large extent. Eicosanoids (members of the omega-6 family), which are produced by AA, are pro-inflammatory in nature. As an example, PGE2, TXA2, and LTB4 are strong inflammatory, vasoconstricting, and platelet-aggregating mediators. Conversely, mediators that are produced by EPA and DHA contain no inflammatory or inflammatory-resolving properties. COX and LOX enzymes convert EPA into E-series resolvins, and DHA into D-series resolvins, protectins, and maresins, respectively, which mediate the resolution of inflammation and tissue repair. The contradictory effects of these results highlight the biological significance of the EPA/DHA ratio to AA. Excessive consumption of omega-6 PUFAs in relation to omega-3s may imbalance eicosanoid production towards pro-inflammatory pathways, which have a role in the pathogenesis of chronic disease, including CVD, arthritis, and neurodegeneration. Competitive inhibitory effects of dietary AA metabolism may be achieved through increased intake of omega-3, which replaces AA in membrane phospholipids, and competes with the same enzymes (COX and LOX), thereby preventing the production of pro-inflammatory eicosanoids. Surprisingly, even eicosanoids that are produced out of omega-6 PUFAs, such as lipoxins (e.g., LXA4), can be found to have antiinflammatory and pro-resolving effects. These LOXs are produced through the transcellular pathway synthesis between cell types and LOX isoforms interactions. It is possible that not all omega-6-derived eicosanoids are pathogenic, and lipoxins assist in dampening neutrophil recruitment and enhancing the actions of macrophages in clearing cellular debris. Eicosanoids are also complexed by the receptor-mediated signaling. The effects of eicosanoids are achieved by attaching to receptors in target cells that are linked to G-proteins. As an illustration, PGE2 interacts with four EP receptors (EP1 to EP4), with each one signaling biochemical activity through it in different cells based on the location and the signal involved. In the same way, GPCRs such as ChemR23, ALX/FPR2, and GPR32 are bound by resolvins and protectins to trigger pro-resolving pathways (Krishnamoorthy et al., 2010). Deregulated eicosanoid signaling may aggravate disease in pathological states. As an example, asthma and allergic disorders are linked to overproduction of leukotrienes, and chronic pain and cancer development to the overproduction of prostaglandin.

3.1.4 Health impacts of individual polyunsaturated fatty acids

3.1.4.1 Eicosapentaenoic acid

EPA (20:5 n-3), a long-chain omega-3 PUFA is also famous for its antiinflammatory and cardioprotective effects. Being a precursor of eicosanoids such as the prostaglandin E3 (PGE3) and leukotrienes B5 (LTB5) is less inflammatory than that of AA. Research has also defined that EPA supplementation has the capability to reduce systemic markers of inflammation, such as C-reactive protein (CRP) and interleukin-6 (IL-6) in individuals with cardiovascular and metabolic diseases. Moreover, the REDUCE-IT trial demonstrated that EPA, at high doses as icosapent ethyl, massively decreased cardiovascular events in patients who have high levels of triglycerides (Bhatt et al., 2019). In addition, to the known cardiovascular protective impact, EPA has a neuroprotective effect due to the regulation of serotonin and dopamine neurotransmission that is essential as far as mood regulation and depression treatment are concerned. Moreover, EPA has proven to be a successful additional intervention in mood disorders, especially in individuals with an increased level of inflammatory markers. Fig. 3.3. illustrates the key physiological roles, including cardiovascular protection, antiinflammatory effects, membrane stability, and neurological development.

3.1.4.2 Docosahexaenoic acid

The most common omega-3 fatty acid present in the human brain and retina is the DHA (22:6 n-3). It contains over 90% of omega-3 fatty acids in such neural tissue. This is a very vital fatty acid that is important to the growth of the brain, particularly in the third trimester of pregnancy and during early childhood. Infants have been shown to have enhancement in cognitive and visual perception (Meldrum et al., 2015). Moreover, in adults, the DHA is believed to keep the brain functioning and protect it, potentially decreasing neurodegenerative diseases, such as Alzheimer's disease. One of the roles of DHA is that it is included in the membrane of the synapses, and this allows it to sustain the membrane fluidity, neurotransmission, and activation of signaling pathways that keep cells alive. It also leads to the expression of

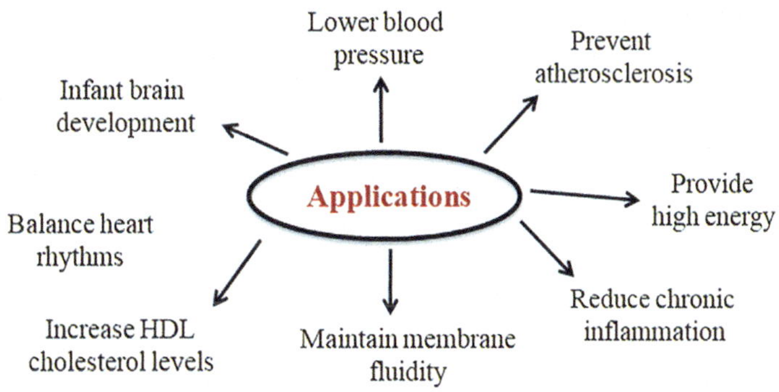

FIGURE 3.3 Applications of fatty acids in human health.

neuroprotectin D1, a specialized pro-resolving mediator that suppresses oxidative stress and inflammation in the central nervous system (Bazan et al., 2012). DHA, which is a structure of photoreceptor cells, is important in the development and functioning of the retina. Thus the shortage of DHA is associated with vision issues.

3.1.4.3 *Alpha-linolenic acid*

ALA (18:3 n-3) is the major plant-omega-3 fatty acid (also known as omega-3 fatty acid), which is found in foods such as flaxseeds, chia seeds, walnuts, and canola oil. Despite its vitality and beneficial nature to cardiovascular health, the biological activity of ALA depends on whether it is transformed to EPA and DHA, and such conversion is extremely poor in humans, with less than 10% being converted to EPA and less than 1% converted to DHA (Brenna et al., 2009). Nonetheless, the use of ALA has been associated with the reduction of cardiovascular risk, which can probably be attributed to using ALA because of its lipid-lowering, antithrombotic, and antiinflammatory properties. Epidemiological studies show that increased intake of ALA is associated with lower prevalence rates of stroke and coronary heart disease (CHD), particularly in groups with a low dietary intake of seafood (de Goede et al., 2011). Moreover, ALA has the potential to enhance any metabolic profiles, such as insulin sensitivity and adiponectin. This would result in an improved control of blood sugar and the risk of type 2 diabetes decreasing. However, like its limited conversion into EPA and DHA, ALA, alone, perhaps, cannot fully mimic the benefits of the marine-derived omega-3 fatty acids, especially in neural and retinal tissues.

3.1.4.4 *Arachidonic acid*

The omega-6 PUFA, AA (20:4 n-6), has numerous implications on human health. AA, which is an essential component of the membrane phospholipids, is released and results in the synthesis of numerous bioactive eicosanoids when the cells are stimulated. These eicosanoids are prostaglandins, thromboxanes, and leukotrienes, which are important in the regulation of inflammation, pain, and fever. Although commonly associated with the pro-inflammatory processes, AA-derived mediators also play a role in controlling immune activity, which is critical in the resolution of inflammation under standard conditions. Moreover, relative to DHA, AA is the second most common in the neuronal membranes in the context of brain development, thus playing a role in synaptic plasticity, neurogenesis, and signal transduction. AA is crucial in terms of optimal growth and development, and thus its addition to many infant formulas, in conjunction with DHA is aimed at promoting neural and visual development (Hadley et al., 2016). Similarly, AA plays an important role in the physiology of muscles; it regulates the synthesis of proteins and repair of muscles; therefore it is especially significant among athletes and patients during their growth or rehabilitation periods. An optimal ratio of AA to EPA as well as DHA in the diet is essential; a higher intake of AA might potentially increase chronic low-grade inflammation, and a deficit in the diet may impair some of the most important physiological functions (Innes & Calder, 2018). Thus nutritionists suggest balance and an appropriate omega-6 and omega-3 ratio to maintain an ideal immune and inflammatory balance.

3.1.4.5 *Linoleic acid)*

The major essential omega-6 fatty acid in the human diet is LA (18:2 n-6), a precursor of AA. Soybean, corn, and sunflower oils are some of the vegetable oils that have this fatty acid. LA cannot be substituted in keeping the skin barriers intact, in cell wall structure, and normal development, especially in early life. An LA deficiency may lead to scaly skin, retarded growth, and infertility (Kris-Etherton et al., 2021). On the other hand, although LA is a crucial nutrient, its overconsumption is a widespread case in the western diet, which could possibly increase the generation of pro-inflammatory eicosanoids unless it is replaced by omega-3 fatty acid consumption. High intake of dietary LA was highlighted to be associated with a greater amount of AA in membrane phospholipids, but this association does not always relate to systemic inflammation, thus showing the existence of a more complicated interaction (Johnson & Fritsche, 2012). In comparison, moderate consumption of LA is linked to cardiovascular effects, including the decrease of LDL cholesterol and the endothelial functionality. In essence, LA is important in ensuring that the skin is healthy, the performance of the immune system, and the metabolic balance. Nevertheless, the imbalanced consumption of these fatty acids in comparison to the omega-3 ones might predispose to the inflammatory and chronic disorders, which is why the recommendations should prioritize the augmentation of the intake of the former over a significant diminution of the latter.

3.1.5 Clinical and epidemiological evidence

In the past two decades, clinical and epidemiological evidence has continued to support the importance of PUFAs in human health. Research has focused much on the role of omega-3 fatty acids (including EPA and DHA) and, to a lesser extent, omega-6 fatty acid supplementation in the prevention and treatment of CVD, metabolic disorders, inflammatory disease, and mental health problems. Regardless of the major advances, the field still raises some complications due to the differences in the designs of the trials, the nature of the study population, and the type of PUFA formulations used. Numerous randomized controlled trials (RCTs) have been conducted to test the impact of PUFA supplementation on cardiovascular health. In high-risk patients with high triglycerides, the REDUCE-IT trial (2019) demonstrated that icosapent ethyl, a pure EPA ethyl ester, at 4 g/day was a major cardiovascular event reducer (by 25%). Such was the case despite the fact that such patients were already taking statin medications (Bhatt et al., 2019). On the same note, the JELIS trial in Japan established that the coronary events were reduced among the individuals on statin therapy, who were given 1.8 g/day of EPA. Nevertheless, other trials, such as VITAL (Manson et al., 2019) and ASCEND (Bowman et al., 2018), which were lower doses (approximately 1 g/day of EPA+DHA), did not provide the same or clear results, which indicated the potential association between the dosage of PUFAs and their efficacy. These mixed findings have been lumped together in metaanalyzes and have resulted in more comprehensive findings. In addition, a metaanalysis of studies by Hu et al. showed a significant relationship between omega-3 supplementation and a decrease in the likelihood of myocardial infarction and CVD morbidity and mortality when the supplements were used at high dosages and over a long duration of time. On the other hand, in their review of the data of the Omega-3 Treatment Trialists concluded that low-dose supplementation only offered slight benefits in high-income countries characterized by a high level of statin use. The cardioprotective relationship of increased intake of omega-3 has been generally supported by observational studies. On the other hand, the underlying limitations of observational studies are residual confounding and the complicated nature of diet–disease interactions, thus preventing causal relationships. In neurological and psychiatric conditions, PUFA supplementation has been shown to have potential, but the outcomes are conflicting. DHA plays a vital role in the brain structure and the brain functions; a lack of DHA is associated with cognitive decline and neurodegeneration. There have been inconsistent results in clinical trials of interventions in Alzheimer's disease: some studies have found cognitive stabilization with DHA-rich interventions, others, including the ADCS DHA trial, have not. On depression, metaanalyzes suggest EPA-dominant preparations are more effective than DHA, particularly in those with clinical depression or in those receiving antidepressant therapy. Clinical trials on Alzheimer's disease have had mixed results; some studies have found cognitive stabilization with DHA-rich preparations, whereas others, including the ADCS DHA trial, did not. In the case of depression, according to metaanalyzes, formulations containing EPA only show a higher level of efficacy over treatments based on DHA alone, particularly in patients with clinical depression or undergoing antidepressant treatment. Moreover, the omega-3 fatty acids have been found to be effective in improving the lipid profiles, insulin sensitivity, and inflammatory markers in the presence of metabolic and inflammatory conditions. In their metaanalysis, Hartweg et al., 2008) determined that omega-3 supplementation slightly lowered the levels of triglycerides and CRP of individuals with type 2 diabetes. Moreover, the recent studies also indicate that omega-3 fatty acids could lower the possibility of nonalcoholic fatty liver disease by enhancing liver fat metabolism levels and reducing fat accumulation (Jump et al., 2012). The clinical studies in this field, though, have been small and have been varied. This is particularly in individuals who have high triglycerides. This has in turn led to an upward adjustment of the therapeutic threshold since lower dosages of about 1 g/day which have been used in earlier studies, as well as are found over the counter in nutritional supplements, may not be sufficient to induce a clinical effect. Moreover, the availability and formulation of PUFAs, in particular, ethyl ester forms as opposed to triglyceride forms, is also known to affect the absorption and the effectiveness of PUFAs. This complicates the comparison of outcomes of various studies (Ghasemifard et al., 2014). The contribution of omega-6 fatty acids (particularly, LA) is a controversial issue. Despite the past links to pro-inflammatory effects, current studies indicate that an increased consumption of LA is not correlated with a greater level of inflammation in most populations and, in fact, it can decrease the risk of cardiovascular disease (Johnson & Fritsche, 2012; Marklund et al. (2019) performed a metaanalysis and found that there was an inverse relationship between LA consumption and risk of CHD. This perspective disputes previous assumptions, indicating that the general pattern of diet and the proportion of PUFAs are more significant than the amount of omega-6 that is taken in as one of the determinants of disease risk. The inconsistency of the results has been attributed to differences in the participants of the studies (between the disease prevention and the treatment groups), differences in the baseline levels of omega-3, inconsistencies in using the placebo controls, and the absence of standard biological markers. The lipid levels or inflammatory markers potentially limiting the utility of the research findings and some complicating the assessment, in turn, the effects of diet, such as the total amount of fat, the omega-6/omega-3 ratio, and the pattern of diet, such as the Mediterranean and Western diets, are under investigation, to determine the possible impact it has on the results of supplementation. An example is that the EPA and DHA supplementation can prove to have stronger effects in the groups with low fish intake or high inflammatory load, which means that contextual dietary factors are critical to the overall interpretation of efficacy. The supporting clinical and epidemiological evidence of supporting PUFA supplementation suggests that there are slight but significant changes in the risk of CVDs, and inflammatory diseases, particularly when larger amounts of EPA and DHA are used. At present, the study results depend on the particular context and methods, and the tendencies have been inclined toward an agreement on the significance of the given ratio as well as the number of PUFAs to predict the clinical outcomes. Thus future research has to employ specific groups of participants to enhance the existing recommendations and maximize the health effects of PUFA interventions. These groups are supposed to be separated according to the genetic factors, the initial levels of the PUFAs, and the diets.

3.1.6 Emerging research and therapeutic applications

The importance of PUFAs has expanded significantly over recent years beyond the conventional dietary recommendations. Their incorporation into functional foods and nutraceuticals, their therapeutic importance in the treatment of complex diseases, and their production by biotechnological progress and discoveries have conferred on the PUFAs a focal interest in modern nutritional science. Moreover, contemporary studies are also paying growing attention to the exploration of individualized approaches toward the metabolism of PUFA, and the aim is to increase the health outcomes based on the individual genetic and metabolic peculiarities. Another potentially interesting use of PUFAs is their addition to preventive health foods and nutraceuticals, which is a growing trend due to the growing interest of consumers in the topic of prevention. As a result, there has been a widespread distribution of functional products such as omega-3 fortified milk, eggs, yogurt, and plant-based alternatives. The incorporation of the EPA and DHA has shown effectiveness in reducing serum triglyceride levels and enhancing the functioning of the endothelium, which justifies their usage as beneficial components in functional foods developed to support cardiovascular health. In addition, the increased application of food-grade PUFA supplements in pediatric, geriatric, and sports nutrition is a reflection of the flexibility of PUFAs across the lifespan. In addition, to their well-known disease-preventive role, PUFAs are now being investigated as potential therapies for neurodegenerative diseases, including those of Alzheimer's disease and Parkinson's disease. The primary omega-3 fatty acid in the brain is DHA, which is necessary to preserve the structure of neuronal membranes. It is also involved in neurogenesis and plasticity of synapses. In recent studies, there has been an indication that DHA supplementation has the potential to alleviate the cognitive decline in individuals with mild cognitive impairment. Besides that, omega-3 PUFAs facilitate resolving neuroinflammation through resolvins and protectins as examples of neuroprotective lipid mediators formed by EPA and DHA. Supplementation of omega-3 has been shown to reduce neurodegeneration and oxidative stress in an animal model of Parkinson's disease. On the other hand, the outcomes of the clinical trials that have been carried out on human subjects have given mixed results, hence requiring more comprehensive research to determine the exact demographics of the patient groups that would benefit most from this form of treatment. These factors may control the process of cancer progression by changing cell membrane fluidity, controlling the expression of genes, and blocking the pathways of inflammation via eicosanoids. It has been discovered that EPA and DHA have the ability to retard the proliferation of breast, colorectal, and prostate cancer. The effect witnessed is a product of a series of processes. These include induction of apoptosis in cancer cells, inhibition of angiogenesis, and inhibition of NF-κB signaling pathways (Gerber, 2012). According to the clinical studies, omega-3s may be used to supplement cancer treatment, making chemotherapy more effective and decreasing the side effects such as loss of weight and inflammation (Laviano et al., 2013). On the other hand, the effectiveness of this treatment depends on the type of cancer, the dosage used, and the nutritional status of the patient, hence the complexity of PUFAs and cancer interaction. Moreover, PUFAs are also being tested as potentially useful in the future treatment of autoimmune diseases, such as rheumatoid arthritis, inflammatory bowel disease, and multiple sclerosis. Omega-3 PUFAs have been demonstrated to reduce the production of pro-inflammatory cytokines, including TNF-alpha, IL-1b, and IL-6, and also promote the change in the profile of the immune response to a less inflammatory state. Researchers, in turn, have designed oilseed crops, including Camelina sativa and Brassica napus, to yield EPA and DHA. Moreover, microalgae, which are the major producers of omega-3 fatty acids in marine life, are currently grown under controlled conditions to enable the extraction of PUFA. The emerging research trends and therapeutic applications of PUFAs across different health conditions are presented in Table 3.2. The developments offer alternative, plant-based sources of omega-3 fatty acids, and this facilitates sustainability and also mitigates the chances of heavy metal contamination. Furthermore, engineered strains of the yeast and fungi are underway for large-scale engineering of PUFAs, which could have applications in the pharmaceutical and food sectors. Personalized nutrition will be the next stage of PUFAs research. The method is personalized in terms of dietary recommendations based on individual variability, such as genetic variations, the effects of gut microbiomes, and metabolic features. The genetic variations that govern the activity of significant enzymes, including the FADS1 and FADS2 (fatty acid desaturases), have a major influence on the ability of an individual to convert ALA to EPA and DHA. As an illustration, individuals harboring some FADS gene mutations may lack the capacity to synthesize long-chain omega-3 fatty acids in their bodies. They can therefore be required to obtain these fatty acids through their diet to ensure that they have healthy levels in their

TABLE 3.2 Emerging research and therapeutic applications of polyunsaturated fatty acids (*PUFAs*).

PUFA/derivative	Emerging research focus	Mechanism of action	Research status	References
Alpha-linolenic acid	Role in cardiometabolic health and inflammation modulation	Conversion to EPA and DHA (limited efficiency); modulation of lipid metabolism	Epidemiological studies and dietary intervention trials	Calder, (2020)
Eicosapentaenoic acid (EPA)	Antiinflammatory and cardioprotective potential	Production of resolvins and inhibition of pro-inflammatory eicosanoids	Approved pharmaceutical formulations; ongoing clinical trials	Calder, (2015)
Docosahexaenoic acid (DHA)	Neurodevelopment and cognitive health	Structural role in neuronal membranes; neuroprotective signaling	Extensive clinical and experimental studies	Liu et al. (2015); Calder (2020)
Linoleic acid	Skin health and metabolic regulation	Precursor of arachidonic acid; membrane phospholipid synthesis	Nutritional and mechanistic studies	
Arachidonic acid	Immune signaling and inflammation	Precursor of prostaglandins, leukotrienes, and thromboxanes	Experimental and clinical research	Calder, (2020)
Specialized pro-resolving mediators	Resolution of chronic inflammation	Termination of inflammation via receptor-mediated pathways	Preclinical and early clinical research	

tissues. Besides, sex, age, electrophrone concentration, and diet (high levels of omega-6 fatty acids) are also factors that affect the processing of PUFAs. Thus the joint omics techniques are typically employed to give the dietary recommendations of the PUFAs, considering genetic and metabolic aspects (Minihane et al., 2015). Not all studies disapprove the possibility that omega-3 fatty acids may stimulate the proliferation of positive microorganisms, including Bifidobacterium and Lactobacillus, and this may increase their antiinflammatory property.

3.2 Conclusion

PUFAs are important to human health because of their antiinflammatory, neuroprotective, and cardiometabolic benefits, which include omega-3 fatty acids, namely, EPA, DHA, and ALA. On the other hand, the omega-6 fatty acids (LA and AA) are essential in growth, skin health, and immune system functionality, but an excess of the former over the latter may exacerbate inflammation. Enzymatic processes have tight regulation in the synthesis and metabolism of these fatty acids, such as desaturases and elongases, which are regulated by genetic factors, age, sex, dietary habits, and exposure to the microbiome. The PUFAs form an important aspect of nutritional sciences, and it has great implications in the prevention of diseases and health promotion. Their potential is entirely untapped, and further interdisciplinary research is an inevitable way to achieve this goal and use evidence-based strategies to improve the health of individuals and the population.

References

Arad, M., Waldman, M., Abraham, N. G., & Hochhauser, E. (2020). Therapeutic approaches to diabetic cardiomyopathy: Targeting the antioxidant pathway. *Prostaglandins & Other Lipid Mediators, 150*, 106454. https://doi.org/10.1016/j.prostaglandins.2020.106454.

Astrup, A., Magkos, F., Bier, D. M., Brenna, J. T., de Oliveira Otto, M. C., Hill, J. O., King, J. C., Mente, A., Ordovas, J. M., Volek, J. S., Yusuf, S., & Krauss, R. M. (2020). Saturated fats and health: A reassessment and proposal for food-based recommendations. *Journal of the American College of Cardiology, 76*(7), 844–857. https://doi.org/10.1016/j.jacc.2020.05.077.

Back, M., & Powell, W. S. (2016). Leukotriene receptors: Crucial components in vascular inflammation. *Science Signaling, 9*, 416.

Bazan, N. G., Molina, M. F., & Kim, J. H. (2012). Neuroprotectin D1: A DHA-derived mediator that promotes cell survival and resolves inflammation. *Biochimie, 94*(1), 114–122.

Bhatt, D. L., Steg, P. G., Miller, M., Brinton, E. A., Jacobson, T. A., Ketchum, S. B., Doyle, R. T., Juliano, R. A., Jiao, L., Granowitz, C., Tardif, J.-C., & Ballantyne, C. M. (2019). Cardiovascular risk reduction with icosapent ethyl for hypertriglyceridemia. *New England Journal of Medicine, 380*(1), 11–22. https://doi.org/10.1056/nejmoa1812792.

Borghi, C., & Cicero, A. F. G. (2006). Recent evidence of the role of omega-3 polyunsaturated fatty acids on blood pressure control and hypertension-related complications. *Future Lipidology, 1*(5), 569–577.

Bowman, L., Mafham, M., Karl, W., Stevens, W., Buck, G., Barton, J., Murphy, K., Aung, T., Haynes, R., Cox, J., Murawska, A., Young, A., Lay, M., Chen, F., Sammons, E., Waters, E., Adler, A., Bodansky, J., Farmer, A., & Armitage, J. (2018). Effects of n−3 Fatty Acid Supplements in Diabetes Mellitus. *New England Journal of Medicine, 379*(16), 1540–1550. https://doi.org/10.1056/nejmoa1804989.

Brenna, J. T. (2002). Efficiency of conversion of alpha-linolenic acid to long chain n-3 fatty acids in man. *Current Opinion in Clinical Nutrition and Metabolic Care, 5*(2), 127–132. https://doi.org/10.1097/00075197-200203000-00002.

Brenna, J. T., Salem, N., Sinclair, A. J., & Cunnane, S. C. (2009). α-Linolenic acid supplementation and conversion to n-3 long-chain polyunsaturated fatty acids in humans. *Prostaglandins, Leukotrienes, and Essential Fatty Acids, 80*(2-3), 85–91. https://doi.org/10.1016/j.plefa.2009.01.004.

Burdge, G. C., & Calder, P. C. (2005). Conversion of α-linolenic acid to longer-chain polyunsaturated fatty acids in human adults. *Reproduction, Nutrition, Development, 45*(5), 581–597. https://doi.org/10.1051/rnd:2005047.

Burdge, G. C., & Wootton, S. A. (2002). Conversion of α-linolenic acid to eicosapentaenoic, docosapentaenoic and docosahexaenoic acids in young women. *Journal of Nutrition, 88*(4), 411–420. https://doi.org/10.1079/bjn2002689, http://journals.cambridge.org/BJN.

Calder, P. C. (2008). Polyunsaturated fatty acids, inflammatory processes and inflammatory bowel diseases. *Molecular Nutrition and Food Research, 52*(8), 885–897. https://doi.org/10.1002/mnfr.200700289UnitedKingdom, http://www3.interscience.wiley.com/cgi-bin/fulltext/119426241/PDFSTART.

Calder, P. C. (2020). Nutrition, immunity and COVID-19. *BMJ Nutrition, Prevention & Health, 3*(1), 74–92.

Calder, P. C. (2017). Omega-3 fatty acids and inflammatory processes: from molecules to man. *Biochemical Society Transactions, 45*(5), 1105–1115. https://doi.org/10.1042/bst20160474.

Calder, P. C. (2015). Marine omega-3 fatty acids and inflammatory processes: Effects, mechanisms and clinical relevance. *Biochimica et Biophysica Acta (BBA) - Molecular and Cell Biology of Lipids, 1851*(4), 469–484. https://doi.org/10.1016/j.bbalip.2014.08.010.

de Goede, J., Verschuren, W. M. M., Boer, J. M. A., Kromhout, D., & Geleijnse, J. M. (2011). Alpha-linolenic acid intake and 10-year incidence of coronary heart disease and stroke in 20,000 middle-aged men and women in the Netherlands. *PLOS ONE, 6*(3), e17967. https://doi.org/10.1371/journal.pone.0017967.

Dyall, S. C. (2015). Long-chain omega-3 fatty acids and the brain: a review of the independent and shared effects of EPA, DPA and DHA. *Frontiers in Aging Neuroscience, 7*. https://doi.org/10.3389/fnagi.2015.00052.

Furse, S., de Roover, C., & Koulman, A. (2022). Omega-3 fatty acids and their lipid mediators in health and disease. *Annual Review of Nutrition, 42*, 331–355.

Gerber, M. (2012). Omega-3 fatty acids and cancers: a systematic update review of epidemiological studies. *British Journal of Nutrition, 107*(S2), S228–S239. https://doi.org/10.1017/s0007114512001614.

Ghasemifard, S., Turchini, G. M., & Sinclair, A. J. (2014). Omega-3 long chain fatty acid "bioavailability": A review of evidence and methodological considerations. *Progress in Lipid Research, 56*, 92–108. https://doi.org/10.1016/j.plipres.2014.09.001.

Gladine, C., Newmann, J. W., Durand, T., Pedersen, T. L., Galano, J.-M., Demougeot, C., Berdeaux, O., Pujos-Guillot, E., Mazur, A., & Comte, B. (2014). Lipid pofiling following intake of the omega 3 fatty acid DHAIdentifies the peroxidized metabolites F4 neuroprostanes as the best predictors of atherosclerosis prevention. *PLoS ONE*. https://doi.org/10.1371/journal.pone.0089393.

Goyens, P. L. L., Spilker, M. E, Zock, P. L, Katan, M. B., & Mensink, R. P. (2006). Conversion of α-linolenic acid in humans is influenced by the absolute amounts of α-linolenic acid and linoleic acid in the diet and not by their ratio. *The American Journal of Clinical Nutrition, 84*(1), 44–53. https://doi.org/10.1093/ajcn/84.1.44.

Gunstone, F. D. (2009). *The chemistry of oils and fats: sources, composition, properties and uses*. John Wiley & Sons.: Blackwell Publishing.

Hadley, K., Ryan, A., Forsyth, S., Gautier, S., & Salem, N. (2016). The essentiality of arachidonic acid in infant development. *Nutrients, 8*(4), 216. https://doi.org/10.3390/nu8040216.

Hartweg, J., Perera, R., Montori, V., Dinneen, S., Neil, H. A., Maayan, N., & Farmer, A. (2008). Omega-3 polyunsaturated fatty acids (PUFA) for type 2 diabetes mellitus. *Cochrane Database of Systematic Reviews*(1).

Imig, J. D. (2016). *Advances in pharmacology, endothelium*. Elsevier, 105–141. https://doi.org/10.1016/bs.apha.2016.04.003.

Innes, J. K., & Calder, P. C. (2018). Omega-6 fatty acids and inflammation. *Prostaglandins, Leukotrienes and Essential Fatty Acids, 132*, 41–48. https://doi.org/10.1016/j.plefa.2018.03.004.

Innes, J. K., & Calder, P. C. (2020). Marine omega-3 (n-3) fatty acids for cardiovascular health: An update. *Nutrients, 12*(4), 1–15.

Johnson, G. H., & Fritsche, K. (2012). Effect of dietary linoleic acid on markers of inflammation in healthy persons: a systematic review of randomized controlled trials. *Journal of the Academy of Nutrition and Dietetics, 112*(7), 1029–1041.e15. https://doi.org/10.1016/j.jand.2012.03.029.

Jump, D. B., Depner, C. M., & Tripathy, S. (2012). Omega-3 fatty acid supplementation and cardiovascular disease. *Journal of Lipid Research, 53*. https://doi.org/10.1194/jlr.R027904.

Kris-Etherton, P. M., Grieger, J. A., & Etherton, T. D. (2021). Dietary reference intakes for DHA and EPA. *Prostaglandins, Leukotrienes, and Essential Fatty Acids, 88*(1), 99–102.

Krishnamoorthy, S., Recchiuti, A., Chiang, N., Yacoubian, S., Lee, C.-H., Yang, R., Petasis, N. A., & Serhan, C. N. (2010). Resolvin D1 binds human phagocytes with evidence for proresolving receptors. *Proceedings of the National Academy of Sciences, 107*(4), 1660–1665. https://doi.org/10.1073/pnas.0907342107.

Laviano, A., Rianda, S., Molfino, A., & Fanelli, F. R. (2013). Omega-3 fatty acids in cancer. *Current Opinion in Clinical Nutrition and Metabolic Care, 16*(2), 156–161. https://doi.org/10.1097/mco.0b013e32835d2d99.

Lemaitre, R. N., Fretts, A. M., Sitlani, C. M., Biggs, M. L., Mukamal, K., King, I. B., Song, X., Djoussé, L., Siscovick, D. S., McKnight, B., Sotoodehnia, N., Kizer, J. R., & Mozaffarian, D. (2015). Plasma phospholipid very-long-chain saturated fatty acids and incident diabetes in older adults: the Cardiovascular Health Study. *The American Journal of Clinical Nutrition, 101*(5), 1047–1054. https://doi.org/10.3945/ajcn.114.101857.

Leonard, A. E., Pereira, S. L., Sprecher, H., & Huang, Y. S. (2004). Elongation of long-chain fatty acids. *Progress in Lipid Research, 43*(1), 36–54. https://doi.org/10.1016/S0163-7827(03)00040-7, www.elsevier.com/locate/plipres.

Liu, J. J., Green, P., John Mann, J., Rapoport, S. I., & Sublette, M. E. (2015). Pathways of polyunsaturated fatty acid utilization: Implications for brain function in neuropsychiatric health and disease. *Brain Research, 1597*, 220–246. https://doi.org/10.1016/j.brainres.2014.11.059.

Manson, JoA. E., Cook, N. R., Lee, I-M., Christen, W., Bassuk, S. S., Mora, S., Gibson, H., Albert, C. M., Gordon, D., Copeland, T., D'Agostino, D., Friedenberg, G., Ridge, C., Bubes, V., Giovannucci, E. L., Willett, W. C., & Buring, J. E. (2019). Marine n–3 fatty acids and prevention of cardiovascular disease and cancer. *New England Journal of Medicine, 380*(1), 23–32. https://doi.org/10.1056/nejmoa1811403.

Meldrum, S., Dunstan, J., Foster, J., Simmer, K., & Prescott, S. (2015). Maternal fish oil supplementation in pregnancy: A 12 year follow-up of a randomised controlled trial. *Nutrients, 7*(3), 2061–2067. https://doi.org/10.3390/nu7032061.

Minihane, A. M., Vinoy, S., Russell, W. R., Baka, A., Roche, H. M., Tuohy, K. M., Teeling, J. L., Blaak, E. E., Fenech, M., Vauzour, D., McArdle, H. J., Kremer, B. H. A., Sterkman, L., Vafeiadou, K., Benedetti, M. M., Williams, C. M., & Calder, P. C. (2015). Low-grade inflammation, diet composition and health: current research evidence and its translation. *British Journal of Nutrition, 114*(7), 999–1012. https://doi.org/10.1017/s0007114515002093.

Marklund, M., Wu, J. H. Y., Imamura, F., Del Gobbo, L. C., Fretts, A., de Goede, J., Shi, P., Tintle, N., Wennberg, M., Aslibekyan, S., Chen, T.-A., de Oliveira Otto, M. C., Hirakawa, Y., Eriksen, H. H., Kröger, J., Laguzzi, F., Lankinen, M., Murphy, R. A., Prem, K., & Risérus, U. (2019). Biomarkers of Dietary Omega-6 Fatty Acids and Incident Cardiovascular Disease and Mortality. *Circulation, 139*(21), 2422–2436. https://doi.org/10.1161/circulationaha.118.038908.

Tao, H., & Abe, I. (2021). Enzymology and biosynthesis of the orsellinic acid derived medicinal meroterpenoids. *Current Opinion in Biotechnology, 69*, 52–59. https://doi.org/10.1016/j.copbio.2020.11.016.

Chapter 4

Sourcing polyunsaturated fatty acid-rich ingredients: superfoods, microbial sources, and market integration

Prajwal Jakhmola[1], Karan Saini[1], Yograj Neha[1,2], and Vidyashankar Srivatsan[1,2]

[1]*Applied Phycology and Food Technology Laboratory, Dietetics and Nutrition Technology Division, CSIR-Institute of Himalayan Bioresource Technology, Palampur, Himachal Pradesh, India,* [2]*AcSIR-Academy of Scientific and Innovative Research, Ghaziabad, Uttar Pradesh, India*

4.1 Introduction

Fatty acids are hydrophobic biomolecules of plant and animal cells and represent the primary building blocks, fundamental constituents, and structural units of lipids. Structurally, they are made of a straight hydrocarbon chain with a terminal carboxyl (–COOH) group and typically contain even numbers of carbon atoms ranging from C4 to C28. Fatty acids are classified into saturated fatty acids (SFA), fully hydrogenated (no double bonds), completely saturated fatty acids, or unsaturated fatty acids (UFA) (double bonds present), with the latter further divided into monounsaturated fatty acids (MUFA) and polyunsaturated fatty acids (PUFA). SFAs, such as lauric acid, myristic acid, palmitic acid (PA), and stearic acid (SA), are prevalent in tropical oils, including cocoa, palm, and palm kernel oils (Qi et al., 2004). Further, UFA contain one or more double bonds, where MUFAs consist of a single double bond, and PUFAs contain two or more. Oleic acid (OA) (18:1 n-9) is the most predominant MUFA in animal fats and plant seeds such as maize (Fahs et al., 2010). SFA and MUFA primarily function as energy storage molecules, while PUFAs have multiple physiological roles and functions. Some key functions include contribution to the structural integrity of cellular membranes, subcellular organelle stability, and functioning as precursors for various signal transducing molecules such as eicosanoids, prostaglandins, thromboxanes, leukotrienes, and lipoxins (Lee et al., 2016).

In addition to their physiological role, PUFAs have therapeutic properties, specifically antioxidant and antiinflammatory, that offer them myriad bioactivities. PUFAs are considered essential, since their de novo biosynthesis does not occur and they must be acquired from dietary sources. Based on the occurrence of the double bonds, PUFAs can be grouped into two major groups, *viz.*, omega-3 and omega-6 fatty acids (Patel et al., 2019). Predominant PUFAs include linoleic acid (C18:2 n-6, LA) and α-linolenic acid (C18:3 n-3, ALA) that act as precursors for further long-chain PUFAs (LC-PUFAs) such as eicosapentaenoic acid (EPA), docosapentaenoic acid (DPA), and docosahexaenoic acid (DHA). LA is a omega-6 fatty acid, primarily obtained from plant oils (vegetable oils) such as soybean, sunflower, safflower, cottonseed, etc., while ALA is an omega-3 fatty acid present abundantly in both plants (chia, flax, and perilla seeds) and microbial sources (algae, fungi, and bacterial sources) (Qi et al., 2004). LC-PUFAs such as DPA, EPA, and DHA are predominantly obtained from marine sources, primarily fish and algal sources. Although humans can biotransform ALA into EPA, DPA, and DHA, this conversion occurs at a very limited rate, making LC-PUFAs an important dietary component (Patel et al., 2022). LC-PUFAs have a restricted supply owing to their limited availability only from marine sources. With the increasing global demand for LC-PUFAs, predominantly as dietary supplements and feed ingredients, there is a considerable interest in the industrial biosynthesis of PUFAs.

Microorganisms consisting of abundant concentrations of PUFAs, called single-cell oils (SCO), have been explored for commercial production (Ochsenreither et al., 2016). The global market for LC-PUFAs, particularly omega-3 fatty acids, is estimated at USD 13 billion with a compounded growth of 8% annually. Currently, the cost of microbial-derived SCOs is estimated at USD 500 per kg and reaches much higher depending on the PUFA composition. In the case of omega-6

Omega-3 and Omega-6 Polyunsaturated Fatty Acids in Food Systems. DOI: https://doi.org/10.1016/B978-0-443-43810-3.00004-X

PUFA arachidonic acid (ARA), the global demand is estimated at 400,000 tonnes per year, and the market is estimated to be more than USD 2 billion (Nandoskar et al., 2026). The growing demand for PUFA production is driven by their therapeutic properties. LC-PUFAs, particularly EPA and DHA, have been used in the management of dyslipidaemia, obesity, diabetes, and cognitive health (Cardoso et al., 2016). Further, PUFAs contribute to cholesterol reduction and decrease the risk of atherosclerosis and coronary artery disease. In addition, LC-PUFAs play a vital role in cognition, brain development, and visual acuity in infants (Katiyar & Arora, 2020). Some commercially exploited microorganisms for the production of PUFAs are *Mucor circinelloides* for gamma linolenic acid (GLA), *Mortierella alpina* for ARA, *Yarrowia lipolytica* for EPA, and *Schizochytrium* spp. for DHA (Zhang et al., 2022). These microbial resources have been considered as environmentally sustainable alternatives to traditional, marine sources such as fish. By 2050, the global population is expected to reach 9 billion, and the demand for dietary ingredients is expected to increase continuously; there is a need for identifying sustainable sources of PUFAs (Martínez-Córdova et al., 2017). This necessitates the identification of superfoods and novel microorganisms for PUFA production and the development of sustainable bioprocesses for low-cost biomanufacturing of PUFAs. In this context, the present chapter systematically describes the different bioresources and the recent innovations in the bioprocessing of PUFAs. Although the chapter provides a summary of information on the various bioresources, special attention is given to microalgae as a sustainable resource for PUFA production.

4.2 Structure and biosynthesis of polyunsaturated fatty acids

Typically, PUFAs have the CH_3–CH_2(n)–COOH skeleton with a long aliphatic chain. The chain length of PUFAs ranges from 16 to 22 carbons, and they are categorized broadly into two types, *viz*., omega-3 (ω-3 PUFAs) and omega-6 (ω-6 PUFAs), based on the position of the first double bond from the methyl end of the aliphatic chain. PUFAs with chain length between 16 and 18 are considered short-chain PUFAs, while PUFAs having chain length above 20 carbons are considered LC-PUFAs. EPA (20:5 n-5, 8, 11, 14, 17), DPA (22:5 n-7, 10, 13, 16, 19), and DHA (22:6 n-4, 7, 10, 13, 16, 19) are some commercially important LC-PUFAs (Barta et al., 2021). Fatty acid biosynthesis (de novo) occurs in the plastids, and they are exported to the endoplasmic reticulum (ER) and cytosol, where they undergo further modifications, including elongation, desaturation, and hydroxylation (Bilbao et al., 2017). Acetyl-CoA serves as the precursor for fatty acid biosynthesis, synthesized by two key enzymes: pyruvate dehydrogenase, which converts pyruvate obtained from glycolysis or the pentose phosphate pathway, and acetyl-CoA synthase, which catalyzes the direct conversion of free acetate to acetyl-CoA (Nethravathy et al., 2021). Two other important enzymes in fatty acid synthesis from acetyl-CoA are acetyl-CoA carboxylase (ACCase) and fatty acid synthase (FAS), the latter being a multienzyme complex located in the stroma of chloroplasts. ACCase regulates the flow of carbon into fatty acid biosynthesis, and a positive correlation has been observed between ACCase activity and fatty acid biosynthesis. There are two types of FAS found in nature: FAS I, present in animals and fungi, and FAS II, which is involved in microalgal fatty acid synthesis. FAS II comprises four subunit proteins: β-ketoacyl-acyl carrier protein (ACP) synthase (KAS), β-ketoacyl-ACP reductase, β-hydroxyacyl-ACP dehydratase (DH), and enoyl-ACP reductase. In the first set of fatty acid synthesis, the acetyl group is transferred to the cysteine group of KAS III (condensing enzyme) and combines with malonyl-ACP to yield acetoacetyl-ACP. This intermediate is then converted to butyryl-ACP in a series of three reduction and dehydration reactions catalyzed by 3-ketoacyl-ACP reductase, 3-hydroxy-ACP DH, and trans-enoyl-ACP reductase (Baba & Shiraiwa, 2013; Jovanovic et al., 2021). After the formation of this four-carbon fatty acid molecule, elongation begins, resulting in the addition of two more carbon units per cycle. The cycle continues until 16–18 carbon units are added. Desaturases present in the chloroplast and ER insert double bonds into these fatty acids, while acyl-ACP thioesterases (TEs) are involved in the termination of fatty acid chains in plastids (Khozin-Goldberg, 2016). Triacylglycerol (TAG), a major lipid storage compound, is synthesized in the ER by the action of acyl transferase and is accumulated as cytoplasmic lipid droplets. The lipid metabolism in plants and microalgae has been reported and is almost similar, with slight differences in algae with respect to the complexity of enzymes and compounds involved. Depending upon the environmental conditions, the PUFAs can be produced by two identified biosynthetic pathways. Aerobic microorganisms such as cyanobacteria, eukaryotic microalgae, and plants exclusively utilize aerobic pathways for PUFA production. In contrast, certain anaerobic organisms, such as *E. coli* and marine microorganisms adapted to high pressure, low temperature, and anoxic environments, depend exclusively on anaerobic pathways for the synthesis of UFA (Tian et al., 2024). LC-PUFAs are synthesized through two distinctive pathways: the conventional aerobic FAS pathway and the anaerobic PUFA synthase (polyketide synthase-like, PKS-like) pathway (Lin & Qu, 2022; Tian et al., 2024). In the FAS aerobic pathway, a sequence of elongation and desaturation is catalyzed by the presence of specific desaturases and elongases (Winwood, 2013). Oxygen is required for desaturases to produce LC-PUFAs from C16 or C18 SFAs, which occurs mainly in microalgae, fungi, and plants (Walsh et al., 2016).

PA, C16:0 is synthesized using acetyl-CoA as a precursor and FAS synthase, with NADPH participating in the process. FAS synthase is a barrel-shaped enzyme complex with multiple catalytic domains, including ACP, malonyl palmitoyl transferase (MPT), ketoacyl synthase (KS), ketoacyl reductase (KR), DH, enoyl reductase (ER), and TE domains (Chi et al., 2022; Jovanovic et al., 2021; Maier, 2017). The MPT domain plays a crucial role in loading the starting unit. The process begins with the KS domain catalyzing substrate condensation to form 3-ketoacyl-ACP. Next, the KR domain catalyzes the reduction of acyl-ACP to form 3-hydroxyacyl-ACP. The DH domain then catalyzes dehydration to form 2-trans-enoyl-ACP, and finally, the ER domain catalyzes the reduction reaction. This four-step process (condensation, reduction, dehydration, and reduction) is repeated seven times to produce PA. SA, C18:0 is produced through an elongation process by specific elongase enzymes (Parsons et al., 2013). The TE domain catalyzes the release of FFAs. Based on this, OA (C18:1) and LA (C18:2) are synthesized step by step using desaturation enzymes (Δ9, Δ12, and Δ15). These desaturases are oxygen-dependent, highlighting the aerobic nature of this pathway (Tian et al., 2024). Two desaturase and elongase pathways have been identified for the synthesis of LC-PUFAs. The conventional Δ6 pathway utilizes Δ6 desaturase to form GLA (C18:3) and stearidonic acid (SDA, C18:4) from LA and ALA, respectively. The Δ6 elongase then extends these intermediates by two carbon atoms to produce dihomo-γ-linolenic acid (DGLA, C20:3) and eicosatetraenoic acid (ETA, C20:4) (Fig. 4.1). This pathway subsequently converts DGLA to ARA (C20:4) and ETA to EPA using Δ5 desaturase, which can also catalyze EPA formation via omega-3 desaturase as shown in Fig. 4.1 (Lippmeier et al., 2009). Alternatively, the Δ8 pathway, mainly found in protist organisms, uses Δ9 elongase to catalyze the extension of LA and ALA by two carbon atoms to yield eicosadienoic acid (EDA, C20:2) and eicosatrienoic acid (C20:3), respectively. These intermediates are then converted by Δ8 desaturase to DGLA and ETA. The subsequent synthesis steps are identical to those in the Δ6 pathway (Li et al., 2011). Microalgae possess remarkable enzymatic diversity, enabling multiple routes to synthesize LC-PUFAs. The anaerobic PUFA synthase pathway is structurally and mechanistically distinct, resembling polyketide synthases (PKS-like). It involves large, multifunctional enzyme complexes that directly assemble LC-PUFAs from malonyl-CoA through iterative condensation, reduction, and dehydration reactions. Unlike the aerobic pathway, this mechanism does not rely on oxygen-dependent desaturases, making it particularly advantageous for organisms inhabiting low-oxygen marine environments. This pathway is considered more energy-efficient and is exploited in biotechnology for microbial production of EPA and DHA (Lin & Qu, 2022).

4.2.1 Regulation of polyunsaturated fatty acid biosynthesis

The regulation of PUFA biosynthesis is a complex phenomenon and is significantly influenced by both genetic factors and environmental conditions. Growth limiting, stressful environmental conditions such as nutrient deprivation, temperature stress, particularly prolonged exposure to cold conditions, high light irradiation, and salinity stress have been reported to modulate lipid metabolism, mainly PUFA biosynthesis. Stressful growth conditions often lead to the accumulation of TAGs in plant and microalgal cells. It is observed that, under stressful growth conditions, citrate is accumulated from the tricarboxylic acid cycle due to the inhibition of NAD-isocitrate dehydrogenase. Citrate is converted to malonyl-CoA by cytosolic ACCase, which further enters the ER for fatty acid elongation. Under extreme, stressful environmental conditions, the cell division rates significantly reduce, thereby reducing the demand for membrane lipid synthesis and consequently fatty acid synthesis. Under such circumstances, fatty acid synthesis is diverted towards the production of storage compounds like TAGs (Bellou et al., 2014). TAGs synthesis acts as a sink and a protective mechanism, scavenging the excess electrons produced during photosynthesis, thereby protecting the thylakoid membrane. Interestingly, microalgae cells accumulate TAG under excess carbon supply beyond the requirement for starch synthesis. This was validated in the starchless mutants in the green unicellular microalgae, *Chlamydomonas, where cells accumulated TAGs under excess carbon supply* compared to the wild-type strain (Nakamura & Li-Beisson, 2016). Advances in genetic engineering strategies have enabled the significant enhancement of PUFA yields in microalgae cells. The strategy of transcription factor manipulation has emerged as a particularly promising method for PUFA enhancement. Understanding the enzymatic mechanisms and biosynthetic regulatory networks would enable effective utilization of microbial biofactories for LC-PUFA production (Tian et al., 2024).

4.3 Sources of polyunsaturated fatty acids

As described earlier, medium-chain PUFAs such as LA and ALA are primarily obtained from angiosperms, particularly seed oils, whereas LC-PUFAs such as ARA, EPA, and DHA are predominantly obtained from microbial sources, such as fungi and microalgae. The current section provides a snapshot of different PUFA sources.

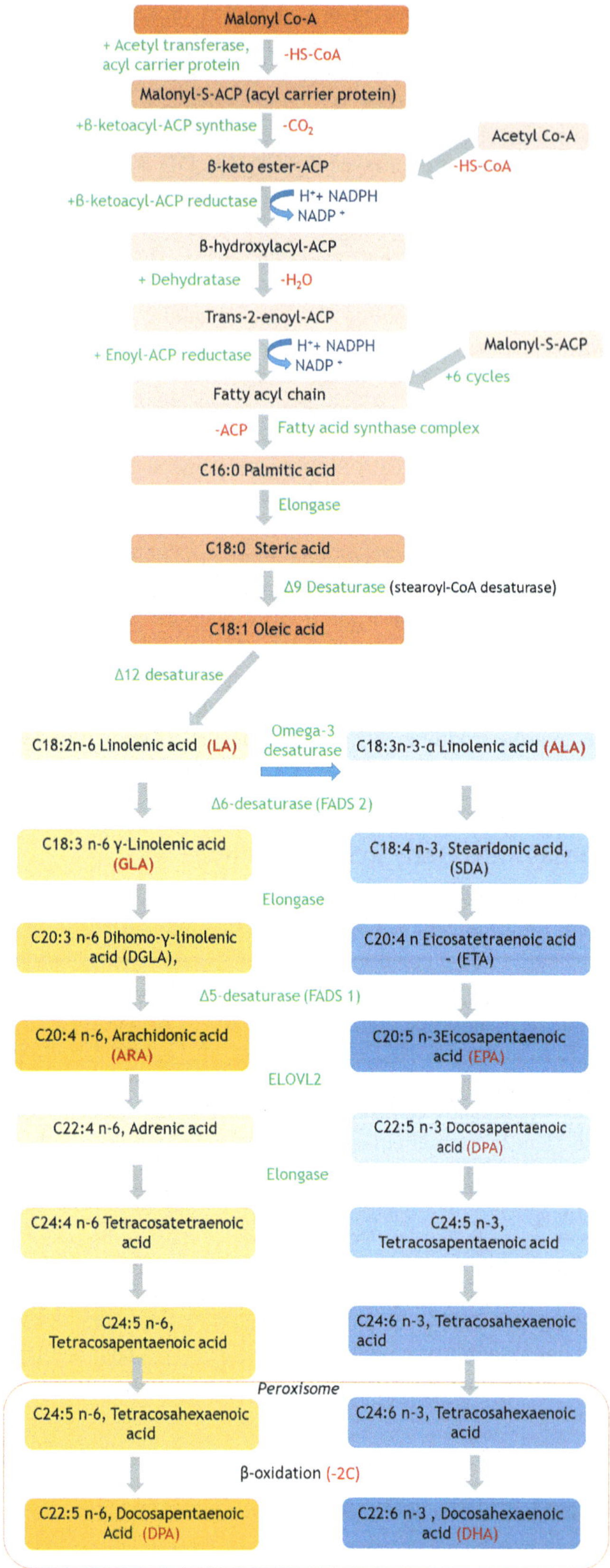

FIGURE 4.1 **Fatty acid biosynthetic pathway (modified from** Jovanovic et al., 2021). Pathway describing the de novo biosynthesis of fatty acids.

4.3.1 Plant-based sources of polyunsaturated fatty acids

Plant-based foods are central to several communities, often providing essential nutrition and bioactive compounds that improve human health. Several plant species can be considered as "superfoods" owing to their ability to provide beyond the basic nutrients such as antioxidants, PUFAs, phytosterols, carotenoids, and other phytochemicals that contribute to their therapeutic properties (Benzie & Wachtel-Galor, 2011). Several terrestrial plant species, particularly oilseed and edible nuts, have been conventionally utilized as a source of dietary PUFAs, and they are listed in Table 4.1 Among these, flaxseed *(Linum usitatissimum L.)*, chia (*Salvia hispanica*), and perilla (*Perilla frutescens*) have been reported to possess high concentrations of omega-3 fatty acid, ALA, constituting anywhere between 40% and 60% of the total fatty acids in the extracted oils (Saini & Keum, 2018). On the contrary, vegetable oils derived from soybean, corn, safflower, and cotton seeds are an abundant source of omega-6, LA, which constitutes 50% to 70% of total fatty acids (Nazir & Zahoor, 2021). In addition to the above sources, novel crops have emerged recently for the large-scale production of PUFA-rich oils. Among the emerging sources, *Plukenetia volubilis* (sacha inchi), a native crop of the Amazon basin, has gained significant attention in recent years owing to its high PUFA content. The sacha inchi seed oil contains up to 80% PUFA, with LA and ALA constituting 35%–40% and 40%–45%, respectively (Wijiani et al., 2026). Similarly, *Perilla frutescens* (Perilla), widely cultivated in East Asian countries, contains ALA up to 60% of total fatty acids, making it a commercially viable source (Guan et al., 2024). Another unique superfood source of PUFAs is *Hippophae rhamnoides* (Sea buckthorn), an indigenous shrub widely grown in the cold desert regions of the Himalayas. Sea buckthorn berry seed oil contains a unique blend of omega-6 GLA and omega-3 ALA in addition to other bioactive molecules such as carotenoids, phytosterols, and polyphenols. The typical fatty acid composition of sea buckthorn oil is saturated fats (PA, SA) constitute 25%–30% of total lipids, monounsaturated fats constituting 25%–30% of total lipids consisting palmitoleic acid (C16:1, n-7), an omega-7 fatty acid and oleic (C18:1, n-9), and PUFAs mainly LA, GLA, and ALA up to 60% of total lipids, where ALA and GLA content are almost equal constituting approximately 30% of total fatty acids (Zielińska & Nowak, 2017a, 2017b). Garden cress (*Lepidium sativum*) has been identified as a potential source of ALA alongside the aforesaid sources. The seed oils possessed ALA up to 40% of total fatty acids with linoleic (8%–11%) and arachidic acid (2%–4%) in lower

TABLE 4.1 Plant-based sources of PUFAs.

Plant source	Oil/lipid content (%)	Major PUFAs	PUFAs (%)	References
Flax	44.8	• ALA • LA	• 43–61 • 15	Ciftci et al. (2012), Aguillón-Páez et al. (2020), Yang et al. (2021)
Perilla	42.8	• ALA • LA	• 65.6–75.85 • 12.5	Zamani Ghaleshahi et al. (2020), Ciftci et al. (2012)
Chia	30.17–32.16	• ALA • LA	• 54.5–64.7 • 16.99–22.5	Ciftci et al. (2012), Melo et al. (2019)
Echium	33.72	• ALA • SDA	• 32.68 • 15.46	Cesconetto-Bisinotto et al. (2025)
Portulaca oleracea L. (purslane)	0.47–0.54	• ALA	• 45.30–51.2	Uddin et al. (2014), Nemzer et al. (2020)
Cannabis sativa (hemp)	25–35	• LA • ALA	• 55.1–63.7 • 15.2–26.2	Shetty and Akhilender (2017)
Lepidium sativum L. (garden cress)	21–24	• ALA	• 30–34	Nehdi et al. (2012)
Amaranthus *cruentus*	6.1	• –	• 44.55	Azri et al. (2025)
Plukenetia volubilis L. (sacha inchi)	33.4–37.6	• LA • ALA	• 35.2–41 • 37.3–44.2	Chirinos et al. (2013)
Sea buckthorn		• LA	• 40.14–57.78	Wirkowska-Wojdyła et al. (2024)

ALA—alpha-linolenic acid, LA—linoleic acid, SDA—stearidonic acid, PUFA—polyunsaturated fatty acids.

quantities. Umesha & Naidu (2015) reported that blending of ALA-rich garden cress oil with sesame, sunflower, and rice-bran oil reduced the omega-6:omega-3 ratio of the blended oils and improved the antioxidant activity as evidenced in in vivo rodent supplementation. The authors observed that continuous supplementation of garden cress oil enhanced the tocopherol content and expression of endogenous antioxidant enzymes in liver of experimental animals. In recent years, *Echium* (*Echium plantagineum)* seed oil has been identified as a potential source of PUFA. The seed oil has a unique fatty acid composition, with the presence of both omega-6 and omega-3 PUFAs such as LA and GLA (omega-6) and omega-3 (ALA and SDA, C18:4, n-3) constituting nearly 60%–65% of total fatty acids (Carlini et al., 2021). The presence of SDA in the Echium oil offers unique health benefits. SDA is an intermediate product of the biosynthetic pathway involving the conversion of ALA to EPA catalyzed by the rate-limiting D6-desaturase enzyme. High concentrations of SDA enable faster conversion to EPA by the activity of elongase and D5 desaturase enzyme. Further, SDA has similar health benefits as those of EPA, such as hypocholesterolemic, hypolipidemia, and antiinflammatory properties, making it a high-value PUFA (Miquel, 2008).

Compared to the conventional seed oils, most of the aforesaid seed oils have excelled omega-6:omega-3 fatty acid ratio, ranging between 3:1 or 2:1, ideal for optimum health. The dietary ratio of omega-6:omega-3 PUFAs is an important determinant of the nutritional quality of an oil. Disproportionate ratios often offset lipid metabolism, promoting inflammation and negatively influencing cardiac health. The ratio recommended for optimal health is between 5:1 and 2:1 (Simopoulos, 2003). However, refined vegetable oils derived from sunflower, safflower, and corn oil possess a highly imbalanced ratio ranging between 15:1 and 25:1, promoting severe inflammatory and cardiometabolic disorders. PUFA-rich seed oils such as that of flax, chia and perilla have exceptionally higher omega-3 content resulting in a ratio of 1:2 to 1:4. Emerging sources such as camelina oil (*Camelina sativa*), hemp seed oil (*Cannabis sativa*) and sea buckthorn seed oil also provide relatively more balanced ratios, between 3:1 and 2:1 closely aligning with the physiological requirements as shown in Table 4.1 (Shetty & Akhilender, 2017; Wirkowska-Wojdyła et al., 2024). Such balanced PUFA ratios in these oils offer them strong antiinflammatory properties. In addition to seed oils, several green leafy vegetable (GLV) crops have been reported to possess omega-3, particularly ALA. *Amaranthus* spp. such as *A. spinosus, A. viridis*, and *A. hypochondrius* have been reported to possess ALA up to 30%–35% of the total fatty acids (Gupta et al., 2024). In addition to ALA, amaranth seeds and leaves also provide a significant amount of phytosterols and squalene that have extensive health benefits, such as antioxidant and antiinflammatory properties (Venskutonis & Kraujalis, 2013). Among the GLVs, purslane (*Portulaca oleracea*) contains high concentrations of PUFAs, up to 40% of total fatty acids (Uddin et al., 2014). Despite the excellent PUFA concentration, the majority of the aforesaid crops are underutilized and undercharacterized. Thus emerging plant seed oil sources and GLVs offer a potential opportunity in the development of next-generation functional foods with high concentrations of PUFAs, making them superfoods. The future research calls for a systematic R&D program on domestication of the aforesaid indigenous crops, developing climate-resilient agrotechnologies, and development of sustainable downstream processing for the production of omega-3 PUFA-rich oils.

4.3.2 Fungi-based polyunsaturated fatty acid production

Fungi are heterotrophic microorganisms and have emerged as sustainable alternatives for the commercial production of bioactive metabolites, including PUFAs. They have been referred to as SCOs and known to accumulate lipids up to 70% of the biomass dry weight. Some oleaginous genera include *Mortierella spp., Mucor spp., Rhodotorula spp., Yarrowa lipolytica,* and *Saccharomyces cerevisiae*. These species accumulate diverse PUFAs such as GLA, ARA, EPA, and DHA and find applications as dietary supplements and nutraceuticals (Xue et al., 2018). Table 4.2 provides a list of oleaginous fungi explored for PUFA production.

Among the several fungal species, *Mortierella alpina*, a filamentous fungus, is most widely studied for the commercial production of omega-6, ARA. *Mortierella alpina* accumulates very high concentrations of TAGs, reaching up to 15 to 20 $g\,L^{-1}$ with ARA constituting 30% to 70% of total fatty acids (Sakuradani, 2010). Other species from the *Mortierella* genus widely used for PUFA production are *M. isabellina* for ARA production, Mortierella alpine Cunninghamella for EPA production (Zhang et al., 2021). In addition, *Mortierella* spp. are widely used for the production of rare PUFAs, particularly omega-6, such as DGLA and GLA (Sakuradani, 2010). Another filamentous fungus finding exceptional use in PUFA production is *Mucor* spp. *Mucor circinelloides* has been identified for efficient production of GLA in high quantities. The lipid content per dry biomass ranges between 15% w/w to 45% w/w, with GLA constituting nearly 20% to 25% of total lipids. The lipid content and GLA concentration vary depending upon the growth medium composition, particularly carbon sources (Fazili et al., 2022). Oleaginous yeasts such as *Lipomyces starkeyi, Yarrowia lipolytica, Aureobasidium melanogenum, Pichia guilliermondii, Candida curvata, Sporidiobolus* spp., *Rhodosporidium toruloides, Rhodotorula glutinis, Rhodotorula mucilaginosa, Cryptococcus spp., Rhodosporidium spp.,* and *Rhodosporidiobolus*

TABLE 4.2 Fungi-based sources of PUFA.

Fungus species	Lipid content (%)	Major PUFA	Major PUFAs %	References
Cunninghamella echinulata	30–48	GLA	16.2–22	Gema et al. (2002), Fakas et al. (2008), Bellou et al. (2012), Alakhras et al. (2015)
Mortierella alpina ST1358	NA	EPA	26.4	Okuda et al. (2015)
Mortierella alpina 1S-4	42.5	ARA	20.3–44	Fujita et al. (2016), Kikukawa et al. (2018), Sakuradani et al. (2013)
		DGLA	4–5.6	
Mortierella alpina	40–52	ARA	9.2–43	Ji et al. (2014), Nie et al. (2014), Vadivelan and Venkateswaran (2014)
Mucor circinelloides	14.7–35.6	GLA	10.8–27.1	Tang et al. (2015)
Thamnidium elegans	10.6–52.7	GLA	6.5–13.6	Bellou et al. (2014), Klempova et al. (2013)
Yarrowia lipolytica	30	EPA	56.5–58	Xue et al. (2013)

ARA—arachidonic acid; DGLA—dihomo-gamma-linolenic acid; GLA—gamma linolenic acid, EPA—eicosapentaenoic acid.

fluvialis accumulate over 50% of their cell dry weight. These all-fungal species are listed in Table 4.2 carbon sources utilized in the growth medium, which play an important role in the lipid yield and productivity of oleaginous yeasts. Glucose is the predominantly used carbon source; in addition, inulin, xylose, glycerol, and starch have been widely used as sources of carbon (Xue et al., 2018). The common production strategies adopted for PUFA production from fungi and oleaginous yeasts are aerobic fermentation (both submerged and solid-state fermentation). Submerged fermentation involves the use of reduced carbon sources such as monosaccharides as a carbon source, and glycine, urea, ammonia salts, and peptone extracts as a source of nitrogen. Solid-state fermentation has also been widely adopted for the cultivation of oleaginous fungi. Growth conditions, mainly carbon/nitrogen ratios, and cultivation temperature affect the lipid productivity in fungi. Manipulation of temperature is an important tool for PUFA biosynthesis, as desaturase enzymes are temperature sensitive and need effective maintenance for achieving optimum yield. Other factors that affect PUFA production in oleaginous fungi are shear force, dissolved oxygen concentration, and culture age. Ageing is an important phenomenon used in the industrial production of ARA from *M. alpina. In* addition to media engineering strategies, random chemical mutagenesis has been used for enhancing lipid and PUFA productivity. Sakuradani et al. (2013) demonstrated that *M. alpina* mutants were able to produce high concentrations of a variety of PUFAs such as mead acid (MA; 20:3n-9; 49% in oil), EDA (20:2n-9; 37%), DGLA (42%), and compared to the wild strain. Further genetic engineering/gene editing techniques have been evaluated to enhance PUFA biosynthesis. Enhancing the expression of 12 and 6 desaturase encoding genes in *M. circinelloides* enhanced PUFA yield (Zhang et al., 2017). Among the several strains of yeasts, *Yarrowa lipolytica* is considered a universal platform for the production of PUFAs owing to its plasticity and quick ability to adapt to wide environmental conditions and exceptional lipid accumulation capabilities. Further, gene editing techniques such as CRISPR-Cas-9, transcription activator-like effector nucleases, and transposons have enabled the enhancement of PUFA productivity in *Y. lipolytica* (Yan et al., 2024).

4.3.3 Microalgae as a source of polyunsaturated fatty acids

Microalgae are photosynthetic microorganisms with wide structural complexity ranging from unicellular to filamentous structures. Microalgae are classified based on their pigment composition and energy storage material, particularly starch-type macromolecules, into cyanobacteria (blue–green algae), rhodophytes (red algae), chlorophytes (green algae), and chromophytes (all other algae). They are distributed in both freshwater and marine environments (Mobin & Alam, 2017). Although they are primarily phototrophic, they have the ability to grow in heterotrophic and photo-heterotrophic (micotrophic) environments with excellent environmental adaptability (Santos-Sánchez et al., 2016). Microalgae are primary producers and accumulate lipids under stressful environmental conditions. Factors such as nutrient (nitrogen and phosphorus) limitation, excess UV radiation, extreme temperatures, and exposure to heavy metals like iron, zinc, copper, and cadmium are known to induce lipid accumulation (Adarme-Vega et al., 2012). Microalgae accumulate both medium and LC-PUFAs, such as LA, ALA, ARA, EPA, and DHA. *Arthrospira platensis, Chlorella vulgaris, Isochrysis spp., Nannochloropsis spp., Tetraselmis spp., Phaeodactylum tricornutum*, and red algae *Porphyrodium sp.* are a few PUFA-accumulating microalgae with lipid contents ranging between 10% and 75% by dry biomass. In addition to the aforesaid photosynthetic microalgal species, heterokonts (heterotrophic, motile algae like strains), including diatoms such as *Nitszchia* spp., *Navicula* spp., *Chaetoceros* spp., *Schizochytrium* spp., *Crypthecodinium cohnii*, are a few oleaginous species explored for PUFA production (Marella et al., 2021).

Lipid content of microalgae is often overestimated due to the lack of specific lipid extraction methods (Bellou et al., 2012). Lipid production may be combined with the production of other bioactive metabolites, such as lutein, beta-carotene, astaxanthin, canthaxanthin, phytosterols, and phycotoxins under specific conditions (Bellou et al., 2014). As discussed earlier, microalgal lipids have a unique composition and possess different PUFAs. Few species and strains of *Chlorella sp., Stichococcus sp., and Tetraselmis suecica* are rich in LA, while species and strains from *Chlorella sp., Asterionella sp., Tetraselmis sp., Dunaliella sp., Rhodomonas sp., Stichococcus sp., Tetradesmus sp., Anacystis sp., Chlamydomonas sp., Dictyosphaerium pulchellum and Sphaerocystis schroeteri* are rich in ALA. Likewise, species such as *Navicula sp., Nannochloropsis sp., Asterionella sp., Pavlova sp., Phaedacturum tricornutum, Nitschia ovalis, Alexandrium sanguiena, Skeletonema costatum, Chlorella ellipsoidea and Heterosigma akasiwo* are rich in EPA while dinoflagellates such as *Amphidinium sp., Prorocentrum sp., Alexandrium sanguiena, Scripsiella trochoidea, Heterocapsa tricuetra*, and heterokonts such as *Schizochytrium limnacium, Crypthecodinium cohnii and Isochrysis galbana* are rich source of DHA. In addition, unique PUFAs such as SDA are reported to be accumulated in species/strains such as *Amphidinium sp., Prorocentrum sp., Rhodomonas sp., Isochrysis sp. and Dunaliella sp.* Cyanobacteria strains such as *Arthrospira platensis, Nostoc* sp., are known to accumulate omega-6 PUFA GLA listed in the Table 4.3 (Lim et al., 2015; Makri et al., 2011; Nalder et al., 2015; Suh et al., 2015). Production of PUFA in microalgae can be modulated and enhanced through optimization of culture conditions, particularly light intensity, photoperiod, culture temperature, growth medium pH, salinity, and agitation speed and carbon and nitrogen concentrations (Wang et al., 2018; Yin et al., 2019). Stressful environmental conditions, such as nutrient deprivation (nitrogen starvation and high salinity), enhance lipid accumulation and consequently PUFA composition (Chen et al., 2017). Genetic engineering/gene editing technologies leading to overexpression of PUFA biosynthesis enzymes in *Phaeodactylum tricornutum* (Xue et al., 2015), overexpression of the long-chain fatty acid elongase genes of *Thalassiosira pseudonana* (Cook & Hildebrand, 2016), or the use of CRISPR/Cas9-based genome-editing on *Nannochloropsis sp.* (Wang et al., 2016) have been reported to enhance the PUFA production in microalgae.

4.3.3.1 Photoautotrophic cultivation and polyunsaturated fatty acid production

Phototrophic/autotrophic cultivation is the most commonly utilized method for industrial-scale microalgae production across diverse applications. Several of the EPA-producing microalgae strains rely on phototrophic growth, with CO_2 being the major source of carbon. *Nannochloropsis* spp. are considered excellent hosts for industrial EPA production. Six species have been identified from *Nannochloropsis* spp., viz., *N. gaditana, N. granulata, N. limnetica, N. oceanica, N. oculata*, and *N. salina* for EPA production, predominantly in autotrophic conditions (Yan et al., 2024). The major advantage behind the autotrophic system of cultivation is the low environmental impact, lower contamination risk, and cost-effectiveness (Saxena et al., 2020). Light intensity plays a major role in biomass and lipid accumulation in *Nannochloropsis* sp. Intensity levels lower than the saturation point enhance biomass accumulation, while beyond the saturation point, biomass production is negatively affected, triggering lipid biosynthesis. In addition to intensity, light wavelength has been reported to enhance PUFA accumulation (Kim et al., 2019). Exposure to blue light enhanced EPA accumulation in *N. oceania* with concentrations up to 5% to 6% dry cell weight and productivity of 12-12 mg L^{-1} day^{-1} in *N. oceania*, much higher than red, yellow, and white light (Chen et al., 2013). Conventional production of Nannochloropsis spp. is achieved through either open raceway ponds or closed photobioreactors. Raceway ponds are open, shallow pond systems with continuous agitation where cultures are exposed to environmental conditions, whereas in closed photobioreactor systems, cells are cultivated in transparent bioreactors where cells receive natural sunlight, but are maintained at a constant pH and dissolved oxygen concentration. Closed photobioreactors often have more controlled conditions compared to open raceway ponds. Further, closed photobioreactors require less area, more accurate operational control, higher surface-to-volume ratio over open raceway ponds. This results in enhanced nutrient uptake, better growth, and biomass productivity (Ren et al., 2022). Although autotrophic cultivation is commercially viable and proven technology, they have several disadvantages, such as photoinhibition, varying yield and productivity owing to fluctuating light intensities, thereby significantly affecting microalgae photosynthetic activity. Excessive irradiance can lead to photoinhibition and damage to the photosynthetic machinery. Likewise, exposure to lower intensity of light and shorter

TABLE 4.3 Microalgae-based sources of PUFA.

Microalgae species	Major polyunsaturated fatty acids	Percentage composition of PUFAs (% w/w total lipids)	References
Arthrospira platensis	• GLA (18:3)	• 34	Yang et al. (2019)
Acutodesmus obliquus	• ALA (18:3)	• 38	Othman et al. (2019)
Aurantiochytrium sp.	• DHA	• 46	Chauhan et al. (2023)
Scenedesmus sp.	• ALA	• 42	
Chlamydomonas reinhardtii	• GLA • ALA • LA • DHA • EPA	• 22 • 44 • 10 • 5.40 • 2.4	James et al. (2011)
Chlorella vulgaris	• LA • ALA	• 24 • 35.5	Othman et al. (2019)
Schizochytrium limacinum	• GLA	• 45	Rodriguez-Espana et al. (2022)
Isochrysis galbana	• DHA • LA • EPA • ALA	• 15.20 • 7.16 • 7 • 2.97	Señoráns et al. (2020)
Chlorella sorokiniana	• ALA • EPA	• 11 • 2.4	Shim et al. (2020)
Crypthecodinium cohnii	• DHA	• 60	Ulmann et al. (2017)
Chaetoceros muelleri	• DHA • EPA • GLA • ARA • LA	• 1.23 • 10.55 • 0.24 • 0.14 • 1.60	de Jesús-Campos et al. (2020)
Heterococcus chodati	• EPA • LA	• 32.60 • 8.10	Lang et al. (2011)
Nannochloropsis sp.	• EPA • ALA	• 33.70 • 17	
Nannochloropsis oceanica	• EPA • ARA • LA	• 27 • 1.63 • 0.68	Wang et al. (2019)
Phaeodactylum tricornutum	• EPA • DHA • ARA • LA	• 35 • 2.8 • 1.02 • 1.13	Hamilton et al. (2014)
Rhodomonas baltica	• GLA • EPA • ALA • LA • ARA	• 3.83 • 6.31 • 15.70 • 11.60 • 0.71	Wang et al. (2019)
Dunaliella sp.	• DHA • GLA • LA	• 21 • 36 • 5.90	Jovanovic et al. (2021)

(Continued)

TABLE 4.3 (Continued)

Microalgae species	Major polyunsaturated fatty acids	Percentage composition of PUFAs (% w/w total lipids)	References
Euglena gracilis	• DHA • GLA • LA	• 9 • 19.30 • 3.50	Lang et al. (2011)

ALA—alpha-linolenic acid, LA—linoleic acid, ARA—arachidonic acid; GLA—gamma linolenic acid, EPA—eicosapentaenoic acid, DHA—docosahexaenoic acid, PUFA—polyunsaturated fatty acids.

photoperiods leads to prolonged dark phase, leading to decreased biomass productivity. Furthermore, photoautotrophic microalgae rely solely on inorganic nutrients such as carbon, nitrogen, and phosphorus for survival and growth (Patel, Singhania, Dong, et al., 2021; Patel, Singhania, Sim, et al., 2021). The nutrient uptake efficiency in microalgae cells may be affected by poor light penetration, turbidity, or unsanitary conditions, resulting in poor biomass productivity (Patel, Singhania, Dong, et al., 2021; Patel, Singhania, Sim, et al., 2021). Since PUFA productivity is strongly linked to both biomass and lipid accumulation, any decline in these parameters directly results in a lower PUFA yield (Chauhan et al., 2023). Thus alternative systems of microalgae biomass production are essential and necessary for sustainable PUFA production.

4.3.3.2 Polyunsaturated fatty acid production from microalgae under heterotrophic conditions

Heterotrophic microalgae can grow in the absence of light by converting organic carbon sources such as glucose, acetate, agricultural flours, and wastewater. This approach allows high cell densities, fast growth, and higher biomass accumulation. However, only a few species can adapt to heterotrophic metabolism, and cultivation is particularly susceptible to contamination by other heterotrophic microorganisms such as bacteria, yeasts, and fungi. Thus complete aseptic conditions are required during heterotrophic cultivation to reduce microbial interference (Morales-Sánchez et al., 2015). Certain microalgal genera, such as *Phaeodactylum* spp. and *Scenedesmus* spp., are obligate autotrophs, while others, such as *Nannochloropsis, Dunaliella, and Tetraselmis*, are capable of utilizing organic substrates as facultative or obligate heterotrophs, similar to the dinoflagellates *Crypthecodinium and Gyrodinium* (Russo et al., 2021). Some species, such as *Galdieria sulphuraria*, accumulate more PUFAs during heterotrophic growth than phototrophic growth, as well as higher levels of saturated and MUFA. Similar patterns were observed in the marine diatom *Cyclotella cryptica*, with glucose-supplemented heterotrophic cultures producing more EPA than autotrophic systems. The availability of easily digested carbon sources, such as glucose, enhances metabolic flow toward lipid biosynthesis (Cupo et al., 2021). Heterotrophic cultivation significantly enhances overall lipid content and biomass concentration. Fermentation-based heterotrophic processes often produce high lipid yields three to four times larger than those achieved through autotrophic growth. For example, *Galdieria sp. USBA-GBX-832* showed improved biomass accumulation and PUFA productivity in heterotrophic culture compared to autotrophic conditions (López et al., 2019). Growth rates under heterotrophy also overcome those that are only supported by photosynthesis, provided adequate nutrients are supplied. Despite its productivity, the economic feasibility of heterotrophic cultivation remains a significant challenge because an alternative is cost-effective. Carbon, nitrogen, and phosphorus are particularly important macronutrients; thus heterotrophic media frequently incorporate glucose as a carbon source, yeast extract or ammonia as nitrogen sources, and phosphates as a phosphorus supplement. In DHA production, glucose alone can account for up to 80% of total production costs. As a result, mixotrophic systems provide an eco-friendly, cost-effective solution by allowing the use of carbohydrate-rich waste streams. Previous research has revealed some heterotrophic microalgae with significant PUFA production capacity. The thraustochytriaceae and crypthecodiniaceae families produce significant amounts of omega-3 PUFA in heterotrophic conditions (Oliver et al., 2020). *Crypthecodinium* species exhibit the greatest levels of omega-3, particularly DHA. Furthermore, *Schizochytrium* and *Ulkenia* from the thraustochytriaceae family have great potential. *Thraustochytrium aureum* strain 28,210 produces 48.3%–58.2% DHA of total fatty acids, whereas strain 38,304 accumulates 41%–75% DHA. *Ulkenia*, on the other hand, produces 5%–13% DHA on average (Oliver et al., 2020). More recently, *Chlorella sp., Planophila sp., and Nannochloropsis* sp. were found to store ALA fractions of around 50%, 36%, and 50% of total fatty acids, respectively (Jain et al., 2022).

4.3.3.3 Polyunsaturated fatty acid production from microalgae under mixotrophic conditions

Mixotrophic microalgae combine photoautotrophic and heterotrophic metabolic characteristics. They use light as an energy source, absorbing CO_2 and organic substrates such as sugars or acids for carbon Source. In contrast to phototrophic cultivation, mixotrophic systems combine both metabolic processes, allowing for increased biomass and lipid accumulation within the same cultivation period. Only certain microalgal species may grow mixotrophically and use both inorganic and organic carbon. Mixotrophic techniques are seen to be very promising for large-scale applications due to their high productivity and carbon sequestration capability (Patel et al., 2020). Because sugars promote accelerated bacterial proliferation, microalgal cultivation in organic carbon–supplemented media requires strict sterilization similar to heterotrophic systems (Ananthi et al., 2021). Mixotrophic conditions significantly support biomass and lipid biosynthesis. For instance, *Scenedesmus obliquus* accumulates considerably higher lipid contents (11.6%–58.6%) under mixotrophic growth compared with photoautotrophic conditions (7.14%). Likewise, *Chlorella vulgaris* grown mixotrophically produces 4.43-fold higher biomass than under phototrophic culture (Katiyar et al., 2018). PUFAs such as ARA (C20:4 n-6), EPA (C20:5 n-3), and DHA (C22:6 n-3) are essential for human health, and interest in their cost-effective production has increased rapidly within nutraceutical and pharmaceutical industries (Jiao et al., 2018). *Nannochloropsis sp.* cultivated mixotrophically with 0.03 mol L^{-1} glucose showed a 1.4-fold increase in biomass compared to phototrophic growth, with slight variations in EPA levels (Sivakumar et al., 2022). PUFAs, particularly EPA, help to improve health outcomes by decreasing neuroinflammatory and cardiovascular risk. Studies on *N. laevis* found that glucose-supported mixotrophic cultivation (5 g L^{-1}) resulted in roughly 50% greater EPA concentrations than heterotrophic growth. Continuous mixotrophic cultivation of *N. gaditana* with glucose (5 g L^{-1}) or glycerol (1 g L^{-1}) significantly increased EPA accumulation compared to autotrophic conditions (Menegol et al., 2019). ARA is especially critical for brain development, making it a valuable PUFA for nutraceutical and medicinal use. Batch cultivation of *Porphyridium purpureum CoE1* under mixotrophic conditions shows a high potential for ARA production. When acetate, glycerol, and glucose were used as carbon sources, ARA content increased by 43% and 52% for acetate (0.25%) and glycerol (0.5%), respectively, when compared to autotrophic cultivation (Castillo et al., 2021).

4.3.4 Macroalgae as a source of polyunsaturated fatty acid

Macroalgae (seaweeds) represent another class of promising, sustainable resources for PUFA production as an eco-friendly alternative to land-based agriculture. Unlike terrestrial crops, macroalgae biomass production does not require arable land, freshwater, synthetic fertilizers, herbicides, or insecticides, thereby being more benign to the environment (Yong et al., 2022). Global models on sustainability indicated that replacing 10% of the human diet with seaweeds could conserve approximately 110 million hectares of arable land (Spillias et al., 2023). Further, seaweeds sequester large amounts of CO_2, and it is reported that approximately 173 Tg C yr^{-1} is being absorbed and fixed by seaweeds, making them a low-carbon-footprint food system (Alleway, 2023). Apart from their environmental benefits, macroalgae have an excellent nutritional profile with a typical composition including carbohydrates (31%–81% dry weight, DW), proteins (5%–22% DW), lipids (2%–13% DW), and dietary fiber (22%–66% DW) (Biris-Dorhoi et al., 2020; Mandalka et al., 2022). Although macroalgae contain comparatively low total lipid levels (2%–10% DW), they are relatively abundant in PUFAs, and their fatty-acid profiles vary among taxa (Shahidi & Ambigaipalan, 2018). Profiling of 17 macroalgal species demonstrated that Rhodophyta contained the highest omega-3 levels (16%–27%), including EPA, DHA, and ALA, followed by Phaeophyta (up to 15%), whereas Chlorophyta showed lower omega-3 contents (1%–9%), except for Ulva, which displayed high ALA (18%) (Pereira et al., 2012). Major macroalgae species producing PUFA are shown in Table 4.4 Phaeophyta, which also displayed remarkable omega-6 fatty acids (23%–44%), including LA and ARA, while Chlorophyta contained moderate amounts (6%–27%). Consistent with these findings, analysis of 27 tropical macroalgae demonstrated considerable PUFA levels, particularly ARA (6.1%–47.0%) and EPA (0.2%–37.0%) in Phaeophyta and Rhodophyta, whereas *Ulva* spp. exhibited lower PUFA contents with medium DHA (0.81%–6.05%) (Kumari et al., 2010). The occurrence of nutritionally essential PUFAs (ALA, LA, EPA, and DHA) despite low total lipid content highlights the potential of macroalgae to enhance the quality of low-fat diets and encourages their use in developing functional foods to enhance human health.

4.4 Downstream processing of polyunsaturated fatty acid

4.4.1 Developing food-grade lipid extraction strategies

Being a nutritionally and pharmaceutically important ingredient, the process of extraction and purification of PUFA must be green, safe, and environmentally friendly. PUFA extraction can be done either dry or wet (Fig. 4.2). A drying

TABLE 4.4 Macroalgae sources of polyunsaturated fatty acid (PUFA).

Macroalgae species	Name of PUFA	Composition of fatty acid (%)	References
Ulvarigida	• Docosahexanoic acid (DHA) • Eicosapentanoic acid (EPA) • Arachidonic acid (ARA) • Alpha-linolenic acid (ALA) • Linoleic acid (LA)	• 4.10 • 1.40 • 1.20 • 10.90 • 1.50	Lopes et al. (2020)
Ulvaprolifera	• DHA • EPA • ARA • ALA • LA	• 0.20 • 2.20 • 1.70 • 0.20 • 22.00	Cardoso et al. (2017)
Codium tomentosum	• LA • ALA • EPA	• 3.40 • 14.00 • 7.90	Lopes et al. (2020)
Laminaria digitata	• LA • ALA • ARA • EPA	• 7.24 • 6.79 • 7.55 • 11.56	Schmid et al. (2016)
Saccharina japonica	• ARA	• 26.93	Susanto et al. (2019)
Palmaria palmata	• EPA	• 41.17	Lopes et al. (2019)
Codium fragile	• LA • ARA • EPA	• 9.21 • 3.41 • 1.48	Pereira et al. (2012)
Cladostephus spongiosus	• LA • ALA • ARA • EPA	• 23.14 • 3.10 • 16.43 • 11.46	Pereira et al. (2012)
Fucus distichus	• LA • ARA • EPA	• 7.70 • 14.70 • 10.90	Khotimchenko et al. (2002)
Porphyra dioica	• LA • ALA • ARA • EPA	• 1.67 • 1.95 • 3.16 • 33.42	Robertson et al. (2015)

pretreatment is required in "the dry method," which is an energy-intensive procedure, making this technique uneconomical in pilot-scale applications. As a result, the wet approach is generally selected to ensure process viability and economy. Wet biomass requires pretreatment to rupture the cell wall, allowing the solvent to reach the lipids. Regardless of the method employed, solvent extraction is used to obtain lipids. Generally, the lipid recovery process can be enhanced in two ways: increasing cell disruption efficiency and minimizing the use of solvents. To date, several cell wall disruption methods have been developed, such as enzymatic treatment, ultrasonication, microwave treatment, bead milling, and pulsed electric field. Among these, enzymatic treatment is considered most gentle with minimal energy requirements (Liang et al., 2012). Owing to the wide variation in cell wall structure and composition, it is vital to select and combine specialized cell wall-degrading enzymes for each species. For example, combining pectinase and papain resulted in a 96.4% ARA-rich lipid recovery from *M. alpina*, which was 1.9 times higher than utilizing Neutrase® protease alone (You et al., 2011). When cellulase and lysozyme were employed jointly, the recovery of EPA-rich lipids from *Nannochloropsis* sp. was greater than with either enzyme alone (Chen et al., 2017). Organic solvent extraction is the most efficient method for extracting microbial PUFAs. It is critical to use food-grade solvents such as hexane, isopropanol, ethanol, butanol, and so on. However, using organic solvents necessitates the creation of explosion-proof workplaces, which raises the expense.

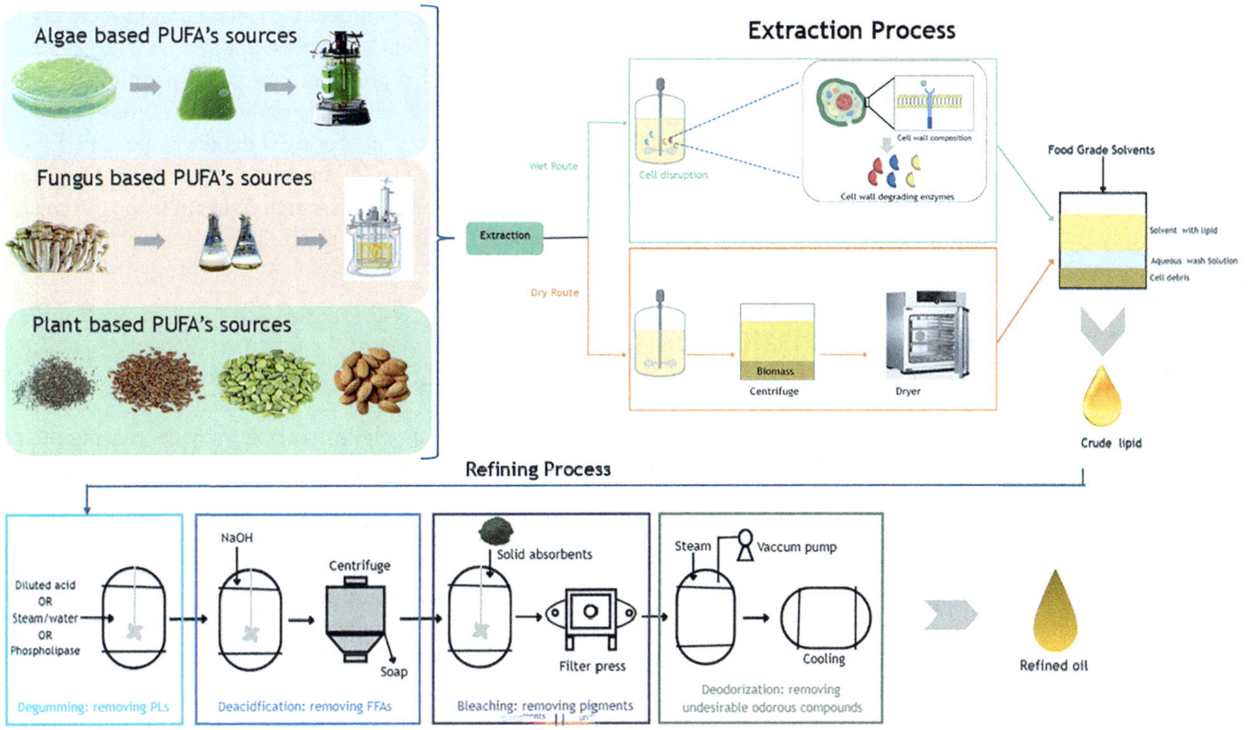

FIGURE 4.2 **Downstream processing for the extraction of** polyunsaturated fatty acids**(PUFAs) from different sources (figure prepared with the help of Biorender software)**. Schematic representation describing different steps in the extraction and purification of PUFAs.

Furthermore, residual solvents can have an impact on the safety of PUFA-containing goods, particularly because some polar solvents are extremely toxic. As a result, numerous unique ways have been developed to remove or significantly minimize the need for organic solvents. Surfactants, which contain both a hydrophobic tail and a hydrophilic head, can interact with cell membranes, causing cell wall disintegration. Surfactants have been found to totally replace polar organic solvents in the extraction of lipids from wet *Nannochloropsis* sp. biomass (Wu et al., 2017). High efficiency of cell wall disruption and high microbial lipid content can enable lipid recovery using a three-phase centrifuge without organic solvents. This simple technology has been successfully used in the industrial extraction of DHA-rich lipids from *Schizochytrium* sp.

4.4.2 Establishing a high-quality lipid-refining process

Lipid-refining operations typically involve multiple operating units, such as degumming, deacidification, bleaching, and deodorization (Fig. 4.2). Water- and acid-based degumming are typically employed to remove hydratable and nonhydratable phospholipids (PLs), respectively. For example, because the majority of PLs in *Chlorella* sp. are nonhydratable, acid-based degumming removed 83% of the PLs, but water-based degumming removed only 19% (Paisan et al., 2017). Traditional degumming cannot ensure residual phosphorus levels of $<10\ mg\ kg^{-1}$, prompting the development of more efficient and environmentally friendly enzymatic degumming.

Phospholipase enzymes can be classified into four major classes based on their hydrolysis sites in PLs: A, B, C, and D, with A/B being acylhydrolases and C/D being phosphodiesterases. Thus the specific enzyme chosen is determined by the makeup of PLs in lipids. Jiang et al. studied the degumming activity of phospholipase A1 and phospholipase C on eight different types of crude lipids. The results revealed that phospholipase A1 was suitable for degumming lipids with a high content of nonhydratable PLs and a low content of starting phosphorus, but phospholipase C provided no evident advantage (Jiang et al., 2015). On an industrial scale, free fatty acids (FFAs) are typically removed using chemical deacidification. In this method, NaOH is used to neutralize the FFAs, and the resultant soap is washed away. However, considerable lipid loss may occur as a result of alkali hydrolysis of triglycerides. Absorption deacidification may be an alternate option because it is simple, safe, and lowers fat loss. When alkali-pretreated microcrystalline cellulose was employed to deacidify microalgal lipids, the acid value was lowered from 25 to 2.5 mg KOH g^{-1}, with a lipid recovery rate of more than 90% (Li et al., 2021). The bleaching process based on solid adsorbents has been applied on a large scale in industry because no solvents and high temperatures are involved. As a result, this procedure requires specific attention in order to retain a high PUFA content while increasing impurity removal. Finally, to eliminate undesired odorous chemicals, high-temperature steam ranging from 180°C to 270°C is utilized on an industrial scale for lipid deodorization, PUFAs are quickly oxidized. PUFA-rich lipids typically have maximum peroxide value (PV) and p-anisidine value (p-AV) limits of 5 and 20 meq kg^{-1}, respectively. Deoxygenated steam may control the PV and p-AV of DHA-rich lipids at 0 and 3.5 meq kg^{-1}, respectively, which is significantly lower than that of nondeoxygenated steam (Yin et al., 2019).

4.5 Health benefits of polyunsaturated fatty acid

4.5.1 Cardiovascular benefits of microalgal polyunsaturated fatty acids

PUFAs derived from microalgae enhance lipid metabolism and reduce circulating cholesterol, thereby decreasing the risk of cardiovascular disorders and stroke Fig. 4.3 (Kutzner et al., 2017). A randomized double-blind trial demonstrated that daily intake of EPA- and DHA-enriched microalgal oil markedly reduced total cholesterol, low-density lipoprotein (LDL), and triglycerides compared with controls (Rao et al., 2020). EPA and DHA modulate lipid homeostasis by decreasing triglycerides and elevating high-density lipoprotein (HDL), while also suppressing platelet aggregation. DHA is more potent than EPA in enhancing vascular function and lowering heart rate and blood pressure (Yamaguchi et al., 2021). Omega-3 fatty acids further inhibit hepatic triglyceride synthesis and reduce circulating very-low-density lipoprotein levels (Koyande et al., 2019). A metaanalysis indicated that *Chlorella* spp. supplementation substantially decreases total cholesterol, reducing cardiovascular risk (Fallah et al., 2018). Clinical studies with DHA-rich microalgal oils have shown greater cardioprotective effects compared with fish oil (Feng et al., 2020). DHA-containing microalgal oil also reduces plasma TAGs and regulates HDL and LDL cholesterol in healthy individuals (Bernstein et al., 2012). Accordingly, the

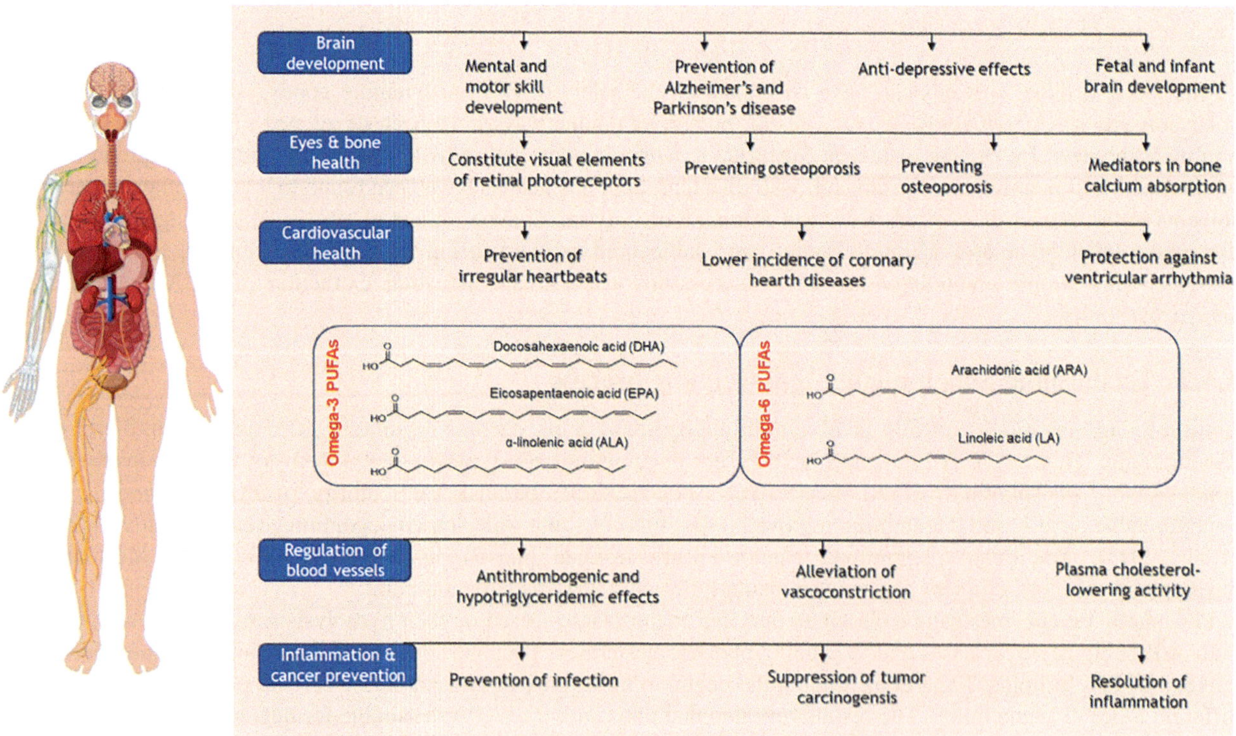

FIGURE 4.3 **Health benefits of polyunsaturated fatty acids (PUFAs) (the figure was prepared with the help of Biorender).** Schematic representation of different health benefits of PUFAs.

European Food Safety Authority advises a daily EPA and DHA intake of 0.2–0.5 g for the general population and 1.0–4.0 g for patients with coronary heart disease to maintain cardiovascular health (Agostoni et al., 2012).

4.5.2 Role of microalgal polyunsaturated fatty acids in diabetes management

Diabetes mellitus is a long-term metabolic disorder characterized by sustained hyperglycemia with disturbances in lipid and protein metabolism (Abutaleb, 2016). Hyperglycemia results from insufficient insulin secretion or reduced tissue responsiveness to insulin (Roglic, 2016). Omega-3 fatty acid supplementation enhances hepatic insulin sensitivity and modulates adipocytokine secretion, thereby mitigating diabetes-related complications (Remize et al., 2021). In murine models, omega-3 intake decreased fasting glucose, improved insulin responsiveness, and reduced pro-inflammatory adipocytokines such as tumor necrosis factor-α, interleukin-6, and plasminogen activator inhibitor-1 (Chacińska et al., 2019). Likewise, zebrafish fed a high-fat diet with microalgal omega-3 showed enhanced glucose tolerance, increased hepatic insulin sensitivity, and reduced adipocytokine production (Ma et al., 2022). Beyond glycaemic control, omega-3 fatty acids promote cardiovascular and metabolic health in diabetic patients by diminishing platelet and leukocyte activity, decreasing blood pressure, inhibiting atherogenesis and thrombosis, and reducing plasma triglycerides, with possible antiarrhythmia effects (McDonald et al., 2013). EPA and DHA supplementation further lowers circulating TAG and cholesterol levels (Zibaeenezhad et al., 2017). Early studies indicated that EPA from *Odontella aurita* reduced metabolic syndrome and diabetes risk in high-fat diet rat models (Haimeur et al., 2012). Moreover, *Chlorella pyrenoidosa* containing GLA attenuated dyslipidaemia and improved insulin-mediated hypoglycemic in streptozotocin-induced diabetic mice (Ramos-Romero et al., 2021).

4.5.3 Antiinflammatory potential of microalgal polyunsaturated fatty acids

The skin acts as the main barrier protecting the body from pathogens and environmental pollutants and is continuously exposed to reactive oxygen species that can initiate inflammatory cascades (Choo et al., 2020). Although inflammation is crucial for defense against infection and tissue injury, dysregulation responses contribute to disease progression (Liu et al., 2023). PUFAs regulate inflammation by influencing catabolic enzymes and mediators, while upregulating proteins such as lipoprotein lipase and fatty-acid-binding proteins that inhibit inflammatory responses (Chacińska et al., 2019). The antiinflammatory capacity of microalgal PUFAs has been shown using extracts from *Phaeodactylum tricornutum*, *Chlorella vulgaris*, *Chlorella ovalis*, *Nannochloropsis oceanica*, *Nannochloropsis oculata*, and *Nannochloropsis granulata*, with EPA playing a pivotal role in regulating the magnitude and duration of inflammation (Tabarzad et al., 2020). EPA is a metabolic precursor of prostaglandin-3, thromboxane-3, and leukotriene-5, which oppose pro-inflammatory eicosanoids and restrain excessive inflammation, thereby promoting immune protection and inflammatory balance Fig. 4.3 (Andrade et al., 2018).

4.5.4 Role of polyunsaturated fatty acid in osteoarthritis management

Osteoarthritis (OA) is a long-term degenerative disorder characterized by metabolic dysregulation in chondrocytes, leading to gradual cartilage breakdown. A key pathological feature is the imbalance between cartilage-degrading matrix metalloproteinases (MMPs) and their natural inhibitors, tissue inhibitors of metalloproteinases (TIMPs). Overactive MMP activity speeds up cartilage breakdown, while inadequate TIMP activity fails to oppose this process. Fatty acids help re-establish this balance by modulating inflammatory mediator synthesis. A 20-carbon fatty acids such as EPA and arachidonic acid (ARA) act as biochemical forerunners of biologically active mediators, including prostaglandins and leukotrienes (Kamolrat & Gray, 2013). Prostaglandins are synthesized by chondrocytes and synoviocytes, whereas leukotrienes derive mainly from inflammatory cells. Although ARA occurs in small amounts, it is crucial for prostaglandin E_2 (PGE_2) production, which controls cartilage metabolism and inflammation. OA is among the most common chronic disorders in the elderly and is acknowledged as a whole-joint disease involving subchondral bone, menisci, ligaments, muscles, capsule, and synovium, not only cartilage (Bocanegra et al., 2009). Its defining feature is gradual cartilage degeneration, resulting in pain, reduced mobility, and joint dysfunction. Clinically, OA is categorized as primary (idiopathic) or secondary, the latter resulting from trauma, inflammation, infection, obesity, deformities, congenital abnormalities, or avascular necrosis (Wall et al., 2010). OA development is affected by obesity, metabolic disorders, joint abnormalities, and genetic predisposition, encouraging growing interest in nutrition and supplementation for prevention and management. Several internally produced and dietary compounds provide clinical relief, slow disease progression, prevent cartilage loss, or stimulate repair (DeFilippis & Sperling, 2006). PUFAs of the n-3, n-6, and n-9 families play important roles in bone and cartilage biology by regulating prostanoid profiles, intercellular signaling, and transcriptional activity (Waldron, 2004). Evidence indicates that fatty acids affect calcium metabolism, where deficiency leads to matrix loss and demineralization, while PUFA supplementation counteracts these effects. Modifying lipid composition in joint tissues may therefore enhance bone strength, prevent osteonecrosis, and improve lubrication (Pritchett, 2007). Additionally, avocado/soybean unsaponifiable derived from lipid extracts stimulates collagen synthesis and exhibits anabolic and antiinflammatory properties, making them potential adjuncts for OA management (Ameye & Chee, 2006).

4.5.5 Role of polyunsaturated fatty acids in obesity regulation

Omega-3 (ω-3) PUFAs safeguard against inflammatory and lipid-related disorders (Cockbain et al., 2012). Chronic inflammation plays a role in diseases such as cancer, diabetes, cardiovascular disease, obesity, neuropsychiatric disorders, and rheumatoid arthritis. Obesity is a multifactorial condition involving an imbalance of the central nervous system (CNS), pancreas, and gastrointestinal tract, and is influenced by genetics, adiposity, and hepatic metabolism. Beyond hypothalamic control of appetite, CNS reward pathways and environmental factors also affect energy balance (Waldron, 2004). Omega-3 fatty acids are beneficial dietary components for obesity prevention and management. Because humans lack omega-3 desaturase enzymes, these PUFAs must be acquired from the diet (Kang et al., 2004). Omega-3 and omega-6 fatty acids exert different, often contrasting, effects on fat accumulation through adipogenesis, lipid homeostasis, brain–adipose signaling, and inflammation. Arachidonic acid (ARA; 20:4 n-6) metabolites stimulate preadipocyte differentiation, whereas omega-3 fatty acids suppress this process at various regulatory levels (Massaro et al., 2006). Omega-6 fatty acids increase triglyceride storage, while omega-3 fatty acids inhibit lipogenic enzymes, decrease fat deposition, and promote β-oxidation in adipose tissue (Ukropec et al., 2003). These fatty acids also selectively regulate adipose signaling and eicosanoid production, thereby governing adipocyte development and tissue expansion. White adipocytes store energy as triglycerides, whereas brown adipocytes expend energy via lipid oxidation. Nutritionally, omega-6 fatty acids are mainly provided as LA from plant seeds and oils such as coconut, cocoa, and palm, while omega-3 fatty acids are chiefly provided as ALA from green leafy plants and seeds including flax, cotton, chia, perilla, and walnuts (Lepperdinger, 2011).

4.5.6 Role of microalgal polyunsaturated fatty acids in autoimmune disorders

Growing accumulating data show that omega-3 PUFAs can alter disease symptoms and treatment-related outcomes in inflammatory and autoimmune disorders, including multiple sclerosis (MS), rheumatoid arthritis, psoriasis, and ulcerative colitis. Autoimmune diseases such as inflammatory bowel disease, MS, asthma, and rheumatoid arthritis respond positively to DHA and EPA through suppression of pro-inflammatory cytokines (Barnett & Prineas, 2004). MS is a chronic demyelinating disease of the CNS in which oligodendrocytes are principle targets. Its disease mechanism involves immunologically driven mechanisms, including activation of T lymphocytes and macrophages (Owens, 2003). Oligodendrocyte apoptosis may occur early, followed by microglial activation and migration of immune cells into lesions (Barnett & Prineas, 2004). Disease progression is associated with excitotoxicity, immune inflammation, and oxidative stress, leading to neuronal and oligodendrocyte damage (Owens, 2003). Altered lipid metabolism is reported in MS patients, with deficiencies of essential PUFAs in erythrocytes and plasma. While LA and GLA may remain normal, subsequent omega-6 fatty acids and omega-3 fatty acids are reduced, indicating defective elongation and desaturation and an adaptive rise in SFAs (Lepperdinger, 2011). Essential fatty acids attenuate experimental autoimmune encephalomyelitis (EAE), an MS model, an effect inhibited by indomethacin, suggesting prostaglandin involvement (Ukropec et al., 2003). Oral GLA- and LA-rich oils mitigate EAE by promoting membrane remodeling, gene transcription, and production of PGE_2 and transforming growth factor-β1 via DGLA and ARA metabolism. Increased PGE_2 shifts cytokine responses from TH1 to TH2, restricting T-cell-mediated autoimmunity (Owens, 2003). Dietary n-6 PUFAs originate mainly from plant seed oils, where LA is elongated and desaturated to GLA, DGLA, and ARA (Massaro et al., 2006). During inflammation, phospholipase A_2 releases ARA, promoting series-2 prostaglandins and thromboxanes, while DGLA forms antiinflammatory series-1 prostaglandins. n-6 PUFAs also affect oligodendrocyte membrane composition and myelin basic protein phosphorylation, a critical step in myelination (Owens, 2003). Clinical supplementation with EPA/DHA in relapsing–remitting MS decreases cytokine and eicosanoid secretion from peripheral mononuclear cells, reinforcing the immunomodulatory role of omega-3 PUFAs in autoimmune disease management (Nkondjock et al., 2003).

4.5.7 Anticancer potential of microalgal polyunsaturated fatty acids

Since the late 1980s omega-3 PUFAs have gained attention for their potential role in cancer prevention and management. Unlike cardiovascular disease, dietary fat composition can influence cancer development at early stages. High saturated fat intake is linked to increased cancer risk, whereas EPA does not promote gastrointestinal malignancies and instead shows protective effects, particularly against colorectal cancer. Long-chain omega-3 PUFAs also suppress prostate tumor growth and exhibit broad anticancer activity as shown in Fig. 4.3 (Augustsson et al., 2003). Lower breast cancer incidence correlates with higher DHA levels in erythrocyte membranes, identifying DHA as a key protective omega-3 PUFA. Oral omega-3 supplementation improves appetite, quality of life, and weight maintenance in cancer patients, while EPA preserves skeletal muscle mass in cancer cachexia (Ryan et al., 2009). Intervention studies show improved chemopreventive outcomes with omega-3 intake, especially DHA. In colorectal cancer, EPA and DHA reduce cell proliferation and promote a balance between apoptosis and growth in colonic tissue. Thus maintaining an appropriate dietary omega-6/omega-3 ratio is important for cancer prevention and therapy (Simopoulos, 2003). Eicosanoids derived from omega-6 fatty acids promote angiogenesis, a process essential for tumor growth and metastasis. Enhanced angiogenesis in solid tumors is associated with poor prognosis and malignant progression. Diets rich in omega-6 fatty acids and total fat correlate with adverse breast cancer outcomes, whereas omega-3 fatty acids inhibit angiogenic signaling (Simopoulos, 2003). Certain fatty acid derivatives also inhibit aromatase, an enzyme involved in hormone-dependent breast cancer progression. Because aromatase is highly regulated in breast tumors, plant sources such as *Brassica campestris* may provide preventive support alongside standard aromatase inhibitor therapies (Fischer & Keller, 2016).

4.6 Market trends and integration of polyunsaturated fatty acid-rich superfoods

As discussed in the previous sections, PUFAs have immense health benefits and contribute to both nutritional and therapeutic requirements. PUFAs are central to the management of several noncommunicable, lifestyle-related disorders. Currently, the global PUFA market, particularly omega-3 fatty acids, is valued at USD 2.1 billion and is projected to reach USD 4.26 billion by 2034, estimated to grow annually at 8.3% (https://www.fortunebusinessinsights.com/industry-reports/omega-3-fatty-acids-market-100248). In another report, the global PUFA market was estimated at USD 6.6 billion and projected to reach USD 11.4 billion by 2035 at a compounded annual growth rate of 5.5%. The Asia Pacific region, followed by North America, registered the highest growth in terms of PUFA demand (Nandoskar et al., 2026). The increasing demand for PUFAs comes from several market segments such as dietary supplements, infant nutrition, pharmaceuticals, pet food, and animal feed. Traditionally, fish oils have led the market, accounting for the major proportion of PUFA sales worldwide, owing to their economic affordability, well-developed supply chains, and high concentrations of EPA and DHA. Fish oil capsules, gelatin capsules, and medical-grade concentrates are widely commercialized for lowering triglycerides, decreasing blood pressure, and enhancing endothelial function, with medical studies supporting their role in heart disease prevention. However, environmental concerns such as excessive fishing, ocean resources decline, and pollution hazards (e.g., heavy metals and long-lasting toxics) have encouraged a transition toward substitute sources (Saini et al., 2021). This necessitates the identification of alternative sources. Plant and microbial-derived PUFAs have found significant market owing to the increased consumer demand for plant-based raw materials, sustainable sourcing, and clean labeled ingredients.

4.6.1 Market integration of polyunsaturated fatty acid products

From a market perspective, fish oils continue to dominate due to affordability and consumer familiarity, but algal oils are increasingly positioned as premium products, particularly in Western markets where plant-based diets are gaining traction. Macroalgae remain a smaller segment but are projected to grow steadily as functional food innovation accelerates, while fungal oils are expected to expand in medical nutrition niches. A list of commercially available PUFA products is presented in Table 4.5.

The first and foremost step in the market integration is the identification of sustainable sources of PUFA. Microbial fermentation and microalgal systems offer a sustainable alternative to conventional marine-derived PUFA. For example, heterotrophic production of DHA from *Schizochytrium* spp., photobioreactor-based production of EPA from *Nannochloropsis*, fermentation-derived production of ARA from *Mucor* spp. and *Morieterella* spp., and seed oil-derived ALA from flax, chia, and perilla offer sustainable and economically viable platforms for essential LC-PUFAs production (Nandoskar et al., 2026). The next important step in market integration is the development of valueadded processes and improvement of the stability of PUFAs. PUFAs are highly susceptible to oxidation owing to the presence of multiple double bonds. Further, they are sensitive to factors such as storage temperature, continuous exposure to light, leading to

TABLE 4.5 Commercially available polyunsaturated fatty acid (PUFA) products.

PUFA	Primary source	Commercial products	Key applications	References
Eicosapentanoic acid (EPA)	*Nannochloropsis oculata*	Almega®PL capsule	Improves atherogenic dyslipidemia by decreasing triglycerides and VLDL cholesterol, which leads to a decrease in the risk of cardiovascular disease	Rao et al. (2020)
Omega fatty acid	*Chlorella sp.*	Algae oil	Alternative omega fatty acid for food supplements	Preechaphonkul et al. (2024)
EPA and docosahexanoic acid (DHA)	*Marine microalgae, Staurosira sp.*	ReNew™ (omega-3 rich oils) human and animal food, whole algae enriched with EPA and DHA (as animal feed)	Improved brain and heart health, having antiinflammatory activity, and support the immunity	http://cellana.com/
DHA	*Schizochytrium sp.*	All-G-Rich™ dehydrated whole algae for poultry nutrition, rich in DHA, biofuels	Support immunity and metabolism, improve brain and heart health, improve bone health, and aging.	https://www.alltech.com/
DHA	*Chlorella sp.*	Golden chlorella, AlgaVia (algal powder, food ingredient line recognized as GRAS), AlgaWise (food oils), AlgaPrime DHA (aquaculture)	Lower the cholesterol having antihyperlipidemic activities	https://www.solazyme.com/
DHA	*Schizochytrium sp.*	DHA gold (oil)	Reduce triglycerides in the blood and decrease thrombosis, prevents cardiac arrhythmias	Ratledge (2004)
PUFA	*Crypthecodinium cohnii*	Life'sDHA® B54–0100 capsule	Improve heart and brain health, improve the infant's cognitive development.	https://www.dsm.com/corporate/home.html
DHA	*Schizochytrium sp.*			
DHA	*Crypthecodinium cohnii, chlorella sp*	DHA3Sure™ DHA algae 35% oil complex, soft gel capsule	Improve the brain, heart health, boost immunity, and improve eye health.	https://gcinutrients.com/
DHA	*Ulkenia sp.*	DHActiveTM oli	Lower triglyceride levels, reduce blood pressure, improve cholesterol levels, and also improve gut health	Ratledge (2004)

Arachidonic acid	*Mortierella alpina.*	ARASCO® oil in infant formula	Reduce hyperglycemia, restore insulin sensitivity, and suppress inflammation	https://www.canada.ca/en/health-canada/services/food-nutrition/genetically-modified-foods-other-novel-foods/approved-products/novel-food-information-dhasco-arasco-sources-docosahexaenoic-acid-arachidonic-acid-infant-formulas.html
EPA	*Ondetolla aurita Nanochloropsissp.*	Alage powder	Improve cardiovascular health, antiinflammatory effects, and overall cellular vitality.	Robertson et al. (2013)
EPA and DHA	*Euphausia Superba*	Superba Krill® oil	Supporting heart health (lowers triglycerides), reducing inflammation and oxidative stress, improving joint mobility, boosting brain function, aiding liver health, and enhancing skin vitality	https://www.superbakrill.com/krill-oil/what-is-krill-oil?__hstc=146130155.39388ee1e9a0489521dbc90aab68c2c2.1769001027247.1769001027247.1769001027247.1&__hssc=146130155.1.1769001027247&__hsfp=6d4667f5d03e2de193187e82df148d2d
VLC-PUFA	Fish	EPAX® Evolve 05 oil	Improve vision, retinal function, skin health, bone density, muscle strength, and male fertility	https://www.stauberusa.com/next-level-omega-3s-epax-evolve-05-makes-waves-at-vitafoods-europe-2025/
EPA and DHA	*Gadus morhua*	Seven sea cod oil capsules	Omega-3s (EPA/DHA), Vitamin A, and Vitamin D, supporting heart health, brain function (learning, memory), joint flexibility, stronger bones (via Vitamin D and calcium absorption), vision, immune function, and skin health, helping fill nutritional gaps and potentially easing inflammation and fatigue.	https://www.seven-seas.com/en_IN/home/product-finder.html

oxidative rancidity and develop off-flavors (Wang et al., 2020). This necessitates the development of stabilization techniques for enhanced shelf life and incorporation into food matrices. Stabilization techniques such as microencapsulation, formation of nanoemulsions, PUFA delivery through liposomes, and spray drying are a few techniques that can be employed for enhancing the shelf life of LC-PUFAs (Islam et al., 2023). Stabilized PUFAs can be incorporated in a variety of food matrices such as beverages, bakery products, snacks, and dairy products. Further advanced processing techniques, termed as "green technologies" such as enzymatic oil recovery, supercritical CO_2 fluid extraction, and membrane purification, enable efficient recovery of PUFAs, preserving the structure and integrity, offering clean label solutions (Marsol-Vall et al., 2022).

In addition to sustainable processing, successful market integration requires a reliable supply chain and agronomic practices for the production of PUFAs, especially for plant resources. Utilization of agri-residues and agri-side streams such as food processing waste, molasses, lignocellulose residues, and fruit pomace as substrate for microbial PUFA production significantly reduces the cost of production and increases the economic viability (Kothri et al., 2020). Further, establishing regulatory and quality frameworks compliant with food safety and labeling requirements of different regulatory agencies is essential for successful market integration. Standardization of parameters such as fatty acid composition, reducing batch variations, and quality parameters such as PV, anisidine value, and total oxidation index are important for market penetration (Bannenberg et al., 2020). Lastly, effective consumer awareness programs and market positioning of PUFA products with clear label claims enable successful market penetration and integration. Branding of PUFA-rich functional foods and superfoods must be backed with scientific evidence of effective market acceptance.

4.7 Conclusion and future perspectives

The future of the PUFA industry lies in two main aspects: affordability and sustainability. Although fish oil-derived PUFAs are cost-effective, the increasing preference for clean labeled, contaminant-free, eco-friendly PUFAs has necessitated the development of alternative PUFA production systems such as fungi and microalgae. Advances in gene editing/genetic engineering technologies have enabled enhanced yield and productivity of algal and fungal PUFAs. Further innovation in fermentation strategies and novel bioreactor technologies enables sustainable PUFA production at economically competitive prices. To meet the growing demand for dietary LC-PUFAs, novel PUFA resources must be identified and characterized. Science-backed product development coupled with compliance to regulatory and quality frameworks is essential for successful market penetration of novel PUFA sources and products. Development of low-cost production processes, use of agri-byproducts as substrates for microbial PUFA production, green extraction and downstream processing technologies such as supercritical fluid extraction, enzyme-based purification, and membrane filtration-based enrichment processes would pave the way for eco-friendly, contaminant-free PUFA products as per market requirements. In conclusion, the PUFA market is a dynamic and rapidly growing sector, underpinned by strong scientific evidence of health benefits and diverse commercial applications.

Funding acknowledgement

The authors thank CSIR-Institute of Himalayan Bioresource Technology (IHBT) for funding from MLP-0204 project. Neha Yograj acknowledges senior research fellowship funding from CSIR No.31/0054(26555)/2026-EMR-I.

Authors contribution: conceptualization

Vidyashankar Srivatsan **manuscript drafting**: Prajwal Jakhmola, Karan Saini, Yograj Neha, Vidyashankar Srivatsan; **data compilation and graphics**: Prajwal Jakhmola, Karan Saini; Yograj Neha **manuscript reviewing:** Vidyashankar Srivatsan; **funding:** Vidyashankar Srivatsan.

References

Abutaleb, M. H. (2016). Diabetes mellitus: An overview. *Pharmacy & Pharmacology International Journal, 4*(5), 406–411.

Adarme-Vega, T. C., Lim, D. K., Timmins, M., Vernen, F., Li, Y., & Schenk, P. M. (2012). Microalgal biofactories: A promising approach towards sustainable omega-3 fatty acid production. *Microbial Cell Factories, 11*(1), 96.

Agostoni, C., Bresson, J. L., Fairweather Tait, S., Flynn, A., Golly, I., Korhonen, H., & Verhagen, H. (2012). Scientific opinion on the tolerable upper intake level of eicosapentaenoic acid (EPA), docosahexaenoic acid (DHA) and docosapentaenoic acid (DPA): EFSA panel on dietetic products, nutrition and allergies (NDA). *EFSA Journal, 10*(7), 1–48.

Aguillón-Páez, Y. J., Romero, L. A., & Diaz, G. J. (2020). Effect of full-fat sunflower or flaxseed seeds dietary inclusion on performance, egg yolk fatty acid profile and egg quality in laying hens. *Animal Nutrition, 6*(2), 179–184.

Alakhras, R., Bellou, S., Fotaki, G., Stephanou, G., Demopoulos, N. A., Papanikolaou, S., & Aggelis, G. (2015). Fatty acid lithium salts from Cunninghamella echinulata have cytotoxic and genotoxic effects on HL-60 human leukemia cells. *Engineering in Life Sciences, 15*(2), 243–253.

Alleway, H. K. (2023). Climate benefits of seaweed farming. *Nature Sustainability, 6*(4), 356–357.

Ameye, L. G., & Chee, W. S. (2006). Osteoarthritis and nutrition. From nutraceuticals to functional foods: A systematic review of the scientific evidence. *Arthritis Research & Therapy, 8*(4), R127 (52).

Ananthi, V., Pugazhendhi, A., & Arun, A. (2021). Efficacy of chemical factors on production and extraction of biodiesel by microalgae. *International Journal of Energy Research, 45*(12), 17080–17093.

Andrade, L. M., Andrade, C. J., Dias, M., Nascimento, C., & Mendes, M. A. (2018). Chlorella and spirulina microalgae as sources of functional foods. *Nutraceuticals, and Food Supplements, 6*(1), 45–58.

Augustsson, K., Michaud, D. S., Rimm, E. B., Leitzmann, M. F., Stampfer, M. J., Willett, W. C., & Giovannucci, E. (2003). A prospective study of intake of fish and marine fatty acids and prostate cancer. *Cancer Epidemiology Biomarkers & Prevention, 12*(1), 64–67 (63).

Azri, A., Debouba, M., Bouajila, J., Yeshitila, M., Cerny, M., Lacroux, E., & Merah, O. (2025). Lipids composition, Fatty Acid and Squalene contents in a wide Amaranth collection. *Journal of Food Composition and Analysis,* 108305.

Baba, M., & Shiraiwa, Y. (2013). *Biosynthesis of lipids and hydrocarbons in algae*. Intech, 978 953.

Bannenberg, G., Rice, H. B., Bernasconi, A., Ferrari, A., Mallon, C., Navarrete, L., ... Ismail, A. (2020). Ingredient label claim compliance and oxidative quality of EPA/DHA omega-3 retail products in the US. *Journal of Food Composition and Analysis, 88*, 103435.

Barnett, M. H., & Prineas, J. W. (2004). Relapsing and remitting multiple sclerosis: Pathology of the newly forming lesion. *Annals of Neurology, 55*(4), 458–468 (60).

Barta, D. G., Coman, V., & Vodnar, D. C. (2021). Microalgae as sources of omega-3 polyunsaturated fatty acids: Biotechnological aspects. *Algal Research, 58*, 102410.

Bellou, S., Makri, A., Sarris, D., Michos, K., Rentoumi, P., Celik, A., & Aggelis, G. (2014). The olive mill wastewater as substrate for single cell oil production by Zygomycetes. *Journal of Biotechnology, 170*, 50–59.

Bellou, S., Moustogianni, A., Makri, A., & Aggelis, G. (2012). Lipids containing polyunsaturated fatty acids synthesized by Zygomycetes grown on glycerol. *Applied Biochemistry and Biotechnology, 166*(1), 146–158.

Benzie, I. F., & Wachtel-Galor, S. (Eds.). (2011). Herbal medicine: Biomolecular and clinical aspects.

Bernstein, A. M., Ding, E. L., Willett, W. C., & Rimm, E. B. (2012). A meta-analysis shows that docosahexaenoic acid from algal oil reduces serum triglycerides and increases HDL-cholesterol and LDL-cholesterol in persons without coronary heart disease3. The. *Journal of Nutrition, 142*(1), 99–104.

Bilbao, P. S., Salvador, G. A., & Leonardi, P. I. (2017). Fatty acids from microalgae: Targeting the accumulation of triacylglycerides. *Fatty Acids, 119*.

Biris-Dorhoi, E. S., Michiu, D., Pop, C. R., Rotar, A. M., Tofana, M., Pop, O. L., & Farcas, A. C. (2020). Macroalgae—A sustainable source of chemical compounds with biological activities. *Nutrients, 12*(10), 3085.

Bocanegra, A., Bastida, S., Benedi, J., Rodenas, S., & Sanchez-Muniz, F. J. (2009). Characteristics and nutritional and cardiovascular-health properties of seaweeds. *Journal of Medicinal Food, 12*(2), 236–258 (47).

Cardoso, C., Afonso, C., & Bandarra, N. M. (2016). Dietary DHA and health: Cognitive function ageing. *Nutrition Research Reviews, 29*(2), 281–294.

Cardoso, C., Ripol, A., Afonso, C., Freire, M., Varela, J., Quental-Ferreira, H., & Bandarra, N. (2017). Fatty acid profiles of the main lipid classes of green seaweeds from fish pond aquaculture. *Food Science & Nutrition, 5*(6), 1186–1194.

Carlini, G. C. G., Roschel, G. G., Ferrari, R. A., Alencar, S. M., Ota, H. C., da Silveira, T. F. F., & Castro, I. A. (2021). Chemical characterization of *Echium plantagineum* seed oil obtained by three methods of extraction. *Journal of Food Science, 86*(12), 5307–5317.

Castillo, T., Ramos, D., García-Beltrán, T., Brito-Bazan, M., & Galindo, E. (2021). Mixotrophic cultivation of microalgae: An alternative to produce high-value metabolites. *Biochemical Engineering Journal, 176*, 108183.

Cesconetto-Bisinotto, M., Chedid, L. D., Gouveia, A. D. S., Ramos, H. J. D. O., Garcia-Moreno, P. J., & Castro, I. A. (2025). Oxidative stability of echium crude oil during the cold-press extraction process. *Italian Journal of Food Science/Rivista Italiana di Scienza degli Alimenti, 37*(2).

Chacińska, M., Zabielski, P., Książek, M., Szałaj, P., Jarząbek, K., Kojta, I., & Błachnio-Zabielska, A. U. (2019). The impact of OMEGA-3 fatty acids supplementation on insulin resistance and content of adipocytokines and biologically active lipids in adipose tissue of high-fat diet fed rats. *Nutrients, 11*(4), 835.

Chauhan, A. S., Patel, A. K., Chen, C. W., Chang, J. S., Michaud, P., Dong, C. D., & Singhania, R. R. (2023). Enhanced production of high-value polyunsaturated fatty acids (PUFAs) from potential thraustochytrid *Aurantiochytrium* sp. *Bioresource Technology, 370*, 128536.

Chen, C. Y., Chen, Y. C., Huang, H. C., Huang, C. C., Lee, W. L., & Chang, J. S. (2013). Engineering strategies for enhancing the production of eicosapentaenoic acid (EPA) from an isolated microalga *Nannochloropsis oceanica* CY2. *Bioresource Technology, 147*, 160–167.

Chen, Q. T., et al. (2017). Influence of a facile pretreatment process on lipid extraction from *Nannochloropsis* sp. through an enzymatic hydrolysis reaction. *RSC Advances, 7*, 53270.

Chi, G., et al. (2022). Production of polyunsaturated fatty acids by *Schizochytrium (Aurantiochytrium)* spp. *Biotechnology Advances, 55*, 107897.

Chirinos, R., Zuloeta, G., Pedreschi, R., Mignolet, E., Larondelle, Y., & Campos, D. (2013). Sacha inchi (*Plukenetia volubilis*): A seed source of polyunsaturated fatty acids, tocopherols, phytosterols, phenolic compounds and antioxidant capacity. *Food Chemistry, 141*(3), 1732–1739.

Choo, W. T., Teoh, M. L., Phang, S. M., Convey, P., Yap, W. H., Goh, B. H., & Beardall, J. (2020). Microalgae as potential anti-inflammatory natural product against human inflammatory skin diseases. *Frontiers in Pharmacology, 11*, 1086.

Ciftci, O. N., Przybylski, R., & Rudzińska, M. (2012). Lipid components of flax, perilla, and chia seeds. *European Journal of Lipid Science and Technology, 114*, 794–800.

Cockbain, A. J., Toogood, G. J., & Hull, M. A. (2012). Omega-3 polyunsaturated fatty acids for the treatment and prevention of colorectal cancer. *Gut, 61*(1), 135–149 (53).

Cook, O., & Hildebrand, M. (2016). Enhancing LC-PUFA production in *Thalassiosira pseudonana* by overexpressing the endogenous fatty acid elongase genes. *Journal of Applied Phycology, 28*(2), 897–905.

Cupo, A., Landi, S., Morra, S., Nuzzo, G., Gallo, C., Manzo, E., & d'Ippolito, G. (2021). Autotrophic vs. heterotrophic cultivation of the marine diatom *Cyclotella cryptica* for EPA production. *Marine Drugs, 19*(7), 355.

de Jesús-Campos, D., López-Elías, J. A., Medina-Juarez, L.Á., Carvallo-Ruiz, G., Fimbres-Olivarria, D., & Hayano-Kanashiro, C. (2020). Chemical composition, fatty acid profile and molecular changes derived from nitrogen stress in the diatom *Chaetoceros muelleri*. *Aquaculture Reports, 16*, 100281.

DeFilippis, A. P., & Sperling, L. S. (2006). Understanding omega-3's. *American Heart Journal, 151*(3), 564–570 (49).

Fahs, C. A., Yan, H., Ranadive, S., Rossow, L. M., Agiovlasitis, S., Wilund, K. R., & Fernhall, B. (2010). The effect of acute fish-oil supplementation on endothelial function and arterial stiffness following a high-fat meal. *Applied Physiology, Nutrition, and Metabolism, 35*(3), 294–302.

Fakas, S., Papanikolaou, S., Galiotou-Panayotou, M., Komaitis, M., & Aggelis, G. (2008). Organic nitrogen of tomato waste hydrolysate enhances glucose uptake and lipid accumulation in *Cunninghamella echinulata*. *Journal of Applied Microbiology, 105*(4), 1062–1070.

Fallah, A. A., Sarmast, E., Dehkordi, S. H., Engardeh, J., Mahmoodnia, L., Khaledifar, A., & Jafari, T. (2018). Effect of *Chlorella* supplementation on cardiovascular risk factors: A meta-analysis of randomized controlled trials. *Clinical Nutrition, 37*(6), 1892–1901.

Fazili, A. B. A., Shah, A. M., Zan, X., Naz, T., Nosheen, S., Nazir, Y., & Song, Y. (2022). Mucor circinelloides: A model organism for oleaginous fungi and its potential applications in bioactive lipid production. *Microbial Cell Factories, 21*(1), 29.

Feng, J., Long, S., Zhang, H. J., Wu, S. G., Qi, G. H., & Wang, J. (2020). Comparative effects of dietary microalgae oil and fish oil on fatty acid composition and sensory quality of table eggs. *Poultry Science, 99*(3), 1734–1743.

Fischer, G. J., & Keller, N. P. (2016). Production of cross-kingdom oxylipins by pathogenic fungi: An update on their role in development and pathogenicity. *Journal of Microbiology, 54*(3), 254–264 (68).

Fujita, T., Kawashima, H., Sakuradani, E., Sakamoto, T., Ando, A., Ogawa, J., & Shimizu, S. (2016). Essential fatty acids for oleaginous fungus *Mortierella alpina*. *Biocatalysis and Agricultural Biotechnology, 8*, 167–170.

Gema, H., Kavadia, A., Dimou, D., Tsagou, V., Komaitis, M., & Aggelis, G. (2002). Production of γ-linolenic acid by *Cunninghamella echinulata* cultivated on glucose and orange peel. *Applied Microbiology and Biotechnology, 58*(3), 303–307.

Guan, L., Zhu, L., Zhang, X., Han, Y., Wang, K., Ji, N., & Lu, S. (2024). Perilla seed oil and protein: Composition, health benefits, and potential applications in functional foods. *Molecules (Basel, Switzerland), 29*(22), 5258.

Gupta, S., Hegde, A. S., Das, S., Joshi, R., & Srivatsan, V. (2024). Bioactive Compounds from Wild Edible Plants of Western Himalayas: Nutritional Profile, UHPLC-QTOF-IMS-Based Phytochemical Characterization, and Their In Vitro Gastrointestinal Digestibility. *ACS Food Science & Technology, 4*(11), 2707–2723.

Haimeur, A., Ulmann, L., Mimouni, V., Guéno, F., Pineau-Vincent, F., Meskini, N., & Tremblin, G. (2012). The role of *Odontella aurita*, a marine diatom rich in EPA, as a dietary supplement in dyslipidemia, platelet function and oxidative stress in high-fat fed rats. *Lipids in Health and Disease, 11*(1), 147.

Hamilton, M. L., Haslam, R. P., Napier, J. A., & Sayanova, O. (2014). Metabolic engineering of *Phaeodactylum tricornutum* for the enhanced accumulation of omega-3 long chain polyunsaturated fatty acids. *Metabolic Engineering, 22*, 3–9.

Islam, F., Imran, A., Nosheen, F., Fatima, M., Arshad, M. U., Afzaal, M., ... Amer Ali, Y. (2023). Functional roles and novel tools for improving-oxidative stability of polyunsaturated fatty acids: A comprehensive review. *Food Science & Nutrition, 11*(6), 2471–2482.

Jain, P., Minhas, A. K., Shukla, S., Puri, M., Barrow, C. J., & Mandal, S. (2022). Bioprospecting indigenous marine microalgae for polyunsaturated fatty acids under different media conditions. *Frontiers in Bioengineering and Biotechnology, 10*, 842797.

James, G. O., Hocart, C. H., Hillier, W., Chen, H., Kordbacheh, F., Price, G. D., & Djordjevic, M. A. (2011). Fatty acid profiling of *Chlamydomonas reinhardtii* under nitrogen deprivation. *Bioresource Technology, 102*(3), 3343–3351.

Ji, X. J., Zhang, A. H., Nie, Z. K., Wu, W. J., Ren, L. J., & Huang, H. (2014). Efficient arachidonic acid-rich oil production by *Mortierella alpina* through a repeated fed-batch fermentation strategy. *Bioresource Technology, 170*, 356–360.

Jiang, X. F., et al. (2015). Application of phospholipase A1 and phospholipase C in the degumming process of different kinds of crude oils. *Process Biochemistry, 50*, 432–437.

Jiao, K., Xiao, W., Xu, Y., Zeng, X., Ho, S. H., Laws, E. A., ... Lin, L. (2018). Using a trait-based approach to optimize mixotrophic growth of the red microalga Porphyridium purpureum towards fatty acid production. *Biotechnology for Biofuels, 11*(1), 273.

Jovanovic, S., Dietrich, D., Becker, J., Kohlstedt, M., & Wittmann, C. (2021). Microbial production of polyunsaturated fatty acids—High-value ingredients for aquafeed, superfoods, and pharmaceuticals. *Current Opinion in Biotechnology, 69*, 199–211.

Kamolrat, T., & Gray, S. R. (2013). The effect of eicosapentaenoic and docosahexaenoic acid on protein synthesis and breakdown in murine C2C12 myotubes. *Biochemical and Biophysical Research Communications, 432*(4), 593–598 (45).

Kang, K., Miyazaki, M., Ntambi, J. M., & Pariza, M. W. (2004). Evidence that the anti-obesity effect of conjugated linoleic acid is independent of effects on stearoyl-CoA desaturase1 expression and enzyme activity. *Biochemical and Biophysical Research Communications, 315*(3), 532–537 (55).

Katiyar, R., & Arora, A. (2020). Health promoting functional lipids from microalgae pool: A review. *Algal Research, 46*, 101800.

Katiyar, R., Bharti, R. K., Gurjar, B. R., Kumar, A., Biswas, S., & Pruthi, V. (2018). Utilization of de-oiled algal biomass for enhancing vehicular quality biodiesel production from Chlorella sp. in mixotrophic cultivation systems. *Renewable Energy, 122*, 80–88.

Khotimchenko, S. V., Vaskovsky, V. E., & Titlyanova, T. V. (2002). Fatty acids of marine algae from the Pacific coast of North California. *Botanica Marina, 45*(1), 17–22.

Kothri, M., Mavrommati, M., Elazzazy, A. M., Baeshen, M. N., Moussa, T. A., & Aggelis, G. (2020). Microbial sources of polyunsaturated fatty acids (PUFAs) and the prospect of organic residues and wastes as growth media for PUFA-producing microorganisms. *FEMS Microbiology Letters, 367*(5), fnaa028.

Khozin-Goldberg, I. (2016). Lipid metabolism in microalgae. In *The physiology of microalgae*. Cham: Springer International Publishing, 413–484.

Kikukawa, H., Sakuradani, E., Ando, A., Shimizu, S., & Ogawa, J. (2018). Arachidonic acid production by the oleaginous fungus *Mortierella alpina* 1S-4: A review. *Journal of Advanced Research, 11*, 15–22.

Kim, S. H., Sunwoo, I. Y., Hong, H. J., Awah, C. C., Jeong, G. T., & Kim, S. K. (2019). Lipid and unsaturated fatty acid productions from three microalgae using nitrate and light-emitting diodes with complementary LED wavelength in a two-phase culture system. *Bioprocess and Biosystems Engineering, 42*(9), 1517–1526.

Klempova, T., Basil, E., Kubatova, A., & Certik, M. (2013). Biosynthesis of gamma-linolenic acid and beta-carotene by Zygomycetes fungi. *Biotechnology Journal, 8*(7), 794–800.

Koyande, A. K., Chew, K. W., Rambabu, K., Tao, Y., Chu, D. T., & Show, P. L. (2019). Microalgae: A potential alternative to health supplementation for humans. *Food Science and Human Wellness, 8*(1), 16–24.

Kumari, P., Kumar, M., Gupta, V., Reddy, C. R. K., & Jha, B. (2010). Tropical marine macroalgae as potential sources of nutritionally important PUFAs. *Food Chemistry, 120*(3), 749–757.

Kutzner, L., Ostermann, A. I., Konrad, T., Riegel, D., Hellhake, S., Schuchardt, J. P., & Schebb, N. H. (2017). Lipid class specific quantitative analysis of n-3 polyunsaturated fatty acids in food supplements. *Journal of Agricultural and Food Chemistry, 65*(1), 139–147.

Lang, I., Hodac, L., Friedl, T., & Feussner, I. (2011). Fatty acid profiles and their distribution patterns in microalgae: A comprehensive analysis of more than 2000 strains from the SAG culture collection. *BMC Plant Biology, 11*(1), 124.

Lee, J. M., Lee, H., Kang, S., & Park, W. J. (2016). Fatty acid desaturases, polyunsaturated fatty acid regulation, and biotechnological advances. *Nutrients, 8*(1), 23.

Lepperdinger, G. (2011). Inflammation and mesenchymal stem cell aging. *Current Opinion in Immunology, 23*(4), 518–524 (59).

Li, M., et al. (2011). Isolation of a novel C18-Δ9 polyunsaturated fatty acid specifc elongase gene from DHA-producing Isochrysis galbana H29 and its use for the reconstitution of the alternative Δ8 pathway in *Saccharomyces cerevisiae. Biotechnology Letters, 33*(9), 1823–1830.

Li, Q. J., et al. (2021). Deacidification of microalgal oil with alka line microcrystalline cellulose. *Applied Biochemistry and Biotechnology, 193*, 952–964.

Liang, K. H., et al. (2012). Enzyme-assisted aqueous extrac tion of lipid from microalgae. *Journal of Agricultural and Food Chemistry, 60*, 11771–11776.

Lim, J. M., Vikramathithan, J., Hwangbo, K., Ahn, J. W., Park, Y. I., Choi, D. W., & Jeong, W. J. (2015). Threonine 286 of fatty acid desaturase 7 is essential for ω-3 fatty acid desaturation in the green microalga *Chlamydomonas reinhardtii. Frontiers in Microbiology, 6*, 66.

Lin, Z., & Qu, X. (2022). Emerging diversity in polyketide synthase. *Tetrahedron Letters, 110*, 154183.

Lippmeier, J. C., et al. (2009). Characterization of both polyunsaturated fatty acid biosynthetic pathways in *Schizochytrium* sp. *Lipids, 44*(7), 621–630.

Liu, S., Hur, Y. H., Cai, X., Cong, Q., Yang, Y., Xu, C., & Fuchs, E. (2023). A tissue injury sensing and repair pathway distinct from host pathogen defense. *Cell, 186*(10), 2127–2143.

Lopes, D., Melo, T., Rey, F., Meneses, J., Monteiro, F. L., Helguero, L. A., Abreu, M. H., Lillebø, A. I., Calado, R., & Domingues, M. R. (2020). Valuing bioactive lipids from green, red and brown macroalgae from aquaculture, to foster functionality and biotechnological applications. *Molecules (Basel, Switzerland), 25*(17), 3883.

López, G., Yate, C., Ramos, F. A., Cala, M. P., Restrepo, S., & Baena, S. (2019). Production of polyunsaturated fatty acids and lipids from autotrophic, mixotrophic and heterotrophic cultivation of *Galdieria* sp. strain USBA-GBX-832. *Scientific Reports, 9*(1), 10791.

Lopes, D., Melo, T., Meneses, J., Abreu, M. H., Pereira, R., Domingues, P., ... Domingues, M. R. (2019). A new look for the red macroalga Palmaria palmata: A seafood with polar lipids rich in EPA and with antioxidant properties. *Marine Drugs, 17*(9), 533.

Ma, K., Chen, S., Wu, Y., Ma, Y., Qiao, H., Fan, J., & Wu, H. (2022). Dietary supplementation with microalgae enhances the zebrafish growth performance by modulating immune status and gut microbiota. *Applied Microbiology and Biotechnology, 106*(2), 773–788.

Maier, T. (2017). Re-engineering biofactories. *Nature Chemical Biology, 13*(4), 344–345.

Makri, A., Bellou, S., Birkou, M., Papatrehas, K., Dolapsakis, N. P., Bokas, D., & Aggelis, G. (2011). Lipid synthesized by micro-algae grown in laboratory-and industrial-scale bioreactors. *Engineering in Life Sciences, 11*(1), 52–58.

Mandalka, A., Cavalcanti, M. I. L. G., Harb, T. B., Toyota Fujii, M., Eisner, P., Schweiggert-Weisz, U., & Chow, F. (2022). Nutritional composition of beach-cast marine algae from the Brazilian coast: Added value for algal biomass considered as waste. *Foods, 11*(9), 1201.

Marella, T. K., Bhattacharjya, R., & Tiwari, A. (2021). Impact of organic carbon acquisition on growth and functional biomolecule production in diatoms. *Microbial Cell Factories, 20*(1), 135.

Marsol-Vall, A., Aitta, E., Guo, Z., & Yang, B. (2022). Green technologies for production of oils rich in n-3 polyunsaturated fatty acids from aquatic sources. *Critical Reviews in Food Science and Nutrition, 62*(11), 2942–2962.

Martínez-Córdova, L. R., Martínez-Porchas, M., Emerenciano, M. G. C., Miranda-Baeza, A., & Gollas-Galván, T. (2017). From microbes to fish the next revolution in food production. *Critical Reviews in Biotechnology, 37*(3), 287–295.

Massaro, M., Habib, A., Lubrano, L., Turco, S. D., Lazzerini, G., Bourcier, T., & De Caterina, R. (2006). The omega-3 fatty acid docosahexaenoate attenuates endothelial cyclooxygenase-2 induction through both NADP (H) oxidase and PKCε inhibition. *Proceedings of the National Academy of Sciences, 103*(41), 15184–15189 (57).

McDonald, D. M., O'Kane, F., McConville, M., Devine, A. B., & McVeigh, G. E. (2013). Platelet redox balance in diabetic patients with hypertension improved by n-3 fatty acids. *Diabetes Care, 36*(4), 998–1005.

Melo, D., Machado, T. B., & Oliveira, M. B. P. P. (2019). Chia seeds: An ancient grain trending in modern human diets. *Food Function, 10*, 3068–3089.

Menegol, T., Romero-Villegas, G. I., López-Rodríguez, M., Navarro-López, E., López-Rosales, L., Chisti, Y., & Molina-Grima, E. (2019). Mixotrophic production of polyunsaturated fatty acids and carotenoids by the microalga *Nannochloropsis gaditana*. *Journal of Applied Phycology, 31*(5), 2823–2832.

Miquel, M. I. R. (2008). Echium oil: A valuable source of n-3 and n-6 fatty acids. *Oléagineux, Corps Gras, Lipides, 15*(4), 252–256.

Mobin, S., & Alam, F. (2017). Some promising microalgal species for commercial applications: A review. *Energy Procedia, 110*, 510–517.

Morales-Sánchez, D., Martinez-Rodriguez, O. A., Kyndt, J., & Martinez, A. (2015). Heterotrophic growth of microalgae: Metabolic aspects. *World Journal of Microbiology and Biotechnology, 31*(1), 1–9.

Nakamura, Y., & Li-Beisson, Y. (Eds.). (2016). *Lipids in plant and algae development*. Cham: Springer International Publishing.

Nalder, T. D., Miller, M. R., & Packer, M. A. (2015). Changes in lipid class content and composition of Isochrysis sp.(T-Iso) grown in batch culture. *Aquaculture International, 23*(5), 1293–1312.

Nandoskar, S. D., Rana, S., & Singh, S. K. (2026). Polyunsaturated fatty acids in biotechnology and health: Sources, Synthesis, Applications, and market trends. *Archives of Microbiology, 208*(3), 142.

Nazir, S., & Zahoor, I. (2021). Oilseed crops as the alternate source of omega fatty acids: A paradigm shift. In *Oil crop genomics*. Cham: Springer International Publishing, 341–352.

Nehdi, I. A., Sbihi, H., Tan, C. P., & Al-Resayes, S. I. (2012). Garden cress (*Lepidium sativum* Linn.) seed oil as a potential feedstock for biodiesel production. *Bioresource Technology, 126*, 193–197.

Nemzer, B., Al-Taher, F., & Abshiru, N. (2020). Phytochemical composition and nutritional value of different plant parts in two cultivated and wild purslane (*Portulaca oleracea* L.) genotypes. *Food Chemistry, 320*, 126621.

Nethravathy, M. U., Mudliar, S. N., RV, S., & Shekh, A. Y. (2021). Network of Metabolic Pathways for Biosynthesis of High-value Products in Microalgae.

Nie, Z. K., Deng, Z. T., Zhang, A. H., Ji, X. J., & Huang, H. (2014). Efficient arachidonic acid-rich oil production by *Mortierella alpina* through a three-stage fermentation strategy. *Bioprocess and Biosystems Engineering, 37*(3), 505–511.

Nkondjock, A., Shatenstein, B., Maisonneuve, P., & Ghadirian, P. (2003). Specific fatty acids and human colorectal cancer: An overview. *Cancer Detection and Prevention, 27*(1), 55–66 (62).

Ochsenreither, K., Glück, C., Stressler, T., Fischer, L., & Syldatk, C. (2016). Production strategies and applications of microbial single cell oils. *Frontiers in Microbiology, 7*, 1539.

Okuda, T., Ando, A., Negoro, H., Muratsubaki, T., Kikukawa, H., Sakamoto, T., & Ogawa, J. (2015). Eicosapentaenoic acid (EPA) production by an oleaginous fungus *Mortierella alpina* expressing heterologous the Δ17-desaturase gene under ordinary temperature. *European Journal of Lipid Science and Technology, 117*(12), 1919–1927.

Oliver, L., Dietrich, T., Marañón, I., Villarán, M. C., & Barrio, R. J. (2020). Producing omega-3 polyunsaturated fatty acids: A review of sustainable sources and future trends for the EPA and DHA market. *Resources, 9*(12), 148.

Othman, F. S., Jamaluddin, H., Ibrahim, Z., Hara, H., Yahya, N. A., Iwamoto, K., & Mohamad, S. E. (2019). Production of α-linolenic Acid by an Oleaginous Green Algae Acutodesmus obliquus Isolated from Malaysia. *Journal of Pure & Applied Microbiology, 13*(3).

Owens, T. (2003). The enigma of multiple sclerosis: Inflammation and neurodegeneration cause heterogeneous dysfunction and damage. *Current Opinion in Neurology, 16*(3), 259–265 (61).

Paisan, S. P., et al. (2017). Assessment of water degumming and acid degumming of mixed algal oil. *Journal of Environmental Chemical Engineering, 5*, 5115–5123.

Parsons, J. B., et al. (2013). Bacterial lipids: Metabolism and membrane homeostasis. *Progress in Lipid Research, 52*(3), 249–276.

Patel, A., Rova, U., Christakopoulos, P., & Matsakas, L. (2019). Simultaneous production of DHA and squalene from Aurantiochytrium sp. grown on forest biomass hydrolysates. *Biotechnology for Biofuels, 12*(1), 255.

Patel, A. K., Chauhan, A. S., Kumar, P., Michaud, P., Gupta, V. K., Chang, J. S., & Singhania, R. R. (2022). Emerging prospects of microbial production of omega fatty acids: Recent updates. *Bioresource Technology, 360*, 127534.

Patel, A. K., Choi, Y. Y., & Sim, S. J. (2020). Emerging prospects of mixotrophic microalgae: Way forward to sustainable bioprocess for environmental remediation and cost-effective biofuels. *Bioresource Technology, 300*, 122741.

Patel, A. K., Singhania, R. R., Dong, C. D., Obulisami, P. K., & Sim, S. J. (2021). Mixotrophic biorefinery: A promising algal platform for sustainable biofuels and high value coproducts. *Renewable and Sustainable Energy Reviews, 152*, 111669.

Patel, A. K., Singhania, R. R., Sim, S. J., & Di Dong, C. (2021). Recent advancements in mixotrophic bioprocessing for production of high value microalgal products. *Bioresource Technology, 320*, 124421.

Pereira, H., Barreira, L., Figueiredo, F., Custódio, L., Vizetto-Duarte, C., Polo, C., & Varela, J. (2012). Polyunsaturated fatty acids of marine macroalgae: Potential for nutritional and pharmaceutical applications. *Marine Drugs, 10*(9), 1920–1935.

Preechaphonkul, N., Sirikwanpong, S., & Maneeruttanarungroj, C. (2024). Freshwater green alga *Chlorella* sp. KLSc59 produced all forms of omega-3 oil: ALA, EPA, and DHA. *Algal Research, 80*, 103532.

Pritchett, J. W. (2007). Statins and dietary fish oils improve lipid composition in bone marrow and joints. *Clinical Orthopaedics and Related Research (1976-2007), 456*, 233–237 (51).

Qi, B., Fraser, T., Mugford, S., Dobson, G., Sayanova, O., Butler, J., & Lazarus, C. M. (2004). Production of very long chain polyunsaturated omega-3 and omega-6 fatty acids in plants. *Nature Biotechnology, 22*(6), 739–745.

Ramos-Romero, S., Torrella, J. R., Pagès, T., Viscor, G., & Torres, J. L. (2021). Edible microalgae and their bioactive compounds in the prevention and treatment of metabolic alterations. *Nutrients, 13*(2), 563.

Rao, A., Briskey, D., Nalley, J. O., & Ganuza, E. (2020). Omega-3 eicosapentaenoic acid (EPA) rich extract from the microalga nannochloropsis decreases cholesterol in healthy individuals: A double-blind, randomized, placebo-controlled, three-month supplementation study. *Nutrients, 12*(6), 1869.

Ratledge, C. (2004). Fatty acid biosynthesis in microorganisms being used for single cell oil production. *Biochimie, 86*(11), 807–815.

Remize, M., Brunel, Y., Silva, J. L., Berthon, J. Y., & Filaire, E. (2021). Microalgae n-3 PUFAs production and use in food and feed industries. *Marine Drugs, 19*(2), 113.

Ren, X., Liu, Y., Fan, C., Hong, H., Wu, W., Zhang, W., & Wang, Y. (2022). Production, processing, and protection of microalgal n-3 PUFA-rich oil. *Foods, 11*(9), 1215.

Robertson, R. C., Guihéneuf, F., Bahar, B., Schmid, M., Stengel, D. B., Fitzgerald, G. F., & Stanton, C. (2015). The anti-inflammatory effect of algae-derived lipid extracts on lipopolysaccharide (LPS)-stimulated human THP-1 macrophages. *Marine Drugs, 13*(8), 5402–5424.4.

Robertson, R., Guihéneuf, F., Schmid, M., Stengel, D. B., Fitzgerald, G., Ross, P., & Stanton, C. (2013). Algae-derived polyunsaturated fatty acids: Implications for human health. *Polyunsaturated Fatty Acids: Sources, Antioxidant Properties and Health Benefits, 2013*, 45–99.

Rodriguez-Espana, M., Mendoza-Sanchez, L. G., Magallon-Servin, P., Salgado-Cervantes, M. A., Acosta-Osorio, A. A., & Garcia, H. S. (2022). Supercritical fluid extraction of lipids rich in DHA from *Schizochytrium* sp. *The Journal of Supercritical Fluids, 179*, 105391.

Roglic, G. (2016). WHO Global report on diabetes: A summary. *International Journal of Noncommunicable Diseases, 1*(1), 3–8.

Russo, G. L., Langellotti, A. L., Oliviero, M., Sacchi, R., & Masi, P. (2021). Sustainable production of food grade omega-3 oil using aquatic protists: Reliability and future horizons. *New Biotechnology, 62*, 32–39.

Ryan, A. M., Reynolds, J. V., Healy, L., Byrne, M., Moore, J., Brannelly, N., & Flood, P. (2009). Enteral nutrition enriched with eicosapentaenoic acid (EPA) preserves lean body mass following esophageal cancer surgery: Results of a double-blinded randomized controlled trial. *Annals of Surgery, 249*(3), 355–363 (66).

Saini, R. K., & Keum, Y. S. (2018). Omega-3 and omega-6 polyunsaturated fatty acids: Dietary sources, metabolism, and significance—A review. *Life Sciences, 203*, 255–267.

Saini, R. K., Prasad, P., Sreedhar, R. V., Akhilender Naidu, K., Shang, X., & Keum, Y. S. (2021). Omega− 3 polyunsaturated fatty acids (PUFAs): Emerging plant and microbial sources, oxidative stability, bioavailability, and health benefits—A review. *Antioxidants, 10*(10), 1627.

Sakuradani, E. (2010). Advances in the production of various polyunsaturated fatty acids through oleaginous fungus *Mortierella alpina* breeding. *Bioscience, Biotechnology, and Biochemistry, 74*(5), 908–917.

Sakuradani, E., Ando, A., Shimizu, S., & Ogawa, J. (2013). Metabolic engineering for the production of polyunsaturated fatty acids by oleaginous fungus *Mortierella alpina* 1S-4. *Journal of Bioscience and Bioengineering, 116*(4), 417–422.

Santos-Sánchez, N. F., Valadez-Blanco, R., Hernández-Carlos, B., Torres-Ariño, A., Guadarrama-Mendoza, P. C., & Salas-Coronado, R. (2016). Lipids rich in ω-3 polyunsaturated fatty acids from microalgae. *Applied Microbiology and Biotechnology, 100*(20), 8667–8684.

Saxena, P., Kumar, M., & Harish (2020). Autotrophic cultivation of microalgae for the production of polyunsaturated fatty acid. *Nutraceutical fatty acids from oleaginous microalgae. A Human Health Perspective*, 165–185.

Schmid, M., Guihéneuf, F., & Stengel, D. B. (2016). Evaluation of food grade solvents for lipid extraction and impact of storage temperature on fatty acid composition of edible seaweeds *Laminaria digitata* (Phaeophyceae) and *Palmaria palmata* (Rhodophyta). *Food Chemistry, 208*, 161–168.

Señoráns, M., Castejón, N., & Señoráns, F. J. (2020). Advanced extraction of lipids with DHA from Isochrysis galbana with enzymatic pre-treatment combined with pressurized liquids and ultrasound assisted extractions. *Molecules (Basel, Switzerland), 25*(14), 3310.

Shahidi, F., & Ambigaipalan, P. (2018). Omega-3 polyunsaturated fatty acids and their health benefits. *Annual Review Of Food Science and Technology, 9*(1), 345–381.

Shetty, U. S., & Akhilender, N. K. (2017). Garden cress (*Lepidium sativum* L.) seed oil: Alternative source for ALA. *The FASEB Journal, 31*, 971 12.

Shim, S. J., Hong, M. E., Chang, W. S., & Sim, S. J. (2020). Repeated-batch production of omega-3 enriched biomass of *Chlorella sorokiniana* via calcium-induced homeoviscous adaptation. *Bioresource Technology, 303*, 122944.

Simopoulos, A. P. (2003). Omega-3 fatty acids and cancer. *Indoor and Built Environment, 12*(6), 405–412 (67).

Simopoulos, A. P. (2003). Fatty Acids: Evolutionary Aspects. Omega-6/omega-3 essential fatty acid ratio: The scientific evidence, 81, 1.

Sivakumar, R., Sachin, S., Priyadarshini, R., & Ghosh, S. (2022). Sustainable production of eicosapentaenoic acid-rich oil from microalgae: Towards an algal biorefinery. *Journal of Applied Microbiology, 132*(6), 4170–4185.

Spillias, S., Valin, H., Batka, M., Sperling, F., Havlík, P., Leclère, D., & McDonald-Madden, E. (2023). Reducing global land-use pressures with seaweed farming. *Nature Sustainability, 6*(4), 380–390.

Suh, S. S., Kim, S. J., Hwang, J., Park, M., Lee, T. K., Kil, E. J., & Lee, S. (2015). Fatty acid methyl ester profiles and nutritive values of 20 marine microalgae in Korea. *Asian Pacific Journal of Tropical Medicine, 8*(3), 191–196.

Susanto, E., Fahmi, A. S., Hosokawa, M., & Miyashita, K. (2019). Variation in lipid components from 15 species of tropical and temperate seaweeds. *Marine Drugs, 17*(11), 630.

Tabarzad, M., Atabaki, V., & Hosseinabadi, T. (2020). Anti-inflammatory activity of bioactive compounds from microalgae and cyanobacteria by focusing on the mechanisms of action. *Molecular Biology Reports, 47*(8), 6193–6205.

Tang, X., Chen, H., Chen, Y. Q., Chen, W., Garre, V., Song, Y., & Ratledge, C. (2015). Comparison of biochemical activities between high and low lipid-producing strains of Mucor circinelloides: An explanation for the high oleaginicity of strain WJ11. *PLoS One, 10*(6), e0128396.

Tian, L., Chi, G., Lin, S., Ling, X., & He, N. (2024). Marine microorganisms: Natural factories for polyunsaturated fatty acid production. *Blue Biotechnology, 1*(1), 15.

Uddin, M. K., Juraimi, A. S., Hossain, M. S., Nahar, M. A. U., Ali, M. E., & Rahman, M. M. (2014). Purslane weed (*Portulaca oleracea*): A prospective plant source of nutrition, omega-3 fatty acid, and antioxidant attributes. *The Scientific World Journal, 2014*(1), 951019 6 page.

Ukropec, J., Reseland, J. E., Gasperikova, D., Demcakova, E., Madsen, L., Berge, R. K., & Sebökova, E. (2003). The hypotriglyceridemic effect of dietary n− 3 FA is associated with increased β-oxidation and reduced leptin expression. *Lipids, 38*(10), 1023–1029 (58).

Ulmann, L., Blanckaert, V., Mimouni, V., X. Andersson, M., Schoefs, B., & Chénais, B. (2017). Microalgal fatty acids and their implication in health and disease. *Mini Reviews in Medicinal Chemistry, 17*(12), 1112–1123.

Vadivelan, G., & Venkateswaran, G. (2014). Production and enhancement of omega-3*fatty acid from Mortierella alpina* CFR-GV15: Its food and therapeutic application. *BioMed Research International, 2014*(1), 657414.

Umesha, S. S., & Naidu, K. A. (2015). Antioxidants and antioxidant enzymes status of rats fed on n-3 PUFA rich Garden cress (*Lepidium Sativum* L) seed oil and its blended oils. *Journal of Food Science and Technology, 52*(4), 1993–2002.

Venskutonis, P. R., & Kraujalis, P. (2013). Nutritional components of amaranth seeds and vegetables: A review on composition, properties, and uses. *Comprehensive Reviews in Food Science and Food Safety, 12*(4), 381–412.

Waldron, M. (2004). The role of fatty acids in the management of osteoarthritis. *Clinical Edge,* 14–16 (50).

Wall, R., Ross, R. P., Fitzgerald, G. F., & Stanton, C. (2010). Fatty acids from fish: The anti-inflammatory potential of long-chain omega-3 fatty acids. *Nutrition Reviews, 68*(5), 280–289 (42).

Walsh, T. A., et al. (2016). Canola engineered with a microalgal polyketide synthase-like system produces oil enriched in docosahexaenoic acid. *Nature Biotechnology, 34*(8), 881–887.

Wang, Q., Lu, Y., Xin, Y., Wei, L., Huang, S., & Xu, J. (2016). Genome editing of model oleaginous microalgae *Nannochloropsis* spp. by CRISPR/Cas9. *The Plant Journal, 88*(6), 1071–1081.

Wang, X., Fosse, H. K., Li, K., Chauton, M. S., Vadstein, O., & Reitan, K. I. (2019). Influence of nitrogen limitation on lipid accumulation and EPA and DHA content in four marine microalgae for possible use in aquafeed. *Frontiers in Marine Science, 6*, 95.

Wang, X., Lin, L., Lu, H., Liu, Z., Duan, N., Dong, T., & Xu, P. (2018). Microalgae cultivation and culture medium recycling by a two-stage cultivation system. *Frontiers of Environmental Science & Engineering, 12*(6), 14.

Wang, C., Sun, C., Lu, W., Gul, K., Mata, A., & Fang, Y. (2020). Emulsion structure design for improving the oxidative stability of polyunsaturated fatty acids. *Comprehensive Reviews in Food Science and Food Safety, 19*(6), 2955–2971.

Wijiani, N., Wardhani, F. A., Firandi, A., Afthoni, M. H., Cahyaningsih, R., Wangchuk, P., & Nugraha, A. S. (2026). Sacha inchi seeds (*Plukenetia volubilis*). In *Underutilized seeds: Sustainable solutions for health, industry, and environment.* Singapore: Springer Nature Singapore, 291–321.

Winwood, R. J. (2013). Recent developments in the commercial production of DHA and EPA rich oils from micro-algae. *Ocl, 20*(6), D604.

Wirkowska-Wojdyła, M., Ostrowska-Ligęza, E., Górska, A., Brzezińska, R., & Piasecka, I. (2024). Assessment of the nutritional potential and resistance to oxidation of sea buckthorn and rosehip oils. *Applied Sciences, 14*(5), 1867.

Wu, C. C., et al. (2017). Surfactants assist in lipid extraction from wet *Nannochloropsis* sp. *Bioresource Technology, 243*, 793–799.

Xue, J., Niu, Y. F., Huang, T., Yang, W. D., Liu, J. S., & Li, H. Y. (2015). Genetic improvement of the microalga *Phaeodactylum tricornutum* for boosting neutral lipid accumulation. *Metabolic Engineering, 27*, 1–9.

Xue, S. J., Chi, Z., Zhang, Y., Li, Y. F., Liu, G. L., Jiang, H., & Chi, Z. M. (2018). Fatty acids from oleaginous yeasts and yeast-like fungi and their potential applications. *Critical Reviews in Biotechnology, 38*(7), 1049–1060.

Xue, Z., Sharpe, P. L., Hong, S. P., Yadav, N. S., Xie, D., Short, D. R., & Zhu, Q. (2013). Production of omega-3 eicosapentaenoic acid by metabolic engineering of *Yarrowia lipolytica. Nature Biotechnology, 31*(8), 734–740.

Yamaguchi, A., Stanger, L., Freedman, C. J., Standley, M., Hoang, T., Adili, R., & Holinstat, M. (2021). DHA 12-LOX-derived oxylipins regulate platelet activation and thrombus formation through a PKA-dependent signaling pathway. *Journal of Thrombosis and Haemostasis, 19*(3), 839–851.

Yan, C. X., Zhang, Y., Yang, W. Q., Ma, W., Sun, X. M., & Huang, H. (2024). Universal and unique strategies for the production of polyunsaturated fatty acids in industrial oleaginous microorganisms. *Biotechnology Advances, 70*, 108298.

Yang, J., Wen, C., Duan, Y., Deng, Q., Peng, D., Zhang, H., & Ma, H. (2021). The composition, extraction, analysis, bioactivities, bioavailability and applications in food system of flaxseed (*Linum usitatissimum* L.) oil: A review. *Trends in Food Science & Technology, 118*, 252–260.

Yang, X., Li, Y., Li, Y., Ye, D., Yuan, L., Sun, Y., & Hu, Q. (2019). Solid matrix-supported supercritical CO_2 enhances extraction of γ-linolenic acid from the cyanobacterium Arthrospira (Spirulina) platensis and bioactivity evaluation of the molecule in zebrafish. *Marine Drugs, 17*(4), 203.

Yin, F. W., et al. (2019). Improving the quality of microalgae DHA-rich oil in the deodorization process using deoxygen ated steam. *Journal of Food Processing and Preservation, 44*, e14602.

Yong, W. T. L., Thien, V. Y., Rupert, R., & Rodrigues, K. F. (2022). Seaweed: A potential climate change solution. *Renewable and Sustainable Energy Reviews, 159*, 112222.

You, J. Y., et al. (2011). Enzymatic hydrolysis and extraction of arachidonic acid rich lipids from *Mortierella alpine. Bioresource Technology, 102*, 6088–6094.

Zamani Ghaleshahi, A., Ezzatpanah, H., Rajabzadeh, G., & Ghavami, M. (2020). Comparison and analysis characteristics of flax, perilla and basil seed oils cultivated in Iran. *Journal of Food Science and Technology, 57*(4), 1258–1268.

Zhang, Y., Luan, X., Zhang, H., Garre, V., Song, Y., & Ratledge, C. (2017). Improved γ-linolenic acid production in *Mucor circinelloides* by homologous overexpressing of delta-12 and delta-6 desaturases. *Microbial Cell Factories, 16*(1), 113.

Zhang, Y., Wang, D., Chen, Y., Liu, T., Zhang, S., Fan, H., et al. (2021). Healthy function and high valued utilization of edible fungi. *Food Science and Human Wellness, 10*(4), 408–420.

Zhang, X. Y., Li, B., Huang, B. C., Wang, F. B., Zhang, Y. Q., Zhao, S. G., ... Wang, Z. P. (2022). Production, biosynthesis, and commercial applications of fatty acids from oleaginous fungi. *Frontiers in Nutrition, 9*, 873657.

Zibaeenezhad, M. J., Ghavipisheh, M., Attar, A., & Aslani, A. (2017). Comparison of the effect of omega-3 supplements and fresh fish on lipid profile: A randomized, open-labeled trial. *Nutrition & Diabetes, 7*(12), 1.

Zielińska, A., & Nowak, I. (2017a). Abundance of active ingredients in sea-buckthorn oil. *Lipids in Health and Disease, 16*(1), 1–11. https://doi.org/10.1186/s12944-017-0469-7.

Zielińska, A., & Nowak, I. (2017b). Abundance of active ingredients in sea-buckthorn oil. *Lipids in Health and Disease, 16*(1), 95.

Chapter 5

Novel sources of polyunsaturated fatty acids: algae, marine, microbial innovations, animal, plants, genetically engineered plants, and other biological sources

Sai Nandhini Ravi, Keerthana Sivakumar, Shivani Mohan, and Yuganthra Balaji
Department of Biotechnology, Vel Tech Rangarajan Dr Sagunthala R&D Institute of Science and Technology, Chennai, Tamil Nadu, India

5.1 Introduction

The essential polyunsaturated fatty acids (PUFAs) include omega-3 as well as omega-6, which assist the human body by supporting cell membranes, managing heart health, and reducing inflammation. Omega-3 fatty acid known as docosahexaenoic acid (DHA) functions as an essential compound for maintaining brain and eye health (Wiktorowska-Owczarek et al., 2015). The consumption of omega-3 PUFAs helps decrease heart-related disease risk and improves diabetes control and depressive symptoms, simultaneously protecting maternal and child health. Studies seeking to determine the effectiveness of omega-3 fatty acids in addressing numerous health situations are still in progress (Shahidi & Ambigaipalan, 2018). The production of PUFAs from microalgae, a novel source, represents a sustainable food source for human nutrition, yet large-scale manufacturing requires overcoming both economic and regulatory obstacles. Advanced technology solutions together with biorefinery strategies need to be implemented for optimizing production techniques and reducing waste alongside product commercialization improvements of microalgae metabolites (Santin et al., 2022). Fermentative production of PUFAs depends on oleaginous microorganisms that construct high amounts of omega-3 fatty acids, including DHA and eicosapentaenoic acid (EPA). The accumulation of lipids increases when microorganisms are grown under specific nitrogen limitation and carbon-to-nitrogen ratio conditions. RNA sequencing allows researchers to improve pathways that produce PUFA. The fermentation method leads to a more sustainable production of PUFAs compared to fish oil extraction because it handles waste substrates while minimizing environmental effects (Kannan et al., 2021). This chapter explores novel sources of PUFAs beyond traditional sources. It covers algal, microbial, plant-based, genetically engineered, and animal-derived PUFAs.

5.2 Algae as a polyunsaturated fatty acid source

PUFAs are not synthesized by human beings; they are still essential for human health because they contain omega-3 (n-3) and omega-6 (n-6) fatty acids, which include DHA, EPA, and arachidonic acid (ARA). These essential fatty acids can only be obtained by humans through diet. High concentrations of PUFAs with balanced omega-6 to omega-3 ratios that meet nutritional requirements can be found in algae. The PUFA profiles of different macroalgae species vary; for example, *Sargassum natans* brown algae primarily show DHA content, while *Gracilaria* sp. red algae have high ARA levels. Since algae don't require land or freshwater, their sustainable qualities ensure that they can serve as a viable food substitute to conventional fish and land animal sources. Consumption of PUFAs from algae brings beneficial health effects due to their antioxidant and antiinflammatory components that help protect against chronic diseases. Algae serve as an effective, sustainable source to deliver essential fatty acids to diets (Shanab et al., 2018).

Omega-3 and Omega-6 Polyunsaturated Fatty Acids in Food Systems. DOI: https://doi.org/10.1016/B978-0-443-43810-3.00005-1

5.2.1 Type of algae for the production of polyunsaturated fatty acids

PUFAs that matter nutritionally exist in the Chlorophyta green algae, together with the Phaeophyta brown algae and Rhodophyta red algae. The scientists examined lipids and fatty acid distributions within 27 tropical macroalgae species for chemotaxonomic identification and different mixture demonstration. The research revealed particular species that provided nutritional value because their n-6/n-3 fatty acid ratios were optimal. According to the research, macroalgae serve competently as alternative PUFA providers for human dietary needs (Kumari et al., 2010). Microalgae contain PUFAs at high levels, among which the essential compounds DHA and EPA are present. Table 5.1 shows the comparative PUFA profiles of different microalgae species. Environmental sustainability allows microalgae production to establish itself as an eco-friendly approach for bioactive compound synthesis. The production of PUFAs by microalgae has received improvements through contemporary biotechnology alongside stress-induction methods. Research shows that microalgae act as an excellent source for developing valuable nutritional products (Ramesh Kumar et al., 2019).

5.2.2 Bio-synthesis of algae for the production of polyunsaturated fatty acid

The enzymatic pathways of $\Delta6$ desaturation during algal PUFA production involve two reactions: first transforming oleic acid (OA) to linoleic acid (LA) before turning it into alpha-linolenic acid (ALA), as shown in Fig. 5.1 The crucial initial step, known as $\Delta6$ desaturation, leads to the production of EPA and DHA, which belong to the category of long-chain PUFAs. The microalgae organism *Emiliania huxleyi* relies on specific enzymes to carry out the catalytic function of $\Delta6$ desaturation that allows fatty acid chains to form double bonds. An 18-carbon PUFA product forms because of this important step that functions as a precursor to longer-chain fatty acids. PUFA biosynthesis in microalgae functions best because these desaturases play an essential role in the system. Marine algae gain improved nutritional properties through this process and support marine food chains because PUFAs act as important agents for aquatic ecological systems (Sun et al., 2024).

The metabolism of PUFAs into unsaturated fatty acids by macroalgae needs the delta-9 desaturase pathway, which functions through desaturase enzyme (DES) activities. A series of enzymatic reactions at the delta-9 position enables macroalgae to produce essential EPA and DHA needed for biological operations, especially regarding inflammation control. As a result of their n-3 and n-6 PUFA synthesis capability, macroalgae serve as essential dietary food sources because mammals do not have the required delta-12DES (Δ12DES). Consuming EPA and DHA provides two advantages to people: reduction of inflammation and proper lipid signal transmission. Macroalgae act as accessible fish oil alternatives that address fish stock depletion, along with fish oil contaminants present in the market. A comprehensive examination of the delta-9 desaturase pathway in macroalgae must occur before extracting human health benefits from the fatty acids (Lupette & Benning, 2020).

5.2.3 Advantage of algae over fish oil

Algae have a significant advantage over fish oil for PUFAs production, because of their sustainability. Farming of microalgae occurs in uninhabited areas, which prevents fish population reduction while ensuring that microalgae do not

TABLE 5.1 Comparative polyunsaturated fatty acids (PUFA) profiles of different microalgae species.

S. no.	Algae class	Species name	Type of PUFAs	References
1.	Microalgae	*Nannochloropsis sp.*	Eicosapentaenoic acid (EPA)	Remize et al. (2021)
2.	Microalgae	*Phaeodactylum tricornutum*	EPA	Remize et al. (2021)
3.	Microalgae	*Schizochytrium* sp.	Docosahexaenoic acid (DHA)	Santin et al. (2021)
4.	Macroalga-e	*Palmaria palmata*	EPA	Van Ginneken et al. (2011)
5	Macroalga-e	*Sargassum natans*	DHA	Van Ginneken et al. (2011)
6.	Microalgae	*Crypthecсdinium cohnii*	DHA	Chen et al. (2023)
7.	Macroalga-e	*Ulva sp.*	Alpha-linolenic acid	Pereira et al. (2012)

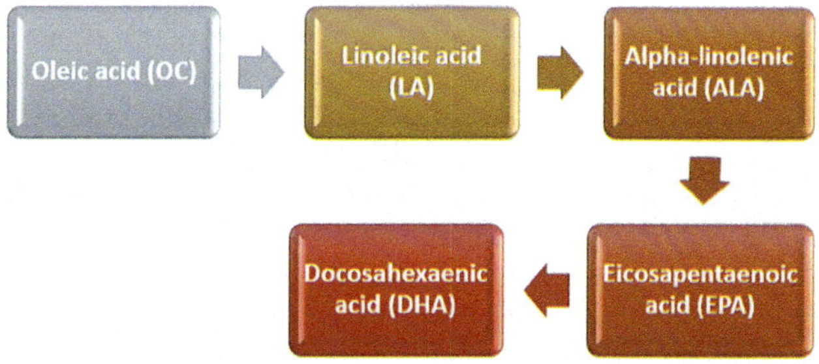

FIGURE 5.1 **Δ6 desaturation pathway in algae for polyunsaturated fatty acid (PUFA) biosynthesis.**

absorb mercury or other harmful components detected in diminished fish supplies. The microalgae provide vegan and vegetarian consumers with sustainable plant-based omega-3 because the microalgae meet the dietary needs of both groups. The selected microalgae strains grow quickly while producing high essential fatty acid levels, which makes their harvesting operations operate efficiently across different cultivation settings. Grouped microalgae provide manufacturers with higher income because many industries, from biofuels to food additives, require their multiple applications serving the market need for sustainable products and health benefits (Adarme-Vega et al., 2012).

5.3 Marine sources for polyunsaturated fatty acid production

Human body health requires omega-3 polyunsaturated fats, namely EPA and DHA, since they support cardiovascular health as well as neurological function. Microalgae serve as an alternative source for extraction methods that work to eliminate contaminants while raising PUFA levels, in addition to keeping oxidative stability high to preserve long shelf-life durations.

5.4 Microbial innovation for the production of polyunsaturated fatty acid and its biosynthesis pathway

Microorganisms, specifically microalgae and yeast, together demonstrate sustainable production of essential PUFAs such as EPA and DHA. Science experts use biotechnology methods to enhance production levels and improve manufacturing procedures. The utilization of microorganisms for health and biotechnology applications will become possible because of measures to close production gaps after manufacturing (Jovanovic et al., 2021). The dietary requirements of vegans can be sustained through microalgae and thraustochytrids since these contain omega-3 PUFAs. Microorganisms provide human beings with necessary fatty acids by substituting traditional harvesting procedures that take place in the wild. A biotechnology approach based on metabolic engineering unlocks better industrial efficiency, and scientific teams have developed commercial EPA and DHA production methods. The preservation time of products increases through microencapsulation methods, and these methods also improve the absorption level of products. Microorganisms should use their production potential for omega-3 fatty acids because the growing vegan food sector and modern biotechnology combine to create this opportunity for environmental benefits and dietary provisions (Saini et al., 2021). The synthesis of PUFAs among microorganisms occurs through two distinct strains: aerobic and anaerobic. PUFAs produced by humans result from the enzymatic activity of desaturases and elongases. The cell requires oxygen together with electron transport chains to perform the desaturation pathway, but the specific electron donor type relies on desaturase location distribution. The bacteria *E. coli*, alongside other bacterial species, deploy metabolic functions through an anaerobic pathway that involves particular enzymatic reactions. The pathways have future possibilities as biotechnology-based tools (Uttaro, 2006).

The innovation of microorganisms now provides sustainable production methods for PUFAs, which replace conventional animal- and plant-based origins. The tiny microbes create essential fatty acids using two different pathways, which include the aerobic desaturase/elongase pathway that functions best in oxygen-rich environments, such as those of *Mortierella alpina* and *Yarrowia lipolytica* (Shah et al., 2022), and the anaerobic PUFA synthase pathway that is oxygen-independent and is utilized by *Schizochytrium* sp. (Guo et al., 2022) for energy-efficient and productive fatty acid synthesis. The combination of CRISPR-Cas9 editing and metabolic engineering, as well as coculturing techniques delivered by modern biotechnology, advances the production of PUFAs and enhances the use of microbial sources (Jovanovic et al., 2021). Agro-industrial waste that is sustainable now gets transformed into nutrient-rich feedstocks, which create lower production expenses and support environmentally friendly manufacturing processes. The microorganisms produce nourishing aquafeeds which aid marine life (Guo et al., 2022) and luxurious omega-rich nutraceuticals for skin health and heart wellness, thereby defining the future of wellness (Sun et al., 2024). Pharmaceutical developers employ drug delivery methods that incorporate PUFA to fight inflammatory diseases with accuracy (Shah et al., 2022). Fig. 5.2 shows the distribution of PUFA content among different microbial species. And the future microbial PUFA production will emerge in the future as the leading force of the omega-3 market because it will join beauty with health and sustainability through hybrid biosynthetic pathways combined with AI-powered strain optimization, while waste valorization is used for these production methods (Allemann et al., 2019; Jovanovic et al., 2021; Shah et al., 2022).

5.5 Animal-derived polyunsaturated fatty acids source and benefits

The combination of PUFAs exists in fatty fish alongside poultry and ruminant items, which consumers can obtain from animal foods. Salmon, mackerel, and sardines from fatty fish catch attention because these fish concentrate long-chain n-3 PUFAs that include EPA and DHA, which deliver diverse health improvements through reduced inflammation while offering better heart health. The inclusion of fish oil or flaxseed supplements in poultry animal diets causes n-3 PUFAs content in poultry food to rise. PHM food and dairy items like omega-6 fatty acids enable consumers to acquire a combination of ALA, omega-3, and omega-6 fatty acids. The PUFA levels in animal products depend directly on the feed the animal receives because PUFA-rich forage consumption boosts PUFA amounts in cow milk, along with cow meat. The animal feed given to animals feeding on oilseed crops containing sunflower, soybean, and corn transmits omega-6 PUFA content to them. The practice of feeding livestock animals controls the extent to which their food products develop PUFA content (Givens, 2005).

5.5.1 Current animal research in the production of n-3 polyunsaturated fatty acids

The scientific community uses rabbits to research how n-3 PUFAs affect the body because multiple key features make their studies advantageous. These laboratory animals stand as the most thoroughly studied nonrodent sample that maintains relevant research findings for human health applications. The metabolic operations along with physiological traits in rabbits provide a complete framework to investigate the impact of dietary n-3 PUFAs on diverse health and reproductive outcomes. The monitoring capabilities of essential human-related endpoints show similarities between rabbit systems and human systems that absorb nutrients in a comparable fashion. Researchers have discovered that dietary modifications in rabbits effectively increase the n-3 PUFA content in their meat, which provides knowledge to create better nutrition plans for both animal and human health (Rodríguez et al., 2019).

Cooked pork and beef liver are important sources of n-3 LC-PUFAs in human nutrition, as these compounds are synthesized in the liver from the plant-derived precursor ALA through natural metabolic processes in animals such as cattle, pigs, and chickens (Gladyshev et al., 2015). Both the metabolic activity of tissue fatty acid biosynthesis and the lipid composition of ingested substances determine the fatty acid profile of animal-derived products, such as eggs, milk, and meat. Monogastric animals, such as pigs, along with poultry and rabbits, demonstrate stronger dietary relationships compared to ruminants due to the ruminant digestive system's ability to transform ingested fats into hydrogenated substances. Recent health trends reveal that consumers better understand why PUFAs are essential for human nutrition. In

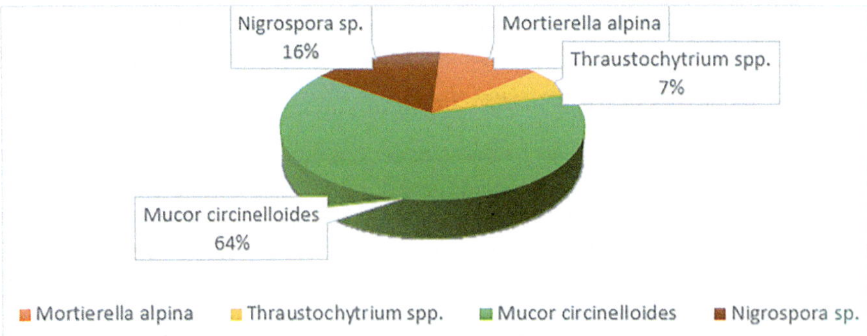

FIGURE 5.2 **Polyunsaturated fatty acid content distribution among microbial species and its biotechnological advancements.**

animal diets, this represents a valid approach to meeting consumer demand for nutritionally beneficial animal products (Kouba & Mourot, 2011). This primarily includes fish—particularly those with high lipid content such as mackerel, salmon, sardine, and herring—eggs (naturally rich in omega-3 fatty acids, including ALA and DHA, or enriched through hens fed ALA-rich diets such as linseed or rapeseed), and meat from birds and mammals (with the highest concentrations found in rabbit, followed by pork and other monogastric animals, and lower levels in polygastric animals such as beef, mutton, and goat). In contrast, butter, milk, dairy products, and cheese are generally low in omega-3 fatty acids. The nature of fatty acids from reserve triglycerides varies mainly because of what the animal eats and depends on its anatomical position, which is equivalent to their placement during butchering.

5.6 Plant-based polyunsaturated fatty acid

Plants offer different key sources of PUFAs that humans can use. The omega-3 fatty acid ALA reaches high levels in seeds and nuts, particularly flaxseeds, chia seeds, and walnuts. The omega-3 and omega-6 PUFAs are abundantly available in numerous oils, including flaxseed oil, hemp oil, and canola oil. The microalgae Spirulina and Chlorella, together with algae, are showing promise as sources for obtaining long chain omega-3 EPA and DHA fatty acids. The essential omega-3 fatty acid compound ALA exists as a minor substance in leafy vegetables, especially purslane. Scientists are looking into genetically modified plant research that focuses on omega-3 enhancement in *Camelina sativa* plants. The plant-based dietary sources provide environmentally friendly solutions for essential fatty acid consumption among vegetarian individuals (Rizzo et al., 2023). The protection against various metabolic disorders functionally belongs to PUFAs, as this composition explores new findings of plant-derived essential fatty acids that prioritize n-3 omega PUFAs. Recent literature has identified algae together with microorganisms and plants that contain stearidonic acid and genetically modified plants as promising sources (Rizzo et al., 2023). An investigation has been conducted to determine marine- and plant-derived omega-3 PUFA (n-3) influences on erythrocyte fatty acid composition and glycolipid metabolic pathways in people who have type 2 diabetes mellitus (Liu et al., 2022).

5.6.1 Natural sources of polyunsaturated fatty acid in plants

Plants offer PUFAs through various seeds and nuts, as well as oil products containing essential fatty acids. Flaxseeds stand out because they possess 39%–64% of their total fat in the form of dietary omega-3 fatty acid ALA. Studies demonstrate that chia seeds function as a nutritional source of ALA while providing substantial omega-3 content to the diet, as explained. The literature shows that hemp seeds possess balanced omega-3 and omega-6 fatty acids, even when these seeds were not mentioned in the provided excerpts. The high content of ALA in walnuts makes these nuts an outstanding choice for consumers. Relevant information about these plant sources of ALA also appears in the text, where the authors discuss cooking with soybean oil and canola oil and mention purslane as a leafy vegetable. These plant-based sources, which supply PUFAs, serve the critical needs of vegetarian and vegan dieters while helping maintain heart health and general wellness (Rizzo et al., 2023). The main objective of this metaanalysis was to evaluate the effects of plant-derived PUFAs on insulin resistance, along with glucose metabolism levels. Randomized controlled feeding trials examined how plant-derived PUFA diets affected insulin resistance markers and glucose metabolism while testing against saturated fatty acid (SFA) and carbohydrate diets. This evidence originates from randomized controlled trials showing that substituting SFA or carbohydrates with plant-derived PUFA consumption probably lowers fasting insulin levels and HOMA-IR values in people without diabetes (Wanders et al., 2019).

5.6.2 Health benefits of plant-based polyunsaturated fatty acid

The plant-based PUFAs bring numerous health benefits to human systems. Omega-3 (ω-3) and omega-6 (ω-6) fatty acids support cardiovascular health, brain function, metabolic wellness, and inflammatory reduction. The heart health benefits and overall physiological balancing properties of ALA, together with other omega-3 fatty acids, have received extensive scientific research. The antiinflammatory activity of omega-3 fats, including ALA, helps decrease cardiovascular inflammation and aids in controlling rheumatoid arthritis according to research (Mititelu et al., 2024). Habitual substitution of saturated fats with PUFAs leads to major decreases in heart attack and stroke occurrences, which makes them vital for sustaining heart health (Mozaffarian et al., 2005). People without easy access to seafood with omega-3 fatty acids use plant-based ALA as their key defense against coronary heart disease. Studies confirm that PUFAs trigger blood pressure reduction together with antiinflammatory effects that help support cardiovascular wellness (Mititelu et al., 2024). PUFAs deliver vital nutrients that aid both body function and the antioxidant defense system. The health advantages of omega-6 and omega-3 fatty acids converge when consumers sustain balanced dietary ratios to avoid adverse effects from excessive omega-6 consumption. In Fig. 5.3, plant-based sources of PUFA as an alternative for essential fatty acids are illustrated.

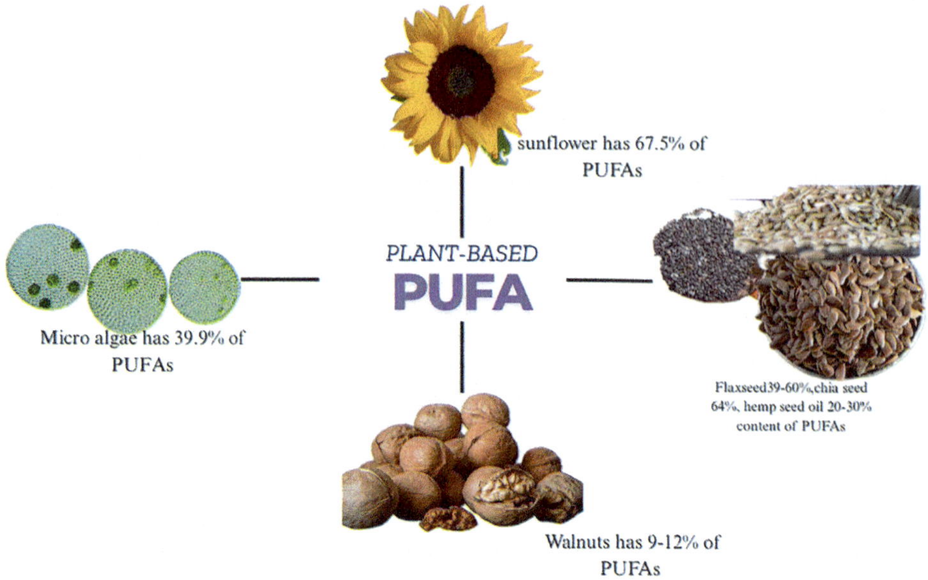

FIGURE 5.3 **Polyunsaturated fatty acid profiles of plant-based sources as sustainable alternatives for essential fatty acids.**

5.7 Genetically engineered plant polyunsaturated fatty acids

Long-chain PUFAs accumulate through genetic modifications in transgenic plants, including *Linum usitatissimum* (linseed) and *Nicotiana tabacum* (tobacco). The modifications bring fatty acyl desaturases and elongases from *Phaeodactylum tricornutum* (algae) and *Mortierella alpina* (fungi), along with *Physcomitrella patens* (moss), into the plants. This allows plant cells to produce DHA and EPA as long-chain PUFAs. The enzymes transform shorter-chain fatty acids into DHA and EPA end products through a production process leading to long-chain PUFAs. The transgenic linseed seeds contain high PUFA levels of very long-chain fatty acids between C20 and C22. Consumers can obtain EPA/DHA through engineered plants such as linseed and rapeseed, which serve as human food products yet maintain fish stocks at sufficient levels (Sprague et al., 2017). The modified version of linseed oil functions as an alternative to fish oil in vegan/vegetarian dietary plans to rectify omega-3 deficiencies. The addition of PUFA-enriched plants, particularly soy and rapeseed, helps to boost the nutritional worth of milk products and meat while producing better eggs. The environmental and nutritional advantages of these products cannot overcome consumer hesitation that persists toward GM products. The precise regulation of genes in GM crops becomes essential because it prevents unintended effects, including seed viability decreases (Patel et al., 2019). The methods of improving PUFA yields include multigene stacking and CRISPR/Cas9 editing combined with microbial coproduction. The genetic engineering workflow for enhancing PUFA production in plants is shown in Fig. 5.4.

Research funded by the Biotechnology and Biological Sciences Research Council demonstrates genetically modified plants serve as a substitute for oily fish to obtain n-3 PUFAs in human diets (West et al., 2021). Scientists used *Thamnidium elegans* to provide the gene sequence for creating the artificial D6D gene, which encodes Δ6DES. A signal sequence from wheat high-molecular-weight glutenin subunit combined with modified codons within the sequence created an expression-optimized wheat gene. The end product of wheat transgenesis with the artificial D6D gene included γ-linolenic acid. Students at the University of Manchester verified γ-linolenic acid in wheat grains of genetically modified plants after they reached maturity at concentrations between 0.04% and 0.32% of total fatty acids. As shown in Table 5.2, microalgae-derived PUFAs exhibit high bioavailability and sustainability.

5.8 Alternative biological sources for polyunsaturated fatty acid production

Black soldier fly larvae (BSFL), mealworms, and silkworm pupae are promising sources to obtain PUFAs. The natural high SFA content in BSFL increases when the larvae consume fish discards and algae-enriched waste which enhances their omega-3 fatty acid content with specific emphasis on EPA and DHA. The PUFA content reached 39.9% when BSFL

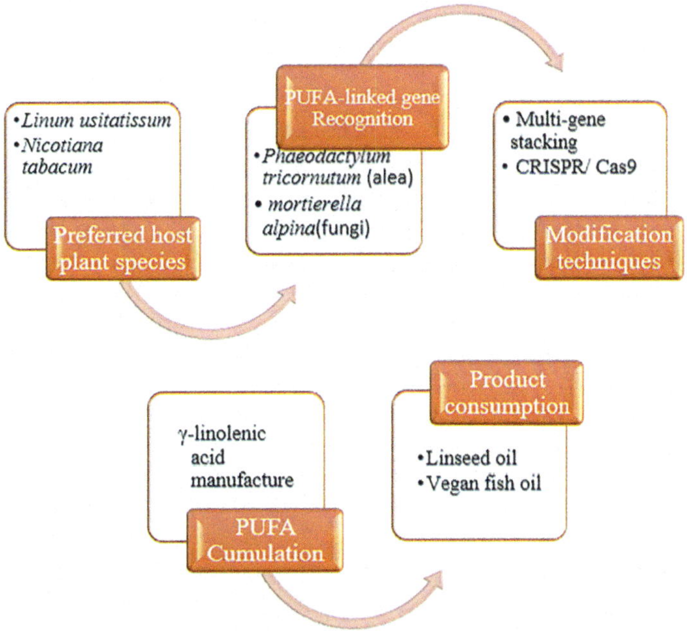

FIGURE 5.4 **Genetic engineering workflow for enhancing polyunsaturated fatty acid (PUFA) production in plants.**

larvae consumed fish discards while their composition primarily consisted of LA and ALA. The utilization of ocean-based material presents production challenges for large-scale industrial operations. The fatty acid profile of mealworms (*Tenebrio molitor*) can be improved through feeding the worms specific dietary substances. The feeding of mealworms with omega-3-rich seeds like flaxseed resulted in omega-3/omega-6 ratios that exceeded 0.5 along with PUFA composition reaching more than 60%, making the insects affordable for animal and human dietary purposes (Fasel et al., 2017). The protein content of silkworm pupae amounts to 55.6% dry weight, while their essential amino acids are balanced, but their PUFA content remains less emphasized compared to their known bioactive peptides and polysaccharides. The therapeutic properties of these proteins and chemicals within insects indirectly promote health benefits to people (Zhou et al., 2022).

The sustainable production of PUFAs can also be achieved through deep-sea fish and symbiotic marine organisms. Dietary addition of algae oil and salmon-byproduct oil revealed promising alternatives to fish oil within European sea bass studies because this supplement increased DHA retention in muscles to 57%–66%, with levels similar to those of traditional fish oil (Marques et al., 2023). The PUFA cycling processes in marine ecosystems heavily depend on sponges and corals because these symbionts encourage symbiotic algae species that produce PUFAs. These organisms do not directly provide PUFAs, but their role in sustainable aquafeed fuels the marine PUFA supply chain (Rix et al., 2016).

5.9 Polyunsaturated fatty acids applications in healthcare

Health risks from heart failure decrease among the number of people consuming high amounts of long-chain omega-3 PUFAS (n-3) through their diet or possess elevated levels of these fatty acids in their bloodstream increase. Evidence indicates that heart failure prevention would benefit from boosting n-3 PUFA dietary consumption. The promotion of n-3 PUFA consumption leads to increased cardiovascular health benefits (Zheng et al., 2022).

Long-chain omega-3 PUFAs to dietary intake should be promoted specifically for people in their middle ages and older adults in order to hinder cognitive deterioration and Alzheimer's disease progression. Dietary interventions need to begin early so cognitive issues do not develop, which supports the response before symptom manifestation. Future research needs to work on maximizing drug dosages with other nutrient combinations to obtain maximum neuroprotective benefits (Wood et al., 2022). During pregnancy, omega-3 PUFAs benefit maternal health by improving metabolic function and insulin sensitivity, and so decrease the occurrence of gestational diabetes together with its related complications. Omega-3 PUFAs help fetal brain development and decrease both preterm delivery and macrosomia rates. A daily intake of

TABLE 5.2 Comparative evaluation of polyunsaturated fatty acid (PUFA) sources based on type, bioavailability, sustainability, and cost-effectiveness.

Source	Primary types of PUFAs	Bioavailability	Sustainability	Cost-effectiveness	References
Algae (microalgae)	Eicosapentaenoic acid (EPA), docosahexaenoic acid (DHA), arachidonic acid (ARA), DPA	The body effectively absorbs EPA and DHA because of their high bioavailability.	The cultivation method shows high sustainability because it can operate on nonarable soil that does not interfere with food agriculture.	The manufacturing and extrusion expenses make this material costly, yet technological advancements are reducing these costs.	Chen et al. (2023); Remize et al. (2021); Santin et al. (2021)
Marine (fish)	EPA, DHA	Its wide consumption along with effective absorption makes this high bioavailability levels.	Environmental sustainability faces two main obstacles, including overfishing along with water pollution issues.	The cost level remains moderate while both fishery resources and processing determine the total expense.	Chen et al. (2023); (Duan et al., 2023)
Microbial innovation	EPA, DHA	Synthetic pathways for production have efficient processes that match fish source bioavailability levels.	This technology uses sustainable methods that prevent depending on fish stocks and has potential for industrial production.	Modern advances in fermentation technology lead to cost reduction.	Chen et al. (2023); Remize et al. (2021); Santin et al. (2021)
Animal source	ALA, EPA, DHA	The bioavailability of enriched products varies across tissues, while these products tend to accumulate in specific tissues.	Sustainability exists at a moderate level depending on the quality of animal feed and farming procedures.	The approach delivers cost-efficient animal feed production, although it cannot match algae's direct efficiency.	Rodríguez et al. (2019)
Plants	ALA, linoleic acid	The bioavailability rate of PUFAs is moderate, while humans have limited ability to change it into long-chain PUFAs such as EPA and DHA.	A highly sustainable crop that grows easily with wide availability and easy cultivation.	Plant oils such as flaxseed and walnuts are easily accessible at affordable prices.	Ramsden et al. (2011); Rizzo et al. (2023)
Genetically engineered plants	EPA, DHA	The bioavailability of PUFAs can be enhanced by genetically modifying their profile	This sustainable system decreases ocean-based resource usage and maximizes agricultural potential.	The initial expenses are elevated since the technology necessitates research and development, yet commercialization will reduce costs	Santin et al. (2021)

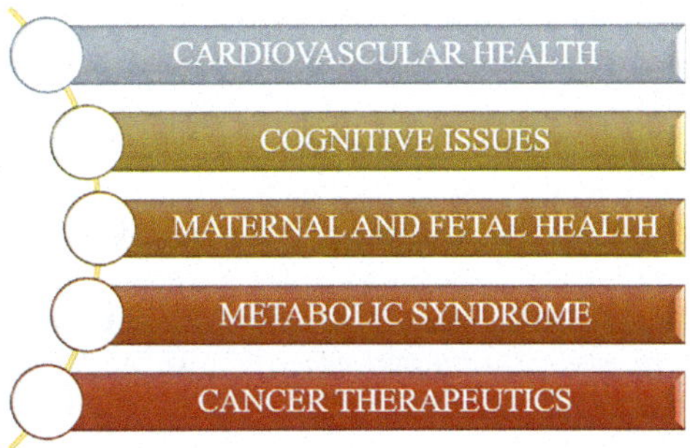

FIGURE 5.5 **Therapeutic roles of eicosapentanoic acid and docosahexanoic acid in supporting human health.**

200–300 mg per day of omega-3 PUFAs provides optimal results (Elshani et al., 2021). The dietary recommendation advises people to lower their dietary intake of SFAs in order to swap these out with PUFAs, viz., n-3 (omega-3) and n-6 (omega-6) to minimize metabolic disorders. High n-6 PUFAs and an elevated n-6/n-3 ratio occur as a result of Western-type dietary patterns. The n-6/n-3 ratio in dietary intake plays a vital role in disease prevention since linolenic acid (LA, 18:3 n-3) along with its longer-chain n-3 PUFAs reduces inflammation (Liput et al., 2021). Integrating PUFAs in place of SFAs results in positive results for insulin sensitivity, together with better glycemic regulation. Dietary substitutions have the potential to deliver special advantages to treatments that aim to prevent type 2 diabetes while improving metabolic health (Telle-Hansen et al., 2019). Tumor cells preferentially absorb fatty acids from PUFAs, which leads to enhanced selective drug delivery that reduces toxicities for healthy tissues (Wang et al., 2012). EPA and DHA have many health benefits as depicted in Fig. 5.5.

5.10 Conclusion

PUFAs play a vital role in the cardiovascular system, nervous system, and inflammation control, yet reliance on marine fish as the primary source is increasingly limited by sustainability, overfishing, and contamination concerns. Sustainable alternatives from microalgae, microbial fermentation, genetically engineered crops, and selected nonmarine sources now offer efficient and scalable solutions for omega-3 fatty acid production, particularly DHA and EPA. Advances in synthetic biology, strain optimization, and fermentation technology have significantly improved production efficiency, purity, and cost-effectiveness. The growing shift toward plant-based and environmentally responsible diets further strengthens the demand for microbe- and plant-derived omega-3 sources. In addition, progress in encapsulation technologies continues to enhance PUFA stability, bioavailability, and shelf life for applications in the food, pharmaceutical, and nutraceutical industries. Future growth of the PUFA market will be driven by AI-assisted strain development, hybrid biosynthetic pathways, and strong industry–academia collaborations, ensuring broad consumer access while maintaining ecological sustainability. Overall, diversification of PUFA sources represents a critical strategy for securing long-term nutritional and environmental health.

References

Adarme-Vega, T. C., Lim, D. K. Y., Timmins, M., Vernen, F., Li, Y., & Schenk, P. M. (2012). Microalgal biofactories: A promising approach towards sustainable omega-3 fatty acid production. *Microbial Cell Factories, 11*. https://doi.org/10.1186/1475-2859-11-96Australia, http://www.microbialcellfactories.com/content/11/1/96.

Allemann, M. N., Shulse, C. N., & Allen, E. E. (2019). Linkage of marine bacterial polyunsaturated fatty acid and long-chain hydrocarbon biosynthesis. *Frontiers in Microbiology, 10*, 702. https://doi.org/10.3389/fmicb.2019.00702.

Chen, W., Li, T., Du, S., Chen, H., & Wang, Q. (2023). Microalgal polyunsaturated fatty acids: Hotspots and production techniques. *Frontiers in Bioengineering and Biotechnology, 11*, 1146881. https://doi.org/10.3389/fbioe.2023.1146881.

Duan, H., Song, W., Zhao, J., & Yan, W. (2023). Polyunsaturated fatty acids (PUFAs): Sources, digestion, absorption, application and their potential adjunctive effects on visual fatigue. *Nutrients, 15*(11), 2633. https://doi.org/10.3390/nu15112633.

Elshani, B., Kotori, V., & Daci, A. (2021). Role of omega-3 polyunsaturated fatty acids in gestational diabetes, maternal and fetal insights: Current use and future directions. *The Journal of Maternal-Fetal & Neonatal Medicine, 34*(1), 124–136. https://doi.org/10.1080/14767058.2019.1593361.

Fasel, N. J., Mene-Saffrane, L., Ruczynski, I., Komar, E., & Christe, P. (2017). Diet induced modifications of fatty-acid composition in mealworm larvae (Tenebrio molitor). *Journal of Food Research, 6*(5), 22. https://doi.org/10.5539/jfr.v6n5p22.

Givens, D. I. (2005). The role of animal nutrition in improving the nutritive value of animal-derived foods in relation to chronic disease. *Proceedings of the Nutrition Society, 64*(3), 395–402. https://doi.org/10.1079/pns2005448.

Gladyshev, M. I., Makhutova, O. N., Gubanenko, G. A., Rechkina, E. A., Kalachova, G. S., & Sushchik, N. N. (2015). Livers of terrestrial production animals as a source of long-chain polyunsaturated fatty acids for humans: An alternative to fish? *European Journal of Lipid Science and Technology, 117*(9), 1417–1421. https://doi.org/10.1002/ejlt.201400449, http://www3.interscience.wiley.com/journal/69502350/home.

Guo, P., Dong, L., Wang, F., Chen, L., & Zhang, W. (2022). Deciphering and engineering the polyunsaturated fatty acid synthase pathway from eukaryotic microorganisms. *Frontiers in Bioengineering and Biotechnology, 10*, 1052785. https://doi.org/10.3389/fbioe.2022.1052785.

Jovanovic, S., Dietrich, D., Becker, J., Kohlstedt, M., & Wittmann, C. (2021). Microbial production of polyunsaturated fatty acids—High-value ingredients for aquafeed, superfoods, and pharmaceuticals. *Current Opinion in Biotechnology, 69*, 199–211. https://doi.org/10.1016/j.copbio.2021.01.009.

Kannan, N., Rao, A. S., & Nair, A. (2021). Microbial production of omega-3 fatty acids: An overview. *Journal of Applied Microbiology, 131*(5), 2114–2130. https://doi.org/10.1111/jam.15034.

Kouba, M., & Mourot, J. (2011). A review of nutritional effects on fat composition of animal products with special emphasis on n-3 polyunsaturated fatty acids. *Biochimie, 93*(1), 13–17. https://doi.org/10.1016/j.biochi.2010.02.027.

Kumari, P., Kumar, M., Gupta, V., Reddy, C. R. K., & Jha, B. (2010). Tropical marine macroalgae as potential sources of nutritionally important PUFAs. *Food Chemistry, 120*(3), 749–757. https://doi.org/10.1016/j.foodchem.2009.11.006.

Liput, K. P., Lepczyński, A., Ogłuszka, M., Nawrocka, A., Poławska, E., Grzesiak, A., Ślaska, B., Pareek, C. S., Czarnik, U., & Pierzchała, M. (2021). Effects of dietary n–3 and n–6 polyunsaturated fatty acids in inflammation and cancerogenesis. *International Journal of Molecular Sciences, 22*(13). https://doi.org/10.3390/ijms22136965, https://www.mdpi.com/1422-0067/22/13/6965/pdf.

Liu, H., Wang, F., Liu, X., Xie, Y., Xia, H., Wang, S., & Sun, G. (2022). Effects of marine-derived and plant-derived omega-3 polyunsaturated fatty acids on erythrocyte fatty acid composition in type 2 diabetic patients. *Lipids in Health and Disease, 21*(1). https://doi.org/10.1186/s12944-022-01630-0.

Lupette, J., & Benning, C. (2020). Human health benefits of very-long-chain polyunsaturated fatty acids from microalgae. *Biochimie, 178*, 15–25. https://doi.org/10.1016/j.biochi.2020.04.022.

Marques, A., Canada, P., Costa, C., Basto, A., Piloto, F., Salgado, M. A., Abreu, H., Dias, J., & Valente, L. M. P. (2023). Replacement of fish oil by alternative n-3 LC-PUFA rich lipid sources in diets for European sea bass (Dicentrarchus labrax). *Frontiers in Marine Science, 10*. https://doi.org/10.3389/fmars.2023.1189319, https://www.frontiersin.org/journals/marine-science#.

Mititelu, M., Lupuliasa, D., Neacşu, S. M., Olteanu, G., Busnatu, Ştefan S., Mihai, A., Popovici, V., Măru, N., Boroghină, S. C., Mihai, S., Ioniță-Mîndrican, C.-B., & Scafa-Udrişte, A. (2024). Polyunsaturated fatty acids and human health: A key to modern nutritional balance in association with polyphenolic compounds from food sources. *Foods, 14*(1), 46. https://doi.org/10.3390/foods14010046.

Mozaffarian, D., Ascherio, A., Hu, F. B., Stampfer, M. J., Willett, W. C., Siscovick, D. S., & Rimm, E. B. (2005). Interplay between different polyunsaturated fatty acids and risk of coronary heart disease in men. *Circulation, 111*(2), 157–164. https://doi.org/10.1161/01.CIR.0000152099.87287.83.

Patel, A., Matsakas, L., Hrůzová, K., Rova, U., & Christakopoulos, P. (2019). Biosynthesis of nutraceutical fatty acids by the oleaginous marine microalgae phaeodactylum tricornutum utilizing hydrolysates from organosolv-pretreated birch and spruce biomass. *Marine drugs, 17*(2), 119. https://doi.org/10.3390/md17020119.

Pereira, H., Barreira, L., Figueiredo, F., Custódio, L., Vizetto-Duarte, C., Polo, C., Rešek, E., Engelen, A., & Varela, J. (2012). Polyunsaturated fatty acids of marine macroalgae: Potential for nutritional and pharmaceutical applications. *Marine Drugs, 10*(9), 1920–1935. https://doi.org/10.3390/md10091920.

Ramesh Kumar, B., Deviram, G., Mathimani, T., Duc, P. A., & Pugazhendhi, A. (2019). Microalgae as rich source of polyunsaturated fatty acids. *Biocatalysis and Agricultural Biotechnology, 17*, 583–588. https://doi.org/10.1016/j.bcab.2019.01.017, http://www.journals.elsevier.com/biocatalysis-and-agricultural-biotechnology/.

Ramsden, C. E., Hibbeln, J. R., & Majchrzak-Hong, S. F. (2011). All PUFAs are not created equal: Absence of CHD benefit specific to linoleic acid in randomized controlled trials and prospective observational cohorts. In In. A. P. Simopoulos (Vol. Ed.), *World review of nutrition and dietetics: Vol. 102*, (pp. 30–43). S. Karger AG. https://doi.org/10.1159/000327789.

Remize, M., Brunel, Y., Silva, J. L., Berthon, J.-Y., & Filaire, E. (2021). Microalgae n-3 PUFAs production and use in food and feed industries. *Marine drugs, 19*(2), 113. https://doi.org/10.3390/md19020113.

Rix, L., De Goeij, J. M., Mueller, C. E., Struck, U., Middelburg, J. J., Van Duyl, F. C., Al-Horani, F. A., Wild, C., Naumann, M. S., & Van Oevelen, D. (2016). Coral mucus fuels the sponge loop in warm-and cold-water coral reef ecosystems. *Scientific Reports, 6*. https://doi.org/10.1038/srep18715, www.nature.com/srep/index.html.

Rizzo, G., Baroni, L., & Lombardo, M. (2023). Promising sources of plant-derived polyunsaturated fatty acids: A narrative review. *International Journal of Environmental Research and Public Health, 20*(3), 1683. https://doi.org/10.3390/ijerph20031683.

Rodríguez, M., G. Rebollar, P., Mattioli, S., & Castellini, C. (2019). n-3 PUFA sources (precursor/products): A review of current knowledge on rabbit. *Animals: An Open Access Journal from MDPI, 9*(10), 806. https://doi.org/10.3390/ani9100806.

Saini, R. K., Prasad, P., Sreedhar, R. V., Naidu, K. A., Shang, X., & Keum, Y. S. (2021). Omega–3 polyunsaturated fatty acids (PUFAs): Emerging plant and microbial sources, oxidative stability, bioavailability, and health benefits—A review. *Antioxidants, 10*(10). https://doi.org/10.3390/antiox10101627, https://www.mdpi.com/2076-3921/10/10/1627/pdf.

Santin, A., Russo, M. T., Ferrante, M. I., Balzano, S., Orefice, I., & Sardo, A. (2021). Highly valuable polyunsaturated fatty acids from microalgae: Strategies to improve their yields and their potential exploitation in aquaculture. *Molecules, 26*(24), 7697. https://doi.org/10.3390/molecules26247697.

Santin, A., Balzano, S., Russo, M. T., Palma Esposito, F., Ferrante, M. I., Blasio, M., Cavalletti, E., & Sardo, A. (2022). Microalgae-based PUFAs for food and feed: Current applications, future possibilities, and constraints. *Journal of Marine Science and Engineering, 10*(7), 844. https://doi.org/10.3390/jmse10070844.

Shah, A. M., Yang, W., Mohamed, H., Zhang, Y., & Song, Y. (2022). Microbes: A hidden treasure of polyunsaturated fatty acids. *Frontiers in Nutrition, 9*, 827837. https://doi.org/10.3389/fnut.2022.827837.

Shahidi, F., & Ambigaipalan, P. (2018). Omega-3 polyunsaturated fatty acids and their health benefits. *Annual Review of Food Science and Technology, 9*(1), 345–381. https://doi.org/10.1146/annurev-food-111317-095850.

Shanab, S. M. M., Hafez, R. M., & Fouad, A. S. (2018). A review on algae and plants as potential source of arachidonic acid. *Journal of Advanced Research, 11*, 3–13. https://doi.org/10.1016/j.jare.2018.03.004.

Sprague, M., Betancor, M. B., & Tocher, D. R. (2017). Microbial and genetically engineered oils as replacements for fish oil in aquaculture feeds. *Biotechnology Letters, 39*(11), 1599–1609. https://doi.org/10.1007/s10529-017-2402-6.

Sun, K., Meesapyodsuk, D., & Qiu, X. (2024). Biosynthetic mechanisms of omega-3 polyunsaturated fatty acids in microalgae. *Journal of Biological Chemistry, 300*(9), 107699. https://doi.org/10.1016/j.jbc.2024.107699.

Telle-Hansen, V. H., Gaundal, L., & Myhrstad, M. C. W. (2019). Polyunsaturated fatty acids and glycemic control in type 2 diabetes. *Nutrients, 11*(5), 1067. https://doi.org/10.3390/nu11051067.

Uttaro, A. D. (2006). Biosynthesis of polyunsaturated fatty acids in lower eukaryotes. *IUBMB Life, 58*(10), 563–571. https://doi.org/10.1080/15216540600920899.

Van Ginneken, V. J., Helsper, J. P., De Visser, W., Van Keulen, H., & Brandenburg, W. A. (2011). Polyunsaturated fatty acids in various macroalgal species from the North Atlantic and tropical seas. *Lipids in Health and Disease, 10*(1), 104. https://doi.org/10.1186/1476-511X-10-104.

Wanders, A. J., Blom, W. A. M., Zock, P. L., Geleijnse, J. M., Brouwer, I. A., & Alssema, M. (2019). Plant-derived polyunsaturated fatty acids and markers of glucose metabolism and insulin resistance: A meta-analysis of randomized controlled feeding trials. *BMJ Open Diabetes Research and Care, 7*(1). https://doi.org/10.1136/bmjdrc-2018-000585, http://drc.bmj.com/.

Wang, J., Luo, T., Li, S., & Zhao, J. (2012). The powerful applications of polyunsaturated fatty acids in improving the therapeutic efficacy of anticancer drugs. *Expert Opinion on Drug Delivery, 9*(1), 1–7. https://doi.org/10.1517/17425247.2011.618183.

West, A. L., Miles, E. A., Lillycrop, K. A., Napier, J. A., Calder, P. C., & Burdge, G. C. (2021). Genetically modified plants are an alternative to oily fish for providing n -3 polyunsaturated fatty acids in the human diet: A summary of the findings of a biotechnology and biological sciences research council funded project. *Nutrition Bulletin, 46*(1), 60–68. https://doi.org/10.1111/nbu.12478.

Wiktorowska-Owczarek, A., Berezińska, M., & Nowak, J. Z. (2015). PUFAs: Structures, metabolism and functions. *Advances in Clinical and Experimental Medicine, 24*(6), 931–941. https://doi.org/10.17219/acem/31243.

Wood, A. H. R., Chappell, H. F., & Zulyniak, M. A. (2022). Dietary and supplemental long-chain omega-3 fatty acids as moderators of cognitive impairment and Alzheimer's disease. *European Journal of Nutrition, 61*(2), 589–604. https://doi.org/10.1007/s00394-021-02655-4.

Zheng, S., Qiu, M., Wu, J. H. Y., Pan, X.-fei, Liu, X., Sun, L., Zhu, H., Wu, J., & Huang, Y. (2022). Long-chain omega-3 polyunsaturated fatty acids and the risk of heart failure. *Therapeutic Advances in Chronic Disease, 13*. https://doi.org/10.1177/20406223221081616.

Zhou, Y., Zhou, S., Duan, H., Wang, J., & Yan, W. (2022). Silkworm pupae: A functional food with health benefits for humans. *Foods, 11*(11), 1594. https://doi.org/10.3390/foods11111594.

Chapter 6

Advances in polyunsaturated fatty acid extraction and purification techniques: innovations in membrane and other technologies

Gokul C.S.[1], Karthikanath P. R.[1,2], Abhiramy D. S.[1], Knawang Chhunji Sherpa[2,3], and Balakumaran Palanisamy Athiyaman[1,2]

[1]*Chemical Sciences and Technology Division, CSIR-National Institute for Interdisciplinary Science and Technology (CSIR-NIIST), Thiruvananthapuram, Kerala, India,* [2]*Academy of Scientific and Innovative Research (AcSIR), Ghaziabad, Uttar Pradesh, India,* [3]*Environmental Technology Division, CSIR-National Institute for Interdisciplinary Science and Technology (CSIR-NIIST), Thiruvananthapuram, Kerala, India*

6.1 Introduction

Fatty acids (FAs) serve as a major fat-soluble component in plants and animals. Based on the presence of double bonds, FAs are broadly categorized as saturated and unsaturated, which are further grouped as monounsaturated or polyunsaturated depending on the degree of unsaturation and chain length (Golijan et al., 2019). With the presence of multiple double bonds, polyunsaturated fatty acids (PUFAs) are a major group of FAs essential for human health, as they constitute the major structural component of cell membranes. They carry out defensive roles against several health conditions such as autoimmune disorders, metabolic complications, fatty liver disease, and other chronic illnesses (Kapoor et al., 2021).

Among the PUFAs, the most essential ones include omega-3 and omega-6 FAs that our human body cannot synthesize and should be taken as diet supplement. Plant oils such as soybean and sunflower oil constitute the primary source of omega-6 FAs, whereas chia, perilla, flax seeds, fatty fish, and marine fish oils are the major sources of omega-3 FAs. Researches are focussing on the key omega-6 FAs such as linoleic acid and arachidonic acid and omega-3 FAs such as eicosapentaenoic acid (EPA), docosahexaenoic acid (DHA), and α-linoleic acid (ALA). Together, these PUFAs play crucial roles in maintaining cardiovascular and neurological health, preventing inflammation, and reducing the risk of certain cancers such as colorectal, breast, and prostate (Kromhout & de Goede, 2014). EPA and DHA are also vital for fetal development. These have been shown to enhance infant immunity and reduce allergy incidence with maternal supplementation (Adarme-Vega et al., 2012). Omega-3 supplementation can regulate cytokine production, thereby better management of autoimmune diseases and improving the quality of life in cancer patients. Altogether, omega-3 and omega-6 FAs among the PUFAs play a profound role in maintaining physiological functions, metabolism, and homeostasis.

Marine fish oil has traditionally been the primary source of EPA and DHA. Even though fish themselves cannot produce these FAs, they depend on microalgae (Sahena et al., 2009). Nowadays, alternative microbial sources, such as bacteria, yeast, filamentous fungi, and especially microalgae, are emerging as a sustainable source for PUFA production (Venegas-Caleron et al., 2010). Among them, microalgae holds a prime position due to its photosynthetic ability, CO_2 fixation, and reduced environmental footprint, making it both an eco-friendly and scalable option (Xue et al., 2013). Species such as *Schizochytrium*, *Aurantiochytrium*, *Thraustochytrium*, and *Crypthecodinium cohnii* have been identified as safe, nonpathogenic producers of PUFAs. DHA from microalgae is already available in markets (Adarme-Vega et al., 2014). In Fig. 6.1, various natural sources of PUFAs are shown along with their broad range of applications.

Omega-3 and Omega-6 Polyunsaturated Fatty Acids in Food Systems. DOI: https://doi.org/10.1016/B978-0-443-43810-3.00006-3

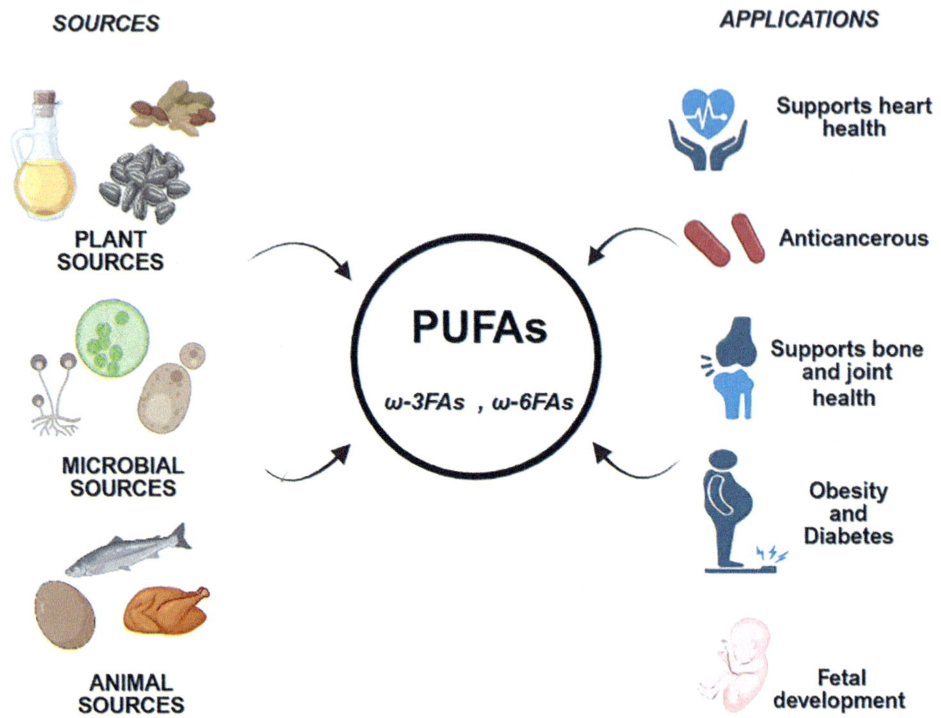

FIGURE 6.1 **Different sources and applications of polyunsaturated fatty acids (PUFAs).** Various natural sources of PUFAs and their importance in human health.
The figure was created with BioRender.com.

Conventional extraction methods are used for separating PUFAs, but they face significant drawbacks such as lengthy processing, high consumption of energy, low yields, and the use of harsh organic solvents. Apart from its consequences in product recovery, these factors may also lead to oxidative degradation of FAs such as omega-3 (Kumar et al., 2020). As a sustainable solution to these, efficient greener alternatives were explored that include the use of supercritical fluids (SCF), eutectic solvents, ionic liquids (ILs), microwave-assisted processes, and enzyme-mediated extraction techniques. By reducing the environmental and economic impact, these emerging methods aim to improve the yield and quality of PUFAs.

The global demand for PUFAs is rising in medical, nutritional, and industrial applications that can only be fulfilled through an innovative, scalable, and sustainable extraction and purification technology. Advancements in membrane-based processes, along with emerging green technologies, provide several opportunities to overcome the drawbacks of traditional methods. This chapter provides insight into advances with more emphasis on membrane-based innovations and complementary approaches that can transform PUFA extraction as well as purification for industrial uses.

6.1.1 Polyunsaturated fatty acids extraction and purification: conventional methods

The potential of PUFAs in preventing various diseases made them an essential supplement for human wellbeing. Increasing demand for these beneficial compounds raised the need for effective methods for extracting PUFAs from their natural sources, such as microalgae, fish oil, and seeds. Conventional methods of PUFA extraction can be categorized into two: mechanical and solvent extraction. Even though these extraction methods have advantages, certain limitations exist regarding the efficiency, cost, and product quality.

6.1.2 Mechanical extraction

Mechanical extraction of oils involves using mechanical, hydraulic, or screw presses, which is one of the oldest methods of oil extraction. By applying compressive forces, mechanical extraction can bring about efficient liquid–solid separation of compounds (Nde & Foncha, 2020). PUFA-rich oil extraction using mechanical methods is a critical, solvent-free approach that can produce high-quality edible oils and nutraceuticals. This method, known as cold pressing or expeller pressing, applies physical pressure to oil-containing sources, such as seeds or microalgae. The pressure causes the release of lipid content through the rupture of the cell walls of the seed or microalgae (Masoodi et al., 2022). However, low extraction efficiency is the major drawback of mechanical extraction, with a notable residual oil content in the solid press-cake (Ali & Watson, 2014). This can only be rectified through the processing of seeds for maximizing the product yield.

6.1.3 Solvent extraction

Liquid–liquid extraction is one of the commonly used conventional extraction methods using solvents for the isolation of PUFA from various sources. This method is usually carried out by effective dissolution of lipids, homogenization of the source material, followed by organic solvent treatment. Many studies have shown hexane as a good solvent choice for frequent oil extraction from high-lipid sources like fish (Sahena et al., 2009). The Bligh and Dyer method is one among the well-known solvent extraction techniques that uses a chloroform and methanol mixture for maximal lipid extraction from various biomass like microalgae (Sharma et al., 2020). Even though high extraction yield can be expected using these techniques, there exist certain limitations. Using toxic and flammable solvents led to environmental and safety concerns. Additionally, the presence of residual solvents added to the concerns regarding human consumption of these products (Rubio-Rodriguez et al., 2010). Later on, researchers were oriented towards developing alternative and sustainable methods that can resolve the existing drawbacks in conventional solvent extraction.

The Soxhlet extraction is an organic solvent extraction technique that employs a Soxhlet apparatus for the extraction of PUFA. In this method, oil contained in the sample is extracted using organic solvents, and the extraction efficiency depends on factors such as reaction time, solvent type, seed size, and processing temperature. In Soxhlet extraction, an enhanced yield of the desired product can be achieved through the repeated contact of samples with the extractant. Soxhlet extraction is adopted as the standard PUFA extraction technique due to its easy operation and cost effectiveness (Zhou, Ding, et al., 2022; Zhou, Wang, et al., 2022). Thermal degradation of lipids was reported in Soxhlet extraction due to the high temperature and prolonged extraction time (Zhang et al., 2018). The application of the Soxhlet method is confined to analytical purposes rather than large-scale PUFA production, mainly due to the reduction in product purity with the presence of residual solvents.

6.2 Urea complexation

Urea complexation is a significant technique used for purifying and concentrating PUFAs, using the difference in molecular shape between saturated, monounsaturated, and the more bent structure of PUFAs. Urea is capable of producing a crystalline lattice with straight-chain molecules. When the FA mixture is cooled with urea, the linear chains of saturated and monounsaturated FAs will get firmly attached to the helical channels in the urea crystal. Whereas the bent structure of unsaturated FAs excludes them from the crystal structure, and they remain in the liquid phase. This selective crystallization results in the unreacted liquid fraction enriched with PUFAs, which can be subjected to further processing. Diagrammatic representation of the urea complexation is depicted in Fig. 6.2.

The effectiveness of PUFA extraction through urea complexation is dependent on several factors, such as reaction time, urea concentration, and the ratio of urea to FAs (Chen & et al., 2023). Several modifications have been attempted in this method, such as urea adduction that could enrich the PUFA yield from seal oil (Zheng et al., 2018). This technique is found to be beneficial as this approach is mild and nondestructive, avoiding harsh chemicals, thereby protecting PUFAs from degradation and oxidation (Shimada et al., 2001). In a recent study, enzymatic oil was extracted from common kilka (*Clupeonella cultiventris),* from which DHA and EPA were concentrated using the urea complexation method. In this study, response surface methodology was used to optimize process variables such as crystallization temperature, crystallization time, and urea-FA ratio in order to increase the yield of DHA and EPA. Through this study, the yield of DHA and EPA increased from 13.32% and 5.39% in crude oil to 58.36% and 12.07% in omega-3 PUFA concentrates (Eskandari et al., 2024). Urea complexation is a promising method for the industrial purification of PUFAs that can be widely used for pharmaceuticals or food supplements.

6.2.1 Molecular distillation

Molecular distillation is an essential technique for purifying and concentrating PUFAs, particularly for producing high-purity omega-3 concentrates. This short-path distillation method operates under a very high vacuum, typically less than 1 Pascal. The low pressure significantly reduces the boiling point of the compounds, which allows separation of the compounds at much lower temperatures than conventional distillation methods. Due to the high degree of unsaturation,

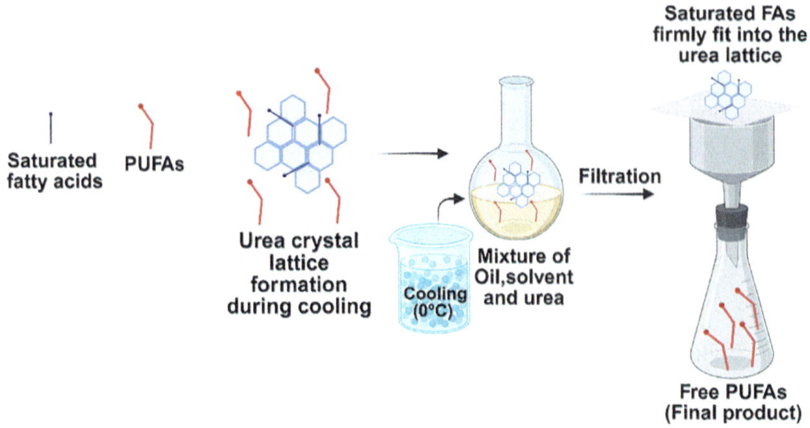
Saturated FAs
firmly fit into the
urea lattice
Saturated
fatty acids
PUFAs
Urea crystal
lattice
formation
during cooling
Filtration
Mixture of
Oil,solvent
and urea
Cooling
(0°C)
Free PUFAs
(Final product)

FIGURE 6.2 **Urea complexation.** Schematic representation of the purification of polyunsaturated fatty acids (PUFAs) through the urea complexation method.
The figure was created with BioRender.com.

PUFAs are extremely susceptible to thermal degradation and oxidation. Thus molecular distillation is an efficient method which reduces damage that can affect the stability of the desired product (Shimada et al., 2001). By operating at low temperatures and with a very short residence time, molecular distillation effectively minimizes damage to the FA molecules.

The separation of PUFAs using molecular distillation is based on the differences in the molecular weight and boiling point of the individual components in the mixture. This technique involves heating the oil and spreading it as a thin film onto a heated surface. Molecules with lower molecular weight, which involve unwanted volatile impurities, evaporate and get condensed on a nearby cooled surface. The remaining heavier, less volatile PUFA-rich fraction persists in the liquid phase, that can be separately collected (Wanasundara et al., 2005). This technique will often be adopted as a final step of concentrating PUFA obtained from other conventional extraction processes (González-Fernández et al., 2017). As molecular distillation can bring about PUFA with high concentration and purity, this auspicious method is adopted for industrial-scale PUFA purification for different applications (Harimana et al., 2016). In a recent study, Meng et al. (2025) used the microalgae *Nanochloropsis gaditana* for the extraction of PUFA, particularly EPA, using molecular distillation combined with subcritical butane. This resulted in a lipid extract with an enhanced EPA content of 58.92% w/w. In their current study, antihyperlipidemic effects of the final extract were studied on mouse models.

6.3 Membrane-based innovations in the extraction and purification of polyunsaturated fatty acids

PUFAs such as EPA, DHA, and ALA are valuable lipids prized in nutrition, pharmaceuticals, and functional foods. However, their tendency to oxidize or degrade under heat, combined with the complex nature of their sources ranging from biomass and microbial cultures to fish and seed oils, poses two main downstream hurdles which includes efficient release of PUFA-rich fractions from their matrices, and selectively purifying or concentrating them from other lipids, polar impurities, and unwanted volatile compounds, without compromising quality (Abdorrezaee & Raisi, 2021; Lv et al., 2020). In recent years, technologies that utilize membrane separation are emerging as a flexible, energy-saving tool that can work together with or can displace traditional solvent extractions, such as distillation and chromatography. This section mainly focuses on the recent revolutions and practical approaches for making use of membranes in the processing of PUFA.

Membrane-based separation methods provide certain advantages, such as improved selectivity and considerable control over the mixing levels of different components (Lv et al., 2020). Membranes are mainly classified as inorganic, organic, or composite. Inorganic membranes—such as ceramic, carbon, and zeolite types—are mainly appraised for their magnificent resistance against harsh acidic and alkaline conditions, along with their ability to tolerate high temperatures, making them a better choice in highly demanded areas. However, their wide applicability is restricted by problems such as brittleness, high cost of production, and difficulties in obtaining optimal structural formation (Ghasemian et al., 2017). On the other hand, polymeric membranes offer superiority in operational flexibility, low production and operating costs, ease in fabrication, and are common attributes in pressure-driven separation processes (Lv et al., 2020). The working of a membrane is largely controlled by factors such as composition of the material, working temperature, flow rate, pressure applied, surface characteristics, and the nature of the raw materials utilized in the production of such membranes (Ghosh, 2007). The pore size of a membrane is the deciding factor in getting superior FAs, as the separation relies upon the molecular dimensions of the components in the mixture. Therefore membrane selection is mainly influenced by pore size or its affinity for the permeating species (Atadashi et al., 2011).

Membrane technologies can be used in nearly all stages of oil processing, which extends solutions to many drawbacks associated with conventional methods. Microfiltration (MF), ultrafiltration (UF), and nanofiltration (NF) contribute as promising alternatives for dewaxing, degumming, and deacidification (and even for bleaching), respectively (Salehi, 2014). In addition, NF, reverse osmosis (RO), and pervaporation (PV) present efficient options for solvent recovery. UF is one of the most common membrane processes for the separation of FAs. The method primarily separates different molecules from a mixture utilizing pressure and is capable of providing high-quality permeates (Benítez et al., 2009). Nowadays, this kind of membrane separation is widely applicable in the fat and oil industry as well, and many studies have been carried out in the recovery of solvent, removal of color from vegetable oils, and for deacidification of oils and phospholipids (Vaisali et al., 2015).

6.3.1 Ultrafiltration and microfiltration

UF is a pressure-driven membrane-based technique in which a porous membrane with a pore size ranging from 2–100 nm enables separation of nanometer-sized particles in the feed of water or conventional organic solvents via a size sieving mechanism under a concentration gradient (Hampu et al., 2020; Mah et al., 2012). This employed hydrophilic flat-sheet polyvinylidene fluoride (PVDF) membranes (MWCO 30 kDa, effective area 0.00146 m^2) in a dead-end stirred cell setup. Prior to use, membranes were soaked, wetted, and compacted under 2 bar nitrogen at room temperature. Experiments were conducted at 60°C and 2 bar with oleic acid (OA) concentrations ranging from 0.003–0.1 g/L. Results showed that OA rejection increased with concentration, reaching upto 98.6% at 0.1 g/L in a 15% glycerol solution (Mah et al., 2012). Ghasemian et al. (2017) concentrated omega-3 PUFA from lantern fish oil using a flat-sheet fluoropolymer/polypropylene UF membrane (ETNA01PP, 1 kDa MWCO) under nitrogen. Using a Box–Behnken design, they optimized temperature, pressure, and stirring, achieving a maximum omega-3 PUFA content of 35.1 wt.% at 36.2°C, 4.8 bar, and 43 rpm. After 3 hours of working, a reduction in omega-3 concentration and oil flux to 7.8% and 32.6% was observed, indicating a stability loss. Tonon et al. in 2016 introduced an UF system with ceramic membranes (10–20 kDa, Pall Corporation), which was coupled with an enzyme hydrolysis unit for separating protein hydrolysates from sardine and shrimp cooking effluents (Tonon et al., 2016).

Ceramic membranes are capable of offering high resistance but suffer from brittleness and are expensive. Comparatively, polymeric substances are inexpensive and flexible but fragile. To overcome these drawbacks, composite membranes with outstanding thermal and chemical stability were discovered. Composite inorganic-organic membranes add on the strengths of both, providing efficient separation (Aliasghari Aghdam et al., 2015). Membrane preparation using the polymer, PVDF, which is a widely used polymer, was attempted due to its excellent mechanical and thermal strength. However, the separation efficiency using PVDF cannot meet industrial requirements. To overcome these drawbacks, PVDF has been coupled with inorganic particles through chemical grafting, physical blending, and surface modification, focusing on its organic-inorganic synergy. Metal oxide additives, such as Al_2O_3, TiO_2, and SiO_2, have been commonly used, among which silica is well known for its high thermal stability, reactivity, and desirable chemical properties (Azmi et al., 2015; Bai et al., 2012). Ghasemian et al. (2017) created asymmetric PVDF/SiO_2 nanocomposite membranes (MWCO 275 kDa) using PVDF and nanoporous silica. Performance of such membranes was assessed for concentrating omega-3 PUFA from lantern fish oil at 4 bar and 30°C under a nitrogen atmosphere in batch mode. Membranes containing 15 wt.% silica achieved a PUFA concentration of 53.9 wt.%, a 19.1% improvement over neat PVDF membranes (34.8 wt. %), while also exhibiting superior antifouling properties. To improve the hydrolysis of oils and fats for FA production, Lv et al. (2018) fabricated a high-temperature-resistant polyethersulfone hollow-fiber UF membrane (MWCO 6 kDa) via gel phase inversion. The process combined membrane separation with atmospheric-pressure hydrolysis of lard using sulfonated cation exchange resin as a heterogeneous catalyst (Lv et al., 2018). This study, conducted by Sallet and his coworkers, investigated concentrating FAs from oil/solvent mixtures obtained via ultrasound-assisted extraction of *Mortierella isabellina* using UF and NF membranes, achieving oil retentions of 45.23%–58.20% and 43.50%–56.00%, respectively, with optimal conditions at 4 bar/40°C (UF) and 12 bar/50°C (NF), producing biodiesel-suitable oil rich in oleic and palmitic acids and demonstrating strong potential for efficient solvent recovery (Sallet et al., 2020).

Over the past decade, covalent organic framework (COF)-based membranes have gained attention for their well-defined crystalline structures and uniform pore size distribution, enabling highly selective separations. They have been applied in gas separation, ion removal, and dye filtration, though their use in organic solvent nanofiltration (OSN) remains relatively unexplored (Asadi Tashvigh & Benes, 2022). A study conducted by Ranasinghe Arachchige and his colleagues reports the first successful use of COF–based mixed matrix membranes for the selective separation of C18 FAs and fatty acid methyl esters (FAMEs) from vegetable oils. Traditional polymeric membranes lack precision due to wide pore size distributions, whereas COFs offer highly ordered, nanometer-scale pores (1.3–3.4 nm) that help in separation based on degrees of unsaturation. COFs were produced, characterized, and incorporated (10–20 wt.%) into a polyepoxy matrix to fabricate membranes. The 1.8 nm COF–epoxy membrane showed the highest selectivity, with methyl stearate permeating 5.9 times faster than methyl linolenate. This technique provides a cost-effective and renewable alternative to conventional methods, supporting efficient production of high purity, biorenewable FAs and FAMEs for industrial uses (Ranasinghe Arachchige et al., 2023).

6.3.2 Nanofiltration and reverse osmosis

NF and RO enable pressure-driven, composition-based separations that surpass simple size exclusion. NF is exquisite for concentrating free FAs and monoglyceride/diglyceride fractions in nonaqueous or solvent-modified streams; it can attain moderate fractionation based on size and charge/polarity variations. RO, which was typically applied to desalination or solvent removal, has been used as a polishing step to desolvate or desalt polar extracts before final PUFA formulation (Ghalamara et al., 2022). OSN, started in the 1990s, has gained attention in pharmaceuticals and fine chemicals for separating, concentrating, and purifying high-value hydrophobic compounds from organic solvents (Marchetti et al., 2014). Utilizing polymeric or ceramic membranes with MWCOs of 100–1000 kDa, OSN specifically operates under pressure-driven mode (30–100 bar), though diafiltration-based concentration has also been applied (Santos-Sánchez et al., 2016).

Membrane processes impart an efficient and sustainable effort for recovering high-value compounds from fish processing effluents, helping in the development of functional ingredients, excluding solvents or adsorbents. NF enables a selective fractionation by the combination of size exclusion and electrostatic (Donnan) effects, which permits partial passage of monovalent salts while retaining larger molecules. Given the size variability of peptides, techniques such as UF, NF, and RO are effective in their separation (Tonon et al., 2016). Kwiatkowski and Cheryan investigated corn oil recovery from ethanol extracts using various NF membranes (DK, TFC-SR1, and TFC-SR2). They achieved oil concentrations above 100 g/L, with results showing that increasing the volume concentration ratio significantly enhanced oil content, demonstrating the effectiveness of NF membranes for concentrating corn oil from ethanol extracts (Kwiatkowski & Cheryan, 2005).

6.3.3 Pervaporation

PV is a membrane-assisted evaporation technique where a selective membrane separates volatile species (e.g., solvents, aroma compounds) from nonvolatiles; volatiles permeate as vapor under a vacuum/permeate sweep (Dawiec et al., 2015). For PUFA processing, PV offers two important applications; first one is the gentle removal of residual solvents after extraction (e.g., ethanol removal) without high temperatures that would oxidize PUFAs, and the second one is the recovery and concentration of desirable volatile bioactives or the removal of low-molecular-weight off-flavors produced during extraction.

PV with organophilic membranes offers an efficient method for separating VOCs, relying on the preferential sorption and diffusion of organic molecules across a dense membrane, followed by desorption under vacuum. This technique is particularly effective at low VOC concentrations and requires no additional chemicals or regeneration steps, making it a clean and sustainable separation technology (Dawiec et al., 2015). Various hydrophobic polymers such as PDMS, poly(1-(trimethylsilyl)- 1-propyne), poly (octylmethylsiloxane), polyether block amide, etc, have been applied for hexane recovery via PV (Castro-Muñoz, 2019). Among these, PDMS is the most widely used due to its strong hydrophobicity, stability (thermal, mechanical, and chemical), high permeability, availability, and low cost.

6.3.4 Membrane liquid–liquid extraction

Membrane liquid–liquid extraction (MLLE) implements selective transport of solutes across an immiscible membrane phase—useful for transferring free FAs, charged lipid derivatives, or polar contaminants between two liquid phases without direct phase mixing. Recent implementations use supported liquid membranes, polymer inclusion membranes, or emulsion membrane systems tailored to FA partitioning behavior.

Medium-chain fatty acids (C6–C12) are high-value compounds widely used in food, feed, pharmaceuticals, cosmetics, fragrances, antimicrobials, and chemical synthesis, traditionally sourced from palm and coconut oils in Southeast Asia and South America. An efficient alternative involves hollow-fiber MLLE with selective extractants, where, using CE as the model system and 3% (w/v) trioctylphosphine oxide in mineral oil, FAs ranging from C5 to C8 were selectively recovered from short-chain fatty acids-rich broths and concentrated into a semibatch alkaline stripping solution for downstream processing (Taiwo et al., 2024). MLLE offers advantages for PUFA processing, such as low energy demand, operation at ambient conditions, and pH-controlled selective transport of ionizable lipids. Coupled MLLE–membrane cascades can offer better removal of polar impurities than NF/RO or adsorption, even though they face challenges such as loss of solvent, emulsion stability, and membrane durability. The application of solvent-resistant supports and green carrier formulations can address these existing problems.

In conclusion, the recovery, purification, and stabilization of PUFAs can be made versatile, energy-efficient, and renewable through membrane-based technologies. Different techniques, including MF, UF, RO, NF, PV and MLLE, offer the selective extraction of target lipid species through size-based fractionation and solvent recovery for the easy removal of volatiles. Different membrane-based techniques employed in PUFA extraction are represented in Fig. 6.3. Polymeric membranes can provide flexibility with low cost in PUFA extraction. On the other hand, inorganic and hybrid composites result in enhanced thermal and chemical stability. Recent advancements, such as COF-based membranes, offer highly

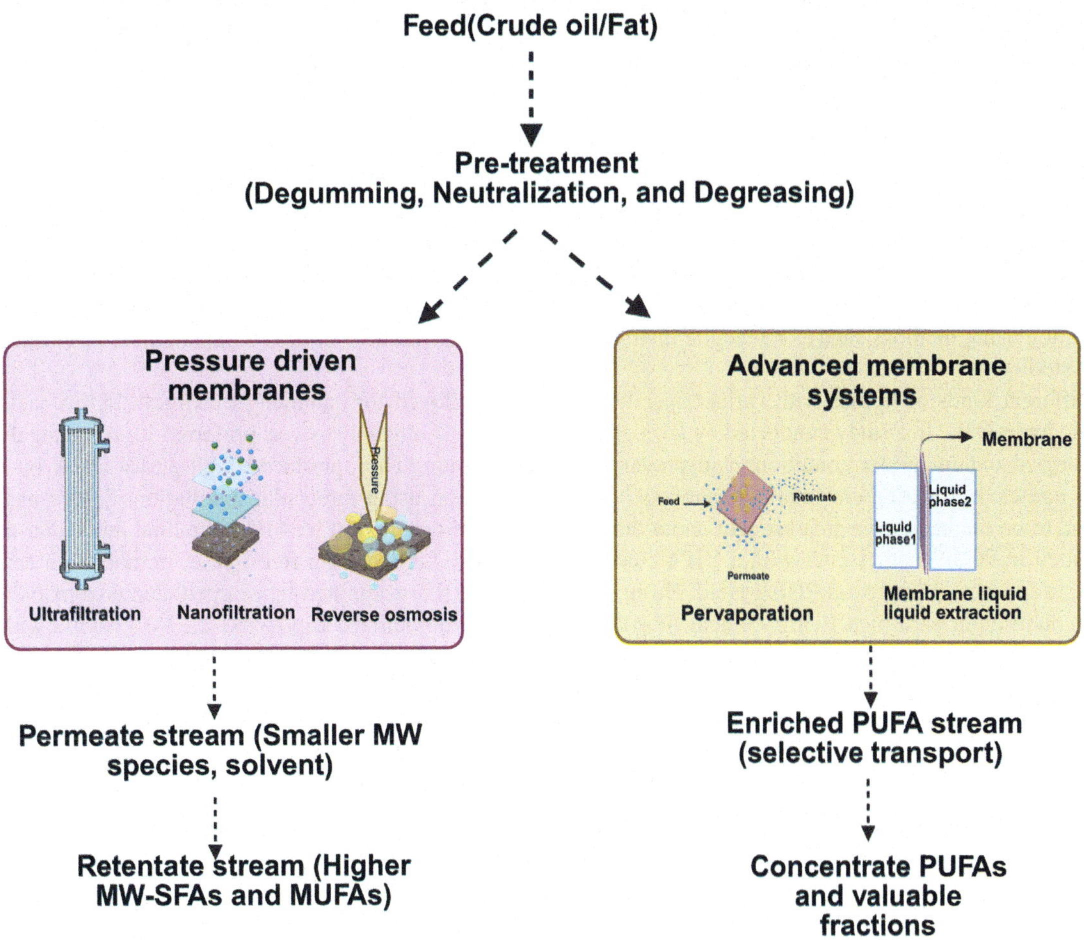

FIGURE 6.3 **Membrane-based separation.** Schematic representation of membrane-based separation of polyunsaturated fatty acids (PUFAs) from crude samples.
The figure was created with BioRender.com.

selective separation. However, these systems face certain limitations, such as fouling, oxidative degradation, and long-term stability issues, which necessitate an integrated process design that combines multiple membrane steps with oxidative control strategies to ensure product quality. Ongoing advances in membrane materials, process optimization, and pilot-scale demonstrations continue to strengthen the potential of these technologies for large-scale PUFA processing in food, pharmaceutical, and nutraceutical industries.

6.4 Other advanced extraction techniques

6.4.1 Microwave-assisted extraction

Microwave-assisted extraction (MAE) is a technique that can extract PUFA in higher yield and quality with comparatively low extraction time. By producing heat through direct microwave conduction to materials, MAE influences subatomic interactions. The generated heat interacts with the water fume arrangement that results in cell disruption, causing an effective intracellular metabolite extraction (Zhou, Ding, et al., 2022; Zhou, Wang, et al., 2022). A study was conducted for the rapid esterification as well as enrichment of omega-3 PUFAs in eggs using MAE. Using microwaves, the esterification efficiency increased from 5.06 to 10.65 times. They also achieved reduced extraction time from 50 to 15 minutes, by incorporating electrically enhanced solid-phase microextraction to MAE (Gu et al., 2024). Studies have also proven that microalgal biomass can become susceptible to the transesterification step after the MAE cycle, even without biomass drying. When the biodiesel recovery using traditional warming took almost 6 hours, MAE was performed in around 15–20 minutes, which reveals MAE as an efficient and affordable strategy for extraction purposes (Kumar et al., 2020). Although microwave extraction is a suitable mode for oil extraction, the feasibility of scaling up using this method should be further analyzed in future work.

6.4.2 Enzyme assisted extraction

The application of enzymes in PUFA concentration is achieved by specific enzymes like lipases, which are capable of catalyzing ethanolysis, transesterification, or hydrolysis of triacylglycerols. The stereospecific activity of certain lipases enables the separation and concentration of omega-3 from the glycerol backbone, resulting in the production of structured lipids. Since using enzymes is simple, inexpensive, and doesn't require high temperatures or organic solvents, it has emerged as a viable substitute for conventional techniques (Rolle, 1998). Enzyme-assisted extraction, followed by PUFA concentration using methods such as molecular distillation, membrane filtration, or urea complexation, has been attempted in many studies.

The different kinds of lipases with variant specificities were employed for achieving maximum PUFA yield through enzymatic hydrolysis. In a study conducted by Li et al. 2024, enzymatic ethanolysis was preferred for microalgal oil which can be carried out in milder conditions and prevents DHA oxidation. They produced high-purity DHA by screening different lipases, optimizing enzymatic ethanolysis, and concentration using molecular distillation. Lipase named UM1 was found to be the best lipase that brought about the highest ethyl ester yield of 95.41%. The final molecular distillation step resulted in 96.52% ethyl ester with a DHA content upto 80.11%. Apart from free lipase, immobilized enzyme was also nurtured to obtain improved PUFA yield. Hasnisa and Jumat (2012) attempted lipase-mediated enzymatic acidolysis to derive palm olein with high PUFA content. For that, they used immobilized Lipozyme TL IM enzyme with reaction conditions such as 50°C, incubation time 24 hours, 10% enzyme, and 1% water in hexane. This resulted in the improved linoleic (24.46%) and α-linolenic acid (3.74%). Sometimes, enzymatic methods are coupled with other methods of concentration to achieve a higher concentration of PUFAs. Nonuse of chemicals and higher PUFA yield were found to be obtained when pretreatment with SCF was done.

6.4.3 Supercritical fluid chromatography

The discovery of SCF is one of the milestones in the process of separating biomolecules. SCFs are defined by pressure, temperature, and density values greater than unity and pressure that is lowered below the threshold required for liquid solidification. The state above this critical point results in a fluid phase that acts as an intermediate between liquid and gas. It can possess density as that of liquids and diffusivity and viscosity comparable to gas (Rubio-Rodríguez et al., 2010). The most widely employed SCF is CO_2 due to its mild critical conditions (P_c: 7.38 MPa and $T_c = 304.15K$) that allow easy processing of thermolabile compounds like omega-3 PUFA. CO_2 can replace the conventional extraction solvents, such as chloroform/hexane, due to its cheap, nontoxic, and nonflammable nature (Davarnejad & Keshavarz, 2012). Supercritical fluid chromatography (SFC) is an alternative to the conventional chromatographic techniques, such as high-pressure liquid chromatography or gas chromatography. The physical properties of SCFs are being utilized as a mobile phase in a column packed with a suitable stationary phase (Kiran et al., 2000). Several methods have been developed for the separation of PUFA, such as omega-3, accounting for its efficient recovery rate because of its high selectivity of both SCF and the stationary phase.

SFC was exploited as a tool for the recovery of DHA and EPA in many studies. Utilizing SFC, an optimal method was developed in a study to obtain DHA-EE and EPA-EE in high purity from tuna oil. Using octadecyl saline as a stationary phase and supercritical carbon dioxide (SC-CO_2) at 65°C and 145 bar, 90% pure DHA-EE with a production of 0.85 g/(kg stationary phase × h) and 50% pure EPA-EE with a production of 0.23 g/(kg stationary phase × h) were obtained (Alkio et al., 2000). Another study was also able to scale up the separation process of the ethyl esters of DHA and EPA at a higher yield and purity from fish oil. The process was already scaled up and installed at production scale in companies like Solutex. Using this technology, they were able to produce omega-3 PUFA at a proportion of 90%, DHA to 80%, and EPA to a concentration of 95% (Yang et al., 2004). Similarly, studies on concentration of EPA-EE from fish oil were conducted with an industrial column filled with porous silicon oxide combined with SC-CO_2 (P = 100–150 bar, T = 40°C–60°C) as mobile phase and (3-aminopropyl)-triethoxysilane as stationary phase, with a flow rate between 4000 and 7000 kg/h. They were able to concentrate EPA-EE from fish oil, from 50% purity to more than 95% purity (Snoey-Elich, 2001).

6.5 Sustainable extraction methods-green solvent extraction methods

The toxicity and hazardous nature of organic solvents used in the extraction of FAs apparently lead to environmental concerns and negative impacts on human health. Green solvents can be considered sustainable alternatives for the extraction of PUFA, which results in lipid extracts with reduced traces of toxic solvents and increased purity. They can also be used for further applications in pharmaceuticals and nutraceuticals. Commonly used green solvents for the purpose of lipid extraction include water, bio-based solvents, liquified gases, SC-CO_2, and natural deep eutectic solvents (NDES)

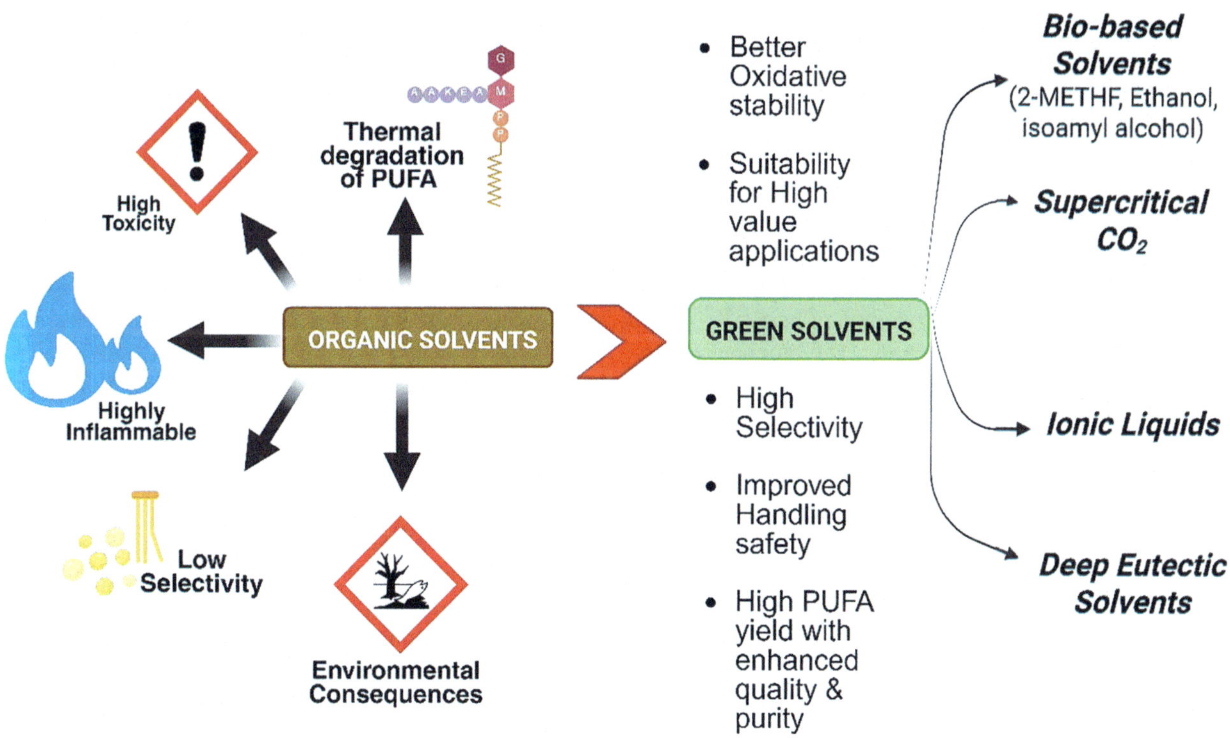

FIGURE 6.4 **Advantages of green solvents in polyunsaturated fatty acid (PUFA) extraction.** Comparison of green solvents with organic solvents used for PUFA extraction.
The figure was created with BioRender.com.

(Hessel et al., 2022). Advantages of green solvent-based extraction over the conventional organic solvent extraction are illustrated in Fig. 6.4.

Bio-based solvents are a class of green solvents that includes certain alcohols, ethers, and esters which are derived from biomass components such as Starch and Cellulose (Alcalde et al., 2023). 2-Methyltetrahydrofuran (2-METHF) is one such bio-based solvent commonly used for the extraction of lipids and proteins. Furfural, contained in renewable sources such as sugarcane and corn cobs, when subjected to hydrogenation, generates this solvent. They serve as an extraction solvent in various conditions due to their lower water solubility, and exhibit a further drop in solubility with increasing temperature. However, the instability of 2-METHF is a major drawback that makes it categorized as a hazardous compound. This can be resolved by the addition of butylated hydroxytoluene, which makes them stable for extraction processes. Fermentation of sugars can lead to the formation of ethanol, which is a low-toxic bio-solvent. Further distillation of ethanol can lead to the production of isoamyl alcohol and 1-propanol in smaller amounts that can also serve as a green solvent for extraction. Still, ethanol was found to be unfavorable for lipid extraction due to its high polarity and solubility in different solvents (Aul & Comanita, 2007). Using SC-CO_2 is one of the emerging renewable PUFA extraction methods that uses SC-CO_2, which is noninflammable and has an easily accessible critical point. Also, the recyclable nature of CO_2 helps to overcome the greenhouse effect to a certain extent. All these advantages make SC-CO_2 extraction a sustainable green extraction method for PUFA (Alcalde et al., 2023).

6.5.1 Supercritical carbon dioxide extraction

Extraction using SC-CO_2 has emerged as a widely used method for isolating PUFAs, with respect to the high susceptibility of PUFAs to thermal degradation. The unique properties of $CO_2$are being exploited in this process by heating and compressing CO_2 beyond its critical point (Tc-31.1°C, Pc-7.38 MPa), making it function as an adaptable solvent suitable for extraction. SC-CO_2 will have gas-like diffusion and liquid-like solvation power (Nozari & Kander, 2025). This method is efficient over other conventional organic solvent methods, as it is nontoxic, noninflammable, with no residual harmful solvents in the final product. Precise adjustment of key parameters, such as temperature, pressure, and flow rate, can improve the selectivity of PUFA extraction. Furthermore, incorporation of ethanol, which is a bio-based solvent, can be crucial to improve the polar lipid solubility and an overall increased yield in high-value PUFAs such as DHA and EPA (Tzima et al., 2023). High-purity concentrate of PUFAs can be obtained by using (SC-CO_2) as it maintains a low operating temperature, preserving the chemical integrity as well as the bioactivity of PUFAs, making it suitable for nutraceutical and pharmaceutical industries.

6.5.2 Ionic liquids and deep eutectic solvents

The high yield of lipids achieved using organic solvents can accompany major safety hazards, including high inflammability, high toxicity, and various other environmental consequences. Considering these aspects, the usage of ILs and NDES has been identified as an alternative to conventional organic solvents. Among the various types of ILs, imidazolium, pyridinium, and cholinium-based ILs constitute the widely studied ones. ILs are represented by robust thermal stability, low vapor pressure, and pronounced ionic conductivity (Saini et al., 2021). Recently, a study evaluated the efficiency of ILs by performing hydrolysis of refined palm olein using a highly efficient liquid enzyme, FG Eversa Transform 2.0, in combination with different CO_2-based alkyl carbamate ILs. Among them, bis(2-ethylhexyl)-ammonium bis(2-ethylhexyl) carbamate (DBCARB) was found to be suitable with desirable hydrophobicity, pH influences, and structural protein optimization. Four percent of DBCARB yielded almost 91 wt.% FA yield, without purification. With purification, 8% DBCARB achieved near maximum equilibrium (95 wt.%) in 8 hours. This study revealed the advantage of using IL in reducing enzyme levels as well as shortening the reaction time (Ng et al., 2023). Similarly, NDES received considerable recognition as a new generation solvent system, accounting its low toxicity, high biodegradability, and easier preparation. NEDS have been exploited in various enzymatic reactions for producing glycolipids, epoxidized oils, and biodiesel. Wang et al. in 2021 attempted the synthesis of n-3 PUFA-rich TAG using immobilized MAS1 lipase and NDES systems. They found that almost a 1.38-fold increase in TAG content was obtained in the enzymatic reaction with the choline chloride/glycerol system compared to the solvent-free system. These data support the promising role of NDES systems in enhanced PUFA recovery.

This chapter comprehensively deals with the advanced extraction techniques for the recovery of PUFAs from different natural resources. Development of sustainable methods for the efficient extraction of PUFAs is notable for various industries, including pharmaceuticals and nutraceuticals. Traditionally, mechanical and solvent-based techniques are dominant in these sectors because of the ease and efficiency of the extraction process. Utilization of harmful organic solvents for the extraction of PUFAs raises concerns about human health, and the consequences can also occur to the environment. In this scenario, innovative membrane-based extraction techniques can enhance the efficiency along with the production of high-purity end products. Additionally, other extraction techniques, including green solvents-based extraction, can be used for the separation of PUFAs, which leads to the production of pure FAs that can be further utilized for the food industry as well. Fig. 6.5 summarizes various traditional and advanced techniques adopted for the extraction and purification of PUFAs. Table 6.1 shows details of different studies conducted to analyze the efficiency of PUFA recovery by using various extraction techniques.

6.6 Future perspectives

Traditionally, solvent extraction and cold pressing have been used for the efficient extraction of PUFA from various sources. However, these methods are inappropriate for the sustainable extraction of PUFAs due to the usage of harmful organic solvents, which raises concerns regarding both the environment and human health. To reduce the negative impacts of these conventional extraction methods, membrane-based methods and green solvent extraction techniques can be considered. Future perspectives of membrane-based separation of PUFAs hold a focus on improvement of selective separation, low cost, and more renewable by adapting advanced and combined technologies. For the recovery of PUFAs, membrane-based systems have immense potential, but they still pose some major drawbacks that need to be addressed to show their full potential. The future of membrane technology lies in adapting to novel solutions that tackle the existing problems. One such effort includes combining organic and inorganic membranes into a hybrid membrane system, which

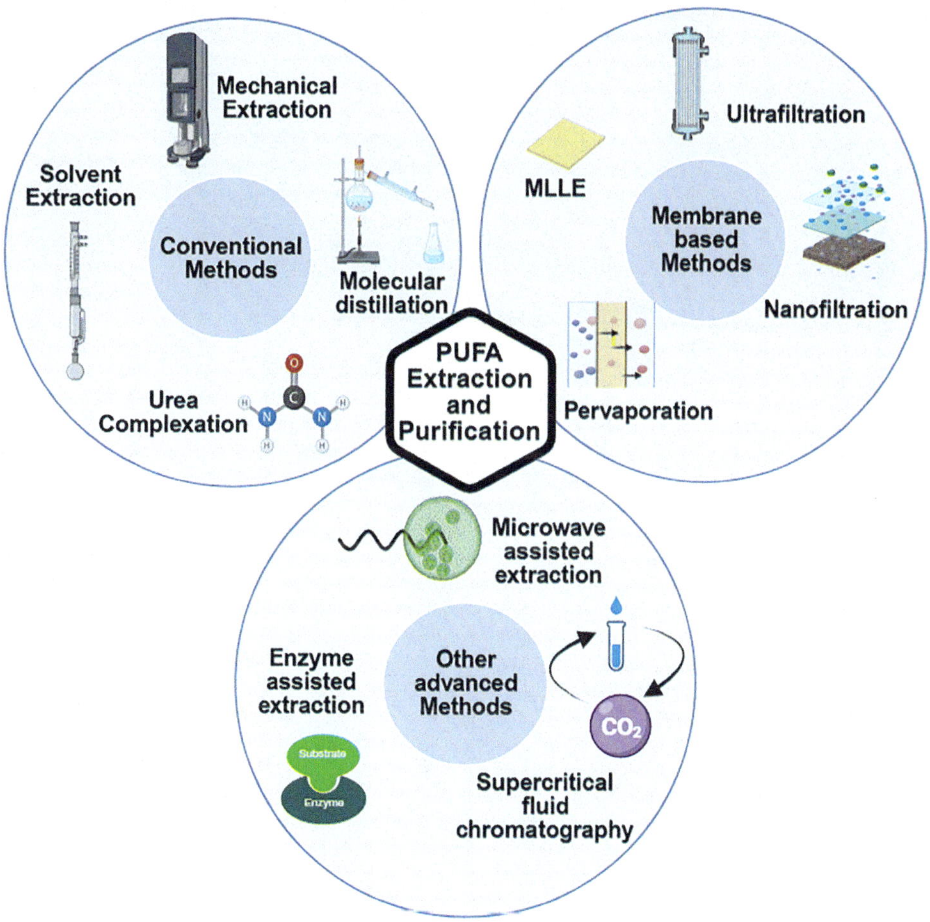

FIGURE 6.5 **Overview of extraction and purification methods of polyunsaturated fatty acids (PUFAs).** Diagrammatic representation of methods used for the extraction and purification of PUFAs.
The figure was created with BioRender.com.

TABLE 6.1 Methods for the extraction and purification of polyunsaturated fatty acids (PUFAs).

Resource of PUFAs		Extraction/purification method	Yield	References
Plant-based resources	Garden cress oil	Solvent extraction	38% PUFA	Olivia et al. (2023)
		Supercritical CO_2 extraction	50% PUFA	
	Crude soybean oil	Solvent extraction followed by PVDF composite NF membrane filtration	80% oil retention, 58% FFA removal	Firman et al. (2013)
Animal-based resources	*Clupeonella cultriventris* (kilka oil)	Urea complexation	EPA and docosahexaenoic acid (DHA) increased 5.39% and 13.32% (crude oil), 12.07% and 58.36% in the omega-3 PUFA concentrate	Eskandari et al. (2024)
	Sardine oil	Enzyme-assisted extraction	37.7% EPA 5.1% ALA	Chakraborty et al. (2010)
	Fish cannery waste	Supercritical extraction	45% of EPA and DHA	Létisse and Comeau (2008)
	Rastrelliger kanagurta	Supercritical fluids	53.6 g/100 of dry sample	Sahena et al. (2010)
	Cod, sardine, salmon, and shark oil	Enzyme-assisted extraction	EPA increased from 16.9% to 30.4%. DHA increased from 6.5% to 9.6%	Aarthy et al. (2016)
	Lantern fish oil	PVDF and nanoporous silica particle used to fabricate a nanocomposite membrane for ultrafiltration	Concentrated omega-3 PUFA upto 53.9%	Ghasemian et al. (2017)
Microbial resources	*Thraustochytrium* sp.	Solvent extraction	DHA of 32.69% of total lipids	Kaliyamoorthy et al. (2023)
	Nannochloropsis gaditana	Molecular distillation with subcritical butane	EPA 58.92% w/w	Meng et al. (2025)
	Microalgae (*Botryococcus* sp., *Chlorella vulgaris*, and *Scenedesmus* sp.)	Solvent extraction	6.8–10.9 g/L	Lee et al. (2010)
		Microwaves	10.0–28.6 g/L	
	Nannochloropsis gaditana	Supercritical CO_2 extraction	EPA-1150 mg/100 g dry biomass	Molino et al. (2019)

promises to overcome limitations of conventional membranes. For instance, those membranes that incorporate COFs, metal organic frameworks, or porous organic polymers are being used because of their superior selectivity, thermal, and chemical stability.

Obtaining a balance between selectivity and permeability is yet another challenge in the recovery of PUFAs. Certain highly selective membranes show low flux, which reduces their productivity. Many advanced membrane materials are still confined to lab-scale studies, which should be scaled upto a commercial level by developing standardized methodologies for the fabrication of membranes, testing, and evaluation. Collaborative efforts should be made between industries, academia, and government sectors to improve the commercialization of innovative membrane technologies.

The high cost of membranes creates problems in their commercialization. In future efforts, an inexpensive membrane should be produced by using more biodegradable and recyclable materials specially made for PUFA recovery. Certain other strategies for reducing maintenance cost and life span of membranes are by creating self-cleaning and antifouling membranes. It can be achieved by introducing modifications in the membrane surface with innovative coatings that repel fouling. For example, introducing external stimuli such as temperature, pH, etc., helps in the self-cleansing of membranes.

The future focus on membrane-based separation techniques should give emphasis on solving problems related to fouling of membranes, enhancing selective separation, scaling up of advanced hybrid membrane systems in a sustainable and cost-effective manner for a wide range of industrial applications. Future innovative membrane systems should align with global goals of sustainability by reducing environmental impacts, which includes the use of renewable materials for membrane fabrication, proper disposal systems, and less chemical inputs in cleansing of membranes, developing long-life membranes, all these helps to reduce the environmental burden. By following these future perspectives, membrane technologies can play a transformative role in improving PUFA separation.

When the conventional studies were focused only on enhanced PUFA yield, they relied on petroleum-based solvents and energy-expensive conventional techniques for achieving maximum yield. However, the concerns on sustainability, safety, overall life-cycle analysis, and product purity have oriented research towards other efficient techniques. The future advancement in PUFA extraction lies in combining these sustainable solvents with advanced technology to bring about high-quality, safe, and environmentally friendly final products while adhering to green chemistry principles. System-level evaluation can contribute to the practical implementation as well as improvement of such green extraction techniques that focus on circular economy models with possibilities of industrial scale-up. PUFA extraction processes can be real-time monitored and precisely executed by incorporating artificial intelligence along with machine learning and sensor-based automation. A collaboration at the global level involving academic, industrial, and government bodies allows establishing regulation, procedures for product identification, and life-cycle assessment.

6.7 Conclusion

PUFAs can be derived in higher quantities as well as purity through different techniques, ranging from mechanical and solvent-based methods to more advanced sustainable methods. While cold methods such as solvent extraction and cold pressing are prominent, drawbacks such as low efficiency and involvement of hazardous chemicals make them inefficient. Innovations in purification techniques were made through methods such as molecular distillation and urea complexation that can address these limitations, minimizing thermal degradation in PUFAs. Advanced techniques such as UF and NF, also later emerged as versatile, efficient techniques that can replace the conventional methods. The selectivity and control provided by these advanced techniques aid in the sustainable impact with efficient recovery and purification of PUFAs. Apart from membrane-based technologies, advanced extraction methods such as MAE, EAE, and SFC also serve as high-quality, effective, and faster alternatives. Adopting green solvents in PUFA extraction, particularly SC-CO_2, helps in transforming the extraction process more sustainable and safer for food and pharmaceutical applications. In total, the sustainable future of PUFA extraction and purification is decided by the advanced techniques and new materials that help to overcome limitations such as thermal and oxidative degradation. In order to meet the global demand for high-purity PUFAs, these advancements in PUFA recovery can help in effective extraction and purification in an economically viable and environmentally sustainable manner.

References

Aarthy, M., Saravanan, P., Ayyadurai, N., Gowthaman, M. K., & Kamini, N. R. (2016). A two step process for production of omega 3-polyunsaturated fatty acid concentrates from sardine oil using Cryptococcus sp. MTCC 5455 lipase. *Journal of Molecular Catalysis B: Enzymatic, 125*, 25–33. https://doi.org/10.1016/j.molcatb.2015.12.013.

Abdorrezaee, Z., & Raisi, A. (2021). A hybrid ultrafiltration/nanofiltration/pervaporation membrane process for intensifying the refining of crude canola oil and solvent recovery. *Chemical Engineering and Processing - Process Intensification, 169*, 108598.

Adarme-Vega, T. C., Lim, D. K. Y., Timmins, M., Vernen, F., Li, Y., & Schenk, P. M. (2012). Microalgal biofactories: A promising approach towards sustainable omega-3 fatty acid production. *Microbial Cell Factories, 11*. Available from: https://doi.org/10.1186/1475-2859-11-96, http://www.microbialcellfactories.com/content/11/1/96.

Adarme-Vega, T. C., Thomas-Hall, S. R., & Schenk, P. M. (2014). Towards sustainable sources for omega-3 fatty acids production. *Current Opinion in Biotechnology, 26*, 14–18. https://doi.org/10.1016/j.copbio.2013.08.003 ISSN 0958-1669.

Alcalde, S., Porcar, R., De La Puente, M. L., Cumming, G. R., Mateos, C., García-Losada, P., Anta, C., Rincón, J. A., & García-Verdugo, E. (2023). Continuous-flow supercritical CO_2 platform for in-situ synthesis and purification of small molecules for drug discovery. *Organic Process Research and Development, 27*(2), 276–285. Available from: https://doi.org/10.1021/acs.oprd.2c00253, http://pubs.acs.org/journal/oprdfk.

Ali, M., & Watson, I. A. (2014). Comparison of oil extraction methods, energy analysis and biodiesel production from flax seeds. *International Journal of Energy Research, 38*, 614–625. https://doi.org/10.1002/er.3066.

Aliasghari Aghdam, M., Mirsaeedghazi, H., Aboonajmi, M., & Kianmehr, M. H. (2015). Effect of ultrasound on different mechanisms of fouling during membrane clarification of pomegranate juice. *Innovative Food Science & Emerging Technologies, 30*, 127–131. https://doi.org/10.1016/j.ifset.2015.05.008.

Alkio, M., Gonzalez, C., Jäntti, M., & Aaltonen, O. (2000). Purification of polyunsaturated fatty acid esters from tuna oil with supercritical fluid chromatography. *Journal of the American Oil Chemists' Society, 77*(3), 315–321. https://doi.org/10.1007/s11746-000-0051-3.

Asadi Tashvigh, A., & Benes, N. E. (2022). Covalent organic polymers for aqueous and organic solvent nanofiltration. *Separation and Purification Technology, 298*, 121589. https://doi.org/10.1016/j.seppur.2022.121589.

Atadashi, I. M., Aroua, M. K., Abdul Aziz, A. R., & Sulaiman, N. M. N. (2011). Membrane biodiesel production and refining technology: A critical review. *Renewable and Sustainable Energy Reviews, 15*(9), 5051–5062. https://doi.org/10.1016/j.rser.2011.07.051.

Aul, R., & Comanita, B. (2007). MeTHF - A green alternative to THF. *Manufacturing Chemist*, 33–34.

Azmi, R. A., Goh, P. S., Ismail, A. F., Lau, W. J., Ng, B. C., Othman, N. H., Noor, A. M., & Yusoff, M. S. A. (2015). Deacidification of crude palm oil using PVA-crosslinked PVDF membrane. *Journal of Food Engineering, 166*, 165–173. https://doi.org/10.1016/j.jfoodeng.2015.06.001.

Bai, H., Wang, X., Zhou, Y., & Zhang, L. (2012). Preparation and characterization of poly(vinylidene fluoride) composite membranes blended with nano-crystalline cellulose. *Progress in Natural Science: Materials International, 22*(3), 250–257. https://doi.org/10.1016/j.pnsc.2012.04.011.

Benítez, F. J., Acero, J. L., Leal, A. I., & González, M. (2009). The use of ultrafiltration and nanofiltration membranes for the purification of cork processing wastewater. *Journal of Hazardous Materials, 162*(2-3), 1438–1445. https://doi.org/10.1016/j.jhazmat.2008.06.036.

Castro-Muñoz, R. (2019). Pervaporation: The emerging technique for extracting aroma compounds from food systems. *Journal of Food Engineering, 253*, 27–39. https://doi.org/10.1016/j.jfoodeng.2019.02.013.

Chakraborty, K., Vijayagopal, P., Chakraborty, R. D., & Vijayan, K. K. (2010). Preparation of eicosapentaenoic acid concentrates from sardine oil by *Bacillus circulans* lipase. *Food Chemistry, 120*(2), 433–442. https://doi.org/10.1016/j.foodchem.2009.10.032.

Chen, et al. (2023). Microalgal polyunsaturated fatty acids: Hotspots and production techniques. *Frontiers in Bioengineering and Biotechnology*.

Davarnejad, R., & Keshavarz, M. (2012). *Gas chromatography application in supercritical fluid extraction process*. InTech. http://doi.org/10.5772/31638.

Dawiec, A., Witek-Krowiak, A., Podstawczyk, D., & Bubała, K. (2015). Mathematical modeling of sorption step in pervaporative aroma compounds recovery from the multicomponent solution. *Chemical Engineering Science, 129*, 78–90. https://doi.org/10.1016/j.ces.2015.02.036.

Eskandari, Z., Hosseini, S. F., & Yaghmur, A. (2024). Production of omega-3 fatty acid concentrates from common kilka oil: Optimization of the urea complexation process. *Molecules (Basel, Switzerland), 29*(11), 2430. https://doi.org/10.3390/molecules29112430.

Firman, L. R., Ochoa, N. A., Marchese, J., & Pagliero, C. L. (2013). Deacidification and solvent recovery of soybean oil by nanofiltration membranes. *Journal of Membrane Science, 431*, 187–196. https://doi.org/10.1016/j.memsci.2012.12.040.

Ghalamara, S., Coscueta, E. R., Silva, S., Brazinha, C., Pereira, C. D., & Pintado, M. E. (2022). Integrated ultrafiltration, nanofiltration, and reverse osmosis pilot process to produce bioactive protein/peptide fractions from sardine cooking effluent. *Journal of Environmental Management, 317*. Available from: https://doi.org/10.1016/j.jenvman.2022.115344, https://www.sciencedirect.com/science/journal/03014797.

Ghasemian, S., Sahari, M. A., Barzegar, M., & Ahmadi Gavlighi, H. (2017). Omega-3 PUFA concentration by a novel PVDF nano-composite membrane filled with nano-porous silica particles. *Food Chemistry, 230*, 454–462. Available from: https://doi.org/10.1016/j.foodchem.2017.02.135, www.elsevier.com/locate/foodchem.

Ghosh, M. (2007). Review on recent trends in rice bran oil processing. *Journal of the American Oil Chemists' Society, 84*(4), 315–324. https://doi.org/10.1007/s11746-007-1047-3.

Golijan, J., Milinčić, D. D., Petronijević, R., Pešić, M. B., Barać, M. B., Sečanski, M., Lekić, S., & Kostić, A. (2019). The fatty acid and triacylglycerol profiles of conventionally and organically produced grains of maize, spelt and buckwheat. *Journal of Cereal Science, 90*. Available from: https://doi.org/10.1016/j.jcs.2019.102845, http://www.elsevier.com/inca/publications/store/6/2/2/8/5/9/index.htt.

González-Fernández, M. J., Ramos-Bueno, R. P., Rodríguez-García, I., & Guil-Guerrero, J. L. (2017). Purification process for MUFA- and PUFA-based monoacylglycerols from edible oils. *Biochimie*. https://doi.org/10.1016/j.biochi.2017.06.002.

Gu, X. C., Zhang, Q. F., Pang, Y. H., & Shen, X. F. (2024). Microwave-assisted esterification and electro-enhanced solid-phase microextraction of omega-3 polyunsaturated fatty acids in eggs. *Food Chemistry, 448*. Available from: https://doi.org/10.1016/j.foodchem.2024.139060, https://www.sciencedirect.com/science/journal/03088146.

Hampu, N., Werber, J. R., Chan, W. Y., Feinberg, E. C., & Hillmyer, M. A. (2020). Next-generation ultrafiltration membranes enabled by block polymers. *ACS Nano, 14*(12), 16446–16471. Available from: https://doi.org/10.1021/acsnano.0c07883, http://pubs.acs.org/journal/ancac3.

Harimana, Y., Korma, S. A., Ali, A. H., Tuyishime, M. A., Habinshuti, I., & Abed, S. M (2016). Extraction, refining and purification of ?-3 PUFA through different techniques - A review. *American Journal of Food Science and Nutrition Research, 4*(1), 18–26.

Hasnisa, H., & Jumat, S. (2012). Enzymatic acidolysis of palm olein with PUFA to improve linoleic and α-linolenic acids ratio (Asidolisis berenzim minyak olein sawit dengan PUFA bagi meningkatkan nisbah asid linoleik dan α-linolenik). *Journal of Tropical Agriculture and Food Science, 40*(Issue 1). https://doi.org/10.1016/j.foodchem.2022.132236, https://cabidigitallibrary.org.

Hessel, V., Tran, N. N., Asrami, M. R., Tran, Q. D., Van Duc Long, N., Escribà-Gelonch, M., Tejada, J. O., Linke, S., & Sundmacher, K. (2022). Sustainability of green solvents-review and perspective. *Green Chemistry, 24*(2), 410–437. Available from: https://doi.org/10.1039/d1gc03662a, http://pubs.rsc.org/en/journals/journal/gc.

Kaliyamoorthy, K., Kandasamy, K., Ponnuvel, M., Kamlangdee, N., Taoka, Y., & Viyakarn, V. (2023). PUFA and carotenoid producing thraustochytrids and their anti-microbial and antioxidant activities. *Frontiers in Marine Science, 10*. https://doi.org/10.3389/fmars.2023.1126452.

Kapoor, B., Kapoor, D., Gautam, S., Singh, R., & Bhardwaj, S. (2021). Dietary polyunsaturated fatty acids (PUFAs): Uses and potential health benefits. *Current Nutrition Reports, 10*(3), 232–242. https://doi.org/10.1007/s13668-021-00363-3.

Kiran, E., Debenedetti, P. G., & Peters, C. J. (Eds.). (2000). *Supercritical fluids*Netherlands: Springer.

Kromhout, D., & de Goede, J. (2014). Update on cardiometabolic health effects of ω-3 fatty acids. *Current Opinion in Lipidology, 25*(1), 85–90. https://doi.org/10.1097/mol.0000000000000041.

Kumar, R., Ghosh, A. K., & Pal, P. (2020). Synergy of biofuel production with waste remediation along with value-added co-products recovery through microalgae cultivation: A review of membrane-integrated green approach. *Science of The Total Environment, 698*, 134169. https://doi.org/10.1016/j.scitotenv.2019.134169.

Kwiatkowski, J. R., & Cheryan, M. (2005). Recovery of corn oil from ethanol extracts of ground corn using membrane technology. *Journal of the American Oil Chemists' Society, 82*(3), 221–227. https://doi.org/10.1007/s11746-005-5175-3.

Lee, J. Y., Yoo, C., Jun, S. Y., Ahn, C. Y., & Oh, H. M. (2010). Comparison of several methods for effective lipid extraction from microalgae. *Bioresource Technology, 101*(1), S75–S77. https://doi.org/10.1016/j.biortech.2009.03.058, http://www.journals.elsevier.com/bioresource-technology/.

Létisse, M., & Comeau, L. (2008). Enrichment of eicosapentaenoic acid and doco- sahexaenoic acid from sardine by-products by supercritical fluid fraction- ation. *Journal of Separation Science, 31*(8), 1374–1380. https://doi.org/10.1002/jssc.200700501.

Li, J., Lin, S., Liu, X., Chen, W., Lan, D., & Wang, Y. (2024). Preparation of high-purity docosahexaenoic acid ethyl ester from algal oil through enzymatic ethanolysis. *Journal of Oleo Science, 73*(8), ess24072. https://doi.org/10.5650/jos.ess24072.

Lv, E., Ding, S., Lu, J., Du, L., Li, Z., Li, J., Zhang, S., & Ding, J. (2018). An integrated process of catalytic hydrolysis and membrane separation for fatty acids production from lard oil. *The Canadian Journal of Chemical Engineering, 96*(9), 2014–2024. https://doi.org/10.1002/cjce.23156.

Lv, E., Ding, S., Lu, J., Yi, W., & Ding, J. (2020). Separation and purification of fatty acids by membrane technology: A critical review. *International Journal of Chemical Reactor Engineering, 18*(9), Available from: https://doi.org/10.1515/ijcre-2019-0224, www.degruyter.com/view/j/ijcre.

Mah, S. K., Leo, C. P., Wu, T. Y., & Chai, S. P. (2012). A feasibility investigation on ultrafiltration of palm oil and oleic acid removal from glycerin solutions: Flux decline, fouling pattern, rejection and membrane characterizations. *Journal of Membrane Science, 389*, 245–256. https://doi.org/10.1016/j.memsci.2011.10.037.

Marchetti, P., Jimenez Solomon, M. F., Szekely, G., & Livingston, A. G. (2014). Molecular separation with organic solvent nanofiltration: A critical review. *Chemical Reviews, 114*(21), 10735–10806. Available from: https://doi.org/10.1021/cr500006j, http://pubs.acs.org/journal/chreay.

Masoodi, L., Gull, A., Masoodi, F. A., Gani, A., Nissar, J., Ahad, T., Nayik, G. A., Mukarram, S. A., Kovács, B., Prokisch, J., El-Ramady, H., & Solberg, S.Ø. (2022). An overview on traditional vs. green technology of extraction methods for producing high quality walnut oil. *Agronomy, 12*(10), Available from: https://doi.org/10.3390/agronomy12102258, www.mdpi.com/journal/agronomy/.

Meng, R., Zhang, Y., Jiang, Y., Li, B., Chen, X., Sun, Z., & Sun, L. (2025). Subcritical fluid and molecular distillation extraction of *Nannochloropsis gaditana* lipid and its metabolic benefits in hyperlipidemic mice. *Frontiers in Nutrition, 12*. https://doi.org/10.3389/fnut.2025.1615332.

Molino, A., Martino, M., Larocca, V., Di Sanzo, G., Spagnoletta, A., Marino, T., Karatza, D., Iovine, A., Mehariya, S., & Musmarra, D. (2019). Eicosapentaenoic acid extraction from nannochloropsis gaditana using carbon dioxide at supercritical conditions. *Marine Drugs, 17*(2), 132. https://doi.org/10.3390/md17020132.

Nde, D. B., & Foncha, A. C. (2020). Optimization methods for the extraction of vegetable oils: A review. *Processes, 8*(2), 209. https://doi.org/10.3390/pr8020209.

Ng, W. Z., Chan, E. S., Tan, Y. S., Liow, M. Y., Ooi, C. W., Tey, B. T., & Song, C. P. (2023). *Hydrolysis of refined palm olein to fatty acids using high strength Fg Eversa® Transform 2.0 along with Co2-based alkyl carbamate ionic liquids. SSRN*. Malaysia SSRN. http://doi.org/10.2139/ssrn.4637708, https://www.ssrn.com/index.cfm/en/.

Nozari, B., & Kander, R. (2025). Supercritical CO_2 technology for biomass extraction: Review. *Industrial Crops and Products, 233*, 121348. https://doi.org/10.1016/j.indcrop.2025.121348.

Olivia, D., Azmeera, T., Eanti, A., & Chakrabarti, P. P. (2023). Garden cress oil as a vegan source of PUFA: Achieving through optimized supercritical carbon dioxide extraction. *Innovative Food Science & Emerging Technologies, 84*, 103283. https://doi.org/10.1016/j.ifset.2023.103283.

Ranasinghe Arachchige, N. P. R., Xiong, N. W., & Bowden, N. B. (2023). Separation of C18 Fatty acid esters and fatty acids derived from vegetable oils using nanometer-sized covalent organic frameworks incorporated in polyepoxy membranes. *ACS Applied Nano Materials, 6*(8), 6715–6725. https://doi.org/10.1021/acsanm.3c00442.

Rolle, R. S. (1998). Review: Enzyme applications for agro-processing in developing countries: An inventory of current and potential applications. *World Journal of Microbiology and Biotechnology, 14*(5), 611–619. https://doi.org/10.1023/a:1008896500986.

Rubio-Rodríguez, N., Beltrán, S., Jaime, I., de Diego, S. M., Sanz, M. T., & Carballido, J. R. (2010). Production of omega-3 polyunsaturated fatty acid concentrates: A review. *Innovative Food Science and Emerging Technologies, 11*(1), 1–12. https://doi.org/10.1016/j.ifset.2009.10.006.

Sahena, F., Zaidul, I. S. M., Jinap, S., Saari, N., Jahurul, H. A., Abbas, K. A., & Norulaini, N. A. (2009). PUFAs in fish: Extraction, fractionation, importance in health. *Comprehensive Reviews in Food Science and Food Safety, 8*(2), 59–74. https://doi.org/10.1111/j.1541-4337.2009.00069.x.

Sahena, F., Zaidul, I. S. M., Jinap, S., Jahurul, M. H. A., Khatib, A., & Norulaini, N. A. N. (2010). Extraction of fish oil from the skin of Indian mackerel using supercritical fluids. *Journal of Food Engineering, 99*(1), 63–69. https://doi.org/10.1016/j.jfoodeng.2010.01.038.

Saini, R. K., Prasad, P., Shang, X., & Keum, Y. S. (2021). Advances in lipid extraction methods—A review. *International Journal of Molecular Sciences, 22*(24), Available from: https://doi.org/10.3390/ijms222413643, https://www.mdpi.com/1422-0067/22/24/13643/pdf.

Salehi, F. (2014). Current and future applications for nanofiltration technology in the food processing. *Food and Bioproducts Processing, 92*(2), 161–177. https://doi.org/10.1016/j.fbp.2013.09.005.

Sallet, D., Fischer, L. T., Ugalde, G., Tres, M. V., Mazutti, M. A., & Kuhn, R. C. (2020). Separation of microbial oil produced by *Mortierella isabellina* using polymeric membranes. *Bioprocess and Biosystems Engineering, 43*(11), 1943–1949. Available from: https://doi.org/10.1007/s00449-020-02383-9, https://rd.springer.com/journal/449.

Santos-Sánchez, N. F., Valadez-Blanco, R., Hernández-Carlos, B., Torres-Ariño, A., Guadarrama-Mendoza, P. C., & Salas-Coronado, R. (2016). Lipids rich in ω-3 polyunsaturated fatty acids from microalgae. *Applied Microbiology and Biotechnology, 100*(20), 8667–8684. Available from: https://doi.org/10.1007/s00253-016-7818-8, link.springer.de/link/service/journals/00253/index.htm.

Sharma, A. K., Chintala, V., Ghodke, P., Prasher, P., & Patel, A. (2020). Extraction and purification of PUFA from microbial biomass. *Nutraceutical Fatty Acids from Oleaginous Microalgae: A Human Health Perspective,* 249–279. https://doi.org/10.1002/9781119631729.ch10.

Shimada, Y., Sugihara, A., & Tominaga, Y. (2001). Enzymatic purification of polyunsaturated fatty acids. *Journal of Bioscience and Bioengineering, 91*(6), 529–538. https://doi.org/10.1016/S1389-1723(01)80169-9.

Snoey-Elich, H (2001). New procedure for the preparation of the ethylic ester of the pentaenoic eicosa acid, (Spanish Patent No. ES 2 159 257 A1). Spanish Patent and Trademark Office..

Taiwo, K. J., Nguyen, H., & Usack, J. G. (2024). Continuous liquid-liquid extraction of medium-chain fatty acids from fermentation broth using hollow-fiber membranes. *Journal of Visualized Experiments : JoVE, 210.* https://doi.org/10.3791/66956.

Tonon, R. V., Dos Santos, B. A., Couto, C. C., Mellinger-Silva, C., Brígida, A. I. S., & Cabral, L. M. C. (2016). Coupling of ultrafiltration and enzymatic hydrolysis aiming at valorizing shrimp wastewater. *Food Chemistry, 198*, 20–27. Available from: https://doi.org/10.1016/j.foodchem.2015.11.094, www.elsevier.com/locate/foodchem.

Tzima, S., Georgiopoulou, I., Louli, V., & Magoulas, K. (2023). Recent advances in supercritical CO_2 extraction of pigments, lipids and bioactive compounds from microalgae. *Molecules (Basel, Switzerland), 28*(3), 1410. https://doi.org/10.3390/molecules28031410.

Vaisali, C., Charanyaa, S., Belur, P. D., & Regupathi, I. (2015). Refining of edible oils: A critical appraisal of current and potential technologies. *International Journal of Food Science and Technology, 50*(1), 13–23. https://doi.org/10.1111/ijfs.12657.

Venegas-Caleron, M., Sayanova, O., & Napier, J. A. (2010). An alternative to fish oils: Metabolic engineering of oil-seed crops to produce omega-3 long chain polyunsaturated fatty acids. *Progress in Lipid Research, 49*, 108–119. https://doi.org/10.1016/j.plipres.2009.10.001.

Wanasundara, U. N., Wanasundara, P. J. P., & Shahidi, F. (2005). Novel separation techniques for isolation and purification of fatty acids and oil by-products. *Bailey's Industrial Oil and Fat Products,* 1–32. https://doi.org/10.1002/047167849X.bio065.pub2.

Wang, X., Zhao, X., Qin, X., Zhao, Z., Yang, B., & Wang, Y. (2021). Immobilized mas1 lipase-catalyzed synthesis of N-3 pufa-rich triacylglycerols in deep eutectic solvents. *Journal of Oleo Science, 70*(2), 227–236. https://doi.org/10.5650/jos.ess20200.

Xue, Z., Sharpe, P. L., Hong, S. P., Yadav, N. S., Xie, D., Short, D. R., Damude, H. G., Rupert, R. A., Seip, J. E., Wang, J., Pollak, D. W., Bostick, M. W., Bosak, M. D., Macool, D. J., Hollerbach, D. H., Zhang, H., Arcilla, D. M., Bledsoe, S. A., Croker, K., ... Zhu, Q. (2013). Production of omega-3 eicosapentaenoic acid by metabolic engineering of *Yarrowia lipolytica. Nature Biotechnology, 31*(8), 734–740. https://doi.org/10.1038/nbt.2622.

Yang, Y. W., Wu, C. J., Wang, X. D., Huang, M., & Ren, Q. L. (2004). Purification of EPA-EE and DHA-EE with supercritical fluid chromatography. *Gao Xiao Hua Xue Gong Cheng Xue Bao/Journal of Chemical Engineering of Chinese Universities, 18*(3), 293–296.

Zhang, Q. W., Lin, L. G., & Ye, W. C. (2018). Techniques for extraction and isolation of natural products: A comprehensive review. *Chinese Medicine, 13*(1), 20. https://doi.org/10.1186/s13020-018-0177-x.

Zheng, Z., Dai, Z., & Shen, Q. (2018). Enrichment of polyunsaturated fatty acids from seal oil through urea adduction and the fatty acids change rules during the process. *Journal of Food Processing and Preservation, 42*(5), Available from: https://doi.org/10.1111/jfpp.13593, http://www.blackwellpublishers.co.uk/journal_new.asp?site=1.

Zhou, J., Wang, M., Saraiva, J. A., Martins, A. P., Pinto, C. A., Prieto, M. A., Simal-Gandara, J., Cao, H., Xiao, J., & Barba, F. J. (2022a). Extraction of lipids from microalgae using classical and innovative approaches. *Food Chemistry, 384*, 132236. https://doi.org/10.1016/j.foodchem.2022.132236.

Zhou, X., Ding, W., & Jin, W. (2022b). Microwave-assisted extraction of lipids, carotenoids, and other compounds from marine resources. In *Innovative and emerging technologies in the bio-marine food sector.* Elsevier, 375–394 https://doi.org/10.1016/B978-0-12-820096-4.00012-2.

Section II

Delivery systems

Chapter 7

Engineering approaches to enhance polyunsaturated fatty acid stability during processing

Fakhreddine Ben Amara[1], Bouthaina Ben Hadj Hmida[2], Khaoula Elhadef[1], Ahlem Chira[3], Sarra Akermi[1], Slim Smaoui[1], and Sonia Jemli[4,5]

[1]*Laboratory of Microbial Biotechnology, Enzymatic and Biomolecules, Centre of Biotechnology of Sfax, Sfax, Tunisia,* [2]*Laboratory of Biochemistry and Enzymatic Engineering of Lipases, National Engineering School of Sfax, University of Sfax, Sfax, Tunisia,* [3]*Laboratory of Biomathematics Lr22es01, Faculty of Sciences of Sfax, Sfax, Tunisia,* [4]*University of Sfax, Sfax, Tunisia,* [5]*Centre of Biotechnology of Sfax, Sfax, Tunisia*

7.1 Introduction

Polyunsaturated fatty acids (PUFAs) are key fatty acids with at least two double bonds in their hydrocarbon chain. These molecules are not only a key part of the structural composition of cells, but also play a vital role in keeping us healthy in lots of ways (Linares-Maurizi et al., 2023). PUFAs remain the main structural constituents of the cell membrane and are considered to play a dynamic role as nutrients in treating autoimmune reactions, nonalcoholic fatty liver disease, and several chronic diseases. Furthermore, reported that the public health benefits of PUFAs have been identified as playing a role in preserving brain function, cholesterol metabolism, and inflammation. Moreover, Calder (2017)indicated that PUFAs act as antioxidants by regulating the inflammatory cycle and modulating antioxidant signaling. Lipid oxidation happens in three steps, starting with initiation, propagation, and finishing with termination. Li, Chen, et al. (2022) revealed that the oxidizing free radicals are fatty acids such as LOO˙, LO˙, and L˙. The trend for PUFAs to pass via oxidation represents an energetic role in maintaining the integrity of the biological membrane of foods (Dessì et al., 2002). Omega-3 (PUFAs),such aseicosapentaenoic acid (EPA) and docosahexaenoic acid (DHA),are known as prevalent and beneficial in safeguarding from various types of metabolic disruptions. However, the PUFAs are the most likely to be oxidized owing to the unsaturated nature of these compounds, which generates various metabolites as well as reactive oxygen species. Additionally, omega-6 PUFAs have the characteristics of initial double bonds at the sixth carbon atom. Linolenic acid (LA) and arachidonic acid (AA) were the most components of omega-6 (Rahman et al., 2024). The omega-6 PUFAs were found typically in western food (Rahman et al., 2024).

PUFAs are more sensitive to the oxidation process, owing to the existence of several unsaturated bonds, which subsequently occur in two forms, namely nonenzymatic and enzymatic oxidation. As a result, cardiac disease, cancer, allergic reactions, and atherosclerosis represent the most undesirable effects of the reactive oxidation products. Therefore the need for appropriate methods to increase the oxidative stability of PUFAs during processing and storage is urgent. Different strategies could be performed to keep the oxidative stability of PUFAs against oxygen, light, moisture, and heat, such as the addition of natural and synthetic antioxidants and encapsulation. Indeed, the production of oil capsules in the agri-food industry could be supplemented to increase the consumption of essential fatty acids such as omega-3 and omega-6. Several techniques of encapsulation, as well as coaxial electrospray, freeze-drying, spray-drying, coacervation, in situ polymerization, melt extrusion, microwave drying, etc., are already being performed for the encapsulation of essential compounds (Albert et al., 2017). In this book chapter, we are interested in the determination of the mechanisms of PUFAs degradation and different strategies for PUFAs stabilization.

Omega-3 and Omega-6 Polyunsaturated Fatty Acids in Food Systems. DOI: https://doi.org/10.1016/B978-0-443-43810-3.00020-8

7.2 Mechanisms of polyunsaturated fatty acid degradation

PUFAs, such as omega-3 (α-linolenic acid [ALA], EPA, DHA) and omega-6 (linoleic acid, arachidonic acid), are vital nutritional components owing to their frequent health benefits, such as cardiovascular protection, antiinflammatory properties, and cognitive support. Recent cohort studies demonstrate that omega-3 supplementation was associated with a 10% reduction in the most important cardiovascular diseases and decreased the risk of cardiac mortality by 35% (Rahman et al., 2024). However, their likelihood to be greatly unsaturated makes them chemically unstable and hence extremely susceptible to oxidative degradation (Musakhanian et al., 2022). Such a process causes rancidity, loss of nutritional value, and the production of potentially harmful compounds implicated in cellular DNA damage and inflammation (Gentile et al., 2017). Oxidative degradation of PUFAs proceeds by three primary related pathways: autoxidation, photooxidation, and enzymatic oxidation. All pathways have a distinct profile of oxidative damage in terms of influencing food quality, shelf life, and safety (Wang et al., 2023).

7.2.1 Oxidation and rancidity pathways

PUFAs are prone to degradation due to their chemical composition of a double bond chain (Mortensen and Ruiz, 2023). The double bonds are very reactive and, under oxidative stress, get converted through a series of reactions to form rancidity and off-flavor (Kasaai, 2025). The primary oxidation mechanisms accountable for PUFA degradation are as follows:

7.2.1.1 Autoxidation (radical chain reaction)

PUFA breakdown occurs mostly by autoxidation, a free-radical chain reaction triggered by heat, light, or metal ions (e.g., Fe^{2+}, Cu^{+}) (Kodali et al., 2020). The response has three stages:

Pro-oxidants (e.g., Fe^{2+}, Cu^{+}, heat ≥60°C) abstract hydrogen from bis-allylic carbons (—CH_2—) of PUFAs to create a lipid radical ($L^{\bullet}$) (Cao et al., 2024):

LH (PUFAs) + Initiator (e.g., $OH^{\bullet}$) → $L^{\bullet}$ + H_2O. For instance, LA produces a pentadienyl radical following the abstraction of hydrogen at C-11. Propagation: lipid radicals take a hydrogen from oxygen to produce peroxyl radicals (LOO-), which add to other PUFAs molecules (Hershelman et al., 2019):

$$L^{\bullet} + O_2 \rightarrow LOO^{\bullet}$$

$$LOO^{\bullet} + LH \rightarrow LOOH + L^{\bullet}$$

Hydroperoxides (LOOH) are the principal oxidation products but degrade into secondary products like aldehydes (Ayala et al., 2014).

Termination:

Radicals dimerize to produce nonreactive species like alcohols, ketones, and aldehydes (Fuloria et al., 2020):

$$LOO^{\bullet} + LOO^{\bullet} \rightarrow \text{Alcohols + ketones + aldehyes (hexanal, MDA)}$$

Rancidity impact:

- Hexanal (>0.05 ppm): Causes grassy off-flavors in oxidized vegetable oils (Majcher and Fahmi, 2025).
- Malondialdehyde: Often employed as a biomarker of lipid peroxidation and oxidative stress (Chira et al., 2022).

7.2.1.2 Photooxidation (light-driven)

Photooxidation of PUFAs is a consequence of the reaction of $^1O_2$ with PUFAs in the presence of photosensitizers like chlorophyll or riboflavin (Aerssens et al., 2022):

$$LH + {}^1O_2 \rightarrow \text{LOOH (conjugated hydroperoxides)}$$

Key characteristics of photooxidation

- Reactivity: Singlet oxygen $^1O_2$ is 22.5 kcal/mol more energetic than triplet oxygen ($^3O_2$) and is able to react with PUFAs directly without free radical initiation (Johnson & Decker, 2015).

Practical Applications: In bottled oils, green glass reduces oxidation by 50% compared to transparent glass (Li, Li, et al., 2022). Titanium dioxide nanoparticles deposited on a polyester (PET) substrate can achieve high UV-blocking levels. PET-TiO_2 fabrics, for example, can achieve ultraviolet protection factor indexes of 50^+, which is comparable to high levels of UV blocking (Cot et al., 2024).

7.2.1.2.1 The rancidity

- Methional: Provides "sunlight flavor" to milk provides "sunlight flavor" to milk, formed by the photosensitization of riboflavin and methionine oxidation when exposed to light (Munoz Insa, 2017).
- 4-Hydroxy-2-nonenal: A photooxidation product that constitutes a toxic aldehyde; a cause of rancid tastes and odors in oxidized fats and oils, ruining food quality (Breitzig et al., 2016).

7.2.1.3 Enzymatic oxidation

Lipoxygenases (LOX) or microbial lipases can be used to catalyze the oxidation of PUFAs at the site-specific level (Hajeyah et al., 2020).

LOX: Tissue of a plant (e.g., soybean) contains LOX, which converts the formation of 13-hydroperoxy-octadecadienoic acid from LA (Singh, Arif, et al., 2022).

The microbial enzymes cleave the triglycerides with the liberation of free PUFAs, which are oxidized more quickly (Patel and Karageorgou, 2020).

The rancidity

- 1-Octen-3-one (>0.1 ppb): Produces mushroom-like flavors in foods like soybeans and mushrooms. Its occurrence is highly related to the process of fungal contamination and lipid oxidation (Xiong et al., 2017).
- Acrolein: A cytotoxic aldehyde that is a byproduct of enzymatic oxidation; it causes food to acquire off-odors and off-flavors, reducing their shelf life and quality (Chang et al., 2022).

7.2.2 Rancidity markers and food impacts

The oxidation of PUFAs yields volatile molecules that are significant rancidity markers (Huo et al., 2024). Below is a discussion of the markers, their chemical origin, their food application, and their threshold of detectability (Table 7.1).

7.3 Environmental factors affecting polyunsaturated fatty acids stability (temperature, oxygen, light, moisture)

PUFAs are prone to oxidation because of their unsaturated structure, and environmental conditions of temperature, oxygen exposure, light, and moisture play a major role in their stability (Harrysson et al., 2021; Wang et al., 2023). These factors must be known to maintain the integrity of PUFAs in food and in supplements (Table 7.2).

7.4 Temperature

Increased temperatures expedite the oxidation of PUFAs by supplying activation energy for free radical generation, adhering to Arrhenius kinetics, with activation energies for n-3 PUFA-rich oils between 82.84 and 96.98 kJ/mol. For example, LA oxidizes tenfold more rapidly at 40°C than at 20°C, but omega-3 fatty acids (ALA, EPA, DHA) exhibit greater susceptibility to oxidation than omega-6 fatty acids (e.g., LA), especially at temperatures exceeding 60°C. Higher temperatures boost molecule mobility and collision frequency, encouraging both temperature-dependent degradation that happens via many pathways:

- Enhancement of the lipid radical production and propagation due to the higher temperatures (Zeis et al., 2019).
- Faster lipolysis and oxidation due to the increase of enzyme activity caused by the elevation of temperature, leading to faster lipolysis and oxidation (Tatiyaborworntham et al., 2022).
- Thermal degradation of fatty acid (Zhuang and Dong, 2022).

Consequently, primary and secondary oxidation products were obtained, which affect the quality and safety process of PUFA-rich diets (Xi et al., 2021). Thus temperature optimization was needed in order to prevent PUFA-rich diets from oxidation. Additionally, both refrigeration at 4°C and freezing from -18°C to -30°C reduce oxidation rates by 2–3 times (Yang and Chiang, 2017) and stop oxidation, respectively, which enables better safeguarding for a long-term period. However, temperature changes, such as thermal cycling between -25°C and -12°C, have been shown to greatly accelerate

TABLE 7.1 Volatile compounds resulting from polyunsaturated fatty acids (PUFAs)oxidation and their impact on rancidity.

Compound	Threshold (ppm)	Odor/flavor	Formation pathway	Common foods	References
Hexanal	0.097	Green and grassy	Linoleic acid hydroperoxide breakdown	Soybean oil, nuts	
2,4-heptadienal	0.25	Fishy and rancid	Omega-3 PUFAs oxidation	Fish oils	
1-octen-3-one	0.00004	Metallic and mushroom	Linoleic acid oxidation	Mushrooms	
Nonanal	0.3	Tallowy and citrus	Oleic acid cooxidation	Olive oil	Yoshitake et al. (2019)
2,6-nonadienal	10	Cucumber-like	ALA oxidation	Algal oils	
Malondialdehyde	-	Painty, and pungent	Secondary oxidation	Processed meats	
2-pentenal	1.6–2.1	Sharp, and apple-like	ALA decomposition	Leafy greens	
4-heptenal	0.1	Creamy and fishy	DHA oxidation	Infant formula	
3-methylbutanal	0.06	Malt-like	Strecker degradation	Stored dairy	
Acrolein	0.25	Acrid and burning	Glycerol pyrolysis	Frying oils	Chang et al. (2022)

TABLE 7.2 Environmental factors affecting polyunsaturated fatty acids (PUFAs) stability and control strategies.

Environmental factor	Effect on PUFAs stability	Control strategies	References
Temperature	Accelerates oxidation, especially at high levels	Refrigeration (4°C), freezing (–20°C or lower), cold-pressing	Pinheiro Pantoja et al. (2024)
Oxygen	Promotes oxidation via radical chain reactions	Vacuum sealing, nitrogen flushing, antioxidant systems (e.g., tocopherols, rosemary extract)	
Light	Induces photooxidation (esp. with chlorophyll)	Amber glass packaging, UV-blocking films, benzophenone additives	
Moisture	Encourages hydrolytic rancidity and microbial growth	Desiccants (silica gel), microencapsulation, lecithin-based nanoemulsions	

lipid oxidation and hydrolysis in herring muscle tissues. Avoiding frequent freezing and thawing is critical for reducing oxidative damage.

7.5 Oxygen exposure

Oxygen generates free radicals, which degrade PUFAs via a series of steps: free radical initiation, propagation, and termination. Peroxyl radicals form when oxygen interacts with PUFAs. Lipid hydroperoxides are the result of a chain reaction initiated by these radicals, which then steal hydrogen atoms from neighboring fatty acid molecules. Metals traces such as iron and copper could enhance the oxidative deterioration of PUFAs. Moreover, these fatty acids are especially susceptible to oxidation due to their high degree of unsaturation (Mititelu et al., 2024). The need to limit this degradation is urgent; thus increasing antioxidant activities and minimizing oxygen exposure were developed, such as nitrogen flushing and vacuum sealing, which can decrease oxygen value in packaging to below 2%, enhancing the stability of PUFA-rich products during the period of conservation (Schirmer et al., 2020).

7.6 Light (photooxidation)

PUFAs' photooxidation was achieved in two main reactions (Assi et al., 2023).

Type I reactions: Interaction between photosensitizers and fatty acid molecules, which begin oxidative reactions (Gutiérrez et al., 2024).
Type II reactions: These photosensitizers produce an electronically excited form of oxygen, which is highly volatile and breaks down the double bonds of PUFA chains (Dessì et al., 2002; Gutiérrez et al., 2024).

For this reason, the incorporation of an effective method, such as packaging, will limit this disorder (Mititelu et al., 2024). For example, the use of amber glass disables about 90% of UV light transmission. In order to reach higher stability of PUFAs, studies have developed the alternative of the introduction of UV-filtering agents in packaging materials such as titanium dioxide or benzophenone derivatives, which absorb harmful wavelengths.

7.7 Moisture and water activity

Moisture and water activity decrease the stability of PUFAs, leading to both hydrolytic and oxidative deterioration. According to, the dissolution of metals like copper and iron in water will increase oxidative rancidity. Additionally, water concentration in oleic acid affects both thermal oxidation levels and the oxidation products. For this reason, the achievement of PUFA stability needs promoting strategies to control the moisture rate and the use of other alternatives like microencapsulation, such as cyclodextrin inclusion complexes.

7.8 Engineering strategies for polyunsaturated fatty acids stabilization

7.8.1 Encapsulation techniques

Due to their polyunsaturated structure, composed of ALA along with DHA and EPA, PUFAs are extremely susceptible to oxidative reduction, which affects their shelf life, bioavailability, and functional performance in food, pharmaceutical, and nutraceutical products. As a result, the search for new alternatives will enhance PUFAs stability and extend shelf life (Du et al., 2022), including protein-polysaccharide complexation (Yiasmin et al., 2025), complex coacervation with spray-drying (Timilsena et al., 2016), and emulsification-spray-drying (Shaw et al., 2007). Microencapsulation was the most powerful technique among these strategies due to its capacity for preservation of the bioactive integrity of PUFAs. The resulting microcapsules facilitate their integration into different matrices such as food and pharmaceuticals. Microencapsulation allows the formation of a powdered form, which enlarges the incorporation of PUFAs in medicinal and culinary compositions with preservation of their biological activities.

The complex coacervation-based microencapsulation technique was achieved following different steps such as polymer solution preparation, emulsion preparation, complex coacervation, charge optimization, and shell hardening (Timilsena et al., 2016).

Various encapsulation methods improve their capacity to protect PUFAs from oxygen and heat, and their use in food applications and dietary supplements. However, different parameters, such as the application area and the sensitivity of the PUFAs, affect the choice of encapsulation technique.

Spray-drying: It is a rapid method based on the emulsification of oils rich in PUFAs and quickly drying them with hot air, which limits oxygen exposure and controls the amount of oil. This technique was used especially for fish oil complexed with proteins and carbohydrates (Venugopalan and Gopakumar, 2021).

Freeze-drying: In contrast, this method was released at freeze temperatures under vacuum to dry emulsions, reducing thermal oxidation and preserving sensitive PUFAs (such as highly fragile oils). It generates higher stable porous microcapsules (Khoshnoudi-Nia et al., 2022).

Microwave drying: It was a rapid drying method based on heating in anaerobic conditions, leading to low porous capsules with good stability against oxidation (Kumar et al., 2024).

Coacervation: It was based on the separation of different polymer phases present in the reaction mixture, which offers the formation of dense microcapsules, a technique for separating polymer phases that forms dense microcapsules, enhancing both their barrier properties against oxygen and their encapsulation efficiency. It was a great method to extend the shelf life of PUFAs.

7.8.2 Antioxidant incorporation

Unfortunately, lipids are susceptible to oxidation, which modifies their taste due to the generation of unsaturated carbonyls and toxic reaction products during the different processes of extraction, storage, and food preparation (Ganesan et al., 2014). For this reason, it was necessary to introduce natural antioxidants derived from plant extracts, synthetic antioxidants (such as DL-α-tocopherol, butylated hydroxytoluene [BHT], butylated hydroxyanisole etc.) to protect PUFAs from oxidative reduction in foods (Nain and Berdal, 2021; Shen and Lu, 2020; Wang et al., 2018). Generally, synthetic and natural tocopherols are the most used antioxidants in meals and dietary supplements (Yui et al., 2016). They play a key role in the reduction of the oxidation rate and in scavenging lipid peroxides in order to stop food damage. Different researchers reported the use of polyphenols, carotenoids, and tocopherols in food preservation (Nain and Berdal, 2021; Shen and Lu, 2020; Wang et al., 2018). For instance, rosemary and green tea extracts (rich in catechins) indicate their effectiveness in the stability of the n-3 PUFAs from flaxseed oil and the DHA-rich oil, respectively, compared to the BHT (Shen and Lu, 2020; Wang et al., 2018). Similarly, chia seed oils have also proved their antioxidant protection due to their rich composition, including carotenoids, tocopherol, and polyphenols (Mikołajczak et al., 2020).

7.8.3 Enzymatic and structural modifications

Fats and oils that haven't been subjected to any alteration processes might lack the required attributes. Hence, the limited availability of these lipids with optimal properties is often due to their high cost. Thus alternative raw materials that can serve as suitable substitutes are developed. These methods change the physico-chemical characteristics of lipids, successfully enhancing properties in foods, namely durability and melting point. Additionally, they can promote consumer health by regulating fatty acid ratios (Zbikowska et al., 2023).

7.8.3.1 Hydrogenation

Hydrogenation is one of the earliest techniques used for transforming oils to improve their utility and extend shelf life. This process involves the saturation of unsaturated fatty acids by incorporating hydrogen gas in the presence of a metal catalyst, generally nickel, at a thermal range extending from 140°C to 200°C (Senanayake & Shahidi, 2020). PUFAs are subjected to hydrogenation when their double bonds interact with hydrogen to produce denser saturated compounds. This method transforms liquid oils into solid or semisolid fats with unique melting points and enhances oxidative stability. Temperature, pressure, and time can be fine-tuned to modify the degree of hydrogenation, enabling either partial or complete hydrogenation based on the characteristics of the target product (Homroy et al., 2024). Despite its effectiveness as a catalyst, nickel can leave hazardous residues and contribute to the creation of trans fatty acid (TFA). Alternative catalysts such as palladium and platinum have been explored. Platinum is less reactive yet generates fewer TFAs, whereas palladium is efficient but susceptible to deactivation (İnanlar & Altay, 2024). However, partial hydrogenation poses significant health risks as it promotes the rearrangement of unsaturated molecules into trans forms instead of complete saturation. Consequently, the creation of TFAs. Due to their correlation with elevated risks of cardiovascular illnesses and overall death rate, these TFAs are being reduced in food products worldwide (Żbikowska et al., 2019). Additionally, moisture in oils can prevent hydrogenation through promoting hydrolysis and the formation of free FA, which can then be saponified in high-temperature hydrogenation settings. To prevent this, oils are usually dried either before or during autoclaving (Senanayake & Shahidi, 2020). Notwithstanding hydrogenation's technological benefits, the nutritional disadvantages—most notably the higher TFA level in partially hydrogenated oils—have made the creation and use of substitute fat modification techniques necessary. Thus the importance of lipase intervention.

7.8.3.2 Enymatic-esterification

These enzymes belong to a variety of organisms, involving animals, plants, and microorganisms, where their primary role is to break down lipids into glycerol, free fatty acids, diacylglycerols (DAGs), and monoacylglycerols (MAGs) (Szymczak et al., 2021). Moreover, lipases are enzymes that facilitate the production of structured triacylglycerols (STAGs). These modified triglycerides are distinctive fat molecules arranged in configurations. DHA may hold one place sn-2 while the other two sites (sn-1 and sn-3) can be filled by other desirable fatty acids. Triacylglycerols (TAGs) with up to 80%–90% DHA, which aren't naturally present in most food sources, can also be produced by these enzymes (Fig. 7.1). TAGs in fish and vegetable oils are usually the source of omega-3 fatty acids, such as DHA, although krill oil contains trace amounts of phospholipids (PLs) that contain DHA and EPA. Because they dissolve more readily in water, PLs are more readily absorbed by the body than TAGs. The EPA and DHA content of PLs can be increased by using a technique known as selective reactions with phospholipases to create omega-3-rich PLs. This strategy enables the regulated insertion of fatty acids at the proper locations within the PL. In a nutshell, lipase-catalyzed esterification is used to improve the stability, bioavailability, and targeted administration of omega-3 fatty acids in TAGs and PLs (Castejón & Señoráns, 2020).

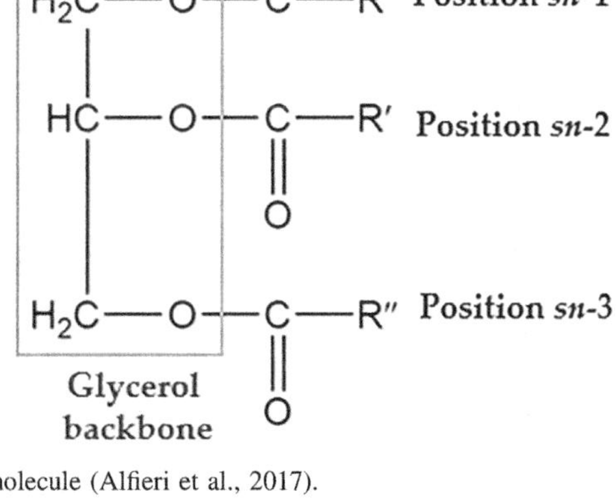

FIGURE 7.1 Structure of a triacylglycerol molecule (Alfieri et al., 2017).

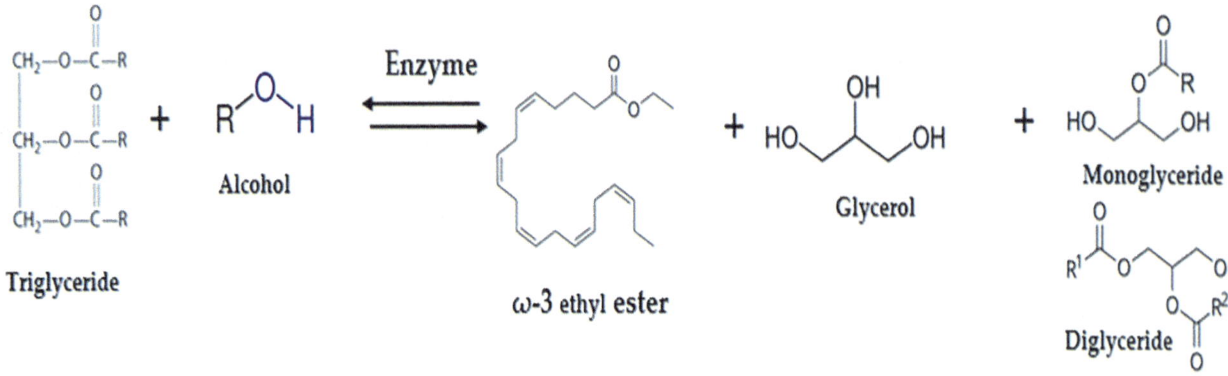

FIGURE 7.2 In the ethanolysis process, a triglyceride is converted into a 2-monoglyceride through the action of an *sn*-1,3-regioselective lipase (Castejón et al., 2020).

7.8.3.2.1 Production of omega-3-rich ethyl ester concentrates

Most commercially available omega-3 concentrates are products derived from omega-3 ethyl esters. Furthermore, the production of structured lipids commonly uses omega-3 fatty acid ethyl esters (FAEE) as intermediates. FAEEs can be synthesized chemically or enzymatically to produce omega-3 concentrates. Due to their mild reaction conditions, good selectivity, few unwanted byproducts, and less oxidation of omega-3 PUFAs, they are a better method, lipases offer a more effective method. Using ethanol (acyl acceptor) and nonspecific lipases, ethanolysis reactions are the main approach for generating omega-3 ethyl esters. TAGs is initially converted into DAGs in this three-step process. DAGs are subsequently transformed into MAGs (DAGs), which are later converted to glycerol and FAEEs (Castejón & Señoráns, 2020) (Fig. 7.2). Various studies have reported the enzymatic production of omega-3 ethyl esters via ethanolysis, examining numerous reaction conditions and the activities of different lipases. TAGs were completely transformed into FAEE with as much as 65% ALA by utilizing an immobilized *Thermomyces lanuginosus* lipase encased in PEG to generate omega-3 FAEE from chia oil. This method showed the new compound's great stability and was ideal for the food sector (Castejón et al., 2019). An extracellular alkaline lipase obtained from Proteus vulgaris (lipase K80) was utilized to produce omega-3 FAEE from menhaden oil, resulting in a pure product (92% FAEEs) (Kim & Kim, 2016).

7.8.3.2.2 Formation of omega-3-enriched 2-monoglycerides

It is widely recognized that the structure of fatty acids in the glycerol backbone of TAGs greatly influences the body's digestion and absorption processes. Fatty acids are consequently located at three distinct positions on TAG molecules, known as sn-1 and sn-3 (outer) and sn-2 (central). Free fatty acids are less readily absorbed than esterified fatty acids in the sn-2 position of TAGs in the form of MAGs. Enzymatic ethanolysis of TAGs is a successful technique that uses a sn-1,3-regioselective lipase to produce 2-MAGs (Ishihara et al., 2019) (Fig. 7.2). According to He et al. (2016), 2-MAGs were produced using Lipozyme TL-IM derived from purified microalgae oil (*Isochrysis galbana* TAGs), yielding a product enriched in 25.2% DHA and 6.9% omega-3 stearidonic acid. Another contribution investigated the regioselective synthesis of 2-MAGs enriched in DHA using three immobilized lipases (RML, CAL-B, and *Alcaligenes* ssp.). The greatest results were obtained when RML was adsorbed onto a hydrophobic substrate (Moreno-Perez and Luna, 2018).

7.8.3.2.3 Production of structured triglycerides enriched in omega-3

TAGs with a distinct rearrangement of various fatty acids throughout the glycerol backbone are typically known as STAGs. With a primary focus on providing functional, structural, and nervous system-related development, particularly for EPA and DHA content -specific food products for infants daily needs and health elements have been designed via the use of lipase-catalyzed reactions. Some researchers have combined lipase-catalyzed processes with new sources of omega-3 to increase the omega -3 content of STAGs for newborn formulae (Fig. 7.3). It has been reported that camelina oil can be used to generate human milk fat replacements. The novel STAG was abundant in palmitic acid in sn-2 and omega-3 fatty acids esterified in sn-1,3. Therefore the created product might be combined with 1,3-dioleoyl-2-palmitoyl-glycerol, the primary TAG of human milk, to create an oil that has an identical composition similar to human milk and contains sufficient amounts of important fatty acids (Faustino et al., 2016). Using a combination of immobilized lipases, the goal of another study was to create TAGs with increased quantities of DHA and ARA at *sn*-2 by modifying commercial new oils

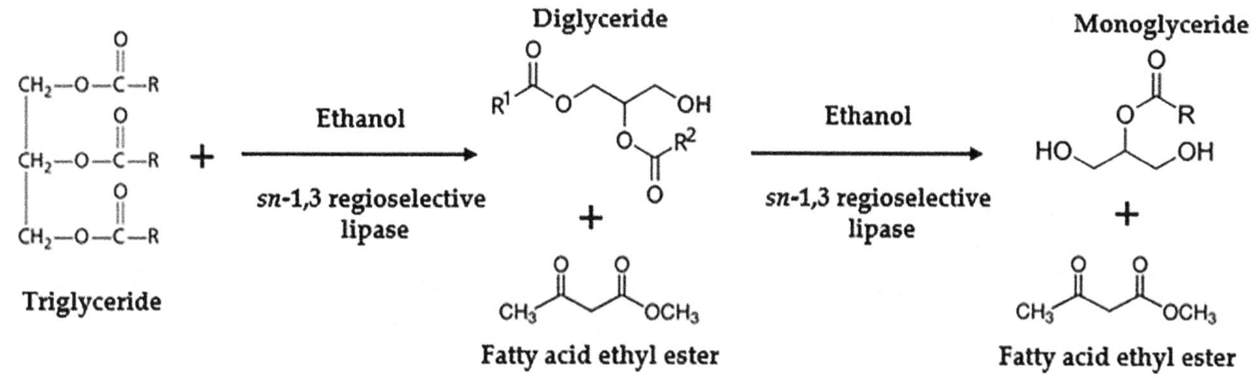

FIGURE 7.3 Transesterification of a triglyceride using ethanol as the acyl acceptor leads to the formation of omega-3 ethyl esters. In the ethanolysis process, a triglyceride is converted into a 2-monoglyceride through the action of an *sn*-1,3-regioselective lipase (Castejón et al., 2020).

from single cell organisms (DHASCO® and ARASCO®) via an enzymatic reaction. The same authors documented that TAGs were produced using caprylic acid at *sn*-1,3 and DHA and ARA at *sn*-2 (48.1% and 35.8%, respectively), creating a product that may be advantageous for kids (Álvarez & Akoh, 2016).

7.8.3.3 Enzymatic interesterification

The World Health Organization states that beneficial oils should contain a balanced mix of saturated, monounsaturated, and polyunsaturated fats, in addition to an adequate amount of essential fatty acids and antioxidants. The optimal ratio for saturated to mono - and polyunsaturated fats is 1:1.5:1, while the recommended ratio for ALA to LA is between 1:5 and 1:10. Nevertheless, this ideal equilibrium is not present in most natural vegetable oils. Certain oils contain a higher concentration of polyunsaturated fats, while others tend to be richer in saturated fats. As a result, no oil satisfies the health advice. Thus the food industry is trying to change oils to tackle this limitation. Enzymatic interesterification is one technique that is gaining popularity. This procedure is implemented to alter the TAG molecule's fatty acid distribution. It modifies the fat's structure without introducing any dangerous ingredients, particularly trans fats. Consequently, it enhances the oil characteristics, including stability, texture, and melting temperature (Singh, Chopra, et al., 2022; Cui et al., 2022). The lipase interestification rate is influenced by several factors, including the enzyme concentration, the temperature and time of the reaction, and the concentration of substrate and fatty acid esters. The effectiveness of this method is determined by the specific types of lipases employed. These biocatalysts are classified according to their regiospecificity. *Candida rugosa* and *Geotrichum candidum* lipases have nonregiospecificity, while others, such as *Mucor miehei* and *Aspergillus niger* lipases, are specific. Accordingly, two scenarios are feasible. The fatty acids are randomly switched to the various locations of the TAG if the lipase interesterification is performed with a nonspecific lipase enzyme. Yet, if the process is performed with *sn*-1,3-specific lipase, the *sn*-1,3 position will be hydrolyzed, leaving the *sn*-2 position unchanged. However, in a real catalytic reaction, acyl migration may occur even during a regiospecific process, leading to the sn-2 fatty acid random redistribution (İnanlar & Altay, 2024; Singh, Arif, et al., 2022). Enzymatic interesterification has several benefits over chemical interesterification, such as improved specificity, less environmental contamination, and simpler postprocessing procedures. Recent research on lipase-catalyzed interesterification has been reported in Table 7.3.

7.8.4 Biopolymer-based delivery systems

Vegetable oils can be encapsulated by trapping liquid oil within a matrix to achieve the required result. The purpose of encapsulating vegetable oils is to enhance their bioavailability, manage their release, improve their oxidative stability, and cover up their flavor, color, and scent. Therefore the liquid oil is either transformed into gels, beads, or powders based on the product's desirability (Pattnaik & Mishra, 2022).

7.8.4.1 Oleogelators

The liquid oil is efficiently trapped and immobilized within a three-dimensional structure by oleogelators, leading to its transformation from a liquid to a solid gel-like structure. It is necessary for the food-grade oleogelators to be Generally

TABLE 7.3 Case studies of enzymatic interesterification.

Case study	Enzymatic interesterification	Main findings	References
Nutritional profile and texture of butter made with milk fat	70°C for 6 h in the presence of 5% lipase	Elevation of the unsaturation level in the oil base	
Investigation of soybean oil interesterified with propylene glycol in supercritical CO_2	Supercritical CO_2 at 276 bars, with 17 g of 1,2-propanediol/unit of oil, 0.3% lipozyme at 70°C for 15 min	Development of more eco-friendly fats with reduced *trans*-fat levels compared to conventional soybean oils	
Producing *trans*-fat-free fats through rice bran oil with fully hydrogenated rice bran oil	Incubation for 24 h at 60°C, 200 rpm with 10% lipozyme.	Generation of novel triacylglycerols with a moderate level of unsaturation and improved functional properties, leading to reduced melting points and lower fat content	
Modification of the margarine properties	Beef Tallow (BT) and coconut oil were melted at 70°C and then mixed to prepare 3 samples (80%, 70% and 60% (w/w)) of BT, with 5% (w/w) Lipozyme at 70°C for 5 h	The margarine exhibited an evenly distributed β′ crystalline form that enhances texture, a diverse fatty acid profile with low-melting triglycerides, and lacked detectable β polymorphs, which helps prevent a gritty mouthfeel	
Production of fats, such as cocoa butter substitutes for chocolate manufacturing.	The mixture of palm oil, palm olein, and palm kernel oil was enzymatically interesterified using 1,3-specific lipase enzymes.	The cocoa butter substitutes formed prominent, small, and dense β′ crystals due to suitable TAG composition, resulting in compound chocolate with ideal hardness, improved texture, and better fracturability.	
Production of human milk fat alternatives from different oils, including important FAs like EPA and DHA.	The sn-1,2-specific lipase enzyme incorporates palmitic acid at the sn-2 position, protecting PUFAs	The mild EIE conditions protected PUFAs while enabling the lipase's sn-2 specificity to incorporate palmitic acid in the desired position, producing a human milk fat substitute.	Ghosh et al. (2016)

Recognized As Safe and have specific characteristics, such as lipophilia, surface activity, thermoreversibility, and nontoxicity. Various oleogelators are available depending on the type of gelling, including:

- Low molecular weight substances, such as PLs (lecithin), phytosterols or sterol esters (sorbitan monostearate, sorbitan tristearate, sitosterol), and fatty acids that create self-assembling fibrous structures (sphingolipids, hydroxy stearic acid);
- polymers include ethyl cellulose, hydroxypropyl methylcellulose, methylcellulose, chitosan, chitin, and proteins like zein and gelatin, and
- crystalline substances, namely plant or natural waxes, MAG, DAG, and policosanol.

Oleogels' structural, thermal, and dynamic properties are influenced by their composition and concentration of oil/oleogelators. The acyl chain length of the vegetable oils and their FA content affect the gelling performance of gel waxes. Consequently, oleogels containing saturated fatty acids and high melting TAGs produce hard gels with high viscosity (Demirkesen & Mert, 2020).

7.8.4.2 Oil beads

Generally speaking, oil beads resemble hydrogel beads with liquid oil as the core material. The fundamental process for making these beads is to dissolve vegetable oil into the wall material solution, then blend the mixture well to create a uniform solution.

Proteins serve as emulsifiers and polysaccharides as structural reinforcing agents to increase the effectiveness of encapsulation. The interaction between soy protein isolate (SPI) and alginate with different oil amounts was investigated. Due to the high viscosity that prevented SPI from moving to the oil-water interface, they discovered that the increase of the alginate, oil, and SPI content to 1.5%, 40%, and 1%, respectively, decreased the emulsion stability. However, higher SPI concentration promoted some aggregation of oil droplets while improving absorption to the oil-water surface. According to, whey protein isolate formed stronger connections with alginate compared to SPI throughout the gel bead formation process by forming hydrogen bonds between polar amino acids and alginate molecules, which assisted in halting the beads' loss of water and sunflower oil. Some researchers have proposed using emulsifiers or the emulsification process in conjunction with ionic gelation to produce oil beads with large oil loading. Therefore using the alginate interaction, da Silva James et al. (2019) showed that the addition of Tween 20 at 1% displayed a stable emulsion. Additionally, they found that the microparticle had a high encapsulation effectiveness (>99.5%) for oil loads of around 75%.

7.8.4.3 Oil powder

The liquid oil that is encapsulated could be converted into stable powders by undergoing numerous phases. (1) The emulsification process involves dispersing the active material (oil) within a solution of wall materials, which is then mixed using a shear blender to create an emulsion. (2) Solvent evaporation is employed to eliminate the solvents utilized to solubilize the wall materials in the solution (Pattnaik & Mishra, 2022). In accordance with Gomes & Kurozawa (2020), when rice protein was utilized for microencapsulation of linseed oil, it showed good emulsion stability following enzymatic hydrolysis by flavorzyme protein hydrolysate, with an ideal encapsulation efficiency of 89.5%. The oxidation process is also controlled by the microcapsules' particle size in addition to the wall materials. Due to a stronger particle-air interface created by a smaller surface-to-volume ratio, Linke et al. (2020) found that smaller particles had more oxidation than bigger ones. By interacting with the oil droplets, the bigger particle-air interface revealed the surface to oxygen and increased oxygen diffusion, which caused negative effects. However, the resistance to oxidation of oil powders may be impacted by altering the encapsulation process, which can vary the particle characteristics (size, density, and porosity).

7.9 Conclusion

Demand for PUFAs has increased due to their health benefits, such as EPA and DHA, which ensure interesting functions in keeping physiological homeostasis. The susceptibility of PUFAs to oxidative degradation has led technologists to question their preservation by encapsulation. The oil could be effectively trapped in a gel or powder matrix by different alternatives such as spray-drying, freeze-drying, microwave drying, coacervation, etc. The encapsulation method needs a good selection of the wall materials, which are mostly a mixture of polysaccharides and proteins. Encapsulation of PUFAs would be a talented method to increase oxidative stability for industrialization and storage. In addition, the fatty acid content was not significantly affected by this incorporation. The resulting oil particles were applied in various areas, as well as in food industries such as dairy, bakery, and meat, where fat replacement or beneficial fatty acid enrichment are major concerns. Encapsulates are accepted by consumers for their taste and flavor attributes when incorporated into food nutrients.

References

Aerssens, D., Cadoni, E., Tack, L., & Madder, A. (2022). A photosensitized singlet oxygen (1O2) toolbox for bio-organic applications: Tailoring 1O2 generation for DNA and protein labelling, targeting and biosensing. *Molecules (Basel, Switzerland), 27*(3), 778. https://doi.org/10.3390/molecules27030778.

Álvarez, C. A., & Akoh, C. C. (2016). Preparation of infant formula fat analog containing capric acid and enriched with DHA and ARA at the sn-2 position. *Journal of the American Oil Chemists' Society, 93*(4), 531–542.

Albert, K., Vatai, G., & Koris, A. (2017). Microencapsulation of vegetable oil-alternative approaches using membrane technology and spray drying. *Hungarian Journal of Industry and Chemistry*, 29–33.

Alfieri, A., Imperlini, E., Nigro, E., Vitucci, D., Orrù, S., Daniele, A., & Mancini, A. (2017). Effects of plant oil interesterified triacylglycerols on lipemia and human health. *International Journal of Molecular Sciences, 19*(1), 104.

Assi, A., Michael-Jubeli, R., Baillet-Guffroy, A., & Tfayli, A. (2023). Characterization of free fatty acids photo-oxidation under UV radiations: A stepwise Raman study. *Journal of Raman Spectroscopy, 54*(1), 24–36. https://doi.org/10.1002/jrs.6449.

Ayala, A., Muñoz, M. F., & Argüelles, S. (2014). Lipid peroxidation: Production, metabolism, and signaling mechanisms of malondialdehyde and 4-hydroxy-2-nonenal. *Oxidative Medicine and Cellular Longevity, 2014*. https://doi.org/10.1155/2014/360438, http://www.landesbioscience.com/journals/oximed.

Breitzig, M., Bhimineni, C., Lockey, R., & Kolliputi, N. (2016). 4-Hydroxy-2-nonenal: A critical target in oxidative stress? *American Journal of Physiology-Cell Physiology, 311*(4), C537. https://doi.org/10.1152/ajpcell.00101.2016.

Calder, P. C. (2017). Omega-3 fatty acids and inflammatory processes: From molecules to man. *Biochemical Society Transactions, 45*(5), 1105–1115.

Cao, H., Xiong, S. F., Dong, L. L., & Dai, Z. T. (2024). Study on the mechanism of lipid peroxidation induced by carbonate radicals. *Molecules (Basel, Switzerland), 29*(5). https://doi.org/10.3390/molecules29051125, http://www.mdpi.com/journal/molecules.

Castejón, N., & Señoráns, F. J. (2020). Enzymatic modification to produce health-promoting lipids from fish oil, algae and other new omega-3 sources: A review. *New Biotechnology, 57*, 45–54.

Castejón, N., Moreno-Pérez, S., Abreu Silveira, E., Fernández Lorente, G., Guisán, J. M., & Señoráns, F. J. (2019). Synthesis of omega-3 ethyl esters from chia oil catalyzed by polyethylene glycol-modified lipases with improved stability. *Food Chemistry, 271*, 433–439. https://doi.org/10.1016/j.foodchem.2018.07.215, www.elsevier.com/locate/foodchem.

Chang, X., Wang, Y., Zheng, B., Chen, Y., Xie, J., Song, Y., Ding, X., Hu, X., Hu, X., & Yu, Q. (2022). The role of acrolein in neurodegenerative diseases and its protective strategy. *Foods, 11*(20), 3203. https://doi.org/10.3390/foods11203203.

Chira, A., Rekik, I., Rahmouni, F., Ben Amor, I., Gargouri, B., & Kallel, C. (2022). Phytochemical composition of Urtica dioica essential oil with antioxidant and anti-inflammatory properties: In vitro and in vivo studies. *Current Pharmaceutical Biotechnology*, (5), 728–739.

Cot, M., Mijas, G., Prieto-Fuentes, R., Riba-Moliner, M., & Cayuela, D. (2024). The influence of titanium dioxide (TiO_2) particle size and crystalline form on the microstructure and UV protection factor of polyester substrates. *Polymers, 16*(4), 475. https://doi.org/10.3390/polym16040475.

da Silva James, N. K., Castro, L. P. S., Freitas, S. P., & Nogueira, R. I. (2019). Increasing energy efficiency in microencapsulation of soybean oil by spray drying. *Brazilian Journal of Development*, (7), 8082–8095.

Demirkesen, I., & Mert, B. (2020). Recent developments of oleogel utilizations in bakery products. *Critical Reviews in Food Science and Nutrition, 60*(14), 2460–2479. https://doi.org/10.1080/10408398.2019.1649243.

Dessì, M. A., Deiana, M., Day, B. W., Rosa, A., Banni, S., & Corongiu, F. P. (2002). Oxidative stability of polyunsaturated fatty acids: Effect of squalene. *European Journal of Lipid Science and Technology, 104*(8), 506–512. https://doi.org/10.1002/1438-9312(200208)104:8<506::AID-EJLT506>3.0.CO;2-1.

Du, Q., Zhou, L., Li, M., Lyu, F., Liu, J., & Ding, Y. (2022). Omega-3 polyunsaturated fatty acid encapsulation system: Physical and oxidative stability, and medical applications. *Food Frontiers, 3*(2), 239–255. https://doi.org/10.1002/fft2.134.

Faustino, A. R., Osório, N. M., Tecelão, C., Canet, A., Valero, F., & Ferreira-Dias, S. (2016). Camelina oil as a source of polyunsaturated fatty acids for the production of human milk fat substitutes catalyzed by a heterologous *Rhizopus oryzae* lipase. *European Journal of Lipid Science and Technology, 118*(4), 532–544. https://doi.org/10.1002/ejlt.201500003, http://www3.interscience.wiley.com/journal/69502350/home.

Fuloria, S., Subramaniyan, V., Karupiah, S., Kumari, U., Sathasivam, K., Meenakshi, D. U., Wu, Y. S., Guad, R. M., Udupa, K., & Fuloria, N. K. (2020). A comprehensive review on source, types, effects, nanotechnology, detection, and therapeutic management of reactive carbonyl species associated with various chronic diseases. *Antioxidants, 9*(11), 1075. https://doi.org/10.3390/antiox9111075.

Ganesan, B., Brothersen, C., & McMahon, D. J. (2014). Fortification of foods with omega-3 polyunsaturated fatty acids. *Critical Reviews in Food Science and Nutrition, 54*(1), 98–114.

Gentile, F., Arcaro, A., Pizzimenti, S., Daga, M., Cetrangolo, G. P., & Dianzani, C. (2017). DNA damage by lipid peroxidation products: Implications in cancer, inflammation and autoimmunity. *AIMS Genetics*, (2), 103–137.

Ghosh, M., Sengupta, A., Bhattacharyya, D. K., & Ghosh, M. (2016). Preparation of human milk fat analogue by enzymatic interesterification reaction using palm stearin and fish oil. *Journal of Food Science and Technology, 53*, 2017–2024.

Gomes, M. H. G., & Kurozawa, L. E. (2020). Improvement of the functional and antioxidant properties of rice protein by enzymatic hydrolysis for the microencapsulation of linseed oil. *Journal of Food Engineering, 267*, 109761.

Gutiérrez, E. L., Sacchetto, J., Boscá, F., Marín, M. L., Massad, W., Montaña, M. P., Miskoski, S., & Ferrari, G. V. (2024). Photosensitized oxygenation reactions as an alternative towards the degradation of fenamates and related pollutants using visible light. *Journal of Water Process Engineering, 60*. https://doi.org/10.1016/j.jwpe.2024.105049, https://www.sciencedirect.com/science/journal/22147144.

Hajeyah, A. A., Griffiths, W. J., Wang, Y., Finch, A. J., & O'Donnell, V. B. (2020). The biosynthesis of enzymatically oxidized lipids. *Frontiers in Endocrinology, 11*. https://doi.org/10.3389/fendo.2020.591819, https://www.frontiersin.org/journals/endocrinology#.

Harrysson, H., Krook, J. L., Larsson, K., Tullberg, C., Oerbekke, A., Toth, G., Pavia, H., & Undeland, I. (2021). Effect of storage conditions on lipid oxidation, nutrient loss and colour of dried seaweeds, *Porphyra umbilicalis* and *Ulva fenestrata,* subjected to different pretreatments. *Algal Research, 56*, 102295. https://doi.org/10.1016/j.algal.2021.102295.

He, Y., Li, J., Kodali, S., Chen, B., & Guo, Z. (2016). The near-ideal catalytic property of *Candida antarctica* lipase A to highly concentrate n-3 polyunsaturated fatty acids in monoacylglycerols via one-step ethanolysis of triacylglycerols. *Bioresource Technology, 219*, 466–478. https://doi.org/10.1016/j.biortech.2016.08.007.

Hershelman, D., Kahler, K. M., Price, M. J., Lu, I., Fu, Y., Plumeri, P. A., Karaisz, F., Bassett, N. F., Findeis, P. M., & Clapp, C. H. (2019). Oxygenation reactions catalyzed by the F557V mutant of soybean lipoxygenase-1: Evidence for two orientations of substrate binding. *Archives of Biochemistry and Biophysics, 674*. https://doi.org/10.1016/j.abb.2019.108082, http://www.elsevier.com/inca/publications/store/6/2/2/7/8/7/index.htt.

Homroy, S., Chopra, R., Singh, P. K., Dhiman, A., Chand, M., & Talwar, B. (2024). Role of encapsulation on the bioavailability of omega-3 fatty acids. *Comprehensive Reviews in Food Science and Food Safety, 23*(1), 1–35. https://doi.org/10.1111/1541-4337.13272, http://onlinelibrary.wiley.com/journal/10.1111/(ISSN)1541-4337.

Huo, J., Peng, W., Ouyang, H., Liu, X., Wang, P., Yu, X., Xie, T., & Li, S. (2024). Exploration of markers in oxidized rancidity walnut kernels based on lipidomics and volatolomics. *Food Research International, 182*, 114141. https://doi.org/10.1016/j.foodres.2024.114141.

İnanlar, B., & Altay, F. (2024). The method that makes oils and fats healthier: Interesterification. *Black Sea Journal of Engineering and Science, 7*(5), 1081–1091.

Ishihara, T., Yoshida, M., & Arita, M. (2019). Omega-3 fatty acid-derived mediators that control inflammation and tissue homeostasis. *International Immunology, 31*(9), 559–567.

Johnson, D. R., & Decker, E. A. (2015). The role of oxygen in lipid oxidation reactions: A review. *Annual Review of Food Science and Technology, 6*, 171–190. https://doi.org/10.1146/annurev-food-022814-015532, http://www.annualreviews.org/journal/food.

Kasaai, M. R. (2025). Oxidative and hydrolytic deteriorations of lipids and several alternative pathways for their protections: An overview. *Food Nutrition Chemistry, 3*(1), 238. https://doi.org/10.18686/fnc238.

Khoshnoudi-Nia, S., Forghani, Z., & Jafari, S. M. (2022). A systematic review and meta-analysis of fish oil encapsulation within different micro/nanocarriers. *Critical Reviews in Food Science and Nutrition, 62*(8), 2061–2082.

Kim, S. J., & Kim, H. K. (2016). Production of Omega-3 fatty acid ethyl esters from menhaden oil using Proteus vulgaris lipase-mediated one-step transesterification and urea complexation. *Applied Biochemistry and Biotechnology, 179*, 347–360.

Kodali, S. T., Kauffman, P., Kotha, S. R., Yenigalla, A., Veeraraghavan, R., Pannu, S. R., Hund, T. J., Satoskar, A. R., McDaniel, J. C., Maddipati, R. K., & Parinandi, N. L. (2020). *Oxidative lipidomics: Analysis of oxidized lipids and lipid peroxidation in biological systems with relevance to health and disease*. Springer Science and Business Media LLC, 61–92. 10.1007/978-3-030-47318-1_5.

Kumar, A., Singh, U., Jaiswal, S. G., Dave, J., Wei, S., & Hailu, G. G. (2024). Recent trends in the encapsulation of functional lipids: Comprehensive review. *Sustainable Food Technology, 2*(6), 1610–1630. https://doi.org/10.1039/d4fb00205a, https://www.rsc.org/journals-books-databases/about-journals/sustainable-food-technology/.

Li, H., Chen, Y., Peng, Q., Tan, X., Chen, G., Zhou, H., & Yan, R. (2022). Flavonoids from bamboo leaves improve the stability of unsaturated fatty acids in the lipids of walnut emulsions. *Industrial Crops and Products, 178*, 114609.

Li, H., Li, Z., Li, N., Zhu, X., Zhang, Y., & Sun, L. (2022). D printed high performance silver mesh for transparent glass heaters through liquid sacrificial substrate electric-field-driven Jet. *Small (Weinheim an der Bergstrasse, Germany)*(17), 2107811.

Linares-Maurizi, A., Reversat, G., Awad, R., Bultel-Poncé, V., Oger, C., Galano, J. M., & Vigor, C. (2023). Bioactive oxylipins profile in marine microalgae. *Marine drugs, 21*(3), 136.

Linke, A., Hinrichs, J., & Kohlus, R. (2020). Impact of the powder particle size on the oxidative stability of microencapsulated oil. *Powder Technology, 364*, 115–122.

Majcher, M., Fahmi, R., Misiak, A., Grygier, A., & Rudzińska, M. (2025). Influence of ozone treatment on sensory quality, aroma active compounds, phytosterols and phytosterol oxidation products in stored rapeseed and flaxseed oils. *Food Chemistry, 469*. https://doi.org/10.1016/j.foodchem.2024.142551 142551.

Mikołajczak, N., Sobiechowska, D. A., & Tańska, M. (2020). Edible flowers as a new source of natural antioxidants for oxidative protection of cold-pressed oils rich in omega-3 fatty acids. *Food Research International, 134*, 109216.

Mititelu, M., Lupuliasa, D., Neacşu, S. M., Olteanu, G., Busnatu, Ş. S., Mihai, A., et al. (2024). Polyunsaturated fatty acids and human health: A key to modern nutritional balance in association with polyphenolic compounds from food sources. *Foods, 14*(1), 46.

Moreno-Perez, S., Luna, P., Señorans, J., Rocha-Martin, J., Guisan, J. M., & Fernandez-Lorente, G. (2018). Enzymatic transesterification in a solvent-free system: Synthesis of sn-2 docosahexaenoyl monoacylglycerol. *Biocatalysis and Biotransformation, 36*(3), 265–270. https://doi.org/10.1080/10242422.2017.1319823.

Mortensen, M. S., Ruiz, J., & Watts, J. L. (2023). Polyunsaturated fatty acids drive lipid peroxidation during ferroptosis. *Cells, 12*(5). https://doi.org/10.3390/cells12050804, https://www.mdpi.com/journal/cells.

Musakhanian, J., Rodier, J. D., & Dave, M. (2022). Oxidative stability in lipid formulations: A Review of the mechanisms, drivers, and inhibitors of oxidation. *AAPS PharmSciTech, 23*(5), 151.

Nain, C. W., Berdal, G., Thao, P. T. P., Mignolet, E., Buchet, M., Page, M., & Larondelle, Y. (2021). Green tea extract enhances the oxidative stability of DHA-rich oil. *Antioxidants, 10*(6). https://doi.org/10.3390/antiox10060982, https://www.mdpi.com/2076-3921/10/6/982/pdf.

Patel, A., Karageorgou, D., Rova, E., Katapodis, P., Rova, U., Christakopoulos, P., & Matsakas, L. (2020). An overview of potential oleaginous microorganisms and their role in biodiesel and omega-3 fatty acid-based industries. *Microorganisms, 8*(3), 2076–2607. https://doi.org/10.3390/microorganisms8030434.

Pattnaik, M., & Mishra, H. N. (2022). Amelioration of the stability of polyunsaturated fatty acids and bioactive enriched vegetable oil: Blending, encapsulation, and its application. *Critical Reviews in Food Science and Nutrition, 62*(23), 6253–6276.

Pinheiro Pantoja, K. R., Melo Aires, G. C., Ferreira, C. P., Lima, M.da C.de, Menezes, E. G. O., & Carvalho Junior, R. N.de (2024). Supercritical technology as an efficient alternative to cold pressing for avocado oil: A comparative approach. *Foods, 13*(15), 2424.

Rahman, M., Usmani, W., Nureen, U., Ullah, A., Masmoum, M. D., Abbas, Z., et al. (2024). Impact of omega-3 fatty acids on cardiovascular disease prevention: An updated meta-analysis of RCTs. *Journal of Advances in Medicine and Medical Research, 6*(36), 240–255.

Schirmer, B.C., Sørheim, O., Skaar, I., & Kure, C.F. (2020). The influence of concentrations of carbon dioxide and residual oxygen on the growth of meat spoilage moulds. FAO.

Senanayake, N., & Shahidi, F. (2020). Modification of fats and oils via chemical and enzymatic methods. In F. Shahidi (Ed.). *In Bailey's industrial oil and fat products* (pp. 1–29). Hoboken, NJ, USA: John Wiley & Sons, Ltd 7th ed.

Shaw, L. A., McClements, D. J., & Decker, E. A. (2007). Spray-dried multilayered emulsions as a delivery method for ω-3 fatty acids into food systems. *Journal of Agricultural and Food Chemistry, 55*(8), 3112–3119.

Shen, Y., Lu, T., Liu, X.-Y., Zhao, M.-T., Yin, F.-W., Rakariyatham, K., & Zhou, D.-Y. (2020). Improving the oxidative stability and lengthening the shelf life of DHA algae oil with composite antioxidants. *Food Chemistry, 313*(3), 126139. https://doi.org/10.1016/j.foodchem.2019.126139.

Singh, P., Arif, Y., Miszczuk, E., Bajguz, A., & Hayat, S. (2022). Specific roles of lipoxygenases in development and responses to stress in plants. *Plants, 11*(7), 979.

Singh, P. K., Chopra, R., Garg, M., Dhiman, A., & Dhyani, A. (2022). Enzymatic interesterification of vegetable oil: A review on physicochemical and functional properties, and its health effects. *Journal of Oleo Science, 71*(12), 1697–1709. https://doi.org/10.5650/jos.ess22118, https://www.jstage.jst.go.jp/article/jos/71/12/71_ess22118/_pdf.

Szymczak, T., Cybulska, J., Podleśny, M., & Frąc, M. (2021). Various perspectives on microbial lipase production using agri-food waste and renewable products. *Agriculture, 11*(6), 540. https://doi.org/10.3390/agriculture11060540.

Tatiyaborworntham, N., Oz, F., Richards, M. P., & Wu, H. (2022). Paradoxical effects of lipolysis on the lipid oxidation in meat and meat products. *Food Chemistry: X, 14*. https://doi.org/10.1016/j.fochx.2022.100317, https://www.journals.elsevier.com/food-chemistry-x.

Timilsena, Y. P., Adhikari, R., Barrow, C. J., & Adhikari, B. (2016). Microencapsulation of chia seed oil using chia seed protein isolate-chia seed gum complex coacervates. *International Journal of Biological Macromolecules, 91*, 347–357. https://doi.org/10.1016/j.ijbiomac.2016.05.058, www.elsevier.com/locate/ijbiomac.

Venugopalan, V. K., Gopakumar, L. R., Kumaran, A. K., Chatterjee, N. S., Soman, V., Peeralil, S., Mathew, S., McClements, D. J., & Nagarajarao, R. C. (2021). Encapsulation and protection of omega-3-rich fish oils using food-grade delivery systems. *Foods, 10*(7). https://doi.org/10.3390/foods10071566, https://www.mdpi.com/2304-8158/10/7/1566/pdf.

Wang, D., Xiao, H., Lyu, X., Chen, H., & Wei, F. (2023). Lipid oxidation in food science and nutritional health: A comprehensive review. *Oil Crop Science, 8*(1), 35–44. https://doi.org/10.1016/j.ocsci.2023.02.002.

Wang, Y. Z., Fu, S. G., Wang, S. Y., Yang, D. J., Wu, Y. H. S., & Chen, Y. C. (2018). Effects of a natural antioxidant, polyphenol-rich rosemary (*Rosmarinus officinalis* L.) extract, on lipid stability of plant-derived omega-3 fatty-acid rich oil. *LWT, 89*, 210–216. https://doi.org/10.1016/j.lwt.2017.10.055, https://www.journals.elsevier.com/lwt.

Xi, Z., Jin, B., & Shan, Z. (2021). Reaction mechanisms involving peroxy radical in the low-temperature oxidation of coal. *Fuel, 300*, 120943.

Xiong, C., Li, Q., Li, S., Chen, C., Chen, Z., & Huang, W. (2017). In vitro antimicrobial activities and mechanism of 1-Octen-3-ol against food-related bacteria and pathogenic fungi. *Journal of Oleo Science, 66*(9), 1041–1049. https://doi.org/10.5650/jos.ess16196.

Yiasmin, M. N., Al Azad, S., Easdani, M., Islam, M. S., Hussain, M., Cao, W., & Hua, X. (2025). The state-of-the-art on exploring polysaccharide-protein interactions and its mechanisms, stability, and their role in food systems. *Food Reviews International*, 1–36.

Yoshitake, M., Kazumi, K., Masahito, K., & Jun, O. (2019). Selective nonanal molecular recognition with nanosheets for lung cancer sensor. *International Journal of Applied Ceramic Technology, 16*(5), 1807–1811.

Yui, Y., Miyazaki, S., Ma, Y., Ohira, M., Fiehn, O., Ikegami, T., McCalley, D. V., & Tanaka, N. (2016). Distinction of synthetic dl-α-tocopherol from natural vitamin E (d-α-tocopherol) by reversed-phase liquid chromatography. Enhanced selectivity of a polymeric C18 stationary phase at low temperature and/or at high pressure. *Journal of Chromatography. A, 1450*, 45–52. https://doi.org/10.1016/j.chroma.2016.04.076.

Zbikowska, A., Onacik-Gür, S., Kowalska, M., Zbikowska, K., & Feszterová, M. (2023). Trends in fat modifications enabling alternative partially hydrogenated fat products proposed for advanced application. *Gels, 9*(6), 453. https://doi.org/10.3390/gels9060453.

Zeis, B., Buchen, I., Wacker, A., & Martin-Creuzburg, D. (2019). Temperature-induced changes in body lipid composition affect vulnerability to oxidative stress in *Daphnia magna. Comparative Biochemistry and Physiology Part - B: Biochemistry and Molecular Biology, 232*, 101–107. https://doi.org/10.1016/j.cbpb.2019.03.008, https://www.journals.elsevier.com/comparative-biochemistry-and-physiology-part-b-biochemistry-and-molecular-biology.

Zhuang, Y., Dong, J., He, X., Wang, J., Li, C., Dong, L., Zhang, Y., Zhou, X., Wang, H., Yi, Y., & Wang, S. (2022). Impact of heating temperature and fatty acid type on the formation of lipid oxidation products during thermal processing. *Frontiers in Nutrition, 9*, 2296–861X. https://doi.org/10.3389/fnut.2022.913297.

Żbikowska, A., Onacik-Gür, S., Kowalska, M., & Rutkowska, J. (2019). Trans fatty acids in polish pastry. *Journal of Food Protection, 82*(6), 1028–1033. https://doi.org/10.4315/0362-028x.jfp-18-497.

Chapter 8

High-pressure processing for retaining polyunsaturated fatty acids nutritional integrity

Sangeetha Karunanithi
Food Technology, Vignan's Foundation for Science, Technology and Research (Deemed to be University), Guntur, Andhra Pradesh, India

8.1 Introduction

8.1.1 Importance of polyunsaturated fatty acids in human nutrition

Polyunsaturated fatty acids (PUFAs) are dietary lipids that are an essential component of the diet and are vital for health, metabolic function, and prevention of disease. PUFAs differ from saturated fatty acids (FAs) by having two or more carbon-carbon double bonds in their hydrocarbon chain, therefore giving them different biochemical and physiological characteristics than saturated FAs. The n-3 (omega-3) and n-6 (omega-6) PUFAs are nutritionally significant for humans because they have a major metabolic regulatory role in human metabolism (Laghari et al., 2026). PUFAs are known as essential FAs because the body does not have the enzymes to make them; therefore must come from food sources. The n-3 PUFA family includes the following: α-linoleic acid (ALA, 18:3 n-3), eicosapentaenoic acid (EPA, 20:5 n-3), and docosahexaenoic acid (DHA, 22:6 n-3) (Keivani & Hosseini, 2023). The ALA sources are mainly from plants: flaxseeds, chia seeds, walnuts, and canola oil. The EPA and DHA are mainly derived from marine animals such as fatty fish (salmon, mackerel, sardines, and tuna), krill oil, and microalgae. The n-6 PUFA family consists of linoleic acid (LA, 18:2n-6) and arachidonic acid (AA, 20:4n-6). LA and AA are mainly obtained from vegetable oils, such as soybean oil, sunflower oil, corn oil, and safflower oil (El-Zenary et al., 2023). There are a variety of ways in which both the n-3 and n-6 PUFA families can positively affect health outcomes.

8.1.2 Oxidative susceptibility of polyunsaturated fatty acids

PUFAs have many health benefits, but because of their multiple double bonds, they are very susceptible to oxidative degradation. The methylene groups located between the double bonds (which are bis-allylic) have relatively low bond dissociation energy and are therefore more likely to be attacked by free radicals. Consequently, PUFAs are much more susceptible to oxidation than monounsaturated and saturated FAs. The oxidation of lipids is a complex process involving free radical chain reactions that results in the formation of undesirable materials, including hydroperoxides, aldehydes, ketones, and volatile hydrocarbons (Musakhanian et al., 2022). Lipid oxidation products contribute to rancidity, color changes, and loss of nutrition to food products. In addition, some secondary oxidation products, such as malondialdehyde (MDA) and 4-hydroxynonenal, have the potential for negative health consequences due to their cytotoxic and mutagenic properties. The oxidation of PUFAs can accelerate in the presence of several factors while food is processed or stored, including contact with oxygen, heat, light, metal ions, or enzymatic activity. Conventional thermal processing methods, including pasteurization, sterilization, frying, and cooking, typically use elevated temperatures, which increase the rate of lipid oxidation reactions. Elevated temperatures not only reduce the nutritional quality of food rich in PUFAs, but they also shorten the shelf life of PUFA-rich food products. Thermal processes applied in completing seafood will result in substantial losses of EPA and DHA, sometimes more than 30%–40%, depending on the processing conditions (Suryati et al., 2022). Likewise, omega-3-fortified dairy and functional products will exhibit oxidative degradation when subjected to heat treatment, resulting in off-flavors typically identified as fishy, metallic, or rancid.

Omega-3 and Omega-6 Polyunsaturated Fatty Acids in Food Systems. DOI: https://doi.org/10.1016/B978-0-443-43810-3.00019-1

8.1.3 Need for nonthermal food processing technologies

Due to the growing interest in less processed foods and maintaining as much of their nutritional value as possible, the food industry has looked into using new processes of cooking that do not apply excessive heat (thermal damage). Among the newer nonthermal methods currently being used are methods of processing food that use high-pressure processing (HPP). This is a method that uses very high levels of water pressure (ranges of 200 to 600 MPa) to kill bacteria and inactivate some enzymes with little to no heat. Since pressure is applied uniformly to all products at once, the product is treated equally (without having one side hotter and another cooler) and causes little to no damage to the nutrients or sensory characteristics of the end-product. HPP preserves the molecular structure of temperature-sensitive compounds, for example, vitamins, antioxidants, and polyunsaturated fats (Enchangan et al., 2025). The bond between the atoms forming these compounds are covalent; therefore, under pressure, the atoms remain in their same position. In addition to lowering the risk of contamination through microbial inactivation, there are many additional benefits associated with HPP, including longer shelf life, higher microbiological safety, and better overall color, flavor, and texture for all products. As a result of these various benefits and attributes, HPP is being adopted commercially by many manufacturers of fruit juices, seafood, meals ready-to-eat, etc.

To support proper development of PUFA in modern nutritional systems, it is important to understand how new food processing techniques affect their preservation. HPP has the potential to maintain nutritional quality in PUFA-rich foods while providing safe, high-quality product. The goal of this in-depth discussion presented in this chapter is to demonstrate how HPP can be used as an effective method for delivering PUFA-rich food items that satisfy modern consumer demands regarding safety, quality, and a low degree of processing.

8.2 Polyunsaturated fatty acids: chemistry and stability

8.2.1 Chemical composition and classification of polyunsaturated fatty acids

PUFAs are long-chain FAs that contain two or more double bonds in their hydrocarbon chains. These double bonds are normally separated by a methylene (-CH_2-) group, thereby establishing a methylene-mediated system, which significantly impacts the chemical reactivity and biological function of these lipids. Double bonds in nature for PUFAs are mainly in the cis form, causing the structure of the molecule to be bend, and therefore increasing the fluidity of membranes and the interactions of lipids in biology. PUFAs, are commonly classified according to where the first double bond is from the methyl end of the FA chain. Following this classification system, PUFAs can be classified into two main categories, such as omega-3 FAs and omega-6 FAs.

8.2.1.1 Omega-3 fatty acids (n-3 polyunsaturated fatty acids)

Omega-3 FAs have their first double bond at the third carbon atom from the methyl end of the FA. Nutritionally important omega-3 FAs include:

- ALA, 18:3 n-3
- EPA, 20:5 n-3
- DHA, 22:6 n-3

ALA must be gotten through the diet (it is an essential fat) (Lim et al., 2023). It is a precursor for EPA and DHA through a series of desaturation and extended-reaction modifications. However, the conversion within the human body from ALA to EPA/DHA is very inefficient (5%–10%), so consuming direct sources of EPA/DHA in the diet (i.e., from marine fish or algal oil) is very important (Roy et al., 2020). Both EPA and DHA are found mainly in marine species (fatty fish, krill, and microalgae), and are essential for brain, eye, heart, inflammation, and overall health. Omega-6 FAs have their first double bond at the sixth carbon from the methyl end of the FA chain. The two primary omega-6 FAs are linoleic acid (LA, 18:2n-6) and arachidonic acid (AA, 20:4n-6).

Essential FAs are FAs needed by the human body but cannot be produced by humans; these essential FAs can be found mostly in vegetable oils (e.g., corn oil, soybean oil, sunflower oil, and safflower oil). Linoleic acid (an omega-6 FA) must be converted to arachidonic acid (also an omega-6 FA) through an extended enzymatic elongation/desaturation process. Arachidonic acid is used in the production of eicosanoids, which modulate the immune system and the body's inflammatory responses (Semenoglou et al., 2025). The ratio of omega-6 to omega-3 FAs must be in balance with one another to maintain the body's homeostasis. High amounts of omega-6 FAs compared to omega-3 FAs can promote absolute inflammation, while an equal intake can assist in improving metabolic and cardiovascular health.

8.2.2 The oxidative deterioration mechanism of polyunsaturated fatty acids

PUFAs are readily oxidized, which is a major drawback in food systems. The presence of multiple double bonds within the PUFA molecules increases the likelihood of free radical reactions, which in turn leads to lipid peroxidation (Laghari et al., 2026). Typically, lipid oxidation occurs via a free-radical chain reaction and can be divided into three major phases, as shown in Fig. 8.1.

8.2.2.1 Initiation

The beginning stage of initiating a reactive chain reaction with a PUFA molecule starts when a reactive species (an oxidizer), such as light, oxygen, or metal ions, removes a hydrogen atom from it. The net result is a lipid radical (L•).

$$LH \rightarrow L\bullet + H\bullet$$

The bis-allylic hydrogens (the hydrogens on carbon atoms that are positioned between two double bonds) that lie between the two double bonds of a PUFA molecule are also extremely vulnerable to the loss of hydrogen because they possess a lower bond dissociation energy than other hydrogen atoms in the same molecule.

8.2.2.2 Propagation

During the propagation stage of the reaction (lipid radical oxidation), the lipid radical competes very quickly with molecular oxygen to produce a lipid peroxyl radical (LOO•).

$$L\bullet + O_2 \rightarrow LOO\bullet$$

After generating the LOO• radical, a LOO• radical removes a hydrogen atom from another PUFA molecule to produce a lipid hydroperoxide (LOOH) and subsequently generate another L• radical. This continues the chain reaction associated with lipid radical oxidation (Campos Espinosa et al., 2022).

$$LOO\bullet + LH \rightarrow LOOH + L\bullet$$

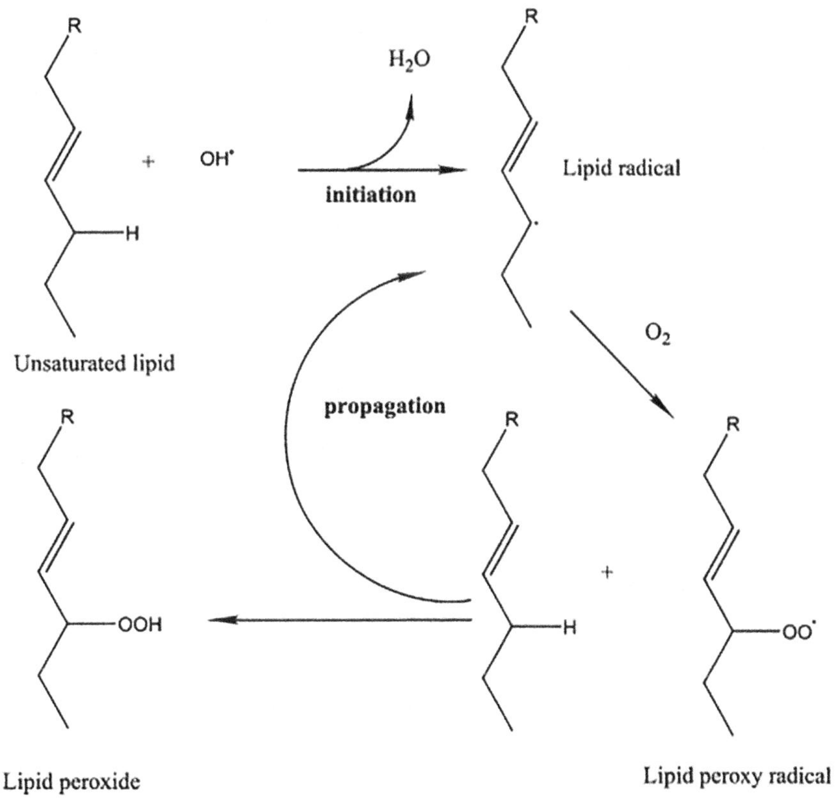

FIGURE 8.1 Mechanism of unsaturated lipid autoxidation (Medina-Meza et al., 2014).

The process will continue in this fashion repeatedly and produce a rapid build-up of oxidation products within PUFA-rich foods throughout the chain reaction.

8.2.2.3 Termination

The end of the lipid radical oxidation chain reaction process occurs when two radicals combine to form nonradical products.

$$L\bullet + L\bullet \rightarrow L\text{–}L$$

$$LOO\bullet + LOO\bullet \rightarrow LOOL + O_2$$

However, the LOOHs formed in the first or second chain reactions may decompose into secondary oxidation products because they are unstable.

8.2.3 Process for creating primary and secondary oxidation products

The most significant products produced from lipid oxidation are LOOHs (the lipid oxidation primary products), which are highly unstable intermediates. These hydroperoxides themselves are not very odoriferous; however, upon decomposition of the hydroperoxides, an array of volatile secondary products is produced which cause the quality of the product to deteriorate (Ismaiel et al., 2025).

Some common examples of secondary oxidation products are:

- Aldehydes (hexanal, propanal, MDA),
- Ketones (2-pentanone, 2-heptanone),
- Alcohols (1-penten-3-ol),
- Hydrocarbons (pentane, ethane).

These secondary oxidation products contribute to undesired sensory characteristics of lipid products, such as rancidity, metallic taste, and fishy flavor. Some oxidation products will also interact with proteins, vitamins, and pigments, which causes a reduction in nutritional value and a change in color.

Lipid oxidation is assessed in food quality using a number of analytical indicators, including:

- Peroxide value (PV)—a measurement of primary oxidation products,
- Thiobarbituric acid reactive substances (TBARS)—an indicator of secondary oxidation products,
- Conjugated dienes and trienes—early indicators of oxidation,
- Analysis of volatile aldehydes—identification of flavor deterioration.

Along with the sensory quality of PUFA-rich foods, the maintenance of low levels of oxidation is vitally important in preserving the nutritional quality of PUFA-rich foods (Laghari et al., 2026).

8.2.4 Factors influencing polyunsaturated fatty acids stability in foods

Several environmental factors, in addition to their composition, affect PUFA oxidative stability in the food system.

1. O_2: As the major reactant in lipid oxidation reactions, O_2 significantly influences PUFA degradation by facilitating reactions oxidizing PUFA during processing, transportation, packaging, and storage. O_2 diffuses into food matrices, where it contributes to the formation of radicals, forming hydroperoxides in food matrices. Various types of packaging technologies (e.g., vacuum packaging and modified atmosphere packaging) have been developed to limit O_2 diffusion into food (Keivani & Hosseini, 2023).
2. Light: PUFA foods containing photooxidation-sensitizing compounds (e.g., chlorophyll, riboflavin, porphyrins) can have their PUFAs oxidized when the respective food becomes exposed to light from the sun or other sources. Light energy is transferred to O_2, resulting in the production of highly oxidizing singlet O_2, which rapidly degrades unsaturated FAs.
3. Temperature: Increased temperature will also influence the oxidation of lipids in food. Lipid oxidation increases with increasing temperature due to an increase in molecular mobility at higher temperatures and a related increase in the rate at which chemical reactions occur in food. Examples of thermal processing techniques include frying, roasting, and sterilization, and the use of these methods can significantly lower PUFA content in food during processing (Li, 2024).
4. Enzymatic activity: The enzymatic activity in plant and animal tissues contains enzymes that accelerate the reaction of lipid oxidation. The two main types of enzymes that are associated with UNA oxidation are lipoxygenase, which will

initiate the addition of oxygen to PUFAs to form hydroperoxides, and lipase, which hydrolyze triglycerides into single FAs, which often will be more prone to oxidation.

5. Food matrix composition: The structural diversity of the matrix can alter the oxidation stability of PUFA. The interaction of lipid, protein, carbohydrate, and water will influence the availability of oxygen or pro-oxidant to be available for reactions. For instance, proteins can be metal chelators and antioxidants against lipid oxidation. The presence of transition metals such as Fe and Cu will catalyze an oxidation reaction. Antioxidant compounds found naturally in food, such as vitamin E (tocopherols), vitamin A (carotenoids), polyphenols, and flavonoids, assist in minimizing lipid oxidation by scavenging free radicals and keeping the lipid molecules stable.

8.2.5 Strategies to enhance polyunsaturated fatty acid stability

There are many different strategies associated with the enhancement of the stability of PUFAs in food systems. These strategies include:

- by integrating natural antioxidants (e.g., BHT, BHA, tocopherols, ascorbic acid, rosemary extract, and Iron E.D.T.A.) into the food matrix;
- microencapsulate the oils that are high in PUFA to reduce their exposure to oxygen;
- using oxygen-barrier packaging to minimize exposure to oxygen;
- store food at controlled temperatures and light conditions, and
- applying nonthermal processing technology, such as HPP, to enhance PUFA stability, as it allows microbial inactivation without the extensive heat exposure that typically accelerates PUFA oxidation (Lie & Nurkhoeriyati, 2025).

8.3 Fundamentals of high-pressure processing

8.3.1 Working principle of high-pressure processing

HPP, also known as high hydrostatic pressure, provides an innovative method for preserving foods without heat by applying high levels of pressure (200–600 MPa) to food products to destroy bacteria but provide food products with an equivalent food quality, including nutrients and flavor, to food products that are thermally preserved (i.e., using heat to destroy bacteria). Unlike conventional processes for preserving foods using heat to destroy bacteria, HPP uses hydrostatic pressure instead to preserve the food by applying hydrostatic pressure uniformly to the food in a liquid rather than using heat from the liquid to destroy the bacteria. HPP uses hydraulic pumps to create the hydrostatic pressure by compressing water in a pressure vessel around the food (Enchangan et al., 2025). All parts of the food will experience the same amount of hydrostatic pressure during HPP since the hydrostatic pressure is applied uniformly across the entire piece of food incorporated within the container. The application of hydrostatic pressure will influence many of the intermolecular forces (such as hydrogen bonds, ionic bonds, and hydrophobic forces) that are responsible for holding protein structures and cellular membranes together, thus causing the breakdown (denaturation) of protein structures and cellular membranes at the molecular level.

Disruption to protein, enzyme, and cellular structures through these interactions causes denaturation of proteins, inactivation of enzymes, and structural modifications on live microbial cells due to HPP. However, covalent bonds are mostly unaffected, allowing essential nutrients such as PUFAs, vitamins, and amino acids to maintain their chemical structure throughout processing. Due to HPP, the permeability of microbial cell membranes increases, thus leaching intracellular components from the cell, thereby inhibiting metabolism of the cells (Tsai et al., 2022). Ribosomes may dissociate from cells, preventing protein synthesis required for cell reproduction; thus the combination of these effects leads to inactivation of the microbes whilst preserving the safety, nutritional, and organoleptic qualities of the finished food products. HPP operates at low temperatures, reducing or minimizing thermal degradation of heat-sensitive compounds such as PUFAs. Consequently, HPP is an ideal method of preserving food products high in PUFAs, which are highly prone to oxidation during conventional heat preservation methods, therefore making HPP an excellent technique for the preservation of food products high in PUFAs.

8.3.2 Isostatic principle (Pascal's law)

Pascal's law of fluid mechanics forms the basis of the isostatic principle, a fundamental concept behind HPP. In simple terms, Pascal's Law states that pressure applied to a confined fluid will be transmitted in all directions equally and instantaneously. HPP uses water to transmit pressure because of its near incompressibility and its ability to provide an even distribution of pressure throughout the chamber. Thus when hydraulic pumps are used to create pressure inside the vessel, the water will transmit this same amount of pressure to every part of the food product within the processing chamber. As a result, even food products with different shapes and compositions will be uniformly processed through isostatic pressure transmission (Roobab et al., 2022). In addition, uniform microbial inactivation will occur throughout any food matrix using HPP due to the isostatic principle, which eliminates the possibility of having unprocessed areas within any food product.

In thermal processing, heat needs to move from the outside part of the food to the inside part of the food, which can create a gradient of temperature differences inside the food. However, pressure is transmitted instantaneously to all parts of the food product at once. Additionally, since pressure is applied uniformly in all directions, the food does not significantly change shape during the processing. Compression is applied to the food at equal rates from all directions, allowing for no mechanical damage or structural damage to occur as a result of this compression (Iftikhar et al., 2026). The importance of this principle is especially significant with respect to very delicate food items, such as fruits, seafood, and ready-to-eat meals. Also, the isostatic principle permits food to be processed in its finished package, resulting in less exposure to contamination postprocessing. Pressure-transmitting flexible packaging, like that used in polyethylene pouches, also provides protection to the food being processed. These properties make HPP an attractive option for commercial food manufacturing operations.

8.3.3 Le Chatelier's principle applied to high-pressure processing

HPP is influenced by another fundamental scientific principle, Le Chatelier's principle, which details how pressure impacts chemical and biochemical reactions. More specifically, Le Chatelier's principle states that if an equilibrium system is subjected to a change from the surroundings (such as a change in pressure, temperature, and concentration), the system will adjust in response to the applied change so as to oppose that change. Therefore when HPP occurs, reactions that produce a decrease in molecular volume are favored, and reactions resulting in an increase in molecular volume are unfavoured. Many biological processes (e.g., enzyme activity, protein folding, and membrane structure) are associated with changes in molecular volume; therefore application of high pressure will alter these processes via shifting the equilibrium to states with lesser molecular volume (Duma-Kocan et al., 2024). For example, tertiary or quaternary structures of proteins are stabilized by hydrophobic interactions and electrostatic forces. When these forces are disrupted by high pressure, the proteins will obstruct those forces, resulting in their unfolding (denaturizing).

Biochemical reactions associated with the deterioration of food are mediated by enzymes whose ability to catalyze reactions is dependent on having a specific three-dimensional shape. These enzymes lose this specific shape and therefore their catalytic ability when exposed to high-pressure conditions. Therefore it takes longer for the biochemical reactions that would cause food spoilage to occur. Pressure has the potential to create structural changes within microbial cells (Tsai et al., 2022). These structural changes disrupt the integrity of the cellular membranes and affect the activity of enzymes involved in metabolism, thereby inhibiting growth. Pressure can alter the phase state of membrane lipids, resulting in an increase in the permeability of the membrane, thus allowing for leakage of intracellular materials from the microbial cell. In addition, ribosomes in microbial cells can dissociate into their constituent subunits as a result of pressure, thus preventing the assembly of ribosomes to form proteins, thus restricting microbial growth (Evrendilek, 2022). In general, small molecules (e.g., FAs, vitamins) form covalent chemical bonds that are minimally affected by the levels of pressure used in food processing. For this reason, essential nutrients in food remain chemically stable during HPP. The selective nature of the effect of HPP on biological structures explains why HPP is an effective means of inactivating microorganisms and preserving the nutritional benefits of food.

8.3.4 High-pressure processing equipment and system components

HPP systems used by the food industry consist of many of the same components as other industrial HPP systems. Each has been designed to create and maintain an extremely high-pressure condition during the food processing cycle in a safe manner. The key component of these systems is the pressure vessel, generally constructed of either very high-strength stainless steel or alloys capable of withstanding a maximum of up to 600 MPa of pressure, as shown in Fig. 8.2. These pressure vessels typically have thick-walls reinforced with structures that can provide sufficient mechanical stability to withstand repeated cycles of great pressure. Another key component of the overall process is the system used to generate the required pressure (the hydraulic system) (Fidalgo et al., 2021). This system utilizes a hydraulic intensifier pump to compress the liquid used as the pressure-transmitting medium. The hydraulic pump converts the mechanical energy from the mechanical power source to hydraulic pressure. Therefore this process allows a gradual build-up of hydraulic pressure inside the pressure vessel. Pressurization usually happens in less than 5 minutes, depending on the desired pressure and the design of the pressurization system. Another key consideration in the process of HPP is that the medium through which

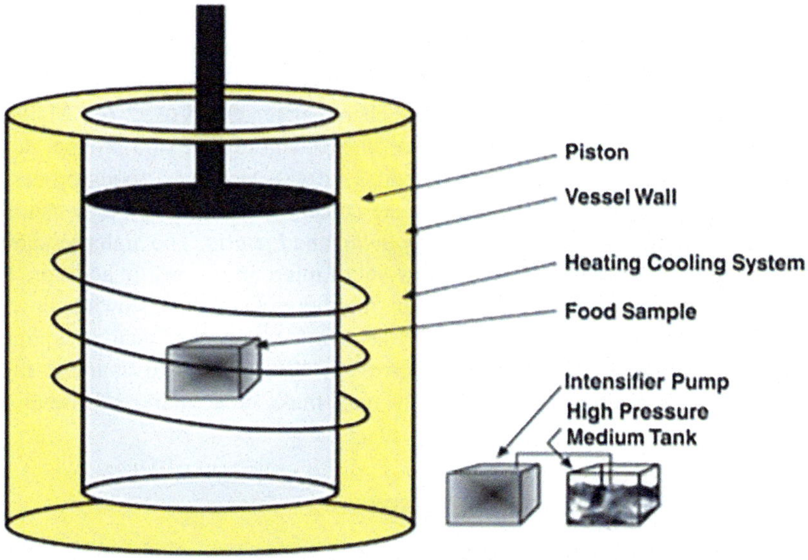

FIGURE 8.2 High-pressure processing equipment (Khaliq et al., 2021).

pressure is transmitted (i.e., the pressure-transmitting medium) is water in most cases, and fills the vessel with food so that the pressure is applied uniformly over the outside of each food product (Roobab et al., 2022). The food product is typically packaged in flexible containers that can transmit pressure and are not damaged by the application of HPP. One other component of HPP equipment is a temperature control system for managing processing conditions. Even though HPP is generally known as a nonthermal technology, the compressive forces in water cause an increase in temperature due to adiabatic heating. Therefore in many systems, cooling systems are included to provide the proper temperatures during processing (Lim et al., 2023). Many of the current HPP systems use an automated monitoring and control system to measure and maintain the pressure intensity, compression rate, holding time, and temperature of the food products being processed. By maintaining consistent processing conditions and automatically controlling each of the processing parameters for various food products, operators can obtain the optimal results of their HPP process.

8.3.5 Relationship between pressure and temperature using a high-pressure process

HPP is generally considered a nonthermal method; however, it increases the temperature of the water product during the process; this occurs through a normal increase in the water temperature for every 100 MPa (10,000 psi) applied. Water will typically increase in temperature between 3°F (2°C) and 5°F (3°C) for every 100 MPa of pressure applied. Therefore if you process food at 300 MPa (300,000 psi), you can expect the food product to experience an average temperature increase of approximately 9°F to 15°F (5°C to 9°C); if you process the food at 600 MPa (600,000 psi), you can expect an average temperature increase of approximately 18°F to 30°F (10°C to 15°C) (Zhu et al., 2022). In addition, the water product will cool back down during expansion; therefore the overall temperature rise and fall during the process should be relatively mild when using HPP versus traditional heat treatments, and will not create major changes in the nutritional composition of the heat-sensitive food products processed with HPP compared to other methods of processing.

While using HPP, a moderate increase in temperature during the processing may allow for more complete inactivation of pathogens and spoilage microorganisms; that type of combined processing of heat and pressure is often referred to as pressure-assisted thermal processing (Duma-Kocan et al., 2024). However, even then, the total time/temperature exposure will still be considerably less than in traditional heat treatment. Because PUFAs are very sensitive to heat (oxidation) during HPP, the relatively low processing temperatures (due to HPP) will help protect the chemical integrity and nutritional value of PUFAs.

8.3.6 Comparison of high-pressure processing to thermal processing

Thermal processing preserves food using methods such as pasteurization and sterilization, which use heat to destroy microorganisms and enzymes. These methods, while effective at controlling microorganisms, can also lead to the destruction of heat-sensitive nutrients, cause changes in sensory attributes of products, or alter how consumers perceive a product. HPP has numerous advantages compared to conventional thermal methods. One key advantage is that it will preserve nutrition (Kumar et al., 2023). HPP operates at low temperatures, reducing the rate of degradation of sensitive compounds such as PUFAs, vitamins, and antioxidants. Another advantage is the preservation of the sensory characteristics of a product. Thermal processing can cause chemical reactions (e.g., the Maillard reaction leading to browned product) and result in altered properties of the color, flavor, and texture of a product due to chemical reactions possibly involving browning or protein coagulation (Evrendilek, 2022). However, foods processed using HPP usually retain their original fresh quality, though HPP-treated foods are considered to be fresh; they can also reduce or eliminate vegetative microorganisms, including Escherichia *coli*, *Salmonella*, and *Listeria*. The high pressure can effectively disrupt cellular membranes and denature enzymes critical to the survival of microorganisms. In addition, HPP increases the shelf life of many foods due to reductions in the populations of microorganisms and slowing down enzymes that would normally cause spoilage (Ramakrishnan et al., 2022). HPP has some drawbacks, such as equipment costs and limited efficacy against bacterial spores without moderate heat; however, HPP's ability to maintain the nutritional value and sensory characteristics of many high-priced food products may make it a viable substitute for traditional thermal processing.

8.3.7 Effect of pressure on lipid oxidation pathways

Lipid oxidation is normally a multistage process consisting of three phases: initiation, propagation, and termination. During the initiation phase, reactive oxygen species/pro-oxidant catalysts react with unsaturated FAs substrates and remove hydrogen atoms to create lipid radicals (L•). Lipid radicals react with oxygen and form lipid peroxyl radicals (LOO•), thus propagating the oxidative chain reaction by means of adjacent lipid molecules. As the propagation phase proceeds, LOOH are formed and, over time, they degrade to produce secondary oxidation products (i.e., aldehydes, ketones, hydrocarbons) that cause quality degradation (Musakhanian et al., 2022). The effects of high pressure on the oxidation of lipids are depicted in Fig. 8.3. The HPP affects lipid oxidation by kinetic (i.e., changing the relative velocity) and structural (i.e., changing the shape and position) factors. In addition, applied pressure does not cleave covalent bonds between molecular constituents forming FAs, using pressures of 200–600 MPa; therefore the primary structure of the PUFAs is mostly unchanged during treatment using high pressure. Pressure impacts the reaction kinetics of chemical reactions by altering their activation volume, and increasing or decreasing the rate of radical (formed by the electron-driven reaction of the oxidant with an oxygen-containing molecule) and the ongoing creation or propagation of radicals (Roobab et al., 2022). In a large number of food systems, pressure stabilizes lipids through reducing lipid oxidation primarily because HPP is done under low to moderate temperature conditions. The reduction in high-energy heat reduces radical formation and the decomposition of hydroperoxide. Studies on fish muscle indicate that applying pressure treatment of between 200 and 300 MPa can slow down the amount of lipid oxidation during frozen storage due to the inactivation of pro-oxidative type enzymes like lipoxygenase and peroxidase (Liu et al., 2021). However, pressure processing will also affect the physical structure of the food matrix, and this can also affect lipid oxidation. Compression of the cellular membranes and/or denaturation of muscle proteins can create conditions that expose lipid molecules to heme iron or other pro-oxidative catalysts. This exposure may initiate oxidation reactions. So the net effect of HPP on lipid oxidation greatly depends on the level of pressure applied, the time of processing, the amount of oxygen in the processing atmosphere, and the composition of the food matrix. Recent studies on sardines processed at 400 to 600 MPa showed that pressure processing maintained the amount of volatiles produced from oxidation, when compared with similarly treated samples, during refrigerated storage. This indicates that properly applied food processing conditions through HPP can maintain lipid stability.

8.3.8 Enzyme inactivation associated with lipid decomposition

In addition to oxidative degradation due to nonenzymatic reactions, enzymatic processes also play an important role in promoting the decomposition of PUFAs found in food. Endogenous enzymes (e.g., lipoxygenase, lipase, phospholipase) catalyze lipid oxidation and increase the potential for oxidative degradation of lipids. Structural changes induced by HPP can inactivate these enzymes by changing their structure and disrupting their catalytic activity.

8.3.8.1 Lipoxygenase

Lipoxygenase is one of the key enzymes responsible for oxidizing PUFAs. This type of enzyme contains nonheme iron and functions by catalyzing the reaction of inserting molecular oxygen into FAs that contain the structural features of cis,cis-1,4-pentadiene, thereby producing LOOHs. The LOOHs produced by the enzymatic reaction described above

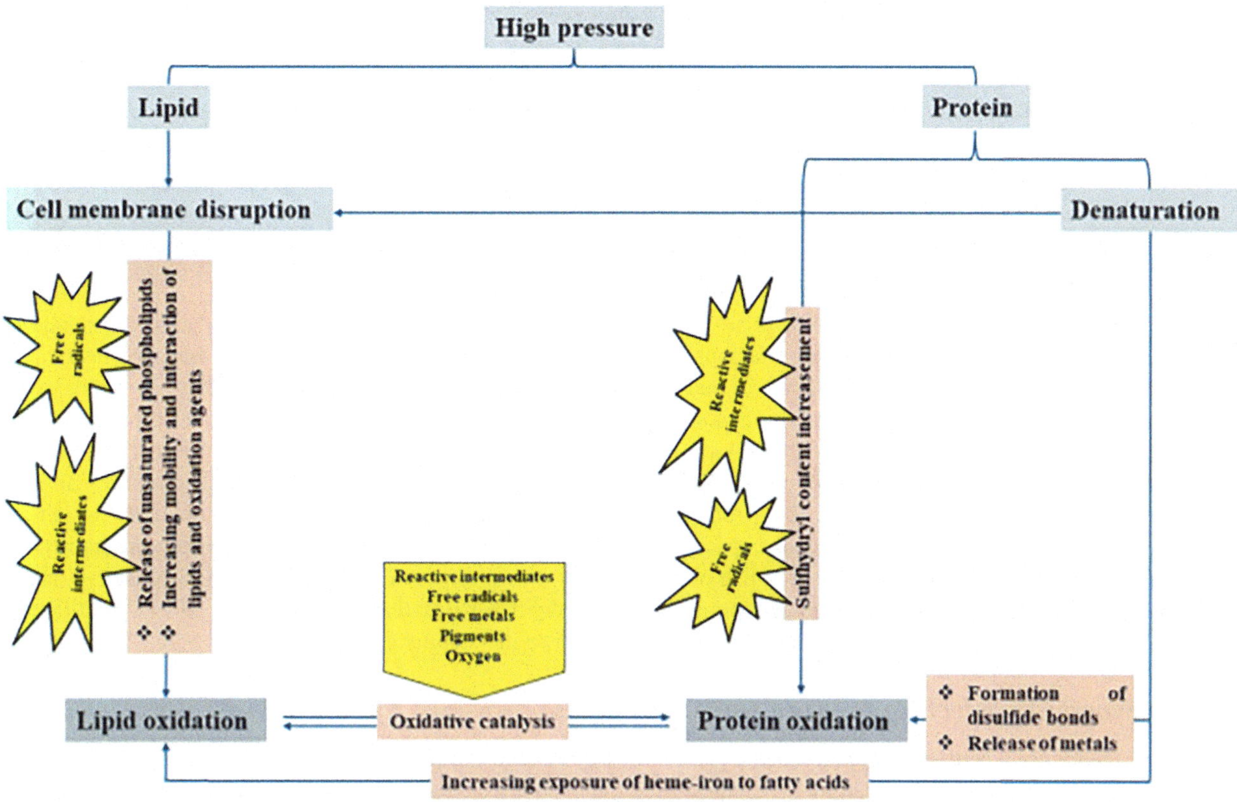

FIGURE 8.3 The effects of high pressure on the oxidation of lipids (Ganjeh et al., 2024).

undergo decomposition, in which they form many volatile compounds (i.e., aldehydes and ketones) (Lie & Nurkhoeriyati, 2025). The presence of volatile compounds creates rancid flavors and deteriorates food quality. High pressure alters the tertiary and quaternary protein structure of lipoxygenase, thereby affecting the hydrogen bond and hydrophobic interactions in the protein and creating conformational modifications to lipoxygenase, leading to decreased enzyme activity. There is growing evidence through experimental data that lipoxygenase activity can be significantly reduced in plant tissues and seafood products above 400 MPa, thereby limiting the preliminary stages of lipid oxidation in food products.

8.3.8.2 Lipase

Lipases catalyze the hydrolysis of triglycerides into free FAs and glycerol. While the activity of lipase does not actually cause lipid oxidation, when free FAs are released into the food matrix, they are more exposed to oxidation and, therefore are more readily degraded through oxidation. The increase in available surface area of the free FAs also makes them more susceptible to oxidation by reactive oxygen species. In addition, if high pressure is applied, lipase activity could be reduced by disrupting the active site of the enzyme and altering the tertiary structure of the enzyme (Truong et al., 2023). Denaturing an enzyme by applying high pressure reduces its ability to bind with substrates and catalyze hydrolysis reactions. Consequently, fewer free FAs are formed, which helps to maintain lipid stability during storage. Thus the combined inactivation of lipoxygenase and lipase is a critical mechanism that HPP uses to preserve the quality of PUFA-rich foods.

8.3.9 Reduction of thermal stress and polyunsaturated fatty acids stability

Thermal stress is one of the primary factors affecting PUFA degradation during conventional food processing. Increased temperatures lead to a greater rate of formation of free radicals, which aids in the process of lipid oxidation and increases the rate of decomposition of LOOHs to other oxidation products. The use of HPP, minimizes thermal stress because the processing occurs at relatively low temperatures (Iftikhar et al., 2026). The pressure medium has a temperature rise from adiabatic heating resulting from compressinon ; however, the temperature exposure of the process is very low compared with conventional heat treatments. Research comparing pressure treatments to those applied through cooking suggests that the amount of omega-3 FAs (EPA and DHA) is greatly reduced from thermal processing (Nagy et al., 2024). However, HPP has no significant effect on altering either the profile of FAs. This difference can primarily be attributed to the fact that heat causes the breaking of chemical bonds and accelerates oxidation reactions, while pressure does not directly cause degradation of FA molecules. Reducing the amount of thermal stress on HPP further assists in preserving other heat-sensitive compounds such as vitamins and natural antioxidants, which help maintain lipid stability (Ismaiel et al., 2025). Therefore the nutritional quality and oxidative stability of pressure-treated foods are superior when compared to thermally treated foods.

8.3.10 Preservation of endogenous antioxidant systems

Naturally occurring antioxidants found in food are essential in properly protecting the natural oxidation degradation of PUFAs, by acting as free radical scavengers. Antioxidants can include tocopherols, carotenoids, polyphenols, and flavonoids. The way these antioxidants work is that they donate hydrogen atoms or electrons to lipid radicals, thus disrupting lipid oxidation chain reactions. Antioxidants are usually significantly degraded by thermal processes, which have a negative effect on the longevity of PUFA-rich foods (Jiang et al., 2022). HPP does not expose the antioxidant to high temperatures for extended periods of time, but rather preserves antioxidants. Moreover, high pressure can cause disruption of the plant cell structure and allow for greater extractability of certain antioxidant compounds, which may contribute to the increased total antioxidant capacity of the food matrix and provide added protection against lipid oxidation. For example, tocopherols present in fish oils have been shown to provide protection against oxidative damage to membrane lipids by stabilizing free radicals produced during lipid peroxidation (Cai & Wang, 2021). Additionally, these antioxidants are also stable through HPP, and help to preserve the stability of PUFA.

8.3.11 Synergistic effects of pressure and antioxidants

Synergistic interactions between the antioxidants present in PUFAs and the pressure treatment during HPP enhance the preservation of the PUFAs from oxidation. When the antioxidants do not degrade through processing, the antioxidants can effectively inhibit free radical chain reactions that are responsible for the oxidation of lipids (Truong et al., 2023). The natural antioxidants tocopherols and polyphenols, for example, will scavenge free radical lipids, thereby terminating the propagation portion of the lipid oxidation pathway. In addition, the polyphenolic antioxidants will chelate the transition metal ions (i.e., iron and copper) that catalyze lipid oxidation reactions (Liu et al., 2021). The use of external antioxidants in conjunction with high pressure has also been shown to increase the oxidative stability of food products that are processed by pressure. For example, various antioxidants, including ascorbic acid, rosemary extract, and polyphenols found in green tea, are used to protect lipids from being oxidized in food systems. The Effect of HPP on PUFA Stability in Food Systems is tabulated in Table 8.1. Therefore the combination of HPP (this) coupled with the use of antioxidant strategies represents a viable approach to maintain the nutritional quality of PUFA-containing foods while providing assurance for the safety of the foods and extending their shelf life.

8.4 Process parameters affecting polyunsaturated fatty acid retention

The efficiency of HPP in the retention of PUFAs is largely dependent upon the processing parameters used during treatment, as tabulated, in Table 8.2. While HPP is considered to be a nonthermal technology, the effects of application/process parameters (pressure applied, holding time, processing temperature, packaging design, and the composition and structure of the food matrix) can play a significant role in controlling lipid stability. These process parameters will determine the extent of inactivation of enzyme activity, structural modification of cell membranes, and the degree of exposure of lipids to pro-oxidative compounds such as iron and oxygen (Luo et al., 2025). If improper process conditions are selected for HPP, then it is possible that some degree of enzyme activity will remain, cell tissue will have been structurally damaged, and lipids will have been excessively exposed to catalytic metallic ions, all of which could result in an increased rate of oxidation (Chmiel et al., 2025). Consequently, careful optimization of processing conditions is necessary to ensure a safe food product from a microbial perspective, while still providing the nutritional and oxidative stability that is required for consumption of PUFA-rich foods such as seafood, meat, dairy, and plant-based functional foods.

8.4.1 Pressure level (MPa)

One of the parameters that greatly affects PUFA retention when subjected to HPP, is the amount of pressure. The commercialized systems of HPP available for use will generally operate within a pressure range of 200–600 MPa,

TABLE 8.1 Effect of high-pressure processing (HPP) on polyunsaturated fatty acid (PUFA) stability in food systems.

Food product/matrix	HPP conditions	Storage conditions	Analytical methods used	Key observations	Effect on PUFA retention/oxidative stability	References
Sardines	400–600 MPa, 1–10 min	Refrigerated storage (4°C)	GC-MS, TBARS, and volatile compound analysis	No significant increase in volatile lipid oxidation compounds after pressure treatment	High retention of EPA and DHA with improved oxidative stability during storage	Ismaiel et al. (2025)
Haddock and mackerel	200–300 MPa, 5 min	Frozen storage (−18°C)	Peroxide value (PV), and GC-FID fatty acid (FA) profiling	Reduction in lipid oxidation due to pressure-induced enzyme inactivation	PUFA oxidation was delayed compared with untreated samples	Lie and Nurkhoeriyati (2025)
Atlantic salmon	300 MPa, 5 min	Refrigerated storage (2°C–4°C)	GC FA analysis, and TBARS	No significant change in EPA and DHA concentrations compared with fresh samples	Improved FA stability compared with thermally cooked fish	Li (2024)
Barramundi fish muscle	150–200 MPa, 5 min	Frozen storage (−20°C)	Conjugated dienes and PV	Pressure treatment delayed the initiation of lipid oxidation reactions	Maintained omega-3 FA composition during storage	Truong et al. (2023)
Herring and mackerel	600 MPa, 10 min	Refrigerated storage	GC-MS lipid analysis, and TBARS	Inhibition of cholesterol oxidation and reduced formation of lipid oxidation products	Significant preservation of PUFA profile during storage	Enchangan et al. (2025)
Tuna muscle	400 MPa, 5 min	Chilled storage (0°C–4°C)	GC-FID FA analysis, and PV	Slight protein denaturation but minimal lipid oxidation	High retention of omega-3 FAs with limited oxidation	Tsai et al. (2022)
Fish oil emulsion	300–500 MPa, 3–5 min	Ambient storage	Oxidative stability index and PV	Pressure had minimal effect on FA composition	PUFA structure remained stable under pressure	Roobab et al. (2022)
Chicken meat	300–400 MPa, 5 min	Refrigerated storage	TBARS assay, and GC FA profiling	Slight increase in oxidation depending on fat composition	PUFA stability was maintained when oxygen exposure was minimized	Iftikhar et al. (2026)

TABLE 8.2 Influence of high-pressure processing (HPP) parameters on polyunsaturated fatty acid (PUFA) stability in different food systems.

Product	Processing conditions tested	Optimized condition	PUFA content observation	Remarks	References
Cow milk	Pressure: 300–500 MPa; holding time: 2–10 min; temperature rise due to adiabatic heating	400 MPa, 5 min	Linoleic acid (LA) and α-linolenic acid (ALA) remained stable	Limited temperature increase prevented PUFA degradation	Lim et al. (2023)
Shrimp muscle	Pressure: 200–400 MPa; holding time: 2–6 min	300 MPa, 4 min	EPA and DHA were maintained with lower peroxide values	Controlled holding time suppressed oxidative enzymes	Zhu et al. (2022)
Fish oil emulsion	Pressure: 250–450 MPa; holding time: 3–8 min	350 MPa, 5 min	EPA and DHA retained with minimal peroxide formation	Emulsion structure provided protection to PUFA	Semenoglou et al. (2025)
Pork loin	Pressure: 200–500 MPa; holding time: 3–10 min; pressure cycles tested	400 MPa, 5 min (single cycle)	LA and arachidonic acid remained stable	Multiple pressure cycles may increase oxidation due to structural disruption	Duma-Kocan et al. (2024)
Atlantic salmon	Pressure: 150–300 MPa; holding time: 5–15 min; chilled storage	300 MPa, 5 min	EPA and DHA are retained during refrigerated storage	Moderate pressure minimized oxidation of omega-3 fatty acids	Fidalgo et al. (2021)
Flaxseed oil emulsion	Pressure: 200–400 MPa; holding time: 3–6 min; antioxidant-rich matrix	320 MPa, 4 min	ALA remained stable	Natural antioxidants enhanced oxidative stability	de Carvalho et al. (2024)
Chicken breast meat	Pressure: 200–500 MPa; holding time: 3–10 min; temperature variation	350 MPa, 5 min	LA showed minimal change	Low processing temperature improved lipid stability	Evrendilek (2022)
Tuna fillets	Pressure: 300–600 MPa; holding time: 2–5 min; packaging: vacuum versus atmospheric	500 MPa, 3 min (vacuum packed)	EPA and DHA are retained during storage	Low oxygen packaging reduced lipid oxidation	Tsai et al. (2022)

depending on the food being processed and the full amount of microbial destruction desired. It is generally accepted that the moderate application of pressure (between 200 and 300 MPa) can partially destroy spoilage microorganisms and also deactivate enzyme systems involved in causing spoilage without significantly disrupting cellular membranes (Arslan et al., 2025). The limited disruption of cellular membrane integrity limits the extent to which there is any lipid oxidation reaction occurring under conditions of moderate pressure. The higher pressure applications (between 400 and 600 MPa) are the most commonly used for commercial pasteurization due to their success in completely destroying the microorganisms and lipid-degrading enzymes such as lipoxygenase and lipase. These enzymes catalyze the oxidation, as well as the hydrolysis, of PUFAs; therefore their destruction provides better stability relative to oxidized lipids during storage (Zhu et al., 2022). However, excessive application of pressure can also affect the structural integrity of muscle proteins in such a way that pro-oxidants are released from heme proteins, which could create the initiating condition for any oxidation reactions.

Numerous studies have shown that applying pressure to PUFA will maintain their stability. For example, when Atlantic salmon was subjected to 300 MPa for 5 minutes, EPA and DHA levels were stable during cold storage. Sardines treated at 400–600 MPa maintained their FA profile and showed less spoilage through microbial activity (Arulkumar et al., 2020). Pork loin treated with 400 MPa had less lipase activity and maintained better lipid stability (Truong et al., 2023). Tuna fillets processed at 500 MPa had an omega 3 FA profile similar to untreated tuna fillets, whereas chicken breast meat processed at 300–400 MPa demonstrated minimal changes to their FA profile. These findings indicate that 300–500 MPa provides an optimal balance of microbial inactivation and PUFA protection.

8.4.2 Holding time and pressure cycles

Holding time refers to how long the food is at the desired pressure in the processing chamber. Holding times range from one to 10 minutes, depending upon the type of food and the level of microbial inactivation needed. In most cases, short holding times will be sufficient to reduce microbial contamination and not cause significant structural changes that contribute to lipid oxidation. Longer periods of holding food at specific temperatures can increase the chance of causing the proteins to lose their shape and causing damage to cell membranes, resulting in the exposure of lipids to oxygen and catalytic metal ions. Pressure cycling (repeatedly cycling food through high and low pressure) has been studied to help inactivate microorganisms; however, if the product is cycled in the presence of oxygen, the risk of cellular damage and the promotion of oxidation increases. Research has shown that fishery products are important examples of how food can be affected by the length of holding time. At a pressure of 400 MPa for 3 minutes, sardine fillets had their FA profile maintained while reducing the number of microorganisms present (Truong et al., 2023). In processing an Atlantic mackerel at 350 MPa for 5 minutes, there was a reduction in the amount of enzymatic oxidation. When shrimp muscle was treated at 300 MPa for 4 minutes, the level of oxidation was significantly lower than in untreated samples (Zhu et al., 2022). In processing smoked salmon at 600 MPa for 3 minutes, the omega-3 FAs remained stable. Also, during storage of cod fillets processed at 400 MPa for 5 minutes, their PUFA content was maintained (Roobab et al., 2022). From these studies, it can be confirmed that holding times for pathogens can generally be controlled within the range of 3–5 minutes while preventing any deterioration of the quality of the available lipids.

8.4.3 Processing temperature and adiabatic heating

Although HPP is classified as an ambient temperature technology, the process of compression transforms the pressure-transmitting medium into thermal energy through the process of adiabatic heating, resulting in an increase in temperature in the pressurization vessel while the product is being processed. The mechanical energy used in the compression is transformed into thermal energy, which will increase the temperature of the pressure vessel. Generally, for every 100 MPa of pressure applied to the pressure vessel, the temperature increase will range from 3°C to 5°C (Arslan et al., 2025). Therefore if the product is processed at 600 MPa, the temperature increase during processing will be approximately 20°C to 30°C (Luo et al., 2025). The increase in temperature has the potential to influence lipid oxidation reactions because elevated temperatures cause the formation of free radicals and increase the rate of hydroperoxides decompose. However, the total thermal exposure experienced by foods during HPP is significantly less than that which would be experienced by the same product processed by traditional heat treatments, such as pasteurization or sterilization. As a result, the degradation of heat-sensitive ingredients, such as PUFAs, is minimal. Studies of various food systems have demonstrated that PUFAs are stable when HPP is used. For example, the FA profile of milk was not significantly affected by processing at 400 MPa despite an increase in temperature (Lim et al., 2023). In addition, salmon fillets, when processed by HPP, had stable EPA and DHA levels. The lipid composition of oysters processed at 300 MPa was maintained, and barramundi fish maintained their FA profile when processed by HPP (Liu et al., 2021). Fish oil emulsions subjected to HPP maintained omega-3 FAs, providing proper temperature control during processing.

8.4.4 Packaging materials and oxygen permeability

Packaging is crucial for preserving PUFA stability during HPP and afterwards. Oxygen is a primary cause of lipid oxidation, so it is imperative to have packaging with low oxygen permeability to keep PUFA-rich foods fresh. In HPP, flexible packaging (polyethylene, polypropylene, or multi-layer polymer films) is typically used because they transmit pressure efficiently without damaging the packaging material (Luo et al., 2025). However, these different types of packaging have varying oxygen barrier properties. When products are packaged with high oxygen permeability, oxygen may be permitted to diffuse into the product, which could cause accelerated lipid oxidation reactions to occur. Using multilayer packaging with oxygen barrier layers such as ethylene vinyl alcohol or polyamide greatly reduces oxygen transmission and helps to preserve the stability of lipids. There are many examples in the literature to illustrate the importance of considering packaging strategies. When vacuum-packaged salmon was processed using HPP, it exhibited significantly lower levels of lipid oxidation than samples stored under atmospheric conditions (Bumbudsanpharoke & Jinkarn, 2022). Packaging tuna with modified atmosphere packaging combined with HPP retained greater amounts of omega-3 FAs levels than did nonmodified atmosphere packaged tuna. Fish packaged in EVOH-based multilayer films exhibited lower PVs throughout storage compared to fish packaged in other packaging materials. HPP-treated and vacuum-packaged shrimp had improved lipid stability, while omega-3-FA-enriched dairy beverages packaged in oxygen barrier packaging maintained their FA stability after being subjected to pressure treatment (Gilstrap et al., 2023).

8.4.5 Food matrix and composition

PUFAs stability during HPP is strongly influenced by the food matrix composition and structure—the most notable being water activity, proteins, lipids distribution, and whether there are antioxidants/pro-oxidants in the matrix. Fish and meat (animals) have lipids attached to cellular membranes, which means that denaturing the protein structures via pressure will expose more lipid to oxygen and to catalytic metal ions that is, iron from heme proteins found in muscle foods (Gilstrap et al., 2023). However, plant-based foods often contain antioxidants that will protect the lipids from oxidative damage. Plant-based antioxidants, such as polyphenols, carotenoids, and tocopherols, are typically protected through high-pressure processes, thereby maintaining PUFA stability. Different studies demonstrate these interactions with different food matrices (i.e., fish muscle tissue using HPP), flaxseed pit preparations where additional phytochemicals (antioxidants) promote PUFA stability, as well as yogurt emulsions using HPP, which maintained lipid distribution/oxidation levels compared to standard processing (Aghababaei et al., 2023). Additionally, almond milk using HPP versus standard processing maintained its lipid quality due to antioxidants provided in the matrix, and functional (enriched with omega-3) beverages formulated with antioxidant compounds improved their PUFA stability by using HPP.

8.5 Sensory and quality attributes of high-pressure processing-treated polyunsaturated fatty acids foods

HPP is well-known to help preserve the nutritional and microbiological qualities of food while keeping desired sensory properties. In contrast, traditional thermal processing uses very high temperatures to create great changes to the characteristics of the product (i.e., flavor, color, texture) while HPP uses lower temperatures, which allows for the preservation of the natural characteristics of food products. The preservation of natural characteristics of PUFA-rich foods (i.e., food that contains large amounts of PUFAs) is particularly important, because lipid oxidation causes an undesirable sensory change through the presence of off-flavors; therefore the sensory attributes of HPP-treated foods are affected by a variety of factors (i.e., pressure intensity, processing time, product formulation, and storage conditions) (Roobab et al., 2022). Furthermore, the preservation of PUFA stability during HPP has a direct correlation to the preservation of sensory attributes (i.e., flavor, aroma, color, texture) of the product. There are many studies that have shown that HPP can help prolong shelf life and preserve sensory acceptability in seafood, meat, dairy, and plant-based products.

8.5.1 Effects on color

Color is a very important quality attribute that affects consumer acceptance of food products. Foods containing PUFAs, such as fish and meat, are often subject to color change due to oxidation processes as well as denaturation of proteins. Thermal processing of these foods may result in pigment alteration and browning reactions, which, in turn, may adversely affect consumer appeal for the final product. The application of high pressure to food products can cause changes in color due to pressure-induced changes in protein structure and pigment stability, particularly in muscle products (fish and meat) (Tsai et al., 2022). Specifically, the application of pressure to muscle products may cause partial denaturation of the myoglobin protein and, therefore have a minor effect on color intensity; however, this effect is likely to be much less than experienced with thermal processing. In a number of studies, the HPP process has been shown to maintain the color of seafood products. For instance, in one study, salmon fillets were treated using HPP at 300 MPa, and almost no change in the color parameters (L*, a*, b*) was observed during 48 hours of refrigerated storage (de Carvalho et al., 2024). Moreover, shrimp processed at 400 MPa also had minimal change in their original pink color due to limited oxidation of their carotenoid pigments (e.g., astaxanthin). In the case of dairy products, HPP treatment usually has little effect on color due to the relatively high stability of milk pigments under pressure.

8.5.2 Effects on texture

Texture is one of the most important sensory properties that can be affected by processing methods. HPP affects the texture of food by changing the structure of proteins and altering the microstructure of the food matrix (Duma-Kocan et al., 2024). In the case of muscle foods, processing with HPP could result in protein denaturation with subsequent gel formation, which in turn could increase the firmness of the muscle product. Research has shown that HPP can enhance the textural stability of seafood. One example would be that Atlantic salmon processed at pressure levels between 300 and 400 MPa exhibit an increase in firmness as a result of pressure-induced aggregation of the proteins. Another example of improved textural properties as a result of pressure is shrimp processed with HPP, which exhibited reduced drip loss during storage compared to shrimp that had been processed without HPP (Evrendilek, 2022). HPP also affects dairy products by altering the structure of casein micelles, resulting in a more viscous product and increased gel formation in yogurt and other fermented dairy products. Plant-based beverages also benefit from HPP, as pressure-induces changes in both proteins and polysaccharides, resulting in improved stability.

8.5.3 Effects on flavor and aroma

Food product flavor is one of the primary factors determining consumer acceptance of products. PUFA oxidation creates volatile compounds (e.g., aldehydes, ketones, and alcohols) that can result in rancid tastes (Iftikhar et al., 2026). HPP helps to preserve flavor by reducing lipid oxidation and maintaining volatile compounds responsible for desirable aroma. In addition, since HPP operates at relatively low temperatures, it inhibits the generation of many heat-induced flavor compounds that could potentially negatively impact the quality of the final product. Research conducted on seafood products demonstrates HPP's ability to maintain the characteristic flavor of fish through the reduction in oxidation product formation (Tsai et al., 2022). For example, HPP studies on processed sardines at 400–600 MPa showed that rancid flavors developed minimally during refrigerated storage. Likewise, HPP-treated tuna fillets possess a flavor profile similar to those processed via thermal methods (Semenoglou et al., 2025).

8.5.4 Consumer acceptance

The acceptance of HPP technology by consumers is widespread because foods treated by this method maintain many of the characteristics of fresh food. Sensory studies conducted using trained panels and consumers have shown that foods processed by high pressure are often rated higher than thermally processed foods in terms of their appearance, flavor, and overall quality (Song et al., 2022). For example, HPP-processed seafood was clearly rated higher than conventional seafood in terms of quality and shelf life when evaluated by consumer panels. Similarly, pressure-treated dairy products and plant-based beverages both received very positive ratings from consumers, largely due to their taste being close to "natural" and having been processed in a very mild manner. With the increased demand for minimally processed foods with a lot of nutritional value, consumers have become increasingly interested in using nonthermal technologies such as HPP for their food processing needs. Overall, HPP is a reliable method for maintaining the sensory and quality of PUFA-rich foods (Nurjati et al., 2025). In addition to inhibiting lipid oxidation and microbial spoilage, HPP preserves the quality of color, texture, and taste. Compared to standard or routine cooking methods (e.g., thermal processing), HPP has superior advantages in preserving food products with their fresh-like characteristics. As a result, there has been increased interest in the application of HPP technology across all types of seafood, meat, dairy products, and plant-based drinks.

8.6 Regulatory aspects and industrial uses of high-pressure processing technology

The broad commercialization of HPP has expanded rapidly in the food industry over the last 20 years due to its ability to provide enhanced safety by preserving nutritional value and sensory characteristics of foods. HPP food preservation is classified as nonthermal (no heat), thus leading to the creation of specific HPP regulations globally by food regulatory agencies for the safe application of HPP technology (i.e., at the food industry level). The regulations focus on microbial inactivation, process validation, product labeling, and quality assurance. Regulatory authorities overseeing PUFA-rich foods, including seafood, dairy products, and functional foods, provide regulatory frameworks that ensure HPP does not decrease the nutritional quality or safety of PUFA-rich foods, specifically with respect to the Food and Drug Administration (FDA), European Food Safety Authority, or the Food Safety and Standards Authority of India (FSSAI) (Barbosa-Canovas et al., 2022). These regulations enable food manufacturers to utilize HPP as a method of preserving food while ensuring the safety of the consumer. Additionally, regulatory authorities have established guidelines for implementing HPP in food processing, which facilitates the innovation of new food preservation technologies and impacts how food manufacturers adopt this technology. Factors impacting whether food manufacturers adopt the technology also include equipment and processing costs, product compatibility with HPP, consumer acceptance of HPP-processed foods, and the ability to implement the technology on a large scale (Nurjati et al., 2025). Currently, HPP is commercially available in food processing industries as a method of preserving food in these sectors: all food segments, such as seafood, meats, juices, dairy drinks, and functional foods containing bioactive components, such as PUFA, have adopted the use of HPP.

8.6.1 Regulating the use of high-pressure processing

While HPP is generally viewed as being a safe and effective means of preserving food, regulatory acceptance of HPP differs greatly around the world. The FDA will allow use of HPP as a substitute for thermal pasteurization in the United States of America, on the precondition that HPP processing has been verified by the manufacturer to provide some level of microbiological reduction or inactivation. Pathogen reduction (inactivation) is one of the primary indications of thermal pasteurization; therefore any food that has been processed by HPP and has been subject to sufficient levels of pathogen reduction or inactivation will be recognized as having been pasteurized. In the European Union (EU), food safety agencies have completed investigations into the safety of HPP-processed foods. They are in agreement with the result of these evaluations: HPP does not cause any harmful chemical changes to the components present in the food when exposed to the HPP process under appropriate conditions (Sorbo et al., 2022). Because of these evaluations, HPP is widely used in the European food industry, especially in seafood, meat, and fruit juices. In India, the FSSAI has also accepted the use of nonthermal technologies such as HPP as emerging food processing methods that will help improve the safety of food and extend the shelf life of food (Chakraborty et al., 2023). Although HPP is still a relatively new technology in India, there is considerable regulatory support and ongoing technological developments that is likely to increase the use of HPP in the food processing industry.

8.6.2 Consumer information and labeling

Food labeling requirements for HPP vary from one regulatory jurisdiction to another. In most countries, HPP is regarded as a processing method, not an additive. Therefore specific labeling requirements are often not enforced. Most manufacturers will still identify the use of HPP in the labeling of their goods because the consumer perceives HPP as an indication of minimally processed, high-quality foods. Despite the absence of regulations concerning the labeling of PUFA-rich foods (e.g., omega-3 fortifications), regulations may contain requirements for manufacturers to provide information on nutritional value and health claims (Nurjati et al., 2025). Health claims for these products must be supported by scientific evidence of the bioactive compounds' presence and stability. The increased consumer demand for clean-label and minimally processed foods has prompted companies to promote HPP technology as a process that preserves the nutrients naturally found in food without using chemical preservatives.

8.6.3 Industrial use of high-pressure processing

Many segments of the food industry have successfully incorporated HPP into their products and methods. The use of HPP in preserving fruit juices and beverages (one of its earliest commercial uses) is an excellent illustration of its effectiveness in inactivating microorganisms while preserving both the taste and nutritional properties of food. HPP is also an accepted practice for making fish and shellfish last longer and still retaining omega-3 FAs (Ismaiel et al., 2025). Also, HPP can help facilitate shucking shellfish (oysters or lobsters) by weakening the adductor muscle, thus increasing the efficiency of processing. In addition, the meat industry has also embraced the use of HPP to increase the safety of ready-to-eat meats (deli and cured meats). HPP is effective at eliminating pathogens without damaging the nutritional value of the products being processed. Dairy products (e.g., milk, yogurt, cheese) can benefit from HPP technology by improving the microbiological safety of the foods while maintaining the sensory quality (Sojecka et al., 2024). HPP is also being used more frequently to process plant-based beverages and functional foods that are fortified with PUFAs to preserve their bioactive ingredients.

8.6.4 Global high-pressure processing market trends and commercialization

Growing interest in safe and minimally processed foods is a key driver of the global HPP market, which has seen significant growth in recent years. North America and Europe are the leading adopters of HPP, due to increasing consumer demand for foods with original flavors, textures, and nutrients. In addition, many large food manufacturers have made capital investments in HPP equipment in order to create premium shelf-stable products. Commercial HPP systems are now capable of processing substantial quantities of packaged products, making them suitable for high-volume commercial production (Knoerzer & Sevenich, 2025). The increasing popularity of functional foods containing omega-3 FAs and other bioactive compounds has increased interest in the application of HPP technology. HPP process preserves the heat-sensitive nutrients in omega-3 FAs and therefore produces a wide range of nutritionally enhanced food products. To enable the large-scale use of HPP in food systems, it must receive regulatory approval and be adopted by industry. HPP has been deemed a safe and effective food preservation method when applied appropriately according to international regulations. Currently, several industries, such as seafood, meat and dairy products, as well as functional beverages, utilize HPP. With demand for minimally processed and nutritionally dense foods at an all-time high, HPP will likely play an increasing role in the food industry (Zhu et al., 2022). HPP's capability of preserving PUFAs and other bioactive components is its significant added value in the creation of functional foods with a greater health benefit.

8.7 Limitations and challenges of high-pressure processing

HPP is a food processing method that has received a great deal of attention recently as an alternative nonthermal food preservation method for PUFA-rich food products. However, many limitations and challenges exist that continue to limit the widespread use of HPP in several food sectors. Challenges exist due to the technological, economic, and biochemical characteristics of working with complex food systems using HPP. Although HPP has been shown to be effective in microbial inactivation and preserving the organoleptic quality of food products, the stability of PUFAs during pressure treatments and during storage may still be affected by oxygen exposure, enzyme activity, and food matrix interactions. Additionally, the capital cost of HPP equipment, lack of continuous processing, and variability in product response under pressure conditions are key factors regarding the industrial implementation of HPP (Roobab et al., 2022). Understanding these limitations will help optimize HPP processing parameters and develop processes to improve the stability of PUFA-rich foods.

8.7.1 High equipment and operational costs

HPP has several disadvantages, including the equipment installation and operating costs, which make HPP systems hard to afford and limit thier factors for small- and medium-scale food processing companies. Commercial HPP systems require highly advanced engineering (compressed air, drilling, etc.) to create a pressure vessel that can withstand an operating pressure of up to 600 MPa, as well as high-quality raw materials (generally 1/2 stainless steel) to withstand multiple cycles of compression while at least 2.8 times heavier than HPP machines (Lim et al., 2023). Therefore the total cost of a commercial HPP system includes capital equipment, maintenance of pumps and pressure maintenance, and inspection or maintenance of HPP equipment. While HPP equipment prices have been decreasing due to technology advances and increased market size, HPP systems have primarily been adopted by large manufacturers of high-value food products such as seafood, ready-to-eat meats, and premium beverages.

8.7.2 Oxidation risks with long-term storage

Despite the benefits offered by HPP in reducing the oxidation of lipids during processing, PUFA-rich products may continue to oxidatively deteriorate during long-term storage. PUFAs contain numerous double bonds and are particularly prone to oxidation via free radicals. This leads to the formation of LOOHs and secondary oxidation products such as aldehydes and ketones. Additionally, pressure treatment may create structural changes in the food matrix that will expose lipids to both atmospheric oxygen and to catalytic metal ions. For instance, with fish and meat, pressure-induced denaturation of proteins may cause iron to be released from heme-containing proteins, facilitating oxidation reactions during long-term storage (Semenoglou et al., 2025). Furthermore, while HPP is effective in inactivating many of the enzymes found in food, there are likely some enzymes responsible for lipid degradation that will maintain a partial level of activity based on the specific processing conditions utilized. Residual enzymatic activity may therefore contribute to lipid oxidation over time, particularly in products that are stored in an oxygen-free atmosphere.

8.7.3 Variance in different food types

Variance in different food types is another major obstacle facing HPP. Food type constitutes yet another major challenge because of variations in food response to processing. A major factor determines the behavior of PUFAs during pressure processing will be dependent upon the structural properties of the food system, as well as the composition of the food system. For instance, seafood products that contain higher amounts of omega-3 FAs will have different responses to pressure than dairy products or plant-based foods (de Carvalho et al., 2024). In fish muscle tissue, lipid molecules are mostly located within cellular membrane and protein structure, both of which are affected by the pressure treatment. Conversely, emulsified foods like some dairy and functional beverages will offer better protection to lipid molecules through emulsification due to the emulsifying ingredients and proteins. Plant-based foods usually have natural antioxidants such as polyphenols and carotenoids, which provide antioxidant activity to lipid molecules, whereas muscle-based foods would have pro-oxidant agents such as heme iron. These factors create challenges in establishing universal processing conditions to optimize PUFA stability among all types of foods.

8.7.4 Limited continuous processing capability

HPP systems that are commercially used usually use batch processes to pack sealed food into flexible packaging, and the food is placed in a vessel, and then it is processed. Although this is a very effective way of protecting food quality and safety, it limits the production throughput compared to other continuous processing technologies like HPP or thermal pasteurization. The use of batches to process food results in longer processing times and lower efficiencies in large-scale manufacturing. Additionally, the requirement that flexible packaging be used with high pressure is often very limited, and materials used in the construction of flexible packages can impose restrictions on the type of food that can actually utilize the packaging (Luo et al., 2025). It is anticipated that in the near future, additional research and development will occur with the purpose of providing a continuous high-pressure system, which will greatly improve these processes and result in substantially reducing production costs. However, as of now, there are no commercially used systems.

8.7.5 Knowledge gaps in long-term polyunsaturated fatty acids stability

Although HPP has been shown in numerous studies to negatively affect the stability of PUFAs in the short term, there is a substantial lack of information about long-term PUFA stability in foods that have undergone HPP. Most studies evaluate either the immediate changes in lipid stability following pressure treatment or lipid stability after several months of storage, but fewer report on the long-term storage effects on lipids (Roobab et al., 2022). Therefore when considering long-term lipid stability in HPP foods, it is critical to clearly understand the interaction of pressure treatment with the food (where the food may be made up of different compounds), the packaging conditions used, and the storage environment throughout the duration of storage (Tsai et al., 2022). In particular, research should focus on assessing the effect of HPP on PUFA oxidation rates, as well as the stability of antioxidants present within HPP foods, and the activity of enzymes in HPP foods, over long-term storage periods. Advances in analytical technology, such as gas chromatography-mass spectrometry (GC-MS), lipidomics, and spectroscopy, may provide further means of studying the long-term behavior of PUFAs in HPP foods.

8.8 Future research directions

HPP may be a useful alternative to conventional thermal processing for retaining the quality of foods that contain polyunsaturated fats. Nature has already made considerable strides in understanding the effects of pressure on the stability of lipids, the inactivation of microorganisms, and the overall quality of food products; however, there are still many areas that require additional research. Future studies should evaluate the optimization of the HPP process, the combination of the use of HPP with other nonthermal preservation technologies, and the examination of novel ways to deliver PUFA-rich functional foods to consumers (Iftikhar et al., 2026). The development and application of advanced analytical methodologies, food engineering, and nanotechnology will be key to improving the efficiency and effectiveness of HPP. Improving on existing studies and increasing the scientific knowledge base of HPP will give researchers the tools necessary to develop new products that are safe and provide superior nutrition when used in the food industry through the use of HPP.

8.8.1 Integration of high-pressure processing with antioxidant strategies

A promising area of research is HPP and antioxidant systems, both natural and synthetic, to provide improved oxidative stability for PUFAs. HPP can significantly reduce the thermal degradation of PUFAs; however, the oxidation process can still take place during storage of the PUFAs from contact with atmospheric oxygen and oxidants. Future studies need to focus on the combined effects of HPP and natural antioxidants (i.e., tocopherols, polyphenols, carotenoids, and extracts from various plants) because these antioxidants can provide stability to lipids through free radical scavenging as well as reducing the rate of propagation of oxidation reactions (Enchangan et al., 2025). Furthermore, by incorporating antioxidant-rich ingredients into food formulations rich in PUFAs, the stability of the lipids will be further improved during storage. Continued research is also needed to determine the optimal combinations of both the pressure treatments and the antioxidant systems to provide the maximum amount of protection against lipid oxidation while also achieving desirable sensory characteristics.

8.8.2 Combination of high-pressure processing with other nonthermal technologies

Combining various nonthermal preservation processes with HPP has been researched and has shown potential for combining multiple technologies to create synergistic effects that provide increased safety in the products while retaining their nutritional value and shelf life (Enchangan et al., 2025). Examples of combinations of multiple technologies include pulsed electric fields, cold plasma, ultrasound, and UV process. These technologies will eliminate microorganisms, reduce enzyme activity, and provide stability to sensitive nutrients as long-chain polyunsaturated fatty acids (LCPUFAs) (Sorbo et al., 2022). Furthermore, hybrid applications of processing methods may provide a lower intensity of the single processing method in comparison to using a single processing technology, thereby reducing the likelihood of food structure damage due to one processing method. Research should continue in order to determine optimized processing parameters from the use of multiple technologies to maximize retention of LCPUFAs and maximize overall product performance.

8.8.3 Nano-encapsulation and polyunsaturated fatty acids delivery systems

Nano-encapsulation technologies are one means to create systems for the delivery of functional PUFAs in food products. Advanced forms of nano-encapsulation may also contribute to the overall stability of PUFAs through creating a physical barrier to limit the PUFA's oxidation potential from environmental exposure (i.e., oxygen or pro-oxidant exposure) (Karunanithi et al., 2024). A multitude of encapsulation techniques (e.g., nanoemulsions, liposomes, and biopolymer-based nanoparticles) have been employed to develop the delivery of bioactive compounds in functional food systems, including (but not limited to) improving omega-3 FA bioavailability and stability during food processing/storage (Srivastav & Karunanithi, 2024). Future research should also investigate the existing interaction between nano-encapsulated PUFA systems and respective HPP conditions, as understanding how pressure relates to the encapsulation structure will ultimately affect the design of long-term stable delivery systems for industrial food applications.

8.8.4 Development of personalized nutrition and functional foods

Personalized nutrition is becoming increasingly popular among consumers as they've discovered new possibilities for creating functional foods containing bioactive compounds (e.g., PUFAs). To make nutritionally fortified foods, HPP will be vital, as it can produce such foods while maintaining the stability of highly sensitive nutrients (Chahdoura et al., 2023). Future research will look into creating custom food products designed for specific health requirements (like cardiovascular health) or for certain benefits (like antiinflammatory benefits). HPP can also help to protect the bioactivity of functional ingredients while providing assurance of microbial safety and extended shelf-life. Furthermore, improvements to ingredient technology and food formulation may help create new PUFA-enriched foods, such as beverages, dairy alternatives, and functional plant-based foods.

8.8.5 Energy efficiency and sustainability

Sustainability is gaining importance for the food processing industry when establishing a new food processing technology. HPP provides many benefits related to quality, but it must also be examined in terms of energy consumption and equipment requirements (Song et al., 2022). Future research should develop HPP systems with improved energy efficiency, reduced operating costs, and processing parameters to enable less environmental impact. Advancements in process optimization, equipment design, and energy recovery systems will most likely contribute to the development of sustainable industrial applications. HPP's usage in conjunction with eco-friendly packaging options and green energy resources will continue to improve the ecological durability of PUFA-abundant foods.

8.9 Summary and conclusions

PUFAs, including omega-3 and omega-6 FAs, provide numerous health advantages, such as preventing cardiovascular incidents, having antiinflammatory attributes, and boosting cognitive performance. The presence of numerous double bonds within the PUFA requires handling with care, due to PUFA being extremely prone to oxidation when traditionally processed and stored. High-heat processing of food increases lipid oxidation, which creates unwanted compounds and alters PUFA quality, flavor/perception, and length of usability once packaged. In contrast to traditional heat methods, HPP is a nonthermal process that can provide a long shelf life while maintaining PUFA's nutrition, as well as bacteria being killed/microorganisms/enzymes inhibited through the concept of boiking (structural alteration of microorganisms/enzymes due to being subjected to very high levels of pressure) instead of heating. This means that many of the heat-sensitive nutrients found in PUFA's are preserved during pressure processing. Inhibiting the thermal breakdown of lipid(s) through the application of pressure can help to minimize the oxidation of lipid(s) caused by nonthermal processes, such as inhibiting the action of lipoxygenase and lipase at high temperatures, as well as aiding in the protection of endogenous antioxidants located within food products.

Research has shows that HPP preserves the FAs found in food systems that are high in PUFAs, including seafood, meat, dairy products, and plant-based foods, while also improving safety through microbial reduction and increasing shelf life. Seafood products with high levels of EPA and DHA have been shown to have improved lipid stability and sensory quality when subjected to HPP. However, several challenges are associated with the use of HPP in the food industry, including high equipment costs, limited batch-processing capacity, variations in food matrix, and the potential for oxidation of products during long-term storage. More research is needed into how to optimize processing parameters and packaging techniques, as well as how to integrate HPP with other technologies such as antioxidant systems and nano-encapsulated products. If successful, HPP will help to create functional foods that are high in PUFAs, while also maintaining their nutritional quality and consumer appeal. As such, HPP is a promising technology for maintaining PUFA stability and ensuring safe, high-quality foods that are beneficial to health.

References

Aghababaei, F., Trujillo, A. J., Juan, B., Capellas, M., & Ferragut, V. (2023). Encapsulating capacity of ultra-high-pressure homogenization (UHPH): Replacement of milk fat by vegetable oils using buttermilk as a functional ingredient in yogurt processing. *LWT, 187*, 115304. https://doi.org/10.1016/j.lwt.2023.115304.

Arslan, M., Zareef, M., Afzal, M., Tahir, H. E., Li, Z., Aalim, H., Abaker, H. M. A., & Zou, X. (2025). Innovative non-thermal processing technologies for shelf life extension and retention of bioactive compounds in liquid foods: Current status and future prospects. *Foods, 14*(17). https://doi.org/10.3390/foods14172953, www.mdpi.com/journal/foods.

Arulkumar, A., Swain, B., & Paramasivam, S. (2020). Shelf life extension of sardines (*Sardinella albella*) using betel leaf (*Piper betle*) incorporated ice. *Food and Bioprocess Technology, 13*(7), 1255–1260.

Barbosa-Canovas, G. V., Bermúdez-Aguirre, D., Franco, B. G., Cando\ugan, K., & Shin, G. Y. (2022). Novel food processing technologies and regulatory hurdles. In *Ensuring global food safety*. Elsevier, 221–228.

Bumbudsanpharoke, N., & Jinkarn, T. (2022). Effect of high-pressure food processing on selected flexible packaging: Structure, physicochemical properties, and migration. *Journal of Food Engineering, 321*, 110970. https://doi.org/10.1016/j.jfoodeng.2022.110970.

Cai, L., & Wang, Y. (2021). Physicochemical and antioxidant properties based on fish sarcoplasmic protein/chitosan composite films containing ginger essential oil nanoemulsion. *Food and Bioprocess Technology, 14*(1), 151–163. https://doi.org/10.1007/s11947-020-02564-0.

Campos Espinosa, G. Y., Udenigwe, C. C., & Tsopmo, A. (2022). Inhibition of low-density lipoprotein oxidation, antioxidative and bile acid-binding capacities of hydrolyzed proteins from carbohydrase-treated oat bran. *Journal of Food Biochemistry, 46*(3), 1–10. https://doi.org/10.1111/jfbc.13675.

Chahdoura, H., Mzoughi, Z., Ziani, B. E. C., Chakroun, Y., Boujbiha, M. A., Bok, S. E., M'hadheb, M. B., Majdoub, H., Mnif, W., Flamini, G., & Mosbah, H. (2023). Effect of flavoring with rosemary, lemon and orange on the quality, composition and biological properties of olive oil: Comparative study of extraction processes. *Foods, 12*(6). https://doi.org/10.3390/foods12061301, www.mdpi.com/journal/foods.

Chakraborty, P., Mukherjee, A., & Kumar, S. (2023). Laws and regulations for emerging food-processing technologies. In *Emerging technologies in food preservation*. CRC Press, 377–387.

Chmiel, M., Świder, O., Roszko, M., Adamczak, L., Cegiełka, A., Pietrzak, D., Florowski, T., Bryła, M., & Florowska, A. (2025). Effect of high-pressure processing and long-time storage on color, lipid oxidation, and free amino acids profile of beef. *Applied Sciences, 15*(5), 2382. https://doi.org/10.3390/app15052382.

de Carvalho, M. D., de Andrade, C. C. P., & Sato, A. C. K. (2024). Dynamic high-pressure microfluidization reduces aggregation and enhances functional properties of flaxseed protein isolates obtained by alkaline extraction. *Innovative Food Science & Emerging Technologies, 96*, 103793.

Duma-Kocan, P., Rudy, M., Gil, M., Żurek, J., Stanisławczyk, R., Krajewska, A., & Dziki, D. (2024). The influence of high hydrostatic pressure on selected quality features of cold-storage pork semimembranosus muscle. *Foods, 13*(13), 2089. https://doi.org/10.3390/foods13132089.

El-Zenary, A. S. A., Boney, J. W., & Harvatine, K. J. (2023). Direct comparison of 18 carbon n–3 and n–6 fatty acids at equal levels in an oil blend on tissue enrichment of long-chain polyunsaturated fatty acid in broiler chickens. *The Journal of Nutrition, 153*(10), 2929–2938.

Enchangan, M. M. G., Seman, M. S., Al-Obaidi, J. R., Zakaria, A. F., Razis, A. F. A., Saari, N., Harith, H. H., & Jambari, N. N. (2025). High-pressure processing (HPP) impacts on indian mackerel meat: Insights into quality attributes, β-parvalbumin antigenicity, and proteomic changes. *Applied Food Research, 5*(1). https://doi.org/10.1016/j.afres.2025.100888, https://www.sciencedirect.com/science/journal/27725022.

Evrendilek, G. A. (2022). High hydrostatic processing of marinated ground chicken breast: Exploring the effectiveness on physicochemical, textural and sensory properties and microbial inactivation. *Food Control, 142*, 109258. https://doi.org/10.1016/j.foodcont.2022.109258.

Fidalgo, L. G., Simões, M. M. Q., Casal, S., Lopes-da-Silva, J. A., Delgadillo, I., & Saraiva, J. A. (2021). Enhanced preservation of vacuum-packaged Atlantic salmon by hyperbaric storage at room temperature versus refrigeration. *Scientific Reports, 11*(1). https://doi.org/10.1038/s41598-021-81047-4.

Ganjeh, A. M., Gomes, A., Barreira, M. J., Pinto, C. A., Casal, S., & Saraiva, J. A. (2024). Effects of pressure-based technologies on food lipids oxidation. *Food Chemistry, 461*. https://doi.org/10.1016/j.foodchem.2024.140768, https://www.sciencedirect.com/science/journal/03088146.

Gilstrap, O., Liu, C., Nindo, C., & Parveen, S. (2023). Pilot scale assessment of high-pressure processing (HPP) to enhance microbiological quality and shelf life of fresh ready-to-eat (RTE) blue crab meat. *Microorganisms, 11*(12), 2909. https://doi.org/10.3390/microorganisms11122909.

Iftikhar, A., Arshad, M. S., Majzoobi, M., Farahnaky, A., & Suleria, H. (2026). Effect of high-pressure processing and Thuja occidentalis leaf powder on the quality, stability, and shelf life of chicken meat patties. *International Journal of Food Science and Technology*. https://doi.org/10.1093/ijfood/vvag002.

Ismaiel, L., Nartea, A., Fanesi, B., Lucci, P., Pacetti, D., Jaeger, H., & Schottroff, F. (2025). Effect of high-pressure processing on color, texture and volatile profile during sardine refrigeration. *Foods, 14*(2), 329. https://doi.org/10.3390/foods14020329.

Jiang, W., Zhang, Y., Julian McClements, D., Liu, F., & Liu, X. (2022). Impact of pea protein-inulin conjugates prepared via the Maillard reaction using a combination of ultrasound and pH-shift treatments on physical and oxidative stability of algae oil emulsions. *Food Research International, 156*, 111161. https://doi.org/10.1016/j.foodres.2022.111161.

Karunanithi, S., Gupta, R. K., Guha, P., & Srivastav, P. P. (2024). Exploring the effects of diverse extraction methods on nanoemulsion formulation using betel leaf essential oil: Assessing antibacterial efficacy against pathogenic microorganisms. *Food and Humanity, 2*. https://doi.org/10.1016/j.foohum.2024.100267, https://www.sciencedirect.com/journal/food-and-humanity.

Keivani, N., & Hosseini, S. F. (2023). Omega-3 polyunsaturated fatty acids: Sources, structural features and health effects. In *Handbook of food bioactive ingredients: Properties and applications*. Italy: Springer International Publishing, 967–995. https://link.springer.com/book/10.1007/978-3-031-28109-9, 10.1007/978-3-031-28109-9_20.

Khaliq, A., Chughtai, M. F. J., Mehmood, T., Ahsan, S., Liaqat, A., Nadeem, M., Sameed, N., Saeed, K., Rehman, J. U., & Ali, A. (2021). High-pressure processing; Principle, applications, impact, and future prospective. In *Sustainable food processing and engineering challenges*. Pakistan: Elsevier, 75–108. https://www.elsevier.com/books/sustainable-food-processing-and-engineering-challenges/galanakis/978-0-12-822714-5, 10.1016/B978-0-12-822714-5.00003-6.

Knoerzer, K., & Sevenich, R. (2025). From concept to commercialization: Unlocking the potential of high-pressure thermal processing. *Food Engineering Reviews, 17*(3), 627–644. https://doi.org/10.1007/s12393-025-09414-9.

Kumar, M., Zhang, B., Potkule, J., Sharma, K., Radha, Hano, C., Sheri, V., Chandran, D., Dhumal, S., Dey, A., Rais, N., Senapathy, M., Natta, S., Viswanathan, S., Mohankumar, P., & Lorenzo, J. M. (2023). Cottonseed oil: Extraction, characterization, health benefits, safety profile, and application. *Food Analytical Methods, 16*(2), 266–280. https://doi.org/10.1007/s12161-022-02410-3, https://www.springer.com/journal/12161.

Laghari, Z. H., Kori, A. H., Mahesar, S. A., & Sherazi, S. T. H. (2026). Overview of conjugated and unconjugated fatty acids and their biological impacts. In *Biology of fatty acids*. Elsevier, 397–414.

Li, L. (2024). Effects of high-pressure thawing on the quality and myofibrillar protein denaturation of Atlantic salmon. *European Food Research and Technology, 250*(6), 1789–1802. https://doi.org/10.1007/s00217-024-04504-0, https://www.springer.com/journal/217.

Lie, R. R., & Nurkhoeriyati, T. (2025). High-pressure processing procedures and effects on fishery products: a review. IOP Conference Series: Earth and Environmental Science. 7551315 1 Institute of Physics Indonesia. https://iopscience.iop.org/journal/1755-1315.1488. 10.1088/1755-1315/1488/1/012106.

Lim, S. H., Chin, N. L., Sulaiman, A., Tay, C. H., & Wong, T. H. (2023). Microbiological, physicochemical and nutritional properties of fresh cow milk treated with industrial high-pressure processing (HPP) during storage. *Foods, 12*(3). https://doi.org/10.3390/foods12030592, www.mdpi.com/journal/foods.

Liu, Y., Ramakrishnan, V. V., & Dave, D. (2021). Enzymatic hydrolysis of farmed Atlantic salmon by-products: Investigation of operational parameters on extracted oil yield and quality. *Process Biochemistry, 100*(July 2020), 10–19. https://doi.org/10.1016/j.procbio.2020.09.019.

Luo, T., Ninan, N., Truong, V. K., He, S., Alhaji, J. H., & Binobead, M. A. (2025). Impact of microwave processing and high-pressure processing on omega-3 fatty acid-enriched snack of microalgae (*Nannochloropsis* sp)–cocoa balls. *International Journal of Food Science and Technology, 60*(1). https://doi.org/10.1093/ijfood/vvaf005, https://academic.oup.com/ijfst/issue.

Medina-Meza, I. G., Barnaba, C., & Barbosa-Cánovas, G. V. (2014). Effects of high pressure processing on lipid oxidation: A review. *Innovative Food Science & Emerging Technologies, 22*, 1–10.

Musakhanian, J., Rodier, J.-D., & Dave, M. (2022). Oxidative stability in lipid formulations: A review of the mechanisms, drivers, and inhibitors of oxidation. *AAPS PharmSciTech, 23*(5), 151.

Nagy, K., Iacob, B.-C., Bodoki, E., & Oprean, R. (2024). Investigating the thermal stability of omega fatty acid-enriched vegetable oils. *Foods, 13*(18), 2961. https://doi.org/10.3390/foods13182961.

Nurjati, S. K., Purnawan, M. A., & Stevviani, R. (2025). High-pressure processing (HPP) energy efficiency and scalability challenges in ultra-processed meat: A review. *Journal of Clean Technology, 2*(1), 45–56.

Ramakrishnan, S. R., Antony, U., & Kim, S. J. (2022). Non-thermal process technologies: Influences on nutritional and storage characteristics of millets. *Journal of Food Process Engineering,* 1–13. https://doi.org/10.1111/jfpe.14215 November.

Roobab, U., Fidalgo, L. G., Arshad, R. N., Khan, A. W., Zeng, X. A., Bhat, Z. F., Bekhit, A. E. D. A., Batool, Z., & Aadil, R. M. (2022). High-pressure processing of fish and shellfish products: Safety, quality, and research prospects. *Comprehensive Reviews in Food Science and Food Safety, 21*(4), 3297–3325. https://doi.org/10.1111/1541-4337.12977, http://onlinelibrary.wiley.com/journal/10.1111/(ISSN)1541-4337.

Roy, V. C., Getachew, A. T., Cho, Y. J., Park, J. S., & Chun, B. S. (2020). Recovery and bio-potentialities of astaxanthin-rich oil from shrimp ((*Peneanus monodon*) waste and mackerel (*Scomberomous niphonius*) skin using concurrent supercritical CO_2 extraction. *Journal of Supercritical Fluids, 159*. https://doi.org/10.1016/j.supflu.2020.104773, https://www.journals.elsevier.com/the-journal-of-supercritical-fluids.

Semenoglou, I., Katsouli, M., Giannakourou, M., & Taoukis, P. (2025). Effect of high-pressure homogenization and wall material composition on the encapsulation of polyunsaturated fatty acids from fish processing. *Molecules (Basel, Switzerland), 30*(7), 1434. https://doi.org/10.3390/molecules30071434.

Sojecka, A. A., Drozd-Rzoska, A., & Rzoska, S. J. (2024). Food preservation in the industrial revolution epoch: Innovative high pressure processing (HPP, HPT) for the 21st-century sustainable society. *Foods, 13*(19), 3028.

Song, Q., Li, R., Song, X., Clausen, M. P., Orlien, V., & Giacalone, D. (2022). The effect of high-pressure processing on sensory quality and consumer acceptability of fruit juices and smoothies: A review. *Food Research International, 157*, 111250. https://doi.org/10.1016/j.foodres.2022.111250.

Sorbo, A., Pucci, E., Nobili, C., Taglieri, I., Passeri, D., & Zoani, C. (2022). Food safety assessment: Overview of metrological issues and regulatory aspects in the European Union. *Separations, 9*(2), 53. https://doi.org/10.3390/separations9020053.

Srivastav, P. P., & Karunanithi, S. (2024). *Emerging methods for oil extraction from food processing waste.*

Suryati, M. A., Azrina, A., Ismail, A., & Nor-Khaizura, M. A. R. (2022). Review on retention of long-chain omega-3 polyunsaturated fatty acids (EPA and DHA) in fish as affected by cooking methods. *International Food Research Journal, 29*(5), 975–990. https://doi.org/10.47836/ifrj.29.5.02, http://www.ifrj.upm.edu.my.

Truong, B. Q., Buckow, R., & Nguyen, M. H. (2023). Effects of high pressure treatment and chitosan coating on selected enzymatic activities and quality indices of Barramundi (*Lates calcarifer*) muscle. *Journal of Aquatic Food Product Technology, 32*(10), 692–706.

Tsai, Y. H., Kung, H. F., Lin, C. S., Hsieh, C. Y., Ou, T. Y., Chang, T. H., & Lee, Y. C. (2022). Impacts of high-pressure processing on quality and shelf-life of yellowfin tuna (*Thunnus albacares*) stored at 4°C and 15°C. *International Journal of Food Properties, 25*(1), 237–251. https://doi.org/10.1080/10942912.2022.2029483, https://www.tandfonline.com/loi/ljfp20.

Zhu, C., Jiao, D., Sun, Y., Chen, L., Meng, S., Yu, X., Zheng, M., Liu, M., Liu, J., & Liu, H. (2022). Effects of ultra-high pressure on endogenous enzyme activities, protein properties, and quality characteristics of shrimp (*Litopenaeus vannamei*) during iced storage. *Molecules (Basel, Switzerland), 27*(19), 6302. https://doi.org/10.3390/molecules27196302.

Chapter 9

Innovations in polyunsaturated fatty acid delivery systems: emulsions, encapsulation, and structured lipids

Bouthaina Ben Hadj Hmida[1], Khaoula Elhadef[2], Fakhreddine Ben Amara[3], Slim Smaoui[3], Mondher Mzoughi[4], and Sameh Ben Mabrouk[1,2,4]

[1]*Laboratory of Biochemistry and Enzymatic Engineering of Lipases, National Engineering School of Sfax, University of Sfax, Sfax, Tunisia,* [2]*Laboratory of Microbial Biotechnology, Enzymatic and Biomolecules, Centre of Biotechnology of Sfax, University of Sfax, Sfax, Tunisia,* [3]*Laboratory of Microbial Biotechnology, Enzymatic and Biomolecules, Centre of Biotechnology of Sfax, Sfax, Tunisia,* [4]*Faculty of Chemical & Metallurgical Engineering, Istanbul Technical University, Dr, Department of Food Engineering, Istanbul, Turkey*

9.1 Introduction

The human body can't synthesize these bioactive compounds; thus they must be included in the daily diet. These powerful nutrients play crucial roles in biological functions, namely, the control of gene expression in cell growth and death, as well as hormone metabolism (Gasa-Falcon et al., 2020). Of all bioactive compounds, Fatty Acids are the most familiar. FAs exist in two forms: saturated (no double bonds) and unsaturated (with double bonds). Hence, unsaturated FAs are further split into monounsaturated (one bond) and polyunsaturated (many bonds) (Islam et al., 2023). Polyunsaturated fatty acids (PUFAs) serve as essential building blocks for cell membranes, and they act as crucial nutrients in managing conditions such as nonalcoholic fatty liver disease, autoimmune disorders, and various chronic diseases.

The most essential PUFAs are omega-3 and omega-6 fatty acids. They are considered essential FAs since they can't be produced inside our bodies. omega-3 and omega-6 are obtained from parent compounds: α-linolenic acids (ALA) and linoleic acid (LA), respectively. To satisfy omega-3 needs, consume plant seeds such as perilla, chia, and flax, fish oil, and cereal products. ALA, eicosapentaenoic acid (EPA), and docosahexaenoic acid (DHA) are crucial omega-3 fatty acids, while LA and arachidonic acid are the sources of omega-6 fatty acids (Balić et al., 2020; Kapoor et al., 2021). Apart from being a major source of energy for the body, PUFAs contribute to blood pressure regulation, supporting immune system function and the absorption of fat-soluble vitamins, modulating the production of antiinflammatory compounds, and safeguarding cardiovascular health (Mititelu et al., 2024).

Despite the numerous advantages of PUFA, their applications are restricted mainly owing to their high sensitivity to oxidation. When they are exposed to different environmental conditions such as light, oxygen, or heating, PUFA are prone to oxidation, isomerization, polymerization, and the release of volatile compounds. Meanwhile, storage and processing lead to the oxidative degradation of PUFA, altering the flavor, value, smell, and color (Islam et al., 2023). Apart from oil damage, PUFA are characterized by low aqueous solubility; therefore they are unable to express their virtue completely. This phenomenon causes weak interaction of PUFA with enzymes in the gastrointestinal system, which decreases the absorption into the blood (Blanco-Llamero et al., 2022). To address these problems, researchers have focused on innovating different stabilized systems to enhance PUFA protection and transportation while avoiding lipid oxidation. Advanced encapsulation and emulsification approaches are investigated to boost the oxidative stability and bioavailability of PUFA by preventing them from degrading and promoting controlled release. They allow PUFA to be diffused in aqueous solutions or dried powders to ensure a safer, sustainable delivery system. Additionally, structured lipids (SLs) provide unique functional characteristics involving absorption amelioration, calorie reduction, and saturated fat level decrease (Homroy et al., 2024).

Omega-3 and Omega-6 Polyunsaturated Fatty Acids in Food Systems. DOI: https://doi.org/10.1016/B978-0-443-43810-3.00016-6

This chapter mainly focuses on understanding the different technologies for PUFA delivery, including emulsification, encapsulation systems, and SLs. Additionally, some examples of the main encapsulated PUFA were delineated in different sectors such as food, medicine, and cosmetics. This chapter also explores the key challenges and future directions in PUFA delivery systems, addressing hurdles such as scalability, cost-effectiveness, and long-term stability.

9.2 Emulsions for polyunsaturated fatty acid delivery

Emulsions represent a commonly adopted strategy for mitigating oxidation of PUFAs, offering the benefits of straightforward preparation and cost-effectiveness. The oxidation rate of PUFAs in emulsions is influenced by the emulsion structure, including the oil phase's degree of unsaturation and the aqueous phase's viscosity and their bis-allylic C-H bond content. Lipid hydroperoxides accumulate at the interface, react with aqueous pro-oxidants, and generate radicals that propagate oxidation into oil droplets. Thus interfacial properties are key determinants of PUFA stability. Lipid hydroperoxides gather at the interface, interact with water-soluble pro-oxidants, and produce radicals that extend oxidation into oil droplets, as explained by Fig. 9.1 (Homroy et al., 2024; Wang et al., 2020).

9.3 Different types of polyunsaturated fatty acid emulsions

Systems for delivering PUFAs can be developed into various emulsion-based formats, including basic and complex emulsions as well as sophisticated nanoscale structures (Fig. 9.2).

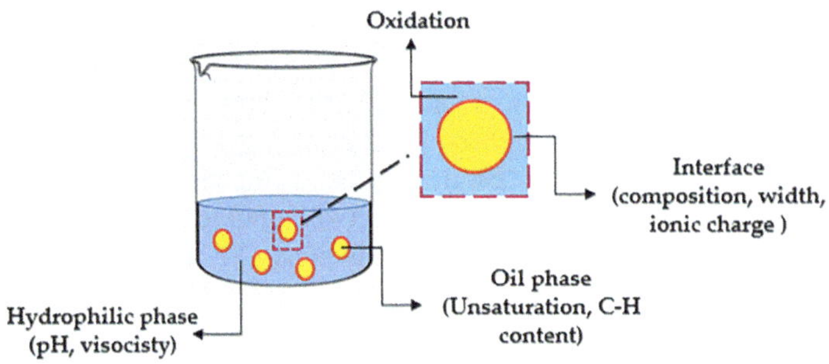

FIGURE 9.1 Lipid oxidation in an emulsion.

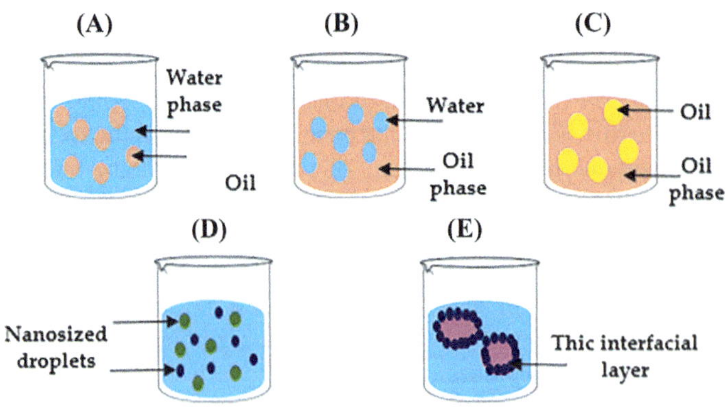

FIGURE 9.2 Different types of emulsions: (A) oil-in-water emulsion, (B) water-in-oil emulsion, (C) oil-in-oil emulsion, (D) nanoemulsions, and (E) Pickering emulsion.

9.4 Simple polyunsaturated fatty acid-based emulsions

Simple emulsions can be categorized into three primary types: oil-in-water (O/W), water-in-oil (W/O), and oil-in-oil (O/O) emulsions, with each type containing one phase distributed within another immiscible liquid. To encapsulate hydrophobic omega–3 PUFAs, O/W emulsions are widely used as a delivery system. As noted by Ghelichi et al. (2023), these emulsions consist of two liquids that do not mix: oil is dispersed as spherical droplets within a continuous water phase. Based on their oil droplet volume fraction, O/W emulsions are classified as either low-fat (<50% oil) or high-fat (>50% oil) systems (Yesiltas et al., 2019). The main benefit of O/W emulsions is that they combine water-soluble and lipid-soluble omega–3 PUFAs in one product, allowing flexible nutrient administration (Vellido-Perez et al., 2021). However, O/W emulsions are inherently unstable from a thermodynamic perspective and are susceptible to degradation due to environmental factors (temperature alterations and mechanical stress), which affects their shelf life (Teixé-Roig et al., 2023). Moreover, oxygen, heat, ions, and UV light can all oxidize the omega–3 PUFAs found in these emulsions. To address this problem, the emulsion's interfacial layer is crucial as it serves as a physical barrier, shielding PUFAs from pro-oxidants found in the air and aqueous phase (Du et al., 2022).

On the other hand, W/O emulsions are composed of droplets of the aqueous phase scattered throughout a continuous lipid phase. In oil-based food matrices, these systems can distribute and encapsulate hydrophilic bioactive substances (proteins, peptides, and minerals) with sustained release (Bao & Pignitter, 2023). However, because the oil phase is always exposed to pro-oxidants, lipid oxidation could occur. This oxidative degradation is impacted by chemical variables such as the fatty acid composition, the presence of lipase and lipoxygenase, and physical variables, namely the emulsion structure, emulsifier features, and processing methods. Food safety is compromised by oxidation at every stage of the supply chain; hence, interfacial engineering plays a crucial role in the stabilization process (Lampi et al., 2020).

Apart from W/O systems, O/O emulsions completely remove water and are referred to as waterless (or water-free) emulsions, anhydrous emulsions, and nonaqueous emulsions; they are essentially blends of incompatible oils. These emulsions are created by dispersing droplets of oil in a nonaqueous liquid that does not mix. Despite the presence of oil in their formulations, oxidation in O/O emulsions has not yet been investigated (Ghelichi et al., 2023).

9.5 Multiple polyunsaturated fatty acid-based emulsions

Various emulsions, referred to as double emulsions, are intricate systems in which one emulsion is distributed within another. The two main kinds of these emulsions are water-in-oil-in-water (W/O/W) and oil-in-water-in-oil (O/W/O). Oil droplets are initially distributed in a continuous water phase in O/W/O emulsions, and this primary emulsion is then distributed into a second exterior oil phase. On the other hand, water droplets are distributed within an oil phase and then subsequently dispersed into a second exterior water phase to generate W/O/W emulsions (Venugopalan et al., 2021). $W_1/O/W_2$ emulsions exhibit a similar appearance and texture compared to the simple PUFA-based emulsion, although with reduced fat content. These emulsions enable the entrapment of hydrophilic bioactive molecules within the internal water phase (W_1), enabling controlled release. $W_1/O/W_2$ preparation involves two key steps: (1) the formation of a primary W_1/O emulsion by homogenizing water and oil phases stabilized with an emulsifier, and (2) the dispersion of this emulsion into a second aqueous phase (W_2) incorporating a water-soluble emulsifier to generate the final $W_1/O/W_2$ structure (Tan & Yoon, Cho, et al., 2021). Like conventional emulsions, multiple emulsions are vulnerable to failure processes such as droplet flocculation, coalescence, Ostwald ripening, and sedimentation. They also have instability challenges, such as interior water droplets expanding, contracting, or ejecting. The main cause of these issues is the difference in osmotic pressure between the W_1 and W_2 phases. Nevertheless, this limitation can be resolved by adding osmotically active solutes (sugars or salts) to the aqueous phases to reduce water diffusion (Leister & Karbstein, 2020). Contrariwise, in $O_1/W/O_2$ emulsions, the inner oil phase is referred to as O_1, while the outer oil phase is known as O_2. Compared to $W_1/O/W_2$ emulsions, $O_1/W/O_2$ emulsions have been the subject of fewer studies over the past 10 years. $O_1/W/O_2$ research is very desirable, though, because it has the potential to replace conventional W/O emulsions, lowering the amount of trans and saturated fats without compromising mouthfeel. Furthermore, $O_1/W/O_2$ emulsions can be used to distribute, protect, and release sensitive bioactive chemicals in a controlled manner (Ghiasi et al., 2024) (Fig. 9.3).

9.6 Multilayer emulsions

They consist of O/W systems where droplets are encased in two or more layers of electrostatically charged biopolymers, created through a process of sequential interfacial deposition. Their synthesis needs to be carefully managed because incorrect polyelectrolyte ratios might lead to instability (bridging or depletion flocculation). These systems exhibit

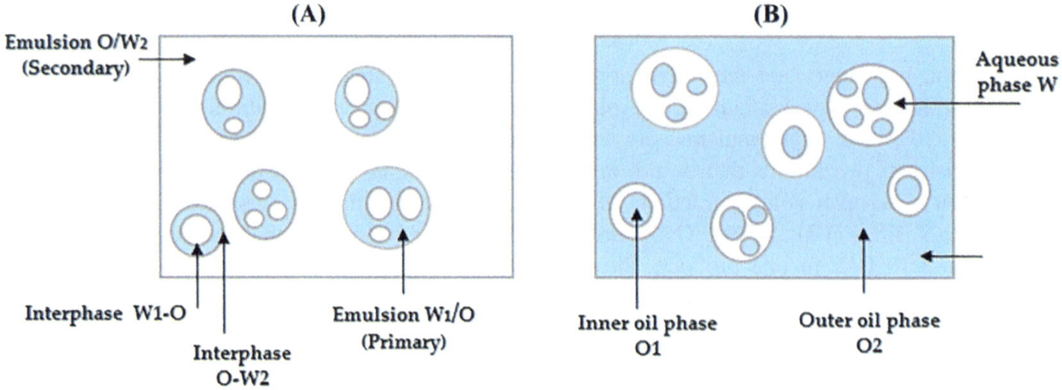

FIGURE 9.3 (A) Illustration of emulsion $W_1/O/W_2$. (B) Emulsion $O_1/W/O_2$.

superior oxidative stability when compared to single-layer emulsions, especially for PUFAs. As a result, the multilayer interfaces may boost antioxidant capacities and serve as a physical barrier to pro-oxidants. For instance, tri-layer configurations offer extra protection by using stronger interfacial coatings to protect lipids from aqueous-phase oxidants, while bilayer emulsions perform better than conventional monolayers (Gasa-Falcon et al., 2020; Wang et al., 2020).

9.7 Nano-emulsions

Nano-emulsions are a class of multiphase colloidal mixtures, especially featuring O/W structures. This emulsion type is composed of immiscible oil droplets suspended in an aqueous phase, with droplet sizes ranging from 50–500 nm. In spite of their nanoscale dimensions, they are widely used to encapsulate PUFA-rich oils, improving oxidative stability, accessibility, and optical transparency. Further, emulsifiers facilitate phase homogenization and move to the oil-water boundary, where they enhance the system's stability by minimizing interfacial tension. Before dispersion occurs, lipophilic bioactive compounds are initially dissolved in the oil phase. To achieve homogenization, either high-energy approaches (high-pressure valve mixers, microfluidizers, ultrasound) or low-energy techniques (self-emulsification or phase inversion) can be employed; the choice of method influences droplet size, cost, and scalability. Due to their improved physical stability and functional effectiveness, the resulting nano-emulsions are particularly effective for delivering omega-3 oils and other nutrients in aqueous food environments (Venugopalan et al., 2021; Islam et al., 2023). In the past few years, the implementation of a self-nanoemulsifying technology for omega-3 PUFA delivery has grown. In a concentrated oil phase, this system blends omega-3 PUFA oil, surfactant, solvents, and additional active ingredients. When dissolved in a water-based solution, it forms unprompted nano-emulsions by thermodynamic energy gain and Gibbs-free energy decrease, producing tiny droplets (less than 200 nm). The self-nanoemulsifying delivery technology improves the oil's oxidation protection and bioavailability while also increasing the product's solubility (Ren et al., 2022).

9.8 Pickering emulsions

Pickering emulsions are created using solid particles (colloidal particles) that attach themselves to the interface between the two emulsion phases. In simpler terms, these solid particles form thick interfacial layers surrounding the droplets, enhancing the stability of Pickering emulsions against coalescence and Ostwald ripening (Peter et al., 2022). To function as effective Pickering stabilizers, colloidal particles must display three key features: (1) intermediate wettability to the oil and aqueous phases for ideal interfacial positioning, (2) moderate surface potential to avoid excessive electrostatic repulsion, and (3) a smaller particle size than the emulsion target to ensure full interfacial coverage (Mwangi et al., 2020). These attributes enable the Pickering colloidal particles to stabilize PUFA through the creation of a robust interfacial layer that provides combined electrostatic barriers, the formation of a 3D percolating network of aggregated particles that limits droplet mobility, and, finally, by inducing a depletion relationship between droplets that enhances stability via restricting their free movement (Yan et al., 2020). Currently, the development of more biocompatible Pickering emulsions is increasingly centered on the use of organic colloidal particles, such as proteins, polysaccharides, and protein–polysaccharide complexes, rather than inorganic particles like silica or titanium dioxide. The organic particles are made from components that are typically considered safe (GRAS, Generally Recognized As Safe.) by the Food and Drug Administration and that are sustainable, plentiful, and cost-effective. The functional properties of these particles can often be customized for use by implementing specific physico-chemical alterations (Tan & Yoon, Cho, et al., 2021).

9.9 Gelled emulsions

They are organized by oil droplets that are emulsified and immobilized within a gel matrix. This is usually achieved by adding thickeners into the main emulsions or by inducing the cross-linking of biopolymers, such as proteins and polysaccharides. These systems enhance the stability of PUFAs by leveraging the advantage of the high viscosity of the gel, which hinders the movement of reactive oxidants. Gelled emulsions serve as effective alternatives to saturated fat by replicating their functional characteristics. Their semisolid structure, produced through a gelled aqueous phase, aids in water retention and allows the encapsulation of bioactive substances, which may further prevent lipid oxidation. (Wang et al., 2020). The mechanical features of the gel are determined by the interactions between the used biopolymers, regulated by their functional groups and conformations. These interactions often lead to an increased elastic modulus (G′). Nonetheless, the effectiveness of such systems hinges on the consistency of the biopolymers used, making careful selection essential to ensure optimal stability and desirable texture (de Carvalho et al.,2025).

9.10 Stabilizers in polyunsaturated fatty acid emulsions

Natural stabilizers such as proteins, polysaccharides, and phospholipids are preferred over synthetic emulsifiers for PUFA delivery due to potential health hazards.

9.11 Proteins

The amphiphilic configuration of proteins is a combination of polar and nonpolar amino acids, leading them to adsorb at oil-water interfaces. Consequently, they contribute to the stabilization of the lipid droplets in emulsions. Due to their larger size, these emulsifiers diffuse more gradually to the interface. Once they achieve the interface, they form a robust viscoelastic film that withstands mechanical stress and offers steric stabilization (Flores-Andrade et al., 2021). Different structures of proteins could provide them with adaptability when they are adsorbed at the oil–water interface of an emulsion. Hence, compact and globular proteins such as β-lactoglobulin generate packed and interconnected interfacial films, while flexible and disordered proteins, namely caseins, produce thicker but less dense interfacial films (Ghelichi et al., 2023). Common milk proteins were applied as food emulsifiers. Cofrades et al. (2020) investigated the performance of sodium caseinate (SC) and whey protein isolate (WPI) as stabilizers for PUFA emulsions. Both proteins were fully adsorbed at oil droplet surfaces, generating protective coatings through spatial and electrostatic repulsion. Yet, SC exceeds WPI in terms of dispersibility due to its disordered and hydrophobic arrangement. This enabled a thicker interfacial layer, enhanced droplet coalescence suppression, and encapsulation success. Padial-Domínguez et al. (2020) showed that hydrolyzed whey protein stabilized omega-3 PUFAs, avoiding modifications in particle size and peroxide values over 10 days of storage, while reducing the formation of unsaturated aldehydes. Conversely, certain studies have concentrated on using plant-derived proteins, including those from peas (Burger & Zhang, 2019), potatoes (García-Moreno et al., 2020), rice (Chen et al., 2020), or winery by-products (Pavlou et al., 2019), to enhance the stability of emulsion-based delivery systems. The use of protein-rich algal extracts as emulsifiers provides an added benefit. According to Silva et al. (2022), emulsions with protein-rich extract from *Arthrospira platensis* as an emulsion proved to possess high emulsifying capability and conserve physical stability for up to 30 days.

9.12 Polysaccharides

These types of emulsifiers typically show potent stability across various pH values, salt levels, and temperatures. However, due to their molecular size, they must be applied in larger quantities to stabilize emulsion-based systems. When polysaccharides are bound at the interface, they produce a thick layer leading to steric repulsion and minor changes in pH and ionic strength, unlike proteins (Teixé-Roig et al., 2023). Polysaccharides with amphiphilic properties proved to be adequate for the stabilization of O/W emulsions individually or in conjunction with other emulsifiers. For instance, Arabic gum has been extensively used due to its ability to lower interfacial tension, generating an emulsion with a particle size of <1 μm. However, it improved flocculation stability across various pH and temperature levels and elevated ionic strength (Flores-Andrade et al., 2021). Polysaccharides derived from *Ulva fasciata* were tested as emulsifiers in β-carotene-fortified emulsions, with particle sizes of 0.8 μm and less than 10% encapsulated component deterioration after 4 days (Shao et al., 2017). Abbasi et al. (2019) have developed a nano-emulsion system formed by protein-sodium alginate to protect the α-linolenic acid during chicken digestion, ensuring targeted delivery to the lower gastrointestinal tract. This boosted omega-3 enrichment in poultry and improved feed efficiency. In another study, the pea protein combined with flaxseed gum was used to stabilize algae oil emulsion, engendering a plant-based DHA delivery system that limits the oxidative rancidity flavors (Sun et al., 2022). Hosseini et al. (2021) designed a chitosan/gelatin bilayer coating for omega-3 PUFA nano-emulsions, boosting their physicochemical stability. This system increased the droplet size, the encapsulation efficacy (from 74% to 81%), and the lipid oxidation.

9.13 Phospholipids and saponins

Phospholipids possess both polar and nonpolar regions within the same molecule, making them amphiphilic configurations able to adhere to oil–water interfaces and stabilize oil droplets. Lecithin is the most used phospholipid-based stabilizer. When it is absorbed, lecithin maintains the emulsion systems via electrostatic repulsion as it delivers a highly negative charge. For example, Gao et al. (2020) reported a low ζ-potential of -70 mV and particle size below 250 nm when soy lecithin was applied at >2% in fractionated coconut oil nano-emulsions. In fact, this emulsifier has been confirmed to be more potent than whey protein or gum Arabic in minimizing interfacial tension, resulting in the smallest particle size when producing O/W nano-emulsions that entrap paprika oleoresin, which was less than 140 nm (Flores-Andrade et al., 2021).

Saponins are gaining attention as a natural substitute for synthetic surfactants. They are composed of a hydrophobic aglycone and a hydrophilic sugar component, which makes them able to offer steric stabilization and form an interfacial layer with robust expansion elasticity. The balance interfacial tension of Quillaja Saponins (QS) can achieve 5.0 mN/m at the interface between medium-chain triglycerides and water. This equilibrium enables QS to exhibit excellent emulsifying features and the ability to create small oil droplets. Nano-emulsions derived from QS can serve as robust carriers for hydrophobic biomolecules, enhancing their dissolution and absorption. Additionally, QS can prevent lipid oxidation in O/W emulsions, which can be utilized to manage flavor retention and release during heating (Xu et al., 2021). Ralla and colleagues explored the emulsifying characteristics of glycyrrhizin acid in O/W emulsions. It has been demonstrated that this emulsion exhibits good stability when subjected to various environmental stresses, such as a broad spectrum of pH levels (5–9), NaCl concentrations (0–200 mM), and high temperatures >60°C (Ralla et al., 2020).

9.14 Encapsulation technologies for polyunsaturated fatty acids

To improve oxidative stability and distribute oils, particularly those that are omega-3-rich, a variety of enhancing techniques have been employed. Preventing deteriorative agents from reaching the bioactive compound is the simplest way to extend the lifespan of oil. Recent technological progress has resulted in the creation of oil encapsulation.

Encapsulation is the process of embedding lipids into a homogeneous or heterogeneous matrix or encapsulating them in a covering. This process can turn liquid oil into tiny capsules that are easier to handle and increase the oil's potential for use in food fortification and nutraceuticals (Banasaz et al., 2020). Researchers are continuously developing and enhancing encapsulation techniques, and studies show that the best encapsulation method for a specific material is influenced by the core's physical and chemical properties as well as the components of the encapsulating shell. This section provides an overview of the typical encapsulation methods and processes illustrated by Fig. 9.4.

9.15 Emulsification

In many processes, emulsification is the initial step, establishing it as a crucial method for encapsulating oils. Emulsion systems are often employed to encapsulate biologically active compounds that are dispersed in water-based solutions. These solutions can be used right away as a liquid emulsion or dried to create a powdered form. Additionally, emulsion droplets can be used as deposition sites during coacervation-based encapsulation or integrated into the product's raw material prior to extrusion. The advantages of encapsulation include reduced production costs and relative ease of preparation. However, because an emulsion loses stability when subjected to severe pH, high solute concentrations, freezing, drying, and heating, functional disadvantages include physical instability and little control over the core release (Homroy et al., 2024). Numerous forms are available for the encapsulation, protection, and controlled release of omega-3 PUFAs, including:

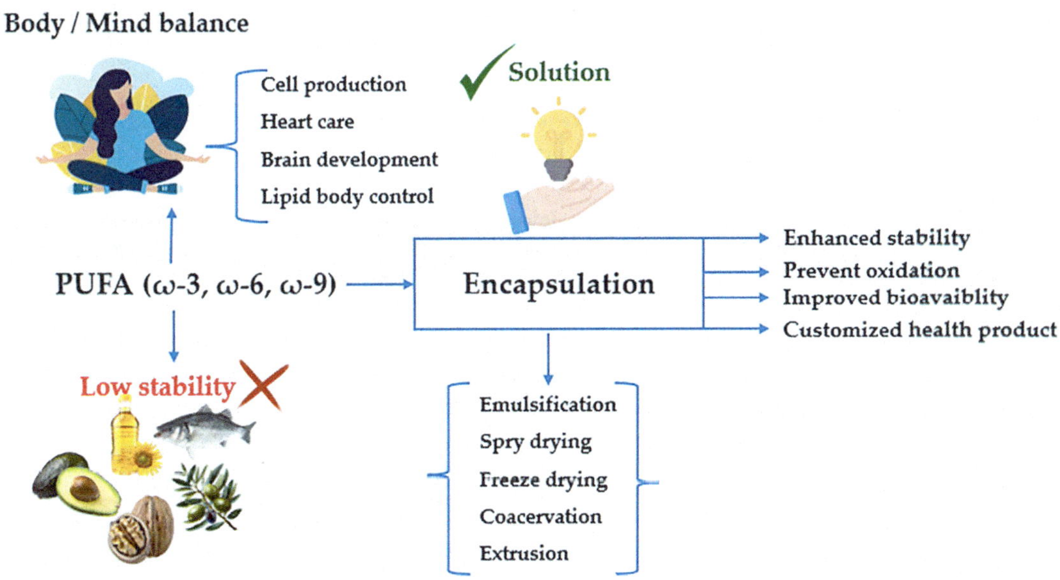

FIGURE 9.4 Amelioration of polyunsaturated fatty acid (*PUFA*)-rich oil stability via encapsulation technologies.

9.16 Liposomes

A liposome is a closed and continuous spherical vesicle made up of one or several phospholipid bilayers. The amphipathic characteristics of phospholipids result in the creation of a spherical bilayer with lipid molecules when they are mixed in a watery environment under certain conditions. Liposomes are beneficial for enclosing lipophilic functional substances. Researchers have developed several techniques to produce liposomes, but the most common method is thin-film hydration, which involves drying organic phospholipids via solvent evaporation and subsequently rehydrating them in an aqueous solution.

Despite this, the technique often results in liposomes that are diverse in shape and size; as a result, it can be combined with microfluidization or sonication to achieve more consistent uniformity in sizes and shapes, which also facilitates the large-scale manufacturing of liposomes (Sarkar & Mackie, 2020).

9.17 Nanoliposomes

One (unilamellar) or multiple (multilamellar) concentric phospholipid bilayers constitute nanoliposomes ($r<100$ nm). They frequently occur by combining physicochemical and mechanical interventions with the hydrophobic effect-driven spontaneous self-assembly of lipid molecules into bilayers. Nanoliposomes could transport hydrophilic and lipophilic phytochemicals, whether individually or in combination. The aqueous polar core can enclose hydrophilic phytochemicals, while the phospholipid bilayers are capable of accommodating hydrophobic (nonpolar tail part) or amphiphilic (interfacial part) phytochemicals. Hydrophilic phytochemicals are generally mixed with the aqueous phase prior to nanoliposome formation, whereas hydrophobic and amphiphilic substances are commonly combined with phospholipids before the formation or added to the complete system later. It has been demonstrated that nanoliposomes can encapsulate and transport phytochemicals, thereby enhancing their stability, regulating their release, and increasing their bioavailability (McClements & Öztürk, 2021).

9.18 Solid lipid nanoparticles and nanostructured lipid carriers

Although the lipid phase of solid lipid nanoparticles (SLNs) and nanostructured lipid carriers (NLCs) is present in fully or partially crystalline states, their structural configuration resembles nanoemulsions. The crystalline nature of these lipid matrices enhances oxidative stability by limiting pro-oxidant diffusion and restricting their contact with encapsulated omega-3 oils. Similar techniques to those used to create emulsions or nanoemulsions can be employed to make SLNs and NLCs; however, homogenization is done past the melting point of the lipid phase. To promote a transition from liquid to solid in the lipid phase, the mixture is then cooled to a temperature below the crystallization point. These systems need to be carefully designed to prevent the buildup or exclusion of the bioactive during droplet crystallization (Venugopalan et al., 2021).

9.19 Hydrogels

Covalent or noncovalent bonds cross-link three-dimensional networks of polymers known as hydrogels, which contain a significant volume of water and withstand breakdown. When hydrophilic groups such as OH, COOH, $CONH_2$, CONH–, and SO_3H expand, they engage with each other to create a gel structure exhibiting substantial mechanical strength. Hydrogels can be utilized as wall materials to shield PUFA from hostile environments such as oxidation, deterioration, or disintegration inside their internal structure. Biopolymeric hydrogels have attracted a lot of interest lately because of their nontoxicity, biodegradability, and biocompatibility. Hydrogels can be classified based on a variety of factors, including their mechanical and structural characteristics (affine or phantom), the type of side groups they contain (neutral or ionic), their physical structure (hydrogen bonded, semicrystalline, amorphous, hydrocolloidal, and super molecular), their preparation method (homo- or copolymer), and their reactivity to stimuli from the physiological environment (ionic strength, pH, electromagnetic radiation, temperature, etc.) (Kwan and Davidov-Pardo, 2018; Jurić et al., 2022).

9.20 Oleo gels

Oleo gels are mainly formed of liquid triglycerides with trace amounts of diglycerides, monoglycerides, fatty acids, and other lipophilic molecules. Some gelators at concentrations from 1% to 10% can be added to solidify their aspect, which crystallizes or interacts with molecules through the hydrogen bonds and van der Waals forces to self-assemble into a 3D network (Li et al., 2022). These forms limit the existence of the FAs while entrapping the oil phase to stimulate the texture of solid fats. Oleo gels have two functional features: firstly, their potential to be used to boost nutritional profiles by substituting fat in food, and secondly employed as delivery systems for the controlled release and enhanced bioavailability of PUFA (Pinto and Martins, 2021).

9.21 Bicelles

Bicelles usually comprise a binary mixture of phospholipids with long and short chains, and they can take on several different shapes. Bicellar nanostructures typically range in diameter from 50 to 500 nm, depending on their form. More recently, designs have emphasized the usage of fatty acids and monoglycerides rather than short-chain phospholipids. The vesicle-like morphology of bicellar nanostructures is helpful for transporting monoglycerides and fatty acids, even though the discoidal aggregate structure is typically linked to bicelles. High monoglyceride fractions can create these structures, and their membrane softening properties can help facilitate mucogenic activities (Tan & Yoon, Cho, et al., 2021).

9.22 Spray drying

Fish oil spray drying involves the following steps: (1) homogenizing an O/W emulsion; (2) mixing the emulsion with wall materials, which can be done before, during, or after homogenization; (3) pumping the emulsion into a hot chamber through a fine nozzle, which creates tiny droplets that dry quickly; and (4) collecting the powder. To increase the dispersibility of the final powders, an extra agglomeration step might occasionally be added. Depending on the use, the type of components and processing conditions employed determine the type of powders that are produced, which must be optimized. Using a variety of wall materials, such as casein, dextrose, maltodextrin, starch, gum arabic, and gelatin, spray drying has been utilized to encapsulate fish oils (Bakry et al., 2016).

9.23 Lyophilization

Another method for turning fluid omega-3 oil compounds into powder is freeze-drying, which involves first freezing the sample to approximately −90 to −40 °C, followed by vacuum dehydration to produce a powder. Freeze-drying is less common in industry than spray drying due to its higher cost, longer turnaround time, and poorer throughput. It does, however, have a few benefits over spray drying that might be useful for applications involving fish oil. Specifically, high temperatures are not required, which lessens the likelihood that the omega-3 oils will oxidize during the microencapsulation process (El-Messery et al., 2020).

9.24 Coaxial electrospray system

Due to the homogeneous size distribution of the particles generated and the maximal maintenance of the core and its bioactivity, this approach exhibits better encapsulation efficiency. In a two-stage electrospray system, the shell solution and core material are concurrently coaxially sprayed into a single nozzle via different feed channels. At the spray nozzle, where the inside oil is held by the outer polymeric solution, a mononuclear encapsulation occurs (Bakry et al., 2016).

9.25 Coacervation

Electrostatic binding between two biopolymers with opposite charges, namely, cationic proteins and anionic polysaccharides, within a specific pH range, is the main mechanism of coacervation. Therefore after mixing the oil droplets with the solution comprising the various biopolymers and going through phase separation, this approach produces oil-holding microgels. Coacervation processes come in two varieties: basic and complex. A single polymer creates the coacervate phase in simple coacervation, which can be precipitated out by adding a nonsolvent, such as ethanol, or by altering the temperature. It can also be salted out by the action of electrolytes. On the other hand, complicated coacervation involves two or more polymers that are oppositely charged. When the medium's pH is lowered below the protein's isoelectric point, the opposite-charged polymers are drawn to one another electrostatically. As a result, the liquid phase and the insoluble coacervate stage separate. As the polymer-dense phase forms around the core droplets and gently cools beneath the gelling temperature, a wall or shell is created. The coacervate shell is heated, dissolved, or cross-linked as needed to strengthen the microcapsules' mechanical and thermal resistance (Homroy et al.,2024).

9.26 Extrusion

To create solidified microcapsules, this technology combines molten wall components with emulsified oil at extreme pressure. The mixture is then forced through a fine nozzle. Although this technique may produce microcapsules on a large scale for commercial use, there are certain drawbacks to using it for fish oil microencapsulation. Specifically, the high temperatures employed during the manufacturing process may encourage the oxidation of fish oil, which entails significant energy and capital expenditures. Centrifugal extrusion, melt-injection, and melt-extrusion are a few extrusion techniques that can be utilized for microencapsulation; these techniques differ in their working principles and the type of microcapsules that are created (Venugopalan et al., 2021). Some examples of encapsulation oil produced through different methods are highlighted in Table 9.1.

9.27 Structured lipids as polyunsaturated fatty acid delivery vehicles

Lipids are vital macronutrients that significantly contribute to physiological functions and overall human health, mainly by providing essential fatty acids. Hence, consuming too much dietary fat is linked to obesity and several metabolic disorders. Following strict low-fat diets can often be difficult for people because of decreased sensory appeal and enjoyment, which often leads to dietary failure and eventual weight regain (Calcaterra et al., 2024). The food science world is buzzing about a breakthrough—fats that pull double duty. These next-generation “smart fats” don't just nourish your body; they might help keep your weight in check. Meet SLs: the custom-designed fats leaving regular oils in the dust when it comes to health benefits. Unlike regular fats, these engineered lipids are easier to digest, contain fewer calories, and have less unhealthy saturated fat. Researchers create SLs by carefully rebuilding natural fat molecules, swapping out different fatty acids to create optimal structures. This molecular tailoring produces fats with better functionality and greater health benefits (Guo et al., 2020).

SLs may be synthesized via different methods, such as chemical, enzymatic, and genetic modification approaches. Among these, the chemical technique remains the most adopted technique at the industrial level due to its low price, operational simplicity, and suitability for scale-up production. Nevertheless, this type presents several drawbacks, namely the lack of reaction specificity, energy requirement, high temperature, and thermal deterioration of substrates and final products. Indeed, the use of heavy chemical processes could lead to the generation of toxic by-products, which pose health risks to consumers. To overcome these challenges, attention has been directed to enzymatic synthesis methods. These biological routes offer various benefits, such as high substrate specificity, milder reaction settings, and decreased harmful compound formation, making them safer. Mu & Porsgaard (2005) have demonstrated that the functional uniqueness of SLs is largely attributed to their specific molecular configuration, which can impact gastric emptying rates and lipid digestion kinetics. Consequently, SLs exhibit distinct physiological benefits that contribute to improved nutritional value

TABLE 9.1 Different encapsulation methods of rich polyunsaturated fatty acid (*PUFA*) oils.

Types of oil	Method	Main results	References
Chia oil	Multilayer emulsion and spray drying	Notable increase in peroxide value (pv) in native oil over a 90-day storage period in comparison to microencapsulated chia oil. After 90 days, the maximum retention of omega3 PUFA was seen in three-layer microcapsules.	Copado et al. (2021)
Fish oil	Nanoemulsion	Improved oxidation stability (lower pv and *p*-anisidine values) in multiple nanoemulsions. As the whey protein isolate concentration increases, the oxidation of fish oil is reduced.	Hwang et al. (2017)
Fish oil	Nanostructured lipid carrier (NLC)	omega-3 oil coencapsulated with α-tocopherol in NLCs exhibited higher oxidative stability than bulk fish oil and NLCs with fish oil alone. NLC encapsulation prevented primary oxidation more than secondary oxidation.	Shahparast et al. (2019)
Krill oil	Nanoemulsions processed by both spray drying and freeze-drying	pv increased over time in all samples but was lower in encapsulates. Those with 2% of krill oil showed the least oxidation. Spray-dried samples exhibited higher pv due to surface oil adsorption and heat exposure.	El-Messery et al. (2020)
Walnut oil	Spry drying	Walnut oil's oxidative stability increased significantly when microencapsulated in 7% 1:1 soy protein-maltodextrin, with 72.2% encapsulation efficiency.	Zhou et al. (2017)
Kilka fish oil	Freeze-drying	Whey powder-sodium caseinate blend effectively stabilizes fish oil against oxidation.	Hosseini et al. (2019)
Algae oil	Emulsion gel	The κ-carrageenan/Tween 80 emulsion gel exhibited reduced lipid oxidation compared to bulk oil following simulated gastrointestinal digestion.	Gayoso et al. (2019)
Sardine oil	Electrospray	Gliadin-pecan husk extract interactions (electrostatic and hydrophobic) enhance fish oil oxidative stability and prolong its shelf-life.	Dórame-Miranda et al. (2021)

and targeted health outcomes. SLs have appeared effective at limiting fat body storage and addressing metabolic disorders, namely fat malabsorption. These features promote the reduction of obesity risk and cardiovascular diseases, while playing an adjuvant function in fetal development and maternal health. Despite these advantages, one of the key challenges associated with SLs is their inherent susceptibility to oxidative deterioration. Although the inclusion of synthetic antioxidants has been used to boost oxidative stability. This strategy frequently conflicts with the principles of clean-label and health-oriented food formulations. For this reason, the development of new food delivery systems customized for SLs is being investigated. These systems aim to protect lipid integrity, prolong shelf life, and amplify the application spectrum of functional fats and oils. Looking ahead, SLs hold considerable potential for incorporation into advanced food technologies involving microencapsulated oils, plastic fats, and structured emulsions, which is in alignment with the high demand for healthy food products. Furthermore, innovative application formats such as aerosolized oils stored in inert gas environments, can provide practical solutions to oxidative instability, emphasizing the broader application of SLs in functional food systems (Lopes et al., 2023). Many studies have focused on the specific nutritional functions of SLs to develop new SLs. In this context, this section highlights recent advances in enzymatic synthesis as a healthy pathway to produce novel SLs, including medium to long-chain triacylglycerols (MLCTs), diacylglycerols (DAGs), triacylglycerols enriched with eicosapentaenoic acid (EPA), and DHA.

9.28 Medium to long-chain triacylglycerol

MLCTs are a novel class of SLs that includes medium-chain fatty acids (MCFAs) (C6–C12) and long-chain fatty acids (LCFAs) (>12) with the same glycerol backbone (Nimbkar et al., 2022). Importantly, MLCTs provide a balance of energy release, efficient digestion, and essential FA supply (Wang et al., 2022). MLTCs are synthesized enzymatically, mainly via lipases-catalyzed reactions involving acidolysis, esterification, and interesterification (Guan et al., 2024). Acidolysis involves the combination of triacylglycerols with free FA, generally with MCFA such as capric, lauric acid, and various vegetable oils such as LCFA. While esterification includes the binding of glycerol to FA produces pure MLCTs. The limitation of this method is the high cost (Kavadia et al., 2018). In contrast, interesterification, an acyl exchange between various triglycerides, is usually selected for its performance and restricted byproduct formation. In more complex systems, a PUFA rich in MLCTs can be synthesized through two enzymatic processes starting with the esterification of the glycerol backbone with PUFA, then acidolysis with MCFA to generate MLM SL with improved nutritional functionality (Lopes et al., 2023).

9.29 Diacylglycerol

It is a specialized lipid constituted by substituting one FA chain on the glycerol backbone with a hydroxyl group. Naturally, it is present in small quantities of oils and fats. DAG can exist in two isomeric forms depending on the position of the hydroxyl group (Arpi et al.,2016). Conversely to triacylglycerol (TAG), DAGs are characterized by their unique structural properties and metabolic benefits. They are associated with lower TAG levels, which reduce body fat storage. Conventionally, DAG is generated using high temperatures. An alternative to work in gentle condition with ensuring selectivity is the enzymatic synthesis (Abd Razak, 2022). Yet, some obstacles are restricting this method, which are the enzyme inhibition caused by the glycerol adsorption, water accumulation, and limited mass transfer between the immiscible glycerol and oil phases. Incorporating organic solvents, ionic liquids, ultrasonic treatment, and specific reactors (to improve substrate interaction) can solve these problems (Lopes et al., 2023).

9.30 Eicosatetraenoic acid and docosahexaenoic acid-enriched triacylglycerol

EPA and DHA are crucial omega-3 PUFA generally present in marine sources, primarily in fish oils, containing about 18% EPA and 12% DHA (Lopes et al., 2023). Research has shown their important roles in fetal development and cardiovascular health due to their antiinflammatory and antithrombotic features (Phang, 2013). Additionally, these FAs have demonstrated promise in sustaining cognitive function and controlling body weight, especially in people with early-stage Alzheimer's disease (Thomas et al., 2015). Demand for highly concentrated EPA and DHA formulations is rising as consumers' understanding of nutrition and health issues increases. Numerous procedures, including physical (low-temperature crystallization), chemical (urea or silver nitrate complexation), and sophisticated ones such as supercritical fluid extraction, can be used to enrich them in oils and fats. To release EPA and DHA in their free acid or ethyl ester forms prior to enrichment, fish oil is usually hydrolyzed or trans-esterified (Lopes et al., 2023).

9.31 Examples of main applications of polyunsaturated fatty acid delivery systems

The different types of PUFA delivery systems allow them to be used across various sectors, including medical treatment, skincare, and enriched functional food (Table 9.2).

9.32 Challenges and/or future perspectives

There are some challenges related to the efficiency and cost-effectiveness of some encapsulation techniques of PUFAs (Hashim et al., 2019). Spray drying is one of the most used techniques for the encapsulation of PUFAs due to its reasonable cost and high production capacity. Challenges regarding its use include the possibility of oxidation of PUFAs due to the high inlet temperatures used in this process (Arab-Tehrany et al., 2012). The contact of oil with air in the drying chamber can also lead to oxidation. Besides, if the moisture level in the drying chamber is high, this can affect the shelf life of the encapsulated PUFAs. In addition, the selection of a coating material that has high water solubility and appropriate viscosity and an effective emulsifier that can stabilize the emulsion before the drying process may be challenging. The quantity of oil that can be loaded into the capsules generally ranges between 20% and 30%, which can be a limitation for the spray drying of PUFAs. These challenges can be overcome in different ways, such as using neutral gas such N_2, dehumidification of the air used for spray drying, using lower inlet temperatures, and a combination of coating materials. Therefore the problems associated with the spray drying process can be solved through appropriate optimization of the product formulation and process conditions (Geranpour et al., 2020). Additionally, freeze-drying, although it can be effective in realizing the oxidative stability of the encapsulated PUFAs, it consumes too much energy and time, is expensive, and has low production capacity at a commercial level. Some techniques are promising in terms of PUFAs

TABLE 9.2 Different application sectors of polyunsaturated fatty acid delivery system.

Application sector	Main results	References
Pharma/medical sector	Docosahexaenoic acid (DHA) emulsions stabilized with egg yolk phospholipid showed swift absorption in neonatal mice, leading to liver metabolism into lysophosphatidylcholine and exhibiting neuroprotective properties.	Kollareth et al.(2020)
	Designed fish oil emulsions with a high DHA/arachidonic acid ratio and low eicosatetraenoic acid (EPA) to lead to the neurodevelopment system in preterm pigs with decreasing EPA-DHA competition.	Molina et al. (2020)
	Topical emulsions of omega-3 (linseed oil), omega-6 (evening primrose oil), and omega-9 (olive oil) significantly accelerate wound healing in rats.	Ishak et al. (2019)
	Pickering emulsions loaded with H9N2 antigens induced a strong humoral and cellular immune response.	Zhang et al. (2023)
Food sector	Development of edible films with ginger oil or curcumin/cinnamon oil nanoemulsions has been demonstrated to prolong the shelf life of chicken fillets.	Li et al. (2020)
	Mutilayer emulsion (whey protein isolate + alginate) significantly boosted the antioxidant activity of curcumin throughout 21 storage days.	Carpenter et al. (2019)
	Multiple emulsions using PGPR and Tween 20 aid in obtaining high stability of β-sitosterol used in functional food and fortified beverages.	Nollet et al. (2018)
	The water-in-oil-in-water double emulsions were efficient for the bioavailability of calcium and vitamin D3 in vitro gastrointestinal models.	Dima and Dima (2020)
Cosmetic sector	*Vellozia squamata* and *Opuntia fcusindica* (L.) Mill hydroglycolic extracts were investigated to create nano-emulsions formulated as antiwrintkle creams.	Ribeiro et al. (2015)
	Liposomes increase the absorption of bioactive ingredients into the skin and offer protection against harmful radiation (UV and blue light), thereby lowering the chances of skin damage.	Bilal and Iqbal (2020)

delivery. However, due to their high cost, their scaling up is challenging. Therefore process optimization is necessary to reduce their cost and to transform their use from lab to large scale (Nejatian et al., 2024).

Another challenge is the fortification of food products with the encapsulated PUFAs. Food properties such as pH, salt content, and composition, and process conditions such as temperature, can affect the stability of emulsions and the integrity of the encapsulated PUFAs. Consequently, this can have a negative impact on the stability and functional properties of PUFAs as well as on the targeted and controlled release of these functional compounds in the food matrix and/or in the human body. The addition of encapsulated PUFAs can change the original physico-chemical and sensory properties of the fortified product itself and reduce its consumer acceptance. For example, encapsulated PUFAs can reduce the water absorption of bread and increase its firmness. In addition, the relatively long shelf life of bakery products makes their fortification with PUFAs more challenging due to the instability of these components and oxidation problems. The fish off-flavor of PUFAs obtained from fish products is another problem facing the addition of these ingredients to some foods such as dairy products. PUFAs obtained from fish may also contain relatively high amounts of toxic compounds, such as mercury and pesticides, due to environmental pollution. Besides, the lack of consumer awareness about the health benefits of PUFAs renders foods enriched with encapsulated PUFAs less attractive to consumers. These problems can be solved using novel, scalable, and cost-effective encapsulation techniques and convenient wall materials to ensure the stability and controlled release of PUFAs and to mask any undesirable flavors prior to fortification, by verifying the levels of toxic compounds in the encapsulated oils, and by increasing consumer awareness about the merits of consuming foods rich in PUFAs. The regulatory standards regarding foods enriched with encapsulated PUFAs also should be followed (Drusch et al., 2012; Hernandez, 2014; Kumar et al., 2024; Patel et al., 2022). Attention should be given to the compatibility between the source of PUFAs and the products to which they are intended to be added. More research should be done by performing sensory analyzes to evaluate the consumer acceptance of foods supplemented with encapsulated PUFAs before their commercialization. In vitro and in vivo studies can be conducted to confirm the bioaccessibility, bioavailability, and health benefits of PUFAs incorporated into food products (Walker et al., 2015; Zhou & Wei, 2023). More studies are needed to assess the efficiency of fortifying foods with encapsulated PUFAs and the possible effects on their physicochemical and sensory properties and stability during storage. Besides, the effect of encapsulation on the bioactivity of PUFAs should be addressed and studied (Nejatian et al., 2024). The incorporation of antioxidants in the oil before its encapsulation can enhance the stability of PUFAs and prevent oxidation during processing and storage (Dias et al., 2017). This can be done using natural low-molecular-weight antioxidant compounds such as plant extracts, phospholipids, and essential oils (Semenova, 2017). Flavor enhancers can also be used to hide any off-flavors caused by the addition of encapsulated PUFAs to foods (Lane & Derbyshire, 2018).

For more sustainable encapsulation of PUFAs, plant proteins can be used as substitutes for animal proteins for the coating of PUFAs. Coencapsulation of PUFAs, such as DHA, with other bioactive compounds, such as antioxidants and probiotics, was found to improve their oxidative stability, digestibility, and bioaccessibility. However, more studies are needed to understand the mechanisms of interaction between PUFAs and such components. Predigestion of PUFAs prior to the encapsulation process is a promising method that can enhance the bioactive properties, the nutritional values, and the digestibility of PUFAs. It can be made using enzymes or fermentation, and it is a good solution for premature infants and people who have gastrointestinal disorders (Jiang et al., 2024).

It is recommended to develop novel emulsifiers that are more efficient in preserving emulsion stability and in protecting PUFAs from oxidation. In addition, further studies should be performed on the emulsion structure design to get better delivery and protection of PUFAs (Wang et al., 2020). Although multiple emulsions, multilayer emulsions, and nanoemulsions are more stable under the stresses of the environment than conventional emulsions, more studies are needed to make their production process less complicated (Vellido-Perez et al., 2021; Chang & Nickerson, 2018).

PUFA-modified SLs represent promising and innovative approaches for the delivery of PUFAs. Yet, further research is needed to make their production process easier and more efficient. Although the production of SLs using chemical methods is relatively cheap, easy to handle, and scale up, it is less specific and less selective, consumes more energy, generates some undesirable side products, and causes thermal damage to reactants and products compared to the enzymatic process (Guo et al., 2020). Enzymatic production of SLs also has limitations that include the complexity of the synthesis process and the challenges related to the production and purification of enzymes. The use of immobilization technology can increase the selectivity of enzymes, giving the possibility to reuse them, and is environmentally friendly and sustainable. However, more studies should be done to improve the performance and selectivity of current enzymes, such as lipases and esterases, using genetic engineering. Technologies such as data science, machine learning, artificial intelligence, and CRISPR/Cas9 can be used to discover new lipases and esterases and to enhance current ones. This can make the production of SLs easier and more cost-effective. Yet, legal, ethical, and safety aspects should be taken into consideration while using these techniques (Hong et al., 2023).

The economic viability and scalability of different delivery systems of PUFAs need to be confirmed before their implementation at a commercial level (Venugopalan et al., 2021). Due to their role in the prevention of various diseases and in promoting physical and mental health, the market demand for PUFAs is continuously increasing. Consequently, PUFAs in different delivery systems are being incorporated in a wider range of food products, such as bakery products, dairy products, beverages, etc. The development of innovative delivery systems will make this fortification more efficient, preserve the original properties of the fortified products, and enhance their consumer acceptance (Kaushik et al., 2015).

Due to the growing demand for PUFAs and PUFAs-fortified foods in the world, conventional sources of PUFAs such as fish oils, are gradually becoming not sufficient to satisfy the market needs for these functional ingredients. Besides, the pollution of seawater has raised the concentration of toxic compounds such as dioxins, heavy metals, organochlorine pesticides, and polychlorinated biphenyls in fish. Thus there is a need to find more sustainable and safer sources of PUFAs (Saini & Keum, 2018). Some vegetable oils and genetically modified plant oilseeds (e.g., *Brassica juncea*, *Arabidopsis thaliana*, and *Camelina sativa*), as well as certain microorganisms, are considered more sustainable sources of PUFAs and represent good alternatives for fish oils. However, growing transgenic plants is limited by some factors such as season, weather, and land availability, as well as public and regulatory concerns about their production. Therefore there is a need to remove these concerns through educating the public about the safety of these plants and by solving regulatory issues. In this context, microorganisms captured more attention due to their ability to produce microbial oils with a profile of fatty acids (including PUFAs) identical to that found in animal and plant sources. Microalgae (e.g., *Crypthecodinium cohnii*) and thraustochytrids are examples of oleaginous microbes that can produce high amounts of PUFAs such as DHA and EPA (Patel et al., 2022; Saini et al., 2021). Various other microbial strains can also be used for PUFAs production. Therefore microorganisms can be used to respond to the increasing demand for PUFAs in the future. However, more studies are needed to improve the performance of these strains through metabolic and genetic engineering and to optimize the extraction of PUFAs from microbial sources (Swetha & Mathanghi, 2024).

9.33 Conclusion

PUFAs are crucial bioactive compounds that play a key role in human health. However, their instability, rapid oxidation, and poor solubility restrict their application and benefits. Hence, new delivery systems such as emulsification, encapsulation, and SLs improve the PUFA protection and controlled release. These advantages allow the effective incorporation of PUFA into functional foods, pharmaceuticals, and cosmetics sectors. Yet, challenges persist in scalability, high cost, and short shelf life of PUFA use. Future research should optimize these approaches for industrial scale while ensuring consumer acceptance and health.

References

Abbasi, F., Samadi, F., Jafari, S. M., Ramezanpour, S., & Shams Shargh, M. (2019). Ultrasound-assisted preparation of flaxseed oil nanoemulsions coated with alginate-whey protein for targeted delivery of omega-3 fatty acids into the lower sections of gastrointestinal tract to enrich broiler meat. *Ultrasonics Sonochemistry, 50*, 208–217. https://doi.org/10.1016/j.ultsonch.2018.09.014, www.elsevier.com/inca/publications/store/5/2/5/4/5/1.

Abd Razak, N. N. B. (2022). Hydrodynamics and kinetics of lipase-catalysed synthesis of diacylglycerols (dag) in batch and continuous flow systems (Doctoral dissertation, Institut National Polytechnique de Toulouse-INPT; Sunway University).

Arab-Tehrany, E., Jacquot, M., Gaiani, C., Imran, M., Desobry, S., & Linder, M. (2012). Beneficial effects and oxidative stability of omega-3 long-chain polyunsaturated fatty acids. *Trends in Food Science & Technology, 25*(1), 24–33. https://doi.org/10.1016/j.tifs.2011.12.002.

Arpi, N., Lubis, Y. M., Supardan, M. D., & Mustapha, W. A. W. (2016). Diacylglycerol-enriched oil production using chemical glycerolysis. *European Journal of Lipid Science & Technology, 118*(12).

Bakry, A. M., Abbas, S., Ali, B., Majeed, H., Abouelwafa, M. Y., Mousa, A., & Liang, L. (2016). Microencapsulation of oils: A comprehensive review of benefits, techniques, and applications. *Comprehensive Reviews in Food Science and Food Safety, 15*(1), 143–182. https://doi.org/10.1111/1541-4337.12179, http://www.interscience.wiley.com/jpages/1541-4337.

Balić, A., Vlašić, D., Žužul, K., Marinović, B., & Bukvić Mokos, Z. (2020). Omega-3 versus omega-6 polyunsaturated fatty acids in the prevention and treatment of inflammatory skin diseases. *International Journal of Molecular Sciences, 21*(3), 741. https://doi.org/10.3390/ijms21030741.

Banasaz, S., Morozova, K., Ferrentino, G., & Scampicchio, M. (2020). Encapsulation of lipid-soluble bioactives by nanoemulsions. *Molecules, 25*(17), 3966. https://doi.org/10.3390/molecules25173966.

Bao, Y., & Pignitter, M. (2023). Mechanisms of lipid oxidation in water-in-oil emulsions and oxidomics-guided discovery of targeted protective approaches. *Comprehensive Reviews in Food Science and Food Safety, 22*(4), 2678–2705.

Bilal, M., & Iqbal, H. M. (2020). New insights on unique features and role of nanostructured materials in cosmetics. *Cosmetics, 7*(2), 24.

Blanco-Llamero, C., Fonseca, J., Durazzo, A., Lucarini, M., Santini, A., Señoráns, F. J., & Souto, E. B. (2022). Nutraceuticals and food-grade lipid nanoparticles: From natural sources to a circular bioeconomy approach. *Foods, 11*(15). https://doi.org/10.3390/foods11152318, www.mdpi.com/journal/foods.

Burger, T. G., & Zhang, Y. (2019). Recent progress in the utilization of pea protein as an emulsifier for food applications. *Trends in Food Science & Technology, 86*, 25–33.

Calcaterra, V., Rossi, V., Magenes, V. C., Baldassarre, P., Grazi, R., Loiodice, M., Fabiano, V., & Zuccotti, G. (2024). Dietary habits, depression and obesity: An intricate relationship to explore in pediatric preventive strategies. *Frontiers in Pediatrics, 12*. https://doi.org/10.3389/fped.2024.1368283, https://www.frontiersin.org/journals/pediatrics.

Carpenter, J., George, S., & Saharan, V. K. (2019). Curcumin encapsulation in multilayer oil-in-water emulsion: Synthesis using ultrasonication and studies on stability and antioxidant and release activities. *Langmuir, 35*(33), 10866–10876.

de Carvalho, M. D., Cavallieri, Â. L. F., & Sato, A. C. K. (2025). Plant proteins in structuring gelled emulsions for saturated fat substitutes: Challenges and opportunities. *Food Research International*, 115753.

Chang, C., & Nickerson, M. T. (2018). Encapsulation of omega 3-6-9 fatty acids-rich oils using protein-based emulsions with spray drying. *Journal of Food Science and Technology, 55*(8), 2850–2861. https://doi.org/10.1007/s13197-018-3257-0, http://www.springerlink.com/content/121580/.

Chen, W., Ju, X., Aluko, R. E., Zou, Y., Wang, Z., Liu, M., & He, R. (2020). Rice bran protein-based nanoemulsion carrier for improving stability and bioavailability of quercetin. *Food Hydrocolloids, 108*, 106042. https://doi.org/10.1016/j.foodhyd.2020.106042.

Cofrades, S., Garcimartín, A., Gómez-Estaca, J., Sánchez-Muniz, F. J., Herranz, B., Macho-González, A., Benedí, J., & Álvarez, M. D. (2020). The effect of emulsifying protein and addition of condensed tannins on n-3 PUFA enriched emulsions for functional foods. *Foods, 9*(11). https://doi.org/10.3390/foods9111589, https://www.mdpi.com/2304-8158/9/11/1589.

Copado, C. N., Julio, L. M., Diehl, B. W. K., Ixtaina, V. Y., & Tomás, M. C. (2021). Multilayer microencapsulation of chia seed oil by spray-drying using electrostatic deposition technology. *LWT, 152*. https://doi.org/10.1016/j.lwt.2021.112206, https://www.journals.elsevier.com/lwt.

Dias, D. R., Botrel, D. A., Fernandes, R. V. D. B., & Borges, S. V. (2017). Encapsulation as a tool for bioprocessing of functional foods. *Current Opinion in Food Science, 13*, 31–37. https://doi.org/10.1016/j.cofs.2017.02.001, http://www.journals.elsevier.com/current-opinion-in-food-science/.

Dima, C., & Dima, S. (2020). Bioaccessibility study of calcium and vitamin D3 co-microencapsulated in water-in-oil-in-water double emulsions. *Food Chemistry, 303*, 125416.

Drusch, S., Regier, M., & Bruhn, M. (2012). Recent advances in the microencapsulation of oils high in polyunsaturated fatty acids. *Novel Technologies in Food Science: Their Impact on Products, Consumer Trends and the Environment*, 1–421. https://doi.org/10.1007/978-1-4419-7880-6.

Du, Q., Zhou, L., Li, M., Lyu, F., Liu, J., & Ding, Y. (2022). Omega-3 polyunsaturated fatty acid encapsulation system: Physical and oxidative stability, and medical applications. *Food Frontiers, 3*(2), 239–255. https://doi.org/10.1002/fft2.134.

Dórame-Miranda, R. F., Gámez-Meza, N., Ovando-Martínez, M., Medina-Juárez, L. A., Cárdenas-López, J. L., Ramírez-Bon, R., Santos-Sauceda, I., Castro-Enríquez, D. D., & Burruel-Ibarra, S. E. (2021). Encapsulation of sardine oil by electrospraying with gliadins and pecan nutshell extracts for its stabilization. *Food and Bioprocess Technology, 14*(3), 457–470. https://doi.org/10.1007/s11947-020-02567-x.

El-Messery, T. M., Altuntas, U., Altin, G., & Özçelik, B. (2020). The effect of spray-drying and freeze-drying on encapsulation efficiency, in vitro bioaccessibility and oxidative stability of krill oil nanoemulsion system. *Food Hydrocolloids, 106*, 105890. https://doi.org/10.1016/j.foodhyd.2020.105890.

Flores-Andrade, E., Allende-Baltazar, Z., Sandoval-González, P. E., Jiménez-Fernández, M., Beristain, C. I., & Pascual-Pineda, L. A. (2021). Carotenoid nanoemulsions stabilized by natural emulsifiers: Whey protein, gum Arabic, and soy lecithin. *Journal of Food Engineering, 290*. https://doi.org/10.1016/j.jfoodeng.2020.110208, http://www.sciencedirect.com/science/journal/02608774.

Gao, W., Jiang, Z., Du, X., Zhang, F., Liu, Y., Bai, X., & Sun, G. (2020). Impact of Surfactants on Nanoemulsions based on fractionated coconut oil: Emulsification stability and in vitro digestion. *Journal of Oleo Science, 69*(3), 227–239. https://doi.org/10.5650/jos.ess19264.

García-Moreno, P. J., Gregersen, S., Nedamani, E. R., Olsen, T. H., Marcatili, P., Overgaard, M. T., Andersen, M. L., Hansen, E. B., & Jacobsen, C. (2020). Identification of emulsifier potato peptides by bioinformatics: Application to omega-3 delivery emulsions and release from potato industry side streams. *Scientific Reports, 10*(1). https://doi.org/10.1038/s41598-019-57229-6, www.nature.com/srep/index.html.

Gasa-Falcon, A., Odriozola-Serrano, I., Oms-Oliu, G., & Martín-Belloso, O. (2020). Nanostructured lipid-based delivery systems as a strategy to increase functionality of bioactive compounds. *Foods, 9*(3), 325. https://doi.org/10.3390/foods9030325.

Gayoso, L., Ansorena, D., & Astiasarán, I. (2019). DHA rich algae oil delivered by O/W or gelled emulsions: Strategies to increase its bioaccessibility. *Journal of the Science of Food and Agriculture, 99*(5), 2251–2258.

Geranpour, M., Assadpour, E., & Jafari, S. M. (2020). Recent advances in the spray drying encapsulation of essential fatty acids and functional oils. *Trends in Food Science and Technology, 102*, 71–90. https://doi.org/10.1016/j.tifs.2020.05.028.

Ghelichi, S., Hajfathalian, M., Yesiltas, B., Sørensen, A. D. M., García-Moreno, P. J., & Jacobsen, C. (2023). Oxidation and oxidative stability in emulsions. *Comprehensive Reviews in Food Science and Food Safety, 22*(3), 1864–1901. https://doi.org/10.1111/1541-4337.13134, http://onlinelibrary.wiley.com/journal/10.1111/(ISSN)1541-4337.

Ghiasi, F., Hashemi, H., Esteghlal, S., & Hosseini, S. M. H. (2024). An updated comprehensive overview of different food applications of W1/O/W2 and O1/W/O2 double emulsions. *Multidisciplinary Foods, 13*(3). https://doi.org/10.3390/foods13030485, www.mdpi.com/journal/foods.

Guan, A., Hou, Y., Yang, R., & Qin, J. (2024). Enzyme engineering for functional lipids synthesis: recent advance and perspective. *Bioresources and Bioprocessing, 11*(1). https://doi.org/10.1186/s40643-023-00723-7.

Guo, Y., Cai, Z., Xie, Y., Ma, A., Zhang, H., Rao, P., & Wang, Q. (2020). Synthesis, physicochemical properties, and health aspects of structured lipids: A review. *Comprehensive Reviews in Food Science and Food Safety, 19*(2), 759–800. https://doi.org/10.1111/1541-4337.12537.

Hashim, N. A., Abdul Mudalip, S. K., Sulaiman, S. Z., & Md Shaarani, S. (2019). Nutritional values and microencapsulation techniques of fish oil from different sources: A mini review. *Materials Today: Proceedings, 42*, 222–228. https://doi.org/10.1016/j.matpr.2020.11.849, https://www.sciencedirect.com/journal/materials-today-proceedings.

Hernandez, E. M. (2014). Issues in fortification and analysis of omega-3 fatty acids in foods. *Lipid Technology, 26*(5), 103–106. https://doi.org/10.1002/lite.201400004, http://www.interscience.wiley.com/jpages/0956-666X.

Homroy, S., Chopra, R., Singh, P. K., Dhiman, A., Chand, M., & Talwar, B. (2024). Role of encapsulation on the bioavailability of omega-3 fatty acids. *Comprehensive Reviews in Food Science and Food Safety, 23*(1), 1–35. https://doi.org/10.1111/1541-4337.13272, http://onlinelibrary.wiley.com/journal/10.1111/(ISSN)1541-4337.

Hong, C. R., Jeon, B. J., Park, K. M., Lee, E. H., Hong, S. C., & Choi, S. J. (2023). An overview of structured lipid in food science: Synthesis methods, applications, and future prospects. *Journal of Chemistry, 2023*. https://doi.org/10.1155/2023/1222373, http://www.hindawi.com/journals/chem/contents/.

Hosseini, H., Ghorbani, M., Jafari, S. M., & Sadeghi Mahoonak, A. (2019). Encapsulation of EPA and DHA concentrate from Kilka fish oil by milk proteins and evaluation of its oxidative stability. *Journal of Food Science and Technology, 56*(1), 59–70. https://doi.org/10.1007/s13197-018-3455-9, http://www.springerlink.com/content/121580/.

Hosseini, S. F., Soofi, M., & Rezaei, M. (2021). Enhanced physicochemical stability of ω-3 PUFAs concentrates-loaded nanoliposomes decorated by chitosan/gelatin blend coatings. *Food Chemistry, 345*, 128865.

Hwang, J. Y., Ha, H. K., Lee, M. R., Kim, J. W., Kim, H. J., & Lee, W. J. (2017). Physicochemical property and oxidative stability of whey protein concentrate multiple nanoemulsion containing fish oil. *Journal of Food Science, 82*(2), 437–444. https://doi.org/10.1111/1750-3841.13591, http://www3.interscience.wiley.com/journal/118509799/issueyear?year=2008.

Ishak, W. M. W., Katas, H., Yuen, N. P., Abdullah, M. A., & Zulfakar, M. H. (2019). Topical application of omega-3-, omega-6-, and omega-9-rich oil emulsions for cutaneous wound healing in rats. *Drug Delivery and Translational Research, 9*(2), 418–433. https://doi.org/10.1007/s13346-018-0522-8, http://www.springer.com/biomed/pharmaceutical+science/journal/13346.

Islam, F., Imran, A., Nosheen, F., Fatima, M., Arshad, M. U., Afzaal, M., Ijaz, N., Noreen, R., Mehta, S., Biswas, S., Rasool, I. F. U., Aslam, M. A., Usman, I., Zahra, S. M., Segueni, N., & Amer Ali, Y. (2023). Functional roles and novel tools for improving-oxidative stability of polyunsaturated fatty acids: A comprehensive review. *Food Science & Nutrition, 11*(6), 2471–2482. https://doi.org/10.1002/fsn3.3272.

Jiang, M., Hu, Z., Huang, Y., Chen, X. D., & Wu, P. (2024). Impact of wall materials and DHA sources on the release, digestion and absorption of DHA microcapsules: Advancements, challenges and future directions. *Food Research International, 191*, 114646. https://doi.org/10.1016/j.foodres.2024.114646.

Jurić, S., Jurić, M., Siddique, M. A. B., & Fathi, M. (2022). Vegetable oils rich in polyunsaturated fatty acids: Nanoencapsulation methods and stability enhancement. *Food Reviews International, 38*(1), 32–69. https://doi.org/10.1080/87559129.2020.1717524, www.tandf.co.uk/journals/titles/87559129.asp.

Kapoor, B., Kapoor, D., Gautam, S., Singh, R., & Bhardwaj, S. (2021). Dietary polyunsaturated fatty acids (PUFAs): Uses and potential health benefits. *Current Nutrition Reports, 10*(3), 232–242. https://doi.org/10.1007/s13668-021-00363-3.

Kaushik, P., Dowling, K., Barrow, C. J., & Adhikari, B. (2015). Microencapsulation of omega-3 fatty acids: A review of microencapsulation and characterization methods. *Journal of Functional Foods, 19*, 868–881. https://doi.org/10.1016/j.jff.2014.06.029, http://www.elsevier.com/wps/find/journaldescription.cws_home/717426/description#description.

Kavadia, M. R., Yadav, M. G., Odaneth, A. A., & Lali, A. M. (2018). Synthesis of designer triglycerides by enzymatic acidolysis. *Biotechnology Reports, 18*. https://doi.org/10.1016/j.btre.2018.e00246, http://www.journals.elsevier.com/biotechnology-reports/.

Kollareth, D. J. M., Deckelbaum, R. J., Liu, Z., Ramakrishnan, R., Jouvene, C., Serhan, C. N., & Zirpoli, H. (2020). Acute injection of a DHA triglyceride emulsion after hypoxic-ischemic brain injury in mice increases both DHA and EPA levels in blood and brain. *Prostaglandins, Leukotrienes, and Essential Fatty Acids, 162*, 102176.

Kumar, A., Singh, U., Jaiswal, S. G., Dave, J., Wei, S., & Hailu, G. G. (2024). Recent trends in the encapsulation of functional lipids: Comprehensive review. *Sustainable Food Technology, 2*(6), 1610–1630. https://doi.org/10.1039/d4fb00205a, https://www.rsc.org/journals-books-databases/about-journals/sustainable-food-technology/.

Kwan, A., & Davidov-Pardo, G. (2018). Controlled release of flavor oil nanoemulsions encapsulated in filled soluble hydrogels. *Food Chemistry, 250*, 46–53.

Lampi, A.-M., Yang, Z., Mustonen, O., & Piironen, V. (2020). Potential of faba bean lipase and lipoxygenase to promote formation of volatile lipid oxidation products in food models. *Food Chemistry, 311*, 125982. https://doi.org/10.1016/j.foodchem.2019.125982.

Lane, K. E., & Derbyshire, E. J. (2018). Omega-3 fatty acids – A review of existing and innovative delivery methods. *Critical Reviews in Food Science and Nutrition, 58*(1), 62–69. https://doi.org/10.1080/10408398.2014.994699.

Leister, N., & Karbstein, H. P. (2020). Evaluating the stability of double emulsions—A review of the measurement techniques for the systematic investigation of instability mechanisms. *Colloids and Interfaces, 4*(1), 8.

Li, L., Liu, G., Bogojevic, O., Pedersen, J. N., & Guo, Z. (2022). Edible oleogels as solid fat alternatives: Composition and oleogelation mechanism implications. *Comprehensive Reviews in Food Science and Food Safety, 21*(3), 2077–2104. https://doi.org/10.1111/1541-4337.12928, http://onlinelibrary.wiley.com/journal/10.1111/(ISSN)1541-4337.

Li, M., McClements, D. J., Liu, X., & Liu, F. (2020). Design principles of oil-in-water emulsions with functionalized interfaces: Mixed, multilayer, and covalent complex structures. *Comprehensive Reviews in Food Science and Food Safety, 19*(6), 3159–3190. https://doi.org/10.1111/1541-4337.12622, http://onlinelibrary.wiley.com/journal/10.1111/(ISSN)1541-4337.

Lopes, P. A., Alfaia, C. M., Pestana, J. M., & Prates, J. A. M. (2023). Structured lipids engineering for health: Novel formulations enriched in n-3 long-chain polyunsaturated fatty acids with potential nutritional benefits. *Metabolites, 13*(10), 22181989. https://doi.org/10.3390/metabo13101060, http://www.mdpi.com/journal/metabolites.

McClements, D. J., & Öztürk, B. (2021). Utilization of nanotechnology to improve the application and bioavailability of phytochemicals derived from waste streams. *Journal of Agricultural and Food Chemistry, 70*(23), 6884–6900.

Mititelu, M., Lupuliasa, D., Neacşu, S. M., Olteanu, G., Busnatu, Ş. S., Mihai, A., & Scafa-Udrişte, A. (2024). Polyunsaturated fatty acids and human health: A key to modern nutritional balance in association with polyphenolic compounds from food sources. *Foods, 14*(1), 46.

Molina, T. L., Stoll, B., Mohammad, M., Mohila, C. A., Call, L., Cui, L., Guthrie, G., Kunichoff, D., Lin, S., Welch-Jernigan, R., Nielsen, J., Premkumar, M., Robinson, J., Smith, V., Teets, H., Obelitz-Ryom, K., Hagan, J., Cruz, S., Lau, P., ... Burrin, D. (2020). New generation lipid emulsions increase brain DHA and improve body composition, but not short-term neurodevelopment in parenterally-fed preterm piglets. *Brain, Behavior, and Immunity, 85*, 46–56. https://doi.org/10.1016/j.bbi.2019.04.031, http://www.elsevier.com/inca/publications/store/6/2/2/8/0/0/index.htt.

Mu, H., & Porsgaard, T. (2005). The metabolism of structured triacylglycerols. *Progress in Lipid Research, 44*(6), 430–448.

Mwangi, W. W., Lim, H. P., Low, L. E., Tey, B. T., & Chan, E. S. (2020). Food-grade pickering emulsions for encapsulation and delivery of bioactives. *Trends in Food Science and Technology, 100*, 320–332. https://doi.org/10.1016/j.tifs.2020.04.020, http://www.elsevier.com/wps/find/journaldescription.cws_home/601278/description#description.

Nejatian, M., Ghandehari Yazdi, A. P., Fattahi, R., Saberian, H., Bazsefidpar, N., Assadpour, E., & Jafari, S. M. (2024). Improving the storage and oxidative stability of essential fatty acids by different encapsulation methods; a review. *International Journal of Biological Macromolecules, 260*. https://doi.org/10.1016/j.ijbiomac.2024.129548, https://www.sciencedirect.com/science/journal/01418130.

Nimbkar, S., Leena, M. M., Moses, J. A., & Anandharamakrishnan, C. (2022). Medium chain triglycerides (MCT): State-of-the-art on chemistry, synthesis, health benefits and applications in food industry. *Comprehensive Reviews in Food Science and Food Safety, 21*(2), 843–867. https://doi.org/10.1111/1541-4337.12926, http://onlinelibrary.wiley.com/journal/10.1111/(ISSN)1541-4337.

Nollet, M., Laurichesse, E., Besse, S., Soubabère, O., & Schmitt, V. (2018). Determination of formulation conditions allowing double emulsions stabilized by PGPR and sodium caseinate to be used as capsules. *Langmuir, 34*(8), 2823–2833. https://doi.org/10.1021/acs.langmuir.7b04085.

Padial-Domínguez, M., Espejo-Carpio, F. J., García-Moreno, P. J., Jacobsen, C., & Guadix, E. M. (2020). Protein derived emulsifiers with antioxidant activity for stabilization of omega-3 emulsions. *Food Chemistry, 329*. https://doi.org/10.1016/j.foodchem.2020.127148, www.elsevier.com/locate/foodchem.

Patel, A., Desai, S. S., Mane, V. K., Enman, J., Rova, U., Christakopoulos, P., & Matsakas, L. (2022). Futuristic food fortification with a balanced ratio of dietary ω-3/ω-6 omega fatty acids for the prevention of lifestyle diseases. *Trends in Food Science and Technology, 120*, 140–153. https://doi.org/10.1016/j.tifs.2022.01.006, http://www.elsevier.com/wps/find/journaldescription.cws_home/601278/description#description.

Pavlou, A., Panayiotou, C., Kalogianni, E. P., Georgiou, D., & Ritzoulis, C. (2019). Fractionation of a hydrocolloid emulsifier reclaimed from winery waste. *Food Chemistry, 301*, 125259. https://doi.org/10.1016/j.foodchem.2019.125259.

Peter, M. J., Lalithapriya, U., Venkatachalapathy, R., & Sukumar, M. (2022). Characterization of an effective drug carrier system for improved oxidative and thermal stability of essential fatty acids: a review. *International Journal of Food Properties, 25*(1), 1753–1772. https://doi.org/10.1080/10942912.2022.2105352.

Phang, M. (2013). Differential effects of long chain omega-3 polyunsaturated fatty acids on platelet aggregation and hemostatic variables in healthy male versus female subjects (Doctoral dissertation, University of Newcastle).

Pinto, T. C., Martins, A. J., Pastrana, L., Pereira, M. C., & Cerqueira, M. A. (2021). Oleogel-based systems for the delivery of bioactive compounds in foods. *Gels, 7*(3). https://doi.org/10.3390/gels7030086, https://www.mdpi.com/journal/gels.

Ralla, T., Salminen, H., Braun, K., Edelmann, M., Dawid, C., Hofmann, T., & Weiss, J. (2020). Investigations into the structure-function relationship of the naturally-derived surfactant glycyrrhizin: Emulsion stability. *Food Biophysics, 15*(3), 288–296. https://doi.org/10.1007/s11483-020-09624-0.

Ren, X., Liu, Y., Fan, C., Hong, H., Wu, W., Zhang, W., & Wang, Y. (2022). Production, processing, and protection of microalgal n-3 PUFA-. *Foods Rich Oil, 11*(9), 1215. https://doi.org/10.3390/foods11091215.

Ribeiro, R. C. D. A., Barreto, S. M. A. G., Ostrosky, E. A., Rocha-Filho, P. A. D., Veríssimo, L. M., & Ferrari, M. (2015). Production and characterization of cosmetic nanoemulsions containing **Opuntia ficus-indica** (L.) Mill extract as moisturizing agent. *Molecules, 20*(2), 2492–2509.

Saini, R. K., & Keum, Y. S. (2018). Omega-3 and omega-6 polyunsaturated fatty acids: Dietary sources, metabolism, and significance—A review. *Life Sciences, 203*, 255–267. https://doi.org/10.1016/j.lfs.2018.04.049, www.elsevier.com/locate/lifescie.

Saini, R. K., Prasad, P., Sreedhar, R. V., Naidu, K. A., Shang, X., & Keum, Y. S. (2021). Omega−3 polyunsaturated fatty acids (PUFAs): Emerging plant and microbial sources, oxidative stability, bioavailability, and health benefits—A review. *Antioxidants, 10*(10). https://doi.org/10.3390/antiox10101627, https://www.mdpi.com/2076-3921/10/10/1627/pdf.

Sarkar, A., & Mackie, A. R. (2020). Engineering oral delivery of hydrophobic bioactives in real-world scenarios. *Current Opinion in Colloid & Interface Science, 48*, 40–52.

Semenova, M. (2017). Advances in molecular design of biopolymer-based delivery micro/nanovehicles for essential fatty acids. *Food Hydrocolloids, 68*, 114–121. https://doi.org/10.1016/j.foodhyd.2016.09.019.

Shahparast, Y., Eskandani, M., Rajaei, A., & Khosroushahi, A. Y. (2019). Preparation, physicochemical characterization and oxidative stability of omega-3 fish oil/α-tocopherol-co-loaded nanostructured lipidic carriers. *Advanced Pharmaceutical Bulletin, 9*(3), 393–400. https://doi.org/10.15171/apb.2019.046, http://apb.tbzmed.ac.ir/.

Shao, P., Qiu, Q., Xiao, J., Zhu, Y., & Sun, P. (2017). Chemical Stability and in vitro release properties of β-carotene in emulsions stabilized by Ulva fasciata polysaccharide. *International Journal of Biological Macromolecules, 102*, 225–231. https://doi.org/10.1016/j.ijbiomac.2017.03.186.

Silva, S. C., Almeida, T., Colucci, G., Santamaria-Echart, A., Manrique, Y. A., Dias, M. M., Barros, L., Fernandes, Â., Colla, E., & Barreiro, M. F. (2022). Spirulina (*Arthrospira platensis*) protein-rich extract as a natural emulsifier for oil-in-water emulsions: Optimization through a sequential experimental design strategy. *Colloids and Surfaces A: Physicochemical and Engineering Aspects, 648*. https://doi.org/10.1016/j.colsurfa.2022.129264, www.elsevier.com/locate/colsurfa.

Sun, M., Li, X., McClements, D. J., Xiao, M., Chen, H., Zhou, Q., Xu, S., Chen, Y., & Deng, Q. (2022). Reducing off-flavors in plant-based omega-3 oil emulsions using interfacial engineering: Coating algae oil droplets with pea protein/flaxseed gum. *Food Hydrocolloids, 122*, 107069. https://doi.org/10.1016/j.foodhyd.2021.107069.

Swetha, N., & Mathanghi, S. K. (2024). Towards sustainable omega-3 fatty acids production – A comprehensive review on extraction methods, oxidative stability and bio-availability enhancement. *Food Chemistry Advances, 4*, 100603. https://doi.org/10.1016/j.focha.2023.100603.

Tan, J. Y. B., Yoon, B. K., Cho, N. J., Lovrić, J., Jug, M., & Jackman, J. A. (2021). Lipid nanoparticle technology for delivering biologically active fatty acids and monoglycerides. *International Journal of Molecular Sciences, 22*(18). https://doi.org/10.3390/ijms22189664, https://www.mdpi.com/1422-0067/22/18/9664/pdf.

Teixé-Roig, J., Oms-Oliu, G., Odriozola-Serrano, I., & Martín-Belloso, O. (2023). Emulsion-based delivery systems to enhance the functionality of bioactive compounds: Towards the use of ingredients from natural, sustainable sources. *Foods, 12*(7), 1502. https://doi.org/10.3390/foods12071502.

Thomas, J., Thomas, C. J., Radcliffe, J., & Itsiopoulos, C. (2015). Omega-3 fatty acids in early prevention of inflammatory neurodegenerative disease: A focus on Alzheimer's disease. *BioMed Research International, 2015*(1), 172801.

Vellido-Perez, J. A., Ochando-Pulido, J. M., Brito-de la Fuente, E., & Martinez-Ferez, A. (2021). Novel emulsions–based technological approaches for the protection of omega–3 polyunsaturated fatty acids against oxidation processes – A comprehensive review. *Food Structure, 27*, 100175. https://doi.org/10.1016/j.foostr.2021.100175.

Venugopalan, V. K., Gopakumar, L. R., Kumaran, A. K., Chatterjee, N. S., Soman, V., Peeralil, S., Mathew, S., McClements, D. J., & Nagarajarao, R. C. (2021). Encapsulation and protection of omega-3-rich fish oils using food-grade delivery systems. *Foods, 10*(7). https://doi.org/10.3390/foods10071566, https://www.mdpi.com/2304-8158/10/7/1566/pdf.

Walker, R., Decker, E. A., & McClements, D. J. (2015). Development of food-grade nanoemulsions and emulsions for delivery of omega-3 fatty acids: Opportunities and obstacles in the food industry. *Food & Function, 6*(1), 42–55. https://doi.org/10.1039/c4fo00723a.

Wang, C., Sun, C., Lu, W., Gul, K., Mata, A., & Fang, Y. (2020). Emulsion structure design for improving the oxidative stability of polyunsaturated fatty acids. *Comprehensive Reviews in Food Science and Food Safety, 19*(6), 2955–2971. https://doi.org/10.1111/1541-4337.12621.

Wang, Y., Zhang, T., Liu, R., Chang, M., Wei, W., Jin, Q., & Wang, X. (2022). Reviews of medium-and long-chain triglyceride with respect to nutritional benefits and digestion and absorption behavior. *Food Research International, 155*, 111058.

Xu, M., Wan, Z., & Yang, X. (2021). Recent advances and applications of plant-based bioactive saponins in colloidal multiphase food systems. *Molecules, 26*(19), 6075.

Yan, X., Ma, C., Cui, F., McClements, D. J., Liu, X., & Liu, F. (2020). Protein-stabilized pickering emulsions: Formation, stability, properties, and applications in foods. *Trends in Food Science and Technology, 103*, 293–303. https://doi.org/10.1016/j.tifs.2020.07.005, http://www.elsevier.com/wps/find/journaldescription.cws_home/601278/description#description.

Yesiltas, B., Torkkeli, M., Almásy, L., Dudás, Z., Wacha, A. F., Dalgliesh, R., García-Moreno, P. J., Sørensen, A. D. M., Jacobsen, C., & Knaapila, M. (2019). Interfacial structure of 70% fish oil-in-water emulsions stabilized with combinations of sodium caseinate and phosphatidylcholine. *Journal of Colloid and Interface Science, 554*, 183–190. https://doi.org/10.1016/j.jcis.2019.06.103, http://www.elsevier.com/inca/publications/store/6/2/2/8/6/1/index.htt.

Zhang, Y., Zhu, T., Xu, S., Gu, P., Cai, G., Peng, S., Liu, Z., Yang, Y., Hu, Y., Liu, J., & Wang, D. (2023). Cationic Nanoparticle-Stabilized Vaccine Delivery System for the H9N2 Vaccine to Promote Immune Response in Chickens. *Molecular pharmaceutics, 20*(3), 1613–1623. https://doi.org/10.1021/acs.molpharmaceut.2c00805.

Zhou, D., Pan, Y., Ye, J., Jia, J., Ma, J., & Ge, F. (2017). Preparation of walnut oil microcapsules employing soybean protein isolate and maltodextrin with enhanced oxidation stability of walnut oil. *LWT - Food Science and Technology, 83*, 292–297. https://doi.org/10.1016/j.lwt.2017.05.029.

Zhou, Q., & Wei, Z. (2023). Food-grade systems for delivery of DHA and EPA: Opportunities, fabrication, characterization and future perspectives. *Critical Reviews in Food Science and Nutrition, 63*(15), 2348–2365. https://doi.org/10.1080/10408398.2021.1974337.

Section III

Health and nutritional benefits

Chapter 10

Nano and microencapsulation of polyunsaturated fatty acids for enhanced stability and bioavailability

Tafadzwa Kaseke[1,2], Sook Chin Chew[3,4], Trust Mukudzeyi Pfukwa[1,2], Faith Seke[1,2], and Olaniyi Amos Fawole[1,2]

[1]*Department of Botany and Plant Biotechnology, South African Chair in Sustainable Postharvest and Agroprocessing Research, University of Johannesburg, Johannesburg, South Africa,* [2]*Postharvest and Agroprocessing Research Centre, Department of Botany and Plant Biotechnology, University of Johannesburg, Johannesburg, South Africa,* [3]*China-ASEAN College of Marine Sciences, Xiamen University Malaysia, Sepang, Selangor, Malaysia,* [4]*Centre of Excellence for Sustainable Technologies for Agricultural Advancement and a Zero-Waste Economy (STARGAZE), Xiamen University Malaysia, Sepang, Selangor, Malaysia*

10.1 Introduction

Polyunsaturated fatty acids (PUFAs) are important fats primarily obtained from dietary sources. Common sources of PUFAs include oil from fish, nuts, and seeds from crops such as canola, corn, soybean, and sunflower, as well as fruits. The most common PUFAs are linoleic acid (ω-6, ω-6) and α-linolenic acid ([ALA], ω-3, ω-3), essential fatty acids (FAs) that the human body cannot synthesize and must be obtained from the diet (Balić et al., 2020). Docosahexaenoic acid (DHA) and eicosapentaenoic acid (EPA) are also vital PUFAs, though they can be synthesized by the human body and are not considered strictly essential (Koop et al., 2022). These FAs play essential roles in various bodily functions and overall health. PUFAs are known to provide protection against various diseases, including osteoarthritis, cancer, and autoimmune disorders. In addition, they can also help reduce low-density lipoprotein cholesterol levels, potentially reducing the risk of heart disease and stroke (Fawole et al., 2021; Mititelu et al., 2024).

PUFAs' health benefits are compromised by their instability under conditions such as oxygen, humidity, light, enzymes, and heat (Kaseke et al., 2021; Saini et al., 2021). The oxidation and degradation of PUFAs can further negatively affect the flavor, taste, color, texture, and potentially the safety of foods, decreasing their marketing quality and shelf-life (Tao, 2015). Additionally, the instability and degradation of PUFAs under the highlighted conditions compromise their bioavailability (Koop et al., 2022). Encapsulation is a common method used to protect PUFAs by providing a coating that enhances their oxidative stability, thermostability, shelf-life, and bioavailability (Nejatian et al., 2024). It can also protect the core material from developing undesirable properties, improving its acceptability and functionality. Encapsulation can be classified based on particle size, with microencapsulation ranging from 1–1000 μm and nanoencapsulation varying from 1–1000 nm (Koop et al., 2022). The size of particles influences the selection of the encapsulation method, the release mechanisms, and the application of the encapsulated material. For instance, nanoencapsulation utilizes very small particles and offers increased bioavailability or targeted delivery (Nejatian et al., 2024). The process of encapsulating PUFAs uses biopolymers, such as proteins and polysaccharides, to prepare an emulsion. This typically includes preparing an aqueous solution of polymers and mixing it with a hydrophobic phase (Kaseke et al., 2024).

Various techniques are employed to produce different types of capsules, depending on the desired product and function. Microencapsulation methods include physical methods such as spray-drying (SD) and freeze-drying (FD), which involve creating a protective shell around a core material. Physicochemical methods, including complex coacervation and ionic gelation, rely on changes in physical properties and interactions between materials (Ozkan et al., 2019). Chemical methods, such as interfacial polymerization, utilize chemical reactions to form the capsule wall. The choice of an encapsulation technique depends on the core material, desired capsule properties such as size, release profile, and stability,

Omega-3 and Omega-6 Polyunsaturated Fatty Acids in Food Systems. DOI: https://doi.org/10.1016/B978-0-443-43810-3.00007-5

and application. Each technique offers distinct advantages and is associated with certain limitations impacting its adoption and application (Kaseke et al., 2024). Nanoencapsulation encompasses various techniques that enclose the core material at the nanoscale, providing protection and controlled release. Common methods include nanoemulsions, which are either oil-in-water (O/W) or water-in-oil (W/O) configurations; nanoliposomes that use lipid bilayers; nanocapsules, characterized by a core-shell structure; solid-lipid nanoparticles (SLN), consisting of solid lipids; and lipid-based nanostructured carriers (Pateiro et al., 2021; Viegas et al., 2023). These diverse characteristics of nanocapsules provide distinct solutions for application in different systems such as drug delivery, cosmetics, and food science, among others.

Encapsulation has become increasingly prevalent in recent years to investigate its impact on the stability, bioavailability, and, consequently, the storage, shelf-life, and utilization of PUFAs by the human body (Kaseke et al., 2024). Therefore this chapter discusses various nano- and microencapsulation techniques for PUFAs, emphasizing how these techniques, along with biopolymers, enhance PUFAs stability, bioavailability, and functionality in various systems. It also highlights the various factors influencing the stability and bioavailability of PUFAs and presents the future possibilities for PUFAs encapsulation.

10.2 Sources and health benefits of polyunsaturated fatty acids

Vegetable oils, marine oils, and essential oils are excellent sources of PUFAs, especially the omega-3 and omega-6 FAs (Bakry et al., 2016). Vegetable oils high in PUFAs are derived from various sources. These include field crops such as sunflower, soybean, and rapeseed; herbal plants such as chia and linseed; nuts such as cashews, macadamia, pecans, pistachios, walnuts, and hazelnuts; and fruit seeds (Fig. 10.1). The omega-3 and omega-6 FAs offer crucial health advantages, including the potential to prevent cardiovascular and nervous system disorders, as well as reduce inflammation. Research also indicates their role in possibly lowering the risk of certain cancers, such as colorectal, breast, and prostate cancers (Fig. 10.1). A balanced ratio of omega-3 to omega-6 FAs is considered essential for maximizing these benefits, with studies suggesting lower omega-6/omega-3 ratios can be beneficial. Regular intake of omega-3 is linked to lowering the risk of cardiovascular disease and reducing inflammation (Kapoor et al., 2021). Apart from this, omega-3 and omega-6 FAs possess strong antiinflammatory and antioxidative properties, linked to improved health, especially in individuals who regularly exercise because of the enhanced generation of reactive oxygen (Bakry et al., 2016). Based on these health advantages, guidelines on omega-3 and omega-6 FAs dietary supplementation have been developed to promote and control their consumption (Balić et al., 2020).

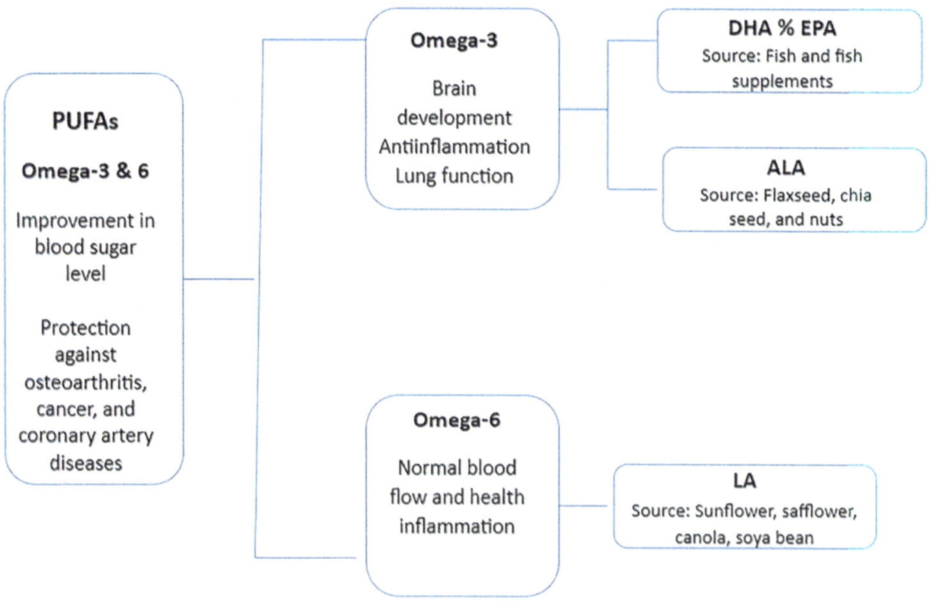

FIGURE 10.1 A summary of the sources, types of polyunsaturated fatty acids (PUFAs), and their biological functions. DHA: docosahexaenoic acid, LA: linoleic acid, and ALA: α-linolenic acid.

10.3 Factors affecting the stability of polyunsaturated fatty acids

The chemical structure of PUFAs, characterized by double bonds, renders them susceptible to oxidative modification by various agents such as oxygen, pH changes, light, metals, and high temperature.

10.3.1 Chemical structure

The stability of PUFAs has a strong negative correlation to the number of multiple bonds they contain (Araujo et al., 2018). Monounsaturated FAs, including oleic acid, are more stable than omega-3 or omega-6 PUFA, such as ALA and arachidonic acid, respectively (Žanetić et al., 2012). Furthermore, the *cis* or *trans* configuration of the double bond influences their susceptibility to oxidation, with the *trans* configuration being more stable compared to the *cis* (Hoekman et al., 2012). The double bonds in PUFAs readily react with oxygen upon exposure, leading to the formation of free radicals. Unmitigated exposure of PUFAs to oxygen promotes the propagation of oxidative reactions, a process called auto-oxidation, that may cause rancidity in food due to the production of off-flavors and unpalatable odors (Geng et al., 2023; Mukwevho et al., 2025).

10.3.2 Light

Exposure to light induces oxidative degradation of PUFAs. In photooxidation, natural sensitizers absorb light energy and transition into an excited state. Natural photosensitizers include compounds such as chlorophyll, curcumin, riboflavin, anthraquinones, and some alkaloids, such as berberine (Kubrak et al., 2022). The collision of excited state photosensitiser and oxygen molecules it energizes them, forming highly reactive oxygen species (ROS) such as singlet oxygen radicals. Singlet oxygen radicals readily react with PUFAs, double bonds, forming lipid hydroperoxides (Bacellar & Baptista, 2019). Minimizing PUFA light exposure, therefore limits the tendency towards photooxidative reactions.

10.3.3 Metal ions

The formation of ROS is also accelerated when PUFAs are contaminated with transition metal ions, including cobalt (Co^{2+}), iron (Fe^{3+}), manganese (Mn^{2+}), and copper (Cu^{2+}). These cations abstract electrons from the double bonds, generating a fatty acyl radical that in turn reacts with oxygen to form lipid hydroperoxides (Repetto et al., 2012). The reaction is further propagated as the lipid hydroperoxides undergo metal cation-catalyzed decomposition, yielding peroxyl radicals that extract hydrogen atoms from other PUFAs (Repetto et al., 2012).

10.3.4 Temperature

Temperature also influences PUFAs stability, with higher temperatures promoting faster degradation compared to lower temperatures (Nagy et al., 2024). The tendency for thermal-induced degradation also increases with the level of unsaturation (Grootveld et al., 2021). Thermal treatment of oils rich in PUFAs leads to peroxidation and formation of lipid oxidation products with cytotoxic and mutagenic potential (Mukwevho et al., 2024; Zhuang et al., 2022). Meanwhile, lower processing and storage temperatures significantly mitigate the degradation of PUFAs-containing products. High temperature promotes higher rates of ROS formation, which prematurely depletes the antioxidant capacity of the system (Réblová, 2012). In addition, it promotes degradation of the antioxidant molecules, which in turn impairs the capacity of the system to mitigate ROS accumulation.

10.3.5 pH

Regarding pH, a lower pH facilitates easier electron donation because in an acidic environment, deprotonation of the antioxidant molecule lowers the ionization potential of the molecule, thereby increasing its radical scavenging capacity (Lemańska et al., 2001). Meanwhile, at higher pH levels, the antioxidant activity is reduced, coupled with an increased tendency towards pro-oxidant activity (Bayliak et al., 2016). The change in pH also forces a change in antioxidant mechanism, where electron donation, rather than hydrogen donation, becomes the main antioxidant mechanism at physiological as well as lower pH environments (Lemańska et al., 2001).

10.3.6 Antioxidants

Exogenous antioxidant compounds act as the primary mechanism for increasing the stability of high PUFA-containing oils during storage and in applications (Yehye et al., 2015). Synthetic exogenous antioxidants such as butylated hydroxyanisole, butylated hydroxytoluene, tert-butylhydroquinone, and propyl gallate have been extensively applied in the food and feed industry (Yehye et al., 2015). However, negative consumer sentiments towards synthetic antioxidants continue to grow due to their potential to cause allergies and cancers (Cömert & Gökmen, 2017). As such, there is increased interest in using plant-derived antioxidants, including carotenoids, vitamin E, vitamin C, and polyphenols, to mitigate PUFAs oxidation.

Antioxidant activities occur via several pathways, including the direct scavenging of ROS, where the antioxidant molecule neutralizes the ROS by donating an electron or a hydrogen atom (Santos-Sánchez et al., 2019). Antioxidants can also have chain-breaking activity, where they disrupt the propagation of radical chain reaction via stabilization of peroxyl radicals formed in the initial oxidative reaction (Grosshagauer et al., 2019). Furthermore, antioxidants also sequester metal cations that catalyze ROS production, thereby slowing down the rate of deleterious reactions (Santos-Sánchez et al., 2019; Yehye et al., 2015). The synergistic activities of antioxidants also act beneficially in systems where antioxidants can regenerate the antioxidant capacity of another antioxidant molecule by reducing it back to its original form. This form of redox recycling has been observed where antioxidants such as ascorbic acid replenish the antioxidant activity of α-tocopherol by donating a hydrogen atom (Çelik et al., 2013; Cömert & Gökmen, 2017). Antioxidant fortification of PUFA-containing oils; therefore greatly enhances their stability. The efficacy of antioxidants in protecting PUFAs is influenced by their chemical structure, environmental conditions, and concentration.

10.4 Factors affecting the bioavailability of polyunsaturated fatty acids

Bioavailability of PUFAs refers to the rate and extent to which these FAs are absorbed from the food or supplements and their availability for use by the body (Kapoor et al., 2021). The understanding of the bioavailability of PUFAs is vital in ensuring adequate intake of these essential FAs. There are a number of factors that influence the bioavailability of PUFAs, which include:

10.4.1 The form and structure of the polyunsaturated fatty acids

The omega-3 PUFAs' bioavailability is influenced by their form. Phospholipid-based forms generally exhibit higher bioavailability compared to triglycerides and ethyl esters (Schuchardt & Hahn, 2013). The delivery method of phospholipids, whether in bulk, emulsions, or liposomes, further impacts absorption. Additionally, whether the PUFAs are free or bound, and the form they exist in (mono, di, or triglycerides) also affects the efficiency of absorption and utilization by the body (Simopoulos, 2006).

10.4.2 Type of diet

The bioavailability of PUFAs varies based on the source, which contains different PUFA types and amounts. Consumption patterns also significantly affect their bioavailability. For example, while fish provides excellent omega-3 PUFAs, plant-based sources are often more widely consumed, influencing overall PUFAs intake. The presence of other components within the PUFAs source also plays a role in how the body absorbs and utilizes these essential FAs (Schlotz et al., 2013).

10.4.3 Gut health and the genetics of individuals

The gut microbiome and genetic factors significantly influence how the body processes PUFAs, particularly omega-3 PUFAs such as ALA, DHA, and EPA. The conversion of ALA into EPA and subsequently DHA is affected by both gut health and individual genetic differences, which impact the bioavailability of these essential nutrients (Kapoor et al., 2021). Research indicates that the gut microbiota plays a role in omega-3 PUFAs metabolism and absorption.

10.4.4 Processing

Processing can severely impact the bioavailability of PUFAs due to oxidation, degradation, and structural changes, which can hinder absorption and utilization. Techniques such as emulsification and encapsulation have been suggested to improve PUFA bioavailability by protecting them from these detrimental effects (Kaseke et al., 2024). This highlights the importance of considering processing methods to maximize the health benefits of PUFAs, particularly omega-6 and omega-3 FAs. Current research focuses on stabilizing PUFAs and enhancing their absorption efficiency (Kaseke et al., 2024).

10.5 Wall materials used in polyunsaturated fatty acids nano and microencapsulation

Biopolymers, derived from natural sources, are widely used for encapsulating PUFAs as a result of their biocompatibility, biodegradability, and biological activities (Abka-khajouei et al., 2022). These materials can be broadly classified into proteins, polysaccharides, and their complexes, each offering unique advantages for PUFA encapsulation (Fig. 10.2).

10.5.1 Proteins

Proteins with strong emulsion and film-forming capabilities are a frequent choice for PUFA encapsulation (Chang et al., 2017). Whey protein isolates (WPI), casein, and gelatin are often used in experiments designed to assess their ability to stabilize emulsions and protect PUFAs from oxidation.

10.5.2 Whey protein

Whey protein contains β-lactoglobulin and α-lactalbumin, which are hydrophobic in nature and are considered binding proteins. These binding proteins, coupled with hydrophobic interactions as well as disulfide bonds, have been reported to help build a protective layer around each oil droplet that keeps out oxygen (Ramos et al., 2012). WPI has been extensively used for encapsulating omega-3 FAs. A study by Duan et al. (2011) demonstrated thatWPI combined with chitosan effectively encapsulated fish oil, significantly reducing lipid oxidation during storage. Rusli et al. (2006) demonstrated that whey protein-based formulations were superior to other wall materials and produced spray-dried powders with greater microencapsulation efficiency. The research highlighted the role WPI played in forming a stable interface layer around oil droplets, guarding against oxidative deterioration.

10.5.3 Casein

Casein is one of the major proteins found in milk, entailing excellent emulsifying ability and gel properties of its own. Casein forms micelles that can encapsulate hydrophobic substances, such as PUFAs (Ghasemi et al., 2021). Caseins make this possible because they stabilize O/W emulsions by hydrophobic interactions and electrostatic repulsion; thus a physical barrier is created against oxygen as well as prooxidants (Semo et al., 2007). Zimet et al. (2011) showed that casein-based nanoparticles effectively encapsulated DHA, effectively preventing any oxidation. The encapsulated DHA was

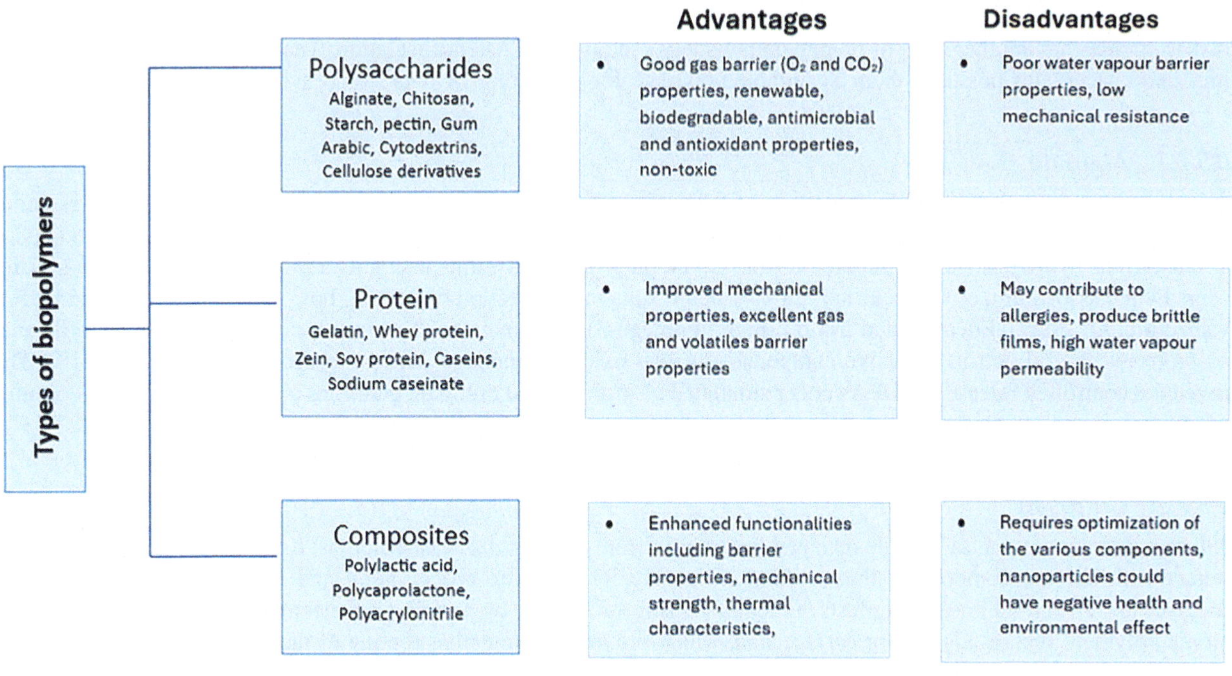

FIGURE 10.2 Biopolymers used in micro and nanoencapsulation of polyunsaturated fatty acids.

comparatively stable and more bioavailable. Casein micelles have also been used to encapsulate fish oil, showing improved oxidative stability and controlled release in simulated gastrointestinal conditions (Ghasemi et al., 2021).

10.5.4 Soy protein

Soy protein offers both a high-quality protein and good emulsifying properties, making it ideal to produce capsules. In encapsulation, its ability to form gels and films often comes in handy. Soy proteins form a network through hydrogen bonds and hydrophobic interactions, stabilizing the PUFAs and providing protection against oxygen exposure (Chen et al., 2018). For example, Wang et al. (2018) used soy protein isolate (SPI) as the carrier for the encapsulation of flax oil, which is rich in omega-3 PUFAs. The encapsulation maintained a higher oxidative stability and controlled release properties thereafter.

10.5.5 Gelatin

Gelatin, a water-soluble protein derived from collagen, possesses excellent film-forming and gelling characteristics. It is widely used in encapsulation due to its ability to form thermoreversible gels, through hydrogen bonding and hydrophobic interactions, effectively entrapping PUFAs (Gómez-Guillén et al., 2011). Fish oil-based films were able to minimize oxidation, significantly improving the oil's shelf-life (Gómez-Estaca et al., 2012). Devi et al. (2012) used gelatin and sodium alginate to encapsulate olive oil, obtaining an efficiency rate of 89%. The results of the experiment showed that gelatin could make coacervates based on the substance, with the tiny balls having a high capacity to contain oils.

10.5.6 Zein

Zein's distinct hydrophobicity enables its application in encapsulating hydrophobic, fat-soluble compounds (Yan et al., 2022). Through self-assembly, zein forms a hydrophobic matrix that protects PUFAs by limiting moisture and oxygen exposure (Luo et al., 2013). Patel et al. (2012) demonstrated that zein-based nanoparticles efficiently encapsulate omega-3 FAs, resulting in enhanced stability and controlled release under simulated gastric conditions.

10.5.7 Polysaccharides

Polysaccharides are another class of biopolymers widely used for PUFAs encapsulation. Their ability to easily form gels, films, and coacervates positions them as suitable polymers for protecting PUFAs from environmental stressors.

10.5.7.1 Alginate

Alginate is a linear polysaccharide consisting of β-D-mannuronic acid (M) and α-L-guluronic acid (G) residues and is obtained from brown seaweeds (Abka-khajouei et al., 2022). Due to the ionic crosslinking with divalent cations (Ca^{2+} etc.), it creates hydrogels, so it is suitable for the enveloping of PUFAs, thus acting as a protective barrier. The gelation occurs by the association of G-blocks and Ca^{2+}, which results in the creation of an "egg box" that immobilizes the PUFAs (Manzoor et al., 2022). Encapsulated fish oil (high in omega-3) in alginate beads showed a high encapsulation efficiency and protected the oil and its bioactive compounds against oxidative damage during storage (Olloqui et al., 2018). This proved the controlled release of PUFAs under simulated gastrointestinal optimal conditions and showed alginate's promise in food and pharmaceutical applications.

10.5.7.2 Chitosan

Chitosan is a cationic polysaccharide obtained from chitin from *crustaceans'* exoskeletons. Its positive charge enables it to interact with anionic compounds, thus making it suitable for complex coacervation and layer-by-layer encapsulation (Dima et al., 2017). Chitosan manifests its encapsulating properties by forming an electrostatic gel or complex with anionic polymers such as alginate or carrageenan, which provides a protective coating of the PUFAs in an acidic milieu. This layer works as a barrier, rejecting oxygen-harmful species (pro-oxidants) (Aranaz et al., 2018). Chew et al. (2015) encapsulated fish oil into chitosan-coated alginate beads. In addition, the chitosan layer increased the oxidative stability of the PUFAs as well as their controlled release in the intestinal condition. The combination of chitosan and alginate was synergistic and resulted in enhanced encapsulation efficiency and stability.

10.5.7.3 Starch

Starch is an inexpensive polysaccharide composed of amylose and amylopectin, which is readily available. Some modified starches have an amphiphilic nature, which is very useful in protecting emulsified PUFAs, with OSA-modified starches being particularly effective (Drusch & Mannino, 2009). By lowering the interfacial tension across the oil-water phases, OSA-modified starch creates stable emulsions. The OSA groups that are hydrophobic interact with the PUFAs, and the starch chains that are hydrophilic serve to stabilize the emulsion in aqueous environments (Drusch & Mannino, 2009). Fallahasghari et al. (2024) covered fish oil rich in omega-3 in OSA-modified starch. Compared to nonencapsulated oil, the OSA-modified starch microcapsules improved the oxidative stability by about three times, thanks to the hydrophobic interactions. This work highlighted the high potential of starch-based encapsulation in different food fortification applications.

10.5.7.4 Pectin

Pectin is an anionic polysaccharide primarily composed of galacturonic acid units and obtained from plant cell walls. In the presence of calcium ions or under acidic conditions, it forms gels, making it suitable for PUFA encapsulation. The gel network, which is formed through hydrogen bonding and ionic interactions, creates a protective matrix around PUFAs (Sai et al., 2024). The gel structure limits oxygen diffusion and protects PUFAs from oxidative degradation. A study by Menin et al. (2018) encapsulated flaxseed oil (rich in omega-3 PUFAs) in pectin-based microcapsules. The encapsulation considerably enhanced the stability of the oil against oxidation, and this can possibly control release properties under simulated gastrointestinal conditions.

10.5.8 Composites

The combination of proteins and polysaccharides can create synergistic effects, improving the encapsulation efficiency and stability of PUFAs. For example, Akhtar et al. (2022) encapsulated Himalayan walnut oil in various pea protein isolate–pectin complex coated lipid oxidation emulsions, exhibiting favorable results with respect to moisture content, color, and density, with a maximum retention of omega FAs (69%). Similarly, Pham et al. (2020) found that complex coacervation of flaxseed protein isolate (FPI) and flaxseed gum (FSG) to encapsulate flaxseed oil produced encapsulated oil that was nine times more stable than nonencapsulated oil. The observed results were attributed to the protective effect of the electron-donating potential of FPI towards the lipid molecules, which were believed to be caused by electrostatic and hydrogen bonding interactions between FPI and FSG. In this respect, Eratte (2016) reported that a SPI-gum Arabic complex microcapsule showed much better stability against oxidation, greater oil microencapsulation efficiency, and lower surface oil content. Electrostatic interactions between the negatively charged gum Arabic and positively charged SPI at pH 4.0 may have induced complex formation and stabilized the coacervate phase. Additionally, the stabilization of fish oil in the gelatin–chitosan complex was related to strong electrostatic interactions between the biopolymers (Hosseini et al., 2021). The polyelectrolyte complex of gelatin and chitosan thus generated a denser matrix around the PUFAs sufficient to prevent oxidation. All these studies suggest that protein–polysaccharide complexes can be used as biopolymers for the encapsulation and stabilization of PUFAs.

10.5.9 Emerging walls materials

Plant-based proteins, such as pea protein, lentil protein, and rice protein, have emerged as eco-friendly alternatives to animal-based proteins for PUFAs encapsulation (Gomes & Sobral, 2022). These proteins are not only cost-effective but also exhibit excellent techno-functional properties, such as emulsification, gelation, and film-forming potential, making them ideal for encapsulation applications. These sources of biopolymers have been recognized for their excellent emulsifying ability, ability to form stable emulsions, greater encapsulation efficiency, and providing stability against oxidation of PUFAs (Aberkane et al., 2014).

10.6 Micro and nanoencapsulation systems

Top-down or bottom-up approaches are normally utilized in micro and nano-encapsulation of food components. The bottom-up approach in micro and nanoencapsulation involves building materials through self-assembly and self-organization of molecules, starting with small structures to create larger particles. Meanwhile, the top-down approach, on the other hand, alters large structured materials (Fig. 10.3) (Ezhilarasi et al., 2013).

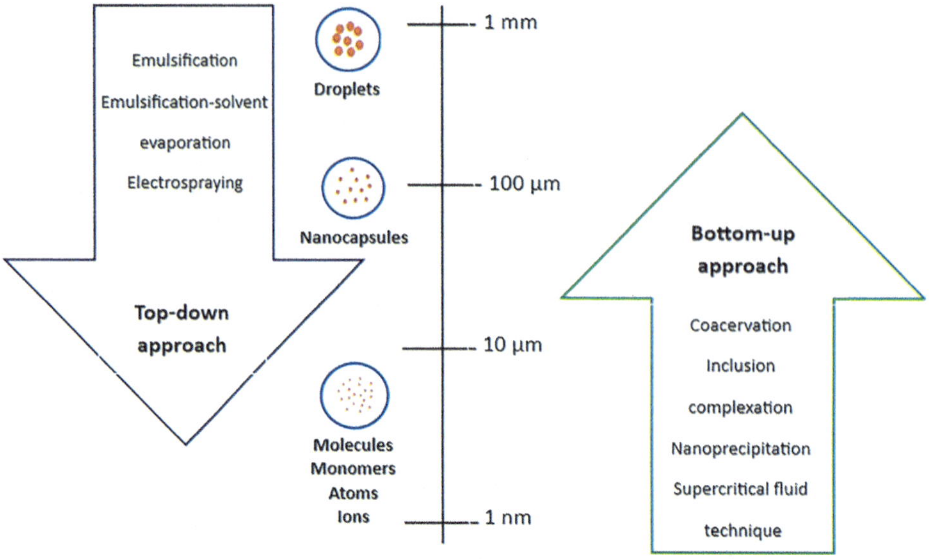

FIGURE 10.3 Bottom-up and top-down approaches in micro and nanoencapsulation of polyunsaturated fatty acids (Ezhilarasi et al., 2013). Image modified with permission from Food and Bioprocess Technology, Springer.

10.6.1 Microencapsulation techniques

Microencapsulation of PUFAs from various sources can be achieved through the use of various techniques such as coacervation, SD, FD, supercritical fluid technology, extrusion, and fluidized bed coating. Microencapsulation has the potential to improve the oxidative stability, thermostability, biological activity, and shelf-life of PUFAs oils. Additionally, it controls the volatility and release properties of essential oils. Emulsion preparation is an important step before microencapsulation.

10.6.1.1 Preparation of emulsion for polyunsaturated fatty acids microencapsulation

Emulsification is a critical process in the microencapsulation of PUFAs, which enables the creation of stable liquid dispersions and creates the foundation for encapsulating active ingredients. Emulsification allows for the generation of various types of emulsions, from simple to multiple, paving the way for controlled release and protection of the active ingredients. Simple emulsions are categorized based on the dispersion of the phase. Water dispersed in oil forms a W/O emulsion. Conversely, oil dispersed in water forms an O/W emulsion (Timilsena et al., 2017). This phase distribution greatly affects the stability and properties of the emulsion. When one phase is proportionally greater than the other, multiple emulsions are formed (Camelo Silva et al., 2022). To further stabilize the emulsion, an emulsifier or surfactant is often added in the continuous phase, and this favors the production of smaller microparticles. In addition, parameters such as pH, viscosity, temperature, and agitation rate during emulsion preparation strongly influence the final size of the microparticles (Timilsena et al., 2017). These complex systems encapsulate droplets within droplets, offering increased stability and bioavailability, and other properties for various applications in the food, drug delivery, and cosmetics. The arrangement of phases dictates the emulsion's overall characteristics and functionality. The selection of emulsifiers and microencapsulation techniques depends on the intended characteristics of the final product and the core material's properties. Various methods, such as high pressure, ultrasound, rotor-stator, and membrane systems, are often used in the formation of emulsions. Emulsification processes often incorporate techniques such as FD, SD, coacervation, extrusion, supercritical fluid, and solvent evaporation to stabilize emulsions (Areekal et al., 2024). These techniques help to remove the dispersing medium (usually water or an organic solvent), solidifying the dispersed phase and creating a stable, powdered or solid product.

10.6.1.2 Spray-drying

SD, a common method used to microencapsulate PUFAs, involves converting a liquid feed, containing the PUFAs, into a dried powder (Fig. 10.4). The PUFAs are typically emulsified or dispersed within a protective wall material, such as

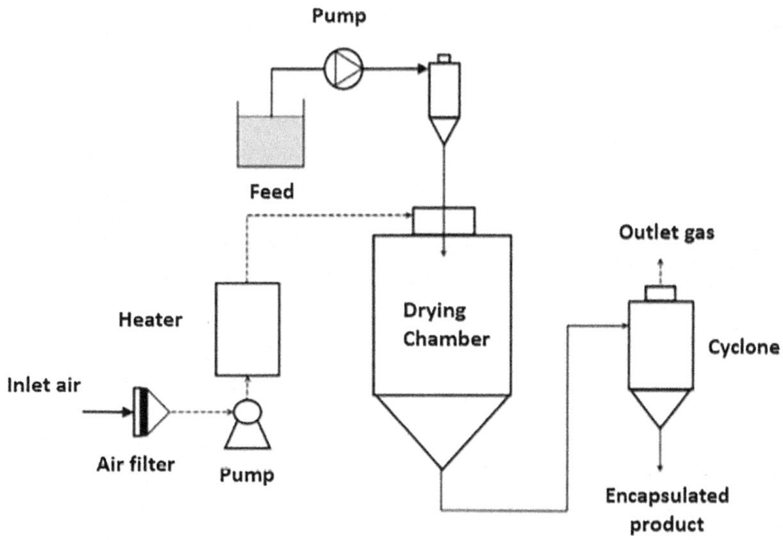

FIGURE 10.4 Illustration of spray-drying microencapsulation (Yakdhane et al., 2021).
Copyrights, Process, MDPI (2021).

carbohydrates or proteins, before being sprayed into a heated chamber (Kaseke et al., 2024). The rapid drying creates microcapsules, which protect the PUFAs from oxidation and degradation, improving their stability for applications in food, pharmaceuticals, and nutraceuticals. However, factors such as inlet and outlet temperatures, feed flow rate, and wall material composition must be carefully considered, as they influence the characteristics of the resulting microcapsules and the encapsulation efficiency of PUFAs (Castejón et al., 2021). SD is often used in combination with wall materials such as maltodextrin, cellulose, protein isolates, and gum Arabic to produce stable PUFAs from various sources of oils such as nuts, field crops, marine, and fruit seed (Kaseke et al., 2024). Research has shown that this technique has been applied to microencapsulate omega-3 FAs extracted from oilseeds and microalgae as well as essential FAs in fish oil, enhancing their bioavailability and oxidative stability (Castejón et al., 2021; Sultana et al., 2023). Spray-dried PUFAs from various oils have been applied in formulating confectionery, dairy, fats and oils, and meat products, providing enhanced qualities to the products (Mangope et al., 2025).

10.6.1.3 Freeze-drying

FD is a low-temperature dehydration process that involves initially freezing the product and then ice removal by sublimation (Makhathini et al., 2023). The primary steps of the FD process involve freezing, primary, and secondary drying. This method is particularly important for heat-labile compounds such as PUFAs (Yang et al., 2024). While offering superior preservation qualities and ease of rehydration, FD is a time-consuming and expensive method. FD has been applied in various areas, including the encapsulation of PUFAs, highlighting its versatility in food processing and preservation. FD encapsulation of kenaf seed oil and pomegranate seed oil has also been shown to preserve bioactive compounds, such as tocopherol and polyphenols, contributing to the delayed degradation of the PUFAs during storage (Chew & Nyam, 2019; Kaseke et al., 2024). This technique is affected by factors such as the type and concentration of the encapsulating material, the oil-to-carrier ratio, and the freezing as well as the drying parameters. Optimization of these parameters is therefore essential to successfully encapsulate and protect the PUFAs during the FD process. FD encapsulation of chia seed oil using a binary blend of whey protein concentrate and modified tapioca starch at a concentration of 25:75 significantly preserved the PUFAs and improved their oxidative and thermal stability (Anand et al., 2024). The study showcases the potential of encapsulation in improving the functionality of PUFAs in various products. Suwannasang et al. (2022) established that the controlled release of PUFAs from encapsulated sacha inchi oil (freeze-dried) significantly improved in fortified yogurt after simulated gastrointestinal digestions, suggesting enhanced bioavailability of the FAs.

10.6.1.4 Coacervation

Coacervation microencapsulation technique uses a coacervating agent, which induces the separation of phases in the polymer solution. This creates a polymer-rich coacervate phase that encapsulates desired components, and a polymer-poor medium (Nezamdoost-Sani et al., 2024). Two coacervation methods are available, namely, simple and advanced coacervation. Simple coacervation involves infusing a polymer solution with a water-soluble desolating agent, causing polymer molecules to separate from the aqueous phase and precipitate as spherical droplets (Fig. 10.5). To form stable microparticles, these droplets are then cross-linked. Meanwhile, advanced coacervation, comprising oppositely charged polymers, proceeds in three phases: phase separation, polymer deposition on a core material, and capsule stabilization (Nezamdoost-Sani et al., 2024). Coacervation is widely used for improving oxidative stability, bioaccessibility, and the controlled release of PUFAs together with biopolymers, including alginate, chitosan, gelatin, and cellulose-derived materials, along with proteins. Cross-linking agents such as glutaraldehyde, genipin, and calcium salts are often used. Coacervation-microencapsulated algae oil showed improved stability against oxidation during storage in comparison with free oil (Mu et al., 2022). Coacervation and SD of pomegranate seed oil using gum arabic and WPI as encapsulants showed superior oxidative and thermal stability when applied to instant coffee beverages (Costa et al., 2022).

10.6.1.5 Extrusion

The emulsion-extrusion technique involves creating microspheres, which encapsulate the active ingredient. The process starts with homogenizing the ingredient in an aqueous polymer solution (Pattnaik & Mishra, 2022). This is followed by spraying into a cross-linker solution (such as $CaCl_2$ or glutaraldehyde) using equipment such as a peristaltic pump or a hypodermic syringe with a specific nozzle size that controls the microparticle size (Perez-Palacios et al., 2022). Microspheres are subsequently formed through cross-linking of the emulsion droplets, followed by hardening through extended incubation in the cross-linker solution (Kaseke et al., 2024). The interfacial surface tension plays a key role in size reduction under constant processing conditions. This method is useful for controlled release and protection of the active ingredient and has been widely applied in drug delivery. Emulsion-extrusion has been applied to microencapsulate various oils, showing great potential to enhance the biological activity and oxidative stability of the PUFAs in the oils (Kaushik et al., 2015).

10.6.1.6 Supercritical fluid

Supercritical fluid encapsulation is a versatile technique for creating micro and nanoparticles using supercritical fluids, typically carbon dioxide, as solvents. The process involves dissolving the core material and coating material in the supercritical fluid, followed by a rapid depressurization (Fig. 10.6). This rapid change causes the coating material to precipitate around the core material, resulting in encapsulated particles. Supercritical fluid encapsulation offers advantages such as precise control over particle size and morphology, the ability to avoid organic solvents, and enhanced stability, as well as controlled release of the encapsulated compounds (Soh & Lee, 2019). The encapsulated product can be incorporated into various applications, such as food, pharmaceuticals, and cosmetics, improving their functionality and controlled release properties. This technique has been used to encapsulate PUFAs in specialty oils such as chia seed and

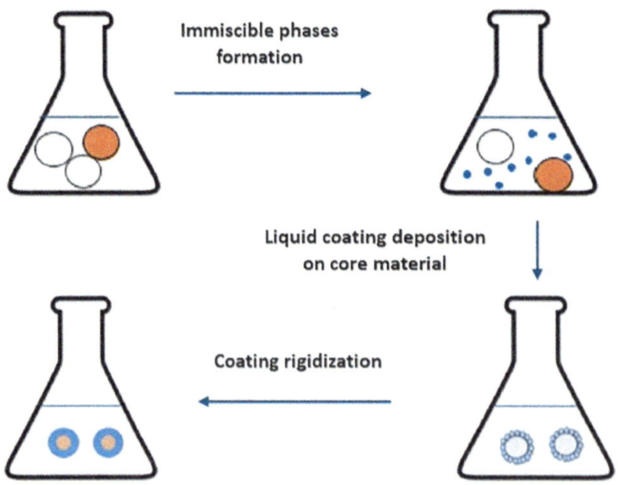

FIGURE 10.5 Illustration of the coacervation technique (Kaseke et al., 2024).
Copyrights, Food and Bioprocess Technology, Springer (2024).

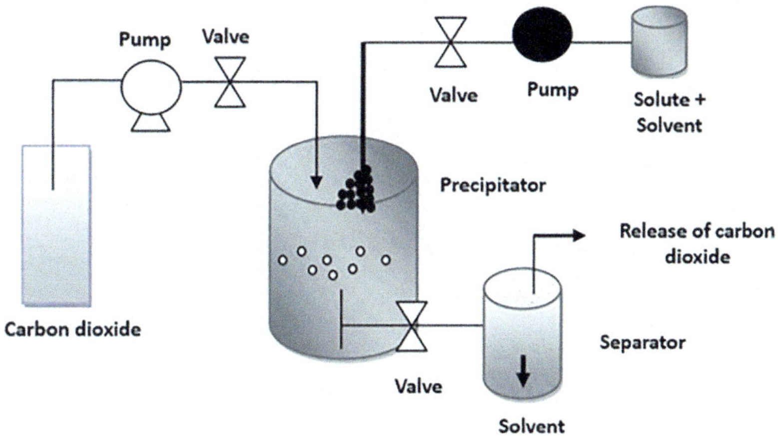

FIGURE 10.6 Illustration of supercritical antisolvent microencapsulation (Karim et al., 2017). Copyrights, Journal of Food and Drug Analysis, Elsevier (2017).

hemp seed oil to prevent oxidation and improve their bioavailability, as well as encapsulating other omega-3-rich oils such as fish oil to increase their stability and delivery in various food functions (Gañan et al., 2020; Gholivand et al., 2024; Karim et al., 2017).

10.6.1.7 *Fluidized bed coating*

Fluidized bed coating involves suspending the seed oil containing PUFAs in a fluidized bed, where coating materials are sprayed onto the droplets, creating microcapsules (Tontul & Topuz, 2015). This process can protect PUFAs from degradation and improve both their bioavailability and stability. This technique can be achieved by using different coating materials, such as proteins or carbohydrates, which form a protective layer around the PUFAs (Singh et al., 2022). This method can improve shelf-life, control release, and mask undesirable flavors or odors associated with PUFAs. Different coating materials and process parameters impact the effectiveness of PUFA encapsulation. Anwar et al. (2010) microencapsulated fish oil using the spray granulation combined with fluidized bed coating using soluble soybean polysaccharide and maltodextrin as encapsulants and reported lower generation of hydroperoxides during storage when compared to free fish oil.

10.6.1.8 *Solvent evaporation*

Solvent evaporation, which is the primary technique for microencapsulation of hydrophilic and hydrophobic materials by a polymeric shell, is carried out by using emulsion-based systems, including w/o/w and o/w double emulsions (Ahangaran, 2022). This technique can be used to effectively disperse the active ingredients (as solute, powder, etc.) in a polymeric solution. The mixture is then dispersed into droplets before evaporating the solvent to form solid microspheres entrapping the active ingredients (Ahangaran, 2022). However, this technology is expensive and difficult to scale up, though it is often used in the pharmaceutical industry to produce microcapsules composed of biodegradable polymers. Some aspects that need to be carefully considered during the solvent evaporation process are the atmospheric pressure, speed of evaporation, and type of emulsion single or double, as these may affect the quality of the microcapsules produced. This technique is mostly applied in drug delivery systems. Jalalizand & Goli, (2021) optimized the fortification of soybean oil with selenium using the solvent evaporation method and mixtures of Arabic and Persian gums. The authors found that solvent evaporation significantly decreased the evolution of oxidation indices, showing the potential of the encapsulated PUFAs in drug delivery systems.

10.6.2 Nanoencapsulation systems

Different nanoencapsulation techniques, including nanocapsules, SLN, nanoemulsions, nanoliposomes, and nanostructured lipid carriers (NLC), have been applied to encapsulate PUFAs with better retention of omega-3 FAs. Fig. 10.7 shows

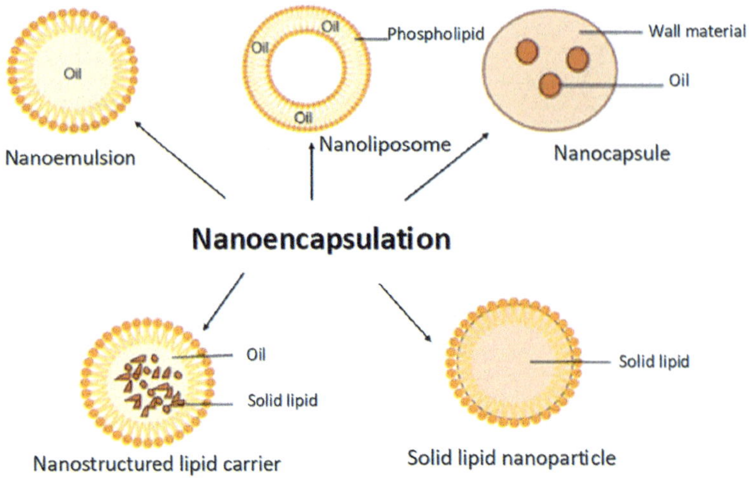

FIGURE 10.7 Nanoencapsulation technologies of polyunsaturated fatty acids.

the schematic illustrations of different nanoencapsulation technologies. Table 10.1 shows the summary of nanoencapsulation of PUFAs in the previous literature.

10.6.2.1 Nanoemulsions

Nanoemulsions are characterized by nano-droplet sizes ranging from 100 to 500 nm. Nanoemulsions are formed by two liquids that cannot mix, such as oil and water. According to Li et al. (2020), a surfactant or emulsifier is used to emulsify oil and water into a single colloidal dispersion system. Nanoemulsion is often used to deliver drugs, compounds, active agents, and nutraceuticals in cosmetics, food and beverages, and pharmaceuticals industries. Compared with conventional emulsions, nanoemulsions presented nano-droplet sizes with a lesser tendency of aggregation between droplets, which results in less flocculation and improved stability and functionalities (Ma et al., 2025). Nanoemulsions are prepared using either low-energy techniques, such as spontaneous emulsification and phase transformation, or high-energy methods such as high-pressure homogenization (HPH), microfluidization, and ultrasonication. Low-energy methods require low equipment requirements, a simple process, and low heat production, while high-energy methods require high equipment requirements and high heat production. However, high-energy methods can prepare the nanoemulsions with nano droplet sizes and higher stability (Ma et al., 2025). These methods have wide applications for industrial production in the food industry (Li et al., 2020).

Currently, HPH is considered one of the most commonly used and efficient technologies in the preparation of nanoemulsions. Previous studies have demonstrated that the bioaccessibility and bioavailability of active ingredients in nanoemulsions could be enhanced (Li et al., 2020). The choice of emulsifier is vital to affect the physical and chemical stability of the nanoemulsion. Proteins, phospholipids, and polysaccharides with high biocompatibility, environmentally friendly, easily available, and high stability are commonly used as emulsifiers (Dammak et al., 2020). Biological macromolecular emulsifiers have been widely studied to promote the stability and bioaccessibility of nanoemulsions. For example, Li et al. (2020) stabilized fish oil nanoemulsions using prepared soybean protein isolate and phosphatidylcholine by HPH at 100 MPa. The study established that the fish oil nanoemulsions produced by phosphatidylcholine and soybean protein isolate presented better storage and oxidative stability compared to Tween 20 nanoemulsions (control). Additionally, the digestibility of fish oil in soybean protein isolate-phosphatidylcholine nanoemulsions was better compared to Tween 20 nanoemulsions. The rate at which free FAs (FFA) were released from soybean protein isolate-phosphatidylcholine nanoemulsions was 86.8% after 2 hours of simulated intestinal digestion.

Ao et al. (2024) encapsulated fish oil and resveratrol in hyaluronic acid-poly(glyceryl)10-stearate nanoemulsions. The nanoemulsions presented better physicochemical stability and oxidative stability. In addition, bioaccessibility and release of FFA were enhanced in this nanoemulsion after in vitro simulated digestion. PUFAs nanoemulsion was prepared with a low-energy technique utilizing sunflower oil (carrier oil) and Tween 85 and isopropanol (surfactant mixture) (Inapurapu et al., 2020). Increased bioaccessibility (53%) was shown in the nanoemulsion compared to the control (34%), which was

TABLE 10.1 Summary of nanoencapsulation techniques of polyunsaturated fatty acids (PUFAs) in the literature.

Nanoencapsulation technique	Preparation method	Physical characteristic	Major findings	References
Nanoemulsion	• Aqueous-titration method and mechanical agitation • Oil phase: Maxepa (300 mg of eicosapentaenoic acid [EPA] and 200 mg of docosahexaenoic acid [DHA]) dissolved in sunflower oil (carrier oil) • Surfactant: Tween 85 and isopropanol	Droplet size: 100–200 nm PDI: less than 0.3 during the 28-day storage	• The omega-3 fatty acids (FAs) content of the nanoemulsions decreased by 5% during 28-day storage at both 4°C and 25°C. • The nanoemulsion improved the bioaccessibility to 53% compared to the plain oils mixed with omega-3 FAs (34%).	Inapurapu et al. (2020)
	• High shear homogenization and high-pressure homogenization • Soy protein isolate: 1%, 2%, 3%, 4%, and 5% w/v • Phosphatidylcholine: 0%, 0.2%, 0.4%, 0.6%, and 1% w/v • Fish oil: 0.5%–3% w/v	Particle size: 245.03–455.33 nm, PDI: 0.23–0.48	• The optimum nanoemulsion was prepared with 2% soy protein isolate, 0.2% phosphatidylcholine, and 1.5% fish oil at 100 MPa homogenization pressure • The nanoemulsions exhibited enhanced oxidative stability and superior resistance to Na^+ ions at concentrations of 0.1–0.5 M. • The nanoemulsions showed droplet aggregation during in vitro gastric digestion and released 86.8% free FAs (FFA) in simulated intestinal digestion (2 h).	Li et al. (2020)
	• A high-energy method was used to prepare an oil-in-water (O/W) nanoemulsion. • 2% evening primrose oil, 2% blackcurrant seed oil, 7% Tween 80, 3% Span 20, and 86% distilled water were blended and ultrasonicated. • 0.29 μL of 20 mg/mL etoposide was dissolved in 99.7 μL of the emulsion above.	Droplet size: 20.7 nm	• Etoposide in PUFAs nanoemulsion presented a greater apoptotic effect and increased efficiency for its anticancer effect. • The etoposide nanoemulsion inhibited the cellular invasion by 55%, while the unencapsulated etoposide inhibited the cellular invasion by 3%.	Alkhatib et al. (2021)
	• The phase inversion temperature method was used to encapsulate fish oil.	Particle size: 155.44 nm (4°C) and 163.04 nm (25°C)	• Fish oil nanoemulsion reduced neutrophil infiltration 24 h after sepsis induction. • The nanoemulsion diet significantly inhibited paw edema in adult female BALB/c mice.	Santos et al. (2021)

(Continued)

TABLE 10.1 (Continued)

Nanoencapsulation technique	Preparation method	Physical characteristic	Major findings	References
			• This demonstrated the antiinflammatory effects of fish oil nanoemulsion in the treatment of inflammatory disorders.	
	• Ultrasonication with a probe • Time: 5 min • Amplitude: 37.26% • Surfactant: 1% Tween 20 • Concentration of surfactant-to-oil ratio: 1.17:1	Encapsulation efficiency: 89.7%, size: 60 nm	• The droplet size of the nanoemulsion increased to 88 nm after storage at 4°C for 28 days. • The nanoemulsion masked the tartness of rosehip oil in yogurt while preserving its linoleic acid content.	Rao et al. (2023)
	• Hyaluronic acid was first esterified with poly(glyceryl)10-stearate and was then used to emulsify and codeliver fish oil and resveratrol.	Encapsulation efficiency: 96.5%–98.2%, loading capacity: 0.445%–0.452%	• The nanoemulsions presented improved physicochemical stability, improved oxidative stability, and antioxidant activity. • The bioaccessibility was enhanced, and a more efficient release of FFA via in vitro simulated digestion.	Ao et al. (2024)
	• O/W emulsification • Porcine gelatin (OG) and a porcine gelatin/isolated whey protein blend (OWG) were used as polymers.	Particle size: 161 nm (OG) and 264 nm (OWG), PDI: 0.11 (OG) and 0.13 (OWG), encapsulation efficiency: 74% (OG) and 83% (OWG)	• There were no cytotoxic effects for free and nanoencapsulated quinoa oil. • Antioxidant activity increased to 50%–63% in neutral medium and 96%–153% in acidic medium. • Nanoemulsions enhanced the inhibition of α-amylase by 5%–7% and amyloglucosidase by 6–9 times, respectively.	Marques et al. (2024)
	• High-pressure microfluidization technique • Surfactants: soy lecithin, flaxseed gum (FSG), and soy protein isolate • Mass fractions of surfactants in aqueous phase: 0.5%, 1.0%, 1.5%, and 2.0% • Mass fraction of flaxseed oil: 5%, 8%, 12%, and 15% • Homogenization pressure: 40, 80, 120, and 160 MPa	Sizes: 300–1000 nm, PDI: 0.1–0.3	• Nanoemulsion presented a lower peroxide value and thiobarbiturate value compared to free flaxseed oil. • Nanoemulsion encapsulation extended the shelf life of flaxseed oil from 35, 33, and 27 days to 55, 48, and 42 days at 20°C, 25°C, and 30°C, respectively. • Oxidative stability of flaxseed oil was enhanced.	Ma et al. (2025)
Nanoliposome	• Sonication • Sunflower oil, lecithin, and glycerol were used to form a nanoliposome to encapsulate fish oil.	Particle size: 409 nm, PDI: 0.557	• The nanoliposomes showed a significant decrease in acidity, peroxide value, and syneresis after 21-day storage, with better protection of oxidative stability.	Ghorbanzade et al. (2017)

			• Fish oil nanoliposomes showed higher retention of DHA and EPA contents in the yogurt. • Sensory evaluation revealed closer qualities between yogurt added with nanoliposomes and the control yogurt.	
	• Sonication • Sunflower oil, lecithin, and glycerol were used to form a nanoliposome to encapsulate fish oil.	Particle size: 339.2 nm, PDI: 0.426, nanoencapsulation efficiency: 90.12 ± 0.27%	• The incorporation of fish oil nanoliposomes did not affect the textural quality and sensory acceptability of bread. • It could improve the nutritional quality of bread and other bakery products.	Ojagh & Hasani (2018)
	• Ultrasonication and microfluidization techniques with 5% w/v lecithin, 2.5% v/v shrimp oil, and 2% v/v glycerol	Particle size: 40–284 nm (ultrasonication) and 214–928 nm (microfluidization), nanoencapsulation efficiency: 93.64% (ultrasonication) and 75.18% (microfluidization)	• Ultrasonication of nanoliposomes presented better centrifugal stability. • Nanoliposomes showed an improvement in stability and better preservation of EPA and DHA, particularly in ultrasonication nanoliposomes. • Nanoliposomes could mask the shrimp oil's fishy odor. • May be applied in foods to enhance the intake of omega-3 FAs and astaxanthin.	Gulzar & Benjakul (2020)
	Sonication technique with 1 mL pistachio oil and 250 μL of 100 mg/mL lecithin.	Particle size: 100–250 nm	Multiple sclerosis patients with nanoliposomes treatment showed an improvement in clinical parameters, a decrease in the level of matrix metallopeptidase-9, and a better quality of life.	Hassanshahi et al. (2022)
	• Grape seed oil-loaded vesicles (80:10:40 mg lecithin/cholesterol/oil) produced by ethanol injection, preheated at 55°C for 20 min, were then subjected to sonication.	Particle size: 180–240 nm	• This nanoliposome-enhanced active film facilitated the controlled release of grape seed oil at low temperatures, delivering potent antioxidant or antimicrobial benefits to preserve meat quality by the successful preservation of chilled mutton for 15 days using this film technology.	Song et al. (2025)
Nanocapsule	• Electrospraying technique • Voltage: 20–25 kV • Flow rate: 0.5–1.0 mL/h	Encapsulation efficiency: 94.0 ± 2.5%	• No significant differences in the average diameter of the nanocapsules at different voltages or flow rates were observed.	Cetinkaya et al. (2021)

(Continued)

TABLE 10.1 (Continued)

Nanoencapsulation technique	Preparation method	Physical characteristic	Major findings	References
	• Shell material: a kafirin isolate (10% w/w) composed of mainly α-kafirins, together with γ- and β-kafirins • 20% w/w of fish oil based on the kafirin content.		• Kafirin can be used as a hydrophobic shell material to produce fish oil nanocapsules. • Fortification of omega-3 FAs into foods.	
	• Omega-3 FAs were emulsified into a surfactant solution: Tween 80, Span 80, and lecithin, and then mixed with gelatin and gum arabicum solution.	NA	• Treatment with omega-3 EPA: DHA nanocapsules to the endothelial cells resulted in increased antiaggregatory effects and an increased production of nitric oxide. • Offer protection to endothelial cells and the cardiovascular system.	Remila et al. (2021)
	• Ultrasonication and lyophilization were used to prepare flaxseed oil nanocapsules with FSG and secoisolariciresinol diglucoside as wall materials.	Particle size: 208.22 nm, encapsulation efficiency: 96%, PDI: 0.131	• The flaxseed oil nanocapsules presented good stability during the 7-days' storage compared to unencapsulated flaxseed oil emulsions.	Fang et al. (2024)
	• Silica-based nanocapsules with linseed oil as the core.	Size: 120 nm	• The nanocapsules showed an oxygen uptake capacity of 13.89 mL/g and an absorption rate of 0.604 mL/g/day at 20°C. • The linseed oil nanocapsules can be added in active food packaging to act as an oxygen scavenger to extend the shelf-life of foods.	Rozo et al. (2024)
Nanoparticle	• Ionotropic gelation: 0.5% w/v chitosan and 0.15% w/v sodium tripolyphosphate (4:1 volume ratio) and pumpkin seed oil.	Size: 20–80 nm	• Dietary supplementation with 1.5–2 mL of nano-encapsulated pumpkin seed oil significantly boosted growth, feed utilization, and disease resistance against *Vibrio parahaemolyticus* infections in whiteleg shrimp. • Dietary supplementation with pumpkin seed oil-loaded chitosan nanoparticles can reverse histological damage in the muscle, hepatopancreas, and intestine caused by *V. parahaemolyticus* infection.	Eissa et al. (2025)
Solid-lipid nanoparticle (SLN)	• Lipid matrix contained resveratrol esterified to stearic acid	Size: 571–1000 nm, PDI: 0.13–0.22	• Incorporation of omega-3 PUFA in human HT-29 colorectal cancer cells	Serini et al. (2018)

	• Emulsifier was a mixture of sodium taurocholate, butanol, and Tween-80		was improved by their encapsulation into SLN. • Cell proliferation was significantly reduced.	
	• Whey protein isolate (2% w/w), palmitic acid (1.25%, 2.50%, and 3.75% w/w), and quercetin (200, 500, and 800 ppm)	Particle size: 90–315 nm, PDI: 0.25–0.60	• The addition of palmitic acid promoted the physical stability of the emulsions by reducing the O/W droplet sizes and PDI. • Quercetin could offer antioxidant activity and increase oxidative stability, while palmitic acid was important in oxidation inhibition.	Azizi et al. (2019)
Nanostructured lipid carrier (NLC)	• High-shear homogenization with cold-pressed blackcurrant, blackberry, raspberry, strawberry, and plum seed oils was used.	Size: 221.0–274.1 nm, PDI 0.13–0.20	• The most stable nanosuspension was achieved using an optimized formulation of 6% lipids (6:2 wax-to-oil ratio), 4% nonionic emulsifiers, and 88% water. • Potential dermal application to facilitate skin supplementing with linoleic acid.	Krasodomska et al. (2016)
	• High shear force hot homogenization plus surfactant (glyceryl stearate and oleic acid, tween 80), and α-tocopherol.	Particle size: 198 nm, PDI: 0.28	• No interaction between the α-tocopherol and the obtained NLCs was observed. • The NLCs potentially offer antioxidant activity to camelina oil.	Sheybani et al. (2023)
	• Melt-emulsification ultrasonic method • Surfactants: 1,2-propylene glycol and Tween 80 • Solid-lipid: glycerol distearate • Liquid lipid: perilla seed oil	PDI: 0.240 ± 0.017 Particle size: 117.5 ± 3.7 nm Encapsulation efficiency: 96.3 ± 0.3%	• The NLCs exhibited sustained release of formononetin for 24 h and better digestibility via in vitro simulated digestion. • The NLC protected the perilla seed oil against oxidation and could be stored at 4°C for 3 months.	Zheng et al. (2023)
	• Copaiba oil: 1%, 5%, and 9% • Precirol®: 1%, 4%, and 7% • Tween®: 0.1%, 0.5%, 0.9%	Particle size: 183;± 1.8 nm PDI: 0.17 ± 0.01	• 6% copaiba oil, 1% Precirol®, and 0.9% Tween® were optimized in the formulation. • Maximum cellular toxicity against MCF-7 cells was observed with the optimized NLC, which inhibited growth by 52.49% at 25 μg/mL	Uchôa et al. (2025)

formed by plain oils blended with PUFAs. Thus the developed nanoemulsions can be used for adjuvant treatments and food applications to increase the intake of PUFAs.

Ma et al. (2025) used high-pressure microfluidization to prepare flaxseed oil nanoemulsion. The findings revealed that the flaxseed oil nanoemulsion was appropriate to store in ceramic containers at low temperature and dark conditions. High-pressure microfluidization can improve the flaxseed oil oxidation stability by extending the storage life of the flaxseed oil in nanoemulsion from 35, 33, and 27 days at 20°C, 25°C, and 30°C to 55, 48, and 42 days at 20°C, 25°C, and 30°C, respectively. Furthermore, tuna oil rich in EPA and DHA was nanoemulsified by chitosan-xanthan gum in Vilanculos et al. (2023). Chitosan and xanthan gum's electrostatic interactions enhanced the steric and stability of the nanoemulsions. In another study, Marques et al. (2024) encapsulated quinoa oil using isolated whey protein and porcine gelatin via O/W emulsification. The nanoemulsion of quinoa oil improved the antioxidant activity of quinoa oil and inhibited 5%–7% and 6–9 times more for the α-amylase and amyloglucosidase enzymes, respectively, as compared to unencapsulated oil. This showed that nanoencapsulation can enhance the antioxidant activity of unsaturated oils with nano-droplet size.

Previous studies revealed that nanoemulsions of unsaturated FAs are suitable for use in food and pharmaceutical applications. In Rao et al. (2023), rosehip oil nanoemulsion was produced by probe ultrasonication with 5 minutes of ultrasonication time, 37.26% of ultrasonication amplitude, and 1% Tween 20 as surfactant with a surfactant to oil ratio of 1.17:1. The rosehip oil nanoemulsion was then incorporated in yogurt and successfully maintained the FAs profile compared to the unencapsulated rosehip oil in yogurt. Moreover, the sensory evaluation showed that rosehip oil nanoemulsion could cover the tartness of rosehip oil when applied to yogurt. Yogurt with rosehip oil nanoemulsion presented admissible pH and acidity and lower peroxide value in comparison to yogurt with unencapsulated rosehip oil and plain yogurt during storage for 28-days. This study confirmed the nanoemulsions' stability and potential application in food products (Rao et al., 2023). Gumus and Gharibzahedi (2021) showed that the addition of omega-3 FAs microcapsules prepared by the emulsion technique to yogurt enhanced its physicochemical, microbiological, rheological, and sensory qualities. These applications can help to enhance the intake of omega-3 FAs for human consumption.

Etoposide was encapsulated in a nanoemulsion consisting of PUFAs (blackcurrant seeds and evening primrose oils) to enhance its antiinvasion and antiproliferation effects against ovarian cancer cells (SK-OV-3 cells) (Alkhatib et al., 2021). The results showed that etoposide in PUFAs nanoemulsion presented a greater apoptotic effect and increased efficiency for its anticancer effect. The etoposide nanoemulsion suppressed the cellular invasion by 55%, while the unencapsulated etoposide suppressed the cellular invasion by 3%. Thus nanoemulsion with PUFAs is suitable for delivering drugs and nutraceuticals for pharmaceutical applications.

10.6.2.2 Nanoliposomes

Nanoliposomes are spherical systems made up of a phospholipid bilayer and a core with sizes less than 1000 nm. Liposomes can be unilamellar (single-layered) or multilamellar (multilayered). Thermal and nonthermal techniques can encapsulate bioactive compounds as core agents. Nanoliposomes can encapsulate hydrophilic or hydrophobic compounds for specific-site delivery. A previous study reported that nanoliposomes of fish oils could deliver higher storage stability, higher retention of omega-3 FAs, and covering of fishy odor (Ghorbanzade et al., 2017). Encapsulation of unsaturated FAs into nanoliposome vesicles can protect the core agents against lipid oxidation (Gulzar & Benjakul, 2020).

Gulzar and Benjakul (2020) prepared the nanoliposomes of shrimp oil using ultrasonication and microfluidization to improve oxidative stability during storage. Shrimp oil is rich in omega-3 FAs and astaxanthin, which are liable to oxygen and temperature conditions during storage. The results revealed that the better nanoencapsulation efficiency of 93.64% was achieved by ultrasonication-nanoliposomes when compared to 75.18% by microfluidization-nanoliposomes. The nanoencapsulation efficiency of ultrasonication-nanoliposomes was maintained constant during the 8 weeks' storage at 30°C. Moreover, ultrasonication-nanoliposomes showed improved oxidative stability with better retention of DHA and EPA during storage compared to unencapsulated oil. The findings showed that nanoliposomes are a good nanoencapsulation technique to protect the unsaturated FAs during storage (Gulzar & Benjakul, 2020).

PUFAs-based nanoliposomes have the potential to be applied in food products to deliver essential FAs with better preservation of nutritional value. Application of fish oil nanoliposomes to yogurt showed that the yogurt with fish oil nanoliposomes presented a lower peroxide value than the yogurt with unencapsulated fish oil (Ghorbanzade et al., 2017). Moreover, Ojagh & Hasani (2018) applied fish oil nanoliposomes (nanoencapsulation efficiency: 90.12%) in bread. The fortification of fish oil nanoliposomes in bread did not affect the textural and sensory qualities of the bread while presenting better oxidative stability. Thus nanoliposomes of PUFAs can act as an additive in functional food products to deliver health benefits.

In addition, nanoliposomes can be applied in active packaging as films to prolong the shelf-life of meat products. Nanoliposomes of grape seed oil were developed using tapioca starch and konjac gum composite vesicles to develop an active film (Song et al., 2025). The compatibility, physicochemical properties, barrier characteristics, mechanical stability, and functionalities of grape seed oil were improved in this nanoliposome. At low temperatures, application of this nanoliposome into the active packaging film could release grape seed oil and deliver its antimicrobial and antioxidant activities to extend the shelf-life of meat. This was shown by the extension of the shelf-life of chilled mutton to 15 days with the application of grape seed oil nanoliposomes packaging film. This study offers suggestions for the advancement of active food packaging with the application of nanoliposomes (Song et al., 2025).

Hassanshahi et al. (2022) investigated the treatment of pistachio oils' PEGylated nanoliposome in the management of multiple sclerosis in a randomized, double-blind, placebo-controlled clinical trial. Pistachio oils with high PUFAs and omega-3 FAs in the form of nanoliposomes were proven to deliver their antiinflammatory activity efficiently to treat multiple sclerosis with no side effects observed. Thus nanoliposomes of PUFAs can be used in pharmaceutical applications.

10.6.2.3 Nanocapsules

Nanocapsules are capsules smaller than 1 μm. Nanocapsules enhance the bioaccessibility and bioavailability, controlled release behavior, and solubility of the encapsulated core agents. High shear homogenization is a common physical technique used to prepare microcapsules currently. However, high shear homogenization does not form nanocapsules from a conventional mixed system. On the other hand, HPH is the common technique used to prepare nanocapsules with expensive equipment and high maintenance costs. Thus ultrasound has been developed as another option to HPH (Rodríguez-Cortina & Hernández-Carrión, 2023). Ultrasound induces cavitation by ultimate turbulence, which helps to form nanocapsules. The combination of high shear homogenization and ultrasonication can prepare nanocapsules in an easier way with lower cost and in a more environmentally friendly manner (Fang et al., 2024).

Cetinkaya et al. (2021) electrosprayed solutions with 10% w/w kafirin and fish oil (20% w/w based on the kafirin content), which resulted in the formation of nanocapsules with sizes ranging from 552 to 861 nm. Kafirin is a cereal prolamin storage protein commonly found in grain sorghum. However, kafirin belongs to the hydrophobic protein, which is interesting to study compared to the common hydrophilic protein. The findings revealed that the nanocapsules presented an encapsulation efficiency of 94% with 20–25 kV voltage and a flow rate of 0.5–1 mL/h. The fish oil was successfully encapsulated within the kafirin shell, which indicates the applicability of the electrospraying technique and the use of kafirin biopolymer. Electrospraying can reduce the quantity of polymer chain entanglements and split up the charged jet expelled from the Taylor cone into nano-droplets. These charged droplets will be evaporated and dried during the travel to the collector to form dried capsules (Cetinkaya et al., 2021). Fang et al. (2024) developed flaxseed oil nanocapsules with FSG and secoisolariciresinol diglucoside as wall materials. The flaxseed oil nanocapsules presented a nanoencapsulation efficiency of 96% and good stability during the 7-days' storage compared to unencapsulated flaxseed oil emulsions. Thus nanoencapsulation is feasible to encapsulate PUFAs to preserve the unsaturated fatty acids content. Furthermore, Haider et al. (2017) prepared the krill oil nanoparticles with chitosan and tripolyphosphate. The results demonstrated that nanoencapsulation improved the oxidative stability of krill oil with lower hydroperoxide content during the 2 weeks' storage at 45°C compared to unencapsulated krill oil.

10.6.2.4 Nanoparticles

Nanoparticles loaded with unsaturated oils can be used as feed additives in aquafarming. Eissa et al. (2025) prepared the pumpkin seed oil-loaded nanoparticles by chitosan as a feed additive for whiteleg shrimp for a 60-day period. The findings demonstrated that dietary intake of 1.5 or 2 mL of pumpkin seed oil-loaded chitosan nanoparticles significantly increased the weight gain, feed conversion ratio, specific growth rate, and survival rate of whiteleg shrimp against *Vibrio parahaemolyticus*. Moreover, dietary intake of chitosan nanoparticles loaded with pumpkin seed oil could help to restore the muscle's histological damage, hepatopancreas, and intestine induced by *V. parahaemolyticus* infection.

Nanoparticles can be applied to advance sustainable food packaging systems. Alvarado et al. (2022) had nano-encapsulated linseed oil into silica nanocapsules as the active oxygen scavengers. These nanoparticles can be incorporated into packaging films as part of active food packaging. The silica-based linseed oil nanocapsules can act as scavengers of oxygen to absorb the remaining oxygen in the environment of the headspace within the food packaging. Thus this can help to preserve the food product shelf-life through reducing the oxidation rate and biochemical changes. Rozo et al. (2024) further studied the oxidation kinetics of linseed oil in oxygen scavenger nanocapsules and reported that linseed oil nanocapsules presented a 13.9 mL/g substantial total oxygen absorption capacity, which is 2–3 times higher than the common nonferrous oxygen scavengers. This result showcases the potential of linseed oil nanocapsules as an oxygen scavenger to prolong the shelf-life of food products.

Since omega-3 PUFAs are correlated with a decrease in the risk of cardiovascular diseases, Remila et al. (2021) had nano-encapsulated EPA and DHA with a ratio of 6:1, followed by gum coating to act as a potent inducer of nitric oxide in the endothelium. The results showed that treatment with omega-3 EPA: DHA nanocapsules to the endothelial cells resulted in increased antiaggregatory effects and an enhanced production of nitric oxide. This formulation proved to enhance and sustain the nitric oxide-dependent relaxations mediated by the endothelium in coronary artery rings and nitric oxide production.

10.6.2.5 Solid-lipid nanoparticles and nanostructured lipid carrier

SLN and NLC are emerging as effective delivery systems for lipophilic compounds. While SLNs consist of crystallized nanoemulsions with a solid-lipid core, NLCs represent an advanced alternative using a blend of solid and liquid lipids. According to Salminen et al. (2013), both methods offer superior encapsulation efficiency, improved controlled release of active ingredient, and stability. A solid matrix protects PUFAs from oxidation by trapping them within a solid-lipid phase. This shields the PUFAs from diffusing to the emulsion surface, where they can be exposed to oxygen and certain pro-oxidants. The use of saturated long-chain phospholipids as emulsifiers further stabilizes the lipid nanoparticles by maintaining the α-subcellular crystals. This phospholipid layer acts as a nucleation site, directing crystallization inward to form organized, repeating triglyceride layers (Salminen et al., 2013).

A previous study encapsulated fish oil in SLN using palmitic acid as a solid-lipid phase and quercetin as an antioxidant into the WPI-stabilized SLN. This formulation showed an improved stability against oxidation of the fish oil and physical stabilization of the emulsions through O/W droplets size reduction (Azizi et al., 2019). Serini et al. (2018) encapsulated omega-3 FAs (DHA and ALA) into resveratrol-based SLN and successfully delivered them into HT-29 colorectal cancer cells through an in vitro study. This decreased cell proliferation and enhanced its growth-inhibitory effects on the cancer cells. Thus SLN is suitable to load with omega-3 FAs to increase the delivery and treatment effects of omega-3 FAs. The current research on SLN-loaded with unsaturated FAs is limited. There are more SLNs have been studied on the saturated FAs and delivery of drug and antioxidant compounds for food, cosmeceutical, and pharmaceutical applications.

NLC is suitable for delivering water-insoluble drugs compared to SLN. This is because of their partially crystalline structure with pores in the core solid shell, offering more drug loading space. Thus this results in higher drug loading efficacy, improved drug stability, and controlled release behavior in NLC (Seabra et al., 2017). Previous studies have utilized NLCs to protect unsaturated FAs and enhance the shelf stability of camelina oil, perilla seed oil, and flaxseed oil (Oskouei et al., 2024; Sheybani et al., 2023; Zheng et al., 2023). Furthermore, Zheng et al. (2023) demonstrated that NLCs coloaded with formononetin and perilla seed oil offered 24-hour controlled release and improved digestibility. Unsaturated FAs can be considered for use as a liquid lipid phase in NLC. For example, Garg and Garg (2024) developed hyaluronic acid-conjugated tacrolimus-loaded NLC using stearylamine and Moringa oleifera seed oil as solid-lipid and liquid lipid, respectively. This formulation showed an improvement in the cellular uptake to enhance its oral absorption and antiinflammatory activity. Furthermore, copaiba oil-loaded NLC was proven to strengthen the cytotoxicity effect against breast cancer cells (Uchôa et al., 2025). Thus NLCs were suitable to be used in pharmaceutical applications to offer antiinflammatory (Garg & Garg, 2024), anticancer (Uchôa et al., 2025), and antimicrobial activities (Seabra et al., 2017).

Seabra et al. (2017) demonstrated that NLCs loaded with DHA enhance bactericidal efficacy against *Helicobacter pylori*, achieving inhibition at 25 μM compared to >100 μM for free DHA. By disrupting bacterial membranes and causing cytoplasmic leakage, this nontoxic formulation offers a promising treatment for *H. pylori* gastric infections. NLCs are also proposed as a protective delivery system for PUFAs, particularly suited for dermal application. Krasodomska et al. (2016) formulated NLCs loaded with fruit seed oils from blackcurrant, blackberry, raspberry, strawberry, and plum. The optimized composition; 4% nonionic emulsifiers, 88% water, and 6% lipids with a 6:2 wax-to-oil ratio, effectively stabilized and protected the sensitive PUFAs in these seeds' oils, enhancing their shelf-life and bioavailability for topical application.

10.6.2.6 Advancements and prospects of polyunsaturated fatty acids encapsulation

Advancements in nanoencapsulation of PUFAs have significantly improved the stability of PUFAs, extension of shelf-life, specific-site delivery, controlled release, bioaccessibility, and bioavailability. Different nanoencapsulation techniques, including nanoliposomes, nanoemulsions, nanocapsules, NLCs, and SLNs, have been developed by emulsification, high-shear homogenization, HPH, electrospraying, ultrasonication, and others (Cetinkaya et al., 2021; Li et al., 2020; Rao et al., 2023).

However, there is a gap in formulating this technology for industrial-scale applications. The limitations of these technologies should be overcome to develop a feasible technology with cost-effective, environmental friendly, and applicable for large-scale production to deliver PUFAs. Different biopolymers have been extensively investigated to enhance the nanoencapsulation efficiency to encapsulate the PUFAs with high stability (Marques et al., 2024; Vilanculos et al., 2023). Incorporating PUFA-loaded nanosystems into foods demands detailed investigation into four key areas: (1) stability within the food matrix, (2) mechanisms of release, (3) interaction with other ingredients, and (4) subsequent bioavailability and bioaccessibility.

Future research should also prioritize cell permeation assays, in vivo models, and human trials to assess both the safety and therapeutic potency of PUFA-based nanosystems (Ao et al., 2024). Additionally, computational models can be generated to elucidate the reaction kinetics, release behavior, and oil oxidation mechanisms of PUFAs in nanosystems. Thus these computational models can be used to simulate the characteristics of these nanosystems in applications under various conditions. A predictive model can be generated to simulate the performance of this PUFAs nanosystem for pharmaceutical, food, and beverage, as well as cosmeceutical applications.

10.7 Conclusions

This chapter has reviewed the potential of nano and microencapsulation in enhancing the stability and bioavailability of PUFAs. The technology has presented a great potential to enhance the stability and bioavailability of PUFAs, especially the omega-3 and omega-6 FAs, leading to improved controlled release and improved efficacy of these FAs in food, pharmaceutical systems, and utilization by the human body. Nano and microencapsulation are actively being leveraged in the food sector to safeguard the benefits of PUFAs and enhance the health benefits and quality of various foods from confectionery, dairy, fats and oils to meat products. Future trends in nano and microencapsulation of PUFAs involve enhancing stability, bioavailability, and therapeutic efficacy through the use of innovative wall materials, advanced encapsulation techniques, and their combinations. These advancements create targeted delivery systems for specific tissues, thereby improving the effectiveness of PUFA-based therapies. This further optimizes the delivery of PUFAs, especially the omega-3 and omega-6 FAs, and enhances their overall impact. However, developing safe, biocompatible, and biodegradable encapsulation systems is crucial for sustainable preservation and utilization of PUFAs. This ensures human and environmental safety while advancing innovation on PUFAs application in pharmaceuticals, food and beverages, and cosmeceuticals.

References

Aberkane, L., Roudaut, G., & Saurel, R. (2014). Encapsulation of fish oil using pea protein: Emulsification and oxidative stability. *Food Chemistry, 145*, 1–8. https://doi.org/10.1016/j.foodchem.2013.08.012.

Abka-khajouei, R., Tounsi, L., Shahabi, N., Patel, A. K., Abdelkafi, S., & Michaud, P. (2022). Structures, properties and applications of alginates. *Marine Drugs, 20*(6), 364. https://doi.org/10.3390/md20060364.

Ahangaran, F. (2022). Microencapsulation: Solvent evaporation. *Principles of Biomaterials Encapsulation: Volume 1, 1*, 377–392. https://doi.org/10.1016/B978-0-323-85947-9.00016-9, https://www.sciencedirect.com/book/9780323859479.

Akhtar, G., Masoodi, F. A., Murtaza, M., & Rather, Z. U. K. (2022). Soy protein isolate-maltodextrin-pectin microcapsules of himalayan walnut oil: Complex coacervation under variable pH systems and characterization. *ACS Food Science and Technology, 2*(8), 1283–1295. https://doi.org/10.1021/acsfoodscitech.2c00125, https://pubs.acs.org/page/afsthl/about.html.

Alkhatib, M. H., Al-Hashemi, S. M., & Gashlan, H. M. (2021). Formulating etoposide in a nanoemulsion containing polyunsaturated fatty acids potentiates its anti-proliferation and anti-invasion activities against the ovarian cancer cells. *Biocell, 45*(3), 695–703. https://doi.org/10.32604/biocell.2021.014349.

Alvarado, J. F., Rozo, D. F., Chaparro, L. M., Medina, J. A., & Salcedo-Galán, F. (2022). Synthesis and characterization of reproducible linseed oil-loaded silica nanoparticles with potential use as oxygen scavengers in active packaging. *Nanomaterials, 12*(18). https://doi.org/10.3390/nano12183257, http://www.mdpi.com/journal/nanomaterials.

Anand, V., Ksh, V., Kar, A., Varghese, E., Vasudev, S., & Kaur, C. (2024). Encapsulation efficiency and fatty acid analysis of chia seed oil microencapsulated by freeze-drying using combinations of wall material. *Food Chemistry, 430*, 136960. https://doi.org/10.1016/j.foodchem.2023.136960.

Anwar, S. H., Weissbrodt, J., & Kunz, B. (2010). Microencapsulation of fish oil by spray granulation and fluid bed film coating. *Journal of Food Science, 75*(6), E359–E371.

Ao, S., Luo, X., Huang, M., Wu, H., Chen, Y., Chen, H., Li, J., Zhou, Y., Yin, X., Cai, T., Yang, Q., Deng, L., & Zhu, K. (2024). Hyaluronic acid-poly (glyceryl)10-stearate nanoemulsion for co-delivery of fish oil and resveratrol: Enhancing bioaccessibility and antioxidant potency. *International Journal of Biological Macromolecules, 273*(Pt 1), 132835. https://doi.org/10.1016/j.ijbiomac.2024.132835.

Aranaz, I., Mengíbar, M., Harris, R., Paños, I., Miralles, B., Acosta, N., & Heras, A. (2018). Functional characterization of chitin and chitosan. *Current Chemical Biology, 3*(2), 203–230. https://doi.org/10.2174/187231309788166415.

Araujo, P., Bjørkkjær, T., Frøyland, L., & Waagbø, R. (2018). Effect of storage time, temperature, antioxidant and thawing on fatty acid composition of plasma, serum and red blood cells – A pilot biobank study. *Clinical Biochemistry, 52*, 94–105. https://doi.org/10.1016/j.clinbiochem.2017.10.004.

Areekal, N. N., Chakkaravarthi, A., & Debnath, S. (2024). Effect of microencapsulation on physical properties of powder developed from blended oils rich in PUFA. *Journal of Food Science and Technology, 61*(12), 2275–2286.

Azizi, M., Li, Y., Kaul, N., & Abbaspourrad, A. (2019). Study of the physicochemical properties of fish oil solid lipid nanoparticle in the presence of palmitic acid and Arre. *Journal of Agricultural and Food Chemistry, 67*(2), 671–679. https://doi.org/10.1021/acs.jafc.8b02246.

Bacellar, I. O. L., & Baptista, M. S. (2019). Mechanisms of photosensitized lipid oxidation and membrane permeabilization. *ACS Omega, 4*(26), 21636–21646. https://doi.org/10.1021/acsomega.9b03244, pubs.acs.org/journal/acsodf.

Bakry, A. M., Abbas, S., Ali, B., Majeed, H., Abouelwafa, M. Y., Mousa, A., & Liang, L. (2016). Microencapsulation of oils: A comprehensive review of benefits, techniques, and applications. *Comprehensive Reviews in Food Science and Food Safety, 15*(1), 143–182. https://doi.org/10.1111/1541-4337.12179, http://www.interscience.wiley.com/jpages/1541-4337.

Balić, A., Vlašić, D., Žužul, K., Marinović, B., & Bukvić Mokos, Z. (2020). Omega-3 versus omega-6 polyunsaturated fatty acids in the prevention and treatment of inflammatory skin diseases. *International Journal of Molecular Sciences, 21*(3), 741. https://doi.org/10.3390/ijms21030741.

Bayliak, M. M., Burdyliuk, N. I., & Lushchak, V. I. (2016). Effects of pH on antioxidant and prooxidant properties of common medicinal herbs. *Open Life Sciences, 11*(1), 298–307. https://doi.org/10.1515/biol-2016-0040.

Camelo-Silva, C., Verruck, S., Ambrosi, A., & Di Luccio, M. (2022). Innovation and trends in probiotic microencapsulation by emulsification techniques. *Food Engineering Reviews, 14*(3), 462-490.

Castejón, N., Luna, P., & Señoráns, F. J. (2021). Microencapsulation by spray drying of omega-3 lipids extracted from oilseeds and microalgae: Effect on polyunsaturated fatty acid composition. *LWT, 148*, 111789.

Çelik, E. E., Gökmen, V., & Fogliano, V. (2013). Soluble antioxidant compounds regenerate the antioxidants bound to insoluble parts of foods. *Journal of Agricultural and Food Chemistry, 61*(43), 10329–10334. https://doi.org/10.1021/jf402523k.

Cetinkaya, T., Mendes, A. C., Jacobsen, C., Ceylan, Z., Chronakis, I. S., Bean, S. R., & García-Moreno, P. J. (2021). Development of kafirin-based nanocapsules by electrospraying for encapsulation of fish oil. *LWT, 136*. https://doi.org/10.1016/j.lwt.2020.110297, https://www.journals.elsevier.com/lwt.

Chang, H., Lv, J., Gao, X., Wang, X., Wang, H., Chen, H., . & Cheng, Y. (2017). Rational design of a polymer with robust efficacy for intracellular protein and peptide delivery. *Nano letters, 17*(3), 1678–1684.

Chen, Y., Zhang, H., Liu, R., Mats, L., Zhu, H., & Tsao, R. (2018). Antioxidant and anti-inflammatory polyphenols and peptides of common bean (Phaseolus vulgaris L.) milk and yogurt in Caco-2 and HT-29 cell models. *Journal of Functional Foods, 45*, 1–10. https://doi.org/10.1016/j.jff.2018.03.031.

Chew, S. C., & Nyam, K. L. (2019). Kenaf (*Hibiscus cannabinus* L.) seed oil. *Fruit Oils: Chemistry and Functionality*, 451–494.

Chew, S. C., Tan, C. P., Long, K., & Nyam, K. L. (2015). In-vitro evaluation of kenaf seed oil in chitosan coated-high methoxyl pectin-alginate microcapsules. *Industrial Crops and Products, 76*, 230–236. https://doi.org/10.1016/j.indcrop.2015.06.055.

Cömert, E. D., & Gökmen, V. (2017). Antioxidants bound to an insoluble food matrix: Their analysis, regeneration behavior, and physiological importance. *Comprehensive Reviews in Food Science and Food Safety, 16*(3), 382–399. https://doi.org/10.1111/1541-4337.12263, http://onlinelibrary.wiley.com/journal/10.1111/(ISSN)1541-4337.

Costa, A. M. M., Gaspar, B. R. A., Calado, V., Tonon, R. V., & Torres, A. G. (2022). Microencapsulation of pomegranate (Punica granatum L.) seed oil by complex coacervation: Stability and application in an instant caffè latte beverage. *Food Chemistry, 381*, 132199.

Dammak, I., Sobral, P. Jd. A., Aquino, A., Neves, M. Ad, & Conte-Junior, C. A. (2020). Nanoemulsions: Using emulsifiers from natural sources replacing synthetic ones—A review. *Comprehensive Reviews in Food Science and Food Safety, 19*(5), 2721–2746. https://doi.org/10.1111/1541-4337.12606, http://onlinelibrary.wiley.com/journal/10.1111/(ISSN)1541-4337.

Devi, N., Hazarika, D., Deka, C., & Kakati, D. K. (2012). Study of complex coacervation of gelatin A and sodium alginate for microencapsulation of olive oil. *Journal of Macromolecular Science, Part A, 49*(11), 936–945. https://doi.org/10.1080/10601325.2012.722854.

Dima, J. B., Sequeiros, C., & Zaritzky, N. (2017). Chitosan from marine crustaceans: production, characterization and applications. *Biological Activities and Application of Marine Polysaccharides*, 39–56. https://doi.org/10.5772/65258.

Drusch, S., & Mannino, S. (2009). Patent-based review on industrial approaches for the microencapsulation of oils rich in polyunsaturated fatty acids. *Trends in Food Science & Technology, 20*(6-7), 237–244. https://doi.org/10.1016/j.tifs.2009.03.007.

Duan, J., Jiang, Y., & Zhao, Y. (2011). Chitosan–whey protein isolate composite films for encapsulation and stabilization of fish oil containing ultra pure omega-3 fatty acids. *Journal of Food Science, 76*(1), C133–C141. https://doi.org/10.1111/j.1750-3841.2010.01905.x.

Eissa, E. S. H., Salama, W. M., Elbahnaswy, S., El-Son, M. A. M., Eldin, Z. E., Amer, S., Almutairi, L. A., Khalil, F. M. A., Bahshwan, S. M. A., AL-Qurashi, M. M., Abd El-Aziz, Y. M., Eissa, M. E. H., Alsaegh, A. A., Mathew, R. T., & Rizk, E. S. T. (2025). Pumpkin seed oil-loaded chitosan nanoparticles enhance growth, digestive enzymes, and immune response in whiteleg shrimp (*Litopenaeus vannamei*): Impacts on histopathology and survival against Vibrio parahaemolyticus. *Aquaculture Reports, 40*. https://doi.org/10.1016/j.aqrep.2024.102599, https://www.sciencedirect.com/science/journal/23525134.

Eratte, D. (2016). Co-encapsulation of Omega-3 Fatty Acids and Probiotic Bacteria Through Complex Coacervation (Doctoral dissertation, Federation University Australia). Accessed 10 March 2025.

Ezhilarasi, P. N., Karthik, P., Chhanwal, N., & Anandharamakrishnan, C. (2013). Nanoencapsulation techniques for food bioactive components: A review. *Food and Bioprocess Technology, 6*(3), 628–647. https://doi.org/10.1007/s11947-012-0944-0.

Fallahasghari, E. Z., Stubbe, P. R., Chronakis, I. S., & Mendes, A. C. (2024). Ethyl cellulose-core, OSA starch-shell electrosprayed microcapsules enhance the oxidative stability of loaded fish oil. *Nanomaterials, 14*(6). https://doi.org/10.3390/nano14060510, http://www.mdpi.com/journal/nanomaterials.

Fang, X., Ge, X.-Y., Qin, Z., He, K., Wang, R.-Y., Cai, X.-S., Liu, H.-M., & Wang, X.-D. (2024). Nanoencapsulation of flaxseed oil: Fabrication, characterization, and storage stability. *LWT, 214*, 117113. https://doi.org/10.1016/j.lwt.2024.117113.

Fawole, O. A., Kaseke, T., & Opara, U. L. (2021). Pomegranate fruit quality and seed drying method: Effect on the chemical composition and bioactivities of the extracted oil. *Processes, 10*(1), 3.

Gañan, N., Bordón, M. G., Ribotta, P. D., & González, A. (2020). Study of chia oil microencapsulation in soy protein microparticles using supercritical CO_2-assisted impregnation. *Journal of CO_2 Utilization, 40*, 101221. https://doi.org/10.1016/j.jcou.2020.101221.

Garg, R., & Garg, A. (2024). Development and evaluation of hyaluronic acid conjugated tacrolimus-loaded nanostructured lipid carriers using moringa oleifera seed oil as liquid lipid. *Journal of Drug Delivery Science and Technology, 95*, 105591. https://doi.org/10.1016/j.jddst.2024.105591.

Geng, L., Liu, K., & Zhang, H. (2023). Lipid oxidation in foods and its implications on proteins. *Frontiers in Nutrition, 10*(June), 1–12. https://doi.org/10.3389/fnut.2023.1192199.

Ghasemi, S., Jafari, S. M., Assadpour, E., & Khomeiri, M. (2021). Encapsulation of DHA in casein micelles: Stability and bioavailability. *Food Chemistry, 345*, 128789. https://doi.org/10.1016/j.foodchem.2020.128789.

Gholivand, S., Tan, T. B., Mat Yusoff, M., Choy, H. W., Teow, S. J., Wang, Y., Liu, Y., & Tan, C. P. (2024). An in-depth comparative study of various plant-based protein-alginate complexes in the production of hemp seed oil microcapsules by supercritical carbon dioxide solution-enhanced dispersion. *Food Hydrocolloids, 153*. https://doi.org/10.1016/j.foodhyd.2024.110001, https://www.sciencedirect.com/science/journal/0268005X.

Ghorbanzade, T., Jafari, S. M., Akhavan, S., & Hadavi, R. (2017). Nano-encapsulation of fish oil in nano-liposomes and its application in fortification of yogurt. *Food Chemistry, 216*, 146–152. https://doi.org/10.1016/j.foodchem.2016.08.022, www.elsevier.com/locate/foodchem.

Gomes, A., & Sobral, P. J. D. A. (2022). Plant protein-based delivery systems: An emerging approach for increasing the efficacy of lipophilic bioactive compounds. *Molecules, 27*(1). https://doi.org/10.3390/molecules27010060, https://www.mdpi.com/1420-3049/27/1/60/pdf.

Gómez-Estaca, J., Montero, P., & Gómez-Guillén, M. C. (2012). Encapsulation of fish oil in gelatin-based films. *Food Hydrocolloids, 27*(2), 1–10. https://doi.org/10.1016/j.foodhyd.2011.08.015.

Gómez-Guillén, M. C., Giménez, B., López-Caballero, M. E., & Montero, M. P. (2011). Functional and bioactive properties of collagen and gelatin from alternative sources: A review. *Food Hydrocolloids, 25*(8), 1813–1827. https://doi.org/10.1016/j.foodhyd.2011.02.007.

Grootveld, M., Percival, B. C., Moumtaz, S., Gibson, M., Woodason, K., Akhtar, A., Wawire, M., Edgar, M., & Grootveld, K. L. (2021). Commentary: Iconoclastic reflections on the 'safety' of polyunsaturated fatty acid-rich culinary frying oils: Some cautions regarding the laboratory analysis and dietary ingestion of lipid oxidation product toxins. *Applied Sciences (Switzerland), 11*(5), 1–34. https://doi.org/10.3390/app11052351, https://www.mdpi.com/2076-3417/11/5/2351/pdf.

Grosshagauer, S., Steinschaden, R., & Pignitter, M. (2019). Strategies to increase the oxidative stability of cold pressed oils. *LWT, 106*(February), 72–77. https://doi.org/10.1016/j.lwt.2019.02.046.

Gulzar, S., & Benjakul, S. (2020). Characteristics and storage stability of nanoliposomes loaded with shrimp oil as affected by ultrasonication and microfluidization. *Food Chemistry, 310*, 125916. https://doi.org/10.1016/j.foodchem.2019.125916.

Gumus, C. E., & Gharibzahedi, S. M. T. (2021). Yogurts supplemented with lipid emulsions rich in omega-3 fatty acids: New insights into the fortification, microencapsulation, quality properties, and health-promoting effects. *Trends in Food Science and Technology, 110*, 267–279. https://doi.org/10.1016/j.tifs.2021.02.016, http://www.elsevier.com/wps/find/journaldescription.cws_home/601278/description#description.

Haider, J., Majeed, H., Williams, P. A., Safdar, W., & Zhong. F. (2017). Formation of chitosan nanoparticles to encapsulate krill oil (Euphausia superba) for application as a dietary supplement. *Food Hydrocolloids, 63*, 27–34. https://doi.org/10.1016/j.foodhyd.2016.08.020.

Hassanshahi, G., Karimabad, M. N., & Jebali, A. (2022). The therapeutic effect of PEGlated nanoliposome of pistachio unsaturated oils and its efficacy to attenuate inflammation in multiple sclerosis: A randomized, double-blind, placebo-controlled clinical trial phase I. *Journal of Neuroimmunology, 362*, 577768. https://doi.org/10.1016/j.jneuroim.2021.577768.

Hoekman, S. K., Broch, A., Robbins, C., Ceniceros, E., & Natarajan, M. (2012). Review of biodiesel composition, properties, and specifications. *Renewable and Sustainable Energy Reviews, 16*(1), 143–169. https://doi.org/10.1016/j.rser.2011.07.143.

Hosseini, S. F., Soofi, M., & Rezaei, M. (2021). Enhanced physicochemical stability of ω-3 PUFAs concentrates-loaded nanoliposomes decorated by chitosan/gelatin blend coatings. *Food Chemistry, 345*, 128865. https://doi.org/10.1016/j.foodchem.2020.128865.

Inapurapu, S. P., Ibrahim, A., Kona, S. R., Pawar, S. C., Bodiga, S., & Bodiga, V. L. (2020). Development and characterization of ω-3 fatty acid nanoemulsions with improved physicochemical stability and bioaccessibility. *Colloids and Surfaces A: Physicochemical and Engineering Aspects, 606*. https://doi.org/10.1016/j.colsurfa.2020.125515, www.elsevier.com/locate/colsurfa.

Jalalizand, F., & Goli, M. (2021). Optimization of microencapsulation of selenium with gum Arabian/Persian mixtures by solvent evaporation method using response surface methodology (RSM): Soybean oil fortification and oxidation indices. *Journal of Food Measurement and Characterization, 15*(1), 495–507. https://doi.org/10.1007/s11694-020-00659-y.

Kapoor, B., Kapoor, D., Gautam, S., Singh, R., & Bhardwaj, S. (2021). Dietary polyunsaturated fatty acids (PUFAs): Uses and potential health benefits. *Current Nutrition Reports, 10*(3), 232–242. https://doi.org/10.1007/s13668-021-00363-3.

Karim, F. T., Ghafoor, K., Ferdosh, S., Al-Juhaimi, F., Ali, E., Yunus, K. B., Hamed, M. H., Islam, A., Asif, M., & Zaidul, I. S. M. (2017). Microencapsulation of fish oil using supercritical antisolvent process. *Journal of Food and Drug Analysis, 25*(3), 654–666. https://doi.org/10.1016/j.jfda.2016.11.017, http://www.elsevier.com/journals/journal-of-food-and-drug-analysis/1021-9498#.

Kaseke, T., Chew, S. C., Magangana, T. P., & Fawole, O. A. (2024). Elucidating the microencapsulation of bioactives from pomegranate fruit waste for enhanced stability, controlled release, biological activity, and application. *Food and Bioprocess Technology,* 1–29.

Kaseke, T., Opara, U. L., & Fawole, O. A. (2021). Oxidative stability of pomegranate seed oil from blanched and microwave pretreated seeds: Kinetic and thermodynamic studies under accelerated conditions. *Journal of Food Processing and Preservation, 45*(10), e15798.

Kaushik, P., Dowling, K., Barrow, C. J., & Adhikari, B. (2015). Microencapsulation of omega-3 fatty acids: A review of microencapsulation and characterization methods. *Journal of Functional Foods, 19*, 868–881.

Krasodomska, O., Paolicelli, P., Cesa, S., Casadei, M. A., & Jungnickel, C. (2016). Protection and viability of fruit seeds oils by nanostructured lipid carrier (NLC) nanosuspensions. *Journal of Colloid and Interface Science, 479*, 25–33. https://doi.org/10.1016/j.jcis.2016.06.041, http://www.elsevier.com/inca/publications/store/6/2/2/8/6/1/index.htt.

Kubrak, T. P., Kołodziej, P., Sawicki, J., Mazur, A., Koziorowska, K., & Aebisher, D. (2022). Some natural photosensitizers and their medicinal properties for use in photodynamic therapy. *Molecules, 27*(4). https://doi.org/10.3390/molecules27041192, https://www.mdpi.com/1420-3049/27/4/1192/pdf.

Koop, B. L., da Silva, M. N., da Silva, F. D., dos Santos Lima, K. T., Soares, L. S., de Andrade, C. J., . & Monteiro, A. R. (2022). Flavonoids, anthocyanins, betalains, curcumin, and carotenoids: Sources, classification and enhanced stabilization by encapsulation and adsorption. Food *Research International, 153*, 110929.

Lemańska, K., Szymusiak, H., Tyrakowska, B., Zieliński, R., Soffers, A. E. M. F., & Rietjens, I. M. C. M. (2001). The influence of pH on antioxidant properties and the mechanism of antioxidant action of hydroxyflavones. *Free Radical Biology and Medicine, 31*(7), 869–881. https://doi.org/10.1016/S0891-5849(01)00638-4.

Li, Y., Li, M., Qi, Y., Zheng, L., Wu, C., Wang, Z., & Teng, F. (2020). Preparation and digestibility of fish oil nanoemulsions stabilized by soybean protein isolate-phosphatidylcholine. *Food Hydrocolloids, 100*, 105310. https://doi.org/10.1016/j.foodhyd.2019.105310.

Luo, Y., Zhang, B., & Whent, M. (2013). Zein nanoparticles for encapsulation of omega-3 fatty acids. *Journal of Food Science, 78*(1), C1–C7. https://doi.org/10.1111/j.1750-3841.2012.02987.x.

Ma, Y., Liu, X., Sun, H., Wang, Y., Bai, G., Guo, Q., Xiao, S., Peng, Y., Song, L., Qiao, M., & Huang, X. (2025). Preparation of flaxseed oil nanoemulsion and its effect on oxidation stability of flaxseed oil and prediction of shelf life. *LWT, 217*, 117404. https://doi.org/10.1016/j.lwt.2025.117404.

Makhathini, N., Kaseke, T., & Fawole, O. A. (2023). Microencapsulation of organic pomegranate peel extract for a food circular economy: Effects of wall materials on powder functional attributes, antioxidant activity and antimicrobial property against foodborne pathogens. *Journal of Agriculture and Food Research, 14*, 100780.

Mangope, K., Kaseke, T., & Fawole, O. A. (2025). Spray-drying microencapsulation of fixed oils: An innovative and sustainable technology to enhance oxidative stability, functionality and application in food systems. *Applied Food Research*, 101200.

Manzoor, A., Dar, A. H., Pandey, V. K., Shams, R., Khan, S., Panesar, P. S., Kennedy, J. F., Fayaz, U., & Khan, S. A. (2022). Recent insights into polysaccharide-based hydrogels and their potential applications in food sector: A review. *International Journal of Biological Macromolecules, 213*, 987–1006. https://doi.org/10.1016/j.ijbiomac.2022.06.044, www.elsevier.com/locate/ijbiomac.

Marques, B. L. M., Passos, T. S., Dantas, A. I., de Lima, M. A. A., Moreira, S. M. G., Rodrigues, V. M., do Nascimento Dantas, M. R., Lopes, P. S., Gomes, A. P. B., da Silva Fernandes, R., Júnior, F. H. X., Sousa Júnior, F. Cd, & de Assis, C. F. (2024). Nanoencapsulation of quinoa oil enhanced the antioxidant potential and inhibited digestive enzymes. *Food Research International, 196*. https://doi.org/10.1016/j.foodres.2024.115066, https://www.sciencedirect.com/science/journal/09639969.

Menin, A., Zanoni, F., Vakarelova, M., Chignola, R., Donà, G., Rizzi, C., Mainente, F., & Zoccatelli, G. (2018). Effects of microencapsulation by ionic gelation on the oxidative stability of flaxseed oil. *Food Chemistry, 269*, 293–299. https://doi.org/10.1016/j.foodchem.2018.06.144.

Mititelu, M., Lupuliasa, D., Neacşu, S. M., Olteanu, G., Busnatu, Ş. S., Mihai, A., & Scafa-Udrişte, A. (2024). Polyunsaturated fatty acids and human health: A key to modern nutritional balance in association with polyphenolic compounds from food sources. *Foods, 14*(1), 46.

Mu, H., Song, Z., Wang, X., Wang, D., Zheng, X., & Li, X. (2022). Microencapsulation of algae oil by complex coacervation of chitosan and modified starch: Characterization and oxidative stability. *International Journal of Biological Macromolecules, 194*, 66–73. https://doi.org/10.1016/j.ijbiomac.2021.11.168.

Mukwevho, P. L., Kaseke, T., & Fawole, O. A. (2024). Ascorbic acid-enriched cactus mucilage coatings maintained quality attributes of roasted 'Wichita'pecan nuts under accelerated storage conditions. *Journal of Agriculture and Food Research, 18*, 101301.

Mukwevho, P. L., Kaseke, T., & Fawole, O. A. (2025). Innovations in biodegradable packaging and edible coating of shelled temperate nuts. *Food and Bioprocess Technology, 18*(9), 7763–7794.

Nagy, K., Iacob, B. C., Bodoki, E., & Oprean, R. (2024). Investigating the thermal stability of omega fatty acid-enriched vegetable oils. *Foods, 13*(18). https://doi.org/10.3390/foods13182961, www.mdpi.com/journal/foods.

Nejatian, M., Yazdi, A. P. G., Fattahi, R., Saberian, H., Bazsefidpar, N., Assadpour, E., & Jafari, S. M. (2024). Improving the storage and oxidative stability of essential fatty acids by different encapsulation methods; a review. *International Journal of Biological Macromolecules, 260*, 129548.

Nezamdoost-Sani, N., Amiri, S., & Khaneghah, A. M. (2024). The application of the coacervation technique for microencapsulation bioactive ingredients: A critical review. *Journal of Agriculture and Food Research*, 101431.

Ojagh, S. M., & Hasani, S. (2018). Characteristics and oxidative stability of fish oil nano-liposomes and its application in functional bread. *Journal of Food Measurement and Characterization, 12*(2), 1084–1092. https://doi.org/10.1007/s11694-018-9724-5, http://rd.springer.com/journal/11694.

Olloqui, E. J., Castañeda-Ovando, A., Contreras-López, E., Hernandez-Sanchez, D., Tapia-Maruri, D., Piloni-Martini, J., & Añorve-Morga, J. (2018). Encapsulation of fish oil into low-cost alginate beads and EPA-DHA release in a rumino-intestinal in vitro digestion model. *European Journal of Lipid Science and Technology, 120*(9). https://doi.org/10.1002/ejlt.201800036, http://onlinelibrary.wiley.com/journal/10.1002/(ISSN)1438-9312.

Oskouei, H. D., Almasi, H., Zeynali, F., Hamishehkar, H., & Amjadi, S. (2024). Improving oxidative stability of flaxseed oil by Zein-Basil seed gum electrospun nanofibers activated by thyme essential oil loaded nanostructured lipid carriers. *Applied Food Research, 4*, 100616. https://doi.org/10.1016/j.afres.2024.100616.

Ozkan, G., Franco, P., De Marco, I., Xiao, J., & Capanoglu, E. (2019). A review of microencapsulation methods for food antioxidants: Principles, advantages, drawbacks and applications. *Food chemistry, 272*, 494–506.

Patel, A. R., Heussen, P. C. M., & Velikov, K. P. (2012). Zein nanoparticles for omega-3 encapsulation. *Journal of Food Science, 77*(1), C1–C7. https://doi.org/10.1111/j.1750-3841.2011.02509.x.

Pattnaik, M., & Mishra, H. N. (2022). Amelioration of the stability of polyunsaturated fatty acids and bioactive enriched vegetable oil: Blending, encapsulation, and its application. *Critical Reviews in Food Science and Nutrition, 62*(23), 6253–6276. https://doi.org/10.1080/10408398.2021.1899127, https://www.tandfonline.com/loi/bfsn20.

Perez-Palacios, T., Ruiz-Carrascal, J., Solomando, J. C., de-la-Haba, F., Pajuelo, A., & Antequera, T. (2022). Recent developments in the microencapsulation of fish oil and natural extracts: Procedure, quality evaluation and food enrichment. *Foods, 11*(20), 3291. https://doi.org/10.3390/foods11203291.

Pham, L. B., Wang, B., Zisu, B., Truong, T., & Adhikari, B. (2020). Microencapsulation of flaxseed oil using polyphenol-adducted flaxseed protein isolate-flaxseed gum complex coacervates. *Food Hydrocolloids, 107*, 105944. https://doi.org/10.1016/j.foodhyd.2020.105944.

Ramos, O. L., Fernandes, J. C., Silva, S. I., Pintado, M. E., & Malcata, F. X. (2012). Edible films and coatings from whey proteins: A review on formulation, and on mechanical and bioactive properties. *Critical Reviews in Food Science and Nutrition, 52*(6), 533–552. https://doi.org/10.1080/10408398.2010.500528.

Rao, S., Radhakrishnan, P., Valiathan, S., & Supriya, M. (2023). Rosehip oil nanoemulsion as a stable delivery system for omega-3 fatty acids to enhance the nutritional value of yogurt. *Food Chemistry Advances, 3*, 100545. https://doi.org/10.1016/j.focha.2023.100545.

Réblová, Z. (2012). Effect of temperature on the antioxidant activity of phenolic acids. *Czech Journal of Food Sciences, 30*(2), 171–177. https://doi.org/10.17221/57/2011-cjfs, http://www.agriculturejournals.cz/publicFiles/60247.pdf.

Remila, L., Belcastro, E., Guenday-Tuereli, N., Park, S., Houngue, U., Vandamme, T., Tuereli, E., Kerth, P., Auger, C., & Schini-Kerth, V. (2021). Nanoencapsulation of the omega-3 EPA:DHA 6:1 formulation enhances and sustains NO-mediated endothelium-dependent relaxations in coronary artery rings and NO formation in endothelial cells. *Journal of Functional Foods, 87*, 104851. https://doi.org/10.1016/j.jff.2021.104851.

Repetto, M., Semprine, J., & Boveris, A. (2012). Lipid peroxidation: Chemical mechanism, biological implications and analytical determination. In A. Catala (Vol. Ed.), *Lipid peroxidation: Vol. 11*, (pp. 3–29). Web of Science. https://www.intechopen.com/books/advanced-biometric-technologies/liveness-detection-in-biometrics.

Rodríguez-Cortina, A., & Hernández-Carrión, M. (2023). Microcapsules of Sacha Inchi seed oil (*Plukenetia volubilis* L.) obtained by spray drying as a potential ingredient to formulate functional foods. *Food Research International, 170*, 113014. https://doi.org/10.1016/j.foodres.2023.113014.

Rozo, D. F., Alvarado, J. F., Chaparro, L. M., Medina, J. A., & Salcedo, F. (2024). Modeling oxidation kinetics of linseed oil in oxygen scavenger nanocapsules to be potentially used in active food packaging. *Food Packaging and Shelf Life, 42*. https://doi.org/10.1016/j.fpsl.2024.101256, https://www.sciencedirect.com/science/journal/22142894.

Rusli, J. K., Sanguansri, L., & Augustin, M. A. (2006). Stabilization of oils by microencapsulation with heated protein-glucose syrup mixtures. *Journal of the American Oil Chemists' Society, 83*(11), 965–972.

Sai, O. S., Aravind, U. K., & Aravindakumar, C. T. (2024). Pectin-based encapsulation systems for bioactive components. In *Biomaterials in microencapsulation*. IntechOpen. http://doi.org/10.5772/intechopen.1004742.

Salminen, H., Helgason, T., Kristinsson, B., Kristbergsson, K., & Weiss, J. (2013). Formation of solid shell nanoparticles with liquid ω-3 fatty acid core. *Food Chemistry, 141*(3), 2934–2943. https://doi.org/10.1016/j.foodchem.2013.05.120.

Saini, R. K., Prasad, P., Sreedhar, R. V., Akhilender Naidu, K., Shang, X., & Keum, Y. S. (2021). Omega– 3 polyunsaturated fatty acids (PUFAs): Emerging plant and microbial sources, oxidative stability, bioavailability, and health benefits—A review. *Antioxidants, 10*(10), 1627.

Santos, D. S., Morais, J. A. V., Vanderlei, Í. A. C., Santos, A. S., Azevedo, R. B., Muehlmann, L. A., Júnior, O. R. P., Mortari, M. R., da Silva, J. R., da Silva, S. W., & Longo, J. P. F. (2021). Oral delivery of fish oil in oil-in-water nanoemulsion: Development, colloidal stability and modulatory effect on in vivo inflammatory induction in mice. *Biomedicine and Pharmacotherapy, 133*. https://doi.org/10.1016/j.biopha.2020.110980, https://www.journals.elsevier.com/biomedicine-and-pharmacotherapy.

Santos-Sánchez, N. F., Salas-Coronado, R., Villanueva-Canongo, C., & Hernandez-Carlos, B. (2019). Antioxidant compounds and their antioxidant mechanism. In E. Shalaby (Ed.). *Antioxidants* (pp. 1). (1st ed.). Intech Open. https://doi.org/10.5772/intechopen.77838.

Schlotz, N., Ebert, D., & Martin-Creuzburg, D. (2013). Dietary supply with polyunsaturated fatty acids and resulting maternal effects influence host–parasite interactions. *BMC Ecology, 13*(1), 41.

Schuchardt, J. P., & Hahn, A. (2013). Bioavailability of long-chain omega-3 fatty acids. *Prostaglandins, Leukotrienes and Essential Fatty Acids, 89*(1), 1–8.

Seabra, C. L., Nunes, C., Gomez-Lazaro, M., Correia, M., Machado, J. C., Gonçalves, I. C., Reis, C. A., Reis, S., & Martins, M. C. L. (2017). Docosahexaenoic acid loaded lipid nanoparticles with bactericidal activity against Helicobacter pylori. *International Journal of Pharmaceutics, 519*, 128–137. https://doi.org/10.1016/j.ijpharm.2017.01.014.

Semo, E., Kesselman, E., Danino, D., & Livney, Y. D. (2007). Casein micelles for DHA encapsulation. *Food Hydrocolloids, 21*(5-6), 1–10. https://doi.org/10.1016/j.foodhyd.2006.07.006.

Serini, S., Cassano, R., Corsetto, P. A., Rizzo, A. M., Calviello, G., & Trombino, S. (2018). Omega-3 PUFA loaded in resveratrol-based solid lipid nanoparticles: Physicochemical properties and antineoplastic activities in human colorectal cancer cells in vitro. *International Journal of Molecular Sciences, 19*(2). https://doi.org/10.3390/ijms19020586, http://www.mdpi.com/1422-0067/19/2/586/pdf.

Sheybani, F., Rashidi, L., Nateghi, L., Yousefpour, M., & Mahdavi, S. K. (2023). Application of nanostructured lipid carriers containing α-tocopherol for oxidative stability enhancement of camelina oil. *Industrial Crops and Products, 202*, 117007. https://doi.org/10.1016/j.indcrop.2023.117007.

Simopoulos, A. P. (2006). Evolutionary aspects of diet, the omega-6/omega-3 ratio and genetic variation: Nutritional implications for chronic diseases. *Biomed Pharmacother, 60*(9), 502–507.

Singh, H., Kumar, Y., & Meghwal, M. (2022). Encapsulated oil powder: Processing, properties, and applications. *Journal of Food Process Engineering, 45*(8), e14047.

Soh, S. H., & Lee, L. Y. (2019). Microencapsulation and nanoencapsulation using supercritical fluid (SCF) techniques. *Pharmaceutics, 11*(1). https://doi.org/10.3390/pharmaceutics11010021, https://www.mdpi.com/1999-4923/11/1/21/pdf.

Song, Z., Zang, Z., Cao, Y., Ma, Y., Li, B., Han, L., & Yu, Q. (2025). Tapioca starch/konjac gum-based composite film incorporated with nanoliposomes encapsulated grape seed oil: Structure, functionality, controlled release and its preservation role for chilled mutton. *Food Chemistry, 463*(Pt 1), 141081. https://doi.org/10.1016/j.foodchem.2024.141081.

Sultana, A., Adachi, S., & Yoshii, H. (2023). Encapsulation of fish oil and essential fatty acids by spray drying. *Sustainable Food Technology, 1*(6), 827–836.

Suwannasang, S., Zhong, Q., Thumthanaruk, B., Vatanyoopaisarn, S., Uttapap, D., Puttanlek, C., & Rungsardthong, V. (2022). Physicochemical properties of yogurt fortified with microencapsulated Sacha Inchi oil. *Lwt, 161*, 113375.

Tao, L. (2015). Oxidation of polyunsaturated fatty acids and its impact on food quality and human health. *Advances in Food Technology and Nutritional Sciences, 1*(6), 135–142.

Timilsena, Y. P., Wang, B., Adhikari, R., & Adhikari, B. (2017). Advances in microencapsulation of polyunsaturated fatty acids (PUFAs)-rich plant oils using complex coacervation: A review. *Food Hydrocolloids, 69*, 369–381. https://doi.org/10.1016/j.foodhyd.2017.03.007, https://www.journals.elsevier.com/food-hydrocolloids.

Tontul, I., & Topuz, A. (2015). Microencapsulation of plant oils rich in alpha-linolenic acid: Effect of processing parameters. *Microencapsulation and Microspheres for Food Applications*, 253–269.

Uchôa, A. F. C., Formiga, A. L. D., Alves, Á. E. F., Cardoso, A. L. M. R., Pereira, G. Md. A., Carvalho, L. M. M., Silva, L. F. Ad, Pereira, P. Sd. S., Souza, P. H. Od, Jales, S. T. L., Silva, A. Le, Souza, R. R. Md, Sobral, M. V., Silva, M. Sd, Barbosa Filho, J. M., & Xavier-Júnior, F. H. (2025). Optimization and functionalization of copaiba oil-loaded nanostructured lipid carriers to improve cytotoxicity against breast cancer cells. *Journal of Drug Delivery Science and Technology, 105*. https://doi.org/10.1016/j.jddst.2024.106575, https://www.sciencedirect.com/science/journal/17732247.

Vilanculos, J. R. Z., de Farias, B. S., Engelmann, J. I., Ribeiro, E. S., de Oliveira, P. D., Jr, T. R. S. A. C., Pinto, L. A., & de, A. (2023). Physicochemical evaluation of chitosan-xanthan gum nanoemulsions as polyunsaturated enriched lipid-carrier. *Journal of Molecular Liquids, 386*, 122533. https://doi.org/10.1016/j.molliq.2023.122533.

Wang, Y., Li, J., & Zhou, B. (2018). Soy protein isolate for flaxseed oil encapsulation. *Food Chemistry, 245*, 1–10. https://doi.org/10.1016/j.foodchem.2017.10.092.

Yan, X., Li, M., Xu, X., Liu, X., & Liu, F. (2022). Zein-based nano-delivery systems for encapsulation and protection of hydrophobic bioactives: A review. *Frontiers in Nutrition, 9*. https://doi.org/10.3389/fnut.2022.999373.

Yang, M., Li, L., Zhu, X., Liang, L., Chen, J., Cao, W., Liu, W., Duan, X., Ren, G., & Liu, Z. (2024). Microencapsulation of fish oil by spray drying, spray freeze-drying, freeze-drying, and microwave freeze-drying: Microcapsule characterization and storage stability. *Journal of Food Science, 89*(6), 3276–3289. https://doi.org/10.1111/1750-3841.17098.

Yehye, W. A., Rahman, N. A., Ariffin, A., Abd Hamid, S. B., Alhadi, A. A., Kadir, F. A., & Yaeghoobi, M. (2015). Understanding the chemistry behind the antioxidant activities of butylated hydroxytoluene (BHT): A review. *European Journal of Medicinal Chemistry, 101*, 295–312. https://doi.org/10.1016/j.ejmech.2015.06.026, http://www.journals.elsevier.com/european-journal-of-medicinal-chemistry/.

Žanetić, M., Cerretani, L., Škevin, D., Perica, S., Vitanović, E., & Špika, M. J. (2012). Relationship between phenolic content and oxidative stability in Dalmatian virgin olive oils. In CEFood 2012 – Proceedings of the 6th Central European Congress on Food (pp. 74–79). University of Novi Sad, Faculty of Technology, Croatia.

Zheng, L., Xu, H., Zhang, H., Shi, C., Zhou, W., & Zhang, X. (2023). Nanostructured lipid carrier as a strategy for encapsulation of formononetin and perilla seed oil: In vitro characterization and stability studies. *Food Bioscience, 53*, 102707. https://doi.org/10.1016/j.fbio.2023.102707.

Zhuang, Y., Dong, J., He, X., Wang, J., Li, C., Dong, L., Zhang, Y., Zhou, X., Wang, H., Yi, Y., & Wang, S. (2022). Impact of heating temperature and fatty acid type on the formation of lipid oxidation products during thermal processing. *Frontiers in Nutrition, 9*. https://doi.org/10.3389/fnut.2022.913297.

Zimet, P., Rosenberg, D., & Livney, Y. D. (2011). Casein nanoparticles for DHA encapsulation. *Food Hydrocolloids, 25*(5), 1–10. https://doi.org/10.1016/j.foodhyd.2010.10.003.

Chapter 11

Docosahexaenoic acid and eicosapentaenoic acid in cardiovascular health: implications for functional food development

Monisha Prasad[1], Kalaiselvi Krishnamoorthy[2], Manoj Kumar Srinivasan[3], and Muthu Thiruvengadam[4]

[1]*Molecular Nutrition and Genomics Laboratory, Department of Community Medicine, Saveetha Medical College and Hospital, Saveetha Institute of Medical and Technical Sciences, Saveetha University, Chennai, Tamil Nadu, India,* [2]*Centre for Herbal Pharmacology and Environmental Sustainability, Chettinad Hospital and Research Institute, Chettinad Academy of Research and Education, Chennai, Tamil Nadu, India,* [3]*Saveetha Medical College, Saveetha Institute of Medical and Technical Science (SIMATS), Chennai, Tamil Nadu, India,* [4]*Department of Crop Science, College of Sanghuh Life Science, Konkuk University, Seoul, Republic of Korea*

11.1 Introduction

Cardiovascular diseases (CVDs) are the leading cause of death and illness across the world, and they claim millions of lives each year while continuing to be a major public health issue (Cesare et al., 2024; Global, regional, and national burden of cardiovascular diseases and risk factors in 204 countries and territories, 2025; Netala et al., 2024). In 2021, CVDs were responsible for nearly 20.5 million deaths, which is close to one-third of all deaths worldwide. This points to the growing burden of the disease on many different population groups (Cesare et al., 2024). Though CVDs were considered a problem of developed countries in the past, today more than 75% of CVD-related deaths are accounted for in low- and middle-income countries. This is because these areas have less access to health care, less effective preventive strategies, and are also exposed to more risk factors such as high blood pressure, diabetes, obesity, and smoking, which in combination contribute to this disproportionate distribution (Cesare et al., 2024; Netala et al., 2024). Apart from being a health problem, CVDs also impose a huge economic burden as they increase the cost of health care, reduce productivity, and pose an economic burden on families and countries (Netala et al., 2024).

In this situation, nondrug measures such as dietary and lifestyle changes have become important for preventing and managing CVD (Saina et al., 2023). Nutrition is known as one of the strongest factors affecting premature CVD outcomes, even more than quitting smoking or staying active (Yanru et al., 2025). Global dietary guidelines encourage the intake of fruits, vegetables, whole grains, legumes, and fish and advise limiting processed meats, saturated fats, and refined foods to lower cardiovascular risk (Yanru et al., 2025; Kerver et al., 2003). Plant-based foods, including fiber, nuts, fruits, and vegetables, consistently show protective effects. The Mediterranean diet is considered one of the best-supported eating patterns for reducing CVD risk factors and improving health outcomes (Chen et al., 2023).

Among targeted nutritional strategies, omega-3 polyunsaturated fatty acids (PUFAs), especially eicosapentaenoic acid (EPA) and docosahexaenoic acid (DHA) have gained strong scientific interest for their possible heart-protecting properties (Abdul Jabbar et al., 2026; Janani et al., 2023). These long-chain omega-3 fatty acids mainly come from marine food supplements and certain pharmaceutical products. Prospective cohort studies have linked them to reduced chances of coronary heart disease (CHD), heart attack, and death from heart conditions. They help improve triglyceride levels, inflammation, platelet function, and blood vessel health, which all contribute to these protective effects (Abdul Jabbar et al., 2026). However, the effectiveness of omega-3 supplementation in lowering major heart-related events is still debated. Randomized controlled trials and metaanalyses report mixed results and raise questions about dosage

Omega-3 and Omega-6 Polyunsaturated Fatty Acids in Food Systems. DOI: https://doi.org/10.1016/B978-0-443-43810-3.00008-7

formulation, initial dietary intake, and population-specific effects (Abdelhamid et al., 2018; Bernasconi et al., 2020; Le et al., 2023). The goal of this chapter is to explore the role of omega-3 PUFAs in heart health. It will evaluate current evidence on the ways they protect the heart and their effectiveness in treatment. Additionally, it clarifies how these fatty acids may be used in preventing and managing cardiovascular disease.

The biochemical profiles of DHA and EPA omega-3 and omega-6 fatty acids are two essential types of PUFAs needed for human health, and among omega-3s, EPA and DHA are considered the most important ones (Pal et al., 2020; Tomczyk et al., 2023). EPA and DHA are long-chain PUFAs, and they each have their first double bond located at the third carbon from the methyl end, which is typical of all n-3 PUFAs (Tomczyk et al., 2023). This specific structure allows them, once they are esterified, to fit into membrane phospholipids where they help change lipid raft dynamics, affect oxidative susceptibility, and influence cellular signaling and distribute cholesterol within cell membranes (Qin et al., 2023). Because humans lack the enzymes needed to create a double bond at the omega-3 position, these fatty acids must come from the diet. Alpha-linolenic acid (ALA), which is found in green leafy plants, nuts, seeds, and vegetable oils, acts as the precursor for EPA and DHA, yet the conversion process through several steps of desaturation and elongation is limited in humans (Sun et al., 2024; Tomczyk et al., 2023; Tocher et al., 2019). Marine algae are the main source of long-chain omega-3s, and these omega-3s accumulate in fish, which become the primary dietary source of EPA and DHA for humans (Harwood et al., 2019; Marrero et al., 2021). While both fish and humans can produce EPA and DHA in their bodies, the amount created is not enough to satisfy their needs, especially for DHA. The body creates DHA from EPA through the Sprecher pathway that includes elongation to a 24-carbon intermediate followed by chain shortening through beta oxidation (Tocher et al., 2019; Harwood et al., 2019).

Despite belonging to the same biochemical family, EPA and DHA differ greatly in how they are metabolized, distributed, and in their physiological functions (Choi & Calder, 2024; Russell & Bürgin-Maunder, 2012). Both compete to be included in membrane phospholipids, and this process pushes out omega-6 PUFAs that are common in Western diets, and the competition affects the production of inflammatory mediators and cell signaling (Pal et al., 2020). DHA is concentrated in brain and eye tissues, where it is essential for cognitive development and vision, while EPA cannot take on these roles (Tomczyk et al., 2023). Cardiovascularly, EPA and DHA help lower triglycerides, reduce blood pressure, improve endothelial function, and have antiinflammatory effects. They act as precursors to specialized pro-resolving mediators (SPMs), and these mediators boost macrophage phagocytic activity, help with clearing microbes, and promote tissue repair by resolving inflammation (Jo et al., 2025; Tomczyk et al., 2023). Omega-3 fatty acids, including EPA and DHA, also support angiogenesis by stimulating vascular endothelial cell growth and increasing levels of angiogenic factors like VEGF, bFGF, and angiopoietin 2 (Jo et al., 2025). Metabolically, EPA is less conserved since it converts to DHA and is more susceptible to beta oxidation or eicosanoid synthesis. In contrast, DHA is often retained in tissues and is more resistant to breakdown (Willora et al., 2020). Both fatty acids help protect the cardiovascular system, but recent studies suggest that DHA may be better than EPA at improving certain cardiometabolic risk markers, emphasizing the need to understand their individual biological effects (Choi & Calder, 2024; Tomczyk et al., 2023).

11.2 Mechanisms of action in cardiovascular protection

Omega-3 fatty acids display antiinflammatory actions through various molecular and cellular mechanisms, which are of great interest in cardiovascular protection (Table 11.1). After being incorporated into phospholipid membranes, omega-3 fatty acids alter the microdomain structure of membranes, affecting receptor aggregation and subsequent signaling pathways such as NF-κB, MAPK, and JAK/STAT activation. This results in decreased transcription of pro-inflammatory cytokines, adhesion molecules, and chemokines that mediate endothelial activation and leukocyte adhesion. Concomitantly, omega-3 fatty acids bind to nuclear receptors such as peroxisome proliferator-activated receptors (PPARs) and other lipid-sensing transcription factors, thus reprogramming gene expression to an antiinflammatory and cytoprotective phenotype. They also inhibit inflammasome and oxidative stress signaling, which limits vascular injury and smooth muscle cell proliferation. By modulating these cellular pathways, omega-3 fatty acids inhibit chronic vascular inflammation and interrupt atherogenesis at several critical steps (Fig. 11.1).

11.2.1 Antiinflammatory effects

DHA and EPA provide protection for the heart through several related mechanisms that affect the main physiological pathways involved in cardiovascular disease, but the way they act is not always fully clear (Fig. 11.1). Their strong antiinflammatory effects are important since chronic low-grade inflammation is a major factor in atherosclerosis and other heart issues (Netala et al., 2024). EPA and DHA influence inflammatory processes by competing with arachidonic acid for

TABLE 11.1 Cardioprotective mechanisms of eicosapentaenoic acid (EPA) and docosahexaenoic acid (DHA).

Mechanism	EPA/DHA effects	Outcome in cardiovascular health	References
Antiinflammatory activity	Compete with arachidonic acid; produce less inflammatory eicosanoids; form SPMs.	Reduces chronic inflammation and atherosclerosis progression.	Janani et al. (2023), Jo et al. (2025), Innes and Calder (2020)
Lipid modulation	↓ Triglycerides, ↑ HDL, and DHA increase LDL particle size.	Improves dyslipidemia and reduces atherogenic risk.	Choi and Calder (2024), Innes and Calder (2020)
Antithrombotic effect	Produces thromboxane A_3, a weak platelet aggregator.	Lowers thrombosis risk and prevents MI and stroke.	Janani et al. (2023), Innes and Calder (2020)
Vasodilation	Enhances nitric oxide availability and vasodilatory eicosanoids.	Improves vascular tone and reduces blood pressure.	Innes and Calder (2020)
Heart rate and arrhythmia control	Stabilizes myocardial membranes; reduces excitability.	Reduces risk of malignant arrhythmias and sudden cardiac death.	Innes and Calder (2020)
Endothelial protection and plaque stabilization	↓ Oxidative stress; ↑ collagen synthesis.	Stabilizes atherosclerotic plaques and prevents rupture.	Netala et al. (2024), Innes and Calder (2020)

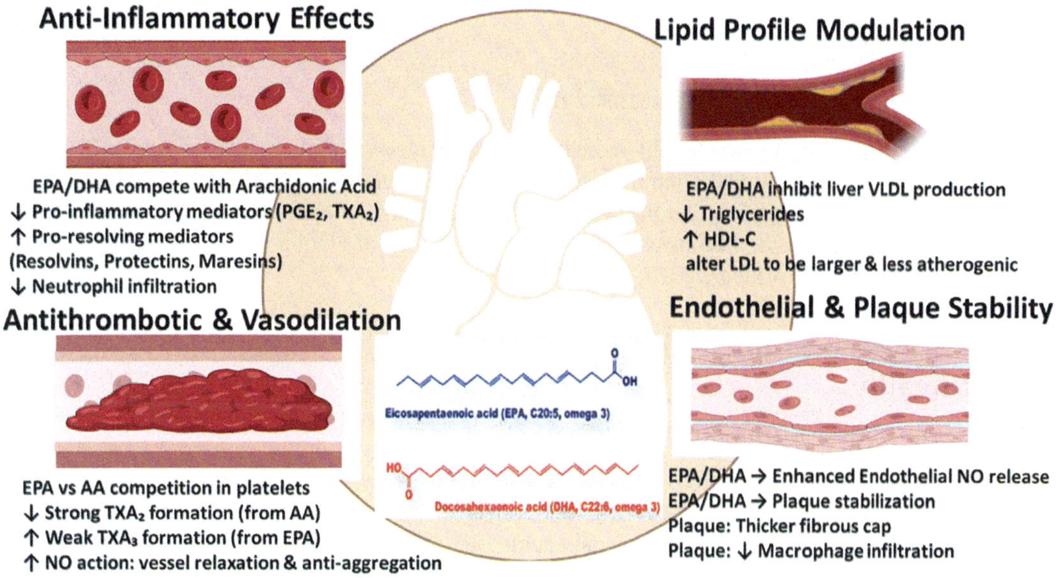

FIGURE 11.1 The synergistic cardioprotective effects of omega-3 fatty acids (eicosapentaenoic acid [EPA] and docosahexaenoic acid [DHA]) reduce overall cardiovascular risk. Some of these processes are the stabilization of cardiac electrophysiology, lipid-modulating activities, antithrombotic and vasodilatory properties, antiinflammatory effects, and improvements in endothelial function and plaque stability.

cyclooxygenase and lipoxygenase enzymes, and this competition shifts the production of eicosanoids from the pro-inflammatory thromboxane A2 and prostaglandin E2 to the less inflammatory thromboxane A3, prostaglandin E3 (Janani et al., 2023; Tomczyk et al., 2023). They also serve as starting points for SPMs such as resolvins, protectins, and maresins, which help to resolve inflammation by promoting debris clearance, reducing neutrophil infiltration, and improving tissue repair (Jo et al., 2025). Also, omega-3 fatty acids influence gene expression by activating PPARs, a process that suppresses pro-inflammatory genes and increases the activity of anti-inflammatory pathways (Janani et al., 2023).

11.2.2 Lipid profile modulation

EPA and DHA significantly improve dyslipidemia, which is a major risk factor for cardiovascular issues, but the degree of improvement can vary between individuals (Fig. 11.1). They lower plasma triglycerides by reducing hepatic VLDL production and increasing triglyceride clearance through improved lipoprotein lipase activity (Janani et al., 2023; Choi & Calder, 2024). Additionally, they raise HDL cholesterol, which helps transport cholesterol away from the arteries, and DHA often has a stronger effect than EPA in this area (Choi & Calder, 2024). While DHA may slightly increase LDL cholesterol, it changes the LDL particles into a larger and less harmful form, which in turn lowers the overall cardiovascular risk (Choi & Calder, 2024).

11.2.3 Antithrombotic and vasodilatory properties

Omega-3 fatty acids lower the risk of thrombosis by reducing platelet aggregation, although the extent of this effect may differ in some cases. EPA competes with arachidonic acid in platelet membranes, which results in the formation of thromboxane A3, a compound that is a much weaker platelet aggregator than thromboxane A2 and therefore reduces the chance of clot formation that can lead to myocardial infarction or stroke (Janani & Gopalakrishnan, 2023; Innes & Calder, 2020). DHA and EPA also help widen blood vessels by increasing the production of vasodilatory eicosanoids and improving the availability of nitric oxide, and this enhances vascular tone while lowering blood pressure (Innes & Calder, 2020).

11.2.4 Effects on heart rate and arrhythmias

EPA and DHA have a positive effect on heart function. They lower resting heart rate, stabilize heart cell membranes, and reduce stroke risk (Janani et al., 2023; Innes & Calder, 2020). Their interaction with heart ion channels reduces electrical excitability and decreases the chances of serious ventricular arrhythmias, which helps to lower the risk of sudden cardiac death (Innes & Calder, 2020).

11.2.5 Endothelial function and plaque stabilization

Omega-3 fatty acids improve endothelial function by increasing nitric oxide availability and lowering oxidative stress, this leads to better vascular relaxation and limits inflammatory cell adhesion (Innes & Calder, 2020). They also help stabilize plaque by reducing inflammation in atherosclerotic lesions, slowing down smooth muscle cell growth, and boosting collagen production. This strengthens the fibrous cap and lowers the chance of plaque rupture, which is a major cause of acute cardiovascular events (Innes & Calder, 2020; Netala et al., 2024).

11.3 Clinical evidence of docosahexaenoic acid and eicosapentaenoic acid in cardiovascular health

11.3.1 Epidemiological and prospective evidence

The cardioprotective potential of EPA and DHA has been studied thoroughly in clinical and population-based research, and this work provides a detailed understanding of their role in heart health. Long-term cohort studies consistently show that higher intake of fish, fatty fish, or marine omega-3 fatty acids EPA + DHA, along with higher blood or tissue levels of these fatty acids, is linked to lower risk of developing cardiovascular disease, including conditions such as CHD, heart attack, and overall cardiovascular death (Janani & Gopalakrishnan, 2023; Innes & Calder, 2020). These benefits come mainly from improvements in established cardiovascular risk factors, which include lowering triglycerides, reducing blood pressure, improving heart rate variability, decreasing platelet aggregation, enhancing endothelial function, and reducing chronic inflammation (Innes & Calder, 2020). However, these observational findings may be influenced by other lifestyle factors linked to high fish consumption, like better socioeconomic stability or healthier dietary habits, and this shows the complexity of proving direct cause and effect (Abdelhamid et al., 2018). Despite these factors, not eating enough seafood-based omega-3 fatty acids has been estimated to add significantly to the global burden of ischemic heart disease, highlighting their importance for public health (Abdelhamid et al., 2018).

11.3.2 Randomized clinical trials

Randomized clinical trials (RCTs) provide the highest level of clinical evidence; they have looked at EPA and DHA supplementation for both primary prevention of people without established CVD and secondary prevention of patients with known CVD or those at higher risk. Early RCTs showed clear cardiovascular benefits from omega-3 supplementation (Elagizi et al., 2021). However, more recent trials and metaanalyses have produced inconsistent results. This has led to ongoing debate about their effectiveness (Le et al., 2023; Tutor et al., 2024). Variability in outcomes is partly linked to factors like suboptimal dosing, often less than 1 g/day of EPA and DHA, and the common use of modern heart-protecting medications among trial participants (Elagizi et al., 2021). Targeted clinical trials in patients with diabetes, prediabetes, high cardiovascular risk, or existing CHD show potential benefits for both primary and secondary prevention outcomes (Natarajan et al., 2024; Tutor et al., 2024). Importantly, increasing evidence points to different physiological effects of EPA and DHA. Both reduce triglycerides and increase HDL cholesterol. However, DHA may lead to larger increases in HDL but can also raise LDL cholesterol; this happens while shifting towards larger, less harmful LDL particles. In contrast, EPA tends to have a neutral effect on LDL levels (Choi & Calder, 2024).

11.3.3 Metaanalyses and systematic reviews

Several large-scale RCTs, including STRENGTH and OMEMI, reported no significant reductions in major adverse cardiovascular events with EPA plus DHA supplementation. This is especially true at moderate doses of about 1.5 g/day, which continues to fuel ongoing controversy (Khan et al., 2021; Tutor et al., 2024). Some evidence suggests that trials using EPA alone lead to greater reductions in relative risk compared to those using combinations of EPA and DHA. This trend influenced recent clinical guidelines and gained attention following studies on purified EPA ethyl esters (Bhatt, 2022; Khan et al., 2021). However, conflicting results continue; several large-scale RCTs, including STRENGTH and OMEMI, reported no significant reductions in major adverse cardiovascular events with EPA + DHA supplementation, especially at moderate doses of about 1.5 g/day, this has led to ongoing debate (Khan et al., 2021; Tutor et al., 2024). In contrast, high-dose purified EPA 4 g/day led to a significant reduction in cardiovascular events, this suggest that dosage and formulation play a crucial role in treatment results (Bhatt, 2022; Elagizi et al., 2021; Yu et al., 2022).

11.3.4 Dosage considerations and safety profiles

Determining the best clinical dosage is crucial for getting the cardioprotective effect. Evidence shows that EPA and to some extent DHA produce more consistent benefits when given at higher doses, usually 2 g or more per day. This level has been linked to positive changes in cardiovascular risk markers (Choi & Calder, 2024; Tutor et al., 2024; Yan et al., 2022; Visioli & Poli, 2020). While omega-3 fatty acids are generally safe, high doses of 3 g or more per day can raise the risk of bleeding, especially in people on anticoagulant therapy; this situation needs careful clinical monitoring (Abdelhamid et al., 2018; Suwan, 2015). Most side effects are mild and relate to the stomach, such as nausea, diarrhea, and a fishy aftertaste. People with fish or shellfish allergies should be careful when using supplements made from marine sources (Barry et al., 2022). Overall, current clinical evidence shows that DHA and EPA can be helpful for heart health, though their effectiveness depends on the dose formulation and individual patient factors.

11.4 Functional food development: fortification with docosahexaenoic acid and eicosapentaenoic acid

11.4.1 Overview and rationale for fortification

The known health benefits of DHA and EPA, along with the common lack of omega-3 fatty acids in diets around the world, have spurred interest in adding EPA and DHA to functional foods as a public health strategy (Damerau et al., 2022; Hasan et al., 2023). Foods enriched with marine omega-3s offer an easy alternative to eating fish or taking supplements; they provide a simple way to boost daily intake through foods people regularly eat (Damerau et al., 2022). As consumer awareness of health-promoting foods continues to rise, the demand for omega-3-enriched products has expanded rapidly across international markets (Hasan et al., 2023).

11.4.2 Types of functional foods

Functional foods are a wide range of nutritional products that have physiological benefits beyond their nutritional value due to the actions of bioactive compounds in readily bioavailable and metabolically active forms. These foods can be naturally rich in health-promoting compounds, supplemented with targeted nutrients, or designed to improve functional properties by processing and technological manipulation. The biological activities of these foods are mediated through a variety of mechanisms, such as modulation of metabolism, improvement of gut microbiota, regulation of redox balance, and modulation of immune and endocrine systems. By combining bioactive lipids, peptides, probiotics, vitamins, minerals, and phytochemicals in familiar foods, the functional food groups provide a useful dietary approach to disease prevention, metabolic management, and sustained health maintenance (Fig. 11.2).

A wide variety of food products has been successfully used for DHA and EPA fortification to meet different consumer preferences (Table 11.2). Dairy items like milk and yogurt are a common choice because they are compatible and well accepted by consumers. Beverages such as fruit juices and drinkable mixes have also been effectively fortified (Castejón et al., 2021; Damerau et al., 2022; Hasan et al., 2023). Moreover, cereal and bakery products like bread, breakfast cereals, and cookies are becoming more popular for omega-3 enrichment (Hasan et al., 2023; Ye et al., 2018). Other fortified products include spreads, sauces, and special formulas like infant formulas. This shows the variety of food systems that can deliver omega-3 (Liu et al., 2022; Lv & Xu, 2022). The increasing availability of these fortified items highlights the growing market for n-3 PUFA products (Fig. 11.2) (Hasan et al., 2023).

11.4.3 Microencapsulation and delivery systems

A major challenge in adding DHA and EPA to food is their high vulnerability to oxidation, which can cause nutrient loss off-flavors, and possibly harmful byproducts (Damerau et al., 2022; Wang et al., 2021; Venugopalan et al., 2021; Wang, Ossemond, et al., 2022; Wang, Zheng, et al., 2022). To tackle this issue, microencapsulation technologies are crucial in protecting omega-3 fatty acids. Microencapsulation coats omega-3 oils in a protective shell, which keeps them safe from oxygen, light, and metal ions. As a result, it improves oxidative stability, extends shelf life, and hides unpleasant sensory qualities (Castejón et al., 2021; Comunian & Fávaro-Trindade, 2016; Pérez-Palacios et al., 2022). It also allows the conversion of liquid oils into powder form, which improves how well they mix into different food products and makes them easier to use on a large scale (Comunian & Fávaro-Trindade, 2016; Kumar et al., 2024; Venugopalan et al., 2021). Spray drying is the most common industrial method because it is cost-effective and works well with heat-sensitive compounds (Kaushik et al., 2014; Melgosa et al., 2020). In addition to microencapsulation, nanoencapsulation, and emulsification, create smaller, more stable particles or oil-in-water mixtures. These techniques improve the solubility, stability, and bioaccessibility of omega-3s (Henao-Ardila et al., 2024; Venugopalan et al., 2021). Emulsion-based systems are especially useful for adding DHA-rich oils to water-based food products. They can also be spray dried for easier storage (Venugopalan et al., 2021; Wang, Ossemond, et al., 2022; Wang, Zheng, et al., 2022). The choice of wall

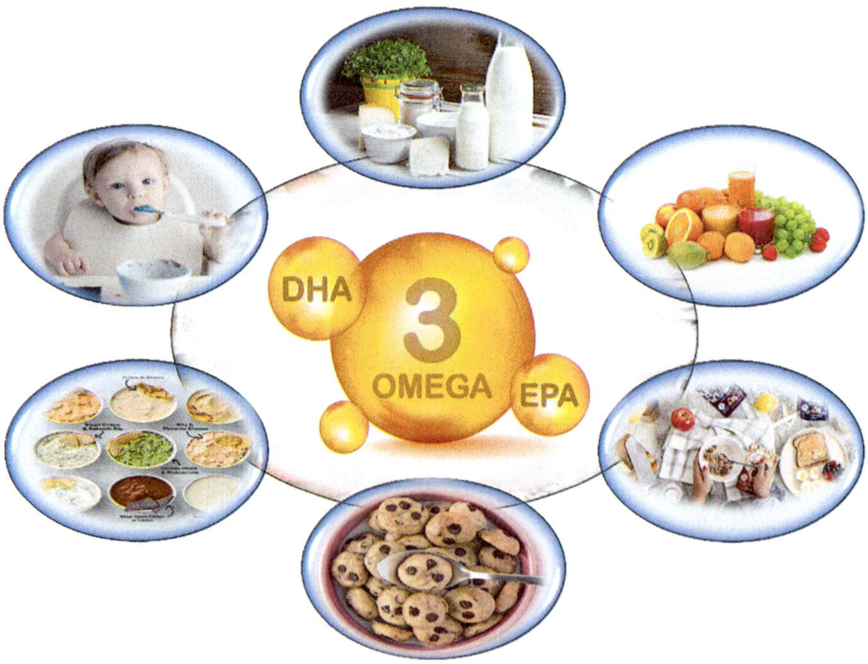

FIGURE 11.2 Different forms of food enriched with docosahexaenoic acid (DHA) and eicosapentaenoic acid (EPA). Foods like milk, yogurts, fresh fruit juices, bakery products, spreads, sauces, and special formulas like infant formulas are fortified with EPA and DHA.

TABLE 11.2 Functional food applications of docosahexaenoic acid (DHA) and eicosapentaenoic acid (EPA).

Category	Types of products	Advantages	Challenges	References
Dairy products	Milk and yogurt	Good incorporation; high consumer acceptance.	Oxidation risk and flavor issues.	Hasan et al. (2023), Damerau et al. (2022), Castejón et al. (2021)
Beverages	Juice-based drinks and emulsions	Easy fortification using emulsifiers.	Poor water solubility of DHA.	Castejón et al. (2021), Lv and Xu (2022)
Bakery and cereals	Bread, cookies, and cereals	Stable when microencapsulated.	Requires strong encapsulation.	Ye et al. (2018), Melgosa et al. (2020)
Infant formulas	DHA-rich algal oils	Supports brain and retinal development.	High production cost.	Lv and Xu (2022), Sehl et al. (2022)
Specialized health foods	Bars, spreads, and fortified powders	High stability and convenience.	Sensory masking required.	Pérez-Palacios et al. (2022), Kumar et al. (2024)
Encapsulated powders	Spray-dried DHA/EPA microcapsules	High shelf life and easy mixing with foods.	Expensive microencapsulation technologies.	Kumar et al. (2024)

materials, often proteins or polysaccharides, greatly affects encapsulation efficiency and oxidative resistance. This makes formulation science an important part of product development (Damerau et al., 2022; Du et al., 2022).

11.4.4 Stability, bioavailability, and sensory challenges

Despite the technological advancements, stability and sensory problems remain major issues in the addition of DHA and EPA to food. This is because they are highly prone to oxidation due to their polyunsaturated chemical nature, which results in off-flavors and rancidity, thus affecting consumer acceptance (Damerau et al., 2022; García-Moreno, 2017; Venugopalan et al., 2021). It has been observed in various studies that the oxidation levels are high in commercial fish oil supplements, thus pointing towards the need for improved stability strategies (Venugopalan et al., 2021). Food processing, such as frying, also results in increased oxidation and reduced bioavailability (Alijani et al., 2024). Sensory challenges such as a typical "fishy" smell and taste create extra obstacles, especially in foods with neutral or delicate flavors (Damerau et al., 2022; Wang, Ossemond, et al., 2022; Wang, Zheng, et al., 2022). How much of a nutrient gets absorbed can vary based on food structure, how it is packaged, and the level of oxidation. This makes improving the delivery systems important (Alijani et al., 2024; Venugopalan et al., 2021). Water solubility adds to the limitations since DHA does not mix well with water; this makes it hard to add to drinks and other water-based products (Lv & Xu, 2022). Changing oils into a powder form through encapsulation helps with handling, storage, and mixing into various food products (Venugopalan et al., 2021).

11.4.5 Regulatory frameworks and health claims

Fortification with DHA and EPA is controlled by strict regulations to protect consumers and ensure the scientific validity of health claims. Organizations like the European Food Safety Authority (EFSA) and the U.S. Food and Drug Administration (FDA) review and approve claims about omega-3 benefits (Liu & Lin, 2024). In the EU, foods can label themselves as a "source of omega-3 fatty acids" if they have at least 40 mg of EPA and DHA per 100 g and per 100 kcal. They can also use the approved health claim "EPA and DHA contribute to the normal function of the heart" with a daily intake of 250 mg EPA + DHA (Elvevoll et al., 2023). The FDA permits some qualified health claims that associate omega-3 consumption with a reduced risk of CHD, but these health claims must be drafted very carefully because of the scientific variability that is involved (Hasan et al., 2023). Obtaining regulatory approval requires scientific evidence that ensures the health claims are a true reflection of the scientific benefits (Kušar et al., 2021; Liu & Lin, 2024). Still, the whole regulatory process can be expensive and time-consuming for manufacturers, especially since the guidelines have to continuously change with new research coming out (Hasan et al., 2023; Kušar et al., 2021). Given widespread suboptimal omega-3 intake, ongoing efforts to strengthen compliance and update labeling standards remain a high priority in global nutrition policy (Fuentes et al., 2024).

11.5 Emerging trends and innovations

11.5.1 Plant-based and algal docosahexaenoic acid/eicosapentaenoic acid sources

Growing demand for omega-3 fatty acids, along with concerns about marine resource sustainability, environmental pollutants, and the rising popularity of plant-based diets, has sparked significant interest in alternative sources of DHA and EPA (Derbyshire et al., 2024; Sehl et al., 2022). Microalgae, the main producers of omega-3 PUFAs in marine ecosystems, are one of the most promising sustainable and vegan sources of high-quality DHA and EPA (Oliver et al., 2020; Rizzo et al., 2025). Cultivated in controlled conditions, microalgae reduce oxidative damage and eliminate the variability and contamination risks linked to fish oils (Derbyshire et al., 2024; Kunj et al., 2025; Sehl et al., 2022). Developments in biotechnology, including genetic engineering, are increasing algal yields and lowering production costs. This strengthens their potential as large-scale sources of omega-3 (Kunj et al., 2025; Qin et al., 2023). Microalgal oils also solve the supply issues of capture fisheries and tackle environmental and sustainability concerns (Qin et al., 2023). Genetically modified oilseed plants that can synthesize EPA and DHA directly are becoming an important source to overcome the limitations of traditional plant-based omega-3s like ALA, which is not efficiently converted to long-chain PUFAs in humans (Bailey et al., 2024). Yeasts and fungi also provide alternative biotechnological options for sustainable omega-3 production (Rollin et al., 2023). These innovations are crucial for addressing increasing global nutritional demands, especially as fishery outputs level off and the population grows quickly (Bailey et al., 2024).

11.5.2 Nanotechnology and emulsification in food matrices

As DHA and EPA are very sensitive to oxidation and do not dissolve well in water-based food systems, new nanotechnology and emulsification methods are important for improving their stability, bioavailability, and function in fortified foods (Henao-Ardila et al., 2024; Prieto & Lagaron, 2024). Nanoencapsulation, which involves enclosing omega-3 oils in nanoparticles, offers better protection against oxidation; it also hides unwanted tastes, improves how these nutrients are released, and boosts their bioavailability in food, nutraceutical, and pharmaceutical uses (McClements & Öztürk, 2021; Prieto & Lagaron, 2024). Beyond nanoencapsulation, new emulsion systems are also becoming important. These include simple and multiple lipid emulsions, solid lipid nanoparticles, and self-assembling delivery systems. These systems aim to incorporate lipophilic omega-3 fatty acids into water-based foods while improving dispersion and stability (Perez et al., 2021). Better emulsification allows DHA and EPA to mix well in water-based products, which expands the types of food that can be fortified (Henao-Ardila et al., 2024). Additionally, turning emulsion-based or colloidal systems into powder using methods like spray drying makes handling, storage, and shelf stability easier, which helps with commercial use (Venugopalan et al., 2021).

11.5.3 Personalized nutrition and nutrigenomics

Personalized nutrition, which customizes dietary advice based on a person's genetic and physical traits, is changing the future of omega-3 research and dietary guidance (Lagoumintzis & Patrinos, 2023). Nutrigenomics studies how genetic differences affect nutrient metabolism. This shows a significant range of individual responses to omega-3 supplementation (Lagoumintzis & Patrinos, 2023; Wang, Ossemond, et al., 2022; Wang, Zheng, et al., 2022). Polymorphisms in genes that encode fatty acid desaturase FADS and elongase ELOVL enzymes play a key role in producing long-chain PUFA and influencing levels of DHA and EPA in the blood. These genetic differences can affect lipid responses such as the reduction of triglycerides after omega-3 intake (Babu et al., 2024; Hong et al., 2023; Keathley et al., 2022a, 2022b). As we learn more about these gene nutrient interactions, personalized nutrition strategies based on genotype are becoming more common. These strategies can provide tailored recommendations for EPA and DHA, which may help prevent and manage chronic diseases like cardiovascular disease CVD (Jujjavarapu et al., 2024; Wang, Ossemond, et al., 2022; Wang, Zheng, et al., 2022). Multiomics approaches that combine genomic, metabolomic, and lipidomic profiles are being studied to better predict how individuals respond to supplementation (Morin-Bernier et al., 2024). Despite its potential, challenges exist; there is a need for scientifically validated nutrigenetic tests and easy-to-understand interpretation tools for consumers and clinicians, which hinder widespread adoption (Almeida et al., 2019; Keathley et al., 2022a, 2022b).

11.5.4 Sustainability and consumer acceptance

Sustainability and consumer views are increasingly influencing omega-3 production and product development. Environmental issues linked to the usual marine omega-3 sources, including overfishing, habitat loss, and contamination from pollutants like heavy metals and microplastics have shown the need for more sustainable options (Bhashira & Gopalakrishnan, 2025; Derbyshire et al., 2024; Karageorgou et al., 2023). At the same time, rising consumer interest in ethically sourced, eco-friendly, and health-boosting products has pushed the shift toward plant-based and algal omega-3 sources (Nazzaro et al., 2025; Sehl et al., 2022). Consumer health awareness, together with the rise of vegetarianism and veganism, is raising the demand for sustainably sourced functional foods that contain EPA and DHA (Subramani et al., 2023). The global omega-3 market is expected to grow, with much of this growth likely coming from newer sustainable sources like algal oils, fungal oils, and engineered plants (Oliver et al., 2020; Rollin et al., 2023). Clear and trustworthy labeling, along with scientifically backed health information, plays a key role in shaping buying habits and building consumer trust (Nazzaro et al., 2025). Consumers are likely to spend more on functional foods if they perceive the health benefits as credible, although more research is required to identify the factors that influence consumer choices with regard to sustainability (Subramani et al., 2023).

11.6 Challenges and future directions

11.6.1 Bioavailability enhancement

Bioavailability optimization of DHA and EPA remains a large challenge even with the latest developments in delivery technologies. The absorption process can differ depending on a number of variables, such as the chemical structure, for example, triglycerides and ethyl esters, food interactions, processing, and the presence of any dietary fat at the time of administration (Alijani et al., 2024; Chuang et al., 2023). Microencapsulation and nanoencapsulation techniques are crucial in protecting omega-3 fatty acids from oxidation. The techniques are also useful in concealing any undesirable sensory properties and improving the delivery and stability of omega-3s in fortified foods (Homroy et al., 2023; Kumar et al., 2024). The technologies convert unstable oils into more stable food-grade products for various applications (Venugopalan et al., 2021). Emulsification systems, including self-emulsifying drug delivery systems, have demonstrated promising outcomes in enhancing the digestion and absorption of omega-3 fatty acids in the gastrointestinal tract (Chuang et al., 2023). Future research will probably concentrate on newer encapsulation and controlled release technology to ensure maximum absorption and prevent degradation during processing, storage, and digestion (Homroy et al., 2023; Lv & Xu, 2022). Omega-3 bioavailability enhancement is essential to ensure that fortified foods offer clinical benefits.

11.6.2 Consumer education and labeling

Consumer acceptance and understanding of omega-3 fortified foods remain a factor in their market success. Although awareness about the health benefits of long-chain omega-3 PUFAs is on the rise, their consumption remains low in many segments due to a lack of consumer facts (Derbyshire et al., 2024). Consumers are more likely to adopt and use functional ingredients if they are aware of the health relevance and know the source of the nutrient (Ramalho et al., 2021). Health claim regulations, such as those by EFSA and FDA, ensure that these claims are scientifically valid and communicated accurately. This helps avoid the spread of misinformation and helps build consumer trust (Fuentes et al., 2024). As new scientific evidence emerges, these regulations and health claims must be regularly updated to reflect the current status of evidence and maintain transparency in labeling (Hasan et al., 2023; Karapanou et al., 2024). Initiatives for front-of-pack labeling are also being pilot-tested to enable consumers to make more informed choices and promote healthier purchasing practices. This remains an important area for future public health action (Penzavecchia et al., 2022; Sumathy & Gopalakrishnan, 2022). Communication and consistent messaging are critical to counter misinformation and improve public understanding of the health benefits of omega-3 fatty acids.

11.6.3 Cost-effectiveness in product development

Economic hurdles remain a significant challenge in the inclusion of DHA and EPA in food items. Conventional marine-derived omega-3 and other novel sources, such as microalgae, are often associated with high production costs, which is a significant barrier to their use (Qin et al., 2023). Studies on microalgae biodiesel and oil production can often reveal high production costs, thus indicating the need for better production systems (Javed et al., 2019). Novel biorefinery concepts that can isolate high-value omega-3 oils from microalgal biomass and utilize the remaining parts for lower-value applications, such as animal feed ingredients, provide novel approaches to improve economic viability (Sarker et al., 2020). Ensuring that omega-3 production is both sustainable and economically viable is crucial, as the demand for these compounds continues to rise with increased pressure on marine resources (Rollin et al., 2023; Shepon et al., 2022). Process optimization approaches, such as integrating supercritical fluid extraction into production processes that also isolate multiple products, may provide approaches to make these alternative production methods more competitive by increasing efficiency and value recovery (Maschmeyer et al., 2020).

11.6.4 Integration with other nutraceuticals for synergistic effects

Nutrient synergy is an area that needs to be explored further. A combination of bioactive compounds could potentially offer better health benefits than individual nutrients. A combination of omega-3 fatty acids with complementary nutraceuticals could potentially enhance bioavailability, stability, and biological activity (Leena et al., 2020). For instance, a combination of fish oil-derived omega-3 fatty acids with polyphenols has been found to have enhanced antioxidant and antiinflammatory properties. This is an indication that they may potentially offer more significant metabolic and cardiovascular benefits (Méndez & Medina, 2021). A combination of omega-3 fatty acids with extended-release niacin has also been found to have enhanced effects on lipid profiles, indicating potential benefits in reducing cardiovascular risk (Townsend et al., 2023). Furthermore, marine-derived bioactive compounds such as peptides, polysaccharides, and carotenoids have been found to have additive or synergistic effects with omega-3 fatty acids in reducing markers of oxidative stress, inflammation, and obesity (Ebrahimi et al., 2023). Further research and development in synergistic formulation may lead to the development of more potent multitargeted functional foods that may potentially address complex chronic diseases such as cardiovascular disease and metabolic syndrome. This is a promising frontier for next-generation nutraceutical development and functional food innovation.

11.7 Conclusion

EPA and DHA are very well known for their importance to heart health. Many studies have shown that they can reduce inflammation, improve lipid profiles, help blood vessel function, and prevent blood clots, all of which can help reduce the risk of serious heart issues. However, despite these benefits, the worldwide consumption of EPA and DHA is still not enough, which is a serious public health concern. Food fortification with omega-3 fatty acids is a simple way to address this nutritional deficiency, and there is a growing consumer interest in simple health-promoting products. However, there are still a few challenges that need to be addressed, such as the instability of these fatty acids when they are exposed to air, which requires technologies such as microencapsulation to maintain their quality and efficacy. In the future, sustainable sourcing from microalgae, improved delivery systems, personalized nutrition plans, and combining them with other health products could bring about some exciting new developments. Improving consumer education and clear labeling will also help more people accept and benefit from omega-3 fortified foods.

References

Abdelhamid, A. S., Brown, T. J., Brainard, J. S., Biswas, P., Thorpe, G. C., Moore, H. J., Deane, K. H. O., AlAbdulghafoor, F. K., Summerbell, C. D., Worthington, H. V., Song, F., & Hooper, L. (2018). Omega-3 fatty acids for the primary and secondary prevention of cardiovascular disease. *Cochrane Database of Systematic Reviews, 7*(7). https://doi.org/10.1002/14651858.cd003177.pub3.

Abdul Jabbar, A. B., Naeem, U., Zulfiqar, K., Ahmed, S., Inam, M., Hinkamp, C., et al. (2026). Highlights of cardiovascular disease prevention studies presented at the 2025 American Heart Association Scientific Sessions. *Current Atherosclerosis Reports, 28*, 7. https://doi.org/10.1007/s11883-025-01376-x.

Alijani, S., Hahn, A., Harris, W., & Schuchardt, J. P. (2024). Bioavailability of EPA and DHA in humans – A comprehensive review. *Progress in Lipid Research, 97*, 101318. https://doi.org/10.1016/j.plipres.2024.101318.

Almeida, V. A., Littlejohn, P., Cop, I., Brown, E., Afroze, R., & Davison, K. M. (2019). Comparison of nutrigenomics technology interface tools for consumers and health professionals: A sequential explanatory mixed methods investigation. *Journal of Medical Internet Research, 21*(6), Available from https://doi.org/10.2196/12580, https://www.jmir.org/2019/6/e12580/PDF.

Babu, S. V., Ramya, P., & Gracewell, J. (2024). Revolutionizing heart disease prediction with quantum-enhanced machine learning. *Scientific Reports, 14*, 7453. https://doi.org/10.1038/s41598-024-55991-w.

Bailey, E., Wojcik, J., Rahn, M., Roos, F., Spooren, A., & Koshibu, K. (2024). *Microalgal oil as an alternative source of essential nutrients omega-3 DHA and EPA*. undefined: Research Square. Available from https://doi.org/10.21203/rs.3.rs-5111519/v1, https://www.researchsquare.com/browse.

Barry, A. R., Bishop, K. E., Pearson, G. J., Koshman, S. L., et al. (2022). Omega-3 fatty acids for cardiovascular disease prevention: A practice tool for pharmacists. *Canadian Pharmacists Journal / Revue des Pharmaciens du Canada, 155*(3), 169–174. 10.1177/17151635221087639.

Bernasconi, A., Wiest, M. M., Lavie, C. J., Milani, R. V., & Laukkanen, J. A. (2020). Effect of omega-3 dosage on cardiovascular outcomes. *Mayo Clinic Proceedings, 96*(2), 304. https://doi.org/10.1016/j.mayocp.2020.08.034.

Bhashira, R., & Gopalakrishnan, S. (2025). The association between seafood consumption and non-seafood consumption with serum levels of non-HDL cholesterol. *Romanian Journal of Diabetes, Nutrition and Metabolic Diseases, 32*(2), 180–186. Available from https://doi.org/10.46389/rjd-2025-1610, http://www.rjdnmd.org/index.php/RJDNMD/article/view/1610.

Bhatt, D. L. (2022). Substantial impact of eicosapentaenoic acid on cardiovascular outcomes in the REDUCE-IT Trial. *CardioMetabolic Syndrome Journal, 2*(1), 22. https://doi.org/10.51789/cmsj.2022.2.e3.

Castejón, N., Luna, P., & Señoráns, F. J. (2021). Microencapsulation by spray drying of omega-3 lipids extracted from oilseeds and microalgae: Effect on polyunsaturated fatty acid composition. *LWT, 148*, 111789. https://doi.org/10.1016/j.lwt.2021.111789.

Chen, W., Zhang, S., Hu, X., Chen, F., Li, D., et al. (2023). A review of healthy dietary choices for cardiovascular disease: From individual nutrients and foods to dietary patterns. *Nutrients, 15*(23), 4898. 10.3390/nu15234898.

Cesare, M. D., Perel, P., Taylor, S., Kabudula, C., Bixby, H., Gaziano, T. A., et al. (2024). The heart of the world. *Global Heart, 19*(1). https://doi.org/10.5334/gh.1288.

Choi, G. Y., & Calder, P. C. (2024). The differential effects of eicosapentaenoic acid and docosahexaenoic acid on cardiovascular risk factors: An updated systematic review of randomized controlled trials. *Frontiers in Nutrition, 11*. Available from https://doi.org/10.3389/fnut.2024.1423228, journal.frontiersin.org/journal/nutrition.

Chuang, J., Briskey, D., Dang, J., Rajgopal, A., Rao, A., et al. (2023). A randomized double-blind trial to measure the absorption characteristics of eicosapentaenoic acid and docosahexaenoic acid rich oil blend with natural lipid-based delivery system. *Food Science and Biotechnology, 33*(8), 1957. https://doi.org/10.1007/s10068-023-01466-z.

Comunian, T. A., & Favaro-Trindade, C. S. (2016). Microencapsulation using biopolymers as an alternative to produce food enhanced with phytosterols and omega-3 fatty acids: A review. *Food Hydrocolloids, 61*, 442–457. 10.1016/j.foodhyd.2016.06.003.

Damerau, A., Mustonen, S. A., Ogrodowska, D., Varjotie, L., Brandt, W., Laaksonen, O., Tańska, M., & Linderborg, K. M. (2022). Food fortification using spray-dried emulsions of fish oil produced with maltodextrin, plant and whey proteins—effect on sensory perception, volatiles and storage stability. *Molecules, 27*(11), 3553. https://doi.org/10.3390/molecules27113553.

Derbyshire, E. J., Birch, C. S., Bonwick, G. A., English, A., Metcalfe, P., & Li, W. (2024). Optimal omegas – barriers and novel methods to narrow omega-3 gaps. A narrative review. *Frontiers in Nutrition, 11*. https://doi.org/10.3389/fnut.2024.1325099.

Du, Q., Zhou, L., Li, M., Lyu, F., Liu, J., Ding, Y., et al. (2022). Omega-3 polyunsaturated fatty acid encapsulation system: Physical and oxidative stability, and medical applications. *Food Frontiers, 3*(2), 239–255. 10.1002/fft2.134.

Ebrahimi, B., Baroutian, S., Li, J., Zhang, B., Ying, T., & Lu, J. (2023). Combination of marine bioactive compounds and extracts for the prevention and treatment of chronic diseases. *Frontiers in Nutrition, 9*. https://doi.org/10.3389/fnut.2022.1047026.

Elagizi, A., Lavie, C. J., O'keefe, E., Marshall, K., O'keefe, J. H., & Milani, R. V. (2021). An update on omega-3 polyunsaturated fatty acids and cardiovascular health. *Nutrients, 13*(1), 1–12. Available from https://doi.org/10.3390/nu13010204, https://www.mdpi.com/2072-6643/13/1/204/pdf.

Elvevoll, E. O., Eilertsen, K. E., Aschan, M., & Bandarra, N. M. (2023). New marine low trophic resources as food: Nutritional and food safety aspects. *Frontiers in Aquaculture, 2*. Available from https://doi.org/10.3389/faquc.2023.1254038, www.frontiersin.org/journals/aquaculture.

Fuentes, J. B., Beara, I., & Torović, L. (2024). Regulatory compliance of health claims on omega-3 fatty acid food supplements. *Foods, 14*(1), 67. https://doi.org/10.3390/foods14010067.

Global, regional, and national burden of cardiovascular diseases and risk factors in 204 countries and territories. (2025). 1990–2023. *Journal of the American College of Cardiology*. https://doi.org/10.1016/j.jacc.2025.08.015.

Hasan, D. S., Arief, Y. S., & Sangadji, S. S. (2023). Functional foods and their implications for health promotion. *Journal of Nutrition Education and Behavior, 55*(10), 769. https://doi.org/10.1016/j.jneb.2023.07.001.

Harwood, J. (2019). Algae: Critical sources of very long-chain polyunsaturated fatty acids. *Biomolecules, 9*(11), 708. 10.3390/biom9110708.

Henao-Ardila, A., Quintanilla-Carvajal, M. X., & Moreno, F. L. (2024). Emulsification and stabilisation technologies used for the inclusion of lipophilic functional ingredients in food systems. *Heliyon, 10*(11). https://doi.org/10.1016/j.heliyon.2024.e32150.

Homroy, S., Chopra, R., Singh, P. K., Dhiman, A., Chand, M., & Talwar, B. (2023). Role of encapsulation on the bioavailability of omega-3 fatty acids. *Comprehensive Reviews in Food Science and Food Safety, 23*(1). https://doi.org/10.1111/1541-4337.13272.

Hong, B. V., Agus, J. K., Tang, X., Zheng, J. J., Romo, E. Z., Lei, S., & Zivkovic, A. M. (2023). Precision nutrition and cardiovascular disease risk reduction: The promise of high-density lipoproteins. *Current Atherosclerosis Reports, 25*(10), 663–677. Available from https://doi.org/10.1007/s11883-023-01148-5, https://www.springer.com/journal/11883.

Innes, J. K., & Calder, P. C. (2020). Marine omega-3 (N-3) fatty acids for cardiovascular health: An update for 2020. *International Journal of Molecular Sciences, 21*(4), Available from https://doi.org/10.3390/ijms21041362, https://www.mdpi.com/1422-0067/21/4/1362/pdf.

Janani, J., Lakshmanan, K., & Gopalakrishnan, S. (2023). Unveiling the atherogenic lipoprotein particle: A case-control study. *Romanian Journal of Diabetes, Nutrition and Metabolic Diseases, 30*(4), 398–402. Available from https://doi.org/10.46389/rjd-2023-1384, http://www.rjdnmd.org/index.php/RJDNMD/article/view/1384/837.

Javed, F., Aslam, M., Rashid, N., Shamair, Z., Khan, A. L., Yasin, M., Fazal, T., Hafeez, A., Rehman, F., Rehman, M. S. U., Khan, Z., Iqbal, J., & Bazmi, A. A. (2019). Microalgae-based biofuels, resource recovery and wastewater treatment: A pathway towards sustainable biorefinery. *Fuel, 255*, 115826. https://doi.org/10.1016/j.fuel.2019.115826.

Jo, S., Hwangbo, H., Francis, N., Lee, J. Y., Pei, M., & Kim, G. H. (2025). Fish-derived biomaterials for tissue engineering: Advances in scaffold fabrication and applications in regenerative medicine and cancer therapy. *Theranostics, 15*(12), 5666–5692. https://doi.org/10.7150/thno.109186.

Jujjavarapu, M., Narasimhan, M., Rathinam, S., & Balasubramanian, S. (2024). Screening for chronic obstructive pulmonary disease in patients with coronary artery disease at a tertiary care hospital. *International Journal of Experimental Research and Review, 41*(Spl Vol), 120–129. https://doi.org/10.52756/ijerr.2024.v41spl.010.

Kerver, J. M., Yang, E. J., Bianchi, L., Song, W. O., et al. (2003). Dietary patterns associated with risk factors for cardiovascular disease in healthy US adults. *The American Journal of Clinical Nutrition, 78*(6), 1103–1110. 10.1093/ajcn/78.6.1103.

Karageorgou, D., Rova, U., Christakopoulos, P., Katapodis, P., Matsakas, L., & Patel, A. (2023). Benefits of supplementation with microbial omega-3 fatty acids on human health and the current market scenario for fish-free omega-3 fatty acid. *Trends in Food Science and Technology, 136*, 169–180. Available from https://doi.org/10.1016/j.tifs.2023.04.018, http://www.elsevier.com/wps/find/journaldescription.cws_home/601278/description#description.

Karapanou, V., Arndt-Bascle, C., & Toktosunova, F. (2024). Regulatory governance of large-scale food fortification. *OECD. Regulatory Policy Working Papers*. https://doi.org/10.1787/b1e00dfb-en.

Kaushik, P., Dowling, K., Barrow, C. J., & Adhikari, B. (2014). Microencapsulation of omega-3 fatty acids: Review of microencapsulation and characterization methods. *Journal of Functional Foods, 19*, 868. https://doi.org/10.1016/j.jff.2014.06.029.

Keathley, J., Garneau, V., Marcil, V., Mutch, D. M., Robitaille, J., Rudkowska, I., et al. (2022a). Nutrigenetics, omega-3 and plasma lipids/lipoproteins/apolipoproteins with evidence evaluation using the GRADE approach: A systematic review. *BMJ Open, 12*(2). https://doi.org/10.1136/bmjopen-2021-054417.

Keathley, J., Garneau, V., Marcil, V., Mutch, D. M., Robitaille, J., Rudkowska, I., et al. (2022b). Clinical practice guidelines using GRADE and AGREE II for the impact of genetic variants on plasma lipid/lipoprotein/apolipoprotein responsiveness to omega-3 fatty acids. *Frontiers in Nutrition, 8*, 768474. https://doi.org/10.3389/fnut.2021.768474.

Khan, S. U., Lone, A. N., Khan, M. S., Virani, S. S., Blumenthal, R. S., Nasir, K., Miller, M., Michos, E. D., Ballantyne, C. M., Boden, W. E., & Bhatt, D. L. (2021). Effect of omega-3 fatty acids on cardiovascular outcomes: A systematic review and meta-analysis. *eClinicalMedicine, 38*. Available from https://doi.org/10.1016/j.eclinm.2021.100997, www.thelancet.com/journals/eclinm/issue/current.

Kumar, A., Singh, U., Jaiswal, S. G., Dave, J., Wei, S., & Hailu, G. G. (2024). Recent trends in the encapsulation of functional lipids: Comprehensive review. *Sustainable Food Technology, 2*(6), 1610–1630. Available from https://doi.org/10.1039/d4fb00205a, https://www.rsc.org/journals-books-databases/about-journals/sustainable-food-technology/.

Kunj, P., Sahu, S., Singh, G., & Arya, S. K. (2025). A review on algal oils as a sustainable source of essential omega-3 fatty acids. *Bioresource Technology Reports, 30*, 102154. https://doi.org/10.1016/j.biteb.2025.102154.

Kušar, A., Žmitek, K., Lähteenmäki, L., Raats, M. M., & Pravst, I. (2021). Comparison of requirements for using health claims on foods in the European Union, the USA, Canada, and Australia/New Zealand. *Comprehensive Reviews in Food Science and Food Safety, 20*(2), 1307–1332. https://doi.org/10.1111/1541-4337.12716.

Lagoumintzis, G., & Patrinos, G. P. (2023). Triangulating nutrigenomics, metabolomics and microbiomics toward personalized nutrition and healthy living. *Human Genomics, 17*(1), Available from https://doi.org/10.1186/s40246-023-00561-w, https://humgenomics.biomedcentral.com/.

Le, V. T., Knight, S., Watrous, J. D., Najhawan, M., Dao, K., McCubrey, R. O., Bair, T. L., Horne, B. D., May, H. T., Muhlestein, J. B., Nelson, J. R., Carlquist, J. F., Knowlton, K. U., Jain, M., & Anderson, J. L. (2023). Higher docosahexaenoic acid levels lower the protective impact of eicosapentaenoic acid on long-term major cardiovascular events. *Frontiers in Cardiovascular Medicine, 10*. Available from https://doi.org/10.3389/fcvm.2023.1229130, www.frontiersin.org/journals/cardiovascular-medicine.

Leena, M. M., Silvia, M. G., Vinitha, K., Moses, J. A., & Anandharamakrishnan, C. (2020). Synergistic potential of nutraceuticals: Mechanisms and prospects for futuristic medicine. *Food and Function, 11*(11), 9317–9337. Available from https://doi.org/10.1039/d0fo02041a, http://pubs.rsc.org/en/journals/journal/fo.

Liu, C. C., & Lin, H. C. (2024). Are health claims in aging-related functional food packages different from those of general functional foods? Content analysis of food packaging from Taiwan. *Frontiers in Public Health, 12*. Available from https://doi.org/10.3389/fpubh.2024.1402969, http://journal.frontiersin.org/journal/public-health/section/public-health-education-and-promotion#archive.

Liu, Y., Ren, X., Fan, C., Wu, W., Zhang, W., & Wang, Y. (2022). Health benefits, food applications, and sustainability of microalgae-derived N-3 PUFA. *Foods, 11*(13), 1883. https://doi.org/10.3390/foods11131883.

Lv, W., & Xu, D. (2022). Docosahexaenoic acid delivery systems, bioavailability, functionality, and applications: A review. *Foods, 11*(17), 2685. https://doi.org/10.3390/foods11172685.

Maschmeyer, T., Luque, R., & Selva, M. (2020). Upgrading of marine (fish and crustaceans) biowaste for high added-value molecules and bio(nano)-materials. *Chemical Society Reviews, 49*(13), 4527. https://doi.org/10.1039/c9cs00653b.

McClements, D. J., & Öztürk, B. (2021). Utilization of nanotechnology to improve the handling, storage and biocompatibility of bioactive lipids in food applications. *Foods, 10*(2), 1–17. Available from https://doi.org/10.3390/foods10020365, https://www.mdpi.com/2304-8158/10/2/365/pdf.

Marrero, M., Monroig, Ó., Betancor, M., Herrera, M., Pérez, J. A., Garrido, D., Galindo, A., Giráldez, I., Rodríguez, C., et al. (2021). Influence of dietary lipids and environmental salinity on the n-3 long-chain polyunsaturated fatty acids biosynthesis capacity of the marine teleost Solea senegalensis. *Marine Drugs, 19*(5), 254. 10.3390/md19050254.

Melgosa, R., Sanz, M. T., & Beltrán, S. (2020). Supercritical CO_2 processing of omega-3 polyunsaturated fatty acids – Towards a biorefinery for fish waste valorization. *The Journal of Supercritical Fluids, 169*, 105121. https://doi.org/10.1016/j.supflu.2020.105121.

Morin-Bernier, J., de Toro-Martín, J., Barbe, V., San-Cristobal, R., Lemieux, S., Rudkowska, I., Couture, P., Barbier, O., & Vohl, M. C. (2024). Revisiting multi-omics-based predictors of the plasma triglyceride response to an omega-3 fatty acid supplementation. *Frontiers in Nutrition, 11*. Available from https://doi.org/10.3389/fnut.2024.1327863, journal.frontiersin.org/journal/nutrition.

Méndez, L., & Medina, I. (2021). Polyphenols and fish oils for improving metabolic health: A revision of the recent evidence for their combined nutraceutical effects. *Molecules, 26*(9), 2438. https://doi.org/10.3390/molecules26092438.

Natarajan, K., Vinoth Kumar, V., Mahesh, T. R., Abbas, M., Kathamuthu, N., Mohan, E., & Annand, J. R. (2024). Efficient heart disease classification through stacked ensemble with optimized firefly feature selection. *International Journal of Computational Intelligence Systems, 17*(1). https://doi.org/10.1007/s44196-024-00538-0.

Nazzaro, C., Uliano, A., Lerro, M., & Stanco, M. (2025). From claims to choices: How health information shapes consumer decisions in the functional food market. *Foods, 14*(4), 699. https://doi.org/10.3390/foods14040699.

Netala, V. R., Teertam, S. K., Li, H., & Zhang, Z. (2024). A comprehensive review of cardiovascular disease management: Cardiac biomarkers, imaging modalities, pharmacotherapy, surgical interventions, and herbal remedies. *Cells, 13*(17), Available from https://doi.org/10.3390/cells13171471, https://www.mdpi.com/journal/cells.

Oliver, L., Dietrich, T., Marañón, I., Villarán, M. C., & Barrio, R. J. (2020). Producing omega-3 polyunsaturated fatty acids: A review of sustainable sources and future trends for the EPA and DHA market. *Resources, 9*(12), 1–15. Available from https://doi.org/10.3390/resources9120148, https://www.mdpi.com/2079-9276/9/12/148.

Pal, A., Metherel, A. H., Fiabane, L., Buddenbaum, N., Bazinet, R. P., & Shaikh, S. R. (2020). Do eicosapentaenoic acid and docosahexaenoic acid have the potential to compete against each other? *Nutrients, 12*(12), 1–12. Available from https://doi.org/10.3390/nu12123718, https://www.mdpi.com/2072-6643/12/12/3718/pdf.

Penzavecchia, C., Todisco, P., Muzzioli, L., Poli, A., Marangoni, F., Poggiogalle, E., Giusti, A. M., Lenzi, A., Pinto, A., & Donini, L. M. (2022). The influence of front-of-pack nutritional labels on eating and purchasing behaviors: A narrative review of the literature. *Eating and Weight Disorders, 27*(8), 3037–3051. Available from https://doi.org/10.1007/s40519-022-01507-2, https://www.springer.com/journal/40519.

Perez, J. A. V., Ochando-Pulido, J. M., de la Fuente, E. B., & Martínez-Férez, A. (2021). Novel emulsions-based technological approaches for the protection of omega-3 polyunsaturated fatty acids against oxidation processes – A comprehensive review. *Food Structure, 27*, 100175. https://doi.org/10.1016/j.foostr.2021.100175.

Prieto, C., & Lagaron, J. M. (2024). Nanoencapsulation and nanocoating of bioactives of application interest in food, nutraceuticals and pharma. *Nanomaterials, 14*(3), 313. https://doi.org/10.3390/nano14030313.

Pérez-Palacios, T., Ruiz, J., Solomando, J. C., de-la-Haba, F., Pajuelo, A., & Antequera, T. (2022). Recent developments in the microencapsulation of fish oil and natural extracts: Procedure, quality evaluation and food enrichment. *Foods, 11*(20), 3291. https://doi.org/10.3390/foods11203291.

Qin, J., Kurt, E., LBassi, T., Sa, L., & Xie, D. (2023). Biotechnological production of omega-3 fatty acids: Current status and future perspectives. *Frontiers in Microbiology, 14*. https://doi.org/10.3389/fmicb.2023.1280296.

Ramalho, A., Altintzoglou, T., Mendes, J., Nunes, M. L., Dinis, M. T., & Dias, J. (2021). Farmed fish as a functional food: Perception of fish fortification and the influence of origin – Insights from Portugal. *Aquaculture, 501*, 22. https://doi.org/10.1016/j.aquaculture.2018.11.002.

Rizzo, M. G., Briglia, M., Zammuto, V., Morganti, D., Faggio, C., Impellitteri, F., Multisanti, C. R., & Graziano, A. C. E. (2025). Innovation in osteogenesis activation: Role of marine-derived materials in bone regeneration. *Current Issues in Molecular Biology, 47*(3), 175. https://doi.org/10.3390/cimb47030175.

Rollin, S., Gupta, A., Franco, C. M. M., Singh, S., & Puri, M. (2023). Development of sustainable downstream processing for nutritional oil production. *Frontiers in Bioengineering and Biotechnology, 11*. Available from https://doi.org/10.3389/fbioe.2023.1227889, http://journal.frontiersin.org/journal/bioengineering-and-biotechnology#archive.

Russell, F. D., & Bürgin-Maunder, C. S. (2012). Distinguishing health benefits of eicosapentaenoic and docosahexaenoic acids. *Marine Drugs, 10*(11), 2535–2559. https://doi.org/10.3390/md10112535 Available from: http://www.mdpi.com/1660-3397/10/11/2535/pdf.

Saina, S., Senthil, P., & Prakash, O. (2023). Burden of illness, risk factor and physical activity in cardiovascular disease-A review. *Biomedicine, 43*(4), 1080–1093. https://doi.org/10.51248/.v43i4.2139.

Sarker, P. K., Kapuscinski, A. R., McKuin, B., Fitzgerald, D. S., Nash, H. M., & Greenwood, C. (2020). Microalgae-blend tilapia feed eliminates fishmeal and fish oil, improves growth, and is cost viable. *Scientific Reports, 10*(1), Available from https://doi.org/10.1038/s41598-020-75289-x, www.nature.com/srep/index.html.

Sehl, A., Caderby, E., Bouhouda, S., Rébeillé, F., Griffiths, H., & Da Rocha Gomes, S. (2022). How do algae oils change the omega-3 polyunsaturated fatty acids market? *OCL, 29*, 20. https://doi.org/10.1051/ocl/2022018.

Shepon, A., Makov, T., Hamilton, H. A., Müller, D. B., Gephart, J. A., Henriksson, P. J. G., Troell, M., & Golden, C. D. (2022). Sustainable optimization of global aquatic omega-3 supply chain could substantially narrow the nutrient gap. *Resources, Conservation and Recycling, 181*. Available from https://doi.org/10.1016/j.resconrec.2022.106260, www.elsevier.com/locate/resconrec.

Subramani, S., Varshney, N., Anand, M. V., Soudagar, M. E. M., Al-keridis, L. A., Upadhyay, T. K., Alshammari, N., Saeed, M., Subramanian, K., Anbarasu, K., & Rohini, K. (2023). Cardiovascular diseases prediction by machine learning incorporation with deep learning. *Frontiers in Medicine, 10*. Available from https://doi.org/10.3389/fmed.2023.1150933, journal.frontiersin.org/journal/medicine.

Sumathy, S., & Gopalakrishnan, S. S. (2022). Study to estimate the role of blood groups in the development of cardiovascular complications among SARS Cov 2 patients – A cross-sectional study. *Romanian Journal of Diabetes, Nutrition and Metabolic Diseases, 29*(2), 183–187. Available from https://doi.org/10.46389/rjd-2022-1090, http://www.rjdnmd.org/index.php/RJDNMD/article/view/1113/719.

Sun, K., Meesapyodsuk, D., & Qiu, X. (2024). Biosynthetic mechanisms of omega-3 polyunsaturated fatty acids in microalgae. *Journal of Biological Chemistry, 300*(9), 107699. https://doi.org/10.1016/j.jbc.2024.107699.

Tomczyk, M., Heileson, J. L., Babiarz, M., & Calder, P. C. (2023). Athletes can benefit from increased intake of EPA and DHA—Evaluating the evidence. *Nutrients, 15*(23), Available from https://doi.org/10.3390/nu15234925, http://www.mdpi.com/journal/nutrients/.

Tocher, D., Betancor, M., Sprague, M., Olsen, R., Napier, J., et al. (2019). Omega-3 long-chain polyunsaturated fatty acids, EPA and DHA: Bridging the gap between supply and demand. *Nutrients, 11*(1), 89. 10.3390/nu11010089.

Townsend, J. R., Kirby, T. O., Sapp, P. A., Gonzalez, A. M., Marshall, T. M., & Esposito, R. (2023). Nutrient synergy: Definition, evidence, and future directions. *Frontiers in Nutrition, 10*. Available from https://doi.org/10.3389/fnut.2023.1279925, journal.frontiersin.org/journal/nutrition.

Tutor, A., O'Keefe, E. L., Lavie, C. J., Elagizi, A., Milani, R., & O'Keefe, J. (2024). Omega-3 fatty acids in primary and secondary prevention of cardiovascular diseases. *Progress in Cardiovascular Diseases, 84*, 19–26. Available from https://doi.org/10.1016/j.pcad.2024.03.009, https://www.sciencedirect.com/science/journal/00330620.

Venugopalan, V. K., Gopakumar, L. R., Kumaran, A. K., Chatterjee, N. S., Soman, V., Peeralil, S., Mathew, S., McClements, D. J., & Nagarajarao, R. C. (2021). Encapsulation and protection of omega-3-rich fish oils using food-grade delivery systems. *Foods, 10*(7), Available from https://doi.org/10.3390/foods10071566, https://www.mdpi.com/2304-8158/10/7/1566/pdf.

Visioli, F., & Poli, A. (2020). Fatty acids and cardiovascular risk. evidence, lack of evidence, and diligence. *Nutrients, 12*(12), 3782. 10.3390/nu12123782.

Wang, F., Zheng, J., Cheng, J., Zou, H., Li, M., Deng, B., et al. (2022). Personalized nutrition: A review of genotype-based nutritional supplementation. *Frontiers in Nutrition, 9*. https://doi.org/10.3389/fnut.2022.992986.

Wang, J., Han, L., Wang, D., Sun, Y., Huang, J., Shahidi, F., et al. (2021). Stability and stabilization of omega-3 oils: A review. *Trends in Food Science & Technology, 118*, 17–35. 10.1016/j.tifs.2021.09.018.

Wang, J., Ossemond, J., Jardin, J., Briard-Bion, V., Henry, G., Gouar, Y. L., et al. (2022). Encapsulation of DHA oil with heat-denatured whey protein in Pickering emulsion improves its bioaccessibility. *Food Research International, 162*, 112112. https://doi.org/10.1016/j.foodres.2022.112112.

Willora, F. P., Grønevik, B., Liu, C., Palihawadana, A. M., Sørensen, M., & Hagen, Ø. (2020). Total replacement of marine oil by rapeseed oil in plant protein rich diets of juvenile lumpfish (*Cyclopterus lumpus*): Effects on growth performance, chemical and fatty acid composition. *Aquaculture Reports, 19*, 100560. https://doi.org/10.1016/j.aqrep.2020.100560.

Yan, J., Liu, M., Yang, D., Zhang, Y., & An, F. (2022). Efficacy and safety of omega-3 fatty acids in the prevention of cardiovascular disease: A systematic review and meta-analysis. *Cardiovascular Drugs and Therapy, 38*(4), 799. https://doi.org/10.1007/s10557-022-07379-z.

Yanru, L., Ulaganathan, V., Gunasekaran, B., Bhattacharya, T., et al. (2025). Recent nutraceutical interventions for hypertension: A comprehensive review of randomized clinical evidence. *Current Nutrition Reports, 14*(1). 10.1007/s13668-025-00681-w.

Ye, Q., Nicolas, G., & Selomulya, C. (2018). Microencapsulation of active ingredients in functional foods: From research stage to commercial food products. *Trends in Food Science & Technology, 78*, 167. https://doi.org/10.1016/j.tifs.2018.05.025 ?.

Yu, F., Qi, S., Ji, Y., Wang, X., Fang, S., & Cao, R. (2022). Effects of omega-3 fatty acid on major cardiovascular outcomes: A systematic review and meta-analysis. *Medicine, 101*(30), e29556. https://doi.org/10.1097/md.0000000000029556.

Chapter 12

Docosahexaenoic acid and eicosapentaenoic acid in inflammation regulation: opportunities in functional and nutraceutical foods

M.J. Rekha[1,*], K.L. Madhukala[1], and Bharathi Suresh[2]

[1]*Department of Life Sciences, Acharya Bangalore B-School, Lingadheeranahalli, Andrahalli, Bengaluru, Karnataka, India,* [2]*Graduate School of Biomedical Science and Engineering, Hanyang University, Seoul, South Korea*

12.1 Introduction

Life expectancy is rising worldwide, yet there is a surge in ageing that has accompanied this demographic shift and lifestyle-related noncommunicable diseases (NCDs), which include cardiovascular disease, type 2 diabetes mellitus, obesity, neurodegenerative disorders, chronic kidney disease, and certain cancers (Calder, 2017; Hajat & Stein, 2018). These noncommunicable disease conditions are increasingly recognised as they share a common pathophysiological mechanism, such as chronic low-grade inflammation. According to WHO data, these diseases are among the main causes of death worldwide. Inflammation leads to multimorbidity that burdens both healthcare and social systems, and this could intensify the global disease burden in the coming decades (Soares et al., 2023). In aggregate, undernutrition and overnutrition will significantly increase the risk of NCDs. This underscores the urgent need for scientific evidence on dietary and nutritional interventions that mitigate inflammatory pathways .

In this chapter, dietary bioactive compounds have emerged as a cornerstone of preventive and therapeutic nutrition. Among the most rigorously studied are the omega-3 long-chain polyunsaturated fatty acids (LC-PUFAs))—particularly eicosapentaenoic acid (EPA, 20:5 n-3) and docosahexaenoic acid (DHA, 22:6 n-3)—predominantly derived from marine oils and fatty fish (Calder, 2020). Thus these PUFAs exhibit well-characterised pleiotropic antiinflammatory and pro-resolving activities at the cellular and molecular levels, positioning them as high-value candidates for nutraceutical and functional food development. In recent years, the sale of omega-3 ingredients has globally increased by 4 billion US dollars, and it is also expected to grow at an annual growth rate (CAGR) of more than 8% through 2030 (GOED, 2022), reflecting both market momentum and an expanding scientific literature supporting their therapeutic relevance.

Despite decades of research, however, translating laboratory findings into clinically effective nutraceutical products remains considerably challenging. Critical issues that continue to limit the full therapeutic exploitation of these fatty acids are bioavailability, optimal dosing, molecular form (triglyceride vs ethyl ester vs phospholipid), oxidative stability, and interindividual response variability (Schuchardt & Hahn, 2013). Furthermore, the biochemical distinction between EPA and DHA—long obscured by the widespread use of combined fish oil supplements—has gained increasing recognition as essential to understanding their differential mechanisms of action in inflammatory disease (Byelashov et al., 2015). Alongside omega-3 PUFAs, growing attention is being directed toward the broader landscape of bioactive lipids and targeted nutritional formulae as means of improving patient outcomes and reducing healthcare expenditures(van der Wurff et al., 2020).

[*] Corresponding author.

Omega-3 and Omega-6 Polyunsaturated Fatty Acids in Food Systems. DOI: https://doi.org/10.1016/B978-0-443-43810-3.00030-0

Thus the present chapter aims: (1) to elucidate the cellular and molecular mechanisms of inflammation. (2) To understand the unresolved inflammation and the limitations of conventional pharmacological approaches, such as non-steroidal anti-inflammatory drugs (NSAIDs). (3) To evaluate current nutraceuticals and their classifications, focusing on dietary lipids and biological significance in regulating inflammation and other diseases. (4) To outline applications and strategies in developing omega-3 fatty acids as functional foods. (5) To project the future research and commercial perspectives for omega-3 PUFAs and related bioactive lipids in the management of inflammation-driven diseases.

12.2 Inflammation and its mechanism

Inflammation plays an essential role in the immune system by triggering a destructive response to pathogenic microbes, harmful chemicals, or injured cells. It eliminates these harmful reactions and introduces therapeutic progression (Fig. 12.1). Nevertheless, the failure of this response to resolve efficiently marks in chronic inflammatory conditions, which are the vital cause of numerous serious ailments, including cardiovascular diseases (CVD), metabolic syndrome, neurodegenerative disorders, and autoimmune diseases (Furman et al., 2019).

12.3 Inflammatory response and cellular equilibrium

The foremost cause of the inflammatory response is to restore cellular balance and overcome the detrimental effects. The physiological condition of homeostasis is closely linked to the process that initiates inflammation (Ahmed, 2011b). Therefore inflammation is termed an "adaptive response" to any negative impact that endangers cellular equilibrium. The longer this reaction continues, the more detrimental the effects will be for the host. To prevent worsening of its adverse conditions, the inflammatory response must be as short-lived as possible, despite its protective role in cellular physiology (Medzhitov, 2010).

12.4 Mechanism of inflammation

The inflammatory response is activated by both innate and adaptive immune mechanisms to combat pathological conditions; thus inflammation is a beneficial event that plays a significant role in human health (Chen et al., 2018; Dunkelberger & Song, 2009). The cardinal signs of inflammation, including pain, swelling, redness, and heat, are known to humankind and are observed in response to injury or microbial infection at the cellular and vascular levels (Ahmed, 2011a). The classical pathway of inflammation is the arachidonic acid (AA)-mediated pathway, resulting in the production of leukotrienes and prostaglandins by the action of lipoxygenases and cyclooxygenase-2 (COX-2) (Fig. 12.2).

The levels of inflammatory mediators in the local tissue are regulated by the colonic initiation of signalling pathways that draw inflammatory cells from the circulation, a process termed the inflammatory response (Chen et al., 2018). This response is triggered by appropriate stimuli, such as pathogenic microorganisms, foreign invaders, internal and external irritants, and many others. Inflammation is stimulated within a few minutes of exposure by host cells through the innate immune mechanism. The key immune cells that are instrumental in this process are dendritic cells, mast cells, neutrophils,

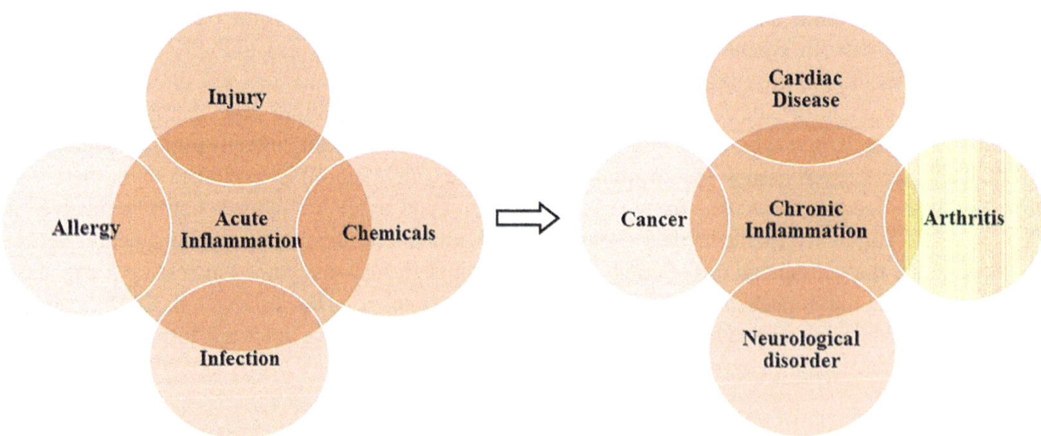

FIGURE 12.1 Causes of acute inflammation and consequences of chronic inflammation.

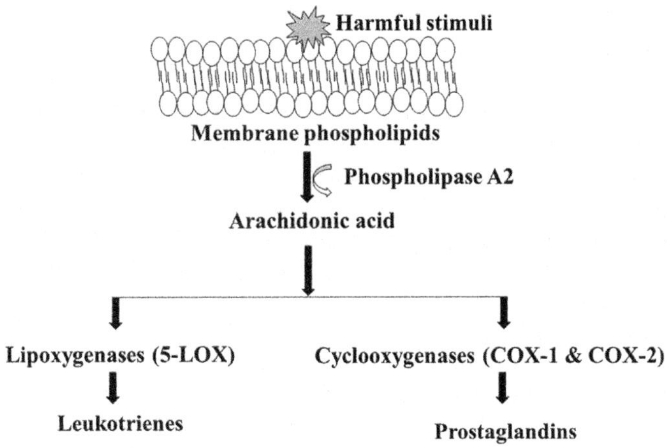

FIGURE 12.2 Arachidonic acid-mediated inflammatory pathway.

macrophages, and lymphocytes (Akira et al., 2006). In addition to immune cells, the inflammatory response is also facilitated by nonimmune cells, such as epithelial, endothelial, and fibroblast cells. Both of these target tissues and inflammatory pathways, and they differ greatly depending on the composition of the stimulants.

12.5 Cellular components of inflammation

The cellular mechanism of inflammation orchestrates a dynamic, multiphase role in initiating, sustaining, and resolving the inflammatory response. The various cellular and vascular events of the inflammatory cascades include the migration of leukocytes from their natural sites, fluid accumulation, and plasma accumulation at the place of inflammation (Abdulkhaleq et al., 2018). Numerous inflammatory mediators and signalling molecules, such as prostaglandins, leukotrienes, eicosanoids, histamines, and free radicals, are secreted by immune cells and are predominantly involved in inflammation (Soares et al., 2023).

Neutrophils, which are termed phagocytes, are characterised by their complexity and heterogeneity, responding to tissue signals and playing a role in recruiting other immune cells that stimulate chronic inflammation (Nathan, 2006). These cells employ multiple mechanisms, such as degranulation, phagocytosis, and neutrophil extracellular traps (NETs), to fight pathogens (He et al., 2025). Macrophages derived from monocytes exhibit notable elasticity in response to stimuli such as IL-4 and TGF-β, and can reform in directing the tissue therapeutic phenotype (Li et al., 2023). Dendritic cells continue to serve as key protectors that process antigens and trigger adaptive immune responses, but new studies reveal that metabolic conditions influence their roles in inflammation and tolerance (Jin et al., 2025). Mast cells of the immune system play a vital role in acute inflammation by rapidly secreting histamine, cytokines, and proteases in response to allergens and pathogenic organisms (Mukai et al., 2018). Basophils and eosinophils are best known for their roles in allergic and parasitic defence; however, they can also influence inflammatory settings through granule release and key signalling molecules—IL-4, IL-5, and IL-3, which are part of type 2 immune responses (Stone et al., 2010). Finally, T and B lymphocytes support adaptive immunity: CD4+ T helper cell subsets control inflammatory mediators, whereas antibody and cytokine production induce inflammation by B cells. These immune cells work together to generate the complex network that causes, maintains, and reduces inflammatory conditions. Several inflammatory sequences are identified, triggered by various factors and regulated by diverse mechanisms. Owing to its widespread nature, inflammation is thought to affect normal physiology and the body's pathology significantly. The current understanding of inflammation has been significantly expanded by the massive expansion of scientific fields in various directions. Because of this, it is still a long way to understanding the full impact of inflammation on human health and illness (Ahmed, 2011a).

However, studies have shown that the inflammatory response is a cascade of reactions observed at the cellular and molecular levels that effectively reduces damage at the infection or injury site (Chen et al., 2018). These alleviatory events effectively repair tissue and restore equilibrium, thereby resolving the acute inflammatory response and being mediated by the innate immune system. The uninhibited condition of acute inflammatory response will result in chronic inflammation, thus leading to various types of disorders like Alzheimer's, cancer, rheumatoid arthritis, respiratory ailments, in addition to others (Leyva-López et al., 2016). Therefore combating the inflammatory mechanism that plays a notable role in reducing chronic inflammation by targeting multiple pathways, with effective drugs, minimal side effects, and unfavorable compensatory mechanisms (Koeberle & Werz, 2014).

Presently, conventional pharmacological interventions to regulate inflammation often depend on NSAIDs like diclofenac, naproxen, celecoxib, and glucocorticoids that are potent inhibitors of inflammatory enzymes, which operate through diverse mechanisms and primarily target inflammatory pathways (Reichardt et al., 2021; Ribeiro et al., 2022). These drugs are widely used but are frequently associated with several deleterious side effects, such as serious gastrointestinal problems, ulcers, and cardiovascular issues (Fosslien, 1998; Wright, 2002; Vane & Botting, 1998). Thus warrants the exploration of natural inflammation regulatory agents, particularly dietary sources with minimal side effects.

12.6 Vital strategic opportunity routes

The massive development of the worldwide nutraceutical and functional food market is driven by the critical need to address the global omega-3 fatty acid deficiency. Long-chain omega-3 polyunsaturated fatty acids (LCPUFAs)—DHA and EPA have been established to mitigate the inflammatory response and facilitate its resolution, highlighting their therapeutic benificial across diverse health conditions (Troesch et al., 2020). Thus DHA and EPA may prevent and treat disease in several areas, including age-related muscle loss, cancer, perioperative care, and cognitive health. Currently, global research indicates that approximately 76% of the world's population fails to meet the recommended dietary intake of omega-3 fatty acids EPA and DHA, revealing an important public health gap in crucial nutrient intake (Calder et al., 2025). This prevalent shortage is associated with inconsistent, widespread recommendations and lower marine food consumption, which emphasise the need for rapid availability and advanced solutions such as enriched, efficient nutrients and supplements (Hitl et al., 2025). Strategic opportunities for market differentiation and commercial success hinge on three primary vectors: accurate formulation, an innovative delivery system, and sustainable sources. Therefore the deliberate objective of nutraceuticals interference must shift from merely suppressing inflammatory symptoms (typical of NSAIDs) to vigorously promoting the resolution of inflammation and preserving cellular homeostasis, a process termed immune-resolution (Al-Shaer et al., 2021). The substantial value of dietary lipids like DHA and EPA, with high therapeutic nutraceutical value, is supported by their capacity to initiate the resolution phase.

12.7 Nutraceuticals

In recent times, an increasing variety of nutritional supplements has become more available in hypermarkets, health food stores, and pharmacies. The term "nutraceutical" refers to foods that have nutritional or medicinal functions and aid in the prevention or treatment of health issues (Brower, 1998). Nutraceuticals, also known as designer foods, medical foods, functional foods, phytochemicals, and dietary supplements, comprise a variety of familiar products, such as fortified breakfast cereals and "bio" yoghurts, as well as supplements, plant-based preparations, vitamins, and genetically altered foods (Roberfroid, 2000). Several terms and explanations vary across the globe, which can lead to possible misinterpretations. Nutraceuticals are an inclusive term that encompasses components derived from food sources that offer added health benefits beyond their essential nutritional value (Kalra, 2003).

Treatment with nutraceuticals is one of the nonspecific biological interventions that is designed to enhance overall well-being, prevent malignant progression, and manage symptoms. Recently, nutraceutical compounds have received greater attention due to their potential nutritional health benefits and safety. Several researches have been carried out on these molecules to perform biological functions, such as oxidative defence, cell proliferation, regulating gene expression studies, and also involved in the maintenance of mitochondrial integrity (Hong et al., 2024; Mishra & Kakhlon, 2025). To enhance health status, nutraceuticals can be utilized efficiently to prevent chronic diseases, slow the ageing process, thereby increasing longevity, and preserve the body's functions and integrity. Therefore nutraceuticals are regarded as valuable sources for preventing severe health conditions, including kidney disease, diabetes, gastrointestinal disorders, and various infections (Santini et al., 2017).

There is a wide range of nutraceuticals that have demonstrated a noteworthy role in influencing immune function and vulnerability to specific disease conditions. Some of the findings have shown to indicate diseases associated with oxidative stress, including allergies, neurodegenerative and CVD, cancer, retinal issues, Parkinson's disease, and obesity (Medoro et al., 2023). The fundamental idea of nutraceuticals is to emphasise the importance of prevention. It is often applicable in the context of nutritional complements and functional foods—a framework that directly encompasses the role of long-chain omega-3 fatty acids, particularly EPA and DHA, as key bioactive agents in regulating inflammation and preventing chronic disease (Das et al., 2012).

12.8 Nutritional supplements

Nutritional supplement products are intended to enhance the diet. They may encompass additional dietary constituents, including amino acids, minerals, vitamins, herbs or other botanicals, metabolites, or dietary substances proposed to increase total daily intake. This category also involves concentrates, extracts, or mixtures of these ingredients (Steven H. Zeisel, 1999). Nutritional complements are not designed to manage or cure diseases, whereas nutraceuticals additionally focus on the anticipated therapeutic outcomes of these products. In a nutshell, the therapeutically important nutritional supplements are the long-chain omega-3 PUFAs, specifically EPA and DHA. These fatty acids are available from both marine food sources and concentrated supplement preparations. EPA and DHA represent a critical link between basic nutritional support and targeted antiinflammatory intervention (Kidd, 2007). Several studies have shown that supplementation with these components is associated with a measurable decline in inflammatory cytokines, chemokines, and other mediators, thereby modulating immune responses, making these nutraceuticals highly relevant to the central theme of this chapter (Das et al., 2012; Hong et al., 2024).

12.9 Functional food

As stated by the American Institute of Medicine's Food and Nutrition Board, functional foods are defined as any foods or food ingredients that may offer a health benefit in addition to the traditional nutrients they contain (Ernst, 2001). The concept of functional food refers to the incorporation of food products into the regular diet that offer valuable physiological properties along with other nutritional benefits. Functional foods encompass physiologically active molecules derived from both plant and animal sources (Ernst, 2001).

The concept of nutraceuticals was initially developed in Japan in the 1980s and represents either treated or natural nutrients that positively influence metabolism and overall well-being. Nutraceuticals, medicinal foods, and probiotic foods fall under this category (Sun-Waterhouse, 2011). A balanced diet that is prominent in fruits, vegetables, grains, pulses, seeds, and marine-derived foods has been shown to possess significant health benefits, including antioxidant, antiinflammatory, and cholesterol-lowering effects. There is mounting scientific evidence connecting nutrition to the prevention of chronic illness, which has amplified universal interest in functional foods. Marine-derived functional foods, in particular, serve as rich dietary sources of EPA and DHA—the long-chain omega-3 fatty acids central to this chapter's focus on inflammation regulation (Das et al., 2012; Kidd, 2007).

12.10 Classification

Nutraceuticals and functional foods are categorised based on available sources: natural or conventional, and unnatural or nonconventional as shown in Fig. 12.3 (Hoti et al., 2022). Conventional nutraceuticals are derived from botanical, animal, mineral, or microbial sources, while nonconventional nutraceuticals are products produced through biotechnology (Hoti et al., 2022). The classification of nutraceuticals provides a structured skeleton for understanding the mechanisms of bioactive molecules, the effect of functional lipids (EPA and DHA) as antiinflammatory agents, which are sourced, processed, and delivered through both traditional dietary patterns and modern biotechnological innovation (Bigliardi & Galati, 2013; Demain and V., 2009).

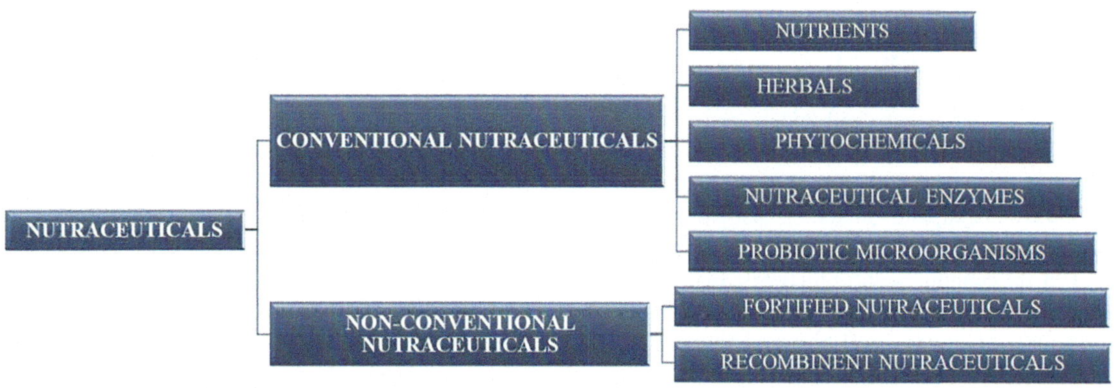

FIGURE 12.3 Demonstrating the spectrum of conventional and nonconventional nutraceuticals.
Modified according to Hoti, G., Matencio, A., Pedrazzo, A.R., Cecone, C., Appleton, S.L., Monfared, Y.K., Caldera, F., & Trotta, F. (2022). Nutraceutical concepts and dextrin-based delivery systems. International Journal of Molecular Sciences, 23(8). https://doi.org/10.3390/ijms23084102MDPI.

12.11 Conventional nutraceuticals

Conventional bioactive compounds are components naturally produced by plants, microbial sources, animals, and minerals that have been shown to deliver beneficial health outcomes beyond basic nutrition. They include nutrients such as vitamins, minerals, amino acids, and omega-3 fatty acids, herbs, plant secondary metabolites, and probiotic microbes (Roberfroid, 2000). These naturally sourced compounds—particularly EPA and DHA—are naturally present in foods without structural or genetic alteration, making them integral to the concept of functional foods that confer measurable physiological benefits in addition to their standard nutritional value (Ernst , 2001; Das et al., 2012).

Among the conventional nutraceuticals, functional lipids—specifically the long-chain omega-3 PUFAs EPA (C20:5) and DHA (C22:6)—have emerged as significant bioactive constituents. These PUFAs play a pivotal role in several critical biological activities, like antioxidant activity, gene modulation, controlling cell division, and maintaining the homeostasis of mitochondria (Hong et al., 2024; Mishra & Kakhlon, 2025). In this perspective, EPA and DHA directly modulate the production of pro-inflammatory mediators, thereby elevating antiinflammatory components and attenuating systemic inflammatory responses (Das et al., 2012); thus these components are positioned as key conventional nutraceutical candidates for managing diseases associated with oxidative stress and chronic inflammation, including cardiovascular disease, neurodegenerative disorders, allergies, and obesity (Medoro et al., 2023).

These natural compounds aid in preventing disease, thereby enhancing immune function, regulating metabolic functions, improving gut health, and lowering inflammation and oxidative stress, thereby improving overall health and well-being without altering the natural structure of food (Das et al., 2012). To achieve disease prevention and health promotion that reflects the fundamental principle underlying nutraceutical science, a noninvasive, food-based approach will be used: that nutrition is a primary and powerful determinant of long-term health outcomes (Kalra, 2003; Santini et al., 2017). As scientific evidence continues to mount linking dietary patterns to the prevention of chronic illness, the role of conventional nutraceuticals—and EPA and DHA in particular—in functional and nutraceutical food formulations has gained substantial global interest (Sun-Waterhouse, 2011).

12.12 Nonconventional nutraceuticals

A biotechnological process has produced nonconventional compounds to improve the nutritional and therapeutic value of foods. These compounds are fortified nutraceuticals, such as vitamin- and mineral-enriched cereals, milk, and juices, and recombinant nutraceuticals, produced using genetic engineering, fermentation, and enzyme technologies (Bigliardi & Galati, 2013; Demain and V., 2009). Biotechnological products aid in antioxidant defence, immune function, and disease prevention, helping reduce the risk of chronic and oxidative stress-related disorders that promote overall health (Medoro et al., 2023).

These nonconventional approaches have been widely applied to enhance the bioavailability of EPA and DHA and to deliver them in functional food matrices. Through microencapsulation, fermentation, and genetic biofortification technologies, it has become possible to enrich everyday food products—including dairy, cereals, and plant-based alternatives—with therapeutically relevant concentrations of these omega-3 fatty acids, thereby extending the antiinflammatory benefits of EPA and DHA to wider populations through routine dietary intake (Demain and V., 2009; Bigliardi & Galati, 2013; Hong et al., 2024).

12.13 Functional lipids

Lipids are one of the diverse and widely distributed biomolecules that perform essential functions in the human body. These lipids act as crucial structural components of cell membranes, significant bases of energy storage, and contributors to cellular signalling pathways that regulate metabolism and other physiological processes (Kidd, 2007). The extent of lipid biomolecule occupancy in cells is also similar to that of proteins, which leads to the precise regulation of metabolic and transport mechanisms. In humans, the nutritional content of dietary fats, rather than their total quantity, is more significant in influencing health outcomes. One of the notable examples of the class of PUFAs includes omega-3 fatty acids such as alpha-linolenic acid (ALA), EPA, and DHA; omega-6 fatty acids (Fig. 12.4); conjugated linoleic acid; medium-chain triglycerides; and phytosterols. The naturally occurring constituents that are obtained from marine foods and conventional nutraceuticals will exemplify the intersection of dietary nutrition and targeted antiinflammatory therapy (Das et al., 2012; Kidd, 2007). Therefore the presence of these nutraceuticals in both natural food sources and fortified functional food products will underscore their dual relevance within the conventional and nonconventional nutraceutical classification frameworks, as described above (Hoti et al., 2022).

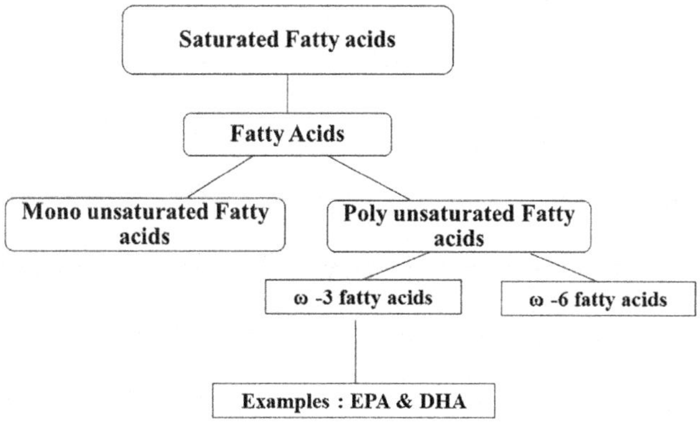

FIGURE 12.4 Flowchart depicting the classification of saturated fatty acids.

12.14 Polyunsaturated fatty acids

PUFAs are a collection of fatty acids that comprise n-6 and n-3 fatty acids. These omega-3 PUFAs, such as EPA (C20:5) and DHA (C22:6), are long-chain omega-3 PUFAs that regulate inflammatory conditions by modulating the production of pro-inflammatory mediators and thereby elevating anti-inflammatory mediators. These fatty acids serve as precursors to specialised pro-resolving mediators (SPMs), such as resolvins, protectins, and maresins, which actively mitigate inflammatory processes and restore tissue homeostasis (Das et al., 2012; Hong et al., 2024). As the central focus of this chapter, EPA and DHA represent the most clinically and nutritionally significant conventional nutraceutical lipids available through both marine food sources and functional food formulations, offering substantial opportunities for the prevention and management of inflammation-driven chronic diseases—spanning cardiovascular disease, metabolic syndrome, neurodegeneration, and immune dysregulation. Thus omega-3 fatty acids are one of the essential bioactive lipids in the transforming landscape of functional nutrition and nutraceutical science (Kidd, 2007; Medoro et al., 2023; Mishra & Kakhlon, 2025).

12.15 Chemical structure of docosahexaenoic acid and eicosapentaenoic acid

12.15.1 Docosahexaenoic acid (cis-4,7,10,13,16,19-docosahexaenoic acid, $C_{22}H_{32}O_2$, 22:6)

DHA is strongly described as an n-3 long-chain PUFA, which consists of 22 carbon atoms and 6 unsaturated double bonds. The initial twin bond is observed at the third carbon atom from the omega end of the carbon chain (Srigley & Rader, 2014). The chemical structure of DHA. DHA in the food rarely occurs as a free fatty acid; however, it occurs in the form of triglyceride in a smaller quantity as phospholipid form (Hirahashi, 2017).

12.15.2 Eicosapentaenoic acid (cis-5,8,11,14,17-eicosapentaenoic acid, $C_{20}H_{30}O_2$, 20:5)

EPA is a type of fatty acid that possesses an additional twelve carbon atoms; thus it belongs to long-chain fatty acids (Srigley & Rader, 2014). The chemical structure of EPA. The important constituent of glycolipids and phospholipids is EPA; it plays a substantial role in altering cell-membrane fluidity. It is the most common fatty acid in marine fats. EPA also acts as a precursor for numerous biological controllers, like signalling molecules and hormones, which are involved in cellular functions (Hitl et al., 2025). EPA production from microbial bases has recently been established through metabolic engineering of microorganisms, and it is expected to develop as a sustainable substitute for fish oil–derived EPA in the near future (Cao et al., 2012).

12.16 Membrane incorporation and cellular function of docosahexaenoic acid and eicosapentaenoic acid

Consequent to dietary absorption, EPA and DHA are combined into the phospholipids of the cell membrane, which leads to variation in membrane fluidity, arrangement of the lipid bundle, and the activity of membrane-associated proteins, including the receptors and ion channels (Calder, 2020). DHA is mainly enriched in neural and retinal tissues, and it accounts for up to 40% of total fatty acids in external segment membranes of photoreceptor (Fliesler & Anderson, 1983).

The greater extent of DHA unsaturation confers exceptional membrane flexibility, which plays a critical role in the rapid signal transduction in neuronal and immune cells (Gutiérrez et al., 2019; Kim et al., 2022).

12.17 The desaturation-elongation cascade

The parent fatty acids are ALA and linoleic acid (LA), respectively, for both omega-3 and omega-6, and these molecules will compete for the same set of enzymes, desaturases and elongases, and, most importantly, the Delta-6 desaturase (FADS2) and Delta-5 desaturase (FADS1). The enzyme-coding genes that are encoded at the FADS1/FADS2 gene cluster are on chromosome 11q12–13 (Mathias et al., 2014). The underlying principle in the reciprocal relationship between the intake of dietary omega-6 and omega-3 PUFA is enzymatic competition. These shared enzymes will saturate as the dietary concentration of LA increases, and they are the rate-limiting steps in the transformation of ALA to DHA and EPA fatty acids. Inherited polymorphisms in the FADS1 and FADS2 genes will significantly modulate the effectiveness of this series of reactions among individuals and populations (Tanaka et al., 2009). Since ancient times, Greenlandic Inuit and Japanese people with omega-3-rich diets are more likely to carry variants of FADS that facilitate the efficient synthesis of long-chain PUFA. In contrast, people with a history of an agrarian diet frequently carry variants associated with maximising the elongation of omega-6 fatty acids. These variances at the population level can lead to tailored nutrition approaches for genetically discrete individuals with the required quantity of preformed DHA/EPA to attain the antiinflammatory effect.

12.17.1 Sources of eicosapentaenoic acid and docosahexaenoic acid

The various sources of DHA and EPA fatty acids are fatty fishes, shellfish, cod liver oil, flax seeds, algal powder, walnuts, etc. (Fig. 12.5). Fish and their oil serve as the most abundant sources of EPA fatty acid, with concentrations varying between 39% and 50% for both freshwater and saltwater fish. EPA serves as a precursor to the series of eicosanoid hormones. DHA is found in fish oil and also in red-brown algae, and it is a significant component of omega-3 fatty acids that are similarly present in the retina. The brain consists of approximately 65% fat, of which 50% is of DHA (Kaur et al., 2012). The DHA and EPA content in marine sources is summarised in Table 12.1

12.17.2 Biological significance of omega-3 fatty acids

Omega-3 fatty acids, predominantly DHA and EPA, have been extensively studied for their significant role in human health. Epidemiological observations, notably among Greenland Eskimos consuming high amounts of seafood-derived fats, revealed a remarkably low incidence of cardiovascular disease, highlighting the protective outcome of omega-3 fatty acids (Zhang et al., 2020). Clinical and experimental studies have shown that omega-3 PUFAs help reduce triglyceride

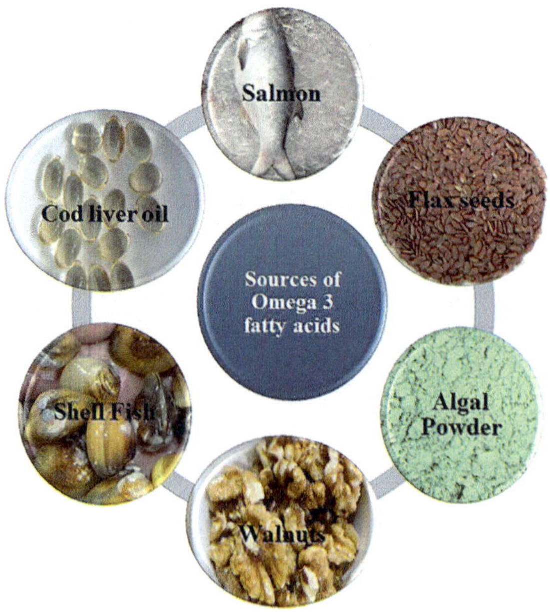

FIGURE 12.5 Diagrammatic representation of various sources of omega-3 fatty acids.

TABLE 12.1 Docosahexaenoic acid (DHA) and eicosapentaenoic acid (EPA) content in some of the selected marine sources (Kris-Etherton et al., 2009; Mohanty et al., 2016).

Fish types	EPA (mg/100 g)	DHA (mg/100 g)
Pacific cod	80	140
Salmo salar	320	1110
Silver salmon	860	1100
Blue fish	250	520
Wild-salmon	430	660
Farmed salmon	360	820
Asian green mussel	159	170
Sardinella longiceps	535	938
Indian oyster	383	377
Cuttlassfish	568	203
Golden masheer	116	202

levels, blood pressure, heart rate, and atherosclerosis risk (Dangardt et al., 2012). EPA and DHA have health benefits ratified by the U.S. Food and Drug Administration (FDA) and provide the supporting evidence for their role in lowering the risk of coronary heart disease (Van Dael, 2021).

Beyond cardiovascular protection, omega-3 fatty acids display antiinflammatory, immunomodulatory, and metabolic benefits (Banaszak et al., 2024; Bodur et al., 2025). They contribute to enhanced cognitive role, concentration, learning, and behavioural regulation, while also supporting mental health (Kidd, 2007). Furthermore, omega-3 PUFAs have been associated with enhanced insulin sensitivity, inhibition of cancer progression, improved wound healing, reduction of joint pain and inflammation, better bone mineral metabolism, and support for weight management through regulation of fat metabolism (Banaszak et al., 2024; Garay et al., 2025). Owing to the above-mentioned diverse health-promoting properties, omega-3 fatty acids are widely recognised as important functional lipids and nutraceuticals.

12.18 Antiinflammatory action of omega-3 fatty acids—molecular mechanisms

12.18.1 Eicosanoid restructuring

The classical interpretations of antiinflammatory activity of omega-3 cores on the competitive shift of AA (20:4 n-6) from phospholipids of the membrane and subsequently in the reduction in the synthesis of pro-inflammatory eicosanoid mediators. These AA mediators, prostaglandin E2 (PGE2), thromboxane A2 (TxA2), and leukotriene B4 (LTB4), are effective pro-inflammatory mediators of acute inflammatory conditions, mediated by COX-2 and 5-lipoxygenase (5-LOX) enzymes. The molecular mechanism underlying acute inflammation is mediated by PGE2-sensitised pain receptors that promote vasodilation, followed by TxA2, which aggregates platelets and causes vasoconstriction, and leukotriene B4. This strong neutrophil chemoattractant also activates leukocyte adhesion molecules.

The alternative substrate for the lipoxygenase (LOX) and COX enzymes is EPA, resulting in the generation of 3-series prostaglandins (PGE3) and thromboxanes A3 (TXA3) and 5- series of leukotrienes (LTB5), and these are generally considered to be biologically less potent than the AA-derived mediators (Calder, 2017; Nelson et al., 2021). This kind of class switching of eicosanoids results in impaired leukocyte chemotaxis, lowered vascular reactivity, and slowed platelet aggregation. Studies have shown that the TxA3 platelet aggregator was approximately 10 times less effective than TxA2. However, the LTB5 reveals that it has almost 10- to 30-fold less power as a chemoattractant than the LTB4 (Nelson et al., 2021).

Studies carried out by Simopoulos in 2002 highlighted the ratio of PUFAs—omega-3 to omega-6 fatty acids in the diet of western countries, which is roughly around 15–20:1, when compared to the evolutionary ratio around 4:1. This research displayed that this western diet significantly contributed to the setting of pro-inflammatory conditions, representing the chronic diseases. Thus restoring the added favourable ratio through enhanced EPA and DHA consumption, thereby offering clear biochemical validation of the antiinflammatory effects of PUFAs supplementation. The results from clinical trials have established that supplementation with 3–4 g/day of EPA and DHA significantly reduced circulating levels of PGE2, TxB2, and LTB4, with a consistent decline in markers of monocyte and neutrophil activation (Calder, 2015).

12.18.2 Nuclear factor-κB signaling pathway modulation

In addition to competing with eicosanoids, EPA and DHA exert direct molecular effects on the expression of inflammatory genes. The key regulator of the production of inflammatory cytokines, including tumour necrosis factor-α (TNF-α), interleukin-6, interleukin-1β, and COX-2, is nuclear factor-κB (NF-κB). At the resting state, NF-κB will be retained in the cytoplasm via its association with inhibitory IκB proteins. During inflammatory stimulation, the IκB kinases (IKKs) phosphorylate IκB, thereby promoting its ubiquitination and proteasomal degradation and releasing NF-κB for nuclear translocation to target transcription of genes (Calder, 2015; Calder, 2017).

A study in 2015 revealed that DHA and EPA together suppress NF-κB activation by various mechanisms, including inhibition of IKK activity, thereby preventing the phosphorylation and degradation of IκB and decreasing nuclear translocation of NF-κB. These effects of DHA and EPA are partly determined by the altered composition of the membrane microdomain, as disruption of lipid raft assembly weakens the colocalization of signalling molecules that is vital for efficient activation of the IKK complex. Furthermore, DHA has been shown to insert directly into lipid rafts of the membrane and to bind to the lipopolysaccharide receptor complex, such as TLR4/CD14/MD-2, thereby reducing endotoxin-stimulated NF-κB activation (Calder, 2015).

The key mediator recognised for omega-3 antiinflammatory signalling is the free fatty acid receptor-4, which is also known as G protein-coupled receptor 120 (GPR120). After the binding of EPA or DHA, GPR120 recruits the adaptor protein beta-arrestin-2, which, in turn, secretes TAB1 (TGF-beta activated kinase 1 binding protein 1). This scaffold protein is essential for the activation of the TAK1 gene, which encodes transforming growth factor-β-activated kinase 1, and thereby downregulates NF-kappaB and c-Jun N-terminal kinases (JNK) signalling. Studies by Oh et al. revealed that mice deficient in GPR120 were entirely unresponsive to the antiinflammatory effects of omega-3 fatty acids, providing convincing in vivo evidence for this receptor-mediated pathway. This finding locates GPR120 receptor as a feasible drug target for the circumstances driven by chronic low-grade inflammation, which includes type 2 diabetes and nonalcoholic steatohepatitis (Oh et al., 2010).

Conversely, this is affected by excessive intake of omega-6 PUFA, mainly AA and its metabolites, in which AA and ceramides, derived from hydrolysis, can drive upregulation of the entire pro-inflammatory transcriptome by activating NF-kappaB (Calder, 2015; Kolesnick & Krönke, 1998). The clear inflammatory resonance of a cell is consequently resolved by the equilibrium between pro-inflammatory omega-6 NF-kappaB activators and antiinflammatory omega-3 NF-kappaB inhibitors—a stability directly dictated by the omega-6:omega-3 ratio of membrane phospholipids (Simopoulos, 2002).

12.18.3 Active resolution of inflammation: specialized pro-resolving mediators

One of the possible and most transformative advances over the previous two decades in the field of functional lipids is omega-3 science, which has led to the discovery of SPMs—a family of bioactive lipid derivatives that actively participate in the resolution of inflammation, separate from simply suppressing the initiation of inflammatory responses. This kind of pattern shift, established at Harvard Medical School by Charles Serhan and his colleagues, primarily reframes the role of omega-3 PUFAs from submissive antiinflammatory substrates to active contributors in the resolution phase of the inflammatory response. These SPMs are derived from EPA and DHA and comprise the E-series resolvins, RvE1 and RvE2, which are produced from EPA via aspirin-modified COX-2 or via cytochrome P450 pathways. Whereas D-series resolvins—RvD1 through RvD6 are generated from DHA, protectins/neuroprotectins (NP)—PD1/NPD1, produced from DHA through 15-LOX, and maresins—MaR1, MaR2, are limited and caused by DHA in macrophages (Serhan, 2017). Discrete resolution actions are produced by each of the SPM family members, which are produced by the biosynthetic route and act on specific G protein-coupled receptors.

Resolution of inflammation is a biosynthetically driven, briefly regulated process that is categorized by: (1) the neutrophil recruitment is terminated to the site of inflammation; (2) the apoptotic neutrophils and cellular debris are removed by the enhanced phagocytosis by macrophages and the process is known as efferocytosis; (3) gets the stimulus for the of lymphatic clearance of inflammatory exudate; (4) finally results in the elevation of tissue renewal and

TABLE 12.2 Outline of key specialized pro-resolving mediator (SPM) classes, their omega-3 precursors, similar receptors, and their biological actions. SPMs that are derived from omega-3 fatty acids eicosapentaenoic acid (EPA) and docosahexaenoic acid (DHA) (Dalli et al., 2016; Serhan & Levy, 2018; Serhan, 2017).

SPM class	Precursor	Receptor	Key biological actions
RvE1, RvE2	EPA	ChemR23	Decreases the neutrophil recruitment, limits the cytokine production, and enhances efferocytosis
RvD1–RvD6	DHA	ALX/FPR2	Promote macrophage phagocytosis, stimulate lymphatic clearance, and reduce TNF-α
PD1/NPD1	DHA	Not yet defined	Neuroprotective, antiapoptotic, inhibit NF-κB, protect retinal cells
MaR1, MaR2	DHA	LGR6, MrgprX4	Accelerate wound healing, inhibit pain sensitization, and enhance tissue regeneration
n-3 DPA-SPMs	DPA	Multiple	Prolonged resolution, cross-talk with EPA/DHA pathways, antifibrotic

reoccurrence to homeostasis is observed (Serhan & Levy, 2018). Each of these steps in inflammation resolution is orchestrated by SPMs via receptor-mediated signalling. E-series resolvin RVE1, which stands in at the ChemR23 counter, regulates the relocation of LTB4-mediated neutrophils. Macrophage efferocytosis efficiency was enhanced two- to threefold by D-series resolvins—RvD1 acting at the site of ALX/FPR2. MaR1 accelerates wound healing and reduces pain sensitization at LGR6. An outline of key SPM classes, their omega-3 precursors, similar receptors, and biological actions is shown in Table 12.2

Disparagingly, unsuccessful or late resolution is now named as resolution deficit. This condition is gradually recognised as a main feature of the pathology of chronic inflammatory diseases, including atherosclerosis, inflammatory bowel disease, chronic obstructive pulmonary disease, and Alzheimer's disease, and is primarily an excess of pro-inflammatory signalling. Thus therapeutic approaches must aim not only to suppress inflammation but also to restore the resolution capacity at the sites of affected tissues; for this purpose, omega-3-derived SPMs are particularly appropriate.

12.19 Omega-3 and omega-6 polyunsaturated fatty acids in the management of disease

12.19.1 Cardiovascular disease

The omega-3 PUFAs' cardiovascular benefits have been the subject of investigation since Dyerberg and Bang's studies in 1970, which showed lower rates of ischemic heart disease among Greenlandic Inuit despite high dietary fat intake. The molecular mechanism of the reduction of triglycerides by DHA and EPA is through PPAR-α mediated reduction of hepatic lipogenesis and greater beta-oxidation, reduction of platelet aggregation through decreased TxA2 and amplified TxA3, lesser resting heart rate, and improved the variability of the heart rate by means of ion channel modulation, thereby reducing the circulating fibrinogen and inflammatory indicators (GISSI-Prevenzione Investigators, 1999).

12.19.2 Neurodevelopment and cognitive health

The dominant omega-3 fatty acid in the human brain and retina is DHA; grey matter fatty acids account for 10%–15% of the brain, and photoreceptor phospholipid fatty acids can reach 50%. The brain gathers DHA at rates of 20–40 mg/day in the pregnancy trimester and in the first two years of postnatal life, a demand that must be met by maternal transfer (placental and lactational) or directly by the infant. DHA is mainly required for normal synaptogenesis, myelination, neurotransmitter receptor function, and the development of visual acuity (Innis, 2008). Deficiencies can be critical in the developmental stages and are related to various issues like decreased cognitive performance, reduced visual acuity, and increased risk of attention deficit hyperactivity disorder.

DHA maintains membrane fluidity at neuronal synapses in the adult and ageing brains, which provides effective signalling through the serotonin and dopamine receptors and produces the NPD1, thereby inhibiting the beta-amyloid peptide-induced apoptotic signalling and lessening the Alzheimer's-associated neuroinflammation, and shields hippocampal neurons from oxidative stress. The biological observational data are steadily linking greater consumption of fish and DHA levels in the blood to reduce the risk of cognitive failure and Alzheimer's disease; nevertheless, clinical trial evidence for supplementation in established dementia remains incomplete.

12.19.3 Inflammatory and metabolic disease

The therapeutic significance of omega-3 fatty acids covers the range of chronic inflammatory conditions. In rheumatoid arthritis, metaanalyses of randomized controlled trials validate that the supplementation of fish oil with 3–5 g/day of EPA+DHA remarkably reduces joint pain, morning stiffness, and also reduces the tender and swollen joints, through the clinically meaningful decrease in the requirement of NSAID (Goldberg & Katz, 2007). EPA and DHA in inflammatory bowel disease attenuate intestinal mucosal inflammation, reduce the generation of colonic PGE2 and LTB4, and promote the integrity of the mucosal barrier. These effects are attributable to both SPM generation and eicosanoid remodelling within the gut-associated lymphoid tissue. Omega-3 fatty acids (DHA and EPA) combat dyslipidemia, macrophage infiltration of adipose tissue, and chronic low-grade inflammation that characterise these conditions in metabolic syndromes and type 2 diabetes. These conditions are achieved by activating the GPR120 receptor in adipocytes and macrophages, and omega-3 fatty acids suppress the activation of JNK and IKK and downregulate insulin receptor substrate (IRS-1) serine phosphorylation, thereby preserving insulin signalling fidelity and improving insulin sensitivity (Oh et al., 2010). The supplementation of omega-3 fatty acids similarly decreases the hepatic de novo lipogenesis. It promotes fatty acid oxidation in nonalcoholic fatty liver disease, thereby reducing liver fat content and circulating liver enzymes.

12.20 Applications as nutraceuticals and a delivery system

12.20.1 Fish oil supplements—a dominant platform and its constraints

One of the dominant nutraceutical forms, EPA and DHA, is encapsulated fish oil, used as a supplement and representing a multibillion-dollar global market anchored by widespread clinical trials. Yet, their hindrance is well-recognised. Since fish oil is extremely vulnerable to lipid oxidation, which is similar to the polyunsaturation that confers biological activity, EPA and DHA are susceptible to peroxidation, resulting in the generation of secondary oxidation mediators like reactive aldehydes, cytotoxic epoxides, and putrid volatile compounds. Oxidised fish oil could be biologically inert or detrimental; so far, consumer surveys indicate that a substantial proportion of commercially available fish oil supplements contain oxidised lipids at levels exceeding voluntary industry limits (Ruxton et al., 2020).

12.21 Fortification approaches and functional foods

Staple foods can be fortified with DHA and EPA, which signifies a promising strategy for distributing population-wide, avoiding dependence on the supplement's availability. There are successful commercial applications, such as DHA-fortified infant formula for the care of premature infants, and omega-3-enriched eggs, which can be achieved by modifying the hen diet with fish meal or algal biomass, thereby increasing DHA content to approximately 150mg per egg from 50 mg. Dairy products like milk, yoghurt, and cheese enriched with omega-3s, and fortified breakfast and cereals could lead to the development of functional foods (Shahidi & Ambigaipalan, 2018).

12.22 Algal oil—a sustainable future of docosahexaenoic acid and eicosapentaenoic acid

The microalgal DHA oil is obtained from the heterotrophic fermentation of *Schizochytrium* sp. and *Thraustochytrid* sp., and has received the governing consent in several markets and is combined into a number of infant formulas, plant-based dairy substitutes, and nutritional supplements (Ryan et al., 2010). The convincing advantages of algal oils are that they bypass the ecological trial of fish-derived fatty acids, which address the concerns about the overfishing disruption of the marine ecosystem, and are entirely free from toxic heavy metals, and it can be suitable for vegetarian consumers.

12.23 Future perspectives

12.23.1 Precision nutrition and customized omega-3 supplementation

One of the major challenges among the population is supplementation with omega-3 fatty acids, which shows extensive inconsistency in individuals' levels of DHA and EPA, their metabolism of these fatty acids, and the resulting clinical effects. The inconsistency in these fatty acids is attributable to the divergence in the fatty acid desaturase (FADS) genes, specifically FADS1 and FADS2, which encode the rate-limiting enzymes Delta 5 and 6 that regulate the biosynthesis of PUFA (Gillingham et al., 2013). Those who carry the insignificant alleles at the FAD loci exhibit a significant reduction in the conversion of ALA to DHA and EPA, which may reveal variance in inflammation responses equivalent to omega-3 supplementation.

The precision diet is one of the evolving fields, by utilizing genomic, metabolomic, lipidomic, and microbiome profiling, promises to reconstruct the supplementation of omega-3 fatty acids from a universal approach to a customized schedule that can be standardized to reference line fatty acid status, FADS genotype, inflammatory biomarker outlines, and gut microbiome composition. The personalized omega-3 dosing processes, based on the dried blood spot or fingerstick omega-3 index measurements (Harris & Von Schacky, 2004), could substantially improve the efficacy and cost-effectiveness of nutraceutical interventions in the management of inflammatory disease.

12.24 The gut microbiome–omega-3 axis

The metabolic and immunological effects of dietary lipids, particularly omega-3 PUFAs, are significantly mediated by the gut microflora. These dietary lipids have exerted bidirectional relations with the gut microflora; thus, the supplementation of omega-3 has been shown to enhance the relative abundance of antiinflammatory genera that include *Bifidobacterium* and *Lactobacillus*, whereas reducing the pro-inflammatory taxa like certain Firmicutes, thereby modulating the microbiome towards a less inflammatory phenotype (Costantini et al., 2017).

The omega-3 fatty acids (DHA and EPA) stimulate the bidirectional interactions with the gut microbiota: omega-3 supplementation has been shown to increase the relative abundance of antiinflammatory genera, including Bifidobacterium and Lactobacillus, while reducing pro-inflammatory taxa such as certain Firmicutes, thus modulating the microbiome toward a less inflammatory phenotype (Costantini et al., 2017). On the other hand, gut bacteria metabolise omega-3 fatty acids to secondary bioactives, such as 10-hydroxy-cis-12-octadecenoic acid (HYA), which have been shown to exert antiinflammatory activity independently in intestinal epithelial cells (Miyamoto et al., 2015).

The mixture of probiotic microbes, prebiotic fibres, and optimally delivered omega-3 fatty acids represents a promising future direction for advancing symbiotic functional foods. These heterogeneous formulations can lead to combinatorial interactions between the gut microbiota and omega-3 fatty acid metabolites, augmenting the biosynthesis of SPM. The SPM mediators strengthen the integrity of the colonic barrier, suppressing the systemic inflammatory response vigorously and continuously, with single-factor supplementation (Moszak et al., 2020).

12.25 Advanced delivery systems and nanoencapsulation

The next-generation delivery system for omega-3 is expected to move beyond traditional microencapsulation toward nanoscale designs capable of targeting specific tissues, cell types, or subcellular compartments. There are several delivery systems, such as nanostructured lipid carriers (NLCs), polymeric nanoparticles, nano-emulsions, and solid lipid nanoparticles, that have been identified as functionalized shuttles, directed by targeting ligands, for the delivery of DHA and EPA to the site of inflammation (Tan et al., 2018).

The coencapsulation of hydrophilic and lipophilic bioactive compounds can be achieved through liposome-mediated formulation, which has been shown to have specific promise for the combination therapy of DHA and EPA with collective antiinflammatory compounds like resveratrol/tocopherols and curcumin. Studies have shown that the combined effects of curcumin and omega-3 in the treatment of osteoarthritis using an in vivo method by downregulating the gene expression of cartilage-degrading enzymes (MP1, MMP3, and MMP13) (Jhun et al., 2025).

12.26 The next-generation therapeutics—resolvin and protectin as mimetics

The findings on SPMs have drawn attention to the production of stable synthetic counterparts of protectins, resolvins, and maresins, which are pharmaceutical-grade, antiinflammatory, and pro-resolving agents (Fig. 12.6). Subsequently, synthetically chemically stabilised mimetics with prolonged biological half-lives are under active development, since these endogenous SPMs in the in-vitro condition will quickly inactivate; chemically stabilised mimetics with prolonged biological half-lives are under active development (Bannenberg & Serhan, 2010). Whereas these agents may be classified as pharmaceuticals rather than nutraceuticals, their expansion is closely connected to the nutritional sciences of PUFAs and dietary amelioration with omega-3 fatty acids, which retain crucial roles in providing the substratum that can result in the biosynthesis of SPMs.

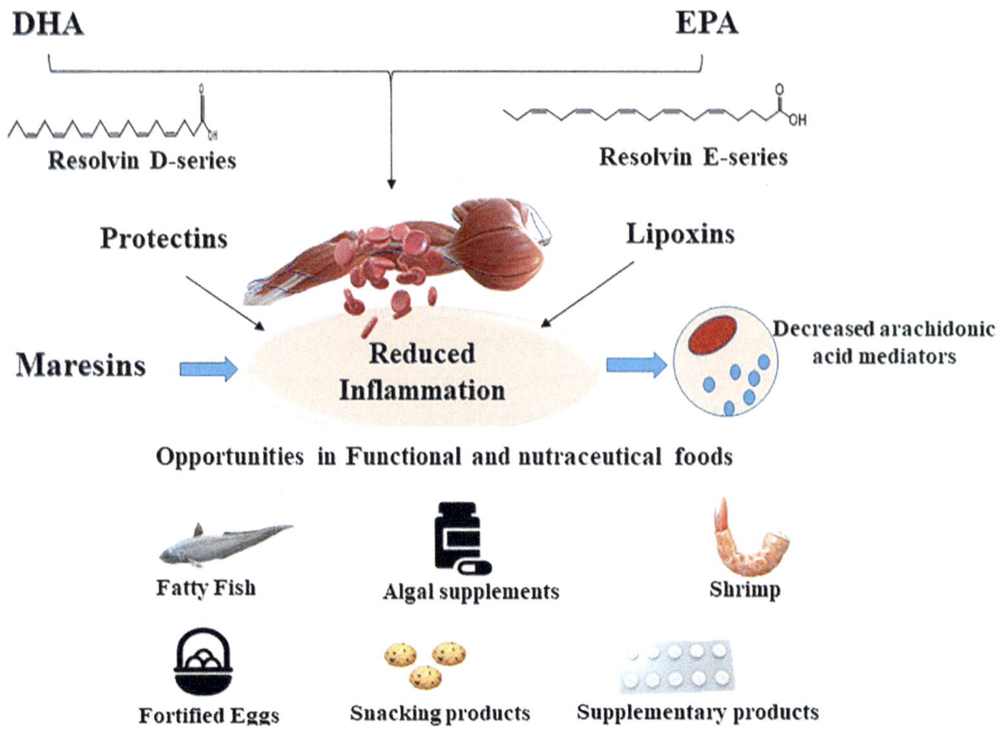

FIGURE 12.6 Schematic illustration of inflammation regulation by functional lipids.

The precision designing of functional foods can be a future for the maximum production of these endogenous SPMs by merging omega-3 fatty acids with the cofactors that are essential in the SPM biosynthesis, like aspirin that acetylates COX-2, thereby enabling the biosynthesis of 18-HEPE and 17-HDHA, and also with the compounds that upregulate the expression of 15-LOX (Serhan, 2017). Thus these methods will epitomise a sophisticated, mechanism-informed approach to functional food design for active metabolic programming, and they move beyond mere substrate delivery.

12.27 Clinical transformation and regulatory outlines

The development of mechanistic omega-3 into accepted health claims and therapeutic applications requires directing the multidimensional regulatory landscapes. The competent health claims of omega-3 PUFAs for reducing the risk of cardiac health disease have the treatment of EPA with a brand name of icosapent ethyl; Vascepa based on the breakthrough REDUCE-IT trial, which has received approval by the U.S. FDA for reducing cardiovascular issues in patients with higher triglyceride levels (Bhatt et al., 2019).

Nevertheless, extending approved claims to inflammatory conditions beyond cardiovascular disease, including neuroinflammation, rheumatoid arthritis, and inflammatory bowel disease, will require robust randomised controlled trials to demonstrate clinical effectiveness at defined doses and in relevant patient populations.

In order to have support for an expanded claim on omega-3 index, EPA + DHA, it is critical to generate clear evidence, and there is a need for the standardization of omega-3 status evaluation as authentic biomarkers for epidemiological studies and clinical trials (Harris & Von Schacky, 2004). The large-scale investment, well-powered trials evaluating EPA and DHA as functional food components for the primary and secondary prevention of inflammatory diseases, remain a high scientific and public health priority. Research on PUFAs remains one of the most urgent scientific and health priorities, with widespread funding and robust studies needed to assess omega-3 fatty acids as an effective dietary ingredient for the prevention of both primary and secondary inflammatory disorders.

12.28 Key challenges and considerations

Although PUFAs (DHA and EPA) have numerous important scientific applications, several challenges need to be addressed to fully understand their potential as nutraceutical agents. The prime most obstacle is their oxidative instability, due to the presence of highly unsaturated EPA and DHA structures that lead to peroxidation, resulting in the production of cytotoxic aldehydes and thereby weakening both safety and efficacy. The vital components of commercial PUFAs are product stabilisation, which can be achieved by mixing with other natural antioxidants such as tocopherols and rosemary extracts, and by encapsulating them in anoxic/nitrogen-blanketed environments. This method can be a cutting-edge system for the effective commercialisation of omega-3 products as functional foods.

The clinical trial outcomes are heterogeneous, as illustrated by the deviation between the outcomes of pure EPA trials (REDUCE-IT) and the insignificant results of EPA + DHA combination trials (ORIGIN and ASCEND). The results of clinical trials highlight the importance of distinguishing between the effects of DHA and EPA and, thus, carefully choosing the appropriate omega-3 for a specific inflammatory disease (Nicholls et al., 2020). The future of product development should be guided by understanding the mechanisms of EPA-specific effects, such as eicosanoid competition and decreased triglyceride levels, in contrast to the DHA-specific effects, such as membrane remodelling, DHA-derived SPMs, and neuroprotection in antiinflammatory pathways.

12.29 Conclusion

The omega-3 fatty acids, DHA and EPA, play an essential role in advancing nutritional science and the development of nutraceutical products, due to their well-characterised role in the mechanism of antiinflammatory properties, such as remodelling of eicosanoid, suppression of NF-κB, antagonists of Toll-like receptor 4 (TLR4), and the inhibition of inflammasome. These scientific potentials of omega-3 nutraceuticals will enable their use in the development of functional foods and dietary supplements that can target inflammatory pathologies. The precision nutrition will be the future of omega-3 nutraceuticals through the innovative delivery systems, engineered plant and sustainable algal-based manufacture, microbiome-informed design approaches, and extended clinical translation. The global scientific community, various food industries, and regulatory bodies should collaborate to overcome residual barriers, such as bioavailability optimisation, the development of clinical data, and regulatory harmonisation. Therefore the next generation of DHA and EPA nutraceutical products will be tailored, sustainably sourced, delivered, and validated mechanistically, and have the potential to lead to a meaningful contribution to the prevention and management of the universal chronic inflammatory diseases.

References

Abdulkhaleq, L. A., Assi, M. A., Abdullah, R., Zamri-Saad, M., Taufiq-Yap, Y. H., & Hezmee, M. N. M. (2018). The crucial roles of inflammatory mediators in inflammation: A review. *Veterinary World, 11*(5), 627–635. https://doi.org/10.14202/vetworld.2018.627-635.

Ahmed, A. U. (2011a). An overview of inflammation: Mechanism and consequences. *Frontiers of Biology in China, 6*(4), 274–281. https://doi.org/10.1007/s11515-011-1123-9.

Ahmed, A. U. (2011b). An overview of in flammation: Mechanism and consequences. *Frontiers in Biology, 6*(4), 274–281. https://doi.org/10.1007/s11515-011-1123-9.

Akira, S., Uematsu, S., & Takeuchi, O. (2006). Pathogen recognition pathogen recognition and innate immunity. *Cell, 124*(4), 783–801. https://doi.org/10.1016/j.cell.2006.02.015.

Al-Shaer, A. E., Buddenbaum, N., & Shaikh, S. R. (2021). Polyunsaturated fatty acids, specialized pro-resolving mediators, and targeting inflammation resolution in the age of precision nutrition. *Biochimica et Biophysica Acta - Molecular and Cell Biology of Lipids, 1866*(7). https://doi.org/10.1016/j.bbalip.2021.158936.

Banaszak, M., Dobrzyńska, M., Kawka, A., Górna, I., Woźniak, D., Przysławski, J., & Drzymała-Czyż, S. (2024). Role of Omega-3 fatty acids eicosapentaenoic (EPA) and docosahexaenoic (DHA) as modulatory and anti-inflammatory agents in noncommunicable diet-related diseases – Reports from the last 10 years. *Clinical Nutrition ESPEN, 63*, 240–258. https://doi.org/10.1016/j.clnesp.2024.06.053, https://www.sciencedirect.com/science/journal/24054577.

Bannenberg, G., & Serhan, C. N. (2010). Specialized pro-resolving lipid mediators in the inflammatory response: An update. *Biochimica et Biophysica Acta (BBA) - Molecular and Cell Biology of Lipids, 1801*(12), 1260–1273. https://doi.org/10.1016/j.bbalip.2010.08.002.

Bhatt, D. L., Steg, P. G., Miller, M., Brinton, E. A., Jacobson, T. A., Ketchum, S. B., Doyle, R. T., Juliano, R. A., Jiao, L., Granowitz, C., Tardif, J.-C., & Ballantyne, C. M. (2019). Cardiovascular Risk Reduction with Icosapent Ethyl for Hypertriglyceridemia. *New England Journal of Medicine, 380*(1), 11–22. https://doi.org/10.1056/nejmoa1812792.

Bigliardi, B., & Galati, F. (2013). Innovation trends in the food industry: The case of functional foods. *Trends in Food Science & Technology, 31*(2), 118–129. https://doi.org/10.1016/j.tifs.2013.03.006.

Bodur, M., Yilmaz, B., Ağagündüz, D., & Ozogul, Y. (2025). Immunomodulatory Effects of Omega-3 Fatty Acids: Mechanistic Insights and Health Implications. *Molecular Nutrition & Food Research, 69*(10). https://doi.org/10.1002/mnfr.202400752.

Brower, V. (1998). Nutraceuticals: Poised for a healthy slice of the healthcare market? *Nature Biotechnology, 16*(8), 728–731. https://doi.org/10.1038/nbt0898-728.

Byelashov, O. A., Sinclair, A. J., & Kaur, G. (2015). Dietary sources, current intakes, and nutritional role of omega-3 docosapentaenoic acid. *Lipid Technology, 27*(4), 79–82. https://doi.org/10.1002/lite.201500013.

Calder, P. C., Cawood, A. L., James, C., Page, F., Putnam, S., & Minihane, A. M. (2025). An overview of national and international long chain omega-3 polyunsaturated fatty acid intake recommendations for healthy populations. *Nutrition Research Reviews, 39*. https://doi.org/10.1017/S0954422425100279, http://journals.cambridge.org/NRR.

Calder, P. C. (2015). Marine omega-3 fatty acids and inflammatory processes: Effects, mechanisms and clinical relevance. *Biochimica et Biophysica Acta - Molecular and Cell Biology of Lipids, 1851*(4), 469–484. https://doi.org/10.1016/j.bbalip.2014.08.010, www.elsevier.com/locate/bbalip.

Calder, P. C. (2017). Omega-3 fatty acids and inflammatory processes: From molecules to man. *Biochemical Society Transactions, 45*(5), 1105–1115. https://doi.org/10.1042/BST20160474, http://www.biochemsoctrans.org/content/45/5/1105.full-text.pdf.

Calder, P. C. (2020). Eicosapentaenoic and docosahexaenoic acid derived specialised pro-resolving mediators: Concentrations in humans and the effects of age, sex, disease and increased omega-3 fatty acid intake. *Biochimie, 178*, 105–123. https://doi.org/10.1016/j.biochi.2020.08.015.

Cao, Y., Cao, Y., & Zhao, M. (2012). Biotechnological production of eicosapentaenoic acid: From a metabolic engineering point of view. *Process Biochemistry, 47*(9), 1320–1326. https://doi.org/10.1016/j.procbio.2012.05.011.

Chen, L., Deng, H., Cui, H., Fang, J., Zuo, Z., Deng, J., Li, Y., Wang, X., & Zhao, L. (2018). Inflammatory responses and inflammation-associated diseases in organs. *Oncotarget, 9*(6), 7204–7218. https://doi.org/10.18632/oncotarget.23208.

Costantini, L., Molinari, R., Farinon, B., & Merendino, N. (2017). Impact of Omega-3 Fatty Acids on the Gut Microbiota. *International Journal of Molecular Sciences, 18*(12), 2645. https://doi.org/10.3390/ijms18122645.

Dalli, J., Colas, R. A., Arnardottir, H., & Serhan, C. N. (2016). Vagal regulation of group 3 innate lymphoid cells and the immunoresolvent PCTR1 controls infection resolution. *Immunity, 46*(1), 92–105. https://doi.org/10.1016/j.immuni.2016.12.009.

Dangardt, F., Osika, W., Chen, Y., Nilsson, U., Gan, L. M., Gronowitz, E., Strandvik, B., & Friberg, P. (2010). Omega-3 fatty acid supplementation improves vascular function and reduces inflammation in obese adolescents. Atherosclerosis, 212(2), 580–585. https://doi.org/10.1016/j.atherosclerosis.2010.06.046.

Das, L., Bhaumik, E., Raychaudhuri, U., & Chakraborty, R. (2012). Role of nutraceuticals in human health. *Journal of Food Science and Technology, 49*(2), 173–183. https://doi.org/10.1007/s13197-011-0269-4.

Demain, A. L., & V., P. (2009). Production of recombinant proteins by microbes and higher organisms. *Biotechnology Advances, 27*(3), 297–306. https://doi.org/10.1016/j.biotechadv.2009.01.008.

Dunkelberger, J. R, & Song, W.-C. (2009). Complement and its role in innate and adaptive immune responses. *Cell Research, 20*(1), 34–50. https://doi.org/10.1038/cr.2009.139.

Ernst, E. (2001). Functional foods, neutraceuticals, designer foods: Innocent fad or counterproductive marketing ploy? *European Journal of Clinical Pharmacology, 57*(5), 353–355. https://doi.org/10.1007/s002280100327.

Fliesler, A. J., & Anderson, R. E. (1983). Chemistry and metabolism of lipids in the vertebrate retina. *Progress in Lipid Research, 22*(2), 79–131. https://doi.org/10.1016/0163-7827(83)90004-8.

Fosslien, E. (1998). Adverse effects of nonsteroidal anti-inflammatory drugs on the gastrointestinal system. *Annals of Clinical and Laboratory Science, 28*(2), 67–81.

Furman, D., Campisi, J., Verdin, E., Carrera-Bastos, P., Targ, S., Franceschi, C., Ferrucci, L., Gilroy, D. W., Fasano, A., Miller, G. W., Miller, A. H., Mantovani, A., Weyand, C. M., Barzilai, N., Goronzy, J. J., Rando, T. A., Effros, R. B., Lucia, A., Kleinstreuer, N., & Slavich, G. M. (2019). Chronic inflammation in the etiology of disease across the life span. *Nature Medicine, 25*(12), 1822–1832. https://doi.org/10.1038/s41591-019-0675-0, http://www.nature.com/nm/index.html.

Garay, M. I., Mazo, T., Ferrero, V., Barotto, N. N., Lagares, C., Granton, M. F., Moreira-Espinoza, M. J., Cremonezzi, D. C., Comba, A., Brunotto, M. N., Tolosa, E. J., Fernandez-Zapico, M. E., & Pasqualini, M. E. (2025). Novel inhibitory effect of Omega-3 fatty acids regulating pancreatic cancer progression. *Carcinogenesis, 46*(1). https://doi.org/10.1093/carcin/bgae081, http://carcin.oxfordjournals.org/.

Gillingham, L. G., Harding, S. V., Rideout, T. C., Yurkova, N., Cunnane, S. C., Eck, P. K., & Jones, P. J. H. (2013). Dietary oils and FADS1-FADS2 genetic variants modulate [13C]α-linolenic acid metabolism and plasma fatty acid composition. *The American Journal of Clinical Nutrition, 97*(1), 195–207. https://doi.org/10.3945/ajcn.112.043117.

GISSI-Prevenzione, Investigators (1999). Dietary supplementation with n-3 polyunsaturated fatty acids and vitamin E after myocardial infarction: results of the GISSI-Prevenzione trial. *The Lancet, 354*(9177), 447–455. https://doi.org/10.1016/s0140-6736(99)07072-5.

Global Organization for EPA and DHA Omega-3s2022. Global EPA & DHA Omega-3 Ingredient Market Report 2020–2021 Data & Forecasts Through 2024.

Goldberg, R. J., & Katz, J. (2007). A meta-analysis of the analgesic effects of omega-3 polyunsaturated fatty acid supplementation for inflammatory joint pain. *Pain, 129*(1-2), 210–223. https://doi.org/10.1016/j.pain.2007.01.020.

Gutiérrez, S., Svahn, S. L., & Johansson, M. E. (2019). Effects of omega-3 fatty acids on immune cells. *International Journal of Molecular Sciences, 20*(20). https://doi.org/10.3390/ijms20205028 MDPI AG.

Hajat, C., & Stein, E. (2018). The global burden of multiple chronic conditions: A narrative review. *Preventive Medicine Reports, 12*, 284–293. https://doi.org/10.1016/j.pmedr.2018.10.008.

Harris, W. S., & von Schacky, C. (2004). The Omega-3 Index: a new risk factor for death from coronary heart disease? *Preventive Medicine, 39*(1), 212–220. https://doi.org/10.1016/j.ypmed.2004.02.030.

He, W., Yan, L., Hu, D., Hao, J., Liou, Y. C., & Luo, G. (2025). Neutrophil heterogeneity and plasticity: Unveiling the multifaceted roles in health and disease. *MedComm, 6*(2). https://doi.org/10.1002/mco2.70063, onlinelibrary.wiley.com/journal/26882663.

Hirahashi, J. (2017). Omega-3 polyunsaturated fatty acids for the treatment of IgA nephropathy. *Journal of Clinical Medicine, 6*(7). https://doi.org/10.3390/jcm6070070, http://www.mdpi.com/2077-0383/6/7/70/pdf.

Hitl, M., Kladar, N., Banović Fuentes, J., Bijelić, K., Đermanović, M., & Torović, L. (2025). Knowledge and consumption patterns of omega-3 fatty acids among the central balkan population—A prospective cross-sectional study. *Nutrients, 17*(1), 122. https://doi.org/10.3390/nu17010122.

Hong, Y., Boiti, A., Vallone, D., & Foulkes, N. S. (2024). Reactive oxygen species signaling and oxidative stress: Transcriptional regulation and evolution. *Antioxidants, 13*(3). https://doi.org/10.3390/antiox13030312, www.mdpi.com/journal/antioxidants.

Hoti, G., Matencio, A., Pedrazzo, A. R., Cecone, C., Appleton, S. L., Monfared, Y. K., Caldera, F., & Trotta, F. (2022). Nutraceutical concepts and dextrin-based delivery systems. *International Journal of Molecular Sciences, 23*(8). https://doi.org/10.3390/ijms23084102 MDPI.

Innis, S. M. (2008). Dietary omega 3 fatty acids and the developing brain. *Brain Research, 1237*, 35–43. https://doi.org/10.1016/j.brainres.2008.08.078.

Jhun, J. Y., Lee, D., Na, H. S., Cho, K. H., Lee, S. Y., Lee, J. S., Lee, Y. J., Kim, S. J., Park, S. H., & Cho, M. L. (2025). Curcumin and omega-3 ameliorate experimental osteoarthritis progression in terms of joint pain and mitochondrial dysfunction. *Journal of Inflammation (United Kingdom), 22*(1). https://doi.org/10.1186/s12950-025-00453-x, https://journal-inflammation.biomedcentral.com/.

Jin, F., Xie, L., Zhang, H., Fan, X., Tian, J., Liu, W., Xiao, Y., & Fan, X. (2025). Dendritic cells: Origin, classification, development, biological functions, and therapeutic potential. *MedComm, 6*(11). https://doi.org/10.1002/mco2.70455, onlinelibrary.wiley.com/journal/26882663.

Kalra, E. K. (2003). Nutraceutical-definition and introduction. *AAPS PharmSci, 5*(3), 27–28. https://doi.org/10.1208/ps050325.

Kaur, N., Chugh, V., & Gupta, A. K. (2012). Essential fatty acids as functional components of foods- A review. *Journal of Food Science and Technology, 51*(10), 2289–2303. https://doi.org/10.1007/s13197-012-0677-0 Springer.

Kidd, P. M. (2007). Omega-3 DHA and EPA for cognition, behavior, and mood: Clinical findings and structural-functional synergies with cell membrane phospholipids. *Alternative Medicine Review, 12*(3), 207–227.

Kim, H. Y., Huang, B. X., & Spector, A. A. (2022). Molecular and signaling mechanisms for docosahexaenoic acid-derived neurodevelopment and neuroprotection. *International Journal of Molecular Sciences, 23*(9). https://doi.org/10.3390/ijms23094635 MDPI.

Koeberle, A., & Werz, O. (2014). Multi-target approach for natural products in inflammation. *Drug Discovery Today, 19*(12), 1871–1882. https://doi.org/10.1016/j.drudis.2014.08.006.

Kolesnick, R. N., & Krönke, M. (1998). Regulation of ceramide production and apoptosis. *Annual Review of Physiology, 60*(1), 643–665. https://doi.org/10.1146/annurev.physiol.60.1.643.

Kris-Etherton, P. M., Grieger, J. A., & Etherton, T. D. (2009). Dietary reference intakes for DHA and EPA. *Prostaglandins, Leukotrienes, and Essential Fatty Acids, 81*(2–3), 99–104. https://doi.org/10.1016/j.plefa.2009.05.011.

Leyva-López, N., Gutierrez-Grijalva, E. P., Ambriz-Perez, D. L., & Heredia, J. B. (2016). Flavonoids as cytokine modulators: A possible therapy for inflammation-related diseases. *International Journal of Molecular Sciences, 17*(6). https://doi.org/10.3390/ijms17060921, http://www.mdpi.com/1422-0067/17/6/921/pdf.

Li, M., Wang, M., Wen, Y., Zhang, H., Zhao, G. N., & Gao, Q. (2023). Signaling pathways in macrophages: Molecular mechanisms and therapeutic targets. *MedComm, 4*(5). https://doi.org/10.1002/mco2.349, onlinelibrary.wiley.com/journal/26882663.

Mathias, R. A., Pani, V., & Chilton, F. H. (2014). Genetic variants in the FADS gene: Implications for dietary recommendations for fatty acid intake. *Current Nutrition Reports, 3*(2), 139–148. https://doi.org/10.1007/s13668-014-0079-1 Current Science Inc.

Medoro, A., Davinelli, S., Colletti, A., Micoli, V., Di, Grandi, E., Fogacci, F., Scapagnini, G., & Cicero, A. F. G. (2023). Nutraceuticals as modulators of immune function: A review of potential therapeutic effects. *Preventive Nutrition and Food Science, 28*(2), 89–107. https://doi.org/10.3746/pnf.2023.28.2.89 Korean Society of Food Science and Nutrition.

Medzhitov, R. (2010). Inflammation 2010: New adventures of an old flame. *Cell, 140*(6), 771–776. https://doi.org/10.1016/j.cell.2010.03.006.

Mishra, K., & Kakhlon, O. (2025). The crucial role of NAD+ in mitochondrial metabolic regulation. *Biocell: Official Journal of the Sociedades Latinoamericanas de Microscopia Electronica, 49*(7), 1101–1123. https://doi.org/10.32604/biocell.2025.061725.

Miyamoto, J., Mizukure, T., Park, S. B., Kishino, S., Kimura, I., Hirano, K., Bergamo, P., Rossi, M., Suzuki, T., Arita, M., Ogawa, J., & Tanabe, S. (2015). A gut microbial metabolite of linoleic acid, 10-hydroxy-cis-12-octadecenoic acid, ameliorates intestinal epithelial barrier impairment partially via GPR40-MEK-ERK pathway. *Journal of Biological Chemistry, 290*(5), 2902–2918. https://doi.org/10.1074/jbc.M114.610733, http://www.jbc.org/content/290/5/2902.full.pdf+html.

Mohanty, B. P., G., S., M., A., S., T., A., R., C., K., P., B., S., D., S., D., J., V., G., M., S., A., K., K., D., M., T., C., S., S., N., D., P., D., P., A., M., V., P., & S., N. (2016). DHA and EPA concentration. *BioMed Research International*, 1–14. https://doi.org/10.1155/2016/4027437.

Moszak, M., Szulińska, M., & Bogdański, P. (2020). You Are What You Eat—The Relationship between Diet, Microbiota, and Metabolic Disorders—A Review. *Nutrients, 12*(4), 1096. https://doi.org/10.3390/nu12041096.

Mukai, K., Tsai, M., Saito, H., & Galli, S. J. (2018). Mast cells as sources of cytokines, chemokines, and growth factors. *Immunological Reviews, 282*(1), 121–150. https://doi.org/10.1111/imr.12634, http://onlinelibrary.wiley.com/journal/10.1111/(ISSN)1600-065X.

Nathan, C. (2006). Neutrophils and immunity: Challenges and opportunities. *Nature Reviews. Immunology, 6*(3), 173–182. https://doi.org/10.1038/nri1785.

Nelson, J. R., Budoff, M. J., Wani, O. R., Le, V., Patel, D. K., Nelson, A., & Nemiroff, R. L. (2021). EPA's pleiotropic mechanisms of action: A narrative review. *Postgraduate Medicine, 133*(6), 651–664. https://doi.org/10.1080/00325481.2021.1921491, http://www.tandfonline.com/loi/ipgm20#.VuKyZLdf2DY.

Nicholls, S. J., Lincoff, A. M., Garcia, M., Bash, D., Ballantyne, C. M., Barter, P. J., Davidson, M. H., Kastelein, J. J. P., Koenig, W., McGuire, D. K., Mozaffarian, D., Ridker, P. M, Ray, K. K., Katona, B. G., Himmelmann, A., Loss, L. E., Rensfeldt, M., Lundström, T., Agrawal, R., Menon, V., Wolski, K., & Nissen, S. E. (2020). Effect of High-Dose Omega-3 Fatty Acids vs Corn Oil on Major Adverse Cardiovascular Events in Patients at High Cardiovascular Risk. *JAMA, 324*(22), 2268. https://doi.org/10.1001/jama.2020.22258.

Oh, D. Y., Talukdar, S., Bae, E. J., Imamura, T., Morinaga, H., Fan, W. Q., Li, P., Lu, W. J., Watkins, S. M., & Olefsky, J. M. (2010). GPR120 Is an omega-3 fatty acid receptor mediating potent anti-inflammatory and insulin-sensitizing effects. *Cell, 142*(5), 687–698. https://doi.org/10.1016/j.cell.2010.07.041, https://www.sciencedirect.com/journal/cell.

Reichardt, S. D., Amouret, A., Muzzi, C., Vettorazzi, S., Tuckermann, J. P., Lühder, F., & Reichardt, H. M. (2021). The Role of Glucocorticoids in Inflammatory Diseases. *Cells, 10*(11), 2921. https://doi.org/10.3390/cells10112921.

Ribeiro, H., Rodrigues, I., Napoleão, L., Lira, L., Marques, D., Veríssimo, M., Andrade, J. P., & Dourado, M. (2022). Non-steroidal anti-inflammatory drugs (NSAIDs), pain and aging: Adjusting prescription to patient features. *Biomedicine & Pharmacotherapy, 150*, 112958. https://doi.org/10.1016/j.biopha.2022.112958.

Roberfroid, M. B. (2000). Concepts and strategy of functional food science: The European perspective. *The American Journal of Clinical Nutrition, 71*(6), 1660S–1664S. https://doi.org/10.1016/S0924-2244(00)88944-X.

Ruxton, C. H. S., Calder, P. C., Reed, S. C., & Simpson, M. J. A. (2020). The impact of long chain n-3 polyunsaturated fatty acids on human health. *Nutrition Research Reviews, 18*(1), 113–129. https://doi.org/10.1079/NRR200497.

Ryan, A. S., Astwood, J. D., Gautier, S., Kuratko, C. N., Nelson, E. B., & Salem, N. (2010). Effects of long-chain polyunsaturated fatty acid supplementation on neurodevelopment in childhood: A review of human studies. *Prostaglandins, Leukotrienes, and Essential Fatty Acids, 82*(4-6), 305–314. https://doi.org/10.1016/j.plefa.2010.02.007.

Santini, A., Tenore, G. C., & Novellino, E. (2017). Nutraceuticals: A paradigm of proactive medicine. *European Journal of Pharmaceutical Sciences, 96*, 53–61. https://doi.org/10.1016/j.ejps.2016.09.003 Elsevier B.V.

Serhan, C. N., & Levy, B. D. (2018). Resolvins in inflammation: Emergence of the pro-resolving superfamily of mediators. *Journal of Clinical Investigation, 128*(7), 2657–2669. https://doi.org/10.1172/JCI97943, https://www.jci.org/articles/view/97943/pdf.

Serhan, C. N. (2017). Treating inflammation and infection in the 21st century: New hints from decoding resolution mediators and mechanisms. *FASEB Journal, 31*(4), 1273–1288. https://doi.org/10.1096/fj.201601222R, http://www.fasebj.org/content/31/4/1273.full.pdf+html.

Shahidi, F., & Ambigaipalan, P. (2018). Omega-3 polyunsaturated fatty acids and their health benefits. *Annual Review of Food Science and Technology, 9*(1), 345–381. https://doi.org/10.1146/annurev-food-111317-095850.

Simopoulos, A. P. (2002). The importance of the ratio of omega-6/omega-3 essential fatty acids. *Biomedicine & Pharmacotherapy, 56*(8), 365–379. https://doi.org/10.1016/s0753-3322(02)00253-6.

Soares, C. L. R., Wilairatana, P., Silva, L. R., Moreira, P. S., Vilar Barbosa, N. M. M., da Silva, P. R., Coutinho, H. D. M., de Menezes, I. R. A., & Felipe, C. F. B. (2023). Biochemical aspects of the inflammatory process: A narrative review. *Biomedicine and Pharmacotherapy, 168*. https://doi.org/10.1016/j.biopha.2023.115764, https://www.journals.elsevier.com/biomedicine-and-pharmacotherapy.

Srigley, C. T., & Rader, J. I. (2014). Content and composition of fatty acids in marine oil omega-3 supplements. *Journal of Agricultural and Food Chemistry, 62*(29), 7268–7278. Available from https://doi.org/10.1021/jf5016973, http://pubs.acs.org/journal/jafcau.

Stone, K. D., Prussin, C., & Metcalfe, D. D. (2010). IgE, mast cells, basophils, and eosinophils. *Journal of Allergy and Clinical Immunology, 125*(2 SUPPL. 2). https://doi.org/10.1016/j.jaci.2009.11.017.

Schuchardt, J. P., & Hahn, A. (2013). Bioavailability of long-chain omega-3 fatty acids. *Prostaglandins, Leukotrienes and Essential Fatty Acids, 89*(1), 1–8. https://doi.org/10.1016/j.plefa.2013.03.010.

Sun-Waterhouse, D. (2011). The development of fruit-based functional foods targeting the health and wellness market: A review. *International Journal of Food Science & Technology, 46*(5), 899–920. https://doi.org/10.1111/j.1365-2621.2010.02499.x.

Tanaka, T., Shen, J., Abecasis, G. R., Kisialiou, A., Ordovas, J. M., Guralnik, J. M., Singleton, A., Bandinelli, S., Cherubini, A., Arnett, D., Tsai, M. Y., & Ferrucci, L. (2009). Genome-wide association study of plasma polyunsaturated fatty acids in the InCHIANTI study. *PLoS Genetics*, (5), 1. https://doi.org/10.1371/journal.pgen.1000338, http://www.plosgenetics.org/article/fetchObjectAttachment.action?uri=info%3Adoi%2F10.1371%2Fjournal.pgen.1000338&representation=PDF.

Tan, C., Xue, J., Abbas, S., Feng, B., & Zhang, X. (2018). Design and fabrication of nanoemulsions for delivery of omega-3 fatty acids: A review of recent advances. *Food Engineering Reviews, 10*(1), 14–29.

Thompson, M., Hein, N., Hanson, C., Smith, L. M., Anderson-Berry, A., Richter, C. K., Stessy Bisselou, K., Kusi Appiah, A., Kris-Etherton, P., Skulas-Ray, A. C., & Nordgren, T. M. (2019). Omega-3 Fatty Acid Intake by Age, Gender, and Pregnancy Status in the United States: National Health and Nutrition Examination Survey 2003–2014. *Nutrients, 11*(1), 177. https://doi.org/10.3390/nu11010177.

Troesch, B., Eggersdorfer, M., Laviano, A., Rolland, Y., Smith, A. D., Warnke, I., Weimann, A., & Calder, P. C. (2020). Expert opinion on benefits of long-chain omega-3 fatty acids (DHA and EPA) in aging and clinical nutrition. *Nutrients, 12*(9), 1–25. https://doi.org/10.3390/nu12092555, https://www.mdpi.com/2072-6643/12/9/2555/pdf.

Van Dael, P. (2021). Role of n-3 long-chain polyunsaturated fatty acids in human nutrition and health: Review of recent studies and recommendations. *Nutrition Research and Practice, 15*(2), 137–159. https://doi.org/10.4162/nrp.2021.15.2.137, https://www.ncbi.nlm.nih.gov/pmc/articles/PMC8007408/pdf/nrp-15-137.pdf.

van der Wurff, I. S. M., Meyer, B. J., & de Groot, R. H. M. (2020). Effect of omega-3 long chain polyunsaturated fatty ccids (n-3 LCPUFA) supplementation on cognition in children and adolescents: A systematic literature review with a focus on n-3 LCPUFA blood values and dose of DHA and EPA. *Nutrients, 12*(10), 3115. https://doi.org/10.3390/nu12103115.

Vane, J. R., & Botting, R. M. (1998). Mechanism of action of antiinflammatory drugs. *International Journal of Tissue Reactions, 20*(1), 3–15.

Wright, J. M. (2002). The double-edged sword of COX-2 selective NSAIDs. *Canadian Medical Association Journal, 167*(10), 1131–1137.

Zeisel, S. H. (1999). Regulation of "nutraceuticals. *Science (New York, N.Y.), 285*(5435), 1853–1855. https://doi.org/10.1126/science.285.5435.1853.

Zhang, B., Xiong, K., Cai, J., & Ma, A. (2020). Fish consumption and coronary heart disease: A meta-analysis. *Nutrients, 12*(8), 1–22. https://doi.org/10.3390/nu12082278, https://www.mdpi.com/2072-6643/12/8/2278/pdf.

Chapter 13

Advancing personalized nutrition: innovative polyunsaturated fatty acids delivery systems for omega-3 and omega-6 fatty acids in functional foods

Amiya Ojha[1,*], Deeplina Das[1], and Tarun Kanti Bandyopadhyay[2]

[1]*Department of Bio Engineering, National Institute of Technology Agartala, Jirania, Tripura, India,* [2]*Department of Chemical Engineering, National Institute of Technology Agartala, Jirania, Tripura, India*

13.1 Introduction

Polyunsaturated fatty acids (PUFAs), especially omega-3 and omega-6 fatty acids, are vital components of the human body since they affect the heart and neurodevelopment, and they are also involved in inflammation. Even though their biological significance is high, modern dietary habits often lack the proper intakes, and innovative approaches should address the need to supplement the PUFA intakes. Fortification of functional foods with bioactive PUFA constituents is one of these promising methods, although the addition of omega-3 and omega-6 fatty acids to food matrices is hindered by various challenges such as oxidative instability, poor solubility, and the development of off-flavors that affect organoleptic quality and shelf life (Ciesielski 2025; Das et al., 2024; Kassem et al., 2025). The encapsulation technique is attracting a lot of attention because people are looking for safe and long-lasting nourishment, and the nutraceuticals, superfoods, and functional food industries are growing at a rapid pace to meet this need (Chang & Nickerson, 2018; Jurić et al., 2020). Scientists and analysts within the nutraceutical industry regularly recommend the charismatic launch of bioactive elements, which is due to their ability to boost bioavailability and therapeutic efficacy. The approach is also beneficial, especially in cases where a long-lasting delivery is needed to ensure physiological concentration levels over prolonged periods. Thus decreasing the frequency of dosage administration and enhancing compliance levels to treatment regimens (Peng et al., 2017). To make the delivery system work better, it should include useful ingredients in food systems that are more stable physically and chemically and have little effect on how the food tastes. Encapsulation methods should also make it possible for chemicals to be taken in more fully when they are eaten and released slowly when certain biological conditions are met (Meyer-Déru et al., 2022). Functional chemicals, which are often hydrophobic, break down quickly in the body or being processed, which means they are not bioavailable. The packaging of these chemicals is very important for their effective delivery. Researchers have been working on new packaging methods that can increase absorption. Functional fats are one of these molecules that stand out because they are good for your health in many ways. Functional lipids, including omega-3 and omega-6 fatty acids, LA (linolenic acid), conjugated LA, carotenoids, and other functional substances, are good for your health in many ways (Kheto et al., 2024). They can help with heart disease, mental illness, and metabolic diseases like diabetes. Vegetables, nuts, meat, fish, algae, and microbes are some natural foods that contain these substances (Saini et al., 2021). In the past, the dietary intake of these fatty acids has been considered a normal constituent of the human diet. However, various studies have shown that direct intake of functional fats is lower than the

[*] Corresponding author: amiya398@gmail.com

Omega-3 and Omega-6 Polyunsaturated Fatty Acids in Food Systems. DOI: https://doi.org/10.1016/B978-0-443-43810-3.00037-3

recommended minimum levels of dietary intake, and this could be because of poor intake, geographical distribution, or low availability.

The chapter is a survey of the state-of-the-art delivery technologies that have been designed to overcome such impediments, hence enabling the effective addition of PUFAs to the functional food products. We discuss high-tech modalities that include nanoemulsions, liposomes, and microencapsulation, which, as a combination, can increase the physicochemical stability, bioavailability, and sensory acceptability of omega-3 and omega-6 fatty acids. Moreover, we also discuss how personalized nutrition can be used in tailoring PUFA-enriched foods to the specifics of an individual's diet, based on advances in nutrigenomics and consumer preference studies. The chapter hopes to provide a broad overview of how new types of delivery systems are transforming personalized nutrition and promoting healthier eating habits by highlighting the recent developments and their implications in the translation.

13.2 Food sources of dietary omega-3 and omega-6 polyunsaturated fatty acids

LA serves as the parent chemical of omega-6 PUFAs and acts as a precursor for the synthesis of long-chain PUFAs, including arachidonic acid (AA) and gamma-linolenic acid (GLA) (Huang et al., 2026; Nath et al., 2025). It is the predominant PUFA found in many plant oils, including soybean, maize, and sunflower, as well as in nuts, seeds, eggs, and meats. Plants are the primary source of omega-3 PUFAs present in both terrestrial and marine environments (Saini et al., 2021). Alpha-linolenic acid (ALA), which is the most prevalent omega-3 PUFA found in a wide range of foods originating from both plants and animals, acts as the precursor for both eicosapentaenoic acid (EPA) and docosahexaenoic acid (DHA) (Fig. 13.1) (Rincón-Cervera et al., 2020). Marine algae mostly carry out the production of these two, and they are also concentrated in the food chain. Therefore fish and fish oils are the most significant sources of EPA and DHA in the food industry; the quantities of these fatty acids can range from several 100 mg to more than 1 g per 100 g of fish (Tocher et al., 2019). A small amount of omega-3 PUFAs may be found in the lipids of cattle, lamb, poultry, and pork (Ponnampalam et al., 2021). As a consequence, meats exhibit a ratio of omega-6:omega-3 that is normally high, whereas the ratio of polyunsaturated to saturated fatty acids (SFAs) is rather low (D'Angelo et al., 2020). LA is the predominant omega-6 fatty acid, while ALA is the predominant omega-3 fatty acid found in meat (Fig. 13.1). Reflective and nonruminant meats have differences in PUFA concentration. ALA comprises 0.7%–1.4% of total fatty acids in beef, pig, and lamb; however, LA is much higher in pork (14.2%) than in beef (2.4%) and lamb (2.7%), resulting in an increased omega-6 to omega-3 ratio in pork. Poultry exhibits a comparable fatty acid profile to pigs, including a substantially

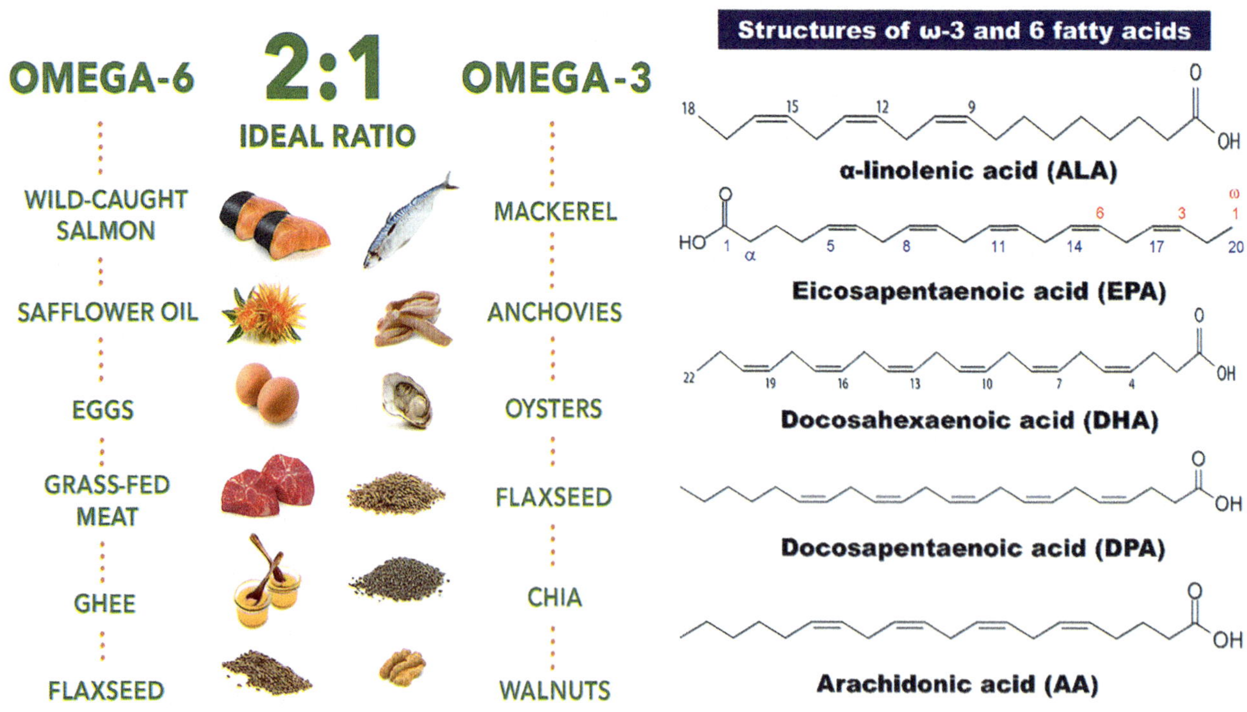

FIGURE 13.1 Different food sources and the structure of omega-3 and omega-6 fatty acids.

elevated concentration of LA. The omega-6:omega-3 ratio in ruminant meat is somewhat more advantageous due to the consumption of grass abundant in ALA; nevertheless, the inefficient conversion of ALA to EPA and DHA constrains the omega-3 fatty-acid levels in the meat (Jeong et al., 2024). Among the several types of fatty acids found in ruminants, conjugated linoleic acids are considered to be vital. Only in moderate quantities (less than 200 mg per 100 g) may AA be found in fish, meat, eggs, poultry, and dairy products. Similar to meat, milk possesses a comparatively low quantity of PUFAs and a low ratio of PUFAs to SFAs, with LA and ALA being the predominant omega-6 (1%–3% w/w) and omega-3 (0.5%–2% w/w) fatty acids in milk fat, correspondingly (Saini et al., 2021).

13.3 Nutritional significance of omega-3 and omega-6 fatty acids

Fatty acids and glycerol are the components that make up triglycerides, which account for about 90% of the fats that we consume via our diet (Menalla et al., 2024). A methyl group is located at one end of a chain of carbon atoms that makes up fatty acids, while an acid group is located at the other end of the chain. Omega-3 and omega-6 fatty acids are both crucial for cell membranes and the production of several other bodily chemicals, including those that control inflammation and blood pressure (Djuricic & Calder, 2021). More and more evidence suggests that omega-3 fatty acids can help protect against heart disease, which can be deadly (Bowen et al., 2016). It is also known that these acids can reduce inflammation, which may be important in this and other illnesses. More and more people are also interested in how omega-3 fatty acids can help avoid diabetes and some types of cancer (Freitas & Campos, 2019). The body can make all but two fatty acids: LA, which is an omega-6 fatty acid, and ALA, which is an omega-3 fatty acid. They are called "essential fatty acids" because you have to get them from food (Alagawany et al., 2022). In addition to being building blocks for other fatty acids, these two are essential for development and repair. For instance, ALA may be used to synthesize EPA and DHA, two omega-3 fatty acids. It is advised to incorporate sources of these into the diet as well, due to the restricted conversion. Plant and seed oils include ALA and LA. Rapeseed and walnut oils are excellent sources of ALA, even though LA levels are often significantly greater. Oily fish, such as salmon, mackerel, and herring, are good sources of EPA and DHA. Meat and egg yolk are two examples of animal products that contain AA (Santos et al., 2020).

LA and ALA compete for metabolism via the enzyme δ-6-desaturase in the human body. It has been proposed that this is crucial for health, since elevated consumption of LA might diminish the availability of δ-6-desaturase for ALA metabolism, thereby heightening the risk of cardiovascular disease. The modern diet often has a high omega-6 to omega-3 ratio (10:1 to 20:1), while a ratio closer to 1:1 or 4:1 is considered optimal for reducing chronic disease risk (Bishehkolaei & Pathak, 2024). Data indicate that over the past 150 years, the consumption of omega-6 has risen while omega-3 intake has declined, coinciding with a surge in heart disease cases (Leung et al., 2019). Consequently, the notion of an "optimal" ratio of omega-6 to omega-3 fatty acids in the diet was established. Nonetheless, the ratio linked to a decreased risk of heart disease remains unidentified, and some experts now propose that the ratio is of little significance; rather, the focus should be on the absolute amounts of consumption. A workshop study in this subject stated that just increasing the quantity of ALA, EPA, and DHA in the diet would accomplish the required rise in changes in the amounts of these fatty acids in the body's organs, and that decreasing the intake of LA and AA was not essential (Ponnampalam et al., 2021). Moreover, the ratio technique fails to differentiate between diets that are sufficient in both omega-6 and omega-3 and those that are lacking in both nutrients.

13.4 Effect of omega-3 and omega-6 polyunsaturated fatty acids on human health

Omega-3 and omega-6 PUFAs, as fundamental structural components of phospholipids, impart liquidity and adaptability to cellular membranes. LA and ALA serve as ancestors for omega-6 and omega-3 PUFAs, respectively. Different types of lipids, like triglycerides and cholesterol esters, as well as very small amounts of phospholipids, store them (Djuricic & Calder, 2021). EPA can be found in all three of these types of lipids, but DHA and AA are more likely to be found in phospholipids. PUFAs change how genes are expressed, how cells talk to each other, how eicosanoid metabolism works, and how the cell membrane is organized (Ali & Szabó, 2023). It has been known for a long time that fatty acids can change the structure of cell membranes and make ingredients for eicosanoid production more or less available. These changes are thought to be caused by the effects of fatty acids on membrane composition and cellular signaling pathways that have been seen.

LA plays an important role in maintaining skin structural integrity and barrier function, as it is a key component of ceramides in the epidermis (You & Liang, 2025). The extracellular matrix, which consists of cholesterol, ceramides, and free fatty acids, forms the permeability barrier of the stratum corneum, with LA being essential for its fluidity. The skin's ability to convert LA to AA is limited due to a lack of necessary enzymes (Fig. 13.2). Fatty acids can be absorbed by the

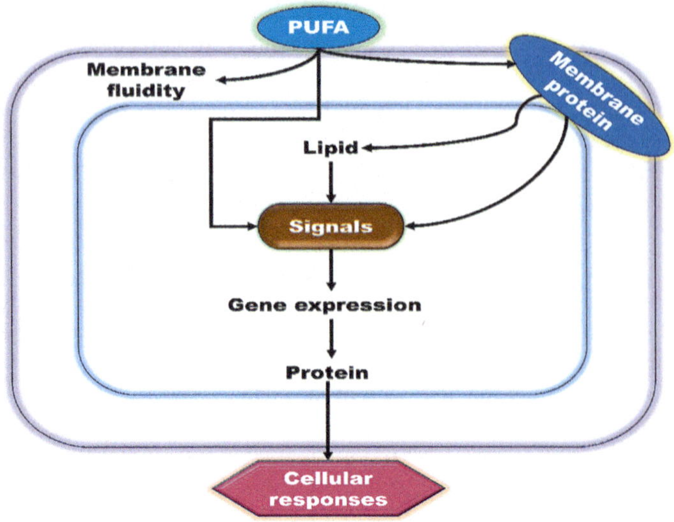

FIGURE 13.2 Significance of polyunsaturated fatty acids (*PUFA*) in the cellular response of the human body.

epidermis and may help protect skin function and appearance while modulating inflammation (Biernacki & Skrzydlewska, 2025). PUFAs can alleviate symptoms of inflammatory skin disorders like atopic dermatitis (AD) and psoriasis by influencing the balance of pro- and antiinflammatory eicosanoids (Olejnik et al., 2023). AD is characterized by a Th2-dominated inflammatory reaction that gradually transforms into other T-cell phenotypes as the disease develops (Krejsgaard et al., 2017). PUFAs have the potential to alleviate cutaneous inflammation as intermediates of lipid mediators and through the regulation of immune pathways. The simultaneous consumption of omega-6 PUFAs (e.g., LA and GLA) and omega-3 PUFAs (e.g., EPA and DHA) may have therapeutic benefits in the treatment of inflammatory dermatoses.

GLA undergoes conversion into dihomo-γ-linolenic acid (DGLA) by the ELOVL-5 enzyme, and then DGLA is embedded into glycerolipids in the cells (Patel et al., 2022). DGLA and its metabolites have various biological effects when they inhibit platelet aggregation, reduce inflammatory reactions, and biosynthesize antiinflammatory eicosanoids like prostaglandin PGE1. Besides that, DGLA increases the expression of E-cadherin, thus inhibiting motility and insensitivity of colorectal cancer cells (Jara-Gutiérrez & Baladron, 2021). Both GLA and DGLA are noted for their ability to suppress oncogenes Her-2/neu and Bcl2 while promoting p53 activity, leading to apoptosis in tumor cells (Hayyan et al., 2025).

LA makes up less than 2% of brain fatty acids and is thought to be functionally insignificant compared to the other fatty acids, AA and DHA that comprise up to 40% of brain fatty acids (Sambra et al., 2021). More than half of cerebral LA is either subject to β-oxidation or is oxidized to oxidized products, whose physiological functions are not completely comprehended but could be involved in the pathophysiology of migraine. Ramsden et al. (2021) showed that over 3 months of consumption of low dietary LA (7% to 2% of total energy intake) and high consumption of EPA and DHA (1.5 g/day) resulted in a decrease in the frequency of migraine and quality of life. Nonetheless, it is not clear whether such benefits are related to reduced LA, increased EPA and DHA, or their interaction; further studies should be done targeting long-term LA depletion.

DHA is an essential omega-3 fatty acid, which is a prerequisite in many physiological processes, especially in the central nervous system and tissue of the retina, where it is highly concentrated. DHA controls the transportation of amino acids, adjusting sodium channels that are voltage-sensitive, and it alters the conformational changes of rhodopsin to photic stimuli, thus supporting neurotransmission, neuroplasticity, and signal transduction. Besides, DHA improves serotonergic and cholinergic neurotransmission and is a precursor of neuroprotective molecules, including neuroprotectin D1 (Sambra et al., 2021). It is essential for the preservation of the brain and visual system, as well as for cognitive and visual development during prenatal and postnatal stages. Although evidence associates maternal omega-3 supplementation during pregnancy with enhanced cognitive scores in early childhood, a comprehensive evaluation of 11 randomized controlled trials revealed a modest overall effect on cognitive, linguistic, or motor development (Gould et al., 2021). The European Food Safety Authority requires the addition of DHA in baby formula due to its critical function.

EPA, an omega-3 PUFA, demonstrates antiinflammatory, antimitotic, and antiallergic properties by diminishing the production of AA through the inhibition of phospholipase A2 (Patel et al., 2022). This facilitates the production of antiinflammatory mediators such as prostaglandin PGE3 and leukotriene B5 through cyclooxygenase-2. The EPA inhibits proinflammatory pathways by suppressing nuclear factor-κB, so reducing IL-1 and TNF-α levels, and by obstructing the

MAPK pathway, which diminishes protein-1 transcription factor activity (da Silva Batista et al., 2024). Evidence indicates that EPA-supplemented meals are effective in treating bipolar depression by modulating microglial activity and chronic inflammation in the brain, hence decreasing the generation of proinflammatory cytokines by microglia and monocytes. Furthermore, EPA promotes presynaptic serotonin release by suppressing PGE2 synthesis.

Since late 2019, COVID-19, induced by SARS-CoV-2, has resulted in a global pandemic characterized by symptoms that vary from mild to life-threatening, influenced by immune-inflammatory reactions and excessive coagulation (Malik et al., 2022). Omega-3 fatty acids, specifically EPA and DHA, are suggested as prospective treatments owing to their antiinflammatory characteristics, capacity to enhance proresolving mediators, and modulation of platelet aggregation and thrombosis. They augment the functioning of innate immune cells (e.g., neutrophils, macrophages) and adaptive immune responses (T-cells, B-cells), facilitating antibody formation and immunological memory. Observational studies associate elevated COVID-19 mortality with places exhibiting a poor omega-3 index (e.g., USA, some areas of Europe), while causality remains unestablished. A pilot research conducted by Asher et al., (2021) showed a 75% reduction in mortality risk among COVID-19 patients with an omega-3 index exceeding 5.7%. A randomized experiment conducted by Doaei et al. (2021) showed that a 14-day intervention including 400 mg of EPA and 200 mg of DHA in severely sick COVID-19 patients enhanced 1-month survival rates (21% vs 3%), renal function, respiratory indicators, and lymphocyte counts, but most outcomes remained unaltered. The moderate dosage indicates the possibility of enhanced effects at increased dosages. Data from a substantial app-based trial with 445,850 users suggest a marginal decrease in COVID-19 infection risk among omega-3 supplement users; nonetheless, the efficacy of omega-3s in preventing infection remains ambiguous.

13.5 Innovative polyunsaturated fatty acid delivery systems

13.5.1 Nanoemulsions

Nanoemulsions are the new methods of delivering PUFAs, and due to the ability of nanoemulsions to increase the solubility, stability, and bioavailability of these lipophilic compounds, the nanoemulsions have attracted much interest. These biphasic (20–500 nm) oil-in-water and water-in-oil submicron dispersions are surfactant-stabilized and confer unique benefits in PUFA delivery in food, pharmaceutical, and nutrition works (Das et al., 2023). The smaller droplet size enables increased digestive systems, decreased light scattering, and therefore better transparency (d <50 nm), reduced aggregation or creaming propensity, and therefore increased product shelf life (Fig. 13.3). In vitro gastrointestinal tests have indicated that lipase hydrolyzes the droplets of nanoemulsions very quickly because of the large surface area and

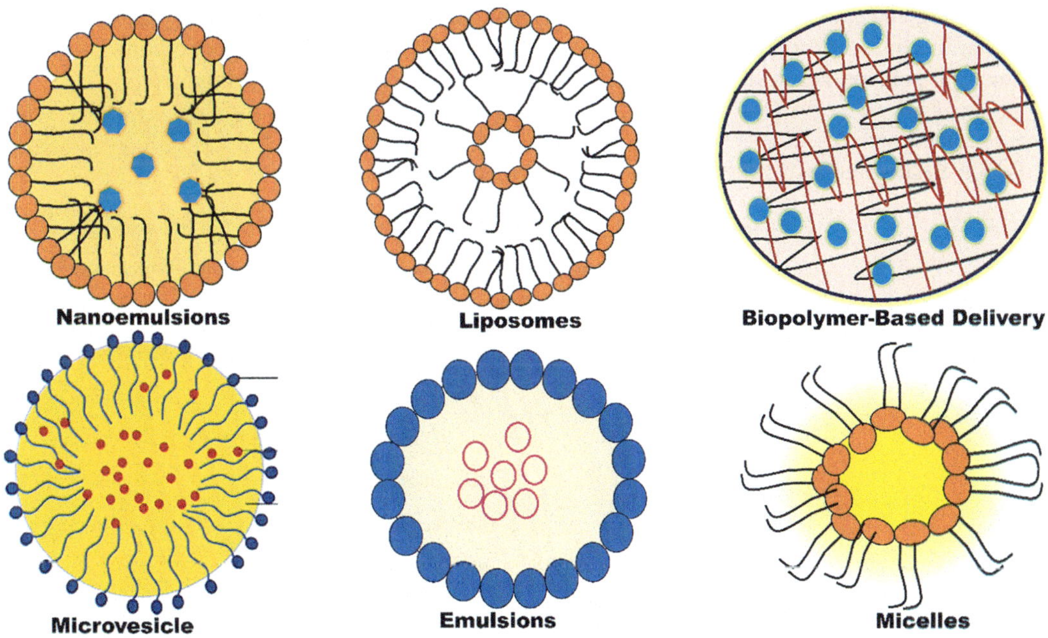

FIGURE 13.3 Different polyunsaturated fatty acids delivery systems.

exposure (Kumar et al., 2021; Ozogul et al., 2022). Even though the PUFA constituents (EPA, DHA) are susceptible to oxidation, the nanoemulsions protect them against outside forces (light, heat, oxygen) and thus ensure the bioactivity. Droplet stability in nanoemulsions is dynamic, which ensures that if the product is stored over extended periods of time, by inhibiting coalescence, creaming, and sedimentation. A study by do Amaral et al., (2025) used nanoemulsions to present omega-3 derivatives as anticancer agents, and they claimed an increased oral bioavailability and tumor regression in murine models. They were formulated using phase-inversion and high-pressure homogenization in order to produce stable droplets of 150 nm diameter (do Amaral et al., 2025). Modern studies are directed to the use of natural emulsifiers (e.g., plant-based proteins, saponins), the use of greener techniques to extract PUFA sources (e.g., green extraction), and the integration of nanoemulsions with ancillary technologies (e.g., microgels) to have controlled release and enhanced gastrointestinal fate.

13.5.2 Liposomes

Liposomes are vesicles that are made of phospholipid bilayers. They also make a good alternative to the delivery of PUFAs since they increase their stability, bioavailability, and specificity, as well as concealing off-taste, as summarized in Table 13.1. These vesicles are characterized by a bubble-like structure that is made up of two concentric layers of phospholipid monolayers, as illustrated in Fig. 13.3. Liposomes stabilize these lipids by trapping PUFAs inside the bilayer, thus preventing oxidative breakdown and, in the process, enhancing their bioavailability (Siddhnath et al., 2024). The lipid composition can be adjusted to adjust the functional properties of liposomal formulations. Addition of fatty acids like the decanoic acid (Lipo -DA) or stearic acid (Lipo-SA) produces membranes that are smaller and less hydrophilic, which stabilizes the entrapment of PUFAs. This change takes place at the molecular level, whereby the fatty-acid methyl chains intercalate with phospholipids, making the bilayer less permeable (Kundu et al., 2020). It is worth mentioning that Lipo-DA has a better storage stability and dissolves bioactive components at a slow rate under conditioned simulated gastrointestinal conditions, and it can be used in food applications (Huang et al., 2024). Adding hydrophobized chitosan (like N-palmitoyl chitosan) and oleic acid to liposomes makes the membranes stiffer and smaller by 30 nm (Abdelbari, 2026). Chitosan coating provides structural integrity and offers protection to PUFAs, thereby increasing their use in nutraceutical and pharmaceutical applications. The amphiphilic palmitoyl groups bind to the bilayer, which inhibits the uptake of water in storage. Superparamagnetic nanoparticles (like nanotex), fluorescent colors (like rhodamine-100), and omega-3 PUFA ethyl esters (omega-3 PUFA-EE) are all mixed in magnetoliposomes, which are made from egg phosphatidylcholine liposomes (Calle et al., 2015). These versatile constructs are used as theranostic agents, which allow delivering therapeutic services and diagnostic imaging at the same time. The liposomes, which are about 200 nm across, are made by hydrating and extruding a lipid film and then using gel filtration chromatography to get rid of the materials that are not inside the liposomes (Girija & Wilson, 2026). High-resolution ^{1}H NMR spectroscopy shows that omega-3 PUFA-EE is mobile, pointing to small, stable structures that can be used to treat inflammation.

TABLE 13.1 Polyunsaturated fatty acids source and their delivery system.

Source	Fatty acid	Delivery system	References
Shellfish	Astaxanthin	Liposomes	(Rincón-Cervera et al., 2020)
Krill oil	EPA/DHA	Capsule	(Attri et al., 2025)
Salmon oil	EPA/DHA	Microcapsule	(Henriques et al., 2014)
Algal oil	DHA	Nanoemulsions	(Czerniel et al., 2025)
Shark liver oil	Squalene	Liposomes	(Zakrzewska et al., 2021)
Seaweed	Fucoxanthin	Liposomes	(Marques et al., 2021)
Pomegranate oil	Punicic acid	Microcapsule	(Adu-Frimpong et al., 2018)
Flaxseed oil	LA, ALA	Nanoemulsions	(Yang et al., 2021)
Sardine oil	EPA/DHA	Liposomes	(Guedes et al., 2020)

13.5.3 Microencapsulation

The term "microencapsulation" describes the method of encasing an active chemical in a covering material. Some common names for encapsulated substances are core material, active component, fill, internal phase, and payload. Capsule, wall material, carrier, membrane, shell, or encapsulation matrix are all terms used to describe the exterior incessant and defensive substance around the core (Elkalla et al., 2023). It also prolongs the shelf life of goods, enhances the efficacy of additives, and broadens the use of nutritionally significant food components, like omega-3 fatty acids. The spray drying of emulsions is a prevalent microencapsulation and drying technique in the food and pharmaceutical sectors due to its flexibility, cost-effectiveness, efficiency, scalability, accessibility of equipment, and production of high-quality powder (Fig. 13.3). The manufacturing of microencapsulated omega-3 oil entails the assortment of core materials and wall materials, formulation design, and the selection of a suitable encapsulation method. Spray-dried fish oil powders were more likely to go bad than fish oil when they were stored. Spray drying is a popular way for businesses to make safe fish oil powders, and researchers are currently working to find ways to make these powders less sensitive to oxygen (Sultana et al., 2023). The mixture is frozen between −90°C and −40°C for freeze drying. It is then dried by redirection under reduced pressure (Fig. 13.3). The best thing about this skill is that it uses low temperatures and removes air, which helps keep products from going bad. Because freeze drying has these benefits, it can be used to microencapsulate ingredients that are very sensitive, like bacteria and PUFAs (Rezvankhah et al., 2020). Another method of microencapsulation that makes use of fluidized bed coating involves applying a coating to powder particles either in a batch operation or in a continuous setting. After being sprayed with a coating substance, the powder elements are deposited in an air stream that is kept at a specified temperature. To keep powdered omega-3 oils from oxidizing while stored, a lipid coating is often applied. Another possible method for microencapsulating omega-3 oils is extrusion. It is possible to make high-density encapsulated goods with this technique. Mixing liquid carriers with omega-3 oils is what it takes, and high pressure lets the mixture go through a die or nozzle (Homroy et al., 2024). In a colloidal solution, coacervation means the splitting of two liquid layers. One phase, called the coacervate phase, has a lot of polymer and is different from the other phase, which does not have any polymer. There is only one polymer in simple coacervation, but two colloids with opposite charges interact in complicated coacervation. In the microencapsulation of omega-3 oils via simple coacervation, the oil component is typically disseminated in a gelatin solution, after which a pH change induces the coacervation of gelatin, resulting in the formation of a coating around the oil droplets (Eratte et al., 2018). Microencapsulated PUFAs are integrated into dairy products (such as yogurt and milk), drinks, and baked goods to augment nutritional content while preserving flavor and shelf stability (Pattnaik & Mishra, 2022). PUFA microcapsules are employed in dietary supplements to enhance bioavailability and conceal fishy aromas, exemplified by Lycored's vegetarian beadlet systems.

13.5.4 Biopolymer-based delivery systems

The biopolymer-based delivery systems take advantage of the biocompatible, biodegradable, and antioxidative biopolymer nanostructures (Kučuk et al., 2023). Fig. 13.3 depicts that electrostatic interactions between oppositely charged biopolymers to produce stable complexes. García-Moreno et al. (2020) looked into how β-lactoglobulin (BLG) and high methoxyl pectin (HMP) could be used to make nanoparticles that could hold LA, which is a type of PUFA. The research found that Mild heat treatment (60°C, 10 minutes) facilitated BLG-LA complexation, but the HMP layer offered a shield to oxidative degradation. The ideal protein–polysaccharide ratios of 1:1 to 2:1 yielded nanoparticles of 337–364 nm with negative pH 4.0 values, making them stable. Fluorimetric studies proved that HMP blocked LA binding sites, hence preventing instability in the long run (García-Moreno et al., 2020). Chitosan is a cationic polysaccharide commonly used together with protein, that is, zein or whey protein isolate (WPI), to protect the PUFAs (Xie et al., 2024). Chitosan-WPI nanoparticles used to deliver DHA had high encapsulation efficiencies of up to 90%, and simulated gastrointestinal conditions demonstrated that they release the payload at a slow rate. This structure has preserved DHA for at least 30 days in storage (Ali et al., 2024). This was possible because chitosan is an antioxidant, and the biopolymer binder is dense. To produce pH-dependent swelling and release profiles, alginate-chitosan hydrogels were produced to entrap DHA. At gastric pH 1.2, the hydrogels showed low release of DHA, but at intestinal pH 6.8, the release was significantly high (Abbasi et al., 2019). Crosslinking of calcium ions enhanced tensile strength, which eliminated PUFA leakages during storage. This method maintained DHA integrity up to 60 days at 25°C (Du et al., 2022). Gharibzahedi et al. (2018) looked into the use of whey protein microgels to give omega-3s. The microgels made by heat gelation and ionic crosslinking were 95% effective at enclosing PUFAs. In vitro processing models showed that the microgels produced PUFAs in the small intestine, which made them 30% more bioavailable than free PUFAs. Dospra et al. (2024) created collagen nanofibers to carry DHA for use in wound repair. Cross-linked with glutaraldehyde, the nanofibers released DHA slowly over 14 days, which reduced oxidative stress in living things. Because the device was biocompatible and biodegradable, it looked like it could be used for topical release. Ali et al. (2024) created lipid-pectin hybrid nanoparticles to release PUFA in systems that stay in the stomach. The nanoparticles, which were made by ionic gelation, were able to surround DHA 85% of the time and stay in the stomach for up to 6 hours, which improved absorption (Ali et al., 2024). The mucoadhesive features of pectin made it easier to target the gut, and the lipid heart kept the PUFAs from going bad.

13.6 Functional foods as polyunsaturated fatty acid delivery platforms

Functional foods effectively provide PUFAs by including bioactive components in daily meals. They improve the nutritional composition of meals while meeting customer demand for health-enhancing goods. PUFAs, particularly omega-3s, are integrated into functional foods to alleviate chronic disease, cardiovascular disease, diabetes, and neurological syndromes (Elagizi et al., 2018). Foods include dairy (yogurt, milk), spreads, baked goods, and chocolate, which are enriched with PUFAs to enhance dietary consumption. Chia seeds, abundant in ALA, along with berries, high in polyphenols, in a breakfast bowl, illustrate a functional meal that utilizes the synergy between PUFAs and antioxidants to diminish inflammation and promote cellular repair (Chen et al., 2024; Djuricic & Calder, 2021). Fish oils, abundant in EPA and DHA, are frequently used in fortified goods; however, plant-based substitutes such as flaxseed and walnuts are more popular owing to sustainability issues (Pandey et al., 2025). Plant proteins derived from legumes, seeds, nuts, tubers, and cereals are increasingly recognized as environmentally viable vehicles for lipophilic substances such as PUFAs. These systems, comprising emulsions, hydrogels, films, and self-assembled structures, safeguard PUFAs against oxidation and enhance their bioavailability. Soy protein-based films, including micro-fibrillated cellulose, have demonstrated improved stability and release of PUFA-rich oils, including clove essential oil, while also displaying antibacterial efficacy against pathogens such as *Escherichia coli* and *Salmonella* spp. (Hu et al., 2025). Microalgae and oleaginous yeasts, such as *Yarrowia lipolytica*, are under investigation for the sustainable synthesis of PUFAs (Jia et al., 2022). These bacteria may biosynthesize EPA and DHA, which are then integrated into functional meals or aquafeed. Advancements in metabolic engineering have enhanced PUFA yields in these systems, mitigating global supply constraints.

13.7 Future directions and emerging trends

Innovations in the future of PUFA delivery include improvement of bioavailability by new encapsulation methods, alternative microbiological production pathways, and designing functional foods and nutraceuticals with PUFAs. Studies are also geared towards optimization of dietary intake, sustainable and cost-effective production, and clarification of PUFA interactions with other food constituents. The nanoemulsions, liposomes, and solid lipid nanoparticles are encapsulation methodologies increasingly used to enhance the stability of PUFA and its bioavailability. These systems protect PUFAs against oxidation, extend shelf life, and allow the ready release in the gastrointestinal tract (Du et al., 2022). As an example, neuroprotective effects are achieved by nanocapsules of EPA and DHA targeted to brain tissues using nanocapsules made with biocompatible polymers or proteins. It is centered around scalable and cost-effective methods of encapsulation using natural biopolymers (e.g., chitosan, alginate) to satisfy consumer requests for clean-label products (Dey et al., 2024). Combining targeted delivery and encapsulation, specifically in the case of gastrointestinal or neurological use, is a strategic goal. Investigations are underway to consider stimuli-responsive nanocarriers that can release PUFAs upon pH or enzyme stimulation.

The use of fish oil as the main source of PUFAs is turning to nonenvironmentally harmful microbial sources, namely microalgae, yeasts, and fungi, due to environmental issues and the preference for vegetarian/vegan products (Saini et al., 2021). *Crypthecodinium cohnii* and *Schizochytrium* sp. strains are being engineered to produce more EPA and DHA. Metabolic engineering and synthetic biology will continue to enhance the production of microbial PUFA. A good avenue can be seen in engineering *Y. lipolytica* to increase PUFA synthase pathways (Jia et al., 2022). Furthermore, the use of organic waste as a culture medium would decrease the expenses and improve sustainability.

Foods fortified with PUFAs, such as dairy products, baked goods, and beverages, are also winning the market position, but oxidative instability remains a major challenge (Islam et al., 2023). Modern trends are focusing on the application of emulsification methodologies to enhance sensory properties and stability. Omega-3 enriched eggs and meat are also gaining commercial momentum, with the main focus of producing PUFA fortified products that reduce sensory aftertastes like fishiness (Ferraz & Silva, 2025). Studies on natural antioxidants (e.g., polyphenols, tocopherols) are aimed at enhancing the stability of PUFA in processing and storage (Blasi & Cossignani, 2020). Additionally, the fortification of plant foods will be in line with the growing vegan market, especially in countries such as India, where sources of microbial PUFA have been authorized to be used as infant food.

The limited absorption of PUFAs, especially omega-3s, presents a significant challenge. Lipid-based delivery methods, including self-emulsifying drug delivery systems and nanostructured lipid carriers, are being engineered to improve absorption (Kesharwani et al., 2023). Research is concentrating on enhancing lipid formulations to augment the solubility and absorption of PUFAs in the gastrointestinal tract. Techniques such as supercritical fluid chromatography and high-performance liquid chromatography are being optimized to yield highly pure PUFA concentrations without heat degradation (Ashraf-Khorassani et al., 2015). The growing popularity of plant-based diets has led to heightened demand for sources of PUFAs such as chia seed oil, flaxseed oil, and algal oil (Saini et al., 2021). These sources are being integrated into supplements and functional meals to accommodate vegan customers. Advancements in extracting PUFAs from botanical and algal sources are anticipated to enhance yield and economic efficiency. Regulatory endorsement, shown by India's FSSAI clearance of microbial DHA and AA for newborn feeding, is propelling industry expansion (Bhupathiraju et al., 2019).

Artificial Intelligence and machine learning are progressively employed to assess multiomics data (genomics, metabolomics, and transcriptomics) to customize PUFA delivery methods according to individual genetic profiles (Ghosh et al., 2025). This facilitates accurate recommendations for omega-3 fatty acids (e.g., EPA and DHA) to enhance health outcomes, including the mitigation of cardiovascular risk or inflammation. Development of AI models that combine genetic variants, such as FADS1/2 alleles, with lifestyle and nutritional factors have been developed to predict the optimum PUFA doses and delivery systems, such as liposomes, emulsions, and supplements (Chilton et al., 2017). By considering single metabolic heterogeneity, such models are likely to increase bioavailability and clinical efficacy. ML algorithms are being explored to predict gene expression changes induced by omega-3 PUFAs, which may support the development of personalized interventions for conditions such as metabolic dysfunction-associated fatty liver disease (Boulos et al., 2025). An artificial intelligence-enhanced wearable sensor and smartphone applications can measure real-time health and nutrition bars in order to measure PUFA intake and metabolism reactions to give individualized dietary counseling. The creation of AI-based applications that combine wearable sensor data with nutrigenomic profiles would allow adjusting PUFA 1-week or daily (through supplements or fortified foods) according to the current physiological variables, such as inflammatory biomarkers and lipid profiles (Pokushalov et al., 2024). New studies highlight the possibility of wearable sensors to personalize nutrition, and future uses can be in the monitoring of PUFA metabolism. Machine learning and artificial intelligence are also used to enhance food processing, maintain the PUFA content, and nutritional value (Gbashi & Njobeh, 2024). As an example, predictive algorithms are used to simulate the effect of cooking factors on the ratio between PUFA and SFA, and machine-learning-inspired processing systems have also been developed to reduce the oxidation of PUFA and improve bioaccessibility. These systems can be characterized by constant monitoring of food quality, based on AI, during the manufacturing process and storage. Besides, the PUFA/SFA ratio of deep-fried fish has risen by 63.05% using genetic algorithms and particle-swarm optimization, which demonstrates the potential of AI in the optimization of food processing (Sadhu et al., 2022).

PUFAs are very prone to lipid peroxidation, resulting in rancidity and reduced shelf life. The joint delivery of natural antioxidants, including rosemary extract and vitamin E, is a modern approach to reduce oxidative decomposition in storage and cooking, including air frying (Siddiqui et al., 2023). New processing modalities are being explored, including cold plasma and pulsed electric fields, to maintain PUFA integrity during food processing (Rathod et al., 2022). Besides this, smart packaging with oxygen absorbers or UV shields is being developed in order to prolong the shelf life of the product.

According to the PUFA market, the rate of growth is estimated to be 5.4% per year between 2023 and 2033 due to the increasing awareness and preference of people toward functional foods and nutraceuticals (Jiménez-Ortega et al., 2025). The United States and India are also major markets, and this is because of rising cases of chronic diseases and conducive regulatory environments for PUFA-enriched products. It is expected that harmonization of international regulatory standards on PUFA-enriched goods and supplements will drive the growth in the market, and research studies are directed at the justification of health claims with clinical trials to enhance the confidence of consumers and to ensure regulatory acceptance.

The high omega-6 to omega-3 ratio of the western diet, which ranges between 8:1 to 25:1, spreads inflammation and supports the need to develop delivery vehicles that emphasize omega-3 fortifications (Mariamenatu & Abdu, 2021). Even though the sources of microbes and algae are viable, their production is very expensive. The technology of bioprocessing will be designed in the future to optimize the methods of manufacturing PUFA delivery systems at a lower cost. Standardized datasets are highly resilient and unnecessary to train strong AI models; future efforts must focus on open-data sharing and joint participation. There is an urgent need to ensure that a wide and representative dataset is curated to reduce bias in AI-based PUFA recommendations, especially in specific demographic groups (Bailey et al., 2024). Implementing AI in nutrigenomics is associated with some issues of privacy and transparency of data that should be ensured with proper protection and ethical standards.

13.8 Conclusion

Innovation of new delivery systems of PUFAs, and in particular, omega-3 and omega-6 fatty acids, is a critical development in individual nutrition and food functionality. These products help in dealing with the most pressing issues regarding oxidative stability, bioavailability, and acceptability to the senses and, therefore, encourage the introduction of PUFAs into various functional food systems. Nanoemulsions, liposomes, microencapsulation, and edible coating techniques of nanotechnology have shown a lot of potential in preserving PUFAs against degradation, enhancing their bioavailability, and hiding unwanted odors, which consequently increases consumer acceptability. The development of personalized nutrition plans, the incorporation of these delivery technologies into them, is consistent with the growing number of people who need individualized diet plans to support their health needs, genetic makeup, and lifestyle habits. Allowing a high level of control over the release rates and dosing of PUFA, these systems are used in the creation of functional foods that can aid cardiovascular health, cognitive activity, and inflammatory control, among other things. Nevertheless, the ongoing challenges that include scalability, cost-effectiveness, and compliance with the regulations need to overcome via collective actions by scientists and industrial actors, as well as the government. Researchers in recent decades have come up with encapsulation techniques that entail the choice of suitable wall materials to employ on the functional lipids to promote bioavailability on oral intake and to stabilize food products. Embedding functional lipids into carrier matrices through various physical and chemical interactions affects the thermal stability of the encapsulated substances, storage stability, and gastrointestinal stability. Encapsulated functional lipids also have superior bioavailability in food systems and physicochemical and functional properties to the food matrix. More studies are needed to consider food safety issues in relation to fortified foods based on encapsulated functional lipids, and a unique literature gap has been demonstrated in relation to the use of novel sources of functional lipids, such as algae, bacteria, and fungi, for the fortification of staple foods through encapsulation methods. All these innovations could change the world of the functional food industry, provide the consumer with knowledge about the right diet, and help to achieve better outcomes in the health of the global population.

References

Abbasi, M., Sohail, M., Minhas, M. U., Khan, S., Hussain, Z., Mahmood, A., Shah, S. A., & Kousar, M. (2019). Novel biodegradable pH-sensitive hydrogels: An efficient controlled release system to manage ulcerative colitis. *International Journal of Biological Macromolecules, 136*, 83–96. https://doi.org/10.1016/j.ijbiomac.2019.06.046, http://www.elsevier.com/locate/ijbiomac.

Abdelbari, M. A. (2026). From anatomy to application: a comprehensive review of nanovesicular systems for otic drug delivery. *AAPS PharmSciTech, 27*(3). https://doi.org/10.1208/s12249-026-03344-3, https://www.springer.com/journal/12249.

Adu-Frimpong, M., Omari-Siaw, E., Mukhtar, Y. M., Xu, X., & Yu, J. (2018). Formulation of pomegranate seed oil: A promising approach of improving stability and health-promoting properties. *European Journal of Lipid Science and Technology, 120*(12). https://doi.org/10.1002/ejlt.201800177.

Alagawany, M., Elnesr, S. S., Farag, M. R., El-Sabrout, K., Alqaisi, O., Dawood, M. A. O., Soomro, H., & Abdelnour, S. A. (2022). Nutritional significance and health benefits of omega-3, -6 and -9 fatty acids in animals. *Animal Biotechnology, 33*(7), 1678–1690. https://doi.org/10.1080/10495398.2020.1869562, http://www.tandf.co.uk/journals/titles/10495398.asp.

Ali, A. H., Hachem, M., & Ahmmed, M. K. (2024). Docosahexaenoic acid-loaded nanoparticles: A state-of-the-art of preparation methods, characterization, functionality, and therapeutic applications. *Heliyon, 10*(9).

Asher, A., Tintle, N. L., Myers, M., Lockshon, L., Bacareza, H., & Harris, W. S. (2021). Blood omega-3 fatty acids and death from COVID-19: A pilot study. *Prostaglandins, Leukotrienes and Essential Fatty Acids, 166*, 102250. https://doi.org/10.1016/j.plefa.2021.102250.

Ali, O., & Szabó, A. (2023). Review of eukaryote cellular membrane lipid composition, with special attention to the fatty acids. *International Journal of Molecular Sciences, 24*(21), 15693. https://doi.org/10.3390/ijms242115693.

Ashraf-Khorassani, M., Isaac, G., Rainville, P., Fountain, K., & Taylor, L. T. (2015). Study of ultrahigh performance supercritical fluid chromatography to measure free fatty acids with out fatty acid ester preparation. *Journal of Chromatography B, 997*, 45–55. https://doi.org/10.1016/j.jchromb.2015.05.031.

Attri, N., Arora, D., Saini, R., Chandel, M., Suthar, P., & Dhiman, A. (2025). Health promoting benefits of krill oil: Mechanisms, bioactive combinations, and advanced encapsulation technologies. *Food Science and Biotechnology, 34*(6), 1285–1308. https://doi.org/10.1007/s10068-024-01737-3.

Bailey, R. L., MacFarlane, A. J., Field, M. S., Tagkopoulos, I., Baranzini, S. E., Edwards, K. M., Rose, C. J., Schork, N. J., Singhal, A., Wallace, B. C., Fisher, K. P, Markakis, K., & Stover, P. J. (2024). Artificial intelligence in food and nutrition evidence: The challenges and opportunities. *PNAS Nexus, 3*(12). https://doi.org/10.1093/pnasnexus/pgae461.

Bhupathiraju, K., Krishnaraju, A. V., Sengupta, K., Golakoti, T., Akolkar, S. K., & Datla, P. (2019). *Nutraceutical and functional food regulations in the United States and around the World*. Elsevier, 445–464. https://doi.org/10.1016/b978-0-12-816467-9.00029-0.

Biernacki, M., & Skrzydlewska, E. (2025). Metabolic pathways of eicosanoids—derivatives of arachidonic acid and their significance in skin. *Cellular & Molecular Biology Letters, 30*(1). https://doi.org/10.1186/s11658-025-00685-y.

Bishehkolaei, M., & Pathak, Y. (2024). Influence of omega n-6/n-3 ratio on cardiovascular disease and nutritional interventions. *Human Nutrition & Metabolism, 37*, 200275. https://doi.org/10.1016/j.hnm.2024.200275.

Blasi, F., & Cossignani, L. (2020). An overview of natural extracts with antioxidant activity for the improvement of the oxidative stability and shelf life of edible oils. *Processes, 8*(8), 956. https://doi.org/10.3390/pr8080956.

Boulos, M., Mousa, R. S., Jeries, N., Simaan, E., Alam, K., Bulus, B., & Assy, N. (2025). Hidden in the fat: Unpacking the metabolic tango between metabolic dysfunction-associated steatotic liver disease and metabolic syndrome. *International Journal of Molecular Sciences, 26*(7). https://doi.org/10.3390/ijms26073448, http://www.mdpi.com/journal/ijms.

Bowen, K. J., Harris, W. S., & Kris-Etherton, P. M. (2016). Omega-3 fatty acids and cardiovascular disease: Are there benefits? *Current Treatment Options in Cardiovascular Medicine, 18*(11), 69.

Calle, D., Negri, V., Ballesteros, P., & Cerdán, S. (2015). Magnetoliposomes loaded with polyunsaturated fatty acids as novel theranostic anti-inflammatory formulations. *Theranostics, 5*(5), 489–503. https://doi.org/10.7150/thno.10069.

Chang, C., & Nickerson, M. T. (2018). Encapsulation of omega 3-6-9 fatty acids-rich oils using protein-based emulsions with spray drying. *Journal of Food Science and Technology, 55*(8), 2850–2861. https://doi.org/10.1007/s13197-018-3257-0.

Chen, J., Wu, G., Zhu, L., Karrar, E., & Zhang, H. (2024). A review of the functional activities of chia seed and the mechanisms of action related to molecular targets. *Food & Function, 15*(3), 1158–1169. https://doi.org/10.1039/d3fo02197a.

Chilton, F. H., Dutta, R., Reynolds, L. M., Sergeant, S., Mathias, R. A., & Seeds, M. C. (2017). Precision nutrition and omega-3 polyunsaturated fatty acids: A case for personalized supplementation approaches for the prevention and management of human diseases. *Nutrients, 9*(11). https://doi.org/10.3390/nu9111165, http://www.mdpi.com/2072-6643/9/11/1165/pdf.

Ciesielski, T. H. (2025). Global Access to Uncontaminated Omega-3 Polyunsaturated Fatty Acids Requires Attention. *AJPM Focus, 4*(4), 100341. https://doi.org/10.1016/j.focus.2025.100341.

Czerniel, J., Gostyńska-Stawna, A., Urbaniak, N., Sommerfeld-Klatta, K., & Stawny, M. (2025). Harnessing algae oil as a sustainable DHA source for parenteral nutrition in vegan patients. *Scientific Reports, 15*(1). https://doi.org/10.1038/s41598-025-03319-7.

da Silva Batista, E., Nakandakari, S. C. B. R., Ramos da Silva, A. S., Pauli, J. R., Pereira de Moura, L., Ropelle, E. R., Camargo, E. A., & Cintra, D. E. (2024). Omega-3 pleiad: The multipoint anti-inflammatory strategy. *Critical Reviews in Food Science and Nutrition, 64*(14), 4817–4832. https://doi.org/10.1080/10408398.2022.2146044, https://www.tandfonline.com/loi/bfsn20.

Das, P., Panda, J. R., Patro, Ch N., Sahu, B., & Patnaik, S. S. (2023). A Comprehensive review of Nanoemulsion applications and their recent advancements. *Current Nanomaterials, 8*(3), 209–223. https://doi.org/10.2174/2405461508666221103121439.

Das, S., Agarwal, P., Mishra, S., Sivamani, Y., Hegde, S., Ganesan, S., & Elayaperumal, S. (2024). *Methods and protocols in food science, fortified foods.* Springer US, 229–261. https://doi.org/10.1007/978-1-0716-4346-4_13.

Dey, B., Prabhakar, M. R., Jayaraman, S., Gujjala, L. K. S., Venugopal, A. P., & Balasubramanian, P. (2024). Biopolymer-based solutions for enhanced safety and quality assurance: A review. *Food Research International, 191.* https://doi.org/10.1016/j.foodres.2024.114723, https://www.sciencedirect.com/science/journal/09639969.

Djuricic, I., & Calder, P. C. (2021). Beneficial outcomes of omega-6 and omega-3 polyunsaturated fatty acids on human health: An update for 2021. *Nutrients, 13*(7), 2421. https://doi.org/10.3390/nu13072421.

do Amaral, S. R., Aires-Fernandes, M., Haddad, F. F., Gini, A. L. R., Scarim, C. B., & Primo, F. L. (2025). Ex Vivo biosafety and efficacy assessment of advanced chlorin e6 Nanoemulsions as a drug delivery system for photodynamic antitumoral application. *Molecules, 30*(3), 544. https://doi.org/10.3390/molecules30030544.

Doaei, S., Gholami, S., Rastgoo, S., Gholamalizadeh, M., Bourbour, F., Bagheri, S. E., Samipoor, F., Akbari, M. E., Shadnoush, M., Ghorat, F., Mosavi Jarrahi, S. A., Ashouri Mirsadeghi, N., Hajipour, A., Joola, P., Moslem, A., & Goodarzi, M. O. (2021). The effect of omega-3 fatty acid supplementation on clinical and biochemical parameters of critically ill patients with COVID-19: A randomized clinical trial. *Journal of Translational Medicine, 19*(1). https://doi.org/10.1186/s12967-021-02795-5, http://www.translational-medicine.com/home/.

Dospra, M., Pavlou, P., Papageorgiou, S., & Varvaresou, A. (2024). Recent studies on the healing properties of eicosapentaenoic acid. *Applied Sciences, 14*(13), 5884. https://doi.org/10.3390/app14135884.

Du, Q., Zhou, L., Li, M., Lyu, F., Liu, J., & Ding, Y. (2022). Omega-3 polyunsaturated fatty acid encapsulation system: Physical and oxidative stability, and medical applications. *Food Frontiers, 3*(2), 239–255. https://doi.org/10.1002/fft2.134.

D'Angelo, S., Motti, M. L., & Meccariello, R. (2020). ω-3 and ω-6 polyunsaturated fatty acids, obesity and cancer. *Nutrients, 12*(9), 2751.

Elagizi, A., Lavie, C. J., Marshall, K., DiNicolantonio, J. J., O'Keefe, J. H., & Milani, R. V. (2018). Omega-3 polyunsaturated fatty acids and cardiovascular health: A comprehensive review. *Progress in Cardiovascular Diseases, 61*(1), 76–85. https://doi.org/10.1016/j.pcad.2018.03.006, http://www.elsevier.com/inca/publications/store/6/2/3/3/2/9/index.htt.

Elkalla, E., Khizar, S., Tarhini, M., Lebaz, N., Zine, N., Jaffrezic-Renault, N., Errachid, A., & Elaissari, A. (2023). Core-shell micro/nanocapsules: From encapsulation to applications. *Journal of Microencapsulation, 40*(3), 125–156. https://doi.org/10.1080/02652048.2023.2178538.

Eratte, D., Dowling, K., Barrow, C. J., & Adhikari, B. (2018). Recent advances in the microencapsulation of omega-3 oil and probiotic bacteria through complex coacervation: A review. *Trends in Food Science and Technology, 71*, 121–131. https://doi.org/10.1016/j.tifs.2017.10.014, http://www.elsevier.com/wps/find/journaldescription.cws_home/601278/description#description.

Ferraz, L. P., & Silva, E. K. (2025). Pulsed electric field-assisted extraction techniques for obtaining vegetable oils and essential oils: Recent progress and opportunities for the food industry. *Separation and Purification Technology, 354.* https://doi.org/10.1016/j.seppur.2024.128833, https://www.sciencedirect.com/science/journal/13835866.

Freitas, R. D. S., & Campos, M. M. (2019). Protective effects of omega-3 fatty acids in cancer-related complications. *Nutrients, 11*(5). https://doi.org/10.3390/nu11050945, https://www.mdpi.com/2072-6643/11/5/945/pdf.

García-Moreno, P. J., Gregersen, S., Nedamani, E. R., Olsen, T. H., Marcatili, P., Overgaard, M. T., Andersen, M. L., Hansen, E. B., & Jacobsen, C. (2020). Identification of emulsifier potato peptides by bioinformatics: Application to omega-3 delivery emulsions and release from potato industry side streams. *Scientific Reports, 10*(1). https://doi.org/10.1038/s41598-019-57229-6, http://www.nature.com/srep/index.html.

Gbashi, S., & Njobeh, P. B. (2024). Enhancing food integrity through artificial intelligence and machine learning: A comprehensive review. *Applied Sciences, 14*(8), 3421. https://doi.org/10.3390/app14083421.

Gharibzahedi, S. M. T., George, S., Greiner, R., Estevinho, B. N., Frutos Fernández, M. J., McClements, D. J., & Roohinejad, S. (2018). New trends in the microencapsulation of functional fatty acid-rich oils using transglutaminase catalyzed crosslinking. *Comprehensive Reviews in Food Science and Food Safety, 17*(2), 274–289. https://doi.org/10.1111/1541-4337.12324, http://www.interscience.wiley.com/jpages/1541-4337.

Ghosh, S., Zhao, X., Alim, M., Brudno, M., & Bhat, M. (2025). Artificial intelligence applied to 'omics data in liver disease: Towards a personalised approach for diagnosis, prognosis and treatment. *Gut, 74*(2), 295–311. https://doi.org/10.1136/gutjnl-2023-331740.

Girija, S., & Wilson, J. (2026). Lipids and liposomes delivery of nutritional components. In *Handbook of nutraceuticals: Science, technology and engineering*. Springer Nature, 739–773. http://doi.org/10.1007/978-3-031-98791-5_26.

Gould, J. F., Roberts, R. M., & Makrides, M. (2021). The influence of omega-3 long-chain polyunsaturated fatty acid, docosahexaenoic acid, on child behavioral functioning: A review of randomized controlled trials of DHA supplementation in pregnancy, the neonatal period and infancy. *Nutrients, 13*(2), 415.

Guedes, M., Costa-Pinto, A. R., Gonçalves, V. M. F., Moreira-Silva, J., Tiritan, M. E., Reis, R. L., Ferreira, H., & Neves, N. M. (2020). Sardine Roe as a source of lipids to produce liposomes. *ACS Biomaterials Science and Engineering, 6*(2), 1017–1029. https://doi.org/10.1021/acsbiomaterials.9b01462, http://pubs.acs.org/journal/abseba.

Hayyan, A., Al-Maari, M. A., Abed, K. M., Alanazi, Y. M., Saleh, J., Gupta, B. S., Kang, D. C. Y., Hizaddin, H. F., & Salleh, M. Z. M. (2025). Enhancing the solubility of dihomo-gamma-linolenic acid using natural deep eutectic solvents for human tumors therapy development. *ChemistrySelect, 10*(8). https://doi.org/10.1002/slct.202405605.

Henriques, J., Dick, J. R., Tocher, D. R., & Bell, J. G. (2014). Nutritional quality of salmon products available from major retailers in the UK: Content and composition of n-3 long-chain PUFA. *British Journal of Nutrition, 112*(6), 964–975. https://doi.org/10.1017/S0007114514001603, http://journals.cambridge.org/BJN.

Homroy, S., Chopra, R., Singh, P. K., Dhiman, A., Chand, M., & Talwar, B. (2024). Role of encapsulation on the bioavailability of omega-3 fatty acids. *Comprehensive Reviews in Food Science and Food Safety, 23*(1), 1–35. https://doi.org/10.1111/1541-4337.13272, http://onlinelibrary.wiley.com/journal/10.1111/(ISSN)1541-4337.

Huang, R., Song, H., Wang, X., Shen, H., Li, X., & Guan (2024). Fatty acids-modified liposomes for encapsulation of bioactive peptides: Fabrication, characterization, storage stability and in vitro release. *Food Chemistry, 440*, 138139. https://doi.org/10.1016/j.foodchem.2023.138139.

Huang, D., Wu, P., Chen, Y., & Zhong, S. (2026). Association between dietary polyunsaturated fatty acids and cardiovascular disease in individuals with rheumatoid arthritis. *European Journal of Medical Research, 31*(1). https://doi.org/10.1186/s40001-026-04085-6.

Hu, Y., Liu, S., & Williams, G. R. (2025). Rationally designed electrosprayed particles for encapsulation of essential oils, flavors, essential fatty acids, and antibacterials. In *Electrospinning and electrospraying encapsulation of food bioactive compounds*. Elsevier, 217–237.

Islam, F., Imran, A., Nosheen, F., Fatima, M., Arshad, M. U., Afzaal, M., Ijaz, N., Noreen, R., Mehta, S., Biswas, S., Rasool, I. F. U., Aslam, M. A., Usman, I., Zahra, S. M., Segueni, N., & Amer Ali, Y. (2023). Functional roles and novel tools for improving-oxidative stability of polyunsaturated fatty acids: A comprehensive review. *Food Science & Nutrition, 11*(6), 2471–2482. https://doi.org/10.1002/fsn3.3272.

Jara-Gutiérrez, Á., & Baladron, V. (2021). The role of prostaglandins in different types of cancer. *Cells, 10*(6), 1487.

Jeong, H. Y., Moon, Y. S., & Cho, K. K. (2024). ω-6 and ω-3 polyunsaturated fatty acids: Inflammation, obesity and foods of animal resources. *Food science of animal resources, 44*(5), 988.

Jia, Y. L., Wang, L. R., Zhang, Z. X., Gu, Y., & Sun, X. M. (2022). Recent advances in biotechnological production of polyunsaturated fatty acids by Yarrowia lipolytica. *Critical Reviews in Food Science and Nutrition, 62*(32), 8920–8934. https://doi.org/10.1080/10408398.2021.1937041, https://www.tandfonline.com/loi/bfsn20.

Jiménez-Ortega, L. A., González-Gómez, J. P., Quiñónez-Angulo, P., Valdez-Baro, O., & Heredia, J. B. (2025). *Interdisciplinary biotechnological advances, bioactive compounds extraction from marine resources and wastes*. Springer Nature Singapore, 31–48. https://doi.org/10.1007/978-981-96-1253-6_2.

Jurić, S., Jurić, M., Siddique, Md Abu B., & Fathi, M. (2020). Vegetable oils rich in polyunsaturated fatty acids: nanoencapsulation methods and Stability enhancement. *Food Reviews International, 38*(1), 32–69. https://doi.org/10.1080/87559129.2020.1717524.

Kassem, J. M., Abdulqahar, F. W., Zaky, A. A., Boulkrane, M. S., Darwish, A., Farouk, A., Ozçelik, B., Magouz, O., Liu, X., & El-Messery, T. M. (2025). Micro and nanoencapsulation of omega-3 fatty acids: functional applications and future perspectives in food systems. *Food Safety and Health, 4*(2), 280–298. https://doi.org/10.1002/fsh3.70071.

Kesharwani, R., Jaiswal, P., Patel, D. K., & Yadav, P. K. (2023). Lipid-based drug delivery system (LBDDS): An emerging paradigm to enhance oral bioavailability of poorly soluble drugs. *Biomedical Materials and Devices, 1*(2), 648–663. https://doi.org/10.1007/s44174-022-00041-0, link.springer.com/journal/44174.

Kheto, A., Adhikary, U., Dhua, S., Sarkar, A., Kumar, Y., Vashishth, R., Shrestha, B. B., & Saxena, D. C. (2024). A review on advancements in emerging processing of whey protein: Enhancing functional and nutritional properties for functional food applications. *Food Safety and Health, 3*(1), 23–45. https://doi.org/10.1002/fsh3.12067.

Krejsgaard, T., Lindahl, L. M., Mongan, N. P., Wasik, M. A., Litvinov, I. V., Iversen, L., & Dum, N. (2017). Malignant inflammation in cutaneous T-cell lymphoma—A hostile takeover.

Kumar, N., Verma, A., & Mandal, A. (2021). Formation, characteristics and oil industry applications of nanoemulsions: A review. *Journal of Petroleum Science and Engineering, 206*, 109042.

Kundu, N., Mondal, D., & Sarkar, N. (2020). Dynamics of the vesicles composed of fatty acids and other amphiphile mixtures: Unveiling the role of fatty acids as a model protocell membrane. *Biophysical reviews, 12*(5), 1117–1131.

Kučuk, N., Primožič, M., Knez, Ž., & Leitgeb, M. (2023). Sustainable biodegradable biopolymer-based nanoparticles for healthcare applications. *International Journal of Molecular Sciences, 24*(4), 3188. https://doi.org/10.3390/ijms24043188.

Leung, H. H., Ng, A. L., Durand, T., Kawasaki, R., Oger, C., Balas, L., Galano, J. M., Wong, I. Y., & Chung-Yung Lee, J. (2019). Increase in omega-6 and decrease in omega-3 polyunsaturated fatty acid oxidation elevates the risk of exudative AMD development in adults with Chinese diet. *Free Radical Biology and Medicine, 145*, 349–356. https://doi.org/10.1016/j.freeradbiomed.2019.10.007, http://www.elsevier.com/locate/freeradbiomed.

Malik, J. A., Ahmed, S., Shinde, M., Almermesh, M. H. S., Alghamdi, S., Hussain, A., & Anwar, S. (2022). The impact of COVID-19 on comorbidities: A review of recent updates for combating it. *Saudi Journal of Biological Sciences, 29*(5), 3586–3599.

Mariamenatu, A. H., & Abdu, E. M. (2021). Overconsumption of Omega-6 polyunsaturated fatty acids (PUFAs) versus deficiency of Omega-3 PUFAs in modern-day diets: The disturbing factor for their "Balanced Antagonistic Metabolic Functions" in the human body. *Journal of Lipids, 2021*, 1–15. https://doi.org/10.1155/2021/8848161.

Marques, F., Lopes, D., da Costa, E., Conde, T., Rego, A., Ribeiro, A. I., Abreu, M. H., & Domingues, M. R. (2021). Seaweed blends as a valuable source of polyunsaturated and healthy fats for nutritional and food applications. *Marine Drugs, 19*(12). https://doi.org/10.3390/md19120684, https://www.mdpi.com/1660-3397/19/12/684/pdf.

Menalla, E., Serna, J. G., Cantero, D., & Cocero, M. J. (2024). Hydrothermal hydrolysis of triglycerides: Tunable and intensified production of diglycerides, monoglycerides, and fatty acids. *Chemical Engineering Journal, 493*. https://doi.org/10.1016/j.cej.2024.152391, https://www.sciencedirect.com/science/journal/13858947.

Meyer-Déru, L., David, G., & Auvergne, R. (2022). Chitosan chemistry review for living organisms encapsulation. *Carbohydrate Polymers, 295*, 119877.

Nath, P. C., Ojha, A., Sharma, M., Inbaraj, B. S., Sridhar, K., Naik, P. K., Dikkala, P. K., & Burla, V. S. S. (2025). *Functional Foods of the Future*. Royal Society of Chemistry, 62–88. https://doi.org/10.1039/9781837673292-00062.

Olejnik, A., Gornowicz-Porowska, J., Jenerowicz, D., Polańska, A., Dobrzyńska, M., Przysławski, J., Sansone, A., & Ferreri, C. (2023). Fatty acids profile and the relevance of membranes as the target of nutrition-based strategies in atopic dermatitis: A narrative review. *Nutrients, 15*(17), 3857. https://doi.org/10.3390/nu15173857.

Ozogul, Y., Karsli, G. T., Durmuş, M., Yazgan, H., Oztop, H. M., McClements, D. J., & Ozogul, F. (2022). Recent developments in industrial applications of nanoemulsions. *Advances in Colloid and Interface Science, 304*, 102685. https://doi.org/10.1016/j.cis.2022.102685.

Pandey, A., Kamran, F., Choudhury, M., Li, L., Rahman, M. S., & Hussain, M. A. (2025). Omega-3 fatty acid fortification of plant-based beverages to enhance their nutritional profile. *Foods, 14*(9). https://doi.org/10.3390/foods14091602, http://www.mdpi.com/journal/foods.

Patel, A., Desai, S. S., Mane, V. K., Enman, J., Rova, U., Christakopoulos, P., & Matsakas, L. (2022). Futuristic food fortification with a balanced ratio of dietary ω-3/ω-6 omega fatty acids for the prevention of lifestyle diseases. *Trends in Food Science and Technology, 120*, 140–153. https://doi.org/10.1016/j.tifs.2022.01.006, http://www.elsevier.com/wps/find/journaldescription.cws_home/601278/description#description.

Pattnaik, M., & Mishra, H. N. (2022). Amelioration of the stability of polyunsaturated fatty acids and bioactive enriched vegetable oil: Blending, encapsulation, and its application. *Critical Reviews in Food Science and Nutrition, 62*(23), 6253–6276. https://doi.org/10.1080/10408398.2021.1899127, https://www.tandfonline.com/loi/bfsn20.

Peng, Y.-C., Yang, F.-L., Subeq, Y.-M., Tien, C.-C., Chao, Y.-F. C., & Lee, R.-P. (2017). Lipid emulsion enriched in omega-3 PUFA accelerates wound healing: A placebo-controlled animal study. *World Journal of Surgery, 42*(6), 1714–1720. https://doi.org/10.1007/s00268-017-4404-x.

Pokushalov, E., Ponomarenko, A., Shrainer, E., Kudlay, D., & Miller, R. (2024). Biomarker-guided dietary supplementation: A narrative review of precision in personalized nutrition. *Nutrients, 16*(23), 4033. https://doi.org/10.3390/nu16234033.

Ponnampalam, E. N., Sinclair, A. J., & Holman, B. W. B. (2021). The sources, synthesis and biological actions of omega-3 and omega-6 fatty acids in red meat: An overview. *Foods, 10*(6), 1358.

Ramsden, C. E., Zamora, D., Faurot, K. R., Macintosh, B., Horowitz, M., Keyes, G. S., Yuan, Z. X., Miller, V., Lynch, C., Honvoh, G., Park, J., Levy, R., Domenichiello, A. F., Johnston, A., Majchrzak-Hong, S., Hibbeln, J. R., Barrow, D. A., Loewke, J., Davis, J. M., ... Mann, J. D. (2021). Dietary alteration of n-3 and n-6 fatty acids for headache reduction in adults with migraine: Randomized controlled trial. *The BMJ, 374*. https://doi.org/10.1136/bmj.n1448, http://www.bmj.com/.

Rathod, N. B., Kulawik, P., Ozogul, Y., Ozogul, F., & Bekhit, A. E. D. A. (2022). Recent developments in non-thermal processing for seafood and seafood products: Cold plasma, pulsed electric field and high hydrostatic pressure. *International Journal of Food Science and Technology, 57*(2), 774–790. https://doi.org/10.1111/ijfs.15392, http://onlinelibrary.wiley.com/journal/10.1111/(ISSN)1365-2621.

Rezvankhah, A., Emam-Djomeh, Z., & Askari, G. (2020). Encapsulation and delivery of bioactive compounds using spray and freeze-drying techniques: A review. *Drying Technology, 38*(1-2), 235–258.

Rincón-Cervera, M.Á., González-Barriga, V., Romero, J., Rojas, R., & López-Arana, S. (2020). Quantification and distribution of omega-3 fatty acids in South Pacific fish and shellfish species. *Foods, 9*(2), 233. https://doi.org/10.3390/foods9020233.

Sadhu, T., Banerjee, I., Lahiri, S. K., & Chakrabarty, J. (2022). Enhancement of nutritional value of fried fish using an artificial intelligence approach. *Environmental Science and Pollution Research, 29*(14), 20048–20063. https://doi.org/10.1007/s11356-021-13548-8, https://link.springer.com/journal/11356.

Saini, R. K., Prasad, P., Sreedhar, R. V., Akhilender Naidu, K., Shang, X., & Keum, Y.-S. (2021). Omega–3 polyunsaturated fatty acids (PUFAs): emerging plant and microbial sources, oxidative stability, bioavailability, and health benefits—a review. *Antioxidants, 10*(10), 1627. https://doi.org/10.3390/antiox10101627.

Sambra, V., Echeverria, F., Valenzuela, A., Chouinard-Watkins, R., & Valenzuela, R. (2021). Docosahexaenoic and arachidonic acids as neuroprotective nutrients throughout the life cycle. *Nutrients, 13*(3), 986. https://doi.org/10.3390/nu13030986.

Santos, H. O., Price, J. C., & Bueno, A. A. (2020). Beyond fish oil supplementation: The effects of alternative plant sources of omega-3 polyunsaturated fatty acids upon lipid indexes and cardiometabolic biomarkers—an overview. *Nutrients, 12*(10), 3159.

Siddhnath, Surasani, V. K. R., Singh, A., Singh, S. M., Hauzoukim, Murthy, L. N., & Baraiya, K. G. (2024). Bioactive compounds from micro-algae and its application in foods: A review. *Discover Food, 4*(1). https://doi.org/10.1007/s44187-024-00096-6, https://www.springer.com/journal/44187.

Siddiqui, S. A., Bahmid, N. A., Taha, A., Khalifa, I., Khan, S., Rostamabadi, H., & Jafari, S. M. (2023). Recent advances in food applications of phenolic-loaded micro/nanodelivery systems. *Critical Reviews in Food Science and Nutrition, 63*(27), 8939–8959. https://doi.org/10.1080/10408398.2022.2056870, https://www.tandfonline.com/loi/bfsn20.

Sultana, A., Adachi, S., & Yoshii, H. (2023). Encapsulation of fish oil and essential fatty acids by spray drying. *Sustainable Food Technology, 1*(6), 827–836.

Tocher, D., Betancor, M., Sprague, M., Olsen, R., & Napier, J. (2019). Omega-3 long-chain polyunsaturated fatty acids, EPA and DHA: bridging the gap between supply and demand. *Nutrients, 11*(1), 89. https://doi.org/10.3390/nu11010089.

Xie, Y., Ding, J., Li, Y., Wei, P., Liu, S., & Yang, R. (2024). The formation of protein–chitosan complexes: Their interaction, applications, and challenges. *Foods, 13*(22), 3572. https://doi.org/10.3390/foods13223572.

Yang, J., Wen, C., Duan, Y., Deng, Q., Peng, D., Zhang, H., & Ma, H. (2021). The composition, extraction, analysis, bioactivities, bioavailability and applications in food system of flaxseed (*Linum usitatissimum* L.) oil: A review. *Trends in Food Science & Technology, 118*, 252–260. https://doi.org/10.1016/j.tifs.2021.09.025.

You, H., & Liang, Y. (2025). Atopic dermatitis: The relationship between immune mediators and skin lipid barrier. *Clinical Reviews in Allergy & Immunology, 68*(1). https://doi.org/10.1007/s12016-025-09057-y.

Zakrzewska, K., Oszajca, K., Zep, W., Piekarska, A., & Sidorkiewicz, M. (2021). The impact of short-term shark liver oil supplementation on the fatty acid composition of erythrocyte membranes. *Nutrients, 13*(10), 3329. https://doi.org/10.3390/nu13103329.

Chapter 14

DHA, EPA, and AA in brain health: brain development, cognition, aging, and depressive disorders through nutritional interventions

Mayssa Hachem[1,2]

[1]Department of Chemistry, College of Engineering and Physical Sciences, Khalifa University of Science and Technology, Abu Dhabi, United Arab Emirates, [2]Food Security and Technology Center, Khalifa University of Science and Technology, Abu Dhabi, United Arab Emirates

14.1 Introduction

Brain health is critical, affecting not only human cognition but also emotional and behavioral responses. Amongst the features influencing brain health, polyunsaturated fatty acids (PUFAs), particularly docosahexaenoic acid (DHA, C22:6 n-3), eicosapentaenoic acid (EPA, C20:5 n-3), and arachidonic acid (AA, C20:4 n-6), have noteworthy gained attention over the last decades in maintaining brain health (Hachem & Nacir, 2022; Hachem et al., 2024; Hachem, Nacir, et al., 2020). In the brain, DHA, EPA, and AA are dynamic in cell membranes and are involved in several aspects of brain function, including neurodevelopment, synaptic plasticity, and inflammation modulation. In recent years, growing evidence has arisen supporting the valuable effects of these fatty acids (FAs) via nutritional involvement, mainly in people at risk of cognitive decay or mood disorders.

DHA, the chief cerebral omega-3 PUFA, is crucial for cells' membrane structure, synaptic function, and neurogenesis. Indeed, DHA is crucial before birth and in early years for brain growth and maturation. The fetus counts severely on maternal DHA, transferred via the placenta, and newborn's DHA is acquired from the mother's breast milk, allowing proper brain development (Tremblay et al., 2020). Additionally, the visual system's development, cognitive skills, and axons' myelination are vastly reliant on adequate DHA levels (Innis, 2008). Besides, DHA supports neurotransmission through receptors' modulation and ion channels, and it is intricated in signaling pathways promoting synaptic plasticity and cognitive function (Gómez-Pinilla, 2008). Although EPA is not as copious as DHA in the brain, it exhibits a harmonizing role in brain health through employing antiinflammatory functions and controlling neuroinflammation. Indeed, chronic inflammation is significant in cognitive decline and neurodegenerative disorders, and EPA's antiinflammatory characteristics would allow its potential consideration as a candidate for preventing or modifying these situations (Chen et al., 2025). Researchers have suggested that DHA and EPA together have beneficial effects on cognition, mostly in aging populations (Loong et al., 2023). While DHA and EPA, naturally produced in fish oils and plant sources, have been widely considered for their neuroprotective characteristics, AA, the primary omega-6 PUFA in the brain, exhibits a harmonizing, brain-diverse function in supporting brain function. AA is a precursor to a diversity of bioactive lipids, including prostaglandins, leukotrienes, and thromboxanes, controlling several mechanisms in the brain, such as inflammation and cell signaling (Zhang et al., 2023). In fact, AA is intricated in synaptic plasticity, neurogenesis, and neuroinflammation, and it is vital for preserving the integrity of neuronal membranes (Rapoport, 2008). Nevertheless, a disproportion between omega-6 and omega-3 PUFA, mainly a high omega-6 to omega-3 ratio, could endorse neuroinflammation and raise the risk of neurodegeneration (Simopoulos, 2002).

Nutritional interventions, including DHA, EPA, and AA, have attracted researchers for further investigation in clinical studies. Indeed, a diet rich in omega-3 PUFA has revealed potential for cognitive function besides delaying the inception

Omega-3 and Omega-6 Polyunsaturated Fatty Acids in Food Systems. DOI: https://doi.org/10.1016/B978-0-443-43810-3.00017-8

of neurodegenerative disorders. Furthermore, clinical studies have shown that omega-3 supplements are beneficial for memory and decrease the risk of Alzheimer's disease in aging populations (Maltais et al., 2022). Additionally, research on depressive diseases has revealed that omega-3 PUFA, mainly EPA, can assist in depression through serotonin and dopamine pathways' modulation and increasing inflammation (Liao et al., 2019).

One of the most interesting areas of research is the investigation of dietary interventions in the inhibition of cognitive decline. Researchers presented that advanced levels of DHA and EPA in the blood were associated with improved cognitive performance and decreased risk of dementia (Saito et al., 2020). This study proves that sustaining an ideal intake of these FAs, through diet and/or supplementation, might have a critical role in maintaining cognitive function with age. Moreover, the profits of maternal DHA consumption in pregnancy have been investigated, and it has been associated with improved neurodevelopmental outcomes in children (Paquet et al., 2024). The actual chapter aims to explore the role of DHA, EPA, and AA in brain development, cognitive function, aging, and mental health, with a focus on depressive syndromes, via dietary and supplementation interventions. Fig. 14.1 covers all areas discussed in the actual book chapter.

14.2 Current scenario/literature review

14.2.1 Docosahexaenoic acid, eicosapentaenoic acid, and arachidonic acid: biochemical overview and sources

Regarding the biochemical aspect, DHA and EPA are biosynthesized from the essential precursor α-linolenic acid (ALA, C18:3 n-3) via elongations and desaturations with a low level of conversion that is inefficient in humans, resulting in the production of less than 10% of DHA (Brenna et al., 2009; Burdge and Calder, 2015). Fig. 14.2 illustrates the biosynthetic pathway of DHA and EPA. DHA's biosynthesis from alimental ALA involves a number of microsomal elongation (ELOVL5) and delta-5 (FADS1) and delta-6 desaturase (FADS2) reactions. The last synthesis of DHA is catalyzed by β-oxidation in peroxisomes. DHA's metabolism produces inflammation-resolving docosanoids.

In the brain, DHA incorporates into phospholipids (PLs) in cells' membranes, influencing membrane fluidity and neurotransmission (Lauritzen et al., 2016). Similarly, it controls synaptic plasticity and neurogenesis and exhibits effective antiinflammatory effects via the bioproduction of specialized pro-resolving mediators (SPMs), including resolvins and neuroprotectins (NPD) (Calder, 2017). EPA, less copious in the brain than DHA, has a role in modulating inflammation via the biosynthesis of E-series resolvins and competing with AA for enzymatic conversion through cyclooxygenase and lipoxygenase (LOX) paths (Duvall & Levy, 2016). Furthermore, EPA affects the behavioral outcomes via variation of neuroinflammation and monoaminergic systems (Mocking et al., 2016). In the brain, besides DHA and EPA, AA is primarily biosynthesised from linoleic acid (LA, C18:2 n-6) and is extremely enhanced in brain PLs. Fig. 14.3 illustrates the biosynthesis of AA from LA.

AA is a precursor for eicosanoids, as well as prostaglandins and leukotrienes, which play a role in immune signaling and vascular tone regulation (Koletzko et al., 2014). Moreover, AA facilitates synaptic role, brain growth, and cellular

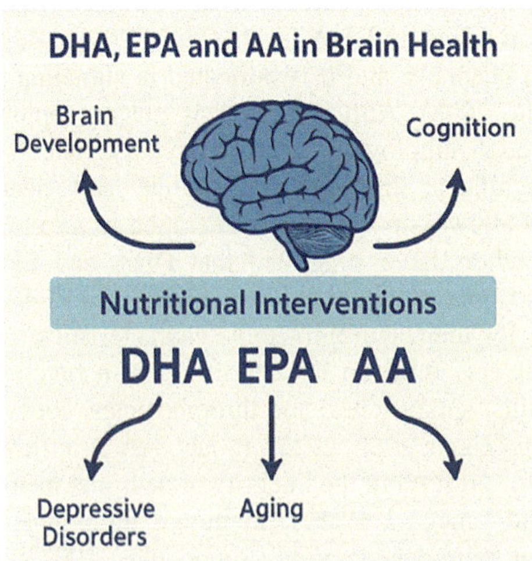

FIGURE 14.1 Docosahexaenoic acid (*DHA*), eicosapentaenoic acid (*EPA*), and arachidonic acid (*AA*) in brain health. These polyunsaturated fatty acids are involved in brain development as well as cognition, aging, and play critical roles in depressive disorders through nutritional interventions.

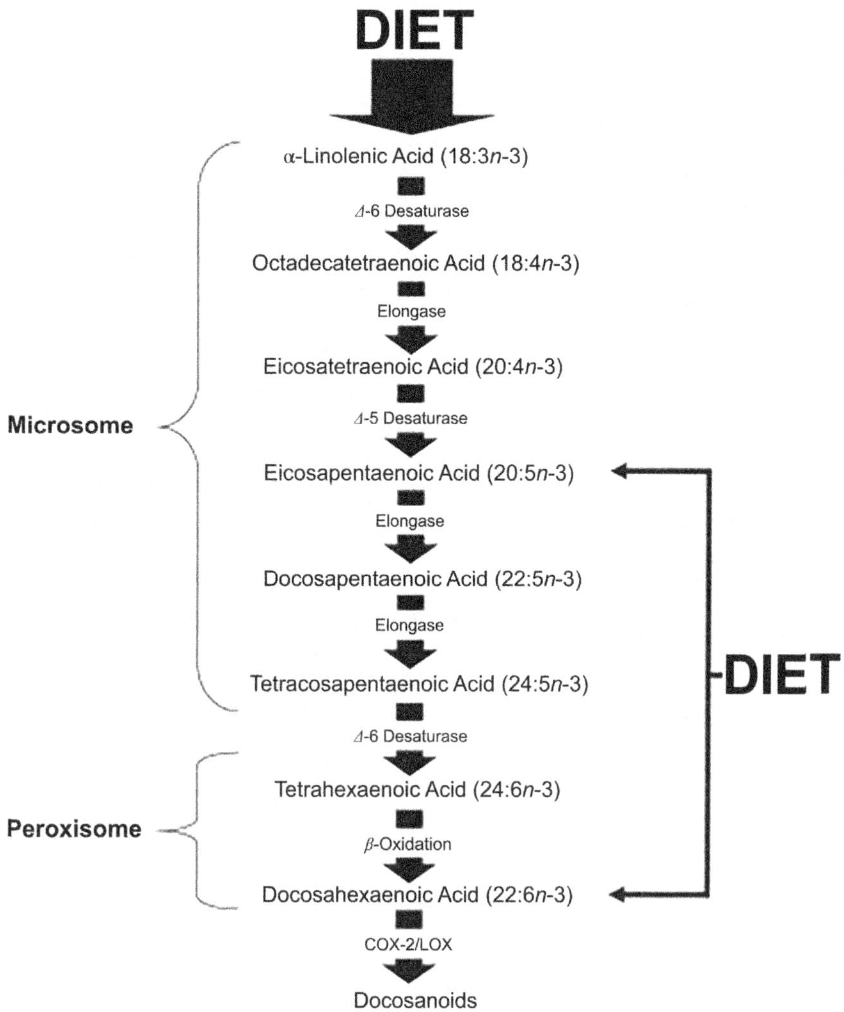

FIGURE 14.2 Illustration showing the biosynthetic path of omega-3 fatty acids (McNamara, 2016). Docosahexaenoic acid (DHA)'s biosynthesis from alimental α-linolenic acid involves a number of microsomal elongation (ELOVL5) and delta-5 (FADS1) and delta-6 desaturase (FADS2) reactions. The last synthesis of DHA is catalyzed by β-oxidation in peroxisomes. DHA's metabolism produces inflammation-resolving docosanoids.

signaling; additionally, unstable AA relative to DHA or EPA may endorse pro-inflammatory responses (SanGiovanni & Chew, 2005). Despite their different functions, the interactions between DHA, EPA, and AA are strongly structured. A well-adjusted supplementation of omega-3 and omega-6 PUFA is required to preserve optimum brain and general health (Hibbeln et al., 2006). When looking to the dietary and endogenous origins of DHA and EPA, both are principally detected in marine sources. The richest natural sources are cold-water fatty fish, for example, salmon, mackerel, sardines, and anchovies. Fish and algal oils are widely used as DHA and EPA supplements needed for pregnant women's, infants', and the elderly's health (Swanson et al., 2012). Likewise, plant seeds, including flaxseed and chia seeds, are rich in ALA, but their conversion to DHA and EPA is limited (Burdge & Wootton, 2002). Furthermore, some microalgae, such as *Schizochytrium*, producing algal oil, are a sustainable alternative source of DHA and are increasingly implemented into infant formulas and fortified nutrients (Liu et al., 2022).

On the other hand, AA is found in animal crops such as meat, eggs, and dairy. Liver and brain tissues are among the richest sources of AA (Koletzko et al., 2008). Similarly, human breast milk is copious in both AA and DHA, underlining their importance in early neurodevelopment (Bernard et al., 2017; Martin et al., 2016; Yehuda et al., 2005). While it is well recognized that AA is endogenously bioproduced from its precursor, LA, several factors, including genetic, hormonal, and nutritional factors, may lead to poor conversion to AA (Weder et al., 2025). Furthermore, advanced bioengineering strategies have fortified crops and livestock feeds with DHA and EPA, supporting the nutritional profiles of animal products (Napier et al., 2015). This practice might cover dietary sufficiency in countries with limited marine resources. Altogether, DHA, EPA, and AA are dynamic components for brain structure and function. While endogenous

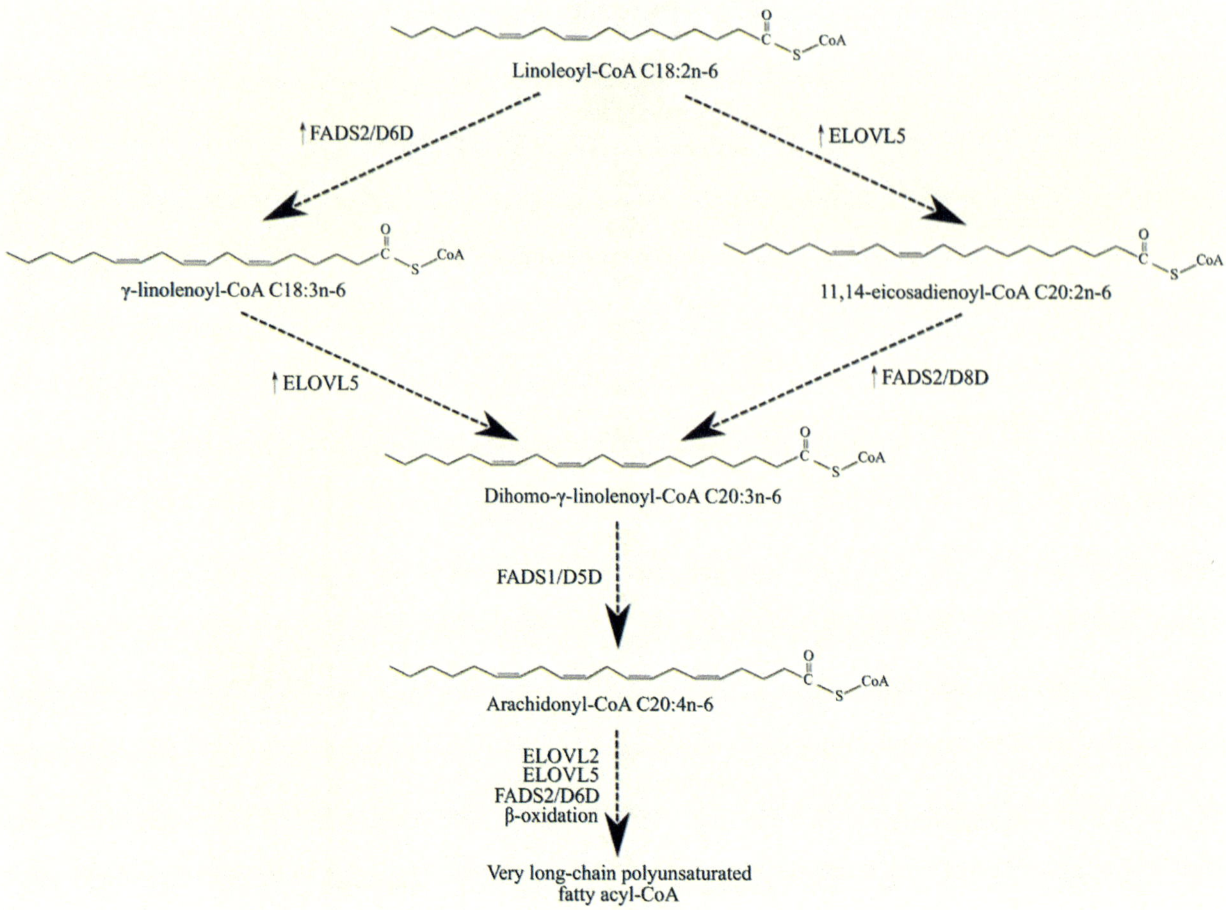

FIGURE 14.3 Arachidonic acid (AA) biosynthesis mechanism (Korbecki Rebacz-Maron, Kupnicka, Chlubek, & Baranowska-Bosiacka, 2023). In humans, AA (C20:4 n-6) is bioproduced from linoleic acid (LA) (C18:2 n-6). Through the action of linoleoyl-CoA, LA undertakes desaturation to γ-linolenoyl-CoA (C18:3 n-6) with FADS2/D6D. This fatty acyl-CoA is transformed to dihomo-γ-linolenoyl-CoA (C20:3 n-6) with ELOVL5 and, lastly, to arachidonyl-CoA (C20:4 n-6) with FADS1/D5D.

synthesis paths are known, the dietary intake of these PUFAs is crucial in order to achieve the best physiological roles. Investigating their biochemical functions and dietary sources is essential for controlling nutritional interventions throughout life stages and in different clinical situations.

14.2.2 Effect of docosahexaenoic acid, eicosapentaenoic acid, and arachidonic acid on brain growth

DHA, EPA, and AA are dynamic components of brain tissue, exhibiting vital functions in neuronal development, myelination, and synaptic plasticity (Fig. 14.4). The human brain gathers these PUFAs quickly throughout gestation and during the first two years of life (Innis, 2014; Koletzko et al., 2014). DHA is the foremost omega-3 PUFA found in the brain's gray matter, with about 10%–20% of total FAs in the cerebral cortex and retina (Lauritzen et al., 2016). DHA's exceptional structure allows high flexibility and supports the fluidity of neuronal membranes, enabling the formation of functional synapses and improving signal transduction (Bazinet & Layé, 2014). Furthermore, DHA supports neurogenesis, dendritic arborization, and the development of several neurotransmitter pathways, including the dopaminergic and serotonergic ones (Guesnet & Alessandri, 2011; Hachem, Belkouch, et al., 2020). Several clinical studies have confirmed that maternal DHA consumption during pregnancy is positively associated with infant cognitive performance and visual acuity (Colombo et al., 2025; Gould et al., 2013; Innis & Friesen, 2008; Rees et al., 2014). Trials have revealed that advanced DHA levels in breast milk or formula are connected with enhanced neurodevelopmental results in infants (Carlson et al., 2013). In animal models, DHA shortage caused a delayed cortical development, impaired learning and memory (Liu et al., 2020; Talamonti et al., 2020).

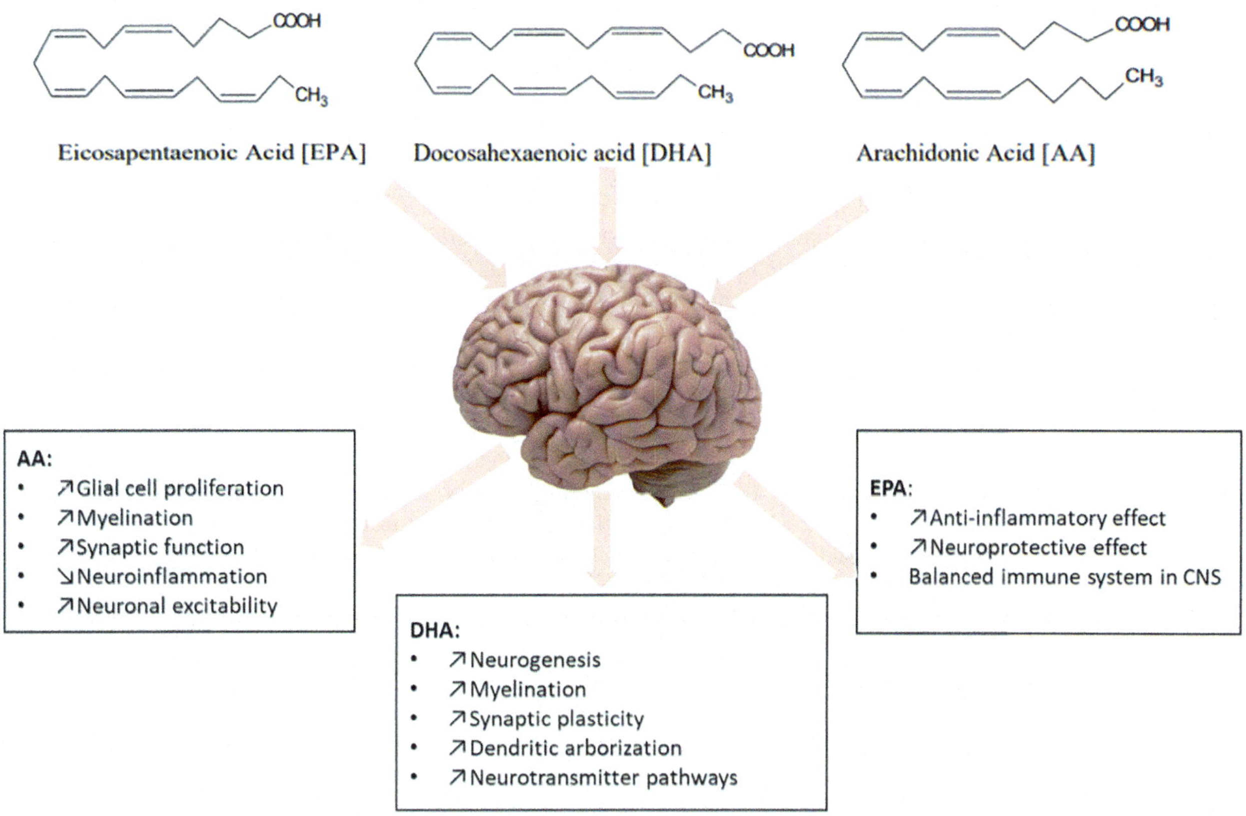

FIGURE 14.4 Docosahexaenoic acid (*DHA*), eicosapentaenoic acid (*EPA*), and arachidonic acid (*AA*) for brain growth. Polyunsaturated fatty acids exhibit vital functions for brain development in addition to neuroprotection function and antiinflammatory effects.

EPA is known for its indirect support of brain development through antiinflammatory and neuroprotective characteristics. Throughout its role in the biosynthesis of resolvins, EPA helps in maintaining a balanced immune system in the central nervous system (Gutiérrez et al., 2019). Besides, EPA impacts brain-derived neurotrophic factor (BDNF) expression, an imperative protein in neuroplasticity and brain development (Vines et al., 2012). Although EPA's incorporation into brain PLs is negligible, it acts as a reservoir for DHA synthesis and allows neurodevelopment via regulation of cytokine production and improving cerebral blood flow (von Schacky, 2021).

In the developing brain, AA is perilous to brain growth, mainly where it aids in glial cell proliferation, myelination, and synaptic function (Wang et al., 2021). AA supports membrane signaling cascades and is a precursor to bioactive eicosanoids, including prostaglandins and leukotrienes, which facilitate neuroinflammation and neuronal excitability (Yehuda et al., 2005). Notably, AA and DHA seem to work synergistically. Researchers have revealed that both AA and DHA supplement in infant formula endorses better cognitive and motor outcomes in comparison to formulas deficient in these PUFAs (Campoy et al., 2011). Human breast milk comprises both AA and DHA, strengthening their vital roles in early life brain development. The optimum development of the brain relies on the accessibility of DHA, EPA, and AA and on the accurate balance between omega-3 and omega-6 PUFAs. A disproportion, mostly an extreme dietary omega-6/omega-3 ratio, might disturb neural signaling and increase vulnerability to neurodevelopmental conditions (Hibbeln et al., 2006). For instance, a lack of DHA throughout gestation and infancy has been connected to lower IQ scores, attention deficits, and low gray matter volume (McNamara & Carlson, 2006; Tanaka et al., 2012). Through rapid brain growth, FA-binding proteins and desaturase enzymes improve PUFA uptake and integration in cells' membranes (Zhang et al., 2018). Moreover, genetic polymorphisms significantly disturb FA metabolism, affecting the need for dietary DHA and AA and proposing a personalized diet in the neurodevelopmental context (Koletzko et al., 2019).

Moreover, in prenatal and early postnatal life, DHA, EPA, and AA are crucial for brain development. Indeed, DHA contributes to the membrane architecture and synaptic function, whereas EPA supports antiinflammatory signaling and vascular regulation, and AA allows cell proliferation and neurotrophic signaling. These PUFAs, combined, form a biochemical foundation for optimal neurodevelopment. Likewise, dietary strategies allowing good intake of these PUFAs via maternal supplement breastfeeding are vital for permanent cognitive and behavioral well-being.

14.2.3 Effect of docosahexaenoic acid, eicosapentaenoic acid, and arachidonic acid on cognitive function

Memory, attention, executive function, and processing speed are a few examples of mental skills involved in cognitive function. From early development through aging, DHA and EPA are crucial for cognitive function, primarily in improving learning abilities, memory, and neuroprotection. Indeed, these PUFAs are vital to neuronal membrane fluidity, signal transduction, synaptic plasticity, and neuroinflammation modulation (Bazinet & Layé, 2014; Lauritzen et al., 2016). Notably, cerebral DHA is greater in synaptic membranes of the cerebral cortex and hippocampus, zones responsible for learning and memory (Cao et al., 2009). Additionally, DHA strengthens synaptic plasticity and long-term potentiation (LTP) through the increase of dendritic spine density and enhancement of neurotransmitter release (Gómez-Pinilla, 2008).

Several studies have suggested a positive correlation between DHA content and cognitive function. In children, advanced prenatal DHA exposure has been connected to improved visual recognition memory and verbal IQ (Helland et al., 2003). In school-aged children, diets with DHA-rich fish oil enhanced reading and memory abilities, predominantly in individuals with learning problems (Richardson & Montgomery, 2005). In older adults, DHA supplements have been correlated with developments in working memory, processing speed, and episodic memory (Yurko-Mauro et al., 2010). Particularly, a randomized controlled trial revealed that 900 mg/day DHA for six months enhanced learning and memory role in age-related cognitive decline (Yurko-Mauro et al., 2010). Indeed, DHA decreases oxidative stress and regulates genes involved in synaptic function (Calder, 2017). Likewise, it increases the expression of BDNF, a significant factor for cognitive resilience and neuroplasticity (Vines et al., 2012).

EPA has a dynamic function in controlling the biochemical environment, encouraging a cognitive role. Because EPA is an antecedent to antiinflammatory lipid mediators, including resolvins and prostaglandins, it resolves neuroinflammation associated with cognitive decline and neurodegenerative diseases (Calder, 2017; Devassy et al., 2016). Furthermore, the EPA might be mainly central in mood-linked features of cognition. For example, EPA supplements have revealed cognitive benefits in persons with depression and mild cognitive impairment (MCI), situations frequently associated with inflammation and oxidative stress (Freeman et al., 2006; Sublette et al., 2011). Although its function in memory and supervisory function is less noticeable than DHA, EPA supports sustaining the cerebral blood flow and endothelial function, indirectly supporting cognitive development (von Schacky, 2021). Additionally, Lin et al. (2012) presented that advanced EPA consumption was meaningfully related to reduced hazard of AD and slower cognitive decay, particularly in those with low levels of omega-3s. Moreover, EPA moderates monoamine neurotransmission, improving dopaminergic and serotonergic pathways intricated in motivation, attention, and emotional regulation (Chalon, 2006).

AA facilitates the synaptic signaling and neurovascular regulation. It is intricated in long-term depression, a process harmonizing with LTP, and essential for synaptic trimming and memory association (Williams et al., 1989). Moreover, AA acts with cannabinoid receptors, disturbing cognitive domains such as learning, memory, and attention (MacCarrone et al., 2011). Some researchers have stressed the synergistic outcome of AA and DHA. Infants nourished with both FAs presented higher cognitive and psychomotor development in comparison to those fed with normal formula (Birch et al., 2000). This recommends that AA is not just a structural component, but also a dynamic biochemical actor in cognition. Table 14.1 summarizes the role of DHA, EPA, and AA in cognitive function.

Finally, the cognitive benefits of PUFAs rely on their total levels and on the ratio of omega-3 and omega-6. An imbalanced ratio has been related to neuroinflammatory progressions and cognitive losses (Hibbeln et al., 2006). An equilibrium between DHA and AA is critical in infancy for ideal neurodevelopment, while in adulthood and aging, preserving DHA and EPA levels is more significant for protecting against cognitive decline and neurodegeneration (Koletzko et al., 2014).

14.2.4 Role of docosahexaenoic acid, eicosapentaenoic acid, and arachidonic acid in aging

A gradual decline in physiological functions, such as neurodegeneration, systemic inflammation, oxidative stress, and impaired cognitive and cardiovascular health, is observed in aging. PUFAs, mainly DHA, EPA, and AA, are essential in controlling these age-related variations. Their contribution to neuroprotection, antiinflammatory signaling, membrane fluidity, and neuronal function makes them pivotal nutrients for healthy aging (Belkouch et al., 2016). With progressing age, DHA in the brain has a tendency to decrease, mainly in areas important for memory such as the hippocampus and prefrontal cortex (McNamara & Carlson, 2006). This decrease is associated with cognitive deterioration, reduced synaptic plasticity, and improved susceptibility to neurodegenerative diseases such as AD (Cunnane et al., 2013). Supplementation with DHA has revealed promise in maintaining cognitive performance and decelerating age-related brain atrophy. Yurko-Mauro et al. (2010) confirmed that older adults with mild memory grievances who consumed DHA with 900 mg/day, 24

TABLE 14.1 Role of docosahexaenoic acid (*DHA*), eicosapentaenoic acid (*EPA*), and arachidonic acid (*AA*) in cognitive function.

PUFA	Role in cognitive function	Effects	References
DHA	– Crucial to neuronal membrane fluidity, signal transduction, synaptic plasticity, and neuroinflammation modulation – Mostly improved in synaptic membranes of the cerebral cortex and hippocampus (learning and memory areas) – Advances in synaptic plasticity and long-term potentiation	– Advances in learning, memory, and neuroprotection – Enhances dendritic spine density and neurotransmitter release – Prenatal DHA is related to enhanced visual recognition memory and verbal IQ in children – DHA-rich fish oil diets improved reading and memory in school-aged children, particularly those with learning difficulties – DHA supplement in older adults is associated with development in working memory, processing speed, and episodic memory – Declines oxidative stress and controls synaptic role genes – Increases brain-derived neurotrophic factor, auxiliary to cognitive resilience and neuroplasticity	(Bazinet & Layé, 2014); (Lauritzen et al., 2016); (Cao et al., 2009); (Gómez-Pinilla, 2008); (Helland et al., 2003); (Richardson & Montgomery, 2005); (Yurko-Mauro et al., 2010); (Calder, 2017); (Vines et al., 2012)
EPA	– Moderates the biochemical environment supporting the cognitive role – Precursor to antiinflammatory lipid mediators (resolvins, prostaglandins) – Supports cerebral blood flow and the endothelial role – Controls monoamine neurotransmission (dopaminergic and serotonergic paths)	– Resolves neuroinflammation related to cognitive failure and neurodegenerative disorders – Displays cognitive assistance in depression and mild cognitive impairment – Advanced EPA consumption is connected to decreased risk of Alzheimer's disease and gentler cognitive decline – Advances motivation, attention, and emotional regulation	(Calder, 2017); Devassy et al., 2016; (Freeman et al., 2006); (Sublette et al., 2011); (von Schacky, 2021); (Lin et al., 2012); (Chalon, 2006)
AA	– Enables synaptic signaling and neurovascular parameters – Intricated in long-term depression, synaptic trimming, and memory association – Interacts with cannabinoid receptors, improving learning, memory, and attention	– Harmonious effect with DHA: infants fed both AA and DHA presented improved cognitive and psychomotor progress in comparison to normal formula-fed infants – Functions as an energetic biochemical actor in cognition	(Williams et al., 1989); (MacCarrone et al., 2011); (Birch et al., 2000)

weeks had noteworthy enhancement in memory and learning responsibilities in comparison to placebo (Yurko-Mauro et al., 2010). Moreover, neuroimaging researchers have stated larger hippocampal volumes and decreased white matter lesions in elderly populations with advanced plasma DHA levels (Pottala et al., 2014). DHA's antiaging effects are partially facilitated by its capability to decrease neuroinflammation and oxidative stress. It is a precursor to NPD-1, illustrated in Fig. 14.5, a specialized pro-resolving lipid mediator that moderates gene expression involved in cell survival, inflammation suppression, and amyloid-beta clearance in the aging brain (Bazan, 2006).

Protectin D1 or europrotectin D-1 (10R, 17S-dihydroxy-docosa-4Z, 7Z, 11E, 13E, 15Z, 19Z-hexaenoic acid) is produced once DHA is free from the membrane PLs through the hydrolytic action of phospholipase A2 (PLA-2), where the enzyme 15-LOX will convert DHA to 17S-hydroperoxy-DHA through a complex process of lipoxygenation. This step is followed by epoxidation and hydrolysis, allowing for the formation of NPD-1.

One of the hallmark characteristics of aging is a chronic low-grade inflammatory system regularly denoted as "inflammaging" (Franceschi et al., 2017). EPA is a potent antiinflammatory biomolecule, resolving inflammation and supporting endothelial and immune function through resolvins and eicosanoids. In older adults, EPA supplements have been related to reduced circulating markers of inflammation such as C-reactive protein (CRP) and interleukin-6 (IL-6) (Wang et al., 2012). These properties are clinically substantial, as systemic inflammation leads to cardiovascular disease, cognitive impairment, sarcopenia, and frailty in the elderly. Still, the EPA has a single role in mood regulation in aging.

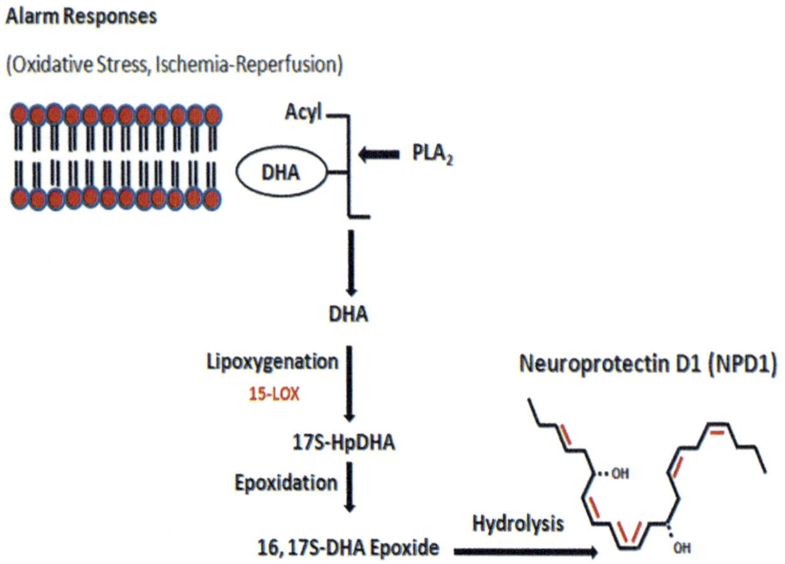

FIGURE 14.5 Illustration showing the biosynthesis of neuroprotectin D-1 (*NPD-1*) from docosahexaenoic acid (*DHA*) (Valenzuela Baez and Valenzuela, 2011). Protectin D-1 or NPD-1 (10R, 17S-dihydroxy-docosa-4Z, 7Z, 11E, 13E, 15Z, 19Z-hexaenoic acid) is produced once DHA is free from the membrane phospholipids through the hydrolytic action of phospholipase A2 (*PLA-2*), where the enzyme 15-lipoxygenase (*15-LOX*) will convert DHA to 17S-hydroperoxy-DHA through a complex process of lipoxygenation. This step is followed by epoxidation and hydrolysis, allowing for the formation of NPD-1.

Depression is predominant in the elderly and frequently cohabits with cognitive decline. EPA has confirmed antidepressant effects, principally in older adults with high levels of inflammatory markers (Freeman et al., 2006; Sublette et al., 2011). This connection is possibly facilitated via the EPA's variation of cytokine.

Although AA exhibits pro-inflammatory characteristics, it has vital physiological functions in aging, together with cell signaling, vasodilation, and neurotrophin activation (Yehuda et al., 2002). Well-adjusted AA levels are essential for preserving synaptic function and neurovascular coupling in older adults. Nevertheless, unbalanced AA metabolism and levels in aging can worsen neuroinflammatory processes and have been involved in the pathogenesis of neurodegenerative diseases such as AD and PD (Farooqui et al., 2007). Therefore sustaining an ideal balance between AA and omega-3 PUFAs is critical for encouraging healthy brain aging. Recent studies suggest that AA might be supportive for cognition when found in proper ratios with DHA (Tian et al., 2025). Both AA and DHA supplementation in elderly animals improved cognitive flexibility and synaptic resilience. Notably, AA participates in moderating the endocannabinoid pathway and neuronal repair mechanisms, which can be protective in aging under precise situations (Qian et al., 2025).

One of the key factors in PUFA-correlated with aging research is the equilibrium between omega-3 and omega-6 PUFAs. The western diet is frequently considered a high omega-6/omega-3 ratio diet, which may intensify inflammation and aging-linked disorders (Simopoulos, 2002). An ideal dietary ratio (~4:1 or less) supports homeostasis and decreases the age-related disease risks. Studies have revealed that dietary interventions that lower this ratio via an amplified omega-3 consumption, mainly DHA and EPA, result in enhancements of cognitive functions, lipid metabolism, and cardiovascular consequences in aging people. Adapted nutritional approaches founded on genotype, dietary behaviors, and inflammatory outlines are progressively being studied to enhance PUFA involvement in the elderly (Minihane et al., 2015).

14.2.5 Docosahexaenoic acid, eicosapentaenoic acid, and arachidonic acid in depressive disorders

Depressive disorders, such as major depressive disorder (MDD), are amongst the most ubiquitous and incapacitating mental health conditions worldwide. Evolving studies have stressed the impact of nutrition and lipid metabolism, mostly the balance of PUFAs, in the pathophysiology and handling of depression. DHA and EPA have been broadly considered for their neuroprotective and antiinflammatory characteristics, while AA is intricated in inflammatory signaling and neurotransmission. Dysregulation of these PUFAs has been connected to alterations in mood, neuroinflammation, and neuronal plasticity in depressive syndromes. Numerous experimental studies have revealed a relationship between poor diets or plasma levels of omega-3 PUFAs and high risk of depression (Grosso, Galvano, et al., 2014; Grosso, Pajak, et al., 2014; Hibbeln, 1998). EPA has substantial antiinflammatory effects and is believed to impact depression through the modulation of cytokine production and neurotransmitter systems, predominantly serotonin and dopamine (Freeman et al., 2006; Su et al., 2015). Sublette et al. (2011) recommended that omega-3 supplementation, mainly EPA-major formulations, is efficient in decreasing depressive symptoms, particularly when applied adjunctively through conventional antidepressants (Sublette et al., 2011). Another inclusive metaanalysis by Liao et al. (2019) showed that high-EPA (≥60% EPA) preparations were further efficient than DHA-rich formulations in lightening depression, signifying different mechanisms of action amongst the two FAs (Liao et al., 2019). One anticipated mechanism is the reduction of pro-inflammatory cytokines such as IL-6, TNF-α, and CRP frequently high in patients with MDD (Miller & Raison, 2016). EPA, especially, gives rise to antiinflammatory eicosanoids and SPMs, including resolvins, which counter neuroinflammation. Moreover, omega-3 PUFAs might decrease cortisol hypersecretion, a mutual feature in depressive disorders (Grosso, Galvano, et al., 2014; Grosso, Pajak, et al., 2014). Neuroimaging research has also indicated that advanced omega-3 consumption is related to higher gray matter volume in mood-related brain areas such as the hippocampus and prefrontal cortex, further supporting their role in maintaining emotional regulation (Conklin et al., 2007). High AA-derived eicosanoids have been detected in patients with depression, showing a latent pro-inflammatory function in mood dysregulation (Yui et al., 2015). Nevertheless, AA is not consistently harmful. In well-adjusted ratios with DHA and EPA, it might support neurodevelopment and emotional steadiness. Yehuda et al. (2005) confirmed that supplementation with a mixture of AA, DHA, and EPA enhanced mood and behavior in patients with marginal personality condition, emphasizing the significance of PUFAs balance rather than a lone deficit or additional (Yehuda et al., 2005). Furthermore, AA-derived endocannabinoids, anandamide (AEA) and 2-arachidonoylglycerol (2-AG), are involved in stress response, emotional regulation, and neuroprotection (McDougle et al., 2014). Dysregulation of this arrangement has been implicated in animal and human models of depression, demonstrating that AA's function is complex and context-dependent. One serious facet of depression is the ratio between omega-6 and omega-3 PUFAs. For instance, in the brain of Flinders Sensitive Line (FSL) rats, an animal model of depression, Green et al. (2005) suggested that in all brain regions, AA level was pointedly advanced in FSL rats mainly in the hypothalamus (increase by 21%), in the nucleus accumbens (increase by 24%), in the prefrontal cortex (increase by 31%), and in the striatum (increase by 23%) (Green et al., 2005). No noteworthy changes were detected for n-3 PUFA, suggesting the existence of reformed brain PUFA arrangement in the animal model of depression (Fig. 14.6).

Values from control (open bars) and FSL (hatched bars) rats are stated as weight percentages (means + SD; n = 5). The percentage rise of AA in the FSL rats.

Furthermore, western diets have a tendency to have an imbalanced ratio (often 15:1 or higher), which endorses a pro-inflammatory state (Simopoulos, 2002). This disproportion might intensify depressive signs. Involvements targeting lowering this ratio, either through reduction of dietary omega-6 consumption or increasing omega-3 uptake, have revealed positive effects on depressive disorders (Sinn et al., 2012). Besides, genetic and enzymatic differences in FA metabolism can affect individual exposure to depressive syndromes by varying the endogenous conversion rates of precursor FAs to

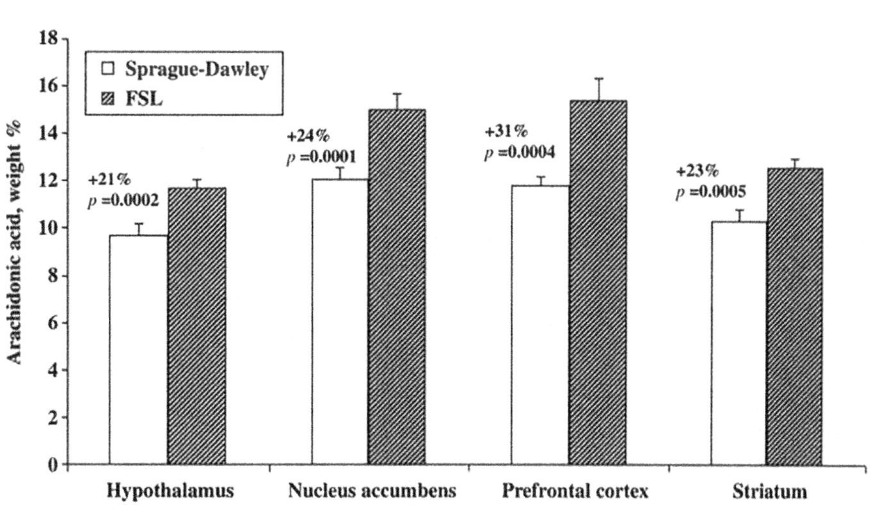

FIGURE 14.6 Arachidonic acid (AA) level of brain areas, including the hypothalamus, nucleus accumbens, prefrontal cortex, and striatum (Green et al., 2005). Values from control (open bars) and Flinders Sensitive Line (*FSL*; hatched bars) rats are stated as weight percentages (means + SD; n = 5). The percentage rise of AA in the FSL rats.

DHA, EPA, or AA (Freeman et al., 2006). The clinical efficacy of DHA, EPA, and AA in handling depressive syndromes relies on their supplementation and on inclusive dietary involvement and specialized nutrition methods. EPA has confirmed reliable antidepressant properties in several randomized controlled trials, with the greatest results detected in persons with high inflammatory markers (Lamon-Fava et al., 2023; Liao et al., 2019). The potential function of AA in emotional parameters, although more debated, might be elucidated through further research into the endocannabinoid system and the context of AA communications with other FAs. Future guidelines comprise biomarker-directed PUFA therapy, gene-diet connections, and personalized PUFA mixtures to enhance treatment efficiency and lessen adverse effects.

14.2.6 Nutritional deficiencies

As previously discussed, DHA, EPA, and AA are primarily found in food (fish/seafood for DHA/EPA and organ meats for AA) or bioproduced in low levels from their precursors (ALA and LA) (Brenna et al., 2009). Deficiencies in these PUFAs can impact neurological health, immune function, as well as general development. Indeed, western diets are often poor in omega-3 and rich in omega-6 PUFA, leading to a nonequilibrated FAs profile impacting negatively the human's health (Simopoulos, 2002). In infancy and early childhood periods, a lack of DHA and EPA is distressing since these PUFAs are vital for neuronal membrane structure, synaptogenesis, as well as visual and cognitive development (Innis, 2007). Moreover, during pregnancy and lactation periods, deficient maternal consumption of DHA is correlated with impaired fetal brain growth, lower IQ scores, and improved hazard of behavioral problems in children (Greenberg, Bell, & Ausdal, 2008). On the other hand, EPA deficiency, although less considered for structural roles, is dynamic for its antiinflammatory properties and variation of mood and cardiovascular health. Yet scarcer in modern diets, AA deficit may rise in the vegetarian population and in those with low desaturase enzyme activity. Indeed, AA is essential for prostaglandin biosynthesis and cell signaling and has a harmonious role with DHA in primary development (Koletzko et al., 2008). Inadequate levels of DHA and AA in preterm infants, who fail the third-trimester intrauterine accretion of PUFAs, are associated with advanced risks of neurodevelopmental delays and inflammatory problems such as necrotizing enterocolitis (Carlson and Colombo, 2016). Lastly, deficiencies in DHA, EPA, and AA can affect neurodevelopment, cognitive function, and immune response throughout life. Guaranteeing suitable diets, principally in critical life phases such as pregnancy, infancy, and aging, is essential for sustaining ideal health.

14.3 Principles/methodology

14.3.1 Biomarkers and cognitive testing for docosahexaenoic acid, eicosapentaenoic acid, and arachidonic acid

In order to understand their roles in brain health and monitoring dietary supplements, nutritional assessment of DHA, EPA, and AA is crucial. These assessments comprise biomarker examination and functional estimations, including cognitive testing. Indeed, biomarkers allow impartial measurement of PUFA levels in different tissues, while cognitive examinations offer data related to nutrient status, mainly in vulnerable people such as infants, children, and the elderly. For instance, FA profiling in plasma, serum PLs, RBC membranes, and adipose tissue is one of those biomarkers. More interestingly, PLs of RBC are considered the gold standard for lengthy status, displaying dietary consumption for many months (Stark et al., 2016). Omega-3 index, known as the sum of RBC EPA and DHA, calculated as a percentage of total FAs, is commonly applied as an authorized predictor of cardiovascular and cognitive results (Harris et al., 2017). AA is classically evaluated together with omega-3s to assess the omega-6 to omega-3 ratio, significant for defining the inflammatory equilibrium of an individual's FA profile (Simopoulos, 2016). Recent developments in lipidomics and metabolomics have improved the sensitivity and specificity of PUFA detection, permitting differentiation of separate isomers and their metabolic derivatives (Hussain et al., 2020). These approaches are mainly valuable in recognizing primary deficits and monitoring the efficiency of dietary interventions in clinical trials.

In parallel with biomarker evaluations, cognitive testing allows efficient validation of PUFA status. In children, the Bayley Scales of Infant Development or the Kaufman Assessment Battery for Children are examples of cognitive and psychomotor performance assessment for DHA and AA contents (Balasundaram and Avulakunta, 2025). Furthermore, in adults and the elderly, the Mini-Mental State Examination and Rey Auditory Verbal Learning Test are frequently applied as neuropsychological batteries (Banks et al., 2024). Additionally, advanced omega-3 indices are consistently associated with enhanced memory, processing speed, and global cognition, primarily in elderly and people at risk of dementia (Cole Ma, & Frautschy, 2009). Briefly, combining FA biomarkers with cognitive testing provides a comprehensive assessment of DHA, EPA, and AA status and their functional significance. This integrative approach is crucial for developing tailored dietary tactics in brain health.

14.3.2 Clinical trials and observational studies on docosahexaenoic acid, eicosapentaenoic acid, and arachidonic acid

Clinical trials have developed our knowledge on the physiological and neurological roles of DHA, EPA, and AA; all known for their implication in neurodevelopment, cognitive function, and inflammatory regulation. In the context of a randomized controlled trial, Mengelberg et al. (2022) investigated the effect of a DHA and EPA diet in the elderly with MCI. For 12 months, in members receiving 1491 mg DHA + 351 mg EPA per day, a slower cognitive decay and greater memory function were observed in comparison with the placebo group, hence suggesting a neuroprotective effect (Mengelberg et al., 2022). Similarly, a vast cohort study from the UK Biobank suggested that higher plasma DHA contents were inversely correlated with dementia, proposing correlations between omega-3 status and brain aging (Sala-Vila et al., 2023).

Moreover, a clinical trial evaluated the outcome of maternal DHA and AA supplements in pregnancy on infant neurodevelopment. Data showed that infants whose mothers had a balanced mixture of DHA and AA (500 mg/day each) had better scores in early language and motor development at 18 months compared to the control group (Guillot et al., 2022). These results feature the importance of balanced n-3 and n-6 consumption for early life outcomes. On the other hand, a 2020 longitudinal trial in Japan revealed that higher erythrocyte AA levels in adults were associated with better executive function and verbal fluency, maybe because of its role in neuroinflammation modulation and synaptic plasticity (Fujino et al., 2023). Contrarily, another study proposed that increases in AA without adequate DHA might endorse pro-inflammatory responses, underlining the importance of ratio over absolute quantity (Wei et al., 2021). Altogether, these studies highlight the importance of DHA, EPA, and AA in cognitive and neurological functions. Likewise, they emphasize the need for equilibrated dietary strategies and further long-term trials to clarify contributory relationships.

14.4 Future perspectives

DHA, EPA, and AA's roles in brain health were investigated, mainly their implication in brain functions, cognitive development, aging, and depressive disorders. Emerging studies highlighted their potential in controlling neurodegenerative conditions (Hachem et al., 2016; Hachem et al., 2020) and stressed their function in primary neural development. A randomized controlled trial confirmed that prenatal diet with DHA and AA meaningfully improved cognitive results in newborn infants, proving a synergetic outcome on neurogenesis and synaptic plasticity (Ogundipe et al., 2018). Moreover, EPA's antiinflammatory characteristics are being examined for their capability to support cognitive roles throughout adolescence, a period marked by significant neural maturation. Additionally, the aging population shows a rising alarm for cognitive decline. A longitudinal study revealed that advanced dietary consumption of DHA and EPA was associated with a decreased risk of MCI and AD in older adults (Wei et al., 2023). These findings suggest that omega-3 PUFAs might exhibit neuroprotective effects through neuroinflammation and oxidative stress, common pathways in elderly cognitive decline. Moreover, PUFAs' implication in mood regulation is progressing. Patients suffering from MDD exhibited lower plasma levels of DHA and EPA compared to healthy controls, and supplementation led to significant developments in depressive disease (Kelaiditis et al., 2023). Thus omega-3 PUFAs may affect neurotransmitter pathways and inflammatory biomarkers associated with depression. Furthermore, genomics and metabolomics research are developing in tailored nutritional interventions. More interestingly, identifying genetic polymorphisms that affect FA metabolism may suggest personalized supplementation strategies to improve brain health. Future research would propose large-scale, longitudinal studies to regulate the optimal dosing treatments. Lastly, deciphering the relationship between PUFAs and other nutrients, such as B vitamins and antioxidants, would allow a better understanding of their supportive outcome on brain health.

14.5 Conclusion

Briefly, DHA, EPA, and AA are vital PUFAs exhibiting various roles and supporting brain health during life. Though DHA supports neural structure and synaptic plasticity, EPA is involved in antiinflammatory balance and mood regulation, whereas AA allows signal transduction and cognitive functions. Together, these PUFAs are a robust biochemical basis for brain growth, effective cognition, aging, and emotional balance. In serious growing stages and throughout the elderly, dietary interventions with suitable consumption of these PUFAs might moderate cognitive decay and depressive symptoms. Emergent studies highlight the therapeutic effect of a well-balanced omega-3 and omega-6 supplement in improving neuroprotection and mental health. While further research is essential to better understand the right dosage and mechanisms of action, prevailing evidence suggests DHA, EPA, and AA as dynamic nutrients for the brain. Finally, future research would allow the development of efficient dietary strategies and therapeutic applications for brain-related diseases, mainly neurodegenerative ones.

References

Bazan, N. G. (2006). Cell survival matters: Docosahexaenoic acid signaling, neuroprotection and photoreceptors. *Trends in Neurosciences, 29*(5), 263–271. https://doi.org/10.1016/j.tins.2006.03.005.

Bazinet, R. P., & Layé, S. (2014). Polyunsaturated fatty acids and their metabolites in brain function and disease. *Nature Reviews. Neuroscience, 15*(12), 771–785. Available from https://doi.org/10.1038/nrn3820, http://www.nature.com/nrn/.

Balasundaram, P., & Avulakunta, I.D. (2025). Bayley Scales Of Infant and Toddler Development StatPearls. Treasure Island (FL) with ineligible companies. Disclosure: Indirapriya Darshini Avulakunta declares no relevant financial relationships with ineligible companies.

Banks, R., Higgins, C., Greene, B. R., Jannati, A., Gomes-Osman, J., Tobyne, S., & Pascual-Leone, A. (2024). Clinical classification of memory and cognitive impairment with multimodal digital biomarkers. *Alzheimers Dement (Amst, 16*(1), e12557. https://doi.org/10.1002/dad2.12557.

Belkouch, M., Hachem, M., Elgot, A., Lo Van, A., Picq, M., Guichardant, M., Lagarde, M., & Bernoud-Hubac, N. (2016). The pleiotropic effects of omega-3 docosahexaenoic acid on the hallmarks of Alzheimer's disease. *The Journal of Nutritional Biochemistry, 38*, 1–11. https://doi.org/10.1016/j.jnutbio.2016.03.002.

Bernard, J. Y., Armand, M., Peyre, H., Garcia, C., Forhan, A., De Agostini, M., Charles, M. A., & Heude, B. (2017). Breastfeeding, polyunsaturated fatty acid levels in colostrum and child intelligence quotient at age 5-6 years. *Journal of Pediatrics, 183*, 43. Available from https://doi.org/10.1016/j.jpeds.2016.12.039, http://www.elsevier.com/inca/publications/store/6/2/3/3/1/1/index.htt.

Birch, E. E., Garfield, S., Hoffman, D. R., Uauy, R., & Birch, D. G. (2000). A randomized controlled trial of early dietary supply of long-chain polyunsaturated fatty acids and mental development in term infants. *Developmental Medicine and Child Neurology, 42*(3), 174–181. https://doi.org/10.1017/S0012162200000311.

Burdge, G. C., & Wootton, S. A. (2002). Conversion of α-linolenic acid to eicosapentaenoic, docosapentaenoic and docosahexaenoic acids in young women. *British Journal of Nutrition, 88*(4), 411–420. Available from https://doi.org/10.1079/bjn2002689, http://journals.cambridge.org/BJN.

Brenna, Salem, J. T., Jr, N., Sinclair, A. J., Cunnane, S. C., International Society for the Study of Fatty, A., & Lipids, I. (2009). alpha-Linolenic acid supplementation and conversion to n-3 long-chain polyunsaturated fatty acids in humans. *Prostaglandins Leukot Essent Fatty Acids, 80*(2-3), 85–91. https://doi.org/10.1016/j.plefa.2009.01.004.

Burdge, G. C., & Calder, P. C. (2015). Introduction to fatty acids and lipids. *World Rev Nutr Diet, 112*, 1–16. https://doi.org/10.1159/000365423.

Calder, P. C. (2017). Omega-3 fatty acids and inflammatory processes: From molecules to man. *Biochemical Society Transactions, 45*(5), 1105–1115. Available from https://doi.org/10.1042/BST20160474, http://www.biochemsoctrans.org/content/45/5/1105.full-text.pdf.

Campoy, C., Escolano-Margarit, M. V., Ramos, R., Parrilla-Roure, M., Csábi, G., Beyer, J., Ramirez-Tortosa, M. C., Molloy, A. M., Decsi, T., & Koletzko, B. V. (2011). Effects of prenatal fish-oil and 5-methyltetrahydrofolate supplementation on cognitive development of children at 6.5 y of age. *American Journal of Clinical Nutrition, 94*(6). https://doi.org/10.3945/ajcn.110.001107, http://www.ajcn.org/content/94/6/1880S.full.pdf+html.

Cao, D., Kevala, K., Kim, J., Moon, H. S., Jun, S. B., Lovinger, D., & Kim, H. Y. (2009). Docosahexaenoic acid promotes hippocampal neuronal development and synaptic function. *Journal of Neurochemistry, 111*(2), 510–521. https://doi.org/10.1111/j.1471-4159.2009.06335.x.

Carlson, S. E., & Colombo, J. (2016). Docosahexaenoic Acid and Arachidonic Acid Nutrition in Early Development. *Advances in Pediatrics, 63*(1), 453–471. https://doi.org/10.1016/j.yapd.2016.04.011.

Carlson, S. E., Colombo, J., Gajewski, B. J., Gustafson, K. M., Mundy, D., Yeast, J., Georgieff, M. K., Markley, L. A., Kerling, E. H., & Shaddy, D. J. (2013). DHA supplementation and pregnancy outcomes. *American Journal of Clinical Nutrition, 97*(4), 808–815. Available from https://doi.org/10.3945/ajcn.112.050021, http://ajcn.nutrition.org/content/97/4/808.full.pdf+html.

Chalon, S. (2006). Omega-3 fatty acids and monoamine neurotransmission. *Prostaglandins, Leukotrienes, and Essential Fatty Acids, 75*(4-5), 259–269. https://doi.org/10.1016/j.plefa.2006.07.005.

Chen, Y., Touboul, R., Chen, Y., & Chang, C. L. (2025). Strategic delivery of omega-3 fatty acids for modulating inflammatory neurodegenerative diseases. *Frontiers in Aging Neuroscience, 17*. Available from https://doi.org/10.3389/fnagi.2025.1535094, https://www.frontiersin.org/journals/aging-neuroscience#.

Cole, G. M., Ma, Q. L., & Frautschy, S. A. (2009). Omega-3 fatty acids and dementia. *Prostaglandins Leukot Essent Fatty Acids, 81*(2-3), 213–221. https://doi.org/10.1016/j.plefa.2009.05.015.

Colombo, J., Shaddy, D. J., Mathis, N., Christifano, D. N., Brown, A. R., Gajewski, B. J., Carlson, S. E., & Gustafson, K. M. (2025). Effects of prenatal DHA dose on infant visual attention. *Developmental Psychobiology, 67*(5), Available from https://doi.org/10.1002/dev.70072, http://onlinelibrary.wiley.com/journal/10.1002/(ISSN)1098-2302.

Conklin, S. M., Gianaros, P. J., Brown, S. M., Yao, J. K., Hariri, A. R., Manuck, S. B., & Muldoon, M. F. (2007). Long-chain omega-3 fatty acid intake is associated positively with corticolimbic gray matter volume in healthy adults. *Neuroscience Letters, 421*(3), 209–212. https://doi.org/10.1016/j.neulet.2007.04.086.

Cunnane, S. C., Chouinard-Watkins, R., Castellano, C. A., & Barberger-Gateau, P. (2013). Docosahexaenoic acid homeostasis, brain aging and Alzheimer's disease: Can we reconcile the evidence? *Prostaglandins, Leukotrienes, and Essential Fatty Acids, 88*(1), 61–70. https://doi.org/10.1016/j.plefa.2012.04.006.

Devassy, J. G., Leng, S., Gabbs, M., Monirujjaman, M., & Aukema, H. M. (2016). Omega-3 polyunsaturated fatty acids and oxylipins in neuroinflammation and management of Alzheimer disease. *Advances in Nutrition, 7*(5), 905–916. Available from https://doi.org/10.3945/an.116.012187, http://advances.nutrition.org/content/7/5/905.full.pdf.

Duvall, M. G., & Levy, B. D. (2016). DHA- and EPA-derived resolvins, protectins, and maresins in airway inflammation. *European Journal of Pharmacology, 785*, 144–155. Available from https://doi.org/10.1016/j.ejphar.2015.11.001, www.elsevier.com/locate/ejphar.

Farooqui, A. A., Horrocks, L. A., & Farooqui, T. (2007). Modulation of inflammation in brain: A matter of fat. *Journal of Neurochemistry, 101*(3), 577–599. https://doi.org/10.1111/j.1471-4159.2006.04371.x.

Franceschi, C., Garagnani, P., Vitale, G., Capri, M., & Salvioli, S. (2017). Inflammaging and 'Garb-aging' *Trends in Endocrinology & Metabolism, 28*(3), 199–212. https://doi.org/10.1016/j.tem.2016.09.005.

Freeman, M. P., Hibbeln, J. R., Wisner, K. L., Davis, J. M., Mischoulon, D., Peet, M., Keck, P. E., Marangell, L. B., Richardson, A. J., Lake, J., & Stoll, A. L. (2006). Omega-3 fatty acids: Evidence basis for treatment and future research in psychiatry. *Journal of Clinical Psychiatry, 67*(12), 1954–1967. Available from https://doi.org/10.4088/JCP.v67n1217, www.psychiatrist.com.

Fujino, H., Suwazono, S., Ueda, Y., Kobayashi, M., Nakayama, T., Imura, O., Matsumura, T., & Takahashi, M. P. (2023). Longitudinal changes in neuropsychological functioning in Japanese patients with myotonic dystrophy type 1: A five year follow-up study. *Journal of Neuromuscular Diseases, 10*(6), 1083–1092. Available from https://doi.org/10.3233/JND-230083, http://www.iospress.nl/journal/journal-of-neuromuscular-diseases/.

Gould, J. F., Smithers, L. G., & Makrides, M. (2013). The effect of maternal omega-3 (n23) LCPUFA supplementation during pregnancy on early childhood cognitive and visual development: A systematic review and meta-analysis of randomized controlled trials1-3. *American Journal of Clinical Nutrition, 97*(3), 531–544. Available from https://doi.org/10.3945/ajcn.112.045781Australia, http://ajcn.nutrition.org/content/97/3/531.full.pdf+html.

Green, P., Gispan-Herman, I., & Yadid, G. (2005). Increased arachidonic acid concentration in the brain of Flinders Sensitive Line rats, an animal model of depression. *Journal of Lipid Research, 46*(6), 1093–1096. https://doi.org/10.1194/jlr.c500003-jlr200.

Greenberg, J. A., Bell, S. J., & Ausdal, W. V. (2008). Omega-3 Fatty Acid supplementation during pregnancy. *Reviews in Obstetrics & Gynecology, 1*(4), 162–169.

Grosso, G., Galvano, F., Marventano, S., Malaguarnera, M., Bucolo, C., Drago, F., & Caraci, F. (2014). Omega-3 fatty acids and depression: Scientific evidence and biological mechanisms. *Oxidative Medicine and Cellular Longevity, 2014*, 1–16. https://doi.org/10.1155/2014/313570.

Grosso, G., Pajak, A., Marventano, S., Castellano, S., Galvano, F., Bucolo, C., Drago, F., Caraci, F., & Malaga, G. (2014). Role of omega-3 fatty acids in the treatment of depressive disorders: A comprehensive meta-analysis of randomized clinical trials. *PLoS One, 9*(5), e96905. https://doi.org/10.1371/journal.pone.0096905.

Guesnet, P., & Alessandri, J. M. (2011). Docosahexaenoic acid (DHA) and the developing central nervous system (CNS) - Implications for dietary recommendations. *Biochimie, 93*(1), 7–12. Available from https://doi.org/10.1016/j.biochi.2010.05.005, www.elsevier.com/locate/biochimie.

Guillot, M., Robitaille, C.-A., Turner, L., Pronovost, E., Caouette, G., Matte-Gagné, C., Olivier, F., Bartholomew, J., Massé, É., Morin, A., Mohamed, I., & Marc, I. (2022). Effects of maternal docosahexaenoic acid supplementation on brain development and neurodevelopmental outcomes of breastfed preterm neonates: Protocol for a follow-up at preschool age of a randomised clinical trial (MOBYDIckPS). *BMJ Open, 12*(5), e057482. https://doi.org/10.1136/bmjopen-2021-057482.

Gutiérrez, S., Svahn, S. L., & Johansson, M. E. (2019). Effects of omega-3 fatty acids on immune cells. *International Journal of Molecular Sciences, 20*(20), Available from https://doi.org/10.3390/ijms20205028, https://www.mdpi.com/1422-0067/20/20/5028/pdf.

Gómez-Pinilla, F. (2008). Brain foods: The effects of nutrients on brain function. *Nature Reviews. Neuroscience, 9*(7), 568–578. https://doi.org/10.1038/nrn2421.

Hachem, M., Ahmmed, M. K., & Nacir-Delord, H. (2024). Phospholipidomics in clinical trials for brain disorders: Advancing our understanding and therapeutic potentials. *Molecular Neurobiology, 61*(6), 3272–3295. Available from https://doi.org/10.1007/s12035-023-03793-y, https://www.springer.com/journal/12035.

Hachem, M., Belkouch, M., Lo Van, A., Picq, M., Bernoud-Hubac, N., & Lagarde, M. (2020). Brain targeting with docosahexaenoic acid as a prospective therapy for neurodegenerative diseases and its passage across blood brain barrier. *Biochimie, 170*, 203–211. https://doi.org/10.1016/j.biochi.2020.01.013.

Hachem, M., Géloën, A., Van, A. L., Foumaux, B., Fenart, L., Gosselet, F., Da Silva, P., Breton, G., Lagarde, M., Picq, M., & Bernoud-Hubac, N. (2016). Efficient docosahexaenoic acid uptake by the brain from a structured phospholipid. *Molecular Neurobiology, 53*(5), 3205–3215. Available from https://doi.org/10.1007/s12035-015-9228-9, http://www.springer.com/biomed/neuroscience/journal/12035.

Hachem, M., Nacir, H., Picq, M., Belkouch, M., Bernoud-Hubac, N., Windust, A., Meiller, L., Sauvinet, V., Feugier, N., Lambert-Porcheron, S., Laville, M., & Lagarde, M. (2020). Docosahexaenoic acid (DHA) bioavailability in humans after oral intake of DHA-containing triacylglycerol or the structured phospholipid AceDoPC® *Nutrients, 12*(1), 251. https://doi.org/10.3390/nu12010251.

Hachem, M., & Nacir, H. (2022). Emerging role of phospholipids and lysophospholipids for improving brain docosahexaenoic acid as potential preventive and therapeutic strategies for neurological diseases. *International Journal of Molecular Sciences, 23*(7), 3969. https://doi.org/10.3390/ijms23073969.

Harris, W. S., Del Gobbo, L., & Tintle, N. L. (2017). The omega-3 index and relative risk for coronary heart disease mortality: Estimation from 10 cohort studies. *Atherosclerosis, 262*, 51–54. Available from https://doi.org/10.1016/j.atherosclerosis.2017.05.007, www.elsevier.com/locate/atherosclerosis.

Helland, I. B., Smith, L., Saarem, K., Saugstad, O. D., & Drevon, C. A. (2003). Maternal supplementation with very-long-chain n-3 fatty acids during pregnancy and lactation augments children's IQ at 4 years of age. *Pediatrics, 111*(1). https://doi.org/10.1542/peds.111.1.e39.

Hibbeln, J. R. (1998). Fish consumption and major depression [9]. *Lancet, 351*(9110), 1213. Available from https://doi.org/10.1016/S0140-6736(05)79168-6, http://www.journals.elsevier.com/the-lancet/.

Hibbeln, J. R., Nieminen, L. R. G., Blasbalg, T. L., Riggs, J. A., & Lands, W. E. M. (2006). Healthy intakes of n-3 and n-6 fatty acids: Estimations considering worldwide diversity. *American Journal of Clinical Nutrition, 83*(6). https://doi.org/10.1093/ajcn/83.6.1483s, http://www.ajcn.org/cgi/reprint/83/6/S1483.

Hussain, G., Anwar, H., Rasul, A., Imran, A., Qasim, M., Zafar, S., Imran, M., Kamran, S. K. S., Aziz, N., Razzaq, A., Ahmad, W., Shabbir, A., Iqbal, J., Baig, S. M., Ali, M., de Aguilar, J.-L. G., Sun, T., Muhammad, A., & Umair, A. M. (2020). Lipids as biomarkers of brain disorders. *Critical Reviews in Food Science and Nutrition, 60*(3), 351–374. https://doi.org/10.1080/10408398.2018.1529653.

Innis, S. M. (2007). Dietary (n-3) fatty acids and brain development. *The Journal of Nutrition, 137*(4), 855–859. https://doi.org/10.1093/jn/137.4.855.

Innis, S. M. (2014). Impact of maternal diet on human milk composition and neurological development of infants. *The American Journal of Clinical Nutrition, 99*(3), 734S. https://doi.org/10.3945/ajcn.113.072595.

Innis, S. M. (2008). Dietary omega 3 fatty acids and the developing brain. *Brain Research, 1237*, 35–43. https://doi.org/10.1016/j.brainres.2008.08.078.

Innis, S. M., & Friesen, R. W. (2008). Essential n-3 fatty acids in pregnant women and early visual acuity maturation in term infants. *American Journal of Clinical Nutrition, 87*(3), 548–557. Available from https://doi.org/10.1093/ajcn/87.3.548, http://www.ajcn.org/cgi/reprint/87/3/548.

Kelaiditis, C. F., Gibson, E. L., & Dyall, S. C. (2023). Effects of long-chain omega-3 polyunsaturated fatty acids on reducing anxiety and/or depression in adults; A systematic review and meta-analysis of randomised controlled trials. *Prostaglandins, Leukotrienes, and Essential Fatty Acids, 192*. Available from https://doi.org/10.1016/j.plefa.2023.102572, http://www.elsevier-international.com/journals/plef/.

Koletzko, B., Boey, C. C. M., Campoy, C., Carlson, S. E., Chang, N., Guillermo-Tuazon, M. A., Joshi, S., Prell, C., Quak, S. H., Sjarif, D. R., Su, Y., Supapannachart, S., Yamashiro, Y., & Osendarp, S. J. M. (2014). Current information and asian perspectives on long-chain polyunsaturated fatty acids in pregnancy, lactation, and infancy: Systematic review and practice recommendations from an early nutrition academy workshop. *Annals of Nutrition and Metabolism, 65*(1), 49–80. Available from https://doi.org/10.1159/000365767, www.karger.ch/journals/anm/anm_jh.htm.

Koletzko, B., Lien, E., Agostoni, C., Böhles, H., Campoy, C., Cetin, I., Decsi, T., Dudenhausen, J. W., Dupont, C., Forsyth, S., Hoesli, I., Holzgreve, W., Lapillonne, A., Putet, G., Secher, N. J., Symonds, M., Szajewska, H., Willatts, P., & Uauy, R. (2008). The roles of long-chain polyunsaturated fatty acids in pregnancy, lactation and infancy: Review of current knowledge and consensus recommendations. *Journal of Perinatal Medicine, 36*(1), 5–14. https://doi.org/10.1515/JPM.2008.001.

Koletzko, B., Reischl, E., Tanjung, C., Gonzalez-Casanova, I., Ramakrishnan, U., Meldrum, S., Simmer, K., Heinrich, J., & Demmelmair, H. (2019). FADS1 and FADS2 polymorphisms modulate fatty acid metabolism and dietary impact on health. *Annual Review of Nutrition, 39*(1), 21–44. https://doi.org/10.1146/annurev-nutr-082018-124250.

Korbecki, J., Rebacz-Maron, E., Kupnicka, P., Chlubek, D., & Baranowska-Bosiacka, I. (2023). Synthesis and Significance of Arachidonic Acid, a Substrate for Cyclooxygenases, Lipoxygenases, and Cytochrome P450 Pathways in the Tumorigenesis of Glioblastoma Multiforme, Including a Pan-Cancer Comparative Analysis. *Cancers (Basel), 15*(3). https://doi.org/10.3390/cancers15030946.

Lamon-Fava, S., Liu, M., Dunlop, B. W., Kinkead, B., Schettler, P. J., Felger, J. C., Ziegler, T. R., Fava, M., Mischoulon, D., & Rapaport, M. H. (2023). Clinical response to EPA supplementation in patients with major depressive disorder is associated with higher plasma concentrations of pro-resolving lipid mediators. *Neuropsychopharmacology: Official Publication of the American College of Neuropsychopharmacology, 48*(6), 929–935. Available from https://doi.org/10.1038/s41386-022-01527-7, https://www.nature.com/npp/.

Lauritzen, L., Brambilla, P., Mazzocchi, A., Harsløf, L. B. S., Ciappolino, V., & Agostoni, C. (2016). DHA effects in brain development and function. *Nutrients, 8*(1), Available from https://doi.org/10.3390/nu8010006, http://www.mdpi.com/2072-6643/8/1/6/pdf.

Liao, Y., Xie, B., Zhang, H., He, Q., Guo, L., Subramanieapillai, M., Fan, B., Lu, C., & McIntyre, R. S. (2019). Efficacy of omega-3 PUFAs in depression: A meta-analysis. *Translational Psychiatry, 9*(1). https://doi.org/10.1038/s41398-019-0515-5.

Lin, P. Y., Chiu, C. C., Huang, S. Y., & Su, K. P. (2012). A meta-analytic review of polyunsaturated fatty acid compositions in dementia. *Journal of Clinical Psychiatry, 73*(9), 1245–1254. Available from https://doi.org/10.4088/JCP.11r07546, http://www.psychiatrist.com/privatepdf/2012/v73n09/v73n0915.pdf.

Liu, J. H., Wang, Q., You, Q. L., Li, Z. L., Hu, N. Y., Wang, Y., Jin, Z. L., Li, S. J., Li, X. W., Yang, J. M., Zhu, X. H., Dai, Y. F., Xu, J. P., Bai, X. C., & Gao, T. M. (2020). Acute EPA-induced learning and memory impairment in mice is prevented by DHA. *Nature Communications, 11*(1), Available from https://doi.org/10.1038/s41467-020-19255-1, https://www.nature.com/ncomms/.

Liu, Y., Ren, X., Fan, C., Wu, W., Zhang, W., & Wang, Y. (2022). Health Benefits, Food Applications, and Sustainability of Microalgae-Derived N-3 PUFA. *Foods, 11*(13). https://doi.org/10.3390/foods11131883.

Loong, S., Barnes, S., Gatto, N. M., Chowdhury, S., & Lee, G. J. (2023). Omega-3 fatty acids, cognition, and brain volume in older adults. *Brain Sciences, 13*(9), Available from https://doi.org/10.3390/brainsci13091278, http://www.mdpi.com/journal/brainsci.

MacCarrone, M., Bernardi, G., Agrò, A. F., & Centonze, D. (2011). Cannabinoid receptor signalling in neurodegenerative diseases: A potential role for membrane fluidity disturbance. *British Journal of Pharmacology, 163*(7), 1379–1390. https://doi.org/10.1111/j.1476-5381.2011.01277.x.

Maltais, M., de Souto Barreto, P., Bowman, G. L., Smith, A. D., Cantet, C., Andrieu, S., & Rolland, Y. (2022). Omega-3 supplementation for the prevention of cognitive decline in older adults: Does it depend on homocysteine levels? *The Journal of nutrition, health and aging, 26*(6), 615–620. https://doi.org/10.1007/s12603-022-1809-5.

Martin, C. R., Ling, P. R., & Blackburn, G. L. (2016). Review of infant feeding: Key features of breast milk and infant formula. *Nutrients, 8*(5), Available from https://doi.org/10.3390/nu8050279, http://www.mdpi.com/2072-6643/8/5/279/pdf.

McDougle, D. R., Kambalyal, A., Meling, D. D., & Das, A. (2014). Endocannabinoids anandamide and 2-arachidonoylglycerol are substrates for human CYP2J2 epoxygenase. *Journal of Pharmacology and Experimental Therapeutics, 351*(3), 616–627. Available from https://doi.org/10.1124/jpet.114.216598, http://jpet.aspetjournals.org/content/351/3/616.full.pdf+html.

McNamara, R. K., & Carlson, S. E. (2006). Role of omega-3 fatty acids in brain development and function: Potential implications for the pathogenesis and prevention of psychopathology. *Prostaglandins, Leukotrienes, and Essential Fatty Acids, 75*(4-5), 329–349. https://doi.org/10.1016/j.plefa.2006.07.010.

Mengelberg, A., Leathem, J., Podd, J., Hill, S., & Conlon, C. (2022). The effects of docosahexaenoic acid supplementation on cognition and well-being in mild cognitive impairment: A 12-month randomised controlled trial. *International Journal of Geriatric Psychiatry, 37*(5). https://doi.org/10.1002/gps.5707.

Miller, A. H., & Raison, C. L. (2016). The role of inflammation in depression: From evolutionary imperative to modern treatment target. *Nature Reviews. Immunology, 16*(1), 22–34. Available from https://doi.org/10.1038/nri.2015.5, http://www.nature.com/nri/index.html.

Minihane, A. M., Vinoy, S., Russell, W. R., Baka, A., Roche, H. M., Tuohy, K. M., Teeling, J. L., Blaak, E. E., Fenech, M., Vauzour, D., McArdle, H. J., Kremer, B. H. A., Sterkman, L., Vafeiadou, K., Benedetti, M. M., Williams, C. M., & Calder, P. C. (2015). Low-grade inflammation, diet composition and health: Current research evidence and its translation. *British Journal of Nutrition, 114*(7), 999–1012. Available from https://doi.org/10.1017/S0007114515002093, http://journals.cambridge.org/BJN.

Mocking, R. J. T., Harmsen, I., Assies, J., Koeter, M. W. J., Ruhé, H. G., & Schene, A. H. (2016). Meta-analysis and meta-regression of omega-3 polyunsaturated fatty acid supplementation for major depressive disorder. *Translational Psychiatry, 6*(3), e756. https://doi.org/10.1038/tp.2016.29.

McNamara, R. K. (2016). Role of Omega-3 Fatty Acids in the Etiology, Treatment, and Prevention of Depression: Current Status and Future Directions. *Journal of Nutrition & Intermediary Metabolism, 5*, 96–106. https://doi.org/10.1016/j.jnim.2016.04.004.

Napier, J. A., Usher, S., Haslam, R. P., Ruiz-Lopez, N., & Sayanova, O. (2015). Transgenic plants as a sustainable, terrestrial source of fish oils. *European Journal of Lipid Science and Technology, 117*(9), 1317–1324. https://doi.org/10.1002/ejlt.201400452.

Ogundipe, E., Tusor, N., Wang, Y., Johnson, M. R., Edwards, A. D., & Crawford, M. A. (2018). Randomized controlled trial of brain specific fatty acid supplementation in pregnant women increases brain volumes on MRI scans of their newborn infants. *Prostaglandins, Leukotrienes, and Essential Fatty Acids, 138*, 6–13. https://doi.org/10.1016/j.plefa.2018.09.001.

Paquet, S. P., Pronovost, E., Simonyan, D., Caouette, G., Matte-Gagné, C., Olivier, F., Bartholomew, J., Morin, A., Mohamed, I., Marc, I., & Guillot, M. (2024). Maternal high-dose docosahexaenoic acid supplementation and neurodevelopment at 5 Years of preterm children. *Clinical Nutrition ESPEN, 64*, 253–262. Available from https://doi.org/10.1016/j.clnesp.2024.09.029, https://www.sciencedirect.com/science/journal/24054577.

Pottala, J. V., Yaffe, K., Robinson, J. G., Espeland, M. A., Wallace, R., & Harris, W. S. (2014). Higher RBC EPA + DHA corresponds with larger total brain and hippocampal volumes: WHIMS-MRI Study. *Neurology, 82*(5), 435–442. https://doi.org/10.1212/WNL.0000000000000080.

Qian, C., Wang, Q., Qiao, Y., Xu, Z., Zhang, L., Xiao, H., Lin, Z., Wu, M., Xia, W., Yang, H., Bai, J., & Geng, D. (2025). Arachidonic acid in aging: New roles for old players. *Journal of Advanced Research, 70*, 79–101. https://doi.org/10.1016/j.jare.2024.05.003.

Rapoport, S. I. (2008). Arachidonic acid and the brain. *Journal of Nutrition, 138*(12), 2515–2520. https://doi.org/10.1093/jn/138.12.2515, http://jn.nutrition.org/cgi/reprint/138/12/2515.

Rees, A., Sirois, S., & Wearden, A. (2014). Maternal docosahexaenoic acid intake levels during pregnancy and infant performance on a novel object search task at 22 months. *Child Development, 85*(6), 2131–2139. https://doi.org/10.1111/cdev.12280.

Richardson, A. J., & Montgomery, P. (2005). Oxford-Durham study: A randomized, controlled trial of dietary supplementation with fatty acids in children with developmental coordination disorder. *Pediatrics, 115*(5), 1360–1366. Available from https://doi.org/10.1542/peds.2004-2164, http://pediatrics.aappublications.org/cgi/reprint/115/5/1360.

Saito, Y., Kim, J. K., Davarian, S., Hagedorn, A., & Crimmins, E. M. (2020). Cognitive performance among older persons in Japan and the United States. *Journal of the American Geriatrics Society, 68*(2), 354–361. Available from https://doi.org/10.1111/jgs.16163, http://onlinelibrary.wiley.com/journal/10.1111/(ISSN)1532-5415.

Sala-Vila, A., Tintle, N., Westra, J., & Harris, W. S. (2023). Plasma omega-3 fatty acids and risk for incident dementia in the UK Biobank Study: A closer look. *Nutrients, 15*(23), Available from https://doi.org/10.3390/nu15234896, http://www.mdpi.com/journal/nutrients/.

SanGiovanni, J. P., & Chew, E. Y. (2005). The role of omega-3 long-chain polyunsaturated fatty acids in health and disease of the retina. *Progress in Retinal and Eye Research, 24*(1), 87–138. https://doi.org/10.1016/j.preteyeres.2004.06.002.

von Schacky, C. (2021). Importance of EPA and DHA blood levels in brain structure and function. *Nutrients, 13*(4), 1074. https://doi.org/10.3390/nu13041074.

Simopoulos, A. P. (2016). An increase in the omega-6/omega-3 fatty acid ratio increases the risk for obesity. *Nutrients, 8*(3), Available from https://doi.org/10.3390/nu8030128, http://www.mdpi.com/2072-6643/8/3/128/pdf.

Simopoulos, A. P. (2002). The importance of the ratio of omega-6/omega-3 essential fatty acids. *Biomedicine & Pharmacotherapy, 56*(8), 365–379. https://doi.org/10.1016/s0753-3322(02)00253-6.

Sinn, N., Milte, C. M., Street, S. J., Buckley, J. D., Coates, A. M., Petkov, J., & Howe, P. R. C. (2012). Effects of n-3 fatty acids, EPA v. DHA, on depressive symptoms, quality of life, memory and executive function in older adults with mild cognitive impairment: A 6-month randomised controlled trial. *British Journal of Nutrition, 107*(11), 1682–1693. Available from https://doi.org/10.1017/S0007114511004788, http://journals.cambridge.org/BJN.

Stark, K. D., Van Elswyk, M. E., Higgins, M. R., Weatherford, C. A., & Salem, N., Jr. (2016). Global survey of the omega-3 fatty acids, docosahexaenoic acid and eicosapentaenoic acid in the blood stream of healthy adults. *Progress in Lipid Research, 63*, 132–152. https://doi.org/10.1016/j.plipres.2016.05.001.

Sublette, M. E., Ellis, S. P., Geant, A. L., & Mann, J. J. (2011). Meta-analysis of the effects of eicosapentaenoic acid (EPA) in clinical trials in depression. *Journal of Clinical Psychiatry, 72*(12), 1577–1584. Available from https://doi.org/10.4088/JCP.10m06634, http://www.psychiatrist.com/privatepdf/2011/v72n12/v72n1202.pdf.

Su, K. P., Matsuoka, Y., & Pae, C. U. (2015). Omega-3 polyunsaturated fatty acids in prevention of mood and anxiety disorders. *Clinical Psychopharmacology and Neuroscience, 13*(2), 129–137. Available from https://doi.org/10.9758/cpn.2015.13.2.129, http://www.cpn.or.kr/journal/download_pdf.php?doi=10.9758/cpn.2015.13.2.129.

Swanson, D., Block, R., & Mousa, S. A. (2012). Omega-3 fatty acids EPA and DHA: Health benefits throughout life. *Advances in Nutrition, 3*(1), 1–7. Available from https://doi.org/10.3945/an.111.000893, http://advances.nutrition.org/content/3/1/1.full.pdf.

Talamonti, E., Sasso, V., To, H., Haslam, R. P., Napier, J. A., Ulfhake, B., Pernold, K., Asadi, A., Hessa, T., Jacobsson, A., Chiurchiù, V., & Viscomi, M. T. (2020). Impairment of DHA synthesis alters the expression of neuronal plasticity markers and the brain inflammatory status in mice. *FASEB Journal, 34*(2), 2024–2040. Available from https://doi.org/10.1096/fj.201901890RR, https://onlinelibrary.wiley.com/journal/15306860.

Tanaka, K., Farooqui, A. A., Siddiqi, N. J., Alhomida, A. S., & Ong, W. Y. (2012). Effects of docosahexaenoic acid on neurotransmission. *Biomolecules and Therapeutics, 20*(2), 152–157. Available from https://doi.org/10.4062/biomolther.2012.20.2.152Singapore, http://pdf.medrang.co.kr/BT/2012/020/BT020-02-03.pdf.

Tian, A., Xu, L., Szeto, I. M.-Y., Wang, X., & Li, D. (2025). Effects of different proportions of DHA and ARA on cognitive development in infants: A meta-analysis. *Nutrients, 17*(6), 1091. https://doi.org/10.3390/nu17061091.

Tremblay, M., Baydala, L., Khan, M., Currie, C., Morley, K., Burkholder, C., Davidson, R., & Stillar, A. (2020). Primary substance use prevention programs for children and youth: A systematic review. *Pediatrics, 146*(3). https://doi.org/10.1542/peds.2019-2747.

Valenzuela Baez, R., & Valenzuela, A. (2011). Docosahexaenoic Acid (DHA), in the Prevention and Treatment of Neurodegenerative Diseases. In R. C.-C. Chang (Ed.). *Neurodegenerative Diseases - Processes, Prevention, Protection and Monitoring*. London: IntechOpen.

Vines, A., Delattre, A. M., Lima, M. M. S., Rodrigues, L. S., Suchecki, D., MacHado, R. B., Tufik, S., Pereira, S. I. R., Zanata, S. M., & Ferraz, A. C. (2012). The role of 5-HT 1A receptors in fish oil-mediated increased BDNF expression in the rat hippocampus and cortex: A possible antidepressant mechanism. *Neuropharmacology, 62*(1), 184–191. https://doi.org/10.1016/j.neuropharm.2011.06.017.

Wang, Q., Liang, X., Wang, L., Lu, X., Huang, J., Cao, J., Li, H., & Gu, D. (2012). Effect of omega-3 fatty acids supplementation on endothelial function: A meta-analysis of randomized controlled trials. *Atherosclerosis, 221*(2), 536–543. https://doi.org/10.1016/j.atherosclerosis.2012.01.006.

Wang, B., Wu, L., Chen, J., Dong, L., Chen, C., Wen, Z., Hu, J., Fleming, I., & Wang, D. W. (2021). Metabolism pathways of arachidonic acids: Mechanisms and potential therapeutic targets. *Signal Transduction and Targeted Therapy, 6*(1), Available from https://doi.org/10.1038/s41392-020-00443-w, www.nature.com/sigtrans.

Weder, S., Müller, S., Dawczynski, C., & Keller, M. (2025). Arachidonic acid as a potentially critical nutrient for vegetarians and vegans – Position paper of the Research Institute for Plant-based Nutrition (IFPE). *Lipids in Health and Disease, 24*(1), Available from https://doi.org/10.1186/s12944-025-02645-z, https://lipidworld.biomedcentral.com/.

Wei, B. Z., Li, L., Dong, C. W., Tan, C. C., & Xu, W. (2023). The relationship of omega-3 fatty acids with dementia and cognitive decline: Evidence from prospective cohort studies of supplementation, dietary intake, and blood markers. *American Journal of Clinical Nutrition, 117*(6), 1096–1109. Available from https://doi.org/10.1016/j.ajcnut.2023.04.001, https://www.sciencedirect.com/journal/the-american-journal-of-clinical-nutrition/about/aims-and-scope.

Wei, Y., Meng, Y., Li, N., Wang, Q., & Chen, L. (2021). The effects of low-ratio n-6/n-3 PUFA on biomarkers of inflammation: A systematic review and meta-analysis. *Food & Function, 12*(1), 30–40. https://doi.org/10.1039/d0fo01976c.

Williams, J. H., Errington, M. L., Lynch, M. A., & Bliss, T. V. (1989). Arachidonic acid induces a long-term activity-dependent enhancement of synaptic transmission in the hippocampus. *Nature, 341*(6244), 739–742. https://doi.org/10.1038/341739a0.

Yehuda, S., Rabinovitz, S., Carasso, R. L., & Mostofsky, D. I. (2002). The role of polyunsaturated fatty acids in restoring the aging neuronal membrane. *Neurobiology of Aging, 23*(5), 843–853. https://doi.org/10.1016/S0197-4580(02)00074-X.

Yehuda, S., Rabinovitz, S., & Mostofsky, D. I. (2005). Essential fatty acids and the brain: From infancy to aging. *Neurobiology of Aging, 26*(1), 98–102. https://doi.org/10.1016/j.neurobiolaging.2005.09.013.

Yui, K., Imataka, G., Nakamura, H., Ohara, N., & Naito, Y. (2015). Eicosanoids derived from arachidonic acid and their family prostaglandins and cyclooxygenase in psychiatric disorders. *Current Neuropharmacology, 13*(6), 776–785. https://doi.org/10.2174/1570159X13666151102103305.

Yurko-Mauro, K., McCarthy, D., Rom, D., Nelson, E. B., Ryan, A. S., Blackwell, A., ... Investigators, M. (2010). Beneficial effects of docosahexaenoic acid on cognition in age-related cognitive decline. *Alzheimer's & Dementia: The Journal of the Alzheimer's Association, 6*(6), 456–464. https://doi.org/10.1016/j.jalz.2010.01.013.

Zhang, W., Chen, R., Yang, T., Xu, N., Chen, J., Gao, Y., & Stetler, R. A. (2018). Fatty acid transporting proteins: Roles in brain development, aging, and stroke. *Prostaglandins, Leukotrienes, and Essential Fatty Acids, 136*, 35–45. Available from https://doi.org/10.1016/j.plefa.2017.04.004, http://www.elsevier-international.com/journals/plef/.

Zhang, Y., Liu, Y., Sun, J., Zhang, W., Guo, Z., & Ma, Q. (2023). Arachidonic acid metabolism in health and disease. *MedComm, 4*(5). https://doi.org/10.1002/mco2.363.

Chapter 15

Global perspectives on docosahexaenoic acid and eicosapentaenoic acid consumption patterns and food industry applications

Kalaiselvi Krishnamoorthy[1], Monisha Prasad[2], and Muthu Thiruvengadam[3]

[1]*Centre for Herbal Pharmacology and Environmental Sustainability, Chettinad Hospital and Research Institute, Chettinad Academy of Research and Education, Chennai, Tamil Nadu, India,* [2]*Molecular Nutrition and Genomics Laboratory, Department of Community Medicine, Saveetha Medical College and Hospital, Saveetha Institute of Medical and Technical Sciences, Saveetha University, Chennai, Tamil Nadu, India,* [3]*Department Crop Science, College of Sanghuh Life Science, Konkuk University, Seoul, Republic of Korea*

15.1 Introduction

Docosahexaenoic acid (DHA) and eicosapentaenoic acid (EPA) are the omega-3 long-chain polyunsaturated fatty acids (n-3 LC-PUFA). Both fatty acids have enormous health benefits, like brain development, eye vision management, cardiovascular disorders (CVD), inflammatory activities, immune system development, and healthy aging mechanisms (Swanson et al., 2012). They support cardiovascular health by reducing plasma triglycerides, improving endothelial function, and lowering the risk of arrhythmias and atherosclerosis. DHA and EPA could be considered as "global nutrition molecules" due to their irreplaceable role in human health and metabolism. Apart from that, in the food technology field, to produce functional foods enriched with fatty acids, DHA and EPA are mainly used. Conventionally, marine sources such as oily fish are predominantly used for DHA and EPA sources, but due to the global demand as well as consumers' food intake options, alternative sources of plant-based polyunsaturated fatty acids (PUFA) are needed in this current decade, which leads to algal oils, krill oils, and microbial fermentation-derived omega-3 productions (Saini et al., 2021; Yeung et al., 2025). These are the alternative sources with nutrition enrichment,this food innovations fulfill the gap between nutritional requirements and ecological responsibility (Martins et al., 2013; Santos et al., 2020; Sprague et al., 2017). Both DHA and EPA are progressively incorporated into the functional foods, infant food products, beverages, and dietary supplements to improve the nutritional enrichment. These incorporations of PUFA into the food industry led to diverse developments in food technology (Derbyshire et al., 2024; Ganesan et al., 2014; Hollander et al., 2019). At the same time, fatty acid combinations are also facing some challenges, like oxidative stability, sensory attributes, and bioavailability, as well as being cost-effective. On the other hand, microencapsulation, nanoemulsion, and liposomal delivery systems have emerged to enhance the stability, solubility, and controlled release of DHA and EPA in fortified products, which helps to overcome the challenges of PUFA as a food product (Tocher et al., 2019).

In the past two decades, global omega consumption has increased due to consumers' awareness of health consciousness (Blasbalg et al., 2011; Nguyen et al., 2019). The Food and Drug Administration (FDA), European Food Safety Authority (EFSA), and Food Safety and Standards Authority of India (FSSAI) are the most important food safety and regulatory authorities. They are raising awareness among consumers of the importance of omega-3 fatty acids and their health benefits. Because these regulatory agencies have validated some health claims and included omega-3 consumption into dietary recommendations, manufacturers are being encouraged to create nutraceutical formulations and fortify basic foods (Banović Fuentes et al., 2024; Gupta et al., 2021). The current chapter covers the overview of the PUFA and their sources, health benefits, specifically DHA and EPA; moreover, the technological innovations involved in the food product manufacturing are explained in detail.

Omega-3 and Omega-6 Polyunsaturated Fatty Acids in Food Systems. DOI: https://doi.org/10.1016/B978-0-443-43810-3.00015-4

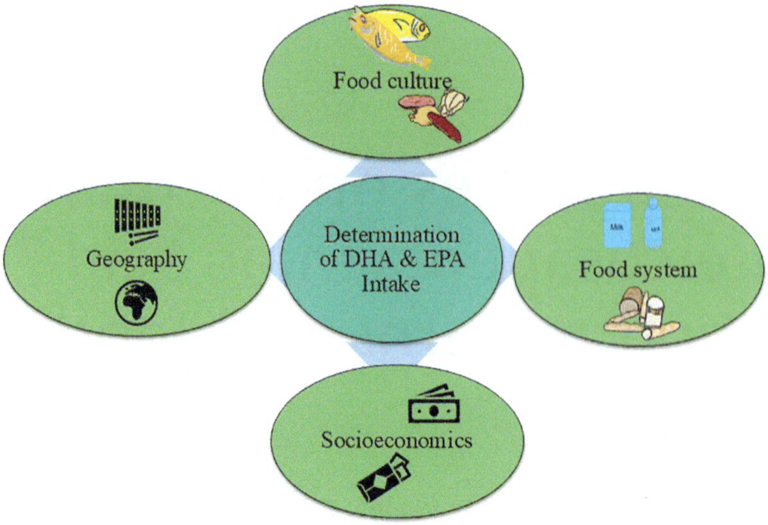

FIGURE 15.1 **Key factors influencing docosahexaenoic acid (DHA) and eicosapentaenoic acid (EPA) consumption.**

15.2 Global consumption patterns of omega

The daily consumption of EPA and DHA, in combination, within the range of 250-500 mg, will protect against CVD and maintain overall human health in adults (Troesch et al., 2020). During pregnancy and lactation, mothers are recommended to consume 100-300 mg of DHA and EPA per day to ensure transmission of the nutrients to the fetus and the infant. However, most of the world's populations unable to accomplish the recommended range of nutrition (Amza et al., 2024; Nguyen et al., 2019). . Countries like Japan, Norway, and Iceland, with potential seafood sources, will naturally get omega-3-rich foods. Likewise, Western countries, Germany, and the United States are considered moderate omega-3-intake countries. South Asian regions are insufficient to achieve the omega-3 intake due to region-based and culture-based food preferences like vegetarianism (Pateiro et al., 2021; Torrissen et al., 2025). Based on this limited omega-rich food consumption, health conditions also affected the lowest and moderate regions, specifically CVD, growth, and development issues. At the same time, sufficient consumption of omega-3 fatty acids in populations leads to a healthy life style and reduced risk of diseases (Rhee et al., 2017; Saini et al., 2021). The consumption of DHA and EPA is interconnected, which can be determined by some factors like geography, food culture, socioeconomics, and food systems (Fig. 15.1). Food consumption patterns differ across regions, for example coastal populations tend to consume fish more frequently, while people in noncoastal or urban areas often have limited access to daily fish consumption (Andrews et al., 2021). Food culture is mainly dominated by traditional behaviors like vegetarianism, non-vegetarian food consumption, for example, seafood is commonly available in Japan and Mediterranean regions, which naturally supports higher omega-3 intake, while vegetarian and cereal-based diet habits are general in South Asia and Africa, where nutrition is insufficient and common in these regions (Byrne et al., 2024; Marrone et al., 2021). Socioeconomic status is another factor, as expenses and procuring authority influence whether people have consumed the fish, nutrition-enhanced supplements, and fortified foods. Nutritional supplements are regularly used by wealthier populations, while lower-income populations often lack access to these types of foods; due to this absence, they are at high risk of chronic disorders. At last, the food system plays an insignificant role here, from food sources to industrial-based products that are developed, such as fish oil capsules and fortified foods (Hergenrader et al., 2022). Consuming DHA and EPA together is essential for bridging the current nutritional gap and is an essential initial step toward resolving this nutritional deficiency in the future.

15.3 Food industry applications of docosahexaenoic acid and eicosapentaenoic acid/ traditional sources of docosahexaenoic acid and eicosapentaenoic acid

Over the past 20 years, consumer acceptance and demand for omega-3 fatty acids have increased, which will influence the food industry. Traditionally, omega-3-rich food sources are marine-based foods and plant-based foods, and both types of oils are used for various processes like food manufacturing, medical purposes, cosmetic product development, etc. Their major sources and their benefits are explained in this section (Fig. 15.2).

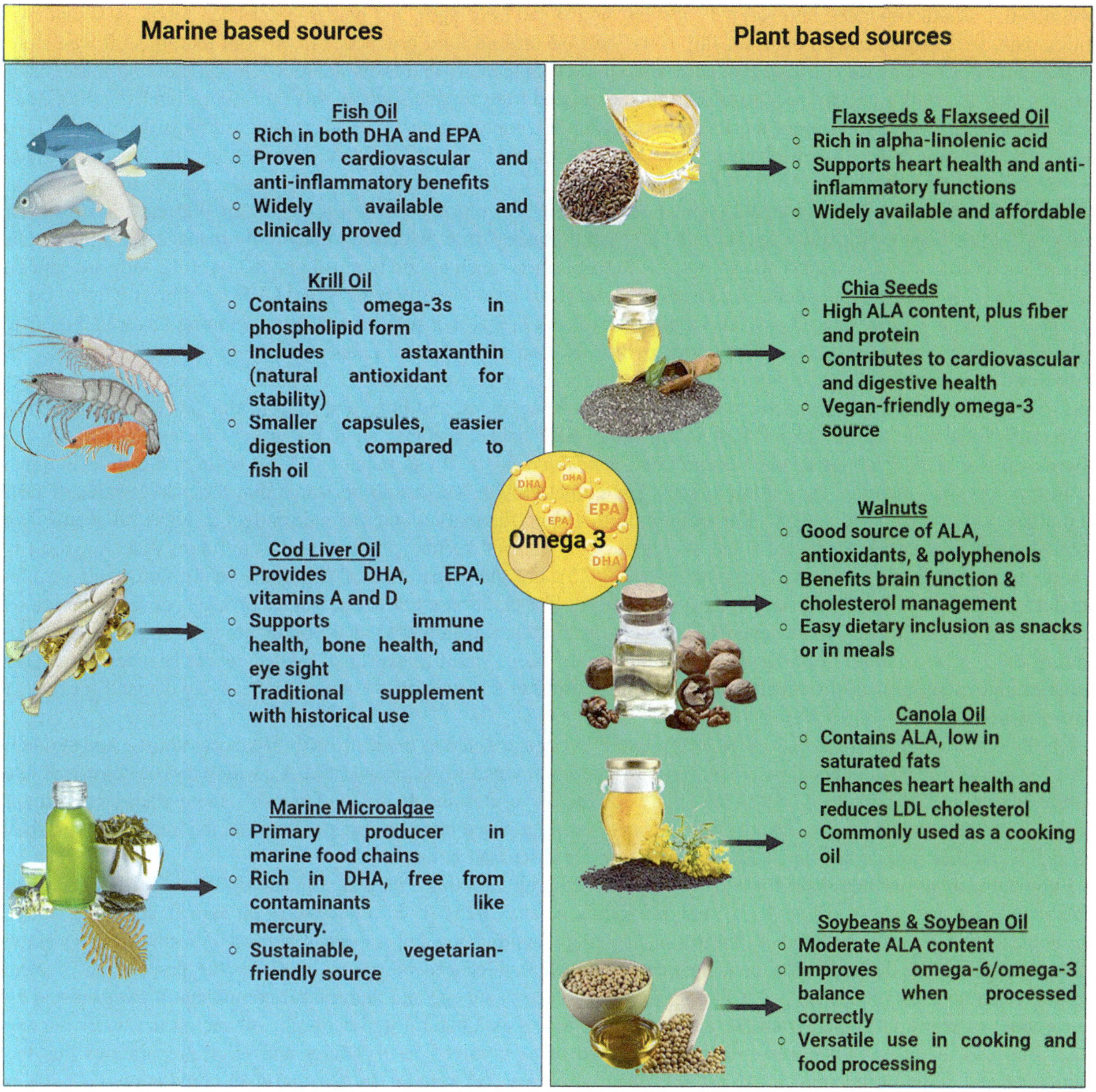

FIGURE 15.2 **Marine-based and plant-based docosahexaenoic acid (DHA) and eicosapentaenoic acid (EPA)-rich sources and their benefits.**

Marine-based food products are naturally rich in omega-3 fatty acid sources; regular consumption is associated with the prevention of numerous disorders like CVD, brain development, and general growth and metabolism (Wei et al., 2025). Fish oil is commonly known for its affordability and availability, as oily and fat-rich fish are regularly used for fish oil production. Fishes like salmon, tuna, shellfish, and krill are used for the oil preparations due to their rich bioactive components. From the perspective of the food industry manufacturers, these sources are used as fish oil, nutraceutical supplements, dairy products, beverages, and infant foods. However, controlled fishing is necessary to preserve a balanced biological ecosystem (Ashraf et al., 2020; Senadheera et al., 2023). Krill (*Euphausia superba*) are very small in size and are called marine crustaceans. It is more expensive compared to fish oil and rich in vitamins A and E, phospholipids, astaxanthin, and flavonoids (Barros et al., 2014; Xie et al., 2019). The DHA content of krill oil is similar to that of fish, but the EPA content is high in level. In 2008, krill oil was authorized by the United States FDA, and later it was officially authorized by the EFSA for use by pregnant and lactating women in 2014 (Colletti et al., 2021). Functional food preparations, fortified product manufacturers, and dietary supplement preparations, such as krill oil, are widely used.

Specifically, it is incorporated into soft gel capsules, nutritional beverages, and omega-3-enriched foods. Astaxanthin, an antioxidant, will help to extend the shelf life of the krill oil-infused food products. Apart from that, this oil was used to prepare infant foods, maternity food products, and sports supplements due to its neurodevelopmental anti-inflammatory activity. Cod liver oil is another important oil source extracted from marine sources, this oil is extracted from the *Gadidae* family of fish in the form of liquid fat. It has anticancer, hepatoprotective, antioxidant, and antifibrosis activities (Dyck et al., 2011; Hünkar et al., 2002; Mohamed et al., 2015; Zachwieja et al., 2025). In the 19th century, this oil was consumed to cure rheumatoid arthritis (Brodziak-Dopierała et al., 2023). Cod liver oil is extracted from the codfish liver, it is rich in vitamins like A, E, and D and omega-3 content, and it's mostly consumed as a supplement in Western diets on a daily basis. Also, this oil is considered a nonsteroidal anti-inflammatory drug, which can potentially manage anti-inflammatory conditions. Fortified food products and nutraceutical preparations such as cod liver oil play a vital role; they are generally incorporated into dietary supplements in capsule form, which is used for osteoporosis and CVD conditions (Global Burden of Cardiovascular Diseases and Risks 2023 Collaborators et al., 2025). Apart from due to its strong flavor and oxidative sensitivity behavior, this oil is used for the microencapsulation methods and mixed with the food products directly, like milk powders, infant foods, health drinks, and fortified food preparations (Jafari et al., 2025). In sports supplements, this cod liver oil is used for muscle recovery, inflammation management, and bone and joint health (Hansen et al., 2021).

Another important marine source rich in omega-3 fatty acids is algae; algal oil was extracted specifically from microalgae varieties *Schizochytrium*, *Ulkenia*, and *Nannochloropsis*. It can maintain CVD, brain and eye development, boost memory, and maintain the gut microbiota. The global growth insights report stated that the market value of DHA-rich algae oil was estimated at USD 840 million in 2024. Yet, the market commercial product of algae oil is still facing some drawbacks, like quick oxidation and stratification in the food sector's production. In the future years, algal oil will emerge as a cutting-edge research area (Tang et al., 2025). For the preparation of functional foods, nutraceuticals, these algal-based oils are utilized, precisely in dairy alternatives like plant-based milk and yogurt products development this oil was used. Compared to fish oil, its neutral sensory character makes it simpler to incorporate into food preparations without adding any food seasonings or preservatives to improve the taste. Significantly, algal oil decreases dependence on marine fisheries and encourages environmental preservation by offering a sustainable response to the rising demand for omega-3 fatty acids.

On the other hand, plant-based sources are generally recognized due to their affordability, accessibility, and suitability for vegetarian and vegan populations. Plant sources are rich in alpha-linolenic acid (ALA), which can be converted into a partial amount of DHA and EPA, which are vitally utilized by vegetarians. In the food industry, these plant-based products are incorporated into beverages, bakery products, dairy product-based alternatives, etc. Some of the important plant-based oil types and their importance in PUFA incorporation are discussed below.

Flaxseed (*Linum usitatissimum* L.) is one of the oilseed crop varieties with a significant amount of PUFA and dietary fibers and rich in vitamins like A, B, and E (Nemli et al., 2025). It has numerous biological activities, such as cardioprotective, anticancer, blood cholesterol management, antidiabetic, hepatoprotective, and anti-inflammatory activity (Duarte et al., 2025; Kajla et al., 2015; Stepień et al., 2025). Flaxseed powder is used for the preparation of bakery products like muffins, bread, and pasta. Flaxseed mucilage acts as an egg and fat replacer component for vegans and low-fat product preparations. Apart from these components, it acts as a natural hydrocolloid, enhancing the water retention, shelf life, and texture of the bakery products. Flaxseed oil is involved in beverages and salad preparations due to its emulsifier and gelling properties; it can act as a plant-based meat alternative. In dairy product preparations, it serve as a texture improver and nutritional value enhancer. Encapsulated flaxseed oil is increasingly incorporated into nutraceuticals, dietary supplements, and infant formulas to deliver stable omega-3 fatty acids (Mohammadkhani et al., 2025). Chia seeds (*Salvia hispanica* L.) belong to the *Lamiaceae* family; they contain rich protein sources, ALA, oleic and linoleic acids, and minerals like potassium, magnesium, and phosphorus. In addition, antioxidants like tocopherols, carotenoids, and phytosterols (Khalid et al., 2022). These substances play a vital role in managing disorders like stroke, depression, Alzheimer's, CVD, antiinflammatories, antidiabetics, and anticancer activity. Compared to the other types of PUFA oils, chia seed oil contains a significant level of α-linolenic acids (Ullah et al., 2016). To improve the nutritional values, shelf life, and texture, chia seeds were progressively used in the food industry, specifically chia seed mucilage can form a gel-like substance when hydrated, this property enables them to act as a natural thickening agent, stabilizer and emulsifier in beverages, dairy products, and sauces. Moreover, chia seed oil is involved in the encapsulations and nutraceutical supplements (Sacco et al., 2021). Chia mucilage used as an egg replacer in gluten-free product preparations can improve the moisture retention and texture. This oil is usually incorporated with bread, cereals, biscuits, and pasta products to improve the fiber content and omega-3 levels (Coronel et al., 2025).

Walnut oil, extracted from the kernels of *Juglans regia*, is another prominent oil type extracted from plant-based sources. This oil contains rich fat content, lipids, proteins, dietary fibers, and carbohydrates (Lopez et al., 2023). Apart from that, walnuts have oleic, linolenic acids, tocopherols, squalene, phytosterols, and polyphenols, which help maintain human health, specifically CVD, blood cholesterol maintenance, obesity conditions, diabetes, metabolic syndrome, and brain functions, and industrial food manufacturing purposes (Hayes et al., 2016). In the food industry, walnut oil is used for functional food productions, health supplements, and nutraceutical preparations (Jahanban-Esfahlan et al., 2019; Liu et al., 2023; Song et al., 2022). Walnut oil is a valuable dietary lipid source and multipurpose ingredient with broad implications for both industrial food manufacturing and health promotion due to its excellent oxidative stability and desirable nutty flavor profile, which makes it suitable for baked products (Li et al., 2023).

Another omega-rich plant source of oil is canola (*Brassica napus*), which belongs to the Brassica family (Petrie et al., 2020). Vegetable-based oils, specifically canola and soy, are effectively being used to substitute for fish oil. Through the mechanical pressing and solvent extraction process, this oil was produced (Ruyter et al., 2019). This oil is rich in vitamins E and K, it has potent anti-inflammatory activities, and it has a light texture and effective flavor. Due to this activity, this oil is mainly used by food product manufacturers (Lin et al., 2022). Similarly, soybean (*Glycine max*) oils have also get more attention in the last few decades, particularly after 1970; they were used as an alternative for animal-based oil products (Blasbalg et al., 2011). This oil is rich in PUFA content, particularly linoleic acid, and vitamin E. Apart from that, soy oil has antioxidant and anti inflammatory potentials (Lemke et al., 2010). For food product manufacturing, processed food preparations, frying, and baking, this soybean oil was used. Regular intake of PUFA-rich soybean oil has been linked to improved endothelial function, lower levels of low-density lipoprotein (LDL) cholesterol, and metabolic health (Harris et al., 2008; Lichtenstein et al., 2006; Messina et al., 2021). The functional qualities, nutritional worth, and technical adaptability of soybean oil ensure its sustained dominance in world food systems. Its contribution to the creation of healthier food items by substituting PUFAs for saturated animal fats has also helped to meet customer expectations for sustainable and heart-healthy dietary alternatives.

15.4 Health and nutritional implications of docosahexaenoic acid and eicosapentaenoic acid

PUFAs such as DHA and EPA are vital for maintaining human health and preventing chronic diseases. Fish oils, algae oils, and fortified foods are the main sources of the PUFAs, specifically, they're famous for their rich nutritional benefits for the heart, brain, eye, and metabolic processes (Fig. 15.3). Over the last few decades, global health professionals have emphasized the importance of DHA and EPA as functional macromolecules that connect nutrition and disease prevention.

15.4.1 Bone and joint health

PUFAs are rich in vital nutrients that improve bone health by controlling the complicated process of bone remodeling. The balanced activity of osteoblasts, which produce new bone cells, and osteoclasts, which cause bone resorption, controls remodeling. PUFAs, especially omega-3 fatty acids, inhibit osteoclastogenesis and inflammatory mediators that cause bone deterioration while promoting osteoblast development and mineralization. These processes allow PUFAs to improve bone density, lower the incidence of osteoporosis and other metabolic bone diseases, and maintain the structural integrity of bone tissue (Kruger et al., 2010; Rozner et al., 2020). A combination of PUFA-enriched foods, calcium, and vitamin D intakes can maintain good bone metabolism and reduce the risk of bone-related disorders, conditions such as osteoporosis and rheumatoid arthritis (Abshirini et al., 2021; Little et al., 2005). It is the most common condition of bone joint disease and a leading cause of disability in older adults. The function of omega-3 fatty acids in preserving bone health is being supported by numerous studies (Kajarabille et al., 2013; Watkins et al., 2000). Through their effects on osteoblast and osteoclast activity, EPA and DHA regulate bone metabolism. They inhibit pro-inflammatory cytokines such as TNF-α, IL-1, and IL-6 that are known to promote bone resorption (Rahman et al., 2009). According to clinical research, consuming enough omega-3 fatty acids improves bone mineral density and lowers the incidence of osteoporosis, especially in women who have gone through menopause (Dou et al., 2021). Furthermore, DHA and EPA provide a natural supplement to traditional treatment by enhancing joint lubrication and reducing cartilage breakdown in people with osteoarthritis conditions (Shawl et al., 2024).

15.4.2 Neuroprotection in aging

DHA and EPA are vital for maintaining the brain structure and function. Parkinson's disease (PD) and Alzheimer's disease (AD) are the most common complicated conditions (Dyall, 2015). Increased consumption of PUFAs, specifically fish and other seafood, has been linked to improved cognitive function and a decreased risk of dementia (Wen et al., 2024). On the other hand, minimal or non-PUFA-rich food consumption is associated with the increased risk of aging-associated

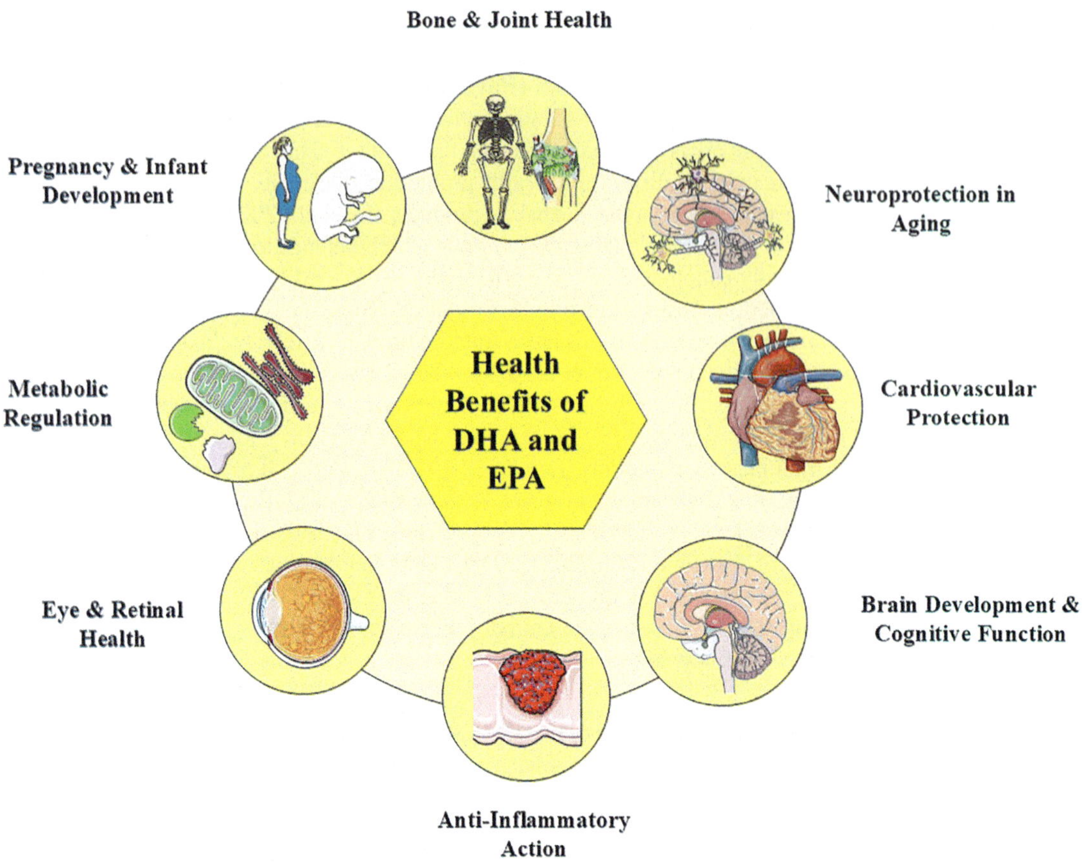

FIGURE 15.3 **Illustration of the health benefits of docosahexaenoic acid (DHA) and eicosapentaenoic acid (EPA).**

cognitive issues, low brain functions, and neurodegenerative disorders due to PD and AD conditions. Specifically, both DHA and EPA act as neuroprotective compounds; these sources can maintain the neurons from apoptosis (Bazan et al., 2011; Fekete et al., 2022). Overall, the proper consumption of the omega-rich products can protect the brain from aging and maintain proper motor abilities.

15.4.3 Cardiovascular (CVD) protection

CVD is one of the leading causes of death worldwide. It is related to the high serum level of triglycerides. Consumption of the regular PUFA-containing foods could reduce the blood level of LDL-cholesterol and triglycerides (TG), which leads to a reduction in CVD conditions. Specifically, a consumption of EPA can improve the cardiovascular system, such as reduced lipid action, plaque stabilization, antiproliferation, vasodilation, and reduction in platelet aggregation, lower TG levels, and improved endothelial function. Apart from that, this EPA has antioxidant and anti-inflammatory activities that improve the endothelial functions. And many research studies stated that the regular food habits of PUFA consumption can manage the CVD condition and its associated complications (Golanski et al., 2021; Oppedisano et al., 2020; Palabiyik & Palabiyik, 2025; Sherratt et al., 2023).

15.4.4 Brain development and cognitive function

Omega-3 fatty acid status is closely linked to mental health, specifically dopaminergic signaling, serotonin receptor activity, and neuronal membrane fluidity, which are all impacted by DHA and EPA. DHA is an essential structural component of neuronal membranes that plays important functions in neurotransmission. It also promotes the development of the visual centers, hippocampus, and cerebral cortex throughout pregnancy and after delivery (Basak et al., 2020; Chalon et al., 2001; Ciappolino et al., 2019). In adults, DHA helps to preserve cognitive performance, and combining DHA and EPA consumption is linked to improved memory retention, learning capacity, and decreased cognitive decline (Lauritzen et al., 2016; Mora et al., 2022; Song et al., 2016). Consuming omega-3-rich foods daily, such as walnuts, flaxseed, fish oil, and marine algae, can improve mental health, reduce depressive symptoms, and boost brain function. Clinical and epidemiological research has demonstrated that communities with a higher omega-3 fish diet had lower rates of dementia and AD, suggesting that these fatty acids have substantial neuroprotective properties (Fotuhi et al., 2009; Ross et al., 2007; Yonezawa et al., 2020).

15.4.5 Anti-inflammatory action

Inflammation is part of the immediate response to infection or injury and is characterized by redness, swelling, heat, and pain (Medzhitov, 2008). These occur because of increased blood flow, increased permeability across blood capillaries, which allows large molecules like antibodies and cytokines to leave the bloodstream and cross the endothelial wall, and increased movement of leukocytes from the bloodstream into the surrounding tissue (Camuesco et al., 2006). Inflammation functions to begin the immunological process, whereas an acute inflammation condition is essential for the healing process; chronic inflammation is involved in various metabolic disorders, such as neurodegenerative conditions, CVD, diabetes, and arthritis. PUFAs are enriched with strong anti-inflammatory activity due to their immune-modulating activity and involvement in molecular signaling regulations (Bodur et al., 2025). Additionally, DHA and EPA prevent oxidative stress and immunological activation by reducing the expression of inflammatory genes controlled by nuclear factor-kappa B. PUFAs promote general physiological homeostasis, protect against chronic inflammation, and preserve immunological stability through these interconnected mechanisms (So et al., 2021; Talero et al., 2015).

15.4.6 Eye and retinal health

The human retina is one of the most metabolically active and lipid-rich organs, depending primarily on PUFAs for eye health, optimum function, and structural integrity. DHA acts as a key structural lipid and is responsible for the light-to-neural signaling transformations; moreover, it protects the retinal cells from oxidative stress. Apart from during the fetal and postpartum period, this DHA is necessary for the maturation of the retina and visual cortex. EPA acts as an inflammation suppressor and supports proper vascular function within the eye (Georgakopoulos et al., 2017; Lafuente et al., 2021; Wang & Ko, 2023). EPA and DHA work together to prevent eye conditions such as age-related macular degeneration, diabetic retinopathy, and dry eye syndrome by increasing tear film stability, enhancing retinal protection, and maintaining overall vision health throughout life (Bettadahalli et al., 2020; Zeppieri et al., 2024).

15.4.7 Metabolic regulation

Metabolic regulations are needed for various mechanisms of functions in the human body, such as maintaining energy, glucose intake, and lipid metabolism via several organs like the liver, pancreas, adipose tissue, and skeletal muscles (Benatti et al., 2004; Risé et al., 2002). The involvement of nutrients plays a vital role in metabolism for PUFAs, specifically DHA and EPA, which have effective bioactive compounds that influence metabolic health at the cellular level. Through the reduction of systemic inflammation and the regulation of adipokine synthesis, they decrease insulin resistance in obesity and metabolic syndrome (Kumar et al., 2019; Suganya et al., 2025). This incorporation, improving membrane flexibility, promotes the optimal arrangement and functioning of membrane-bound receptors such as the insulin receptor and GLUT-4 transporters, which improves glucose uptake and insulin binding efficiency (Sinha et al., 2023). Moreover, the consumption of omega-3 supplements, particularly fish oil, can manage the blood pressure and cholesterol levels, which are majorly involved in the overall metabolism of the human body (Damaiyanti et al., 2023).

15.4.8 Pregnancy

Both DHA and EPA play a vital role in the pregnancy period, such as overall maternal health, placental function, and fetal development (Rasool et al., 2021). The mother transfers DHA to the fetus during pregnancy, particularly in the third trimester when the brain, nervous system, and retina are developed. Longer gestation, a lower risk of premature delivery, and better birth outcomes are all positively correlated with maternal DHA consumption (Basak et al., 2024; Rogers et al., 2013). The visual and cognitive development of infants who receive adequate DHA through nursing or formula fortification is superior. Additionally, improved hand-eye coordination and attention span have been associated with postnatal supplementation. The relevance of omega-3 supplements in maternal nutrition programs is further supported by the fact that they help mothers experience less postpartum depression and inflammatory problems (Basak et al., 2021). EPA is involved in the development of prostaglandin production, nutrient transport, and fetal oxygen supply. Apart from this, both fatty acids reduce the risk of premature birth, infant body weight management, pregnancy-induced hypertension and improve immune tolerance, all of which are involved in a proper situation for fetal development (Carlson et al., 2013).

By regulating neurotransmitter action and inflammatory pathways, a sufficient omega-3 intake leads to the mother's emotional stability and reduces postpartum depression. High-quality DHA and EPA are found in foods like fatty fish, supplements made from algae, chia seeds, flaxseed, and walnuts. These nutrients are vital for supplying the potent nutrients during pregnancy. Overall, consuming a sufficient level of omega-3 PUFAs during pregnancy is essential for mothers' health as well as the development of the fetus's immune system and the child's long-term health benefits (Chowdhury et al., 2022; Rombaldi Bernardi et al., 2012).

15.5 Technological innovations in docosahexaenoic acid/eicosapentaenoic acid integration

The integration of DHA and EPA into food materials, nutraceuticals, and pharmaceutical products leads to the development of technological innovations in the food industry. Although the beneficial health effects of PUFAs have been recognized, incorporating them into consumer-ready formulations is technically challenging due to their oxidative instability, low water solubility, and distinct odor and flavor (Islam et al., 2023; Tocher et al., 2019). Therefore, ongoing technical advancements have focused on enhancing their bioavailability, stability, and sensory quality across the supply chain and manufacturing process. The key technical developments can be characterized by four extensive processes: (1) stabilization strategies, (2) bioavailability optimization, (3) food safety and shelf-life enhancement, and (iv) smart labeling and traceability systems (Fig. 15.4).

15.5.1 Stabilization strategies

Stabilization of the DHA and EPA into the main and subingredients is the foremost challenge in PUFA integration into food materials. The presence of the double bond structure makes them sensitive to heat and light conditions. Stabilization methods have been widely established to keep omega-3 fatty acids from oxidative damage during processing, storage, and digestion (Islam et al., 2023; Zhou & Wei, 2023). Microencapsulation is one of the most effective and broadly used methods for stabilizing omega-3 PUFAs, which are extremely susceptible to oxidative destruction due to their many double bonds (Rasti et al., 2017; Venugopalan et al., 2021). The method creates a protective core-shell structure by trapping lipid droplets inside a covering substance, usually proteins, polysaccharides, and lipids. This barrier reduces lipid peroxidation and the development of rancid smells by limiting oxygen passage, light exposure, and interaction with pro-oxidant metals. During processing and storage, encapsulation stabilizes emulsions and inhibits droplet coalescence by acting as a physical and interfacial barrier. In food and nutraceutical preparations, nanoemulsions provide the most advanced delivery method for improving the functional performance of DHA and EPA (Walker et al., 2015). Nanoemulsions, which are distinguished by droplet sizes that are usually less than 200 nm, offer a kinetically stable

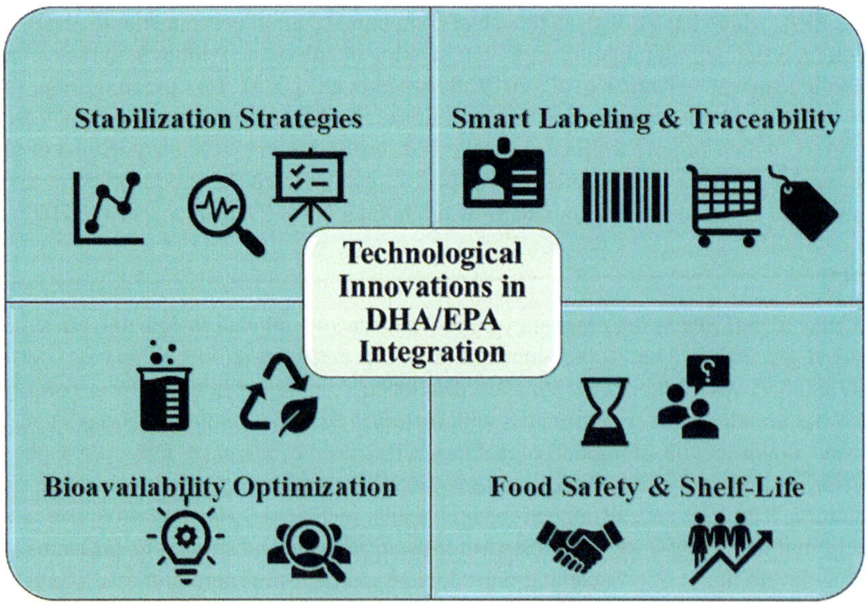

FIGURE 15.4 **Illustration of technology and innovations involved in the omega integration into the food industry.**

distribution that reduces gravitational creaming, phase separation, and coalescence. These submicron droplets' very large surface area enhances their interfacial contact with gastrointestinal lipases, facilitating quick lipid hydrolysis and effective DHA and EPA incorporation into mixed micelles for intestinal absorption. By decreasing the droplet width, the diffusion process of the bile salts and lipolytic enzymes becomes shorter, improving the kinetics of digestion and the bioavailability of omega-3 fatty acids. Lecithin, saponins, and plant-derived proteins are natural emulsifiers that are increasingly used in modern nanoemulsion preparations to meet clean-label and sustainable formulation requirements. By scavenging free radicals and replenishing primary antioxidants in the oil phase, coformulation with antioxidant systems such as tocopherols, ascorbyl palmitate, and rosemary extract offers synergistic oxidative protection (Chen et al., 2017; Venugopalan et al., 2021). Simultaneously, sensory masking technologies have become essential resources for decreasing a particular fishy taste and smell linked to omega-3 fortification, especially in critical applications such as dairy-based products, infant formulas, and drink varieties. Flavor encapsulation and lipid oxidation inhibitors prevent volatile aldehydes from forming, whereas natural aroma compounds and cyclodextrin inclusion complexes physically entrap odor-causing molecules. By binding volatile oxidation products, protein-based encapsulants like whey or pea protein improve taste retention even further and refine the sensory profile (English et al., 2023). The production of flavorful, stable, and bioavailable DHA/EPA-enriched functional meals that satisfy the needs of customers and nutritional efficacy is made possible by the combination of sensory masking techniques with nanoemulsion distribution (Zhou & Wei, 2023).

15.5.2 Bioavailability optimization

The biological efficacy of PUFAs, especially DHA and EPA, is extremely dependent on bioavailability. Their low absorption capacity and poor solubility in water conditions lead to decreased dispersibility during the process of digestion (Cholewski et al., 2018; Li et al., 2023). To overcome these obstacles, a proper delivery system is needed that specifically improves the solubility, absorption in the intestine, and metabolic utilization. Nanotechnology is widely used for the development of drug delivery as a carrier molecule; here, lipid-based nanocarriers gained more attention due to their biocompatibility, protection against oxidation, enhanced absorption, and controlled-release behavior. Solid lipid and nanostructured lipid carriers are widely used as nanocarriers (Cheng et al., 2023). These nanocarriers provide the solid/semisolid lipid matrix that can trap them inside a crystalline core. The lipid matrix allowed the fatty acids to be released in a controlled manner to enhance the pharmacokinetic activity. This is suitable for food and medicine productions due to their effective biocompatibility, and it can easily pass through the biological membrane layers (da Silva Santos et al., 2019; Viegas et al., 2023).

Self-emulsifying drug delivery systems and self-nanoemulsifying drug delivery systems are both innovative techniques used for the drug delivery process. Here, oils, surfactants, and solvents meet gastrointestinal fluids; they naturally create proper emulsions/nanoemulsions (Rehman et al., 2017). Together with phospholipids and bile salts, the resulting submicron droplets speed up micelle production and solubilization, greatly increasing intestinal absorption and bioaccessibility of omega-3s. Their usage in functional food and nutraceutical applications has increased because of their scalability and simplicity of formulation. Furthermore, liposome-based encapsulation is another potential drug delivery method; here, a vesicular phospholipid bilayer was utilized to act as a similar biological membrane, which leads to the bioavailability of the DHA and EPA (Dima et al., 2015; Maiti et al., 2023). Polymeric and biopolymeric coatings like alginate and chitosan prevent early oxidation and provide continuous distribution after ingestion, enabling controlled-release mechanisms. (Edo et al., 2024) This method was specifically used in nutritious, enhanced fortified food preparations. Overall, these novel technological developments are used for the effective PUFA-enriched oil-based food product production.

15.5.3 Food safety and shelf-life considerations

Maintaining quality, nutritional value, and customer trust in contemporary food systems depends on ensuring food safety and extending shelf life. Product stability is decreased, and spoiling is accelerated by elements such as nutritional degradation, lipid oxidation, and microbial contamination (Knorr et al., 2020; Lisboa et al., 2024). Developing technologies like nanomaterials involves active packaging, antioxidant-enhanced encapsulations provide the chances to improve food preservation, control microbial contamination, and reduce the oxidation process. Moreover, the nanosensors act as real-time freshness monitoring in food product manufacturing and storage (Jacinto-Valderrama et al., 2023).

In the food industry, extending shelf life while lowering the usage of chemical additives and preservatives has grown in significance, encouraging advancements in processing techniques, packaging technology, and the development of natural preservative replacements. Specifically, food products are easily getting microbial contaminations, which is caused by the microbes related to the foodborne diseases. This is one of the key challenges in the food industry, facing in food packaging

(Hou et al., 2023). Antimicrobial-based food packaging techniques focus on reducing the growth of pathogens that are present in the food packages and food materials. This antimicrobial-based packaging leads to the control of growth of microbes in food products during packaging, transportation, and consuming stages (Andrade et al., 2025; Balasubramanian et al., 2022). Oxidative stability is another factor that needs to be considered for the food safety process. Naturally, DHA and EPA have a higher level of unsaturated fatty acids. And this is getting very weak in the oxidative breakdown process, which leads to the production of volatile chemicals like aldehydes and lipid peroxides (Islam et al., 2023; Saini et al., 2021). This process reduces the nutritional content and spoils the food's taste. Many natural and synthetic antioxidants are used for their antioxidant properties in food products. Especially tocopherols, ascorbic acid, polyphenols, rosemary extracts, curcumin, green tea catechins, and grape seed polyphenols are widely used (Yanishlieva & Marinova, 2001). These incorporations into food products could improve the nutritional level as well as enhance the shelf life of the products.

15.5.4 Smart labeling and traceability systems

To commercialize the products to market, the proper labeling identification for the products is one of the challenges; to overcome this, some smart technological innovations are widely used in the global market. Proper labeling and identification are key factors for the identification of the products. Clear representation of product details, ingredients, manufacturing details, expiry date, and nutritional values of the ingredients will lead the consumer to understand the product's information, as well as make them believe in the products. Due to the growing population's demand, the DHA and EPA incorporated food product manufacturing, which has increased in recent decades, while at the same time product's reliability is important. To provide detailed information about the products, smart labeling played an important role in novel food products (Nollet, 2024). The QR-based scanning methods are also a good way to learn about the products. Through scanning the QR codes, consumers can get the detailed information about the specific products, like DHA and EPA oils' biological source, extraction methods, shelf-life details, and storage conditions. The integration of sensor-based monitoring and IoT technologies in food product packaging leads to the real-time quality analysis (Singh et al., 2025; Zhou et al., 2025). Those smart sensors continuously track key environmental influences that affect the DHA and EPA oxidation process, temperature, humidity, oxygen exposure, and light intensity, which generally play a vital role in the oxidation process. Furthermore, this sensor-based monitoring improves the product's quality and reduces food contamination. Together, the above innovative technology-based labeling approach and the manufacturing process of the omega-enriched products could reach potential customers as effectively as possible.

15.6 Sustainability and the future of omega-3s

Over the past 20 years, dietary choices have been significantly impacted by growing environmental consciousness and awareness of global health, with a greater emphasis on nutrient-dense and environmentally friendly foods (Kokilaa et al., 2023; Rajasekar & Venmathi, 2021). Modern omega-3 fortification is based on innovative techniques that enhance stability, sensory quality, and bioavailability while shielding DHA and EPA from oxidation (Table 15.1). Omega-3 fatty acids, particularly DHA and EPA, are not just essential nutrients; they have also emerged as hallmarks of sustainable resource management. Human health, environmental stability, and ethical manufacturing are all linked to the sustainability of omega production. The primary worldwide omega-3 fatty acids are fish, specifically small pelagic species, such as anchovies, sardines, and mackerel; however, the dependence on marine sources leads to significant sustainability issues, like ecological imbalances, overfishing, and this leads to climate-based complications in the fish populations (Pateiro et al., 2021). Such demands highlight the need for innovative, environmentally friendly industrial techniques to be developed. The involvement of biotechnology and novel innovative technology can improve the omega-3 production as well as reduce the demand for marine sources. Alternative sources, such as algal culture, microbial fermentation, and modified yeasts, provide a sufficient level of omega-3. Also, these approaches are the zero-waste methods for sustainable omega-3 manufacture, which is supported by turning food system products like algal biomass and fish processing debris into value-added components (Swetha & Mathanghi, 2024). Another transformative progress is the application of synthetic biology and fermentation. Genetically modified yeasts and *oleaginous* microorganisms can produce personalized omega-3 sources at an industrial level. These technology-based products can be resistant to climate change, have minimal ecological footprints, and high productivity in small-scale land productions. Simultaneously, GMO-based camelina, canola, and soybean plant varieties provide enhanced DHA and EPA, which also offer additional diversification of supply chains. Sustainability and product stability are strongly related in the food industry. Reducing waste and boosting commercialization requires improving the oxidative stability and usefulness of omega-3 oils (Betancor et al., 2022; Qin et al., 2023; West et al., 2021).

TABLE 15.1 Docosahexaenoic acid (DHA) and eicosapentaenoic acid (EPA) mechanisms of action and their limitations in food technology.

Innovation and technology	Mechanism of action	Key advantages of EPA and DHA	Food applications	Limitations	References
Microencapsulation	Encapsulates oil droplets within a protective wall material (gum arabic, modified starch, whey proteins)	Protects from oxidation, improves shelf life, dry powder, manages the fishy odor and flavor	Infant formula, bakery mixes, powdered beverages, and clinical nutrition blends	Possible wall material instability under humidity, the cost of high-quality encapsulants	Premi and Sharma (2017); Wangkulangkool et al. (2023)
Nanoemulsions	Formation of nanometer-sized droplets via high-pressure homogenization and ultrasonication	High bioavailability, transparent solutions, improved dispersibility, and fast digestion kinetics	Clear beverages, functional shots, dairy drinks, nutritional waters	Requires surfactants, long-term stability of nanocombined emulsions	Banasaz et al. (2020); Aswathanarayan & Vittal (2019)
Liposomes and vesicular delivery systems	Bilayer vesicles entrap EPA/DHA for targeted delivery	Mimics biological membranes, enhances stability, and targeted release in the GI tract	Medical foods, pharmaceuticals, fortified beverages	High cost, sophisticated formulation equipment	Mankan et al. (2025); Yaghmur et al. (2023)
Cyclodextrin complexation	Inclusion complexes trap hydrophobic omega-3 molecules within cyclodextrin cavities	Excellent sensory masking, good for dry formulations, improves stability	Tablets, capsules, powdered supplements, instant drink mixes	Limited loading capacity, regulatory limits for cyclodextrins in some countries	Yoshikiyo et al. (2019); David et al. (2019)
Protein-polysaccharide conjugates (maillard-based)	Protein-sugar conjugates produce stable interfaces around oil droplets	Superior emulsion stability, enhanced oxidative protection, natural clean-label option	Yogurts, cheese analogs, nutritional beverages	The Maillard reaction can alter color/flavor if not controlled	Kan et al. (2021)
Microalgal bioengineering and high-DHA extracts	Use of engineered microalgae strains with elevated DHA content	Clean vegan source, minimal contaminants, tailored lipid profiles, strong oxidative stability when purified	Infant formula, medical nutrition, premium supplements	High production costs, scale-up energy demand	Deepika et al. (2025); Dalmia and Tumaney (2024)
Antioxidant fortification (natural extracts, polyphenols, rosemary, tocopherols)	Scavenges free radicals, delays lipid oxidation	Enhances stability during processing/storage, supports clean-label positioning	Oils, dressings, baked goods, and encapsulated powders	Interaction with the food matrix may affect flavor	Wang and Fu (2018)
Controlled-release systems (pH-responsive coatings, enteric polymers)	Release triggered by stomach or intestinal conditions	Protects omega-3 during processing and digestion, targeted absorption	Medical nutrition, clinical supplements, fortified pharmaceuticals	Regulatory constraints on polymer types	Zazula et al. (2025); Abdelhafez et al. (2025)

Microencapsulation (Fernandes et al., 2024), spray drying (Castejón et al., 2021), nanoemulsion systems (Walker et al., 2015), and improved lipid carriers (Lacatusu et al., 2013) are among the techniques used to preserve omega-3s from oxidation, increase their integration into varied food components, and improve customer acceptance through sensory masking. The future of omega-3s will be determined by comprehensive sustainability frameworks that include transparent traceability procedures, biotechnology-driven production systems, environmentally conscious sustainable aquaculture, and responsible fisheries management. To ensure long-term availability, a low-impact, diverse supply landscape that includes marine, microbial, and agricultural sources will be crucial (Ji et al., 2015; Shepon et al., 2022). In addition to promoting responsible environmental behavior, these modifications ensure that customers worldwide can continue to benefit from the beneficial nutrients of both EPA and DHA without affecting the safety of the environment.

15.7 Conclusion

The demand for foods and supplements fortified with omega-3 fatty acids is rising quickly as health and well-being become more widely accepted. Both DHA and EPA are essential nutrients for the global industry and overall health. The availability of omega-3-based dietary products, their consumption, and the worldwide degree of omega awareness are all required at the same time. They are essential at various stages of life because of their critical functions in immunological control, CVD protection, brain function, and anti-inflammatory action. Overall, DHA and EPA will play an immense role in influencing future dietary recommendations and food industry innovations. To achieve rising demand while promoting long-term public health, it is essential to further develop worldwide awareness of omega-3s, enhance the sustainability of the supply chain, and increase the variety of ecologically friendly sources of omega-3s.

References

Abdelhafez, A., Khabir, Z., Prestidge, C. A., Garcia-Bennett, A., & Joyce, P. (2025). The impact of formulation design on the oral bioavailability of omega-3 polyunsaturated fatty acids. *Food Research International, 208*, 116171. https://doi.org/10.1016/j.foodres.2025.116171.

Abshirini, M., Ilesanmi-Oyelere, B. L., & Kruger, M. C. (2021). Potential modulatory mechanisms of action by long-chain polyunsaturated fatty acids on bone cell and chondrocyte metabolism. *Progress in Lipid Research, 83*, 101113. https://doi.org/10.1016/j.plipres.2021.101113.

Amza, M., Haj Hamoud, B., Sima, R.-M., Dinu, M.-D., Gorecki, G.-P., Popescu, M., Gică, N., Poenaru, M.-O., Pleş, L., et al. (2024). Docosahexaenoic Acid (DHA) and Eicosapentaenoic Acid (EPA)—Should They Be Mandatory Supplements in Pregnancy? *Biomedicines, 12*(7), 1471. 10.3390/biomedicines12071471.

Andrade, M. A., Barbosa, C. H., Ribeiro-Santos, R., Tomé, S., Fernando, A. L., Silva, A. S., & Vilarinho, F. (2025). Emerging trends in active packaging for food: A six-year review. *Foods, 14*(15). https://doi.org/10.3390/foods14152713, www.mdpi.com/journal/foods.

Andrews, N., Bennett, N. J., Le Billon, P., Green, S. J., Cisneros-Montemayor, A. M., Amongin, S., Gray, N. J., & Sumaila, U. R. (2021). Oil, fisheries and coastal communities: A review of impacts on the environment, livelihoods, space and governance. *Energy Research and Social Science, 75*. https://doi.org/10.1016/j.erss.2021.102009 Available from: http://www.journals.elsevier.com/energy-research-and-social-science/.

Ashraf, S. A., Adnan, M., Patel, M., Siddiqui, A. J., Sachidanandan, M., Snoussi, M., Hadi, S., et al. (2020). Fish-Based Bioactives as Potent Nutraceuticals: Exploring the Therapeutic Perspective of Sustainable Food from the Sea. *Marine Drugs, 18*(5), 265. https://doi.org/10.3390/md18050265.

Aswathanarayan, J. B., & Vittal, R. R. (2019). Nanoemulsions and their potential applications in food industry. *Frontiers in Sustainable Food Systems, 3*. https://doi.org/10.3389/fsufs.2019.00095, www.frontiersin.org/journals/sustainable-food-systems#.

Balasubramanian, D., Girigoswami, A., & Girigoswami, K. (2022). Antimicrobial, pesticidal and food preservative applications of lemongrass oil nanoemulsion: A mini-review. *Recent Advances in Food Nutrition & Agriculture, 13*(1), 51–58.

Banasaz, S., Morozova, K., Ferrentino, G., & Scampicchio, M. (2020). Encapsulation of lipid-soluble bioactives by nanoemulsions. *Molecules, 25*(17), 3966.

Banović Fuentes, J., Beara, I., & Torović, L. (2024). Regulatory compliance of health claims on omega-3 fatty acid food supplements. *Foods (Basel, Switzerland), 14*(1), 67. https://doi.org/10.3390/foods14010067.

Barros, M. P., Poppe, S. C., & Bondan, E. F. (2014). Neuroprotective properties of the marine carotenoid astaxanthin and omega-3 fatty acids, and perspectives for the natural combination of both in krill oil. *Nutrients, 6*(3), 1293–1317. https://doi.org/10.3390/nu6031293.

Basak, S., Mallick, R., Banerjee, A., Pathak, S., & Duttaroy, A. K. (2021). Maternal supply of both arachidonic and docosahexaenoic acids is required for optimal neurodevelopment. *Nutrients, 13*(6), 2061. https://doi.org/10.3390/nu13062061.

Basak, S., Mallick, R., & Duttaroy, A. K. (2020). Maternal docosahexaenoic acid status during pregnancy and its impact on infant neurodevelopment. *Nutrients, 12*(12), 3615. https://doi.org/10.3390/nu12123615.

Basak, S., Mallick, R., Navya Sree, B., & Duttaroy, A. K. (2024). Placental epigenome impacts fetal development: Effects of maternal nutrients and gut microbiota. *Nutrients, 16*(12), 1860. https://doi.org/10.3390/nu16121860.

Bazan, N. G., Molina, M. F., & Gordon, W. C. (2011). Docosahexaenoic acid signalolipidomics in nutrition: Significance in aging, neuroinflammation, macular degeneration, Alzheimer's, and other neurodegenerative diseases. *Annual Review of Nutrition, 31*, 321–351. https://doi.org/10.1146/annurev.nutr.012809.104635.

Benatti, P., Peluso, G., Nicolai, R., & Calvani, M. (2004). Polyunsaturated fatty acids: Biochemical, nutritional and epigenetic properties. *Journal of the American College of Nutrition, 23*(4), 281–302. https://doi.org/10.1080/07315724.2004.10719371.

Betancor, M. B., Sprague, M., González-Silvera, D., Ortega, A., de la Gándara, F., Gong, X., & Mourente, G. (2022). Oils derived from GM crops as sustainable solutions to the supply of Long-chain Omega-3 for on-growing Atlantic Bluefin tuna (*Thunnus thynnus*L.). *Fishes, 7*(6), 366.

Bettadahalli, S., Acharya, P., & Talahalli, R. (2020). Evidence on n-3 fatty acids and oleic acid role in retinal inflammation and microvascular integrity: Insight from a hyperlipidemic rat model. *Inflammation, 43*(3), 868–877. https://doi.org/10.1007/s10753-019-01172-1.

Blasbalg, T. L., Hibbeln, J. R., Ramsden, C. E., Majchrzak, S. F., & Rawlings, R. R. (2011). Changes in consumption of omega-3 and omega-6 fatty acids in the United States during the 20th century. *The American Journal of Clinical Nutrition, 93*(5), 950–962. https://doi.org/10.3945/ajcn.110.006643.

Bodur, M., Yilmaz, B., Ağagündüz, D., & Ozogul, Y. (2025). Immunomodulatory effects of omega-3 fatty acids: Mechanistic insights and health implications. *Molecular Nutrition & Food Research, 69*(10), e202400752. https://doi.org/10.1002/mnfr.202400752.

Brodziak-Dopierała, B., Fischer, A., Chrzanowska, M., & Ahnert, B. (2023). Mercury exposure from the consumption of dietary supplements containing vegetable, cod liver, and shark liver oils. *International Journal of Environmental Research and Public Health, 20*(3), 2129.

Byrne, M. K., Cook, R., Murta, J. C. D., Bressington, D., & Meyer, B. J. (2024). Dietary intakes of long-chain polyunsaturated fatty acids and impulsivity: Comparing non-restricted, vegetarian, and vegan diets. *Nutrients, 16*(6), 875. https://doi.org/10.3390/nu16060875.

Camuesco, D., Comalada, M., Concha, A., Nieto, A., Sierra, S., Xaus, J., Zarzuelo, A., & Gálvez, J. (2006). Intestinal anti-inflammatory activity of combined quercitrin and dietary olive oil supplemented with fish oil, rich in EPA and DHA (n-3) polyunsaturated fatty acids, in rats with DSS-induced colitis. *Clinical Nutrition (Edinburgh, Scotland), 25*(3), 466–476. https://doi.org/10.1016/j.clnu.2005.12.009.

Carlson, S. E., Colombo, J., Gajewski, B. J., Gustafson, K. M., Mundy, D., Yeast, J., Georgieff, M. K., Markley, L. A., Kerling, E. H., & Shaddy, D. J. (2013). DHA supplementation and pregnancy outcomes. *The American Journal of Clinical Nutrition, 97*(4), 808–815. https://doi.org/10.3945/ajcn.112.050021.

Castejón, N., Luna, P., & Señoráns, F. J. (2021). Microencapsulation by spray drying of omega-3 lipids extracted from oilseeds and microalgae: Effect on polyunsaturated fatty acid composition. *Lwt, 148*, 111789.

Chalon, S., Vancassel, S., Zimmer, L., Guilloteau, D., & Durand, G. (2001). Polyunsaturated fatty acids and cerebral function: Focus on monoaminergic neurotransmission. *Lipids, 36*(9), 937–944. https://doi.org/10.1007/s11745-001-0804-7.

Chen, F., Fan, G. Q., Zhang, Z., Zhang, R., Deng, Z. Y., & McClements, D. J. (2017). Encapsulation of omega-3 fatty acids in nanoemulsions and microgels: Impact of delivery system type and protein addition on gastrointestinal fate. *Food Research International (Ottawa, Ont.), 100*(Pt 1), 387–395. https://doi.org/10.1016/j.foodres.2017.07.039.

Cheng, X., Xie, Q., & Sun, Y. (2023). Advances in nanomaterial-based targeted drug delivery systems. *Frontiers in Bioengineering and Biotechnology, 11*, 1177151. https://doi.org/10.3389/fbioe.2023.1177151.

Cholewski, M., Tomczykowa, M., & Tomczyk, M. (2018). A comprehensive review of chemistry, sources and bioavailability of omega-3 fatty acids. *Nutrients, 10*(11), 1662. https://doi.org/10.3390/nu10111662.

Chowdhury, M. H., Ghosh, S., Kabir, M. R., Mamun, M. A. A., & Islam, M. S. (2022). Effect of supplementary omega-3 fatty acids on pregnant women with complications and pregnancy outcomes: Review from literature. *The Journal of Maternal-fetal & Neonatal Medicine, 35*(13), 2564–2580. https://doi.org/10.1080/14767058.2020.1786522.

Ciappolino, V., Mazzocchi, A., Botturi, A., Turolo, S., Delvecchio, G., Agostoni, C., & Brambilla, P. (2019). The role of docosahexaenoic acid (DHA) on cognitive functions in psychiatric disorders. *Nutrients, 11*(4), 769. https://doi.org/10.3390/nu11040769.

Colletti, A., Cravotto, G., Citi, V., Martelli, A., Testai, L., & Cicero, A. F. G. (2021). Advances in technologies for highly active omega-3 fatty acids from krill oil: Clinical applications. *Marine Drugs, 19*(6), 306. https://doi.org/10.3390/md19060306.

Coronel, E. B., Ixtaina, V. Y., & Capitani, M. I. (2025). Correction: Nutritional and functional characterization of chia expeller and gluten-free flours as ingredients for premixes. *Plant Foods for Human Nutrition (Dordrecht, Netherlands), 80*(3), 155. https://doi.org/10.1007/s11130-025-01402-y.

Dalmia, A., & Tumaney, A. W. (2024). Recent biotechnological advances in understanding the omega-3 fatty acid accumulation in algal lipids. *Algal Biotechnology*, 274–283.

Damaiyanti, D. W., Tsai, Z. Y., Masbuchin, A. N., Huang, C. Y., & Liu, P. Y. (2023). Interplay between fish oil, obesity and cardiometabolic diabetes. *Journal of the Formosan Medical Association=Taiwan yi zhi, 122*(7), 528–539. https://doi.org/10.1016/j.jfma.2023.03.013.

David, I., Orboi, M. D., Simandi, M. D., Chirilă, C. A., Megyesi, C. I., Rădulescu, L., & Hădărugă, N. G. (2019). Fatty acid profile of Romanian's common bean (*Phaseolus vulgaris* L.) lipid fractions and their complexation ability by β-cyclodextrin. *PLoS ONE, 14*(11), e0225474.

Deepika, C., Hankamer, B., & Ross, I. L. (2025). Can microalgal omega-3 PUFA production systems remain viable as GM plant sources emerge? *Bioresource Technology, 441*, 133525. https://doi.org/10.1016/j.biortech.2025.133525 Advance online publication.

Derbyshire, E. J., Birch, C. S., Bonwick, G. A., English, A., Metcalfe, P., & Li, W. (2024). Optimal omegas - barriers and novel methods to narrow omega-3 gaps. A narrative review. *Frontiers in Nutrition, 11*, 1325099. https://doi.org/10.3389/fnut.2024.1325099.

Dima, Ş., Dima, C., & Iordăchescu, G. (2015). Encapsulation of functional lipophilic food and drug biocomponents. *Food Engineering Reviews, 7*(4), 417–438.

Dou, Y., Wang, Y., Chen, Z., Yu, X., & Ma, D. (2021). Effect of n-3 polyunsaturated fatty acid on bone health: A systematic review and meta-analysis of randomized controlled trials. *Food Science & Nutrition, 10*(1), 145–154. https://doi.org/10.1002/fsn3.2655.

Duarte, S., Shah, M. A., & Sanches Silva, A. (2025). Flaxseed in diet: A comprehensive look at pros and cons. *Molecules, 30*(6), 1335.

Dyall, S. C. (2015). Long-chain omega-3 fatty acids and the brain: A review of the independent and shared effects of EPA, DPA and DHA. *Frontiers in Aging Neuroscience, 7*, 52. https://doi.org/10.3389/fnagi.2015.00052.

Dyck, M. C., Ma, D. W., & Meckling, K. A. (2011). The anticancer effects of Vitamin D and omega-3 PUFAs in combination via cod-liver oil: One plus one may equal more than two. *Medical Hypotheses, 77*(3), 326–332.

Edo, G. I., Mafe, A. N., Razooqi, N. F., Umelo, E. C., Gaaz, T. S., Isoje, E. F., Igbuku, U. A., Akpoghelie, P. O., Opiti, R. A., Essaghah, A. E. A., Ahmed, D. S., Umar, H., & Ozsahin, D. U. (2024). Advances in bio-polymer coatings for probiotic microencapsulation: Chitosan and beyond for enhanced stability and controlled release. *Designed Monomers and Polymers, 28*(1), 1–34. https://doi.org/10.1080/15685551.2024.2448122.

English, M., Okagu, O. D., Stephens, K., Goertzen, A., & Udenigwe, C. C. (2023). Flavour encapsulation: A comparative analysis of relevant techniques, physiochemical characterisation, stability, and food applications. *Frontiers in Nutrition, 10*, 1019211. https://doi.org/10.3389/fnut.2023.1019211.

Fekete, M., Szarvas, Z., Fazekas-Pongor, V., Feher, A., Csipo, T., Forrai, J., Dosa, N., Peterfi, A., Lehoczki, A., Tarantini, S., & Varga, J. T. (2022). Nutrition strategies promoting healthy aging: From improvement of cardiovascular and brain health to prevention of age-associated diseases. *Nutrients, 15*(1), 47. https://doi.org/10.3390/nu15010047.

Fernandes, B., Oliveira, M. C., Marques, A. C., Dos Santos, R. G., & Serrano, C. (2024). Microencapsulation of essential oils and oleoresins: Applications in food products. *Foods (Basel, Switzerland), 13*(23), 3873. https://doi.org/10.3390/foods13233873.

Fotuhi, M., Mohassel, P., & Yaffe, K. (2009). Fish consumption, long-chain omega-3 fatty acids and risk of cognitive decline or Alzheimer disease: A complex association. *Nature Clinical Practice. Neurology, 5*(3), 140–152. https://doi.org/10.1038/ncpneuro1044.

Ganesan, B., Brothersen, C., & McMahon, D. J. (2014). Fortification of foods with omega-3 polyunsaturated fatty acids. *Critical Reviews in Food Science and Nutrition, 54*(1), 98–114. https://doi.org/10.1080/10408398.2011.578221.

Georgakopoulos, C. D., Makri, O. E., Pagoulatos, D., Vasilakis, P., Peristeropoulou, P., Kouli, V., Eliopoulou, M. I., & Psachoulia, C. (2017). Effect of omega-3 fatty acids dietary supplementation on ocular surface and tear film in diabetic patients with dry eye. *Journal of the American College of Nutrition, 36*(1), 38–43. https://doi.org/10.1080/07315724.2016.1170643.

Global Burden of Cardiovascular Diseases and Risks 2023 CollaboratorsStark, B. A., DeCleene, N. K., Desai, E. C., Hsu, J. M., Johnson, C. O., et al. . (2025). Global, regional, and national burden of cardiovascular diseases and risk factors in 204 countries and territories, 1990–2023. *Journal of the American College of Cardiology, 86*(22), 2167–2243. https://doi.org/10.1016/j.jacc.2025.08.015.

Golanski, J., Szymanska, P., & Rozalski, M. (2021). Effects of omega-3 polyunsaturated fatty acids and their metabolites on haemostasis-current perspectives in cardiovascular disease. *International Journal of Molecular Sciences, 22*(5), 2394. https://doi.org/10.3390/ijms22052394.

Gupta, R. C., Srivastava, A., & Lall, R. (2021). Regulatory guidelines for nutraceuticals in India: An overview. In R. C. Gupta (Ed.). *Nutraceuticals* (pp. 1273–1280). (2nd ed.). Academic Press.

Hansen, M. W., Ørn, S., Erevik, C. B., Bjørkavoll-Bergseth, M. F., Skadberg, Ø., Melberg, T. H., & Kleiven, Ø. (2021). Regular consumption of cod liver oil is associated with reduced basal and exercise-induced C-reactive protein levels; a prospective observational trial: A NEEDED (The North Sea Race Endurance Exercise Study) 2014 sub-study. *Journal of the International Society of Sports Nutrition, 18*(1), 51.

Harris, W. S., Lemke, S. L., Hansen, S. N., Goldstein, D. A., DiRienzo, M. A., Su, H., & George, C. (2008). Stearidonic acid-enriched soybean oil increased the omega-3 index, an emerging cardiovascular risk marker. *Lipids, 43*(9), 805–811.

Hayes, D., Angove, M. J., Tucci, J., & Dennis, C. (2016). Walnuts (*Juglans regia*) chemical composition and research in human health. *Critical Reviews in Food Science and Nutrition, 56*(8), 1231–1241. https://doi.org/10.1080/10408398.2012.760516.

Hergenrader, A., VanOrmer, M., Thompson, M., Slotkowski, R., Freeman, A., Paetz, O., Sweeney, S., Wegner, L., Ali, K., Bender, N., Chaudhary, R., Thoene, M., Hanson, C., & Anderson-Berry, A. (2022). Assessing the impact of socioeconomic status on maternal and cord serum omega-3 polyunsaturated fatty acid levels. *Current Developments in Nutrition, 6*(Suppl_1), 844. https://doi.org/10.1093/cdn/nzac061.044.

Hollander, A., De Jonge, R., Biesbroek, S., Hoekstra, J., & Zijp, M. C. (2019). Exploring solutions for healthy, safe, and sustainable fatty acids (EPA and DHA) consumption in the Netherlands. *Sustainability Science, 14*(2), 303–313. https://doi.org/10.1007/s11625-018-0607-9.

Hou, T., Ma, S., Wang, F., & Wang, L. (2023). A comprehensive review of intelligent controlled release antimicrobial packaging in food preservation. *Food Science and Biotechnology, 32*(11), 1459–1478. https://doi.org/10.1007/s10068-023-01344-8.

Hünkar, T., Aktan, F., Ceylan, A., & Karasu, C. (2002). Effects of cod liver oil on tissue antioxidant pathways in normal and streptozotocin-diabetic rats. *Cell Biochemistry and Function: Cellular Biochemistry and its Modulation by Active Agents or Disease, 20*(4), 297–302.

Islam, F., Imran, A., Nosheen, F., Fatima, M., Arshad, M. U., Afzaal, M., Ijaz, N., Noreen, R., Mehta, S., Biswas, S., Rasool, I. F. U., Aslam, M. A., Usman, I., Zahra, S. M., Segueni, N., & Amer Ali, Y. (2023). Functional roles and novel tools for improving-oxidative stability of polyunsaturated fatty acids: A comprehensive review. *Food Science & Nutrition, 11*(6), 2471–2482. https://doi.org/10.1002/fsn3.3272.

Jacinto-Valderrama, R. A., Andrade, C. T., Pateiro, M., Lorenzo, J. M., & Conte-Junior, C. A. (2023). Recent trends in active packaging using nanotechnology to inhibit oxidation and microbiological growth in muscle foods. *Foods (Basel, Switzerland), 12*(19), 3662. https://doi.org/10.3390/foods12193662.

Jafari, A., Mardani, H., Parsi Nezhad, B., Alaghi, A., & Sahebkar, A. (2025). Beneficial effects of okra (*Abelmoschus esculentus* L.) consumption on anthropometric measures, blood pressure, glycaemic control, lipid profile and liver function tests in randomised controlled trials: A GRADE-assessed systematic review and dose–response meta-analysis. *British Journal of Nutrition, 133*(5). https://doi.org/10.1017/S0007114525000XXX.

Jahanban-Esfahlan, A., Ostadrahimi, A., Tabibiazar, M., & Amarowicz, R. (2019). A comparative review on the extraction, antioxidant content and antioxidant potential of different parts of walnut (*Juglans regia* L.) fruit and tree. *Molecules, 24*(11), 2133. https://doi.org/10.3390/molecules24112133.

Ji, X. J., Ren, L. J., & Huang, H. (2015). Omega-3 biotechnology: A green and sustainable process for omega-3 fatty acids production. *Frontiers in Bioengineering and Biotechnology, 3*, 158. https://doi.org/10.3389/fbioe.2015.00158.

Kajarabille, N., Díaz-Castro, J., Hijano, S., López-Frías, M., López-Aliaga, I., & Ochoa, J. J. (2013). A new insight to bone turnover: Role of ω-3 polyunsaturated fatty acids. *The Scientific World Journal, 2013*, 589641. https://doi.org/10.1155/2013/589641.

Kajla, P., Sharma, A., & Sood, D. R. (2015). Flaxseed—A potential functional food source. *Journal of Food Science and Technology, 52*(4), 1857–1871.

Kan, X., Chen, G., Zhou, W., & Zeng, X. (2021). Application of protein-polysaccharide Maillard conjugates as emulsifiers: Source, preparation and functional properties. *Food Research International, 150*, 110740.

Khalid, W., Arshad, M. S., Aziz, A., Rahim, M. A., Qaisrani, T. B., Afzal, F., Ali, A., Ranjha, M. M. A. N., Khalid, M. Z., & Anjum, F. M. (2022). Chia seeds (*Salvia hispanica* L.): A therapeutic weapon in metabolic disorders. *Food Science & Nutrition, 11*(1), 3–16. https://doi.org/10.1002/fsn3.3035.

Knorr, D., Augustin, M. A., & Tiwari, B. (2020). Advancing the role of food processing for improved integration in sustainable food chains. *Frontiers in Nutrition, 7*, 34. https://doi.org/10.3389/fnut.2020.00034.

Kokilaa, G. L., Chellaiyan, D. V., Rajeshkannan, S., Aarthy, A., Alfred, S. J., & Das, H. (2023). Dietary diversity and nutritional status: An association among the elderly. National Journal of Community Medicine, *14*, 723–729.

Kruger, M. C., Coetzee, M., Haag, M., & Weiler, H. (2010). Long-chain polyunsaturated fatty acids: Selected mechanisms of action on bone. *Progress in Lipid Research, 49*(4), 438–449. https://doi.org/10.1016/j.plipres.2010.06.002.

Kumar, N. G., Contaifer, D., Madurantakam, P., Carbone, S., Price, E. T., Van Tassell, B., Brophy, D. F., & Wijesinghe, D. S. (2019). Dietary bioactive fatty acids as modulators of immune function: Implications on human health. *Nutrients, 11*(12), 2974. https://doi.org/10.3390/nu11122974.

Lacatusu, I., Mitrea, E., Badea, N., Stan, R., Oprea, O., & Meghea, A. (2013). Lipid nanoparticles based on omega-3 fatty acids as effective carriers for lutein delivery. Preparation and in vitro characterization studies. *Journal of Functional Foods, 5*(3), 1260–1269.

Lafuente, M., Rodríguez González-Herrero, M. E., Romeo Villadóniga, S., & Domingo, J. C. (2021). Antioxidant activity and neuroprotective role of docosahexaenoic acid (DHA) supplementation in eye diseases that can lead to blindness: A narrative review. *Antioxidants (Basel, Switzerland), 10*(3), 386. https://doi.org/10.3390/antiox10030386.

Lauritzen, L., Brambilla, P., Mazzocchi, A., Harsløf, L. B., Ciappolino, V., & Agostoni, C. (2016). DHA effects in brain development and function. *Nutrients, 8*(1), 6. https://doi.org/10.3390/nu8010006.

Lemke, S. L., Vicini, J. L., Su, H., Goldstein, D. A., Nemeth, M. A., Krul, E. S., & Harris, W. S. (2010). Dietary intake of stearidonic acid–enriched soybean oil increases the omega-3 index: Randomized, double-blind clinical study of efficacy and safety. *The American Journal of Clinical Nutrition, 92*(4), 766–775.

Li, H., Han, J., Zhao, Z., Tian, J., Fu, X., Zhao, Y., Wei, C., & Liu, W. (2023). Roasting treatments affect oil extraction rate, fatty acids, oxidative stability, antioxidant activity, and flavor of walnut oil. *Frontiers in Nutrition, 9*, 1077081. https://doi.org/10.3389/fnut.2022.1077081.

Lichtenstein, A. H., Matthan, N. R., Jalbert, S. M., Resteghini, N. A., Schaefer, E. J., & Ausman, L. M. (2006). Novel soybean oils with different fatty acid profiles alter cardiovascular disease risk factors in moderately hyperlipidemic subjects. *The American Journal of Clinical Nutrition, 84*(3), 497–504.

Lin, X. L., Baisley, J., Bier, A., Vora, D., & Holub, B. (2022). Transgenic canola oil improved blood omega-3 profiles: A randomized, placebo-controlled trial in healthy adults. *Frontiers in Nutrition, 9*, 847114.

Lisboa, H. M., Pasquali, M. B., dos Anjos, A. I., Sarinho, A. M., de Melo, E. D., Andrade, R., Batista, L., Lima, J., Diniz, Y., & Barro, A. (2024). Innovative and sustainable food preservation techniques: Enhancing food quality, safety, and environmental sustainability. *Foods, 13*(3), 365. https://doi.org/10.3390/su16188223.

Little, C. B., Flannery, C. R., Hughes, C. E., Goodship, A., & Caterson, B. (2005). Cytokine induced metalloproteinase expression and activity does not correlate with focal susceptibility of articular cartilage to degeneration. *Osteoarthritis and Cartilage, 13*(2), 162–170. https://doi.org/10.1016/j.joca.2004.10.014.

Liu, D., Guo, Y., & Ma, H. (2023). Production, bioactivities and bioavailability of bioactive peptides derived from walnut origin by-products: A review. *Critical Reviews in Food Science and Nutrition, 63*(26), 8032–8047. https://doi.org/10.1080/10408398.2022.2054933.

Lopez, C., Rabesona, H., Novales, B., Weber, M., & Anton, M. (2023). Walnut (*Juglans regia* L.) kernel oil bodies recovered by aqueous extraction for utilization as ingredient in food emulsions: Exploration of their microstructure, composition and the effects of homogenization, pH, and salt ions on their physical stability. *Food Research International (Ottawa, Ont.), 173*(Pt 1), 113197. https://doi.org/10.1016/j.foodres.2023.113197.

Maiti, T. K., Parvate, S., Dixit, P., Singh, J., Reddy, V. J., Bhuvanesh, E., & Chattopadhyay, S. (2023). Liposome for encapsulation of essential oil and fatty acids. In *Liposomal encapsulation in food science and technology*. Academic Press, 113–124.

Mankan, E., Karakas, C. Y., Saroglu, O., Mzoughi, M., Sagdic, O., & Karadag, A. (2025). Food-grade liposome-loaded delivery systems: Current trends and future perspectives. *Foods (Basel, Switzerland), 14*(17), 2978. https://doi.org/10.3390/foods14172978.

Marrone, G., Guerriero, C., Palazzetti, D., Lido, P., Marolla, A., Di Daniele, F., & Noce, A. (2021). Vegan diet health benefits in metabolic syndrome. *Nutrients, 13*(3), 817. https://doi.org/10.3390/nu13030817.

Martins, D. A., Custódio, L., Barreira, L., Pereira, H., Ben-Hamadou, R., Varela, J., & Abu-Salah, K. M. (2013). Alternative sources of n-3 long-chain polyunsaturated fatty acids in marine microalgae. *Marine Drugs, 11*(7), 2259–2281. https://doi.org/10.3390/md11072259.

Medzhitov, R. (2008). Origin and physiological roles of inflammation. *Nature, 454*(7203), 428–435. https://doi.org/10.1038/nature07201.

Messina, M., Shearer, G., & Petersen, K. (2021). Soybean oil lowers circulating cholesterol levels and coronary heart disease risk, and has no effect on markers of inflammation and oxidation. *Nutrition, 89*, 111343.

Mohamed, A. A. R., Galal, A. A., & Elewa, Y. H. (2015). Comparative protective effects of royal jelly and cod liver oil against neurotoxic impact of tartrazine on male rat pups brain. *Acta Histochemica, 117*(7), 649–658.

Mohammadkhani, N., Moradnia, M., Mohammadi, M., Ebrahimpour, S., Tabatabaei-Malazy, O., Mirsadeghi, S., & Javar, H. A. (2025). Utilizing the healing power of flaxseed: A narrative review of its therapeutic applications. *Journal of Diabetes & Metabolic Disorders, 24*(1), 128.

Mora, I., Arola, L., Caimari, A., Escoté, X., & Puiggròs, F. (2022). Structured long-chain omega-3 fatty acids for improvement of cognitive function during aging. *International Journal of Molecular Sciences, 23*(7), 3472. https://doi.org/10.3390/ijms23073472.

Nemli, E., Günal-Köroğlu, D., Apak, R., & Capanoglu, E. (2025). Potential of plant-based oil processing wastes/by-products as an alternative source of bioactive compounds in the food industry. *Foods, 14*(15), 2718.

Nguyen, Q. V., Malau-Aduli, B. S., Cavalieri, J., Malau-Aduli, A. E. O., & Nichols, P. D. (2019). Enhancing omega-3 long-chain polyunsaturated fatty acid content of dairy-derived foods for human consumption. *Nutrients, 11*(4), 743. https://doi.org/10.3390/nu11040743.

Nollet, L. M. L., & Ahamad, J. (2024). CRC Press. https://doi.org/10.1201/9781003450719.

Oppedisano, F., Macrì, R., Gliozzi, M., Musolino, V., Carresi, C., Maiuolo, J., Bosco, F., Nucera, S., Caterina Zito, M., Guarnieri, L., Scarano, F., Nicita, C., Coppoletta, A. R., Ruga, S., Scicchitano, M., Mollace, R., Palma, E., & Mollace, V. (2020). The anti-inflammatory and antioxidant properties of n-3 PUFAs: Their role in cardiovascular protection. *Biomedicines, 8*(9), 306. https://doi.org/10.3390/biomedicines8090306.

Palabiyik, A. A., & Palabiyik, E. (2025). Effects of omega-3 fatty acids (n-3 PUFAs) on cardiovascular and muscular health across various populations: A review of supplementation benefits. *Nutrire, 50*, 73. https://doi.org/10.1186/s41110-025-00381-z.

Pateiro, M., Domínguez, R., Varzakas, T., Munekata, P. E. S., Movilla Fierro, E., & Lorenzo, J. M. (2021). Omega-3-rich oils from marine side streams and their potential application in food. *Marine Drugs, 19*(5), 233. https://doi.org/10.3390/md19050233.

Petrie, J. R., Zhou, X. R., Leonforte, A., McAllister, J., Shrestha, P., Kennedy, Y., & Singh, S. P. (2020). Development of a *Brassica napus* (canola) crop containing fish oil-like levels of DHA in the seed oil. *Frontiers in Plant Science, 11*, 727.

Premi, M., & Sharma, H. K. (2017). Effect of different combinations of maltodextrin, gum arabic and whey protein concentrate on the encapsulation behavior and oxidative stability of spray dried drumstick (*Moringa oleifera*) oil. *International Journal of Biological Macromolecules, 105*, 1232–1240.

Qin, J., Kurt, E., LBassi, T., Sa, L., & Xie, D. (2023). Biotechnological production of omega-3 fatty acids: Current status and future perspectives. *Frontiers in Microbiology, 14*, 1280296. https://doi.org/10.3389/fmicb.2023.1280296.

Rahman, M. M., Bhattacharya, A., Banu, J., Kang, J. X., & Fernandes, G. (2009). Endogenous n-3 fatty acids protect ovariectomy induced bone loss by attenuating osteoclastogenesis. *Journal of Cellular and Molecular Medicine, 13*(8B), 1833–1844. https://doi.org/10.1111/j.1582-4934.2009.00649.x.

Rajasekar, H., & Venmathi, E. (2021). Dietary habits among undergraduate medical students in Tamil Nadu; A before and after intervention study. *Journal of Pharmaceutical Research International, 33*(55B), 269–274.

Rasool, A., Alvarado-Flores, F., & O'Tierney-Ginn, P. (2021). Placental impact of dietary supplements: More than micronutrients. *Clinical Therapeutics, 43*(2), 226–245. https://doi.org/10.1016/j.clinthera.2020.11.017.

Rasti, B., Erfanian, A., & Selamat, J. (2017). Novel nanoliposomal encapsulated omega-3 fatty acids and their applications in food. *Food Chemistry, 230*, 690–696. https://doi.org/10.1016/j.foodchem.2017.03.089.

Rehman, F. U., Shah, K. U., Shah, S. U., Khan, I. U., Khan, G. M., & Khan, A. (2017). From nanoemulsions to self-nanoemulsions, with recent advances in self-nanoemulsifying drug delivery systems (SNEDDS). *Expert Opinion on Drug Delivery, 14*(11), 1325–1340.

Rhee, J. J., Kim, E., Buring, J. E., & Kurth, T. (2017). Fish consumption, omega-3 fatty acids, and risk of cardiovascular disease. *American Journal of Preventive Medicine, 52*(1), 10–19. https://doi.org/10.1016/j.amepre.2016.07.020.

Risé, P., Marangoni, F., & Galli, C. (2002). Regulation of PUFA metabolism: Pharmacological and toxicological aspects. *Prostaglandins, Leukotrienes, and Essential Fatty Acids, 67*(2-3), 85–89. https://doi.org/10.1054/plef.2002.0403.

Rogers, L. K., Valentine, C. J., & Keim, S. A. (2013). DHA supplementation: Current implications in pregnancy and childhood. *Pharmacological Research, 70*(1), 13–19. https://doi.org/10.1016/j.phrs.2012.12.003.

Rombaldi Bernardi, J., de Souza Escobar, R., Ferreira, C. F., & Pelufo Silveira, P. (2012). Fetal and neonatal levels of omega-3: Effects on neurodevelopment, nutrition, and growth. *TheScientificWorldJournal, 2012*, 202473. https://doi.org/10.1100/2012/202473.

Ross, B. M., Seguin, J., & Sieswerda, L. E. (2007). Omega-3 fatty acids as treatments for mental illness: Which disorder and which fatty acid? *Lipids in Health and Disease, 6*, 21. https://doi.org/10.1186/1476-511X-6-21.

Rozner, R., Vernikov, J., Griess-Fishheimer, S., Travinsky, T., Penn, S., Schwartz, B., Mesilati-Stahy, R., Argov-Argaman, N., Shahar, R., & Monsonego-Ornan, E. (2020). The role of omega-3 polyunsaturated fatty acids from different sources in bone development. *Nutrients, 12*(11), 3494. https://doi.org/10.3390/nu12113494.

Ruyter, B., Sissener, N. H., Østbye, T. K., Simon, C. J., Krasnov, A., Bou, M., & Berge, G. M. (2019). n-3 Canola oil effectively replaces fish oil as a new safe dietary source of DHA in feed for juvenile Atlantic salmon. *British Journal of Nutrition, 122*(12), 1329–1345.

Sacco, P., Lipari, S., Cok, M., Colella, M., Marsich, E., Lopez, F., & Donati, I. (2021). Insights into mechanical behavior and biological properties of chia seed mucilage hydrogels. *Gels (Basel, Switzerland), 7*(2), 47. https://doi.org/10.3390/gels7020047.

Saini, R. K., Prasad, P., Sreedhar, R. V., Akhilender Naidu, K., Shang, X., & Keum, Y. S. (2021). Omega-3 polyunsaturated fatty acids (PUFAs): Emerging plant and microbial sources, oxidative stability, bioavailability, and health benefits review. *Antioxidants (Basel, Switzerland), 10*(10), 1627. https://doi.org/10.3390/antiox10101627.

Santos, H. O., Price, J. C., & Bueno, A. A. (2020). Beyond fish oil supplementation: The effects of alternative plant sources of omega-3 polyunsaturated fatty acids upon lipid indexes and cardiometabolic biomarkers overview. *Nutrients, 12*(10), 3159. https://doi.org/10.3390/nu12103159.

Senadheera, T. R., Hossain, A., & Shahidi, F. (2023). Marine bioactives and their application in the food industry: A review. *Applied Sciences, 13*(21), 12088.

Shawl, M., Geetha, T., Burnett, D., & Babu, J. R. (2024). Omega-3 supplementation and its effects on osteoarthritis. *Nutrients, 16*(11), 1650. https://doi.org/10.3390/nu16111650.

Shepon, A., Makov, T., Hamilton, H. A., Müller, D. B., Gephart, J. A., Henriksson, P. J., & Golden, C. D. (2022). Sustainable optimization of global aquatic omega-3 supply chain could substantially narrow the nutrient gap. *Resources, Conservation and Recycling, 181*, 106260.

Sherratt, S. C. R., Libby, P., Budoff, M. J., Bhatt, D. L., & Mason, R. P. (2023). Role of omega-3 fatty acids in cardiovascular disease: The debate continues. *Current Atherosclerosis Reports, 25*(1), 1–17. https://doi.org/10.1007/s11883-022-01075-x.

da Silva Santos, V., Badan Ribeiro, A. P., & Andrade Santana, M. H. (2019). Solid lipid nanoparticles as carriers for lipophilic compounds for applications in foods. *Food Research International (Ottawa, Ont.), 122*, 610–626. https://doi.org/10.1016/j.foodres.2019.01.032.

Singh, P. K., Agrawal, N., & Suman, S. (2025). Practices for healthier meat and meat products. In *Healthier meat products*. Cham: Springer Nature Switzerland, 33–47.

Sinha, S., Haque, M., Lugova, H., & Kumar, S. (2023). The effect of omega-3 fatty acids on insulin resistance. *Life (Basel, Switzerland), 13*(6), 1322. https://doi.org/10.3390/life13061322.

So, J., Wu, D., Lichtenstein, A. H., Tai, A. K., Matthan, N. R., Maddipati, K. R., & Lamon-Fava, S. (2021). EPA and DHA differentially modulate monocyte inflammatory response in subjects with chronic inflammation in part via plasma specialized pro-resolving lipid mediators: A randomized, double-blind, crossover study. *Atherosclerosis, 316*, 90–98. https://doi.org/10.1016/j.atherosclerosis.2020.11.018.

Song, C., Shieh, C. H., Wu, Y. S., Kalueff, A., Gaikwad, S., & Su, K. P. (2016). The role of omega-3 polyunsaturated fatty acids eicosapentaenoic and docosahexaenoic acids in the treatment of major depression and Alzheimer's disease: Acting separately or synergistically? *Progress in Lipid Research, 62*, 41–54. https://doi.org/10.1016/j.plipres.2015.12.003.

Song, H., Cong, Z., Wang, C., He, M., Liu, C., & Gao, P. (2022). Research progress on Walnut oil: Bioactive compounds, health benefits, extraction methods, and medicinal uses. *Journal of Food Biochemistry, 46*(12), e14504. https://doi.org/10.1111/jfbc.14504.

Sprague, M., Betancor, M. B., & Tocher, D. R. (2017). Microbial and genetically engineered oils as replacements for fish oil in aquaculture feeds. *Biotechnology Letters, 39*(11), 1599–1609. https://doi.org/10.1007/s10529-017-2402-6.

Stepień, A. E., Trojniak, J., & Tabarkiewicz, J. (2025). Anti-oxidant and anti-cancer properties of flaxseed. *International Journal of Molecular Sciences, 26*(3), 1226.

Suganya, M., Maragatham, S., & Padmapriya, D. (2025). Assessing health-related quality of life using EQ-5D-5L in adolescents with perpetuation of obesity. *Journal of Family Medicine and Primary Care, 14*(5), 1643–1645. https://doi.org/10.4103/jfmpc.jfmpc_1400_24.

Swanson, D., Block, R., & Mousa, S. A. (2012). Omega-3 fatty acids EPA and DHA: Health benefits throughout life. *Advances in Nutrition (Bethesda, Md.), 3*(1), 1–7. https://doi.org/10.3945/an.111.000893.

Swetha, N., & Mathanghi, S. K. (2024). Towards sustainable omega-3 fatty acids production–A comprehensive review on extraction methods, oxidative stability and bio-availability enhancement. *Food Chemistry Advances, 4*, 100603.

Talero, E., García-Mauriño, S., Ávila-Román, J., Rodríguez-Luna, A., Alcaide, A., & Motilva, V. (2015). Bioactive compounds isolated from microalgae in chronic inflammation and cancer. *Marine Drugs, 13*(10), 6152–6209. https://doi.org/10.3390/md13106152.

Tang, W., Wang, R., Liu, W., He, J., & Liu, J. (2025). *A comprehensive review on algae oil: Resources, production, encapsulation and application in food. Food Research International*, 116783.

Tocher, D. R., Betancor, M. B., Sprague, M., Olsen, R. E., & Napier, J. A. (2019). Omega-3 long-chain polyunsaturated fatty acids, EPA and DHA: Bridging the gap between supply and demand. *Nutrients, 11*(1), 89. https://doi.org/10.3390/nu11010089.

Torrissen, M., Gisslevik, E., Gundersen, T. E., Bolstad, T., Eide, O., Rizzo, A. M., Clayton, P., & Robertson, C. (2025). Global variations in omega-3 fatty acid status and omega-6:omega-3 ratios: Insights from > 500,000 whole-blood dried blood spot samples. *Lipids in Health and Disease, 24*(1), 260. https://doi.org/10.1186/s12944-025-02676-6.

Troesch, B., Eggersdorfer, M., Laviano, A., Rolland, Y., Smith, A. D., Warnke, I., Weimann, A., & Calder, P. C. (2020). Expert opinion on benefits of long-chain omega-3 fatty acids (DHA and EPA) in aging and clinical nutrition. *Nutrients, 12*(9), 2555. https://doi.org/10.3390/nu12092555\.

Ullah, R., Nadeem, M., Khalique, A., Imran, M., Mehmood, S., Javid, A., & Hussain, J. (2016). Nutritional and therapeutic perspectives of Chia (*Salvia hispanica* L.): A review. *Journal of Food Science and Technology, 53*(4), 1750–1758. https://doi.org/10.1007/s13197-015-1967-0.

Venugopalan, V. K., Gopakumar, L. R., Kumaran, A. K., Chatterjee, N. S., Soman, V., Peeralil, S., Mathew, S., McClements, D. J., & Nagarajarao, R. C. (2021). Encapsulation and protection of omega-3-rich fish oils using food-grade delivery systems. *Foods (Basel, Switzerland), 10*(7), 1566. https://doi.org/10.3390/foods10071566.

Viegas, C., Patrício, A. B., Prata, J. M., Nadhman, A., Chintamaneni, P. K., & Fonte, P. (2023). Solid lipid nanoparticles vs. nanostructured lipid carriers: A comparative review. *Pharmaceutics, 15*(6), 1593. https://doi.org/10.3390/pharmaceutics15061593.

Walker, R., Decker, E. A., & McClements, D. J. (2015). Development of food-grade nanoemulsions and emulsions for delivery of omega-3 fatty acids: Opportunities and obstacles in the food industry. *Food & Function, 6*(1), 42–55. https://doi.org/10.1039/c4fo00723a.

Wang, W. X., & Ko, M. L. (2023). Efficacy of omega-3 intake in managing dry eye disease: A systematic review and meta-analysis of randomized controlled trials. *Journal of Clinical Medicine, 12*(22), 7026. https://doi.org/10.3390/jcm12227026.

Wang, Y. Z., Fu, S. G., Wang, S. Y., Yang, D. J., Wu, Y. H. S., & Chen, Y. C. (2018). Effects of a natural antioxidant, polyphenol-rich rosemary (*Rosmarinus officinalis* L.) extract, on lipid stability of plant-derived omega-3 fatty-acid rich oil. *LWT, 89*, 210–216.

Wangkulangkool, M., Ketthaisong, D., Tangwongchai, R., Boonmars, T., & Lomthaisong, K. (2023). Microencapsulation of chia oil using whey protein and gum Arabic for oxidation prevention: A comparative study of spray-drying and freeze-drying methods. *Processes, 11*(5), 1462.

Watkins, B. A., Li, Y., Allen, K. G., Hoffmann, W. E., & Seifert, M. F. (2000). Dietary ratio of (n-6)/(n-3) polyunsaturated fatty acids alters the fatty acid composition of bone compartments and biomarkers of bone formation in rats. *The Journal of Nutrition, 130*(9), 2274–2284. https://doi.org/10.1093/jn/130.9.2274.

Wei, W., Cheng, Z., Wang, X., Chang, M., Xie, D., Sun, C., & Li, B. (2025). The potential of marine oils as functional foods: Nutritional composition, health benefits, applications, and future perspectives. *Food Reviews International,* 1–32.

Wen, J., Satyanarayanan, S. K., Li, A., Yan, L., Zhao, Z., Yuan, Q., Su, K. P., & Su, H. (2024). Unraveling the impact of Omega-3 polyunsaturated fatty acids on blood-brain barrier (BBB) integrity and glymphatic function. *Brain, Behavior, and Immunity, 115*, 335–355. https://doi.org/10.1016/j.bbi.2023.10.018.

West, A. L., Miles, E. A., Lillycrop, K. A., Napier, J. A., Calder, P. C., & Burdge, G. C. (2021). Genetically modified plants are an alternative to oily fish for providing *n*-3 polyunsaturated fatty acids in the human diet: A summary of the findings of a Biotechnology and Biological Sciences Research Council funded project. *Nutrition Bulletin, 46*(1), 60–68. https://doi.org/10.1111/nbu.12478.

Xie, D., Gong, M., Wei, W., Jin, J., Wang, X., Wang, X., & Jin, Q. (2019). Antarctic krill (*Euphausia superba*) oil: A comprehensive review of chemical composition, extraction technologies, health benefits, and current applications. *Comprehensive Reviews in Food Science and Food Safety, 18*(2), 514–534.

Yaghmur, A., Ghayas, S., Jan, H., Kalaycioglu, G. D., & Moghimi, S. M. (2023). Omega-3 fatty acid nanocarriers: Characterization and potential applications. *Current Opinion in Colloid & Interface Science, 67*, 101728.

Yanishlieva, N. V., & Marinova, E. M. (2001). Stabilisation of edible oils with natural antioxidants. *European Journal of Lipid Science and Technology, 103*(11), 752–767.

Yeung, A. W. K., Solka, M., Jóźwik, A., Ksepka, N., Matin, M., Wysocki, K., et al. (2025). Omega-3 fatty acids: Dietary components for the promotion of human and animal health. *Animal Science Papers and Reports, 43*(3), 235–260. https://doi.org/10.2478/aspr-2025-0017.

Yonezawa, K., Kusumoto, Y., Kanchi, N., Kinoshita, H., Kanegae, S., Yamaguchi, N., & Ozawa, H. (2020). Recent trends in mental illness and omega-3 fatty acids. *Journal of Neural Transmission (Vienna, Austria: 1996), 127*(11), 1491–1499. https://doi.org/10.1007/s00702-020-02212-z.

Yoshikiyo, K., Yoshioka, Y., Narumiya, Y., Oe, S., Kawahara, H., Kurata, K., & Yamamoto, T. (2019). Thermal stability and bioavailability of inclusion complexes of perilla oil with γ-cyclodextrin. *Food Chemistry, 294*, 56–59.

Zachwieja, A., Pecka-Kiełb, E., Zielak-Steciwko, A., Króliczewska, B., Kaszuba, J., & Kupczyński, R. (2025). Effect of rumen-protected cod liver oil supplementation on fatty acid profile of meat from Limousin and red Angus cattle. *Animals: An Open Access Journal from MDPI, 15*(13), 1856.

Zazula, M. F., Pozzan, R., dos Reis, G. A., Maciel, M., Horlem, T., Banckes, T. N., & Naliwaiko, K. (2025). Advances in oral drug delivery systems for natural polyunsaturated fatty acids: Enhancing bioavailability and therapeutic potential. *Pharmaceutics, 17*(11), 1377.

Zeppieri, M., Gagliano, C., D'Esposito, F., Musa, M., Gattazzo, I., Zanella, M. S., Rossi, F. B., Galan, A., & Babighian, S. (2024). Eicosapentaenoic acid (EPA) and docosahexaenoic acid (DHA): A targeted antioxidant strategy to counter oxidative stress in retinopathy. *Antioxidants (Basel, Switzerland), 14*(1), 6. https://doi.org/10.3390/antiox14010006.

Zhou, Q., & Wei, Z. (2023). Food-grade systems for delivery of DHA and EPA: Opportunities, fabrication, characterization and future perspectives. *Critical Reviews in Food Science and Nutrition, 63*(15), 2348–2365. https://doi.org/10.1080/10408398.2021.1974337.

Zhou, X., Tang, J., Jacobs, T. L., & Saguy, I. S. (2025). Transforming food supply chains through digital tracking and monitoring technologies. *Trends in Food Science & Technology,* 105142.

Section IV

Use in functional foods and product formulation

Chapter 16

Formulation techniques for polyunsaturated fatty acid-enriched foods

R. Rajam[1], Pothiyappan Karthik[1], Billu Abraham[2,3], Plachikkattu Parambil Akhila[2,4], and Karthikeyan Velayutham[1,5]

[1]*Department of Food Technology, Faculty of Engineering, Karpagam Academy of Higher Education, Coimbatore, Tamil Nadu, India,* [2]*Centre for Food Nanotechnology, Karpagam Academy of Higher Education, Coimbatore, Tamil Nadu, India,* [3]*Department of Chemistry, Faculty of Arts, Science, Commerce, and Management, Karpagam Academy of Higher Education, Coimbatore, Tamil Nadu, India,* [4]*Department of Biotechnology, Faculty of Arts, Science, Commerce, and Management, Karpagam Academy of Higher Education, Coimbatore, Tamil Nadu, India,* [5]*Centre for Nanotechnology, Karpagam Academy of Higher Education, Coimbatore, Tamil Nadu, India*

16.1 Introduction

Fatty acids (FAs) of plant and animal sources are composed of long-chain carboxylic acids, and the specific types and proportions of FAs within cell membranes vary across different tissues. This variation enables cells to maintain structural integrity while supporting the function of membrane-associated proteins (Gammone et al., 2018). FAs are broadly classified into saturated and unsaturated based on the presence of a double bond in their hydrocarbon chain (Fig. 16.1). Saturated FAs can be synthesized endogenously from carbohydrates and excess energy by FA synthesis, and their intake from external dietary sources is not essential. FAs with two or more double bonds in the hydrocarbon chain are classified as polyunsaturated fatty acids (PUFAs) and are essential for human health. PUFAs are broadly classified into two major families, omega-3 (n-3) and omega-6 (n-6), based on the position of the first double bond from the methyl (omega) end of the carbon chain. The essential precursors for omega-3 and omega-6 families are α-linolenic acid (ALA; 18:3 n-3) and linoleic acid (LA; 18:2 n-6), respectively. Omega-3 FAs must be obtained through the diet because humans lack the enzymes required for their de novo synthesis. Following ingestion, essential FAs are converted into longer-chain derivatives through a series of desaturation and elongation reactions. Linoleic acid (LA) is converted through enzymatic pathways into arachidonic acid (AA; 20:4 n-6), a primary precursor for eicosanoids involved in inflammatory and immune responses. Conversely, ALA serves as a metabolic precursor for the synthesis of omega-3 FAs such as eicosapentaenoic acid (EPA; 20:5 n-3) and docosahexaenoic acid (DHA; 22:6 n-3), which contribute to cardiovascular, neurological, and antiinflammatory benefits (Gill & Valivety, 1997; Kapoor et al., 2021; Liu et al., 2023). Although the human body can convert ALA into EPA and DHA, the conversion efficiency is relatively low due to the competition between omega-3 and omega-6 FAs for the same desaturase and elongase enzymes. This competitive metabolic pathway significantly limits the endogenous synthesis of long-chain omega-3 PUFAs, with conversion rates typically ranging from 8% to 20% for EPA and less than 10% for DHA. This endogenous conversion of precursor FAs is not sufficient to meet the daily requirement of long-chain PUFAs in the human body, and EPA and DHA must be obtained through dietary sources to maintain health (Timilsena et al., 2017).

Adequate dietary intake of omega-3 FAs reduced the risk of cardiovascular mortality through modulating arrhythmias, blood pressure, and lipid profiles, and by inhibiting platelet aggregation. In addition, omega-3 FAs have shown improvements in metabolic and inflammatory disorders including obesity, type 2 diabetes mellitus, depression, degenerative eye diseases, and arthritis related pain. They also play an important role in maternal health and in reducing the incidence of premature births. Thus, omega-3 FAs must be included in the human diet at approximate intake levels of 1 g per day due to multiple health benefits (Yashodhara et al., 2009). The requirement of EPA and DHA can be met through consumption of marine sources rich in omega-3 FAs or the plant sources that provide their precursors. Marine sources rich in EPA and DHA are fatty fishes (e.g., salmon, mackerel, sardine, tuna), microalgae, and krill oil. In contrast, dietary plant sources provide

Omega-3 and Omega-6 Polyunsaturated Fatty Acids in Food Systems. DOI: https://doi.org/10.1016/B978-0-443-43810-3.00012-9

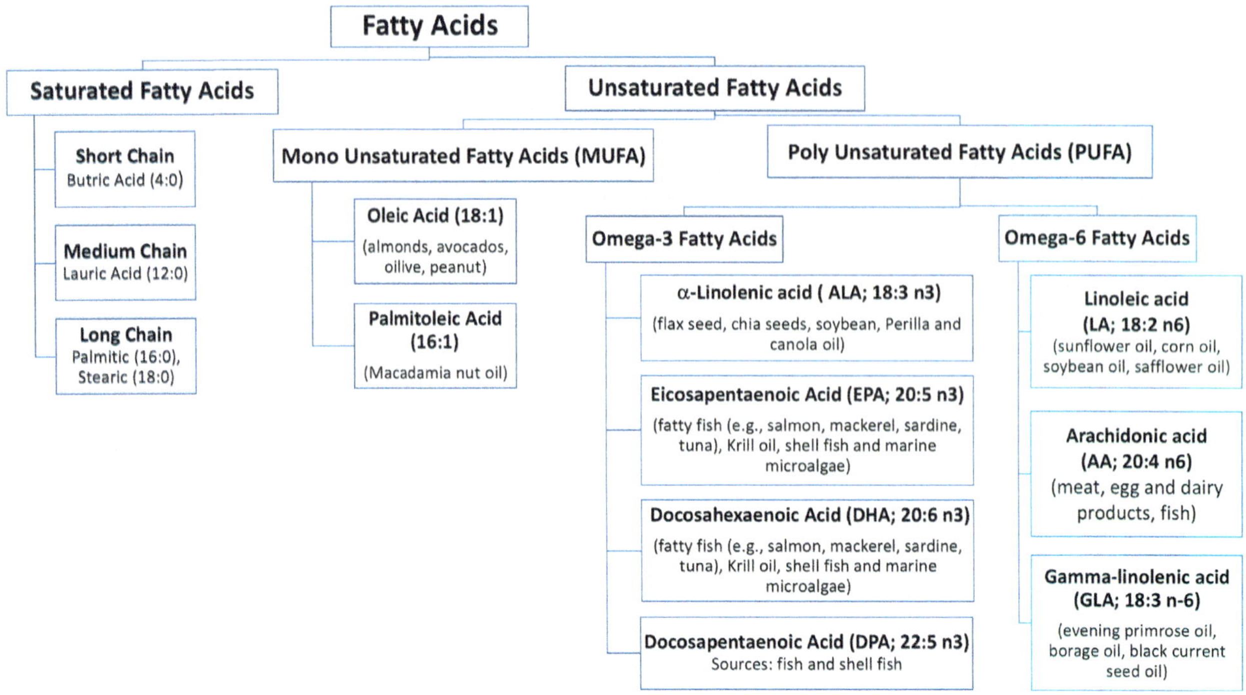

FIGURE 16.1 Classification of fatty acids and their sources.

ALA, a precursor for the formation of long-chain of omega-3 FAs, and are commonly found in soybean, flaxseed, and chia oils. Additionally, omega-6 FAs such as LA and arachidonic acid (AA) are present in corn, rice bran, and peanut oils and in animal products, including eggs and dairy-based products. These plant-based sources are alternatives for individuals with low fish consumption or those following vegetarian or vegan diets (Kapoor et al., 2021; Yashodhara et al., 2009). Dietary supplementation is essential for individuals suffering from the above-mentioned disorders or diseases (Kapoor et al., 2021; Wang et al., 2025; Yashodhara et al., 2009). Omega-3 and omega-6 FAs supplementation in food and pharmaceutical products has been widely approved globally, and various health agencies have published guidelines regarding the supplementation of these FAs. To control cardiovascular mortality, long-chain omega-3 PUFAs are recommended in a regular diet (Kapoor et al., 2021).

Due to their structural characteristics, PUFAs are highly prone to oxidation during processing and storage, which reduces their nutritional value and leads to the formation of unwanted free radicals (Zhu et al., 2025). Various delivery systems, including emulsions, Pickering emulsions, liposomes, hydrogels, and microcapsules, are suggested to prevent oxidative deterioration, improve bioavailability, and enhance controlled release of FAs at the target site. The efficacy of DHA depends on factors such as dose level, duration of supplementation, sex, and age (Arnoldussen & Kiliaan, 2014). The targeted delivery approaches enable the transport and release of active substances at specific sites, resulting in enhanced therapeutic efficacy and improved bioavailability (Zhu et al., 2025). In this context, a recent study reported that higher concentrations of EPA and DHA availability at the target site reduced the release of FAs, which resulted in decreased levels of micellar vesicle formation under in vitro lipolysis conditions; but at the same time, emulsification doubled FA release. Further, in vivo findings confirmed that DHA bioavailability is governed by micelle formation, and EPA uptake is governed by lipolysis. These findings highlight the impact of composition and emulsification on the bioavailability of omega-3 FAs, which is important for designing effective PUFA delivery systems (Abdelhafez et al., 2026).

Different encapsulation approaches are developed for the effective delivery of PUFA-rich oils into the food system. Spray drying and freeze drying are the conventional drying techniques used to transform liquids into powdered form. Shorter residence time in spray drying and low temperature conditions in freeze drying are found to be highly suitable for encapsulating thermally sensitive materials with an acceptable level of encapsulation efficiency. Emulsification reduced droplet size, which in turn improves emulsion stability, which directly influences encapsulation efficiency and improves bioavailability after digestion. Spray freeze drying is an alternative technique that combines the physicochemical properties of spray- and freeze-dried microcapsules. Complex coacervation has also been explored to improve encapsulation efficiency and oxidative stability. This technique forms a dense polymeric coating around oil droplets through electrostatic interactions. Moreover, combinations of methods, such as emulsification followed by spray drying or freeze drying, and coacervation combined with freeze drying, are increasingly being applied to achieve better encapsulation efficiency, improved oxidative stability, and controlled release profiles. Oleogel-based delivery systems are another emerging approach, particularly in bakery applications, where they can replace saturated fats with healthier unsaturated omega-3 and omega-6 FAs by structuring liquid oil into a semisolid network without altering the FA composition. These technological advancements form the basis for the development of omega-3-rich PUFAs fortification in food systems, which are discussed in detail in the following sections.

16.2 Physicochemical and nutritional properties of polyunsaturated fatty acids

PUFAs are essential nutrients that are required for the execution of normal physiological functions and should be obtained from the diet. They are inherently rich in different food sources, mainly in plant and marine sources (Zhu et al., 2025). PUFAs have obtained much attention over the past 40 years with value-added applications in the food, nutrition, and pharmaceutical industries. The increasing interest in PUFAs is mainly due to the evidence gathered for their multimodal benefits in human health (Jacobsen & Let, 2006). PUFAs are vital for maintaining human health, supporting anti-inflammatory responses, enhancing cardiovascular function, improving cognitive performance, and preserving overall cellular integrity (Zakaria et al., 2025). According to the World Health Organization, nearly 41 million deaths were attributed to noncommunicable diseases in 2018 alone. The development of noncommunicable chronic diseases is strongly associated with underlying processes such as inflammation and oxidative stress. PUFAs are known to modulate both antioxidant defense mechanisms and inflammatory signaling pathways, thereby helping mitigate these conditions (Zakaria et al., 2025). The distinctive physical and chemical characteristics of PUFAs arise from the presence of multiple double bonds within their molecular structure. Nevertheless, this makes them especially susceptible to oxidation (Zhu et al., 2025). The presence of multiple double bonds increases their reactivity, leading to the formation of various oxidative metabolites and reactive oxygen species (ROS). Lipid oxidation is detrimental to oils because it decreases nutritional aspects and generates distasteful flavors, resulting in lowered acceptance among consumers. This instance emphasizes the need for appropriate measures to reduce oxidative degradation during processing and storage (Islam et al., 2023; Zhu et al., 2025). Therefore, a sound knowledge of PUFA structure, their oxidation susceptibility, and factors bestowing or limiting bioavailability is necessary for developing suitable PUFA-enriched foods. Hence, emphasizing the need to adopt suitable strategies to limit oxidative damage in processing and storage. Thus, knowledge of PUFA structure, their susceptibility to oxidation, and the factors affecting their availability is essential for designing effective PUFA-enriched food products.

16.2.1 Structural classification and conversion pathways

PUFAs are defined by having two or more double bonds along their hydrocarbon chain. They are mainly grouped into omega-3 (n-3) and omega-6 (n-6) families based on the position of the first double bond from the methyl end of the molecule (Zakaria et al., 2025). Omega-3 FAs include ALA, EPA, and DHA, which are commonly present in sources such as microalgae, bacteria, fish, and other marine organisms. In contrast, omega-6 FAs consist of LA, γ-linolenic acid (GLA), and arachidonic acid (AA) (Wang et al., 2025). ALA acts as the starter molecule for the synthesis of omega-3 FAs, whereas LA acts as the starter molecule for the synthesis of omega-6 FAs in the human body. After ingestion, they are metabolized via three main biochemical pathways. Initially, LA and ALA are integrated into cellular phospholipids, where they function as an energy store. They can also undergo β-oxidation, releasing energy and forming CO_2. Additionally, they are metabolically transformed into physiologically important PUFAs like GLA, ARA, EPA, and DHA (Ruiz-López et al., 2012). The pathway regulating the conversion of omega-3 and omega-6 FAs starts with the enzyme Δ6-desaturase, which adds a double bond to LA and ALA, forming GLA and stearidonic acid as products. These products then undergo chain elongation mediated by elongase-5, resulting in the formation of dihomo-γ-linolenic acid and eicosatetraenoic acid. Later desaturation steps result in the synthesis of ARA and EPA. The FA chains may then undergo further elongation and desaturation reactions promoted by Δ6-desaturase. The last stage, β-oxidation, creates a complete pathway for metabolic docosapentaenoic acid and DHA.

16.2.2 Mechanisms of oxidative degradation

A significant limitation in the application of PUFAs for food and pharmaceutical areas is their significant susceptibility to oxidative deterioration (Jacobsen & Let, 2006). PUFAs are structurally very liable to oxidative degradation owing to the presence of multiple unsaturated bonds (Zhu et al., 2025). A higher number of double bonds means that the FA is more prone to oxidation. DHA, for example, is almost five times as oxidizable as LA (Jacobsen & Let, 2006). This extreme oxidative sensitivity causes challenges for both processing and storage, as these unsaturated bonds easily yield a range of metabolites and ROS. Lipid oxidation can be generally categorized into two groups: enzymatic and nonenzymatic oxidation. Nonenzymatic oxidation involves autoxidation by free-radical mechanisms and photooxidation mediated by ultraviolet light or singlet oxygen (Islam et al., 2023; Zhu et al., 2025). Autoxidation refers to a self-propagating free-radical mechanism with O_2, which starts with initiation, propagation, and ends with termination as principal steps (Jacobsen & Let, 2006). Initiators like heat, metal ions, or protein-derived radicals initiate autoxidation by forming carbon-centered alkyl radicals from unsaturated FAs. This means that in the presence of oxygen, these radicals are propagated through a free radical chain reaction to peroxyl radicals and finally hydroperoxides. Hydroperoxides are the main products of autoxidation, and they are tasteless and odorless. This chain reaction continues until two radicals combine to yield a stable, nonradical compound that eliminates the chain reaction. The cleavage of hydroperoxides leads to secondary species (e.g., alkoxyl and peroxyl radicals), which can perpetuate the chain reaction. These intermediates ultimately undergo thermal decomposition to yield a series of secondary oxidation products, both volatile and nonvolatile. These secondary products are primarily responsible for the deterioration of flavor (Jacobsen & Let, 2006).

Whereas photooxidation occurs only in the presence of light and can be amplified when photosensitizing compounds are present within the food structure. Photooxidation results in the formation of hydroperoxides from unsaturated FAs when they are exposed to light in the presence of photosensitizing agents. In food systems, compounds such as chlorophyll, riboflavin, and hemoproteins act as photosensitizers. These are activated by absorbing visible or near-UV light and interact with unsaturated FAs, forming lipid radicals. The interaction of lipid radicals with oxygen results in peroxyl radicals, which later hydrolyze to hydroperoxides in the type I sensitizer mechanism. Whereas, in the type II sensitizer mechanism, the photosensitizers absorb light, get excited, interact directly with oxygen, and transfer energy. This produces highly reactive singlet oxygen, which interacts with FA double bonds and forms hydroperoxides. These hydroperoxides undergo similar decomposition reactions, such as autoxidation (Jacobsen & Let, 2006). In contrast, enzymatic oxidation is mediated by specific enzymes such as lipoxygenase, naturally present in plant and animal tissues. In addition, oxidation of PUFAs may cause unfavorable flavor changes, and the process may also lead to the development of potentially harmful substances, thus affecting human health. In order to solve the oxidative instability problems associated with PUFAs, different approaches have been developed, for example, antioxidants and delivery systems for the encapsulation of PUFAs (Islam et al., 2023).

16.2.3 Bioavailability

Bioavailability is critically important to the physiological and clinical effects of PUFAs. Bioavailability describes the extent of release from food and digestion, absorption, and distribution in the body (Alijani et al., 2025). In addition, PUFAs constitute a widely studied compound with limited bioavailability that limits optimal absorption into the human body. Studies have shown that omega-6 and omega-3 FAs must be obtained through dietary intake of LA and ALA to ensure sufficient levels in the body. For instance, in the case of ALA, a large proportion is metabolized through β-oxidation after ingestion, producing energy and carbon dioxide, while only a small amount is converted into EPA and DHA (Saini & Keum, 2018; Zhu et al., 2025). The bioavailability of PUFAs is influenced by multiple factors, including molecular structure, concurrent dietary fat intake, processing method, formulation, and the presence of excessive fiber and other drugs, whereas endogenous factors include gastrointestinal health, age, and gender (Alijani et al., 2025). The chemical form of these compounds varies across marine sources, such as fish, algae, krill, and Calanus finmarchicus. For instance, krill oil is frequently promoted with claims that its omega-3 FAs, present in phospholipid form, are absorbed more efficiently than those in fish oil (Alijani et al., 2025).

The low efficiency of ALA to long-chain PUFA conversion rate underscores the importance of adequate dietary intake to achieve effective conversion. Daily intake of 10 g of flaxseed powder substantially enhances circulating ALA levels in healthy young adults; however, a higher intake of 30 g per day is necessary for the EPA production (Edel et al., 2015). Furthermore, the composition of the food may affect the bioavailability of PUFAs, as dietary fat in the matrix can facilitate lipid digestion and absorption. On the other hand, some drugs, such as antibiotics, orlistat, H_2 blockers, and proton pump inhibitors, as well as high dietary fiber, may hinder digestion in the digestive tract. Food processing can also impact the stability of PUFAs, and during frying, EPA and DHA oxidation may be hastened, leading to reduced bioavailability (Alijani et al., 2026).

Another demographic that influences ALA conversion tariffs is gender. Unlike men, women also seem to retain a better capacity for converting ALA into EPA and DHA, which is thought to be related to the stimulation of Δ6-desaturase activity associated with estrogen (Yuan et al., 2022). This conversion efficiency is further enhanced in pregnant women, as their metabolism is adjusted to accommodate the enhanced DHA requirements of the fetus. Numerous health conditions contribute to a reduced capacity of ALA to be used as a precursor for EPA and DHA, linked to diseases such as cardiovascular diseases, obesity, type II diabetes, metabolic syndrome, or nonalcoholic fatty liver (Cholewski et al., 2018). In addition, age is a significant factor in determining ALA metabolism efficiency. A study conducted on the comparison of 38-year-old and 50-year-old males indicated that the older population has a significantly lower capacity to metabolize ALA into EPA and DHA, as the rate of conversion is three to six times lower than in younger individuals. Finally, the imbalance of omega-3 and omega-6 FAs is a relevant variable because they use the same metabolic enzymes in the human body (Yuan et al., 2022). Thus, improving the bioavailability of PUFAs through the production of advanced delivery systems is crucial for them to exert their proper efficacy (Zhu et al., 2025).

16.3 Challenges in polyunsaturated fatty acids-enriched food development

PUFAs, particularly omega-3 and omega-6 FAs, have gained significant interest due to their well-established beneficial effects on cardiovascular health, cognitive development, and metabolic control (Visioli et al., 2026). Thus, the production of functional foods enriched in PUFAs has emerged as a significant area of research in food science and nutrition. However, despite their nutritional value, fortification of foods with PUFAs is technologically challenging due to their chemical instability and potential for oxidative degradation (Islam et al., 2023; Shahidi & Hossain, 2022). The presence of several double bonds in the molecules of the PUFA makes them especially susceptible to lipid oxidation. Exposure to oxygen, light, heat, and metal ions can trigger a series of oxidation reactions that lead to the formation of hydroperoxides and volatile compounds responsible for rancid off-flavors (Shahidi & Hossain, 2022). These oxidative reactions significantly reduce both the nutritional value and sensory quality of PUFA-enriched foods (Ghelichi et al., 2021). Besides oxidative instability, another issue in the formulation of complex food systems containing PUFAs is associated with their hydrophobic character. Most foods contain large amounts of aqueous phases, and PUFAs require effective dispersion systems for stability (Lopes et al., 2023). Processing conditions such as heating, homogenization, oxygen exposure, and mechanical shear can further accelerate lipid oxidation and structural degradation of PUFA molecules (Semenoglou et al., 2025).

16.3.1 Oxidation and sensory attributes

Lipid oxidation is one of the main barriers to the successful use of PUFAs in food systems. Oxidation of unsaturated FAs is a free radical chain reaction that occurs in three steps: initiation, propagation, decomposition, and termination (Halliwell & Chirico, 1993). During the initiation stage, ROS or pro-oxidant metal ions react with PUFA molecules to produce lipid radicals. These lipid radicals react quickly with oxygen to produce lipid peroxyl radicals that can initiate lipid peroxidation by reacting with other lipid molecules. The propagation stage gives rise to the formation of lipid hydroperoxides, which are unstable compounds that degrade to secondary oxidation products, including aldehydes, ketones, and alcohols (Shahidi & Hossain, 2022). These compounds are associated with the formation of unpleasant tastes and odors, which are normally associated with oxidized lipids. For example, volatile aldehydes such as hexanal and propanal are normally used as an indicator for the oxidation of lipids in PUFA-rich systems (Islam et al., 2023). EPA and DHA, which are types of omega-3 FAs, are highly prone to oxidative degradation because of their high level of unsaturation. DHA has six double bonds, which make it highly prone to oxidative degradation compared to saturated or monounsaturated FAs (Swetha & Mathanghi, 2024). Therefore, marine oil that contains EPA and DHA is highly prone to oxidative degradation when incorporated into food products. In addition to affecting the nutritional value, oxidation of PUFAs significantly influences the sensory properties. Even low levels of oxidation byproducts are sufficient to cause off-flavors, which have been described as fishy, metallic, and rancid (Ganesan et al., 2014). The unpalatable sensory properties of PUFA-fortified foods have significant implications for consumer acceptability. Oxidative stability is therefore one of the greatest challenges for technologists seeking to formulate functional foods containing PUFAs.

16.3.2 Food matrix incompatibility

In addition to oxidative instability, another challenge associated with the incorporation of hydrophobic PUFA-rich oils into foods is the incompatibility of these lipids with water. Many foods, such as drinks, dairy, and sauces, have large water contents, and this is a challenge for the incorporation of lipid components, as noted by Islam et al. (2023). The addition of PUFA oil in an aqueous food system can lead to physical instability such as phase separation, creaming, or oil leakage during storage. Such instability in the food system can adversely affect the texture, appearance, and quality of the final food product (Pattnaik & Mishra, 2022). In addition, the distribution of PUFA oil in the food system can lead to variations in the nutritional content of different parts of the food system. These variations are further complicated by the nature of the food processing conditions. Thus, improving sensory quality and enhancing the health benefits of PUFA-enriched food products can be effective strategies to increase consumer acceptability.

16.4 Conventional approaches of polyunsaturated fatty acid delivery

Several strategies have been developed for improving the dietary intake of essential FAs through food fortification. Amongst these strategies, the direct addition of PUFA-rich oil in food formulations is one of the most commonly used methods, owing to its simplicity and cost-effectiveness (Pattnaik & Mishra, 2022). This method requires the incorporation of oil sources of marine or plant origin into food products. Oils rich in PUFAs like fish oil, flaxseed oil, chia seed oil, and algal oil have been extensively used for the formulation of functional food products due to their high omega-3 content (Shahidi & Hossain, 2022). However, despite the simplicity of the method, direct oil incorporation is often characterized by a number of limitations. The direct addition of PUFA-rich oils to food systems is considered to be one of the earliest measures to increase the nutritional value of food products. Marine oils obtained from fish oils and krill oils are known to have high levels of EPA and DHA, whereas flaxseed oil and chia oil have high levels of ALA (Wei et al., 2025). Such oils are generally directly added to food formulations such as dairy products, spreads, bakery items, and infant formula during processing. This method is relatively simple and does not need complex equipment or advanced encapsulation technology. This has enabled the successful development of various PUFA-fortified foods commercially containing these oils (Villamil et al., 2024). However, the addition of PUFA-rich oils in this manner can lead to rapid oxidation and flavor deterioration during storage. In addition, marine oils could impart fishy flavors, which could be detrimental to food acceptability (Wei et al., 2025).

Despite these applications, there are some major technological limitations of conventional incorporation of PUFA, such as oxidative deterioration, lack of sensory stability, and phase separation, which may result in reduced product shelf life and consumer acceptance. The major PUFA-rich oils currently used for food fortification, along with their major technological limitations, are presented in Table 16.1. In recent times, there has been much emphasis on the development of advanced PUFA delivery systems, such as nanoemulsion, microencapsulation, and oleogel technology, for improved stability and bioavailability of PUFA in functional foods (Lazăr et al., 2024).

Abbreviations: EPA, eicosapentaenoic acid; DHA, docosahexaenoic acid; ALA, α-linolenic acid; LA, linoleic acid; PUFA, polyunsaturated fatty acids.

16.5 Emulsion-based polyunsaturated fatty acid delivery systems

Emulsion-based delivery systems have emerged as promising approaches for improving the oxidative stability, bioavailability, and targeted delivery of PUFAs (Wang et al., 2025; Zhu et al., 2025). The composition and structure

TABLE 16.1 Application of polyunsaturated fatty acid (PUFA) rich oils in foods and technological limitations.

PUFA source	Major PUFA	Typical food applications	Technological limitations	References
Fish oil	EPA, DHA	Dairy and spreads	Fishy flavor, oxidation	Turp and Ozuesen (2025)
Krill oil	EPA, DHA	Nutraceutical foods	Oxidative instability	Attri et al. (2024)
Algal oil	DHA	Infant formula	High cost	Liu et al. (2022)
Flaxseed oil	ALA	Bakery products	Thermal instability	Al-Madhagy et al. (2023)
Chia oil	ALA	Functional beverages	Phase separation	Tak et al. (2022)
Perilla oil	ALA	Functional foods	Oxidative degradation	Guan et al. (2024)
Hemp seed oil	ALA, LA	Nutrition bars	Short shelf life	Presa-Lombardi et al. (2023)
Camelina oil	ALA	Salad dressings	Oxidative instability	Mondor and Hernández-Álvarez (2022)
Walnut oil	LA, ALA	Bakery and snacks	Flavor instability	Akhtar et al. (2022)
Soybean oil	LA	Processed foods	Oxidation during storage	Da Rosa et al. (2025)

of emulsions, that is, oil phase, water phase, and interface, significantly contribute to their stability. Thus emulsion-based systems must be designed to improve the oxidative stability of food products containing PUFAs (Wang et al., 2020).

16.5.1 Oil-in-water emulsions

Oil-in-water (O/W) emulsions are well recognized as one of the most effective and widely used systems for incorporating PUFAs. In O/W emulsions, the oil phase of PUFAs is present as a suspension of fine droplets in the aqueous phase (Fig. 16.2). This method is commonly used due to its ease of preparation, cost-effectiveness, and compatibility with various food systems. Unlike other oils, oil-in-water emulsions offer advantages such as oxidative stability, as the emulsifier forms a protective layer on the oil droplets surfaces, thereby slowing oxidation. In addition, surface-active molecules may adsorb at the interface and provide a protective film around the oil droplets. This would provide an additional layer of protection against free radicals, thereby enhancing lipid oxidative stability (Wang et al., 2020).

16.5.2 Nanoemulsions

Nanoemulsion technology represents an advanced approach for improving the delivery and stability of PUFAs. Among several emulsion-based delivery systems, nanoemulsions have gained significant attention due to easy formulation, high stability, small droplet size, and higher bioavailability (Walker et al., 2015). These systems are defined by their less than 100 nm mean particle radii that provide a high surface area and greater aqueous solubility (Wang et al., 2020). However, compared to microemulsions, nanoemulsions exhibit thermodynamic instability. Nanoemulsions are a common formulation in the food and pharmaceutical industry, serving as delivery vehicles for encapsulating, protecting, and delivering bioactive agents (Ezhilarasi et al., 2012). Nanoemulsions have a small particle size, which has both merits and demerits (Walker et al., 2015). Although the underlying principles are still hotly debated, smaller droplets of lipophilic bioactive compounds have been shown to have a generally higher bioavailability than larger droplets. The increased specific surface area of smaller particles enhances enzyme accessibility at the oil-water interface, thereby promoting more efficient lipid digestion. In addition, smaller droplets penetrate the mucus layer with which epithelial cells of the small intestine are covered, providing an increased opportunity for digestion and absorption. These small particles may also traverse the mucus barrier and be directly taken up by epithelial cells. Furthermore, due to curvature effects, smaller droplets can increase the apparent solubility of encapsulated lipophilic compounds in the surrounding aqueous phase near the particle surface, thereby enhancing the driving force for their absorption (Walker et al., 2015). The oxidative stability of PUFAs in such systems is strongly influenced by the properties of the interfacial layer, including its thickness, charge, and composition. Proper design of the emulsion interface can significantly reduce interactions between lipid droplets and pro-oxidants, thereby slowing oxidation reactions. Additionally, structural modifications such as gelation of nanoemulsions have been shown to further enhance stability by reducing peroxide formation during storage. Overall, nanoemulsion-based systems offer improved control over PUFA protection by precisely manipulating interfacial characteristics and system structure (Wang et al., 2020).

16.5.3 Antioxidants and emulsion stability

Antioxidants are crucial for improving the oxidative stability of PUFAs in emulsion-based delivery systems. The addition of antioxidants is one of the main strategies to slow down lipid oxidation. Examples of antioxidants include natural

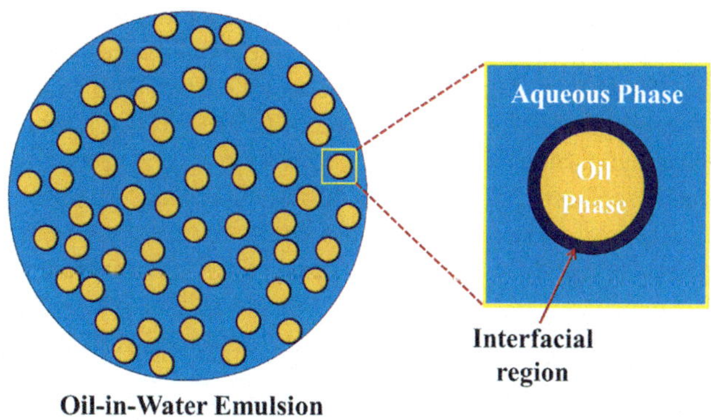

FIGURE 16.2 Oil-in-water emulsion.

compounds like α-tocopherol, followed by synthetic antioxidants such as butylated hydroxytoluene (BHT). Antioxidants primarily act by chelating metal ions and scavenging free radicals (Walker et al., 2015). This process helps prevent the initiation and propagation of lipid oxidation reactions. In emulsion systems, antioxidant efficiency depends on their chemical composition and position within the system, especially at the oil-water interface, where oxidation begins. In addition, emulsifying agents such as protein and phospholipids have inherent antioxidant activities (Karthik & Anandharamakrishnan, 2016b). They have the ability to inactivate free radicals and chelate pro-oxidative metals. Antioxidant activity is significant in nanoemulsion systems, especially given the lipid droplets large surface area, which makes them prone to oxidation. The selection and enhancement of antioxidants are essential for maintaining the stability of PUFA-enriched food products, prolonging shelf life, and maintaining quality (Walker et al., 2015; Wang et al., 2020).

16.6 Micro and nanoencapsulation-based polyunsaturated fatty acid delivery system

Although PUFAs are naturally present in plant, animal, and protist sources, their production, storage, and utilization involve numerous technical challenges (Vera et al., 2026). The main challenge is that these unsaturated FAs are highly vulnerable to oxidative degradation, and their sensory acceptability limits their utilization in food products. To prevent oxidative degradation of PUFAs, microencapsulation is a suitable method to retain the functional properties of the oils as well as to mask the unacceptable flavor (Karthik & Anandharamakrishnan, 2012; Vijaykrishnaraj et al., 2024). Microencapsulation entraps the lipids in protective wall materials, prevents oxidation, and enables targeted release. In recent years, microencapsulation techniques have been widely recognized for controlled delivery of functional ingredients in food materials. Omega -3 FAs have been encapsulated using various techniques such as spray drying (Areekal et al., 2024; Castejón et al., 2021; Ho et al., 2025; Hussain et al., 2025; Karthik & Anandharamakrishnan, 2012), freeze drying (Abdel-Razek et al., 2022; Anwar & Kunz, 2011; Heinzelmann et al., 2000; Koo et al., 2023; Rojas et al., 2019), spray freeze drying (Anand et al., 2024; Karthik & Anandharamakrishnan, 2012), coacervation (Cui et al., 2025; Dabiri Movahed et al., 2024; Mu et al., 2022; Timilsena et al., 2017; Wangsuntornpakdee et al., 2023), and electrospraying/electrospinning (Bisinotto et al., 2026; Natsia et al., 2026; Pires et al., 2023). In addition, emerging and combined approaches, including complex coacervation, emulsification followed by spray drying, emulsification followed by freeze drying, coacervation combined with freeze drying, and oleogelation, have also been explored to improve oxidative stability, controlled release, and improve the bioavailability of omega-3 FAs in the intestinal epithelium (Vera et al., 2026) (see Fig. 16.3).

16.6.1 Spray drying

Among the encapsulation techniques, spray drying is a relatively cost-effective method that provides higher encapsulation efficiency and improved oxidative stability. According to the recent investigation, spray drying is the highly preferred method to encapsulate omega-3 FAs from plant, animal, and protist sources (Figure 16.3 (A), (B), and (C)) (Vera et al., 2026). To meet consumer demand for foods enriched with omega-3 FAs, spray drying is the appropriate method for industrial-scale production (Gharsallaoui et al., 2007). Encapsulation by spray drying transforms the fats and oils into physically and chemically stable, free-flowing powders of micron-sized particles. Entrapment of PUFAs in biopolymer matrices masks the undesirable flavor, prevents oxidative degradation, and enables controlled release of core under specific environmental conditions (Karthik & Anandharamakrishnan, 2012).

To produce spray-dried PUFA-loaded microcapsules, oil-in-water emulsions are first prepared by mixing the oil phase with the aqueous phase containing wall material at an appropriate core-to-wall ratio using high-speed homogenization. To enhance emulsion stability and further lipid particle size reduction, these emulsions can be subjected to two to three cycles of high-pressure homogenization (Karthik & Anandharamakrishnan, 2016a). The stabilized emulsions are immediately spray dried by atomizing into fine droplets in a heated air stream (160°C–180°C), which transforms the liquid form of droplets into free-flowing micron-sized particles (Fig. 16.4). Moisture from the droplets evaporates instantly, resulting in the formation of dried microcapsules. Short residence time during spray drying reduces thermal degradation, which is essential for retaining the functionality of bioactive core compounds. Encapsulation efficiency can be influenced by the type and composition of wall materials, core-to-wall ratio, inlet and outlet air temperatures, feed rate, and hot air flow rate during spray drying (Karthik & Anandharamakrishnan, 2012). Particle size of spray-dried microcapsules is governed by the type of nozzle used for feed atomization, viscosity of feed material, and feed discharge rate (Chang & Nickerson, 2018). Spray-dried microcapsule encapsulation efficiency highly relies on the use of suitable wall materials. Table 16.2 complies with the recently reported studies on encapsulation of PUFA-rich oils using selected wall materials, formulation variables, and spray drying operating conditions for the production of dried microcapsules. Biopolymers such as

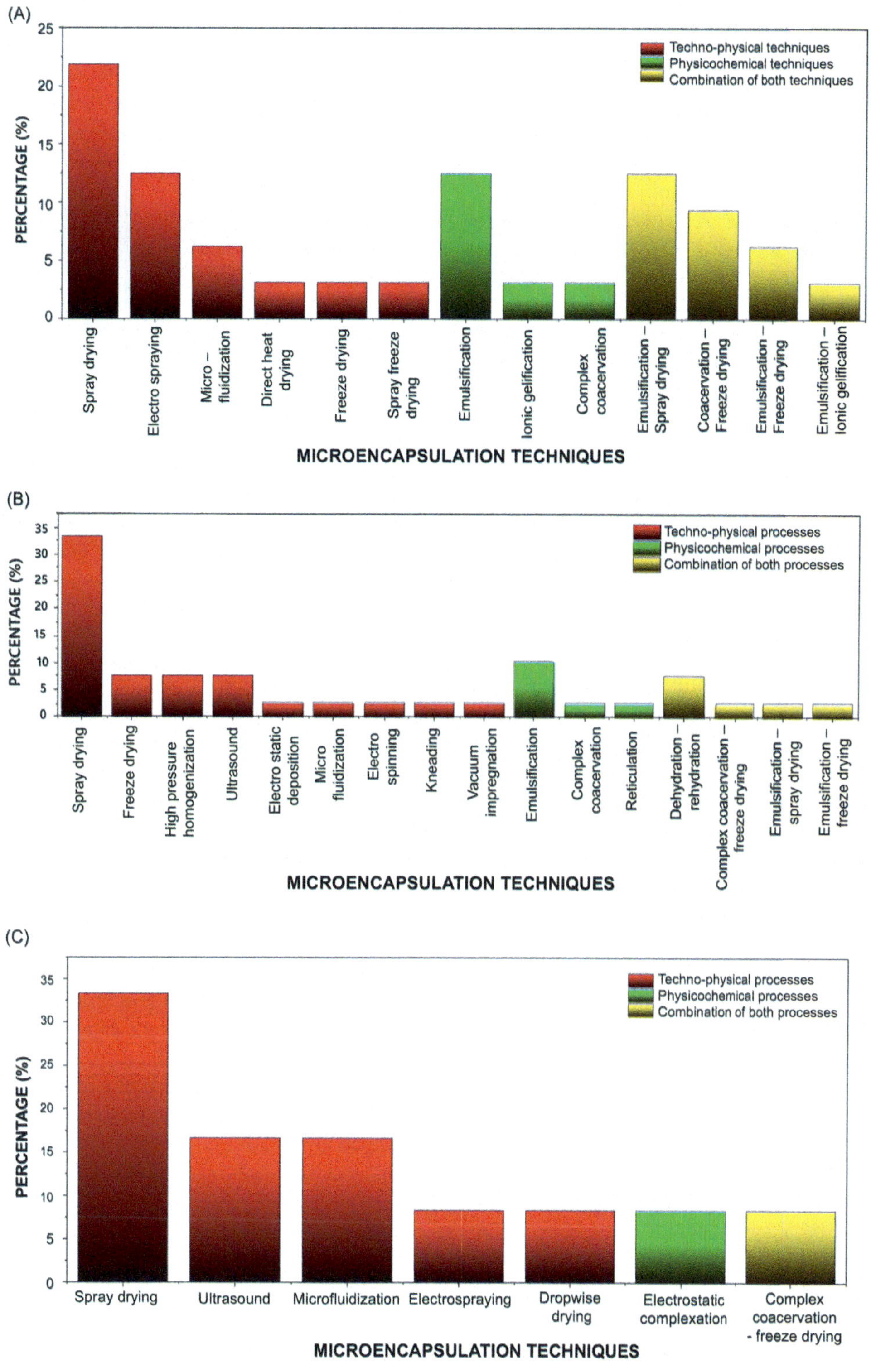

FIGURE 16.3 Most used microencapsulation techniques for the protection of omega-3 from (A) animal sources, (B) plant sources, and (C) protist sources (Vera et al. 2026).

Source: From Vera, W., Muñoz-More, H. D., Ruiz-Flores, L. A., Nole-Jaramillo, J. M., Nolazco-Cama, D. M., & Espinoza-Espinoza, L. A. (2026). Trends and viability of omega-3 fatty acid microencapsulation: A bibliometric and critical analysis. Applied Food Research, 6(1), 101685. https://doi.org/10.1016/j.afres.2026.101685.

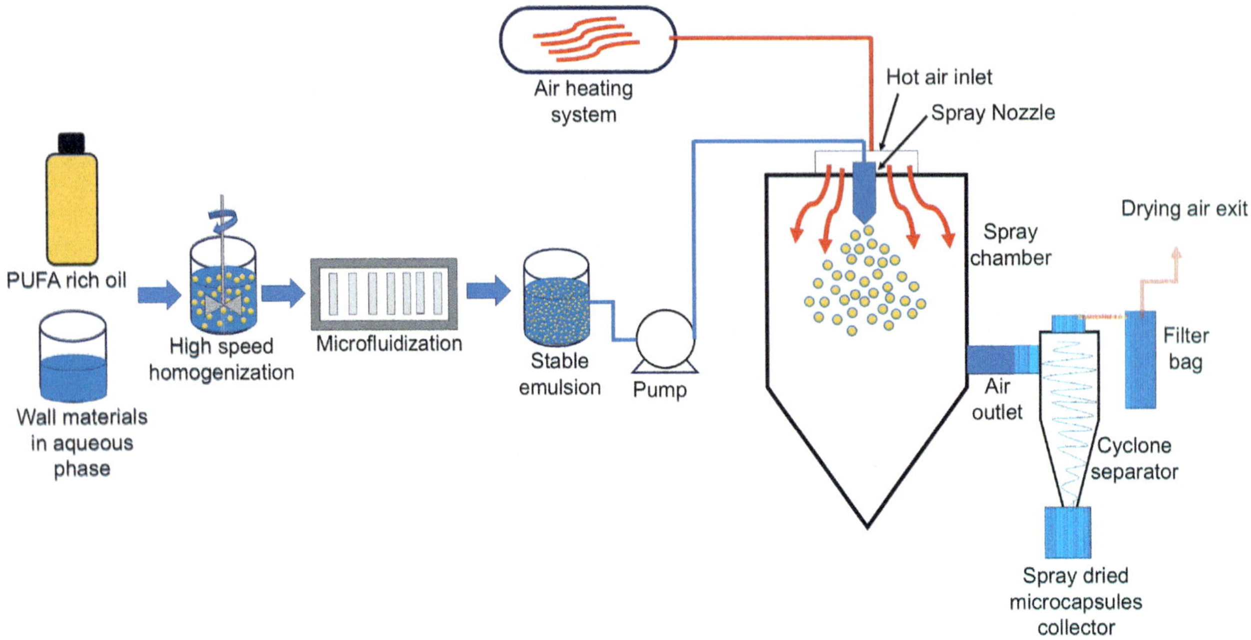

FIGURE 16.4 Microencapsulation of polyunsaturated fatty acid (PUFA) rich oil by the spray drying method.

carbohydrates and proteins in natural and modified form are considered as effective wall materials due to their solubility, film-forming properties that are essential to entrap and protect the PUFAs from external degradation factors during drying and storage. Chang & Nickerson (2018) extensively reviewed the suitability of proteins from animal-based (e.g., sodium caseinate, gelatin, whey protein concentrate, lactose) and plant-based (e.g., chickpea protein isolate, lentil protein isolate, soy protein isolate) sources for the production of spray-dried microcapsules loaded with PUFA-rich oils. Protein and carbohydrates can be used as a single component or blended with each other in different proportions (Chang & Nickerson, 2018). For instance, whey protein isolate was successfully employed to encapsulate DHA using the spray drying method with high encapsulation efficiency (83%) (Karthik & Anandharamakrishnan, 2012). Careful selection and formulation (blends) of wall materials is important to retain the functional properties of PUFAs and release them at the targeted site of the human intestine to achieve the desired health benefits (Vijaykrishnaraj et al., 2024).

To evaluate the stability of omega-3 FAs during spray drying, the pressurized liquid extraction method was adopted to extract PUFA-rich oil from plant sources (chia, camelina, and echium oilseeds) and from microalgae (*Nannochloropsis gaditana*). In addition, chia oil was enzymatically treated to produce chia oil FA ethyl esters. Emulsions of all five PUFA sources were prepared using wall materials, sodium caseinate, and lactose (1:4 core-to-wall ratio), and dried microcapsules (1.5–30 μm) were produced by the spray drying method. The spray drying retained the omega-3 FA profile of microencapsulated extracts, and these results confirmed that the spray drying is a highly suitable method for encapsulation of PUFAs without compromising their functional properties (Castejón et al., 2021).

PUFA-rich flaxseed oil and its blends (flaxseed sesame oil and flaxseed- rice bran oil) were encapsulated in maltodextrin wall matrix using Tween 20 as emulsifier by spray drying method, resulting in encapsulation efficiencies of 73%, 60%, and 80%, respectively (Areekal et al., 2024). To reduce the surface oil content in spray-dried microcapsules, natural or synthetic antioxidants are additionally incorporated during the emulsification step to stabilize the PUFAs in a stable oil-in-water emulsion before spray drying. Lipid oxidation is usually initiated at the oil-water interface, and placing the natural or synthetic antioxidants at this interface may effectively retard the lipid oxidation (Wang et al., 2020). However, in certain cases, the addition of antioxidants becomes challenging due to extra cost and may cause an adverse effect on the final product quality (Gu et al., 2024). To overcome this, emulsions are stabilized by solid particles instead of surfactants by manipulating the interfacial layers, resulting in stable emulsions known as Pickering emulsions. The presence of solid particles acts as a physical barrier that reduces contact between the aqueous and oil phases, thereby limiting oxidation of PUFAs by decreasing interfacial surface area. Spray-dried microcapsules produced from tuna oil Pickering emulsions stabilized by chitosan-ovalbumin polyelectrolyte complexes resulted 8.84% surface oil content and 76.65% encapsulation efficiency (Gu et al., 2024). Omega-3 PUFA-rich spray-dried powders obtained from Pickering emulsion stabilized in cellulose nanocrystals and hydroxypropyl methylcellulose improved the bioavailability and

TABLE 16.2 Spray drying conditions and key outcomes in the microencapsulation of polyunsaturated fatty acid (PUFA)-rich oils.

PUFA source	Wall material	Core to wall	Homogenization	Inlet/outlet temperatures	Key findings	References
Algal oil	Whey protein isolate; Tween 40 (3%, w/w)	1:1	-	120°C/80°C	83% encapsulation efficiency (EE)	Karthik and Anandharamakrishnan (2012)
Chia, camelina, echium oils; *N. gaditana*; chia FAEEs	Sodium caseinate and lactose	1:4	-	170°C/NA	EE: 57.0%–76.9%; highest for chia FAEEs; particle size: 1.5–30 μm	Castejón et al. (2021)
Krill oil	Arabic gum	1:4	-	180°C/80°C; 160°C/80°C	Highest EE at 160°C/ 80°C (42.58%)	Ortiz Sánchez et al. (2021)
CLA (Idesia polycarpa)	Soy protein isolate + maltodextrin; emulsifiers	3:5	10,000 rpm, 30 min	150°C/60°C;	82.38% EE; 781 nm size; 99.34% conversion	Yang et al. (2025)
Flaxseed oil	Hemicelluloses galactoglucomannans and glucuronoxylans	1:3	12,000 rpm, 2 min; High- pressure homogenization 800 bars, 3 cycles	150°C/70°C	Stable at RH 11%–75% (22°C)	Ho et al. (2025)
n-3 MLSLs	Gum Arabic maltodextrin and modified starch (MS)	1:3	-	190°C/100°C	EE: 90.11%; yield: 87.77%	Hussain et al., 2025
Menhaden and Asian swamp eel oils	Maltodextrin,gum Arabic and starch	1:4	700 rpm for 20 h; 20,000 rpm for 5 min high-shear homogenization	180°C–200°C	Maltodextrin+gum Arabic formulation improved oxidative stability	Hashim et al. (2023)
Flax seed oil	Flaxseed meal polysaccharide gum-	NA	18,000 rpm for 5 min	120°C–160°C/ 60°C–80°C	EE: 85.27%–90.78%; highest at 160°C	Shahid et al. (2020)
Algal oil	Buttermilk and maltodextrin	2:1	11,000 rpm for 3 min, high-pressure homogenizer (30 MPa, three cycles)	160°C/80°C	EE decreased at 1:1 core-to-wall than 1:2	Zhang, Pang, et al. (2020)

oxidative stability compared with a conventional emulsifying system (Nyström et al., 2023). Oxidative stability of spray-dried microcapsules of menhaden (*Brevoortia* spp.) and Asian swamp eel (*Monopterus albus*) oil encapsulated in maltodextrin and gum Arabic was studied. Vera et al. (2026) performed a critical bibliometric analysis of scientific trends and advances in the oxidative stability of omega-3 FAs derived from plant, animal, and protist sources between 2010 and 2024. Microencapsulation has been shown to significantly prevent oxidative deterioration for up to 3 months under controlled environments. Among the various microencapsulation techniques, spray drying, complex coacervation, lyophilization, and coaxial electrospraying resulted in acceptable encapsulation efficiency (>60%). PUFA-rich oils entrapped in wall matrices composed of polysaccharides such as maltodextrin, chitosan, gum Arabic, and proteins, including zein, whey isolate, and caseinate, limit oxygen diffusion by forming a semipermeable layer through electrostatic and hydrophobic interactions.

16.6.2 Freeze drying and spray freeze drying

Chia seed oil, baru oil, and pumpkin seed oil were encapsulated using sodium caseinate and stearic acid by the freeze-drying method (−50°C temperature and 100 mmHg pressure). The highest (99%–100%) encapsulation efficiency was obtained for omega-3 and omega-6 FAs of chia seed and baru oils, while 88% encapsulation efficiency was achieved for pumpkin seed oil. The oil entrapped in the solid lipid matrix prevents the migration of oil to the particle's surface due to the affinity between the oil and stearic acid. Furthermore, PUFA concentrations in the freeze-dried microcapsules were 0.29 g/g for chia seed oil, 0.18 g/g for pumpkin, and 0.12 g/g for baru oil, indicating the suitability of microparticles for the development of PUFA-enriched functional foods (Rojas et al., 2019). A study by Anwar and Kunz (2011) suggested that fish oil (33/22 EPA: DHA) was encapsulated in emulsified matrices of soybean soluble polysaccharide (10%) and octenyl succinic anhydride (65%) using freeze drying, and the results were compared with spray drying and spray granulation methods. Extremely porous and irregularly shaped freeze-dried particle morphology resulted in high surface oil content, which leads to reduced oxidative stability during storage. Heinzelmann et al. (2000)investigated the stability of freeze-dried microcapsules prepared from a frozen emulsion composed of fish oil, sodium caseinate, carbohydrate, and water (10:10:10:70). The study concluded that the incorporation of antioxidants and the use of a slower freezing rate are essential for producing freeze-dried microencapsulated fish oil with extended shelf life. In a recent study by Abdel-Razek et al. (2022), also reported the lower protective effect of freeze-dried encapsulates of omega-3-rich oil produced from microfluidized emulsions of blended oil (saturated and polyunsaturated with a desirable ratio of omega-6/omega-3) prepared using whey protein concentrate, maltodextrin, and gum Arabic (8:2:1) as wall materials, when compared to the spray drying method. The similar results were reported by Koo et al. (2023), where the encapsulation efficiency of perilla oil microcapsules produced by the freeze drying method ranged from 51.22% to 85.71%, which was slightly lower than that obtained by spray drying (77.38% to 90.74%). However, this study demonstrated better oxidative stability of freeze-dried microcapsules during storage than spray-dried microcapsules.

To improve the encapsulation efficiency of freeze drying, a novel approach known as spray freeze drying was explored by Karthik and Anandharamakrishnan (2012), in which the bulk liquid of microfluidized emulsion is atomized into fine droplets into the frozen medium, such as cryogenic liquid nitrogen. The cryogenic environment enables rapid freezing of the atomized droplets, which are subsequently lyophilized in a freeze-drier to obtain dried microcapsules. The authors reported that this approach improved the flow properties of microcapsules and enhanced the oxidative stability of DHA-rich oil. In a related study, flaxseed oil enriched with carotenoids was encapsulated using maltodextrin and pectin-wax mixture (6:1 ratio) as wall materials, resulted 70.9% encapsulation efficiency by spray freeze drying, which was comparatively lower than that obtained by spray drying (89.8%) (Elik et al., 2021). Another study compared the effect of different low-temperature drying methods, such as freeze drying, spray freeze drying, and microwave freeze drying with spray drying on the characteristics of fish oil-loaded microcapsules. The results showed that, despite the use of low-temperature drying methods, spray drying resulted in a higher encapsulation efficiency (86.98%) compared to freeze drying (63.29%), spray freeze drying (77.79%), and microwave freeze drying (57.89%). However, the oxidative stability of spray-dried microcapsules was significantly reduced during storage compared to microcapsules produced using low-temperature drying techniques (Yang et al., 2024). For the production of dried microcapsules, omega-3 FAs involve careful optimization of core-to-wall ratio and appropriate encapsulation method. The effect of wall materials on encapsulation efficiency and retention of ALA in chia oil was evaluated using freeze drying with whey protein concentrate and modified tapioca starch as wall materials. An increase in whey protein concentrate in the wall system resulted in higher encapsulation efficiency, whereas a higher proportion of modified tapioca starch in the wall system enhanced ALA retention. The combination of whey protein concentrate and modified tapioca starch (25:75) exhibited higher encapsulation efficiency (97%) and 59.54% ALA content retention and an omega-3 to omega-6 ratio of 3.34

(Anand et al., 2024). Thus, the selection of suitable wall material and its concentration in the wall system, and the method of drying are critical factors influencing the dried particle morphology, encapsulation yield, encapsulation efficiency, and oxidative stability during storage.

16.6.3 Complex coacervation

Complex coacervation is another low-cost method highly suitable for encapsulating hydrophobic substances. Coacervation is a phase separation process induced by modifying the pH and temperature. It is induced in a single polymer system, it is referred to as simple coacervation, and when more than one polymer is involved, it is known as complex coacervation. In complex coacervation, electrostatic interaction among the oppositely charged biopolymers leads to phase separation. Protein and polysaccharides are used to produce complex coacervates suitable to entrap bioactive components. In addition to electrostatic forces, van der Waals intermolecular forces, and hydrophobic interactions are also influencing the coacervation process (Dabiri Movahed et al., 2024; Eghbal & Choudhary, 2018; Timilsena et al., 2017).

To understand the interaction mechanism between the two biopolymers during coacervation, the properties of biopolymers, including molecular weight, concentration, and proportion, as well as optimization of process parameters, including method of emulsion preparation, degree of homogenization, pH, and temperature, are essential. The stability of the coacervates is influenced by pH and temperature, and if these conditions are not favorable, dissociation may occur. Therefore, the complex coacervates are stabilized by crosslinking with synthetic or natural materials (e.g., tannic acid, gallic acid, and glutaraldehyde) (Dabiri Movahed et al., 2024; Timilsena et al., 2017).

Flaxseed oil encapsulated in complex coacervate produced using low-molecular-weight chitosan (1% w/v) and apricot tree (*Prunus armeniaca*) gum extract (0.05%w/v) at a 3:1 ratio, along with tween 20 and potassium hydroxide cross-linking agents, resulted in higher encapsulation efficiency (89%), antioxidant activity (66.32%), lower peroxide value and reduced release rate (Dabiri Movahed et al., 2024). In another study, defatted Antarctic krill oil protein complexed with gum Arabic (3:1 ratio) at pH 3.5, used to entrap the krill oil at a core-to-wall ratio of 0.75:1, resulted 8.022% encapsulation efficiency. The resultant coacervate microcapsules effectively masked the odor of krill oil, which was found to be suitable for food applications without affecting sensory properties (Cui et al., 2025). Walnut oil encapsulated sodium alginate-chitosan complex (1:1 ratio, 1.5% wall material concentration) through complex coacervation (3:2 core to wall ratio) at pH 4 resulted 91.18% encapsulation efficiency and 81.78% encapsulation yield. In addition, the microcapsules exhibited smaller particle size, low hygroscopicity, high thermal stability, and low moisture content, indicating their suitability for storage and food applications (Chen et al., 2025). Recently, Glomm et al. (2023) demonstrated that molecular weight distribution and interfacial tension of polysaccharides influence the encapsulation efficiency and oxidative stability of salmon oil complex coacervate microcapsules. The study concluded that harvesting conditions and the presence of impurities associated with the polysaccharide gum acacia obtained from different sources directly influence its protective effect. To enhance the oxidative stability, soy protein isolate and inulin were used to encapsulate soybean oil enriched with lipophilic antioxidants obtained from Thai rice germ with broken rice pieces (Wangsuntornpakdee et al., 2023). Chitosan and octenyl succinic anhydride-modified starch were used at a 1:3 ratio (w/w) to form the complex coacervates, and the isothermal titration calorimetry method was employed to evaluate the affinity between wall materials. Highest coacervate yield (58.3%) at pH 6.0 and achieved encapsulation efficiency of 93.1%, indicating strong ionic strength between the protein and carbohydrate polymer and effective encapsulation (Mu et al., 2022). These studies confirm that coacervation effectively encapsulates PUFA-rich oils, resulting in more payload, high encapsulation efficiency, improved oxidative stability, and the ability to mask unwanted flavors.

16.6.4 Electrospraying/electrospinning

Electrospinning and electrospraying technologies have gained attention due to their high encapsulation efficiency and suitability for protecting heat-sensitive bioactive components. It is an electrohydrodynamic process, where a high-voltage electric field charges the biopolymer solution at the tip of the capillary tube. The electrically charged liquid droplet forms a jet called a Taylor cone, that stretch, elongate the droplet into breaks into nano-sized particles (electrospraying) Fig. 16.5 or lengthy fibers (electrospinning) (Fig. 16.6), which are deposited on a grounded collector. Due to electrostatic repulsion, the solvent evaporates, resulting in the deposition of nanoscale solid particles or fibers on the surface of the collector plate (Ali et al., 2026; Keshmiri et al., 2025; Pires et al., 2023).

For encapsulation of oils by electrospinning/electrospraying, proteins including soy protein isolate, whey protein isolate, zein, gelatin, and sodium caseinate are found to be suitable, and their electrodynamical properties can be enhanced with the addition of solvents (e.g., acetic acid, water, ethanol) (Pires et al., 2023). The high surface area-to-volume ratio of fibers produced by the electrospinning technique promotes oxidation, resulting in higher initial oxidation levels in

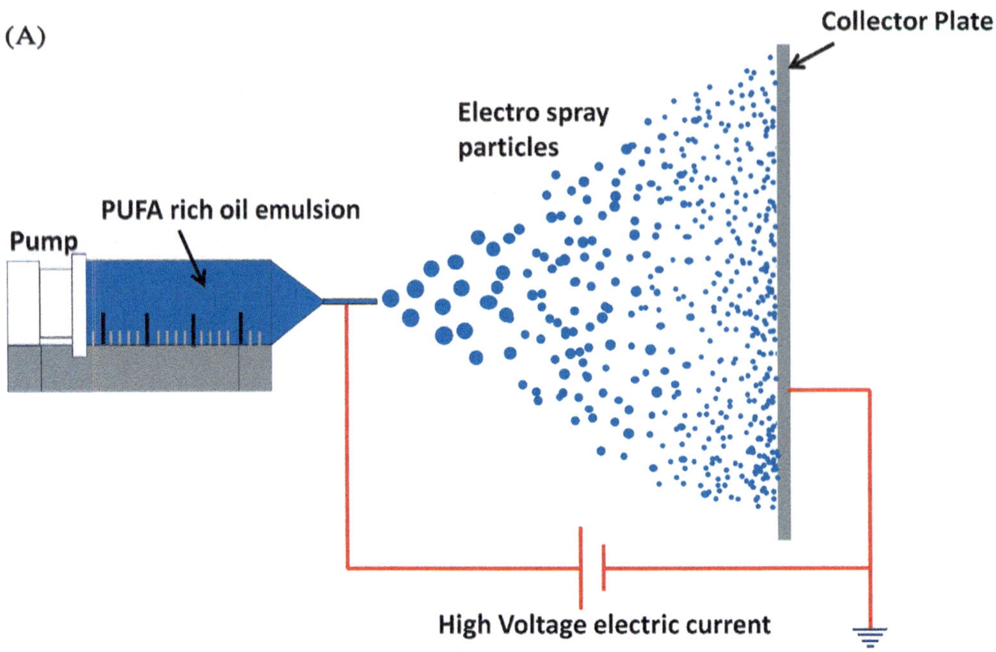

FIGURE 16.5 Production of nanocapsules by the electrospray method.

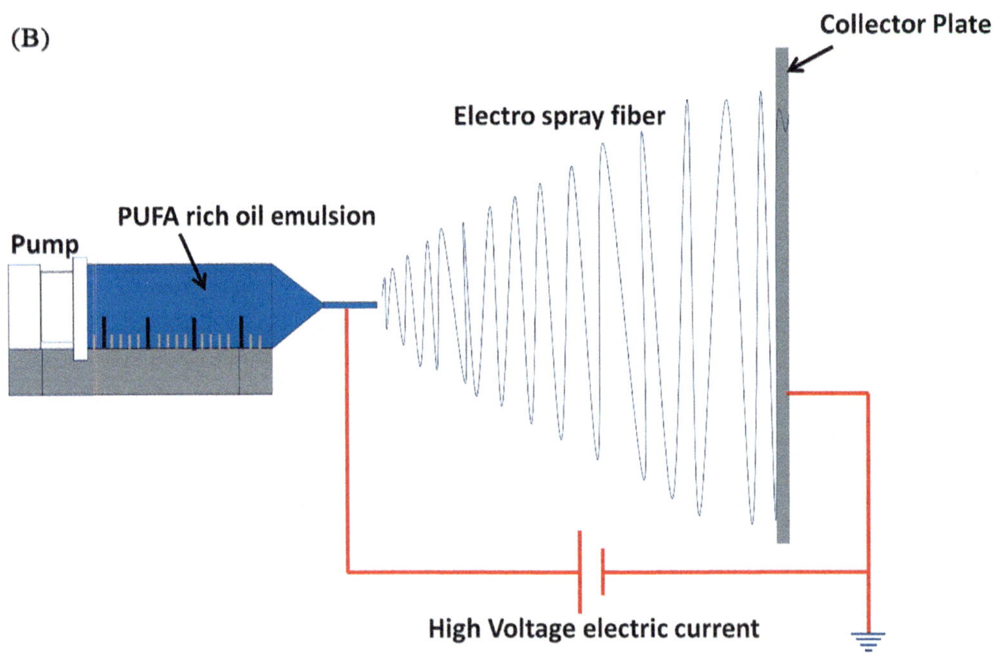

FIGURE 16.6 Production of nanocapsules by the electrospinning method.

encapsulated PUFA-rich oils, such as fish oil and flaxseed oil, compared to the nonencapsulated oils. To mitigate the oxidation issues, synthetic antioxidants like δ-tocopherol, rosemary extract, tannic acid, and BHT are suggested. In a recent study, the electrospraying of hemp seed oil and hemp seed oil bodies emulsions was prepared with hemp seed protein isolate. Electrosprayed microcapsules of hemp seed protein isolate and hemp seed oil body, at a 5:1 ratio, resulted in a 70% lower peroxide value compared to hemp seed oil. The enhanced oxidative stability of oil bodies due to the presence of phospholipid/protein monolayer membrane, which acts as a natural physical barrier against infusion of oxidation promoters (Natsia et al., 2026). Echium oil encapsulated in barley protein hydrolysate by electrospraying (flow rate: 0.1 mL/h, electric current: 18.5 kV, temperature: 23 ± 5°C, and relative humidity 34%–42%). The resulting nano- and microcapsules were spherical in shape, had a narrow range of particle size distribution (<1.5 μm), and high oxygen permeability due to large surface area, which resulted in low encapsulation efficiency (61.1%) (Bisinotto et al., 2026). Polysaccharides and proteins are used to fabricate nanoscale particles/nanofibers with high surface area, and their ability to encapsulate PUFA-rich oils is of growing interest in the area of nutraceutical delivery (Ali et al., 2026).

16.7 Oleogel-based polyunsaturated fatty acid delivery system

Recently, immobilizing the unsaturated FA-rich oils in an oleogel system gained attention due to their ability to mimic the physical properties of conventional solid fats while allowing incorporation of healthier (e.g., omega-3, omega-6) FAs. Edible oleogels are a good choice for replacing trans fats and saturated FAs in the food system. Oleogel consists of two major components: the gelator and the solvent. Oleogels can be prepared either by emulsification or by directly mixing gelator and oil above the gelator's melting point, followed by solidification (Mehany et al., 2025). The self-assembling nature of gelator dispersed in the oil phase forms the three-dimensional network in which the oil phase is stabilized through hydrogen bonding, ionic interactions, and Van der Waals forces (O'Sullivan et al., 2016; Sivakanthan et al., 2022). Oleogelators are classified into low-molecular-weight (200–800 Da) and high-molecular-weight (>1000 Da) gelators (Fig. 16.7). Low-molecular-weight gelators include plant- and animal-based waxes, wax esters, lecithin, phytosterols, oligopeptides, and fatty alcohols. High-molecular-weight gelators, are macromolecules such as proteins (e.g., soy protein isolate, caseinate, gelatin, and whey protein) and polysaccharides (e.g., ethylcellulose, pectin, alginate, xanthan gum, guar gum, and carrageenan), are used individually or in combination for the development of oleogels (Kavya et al., 2024).

In a study, EPA- and DHA-rich fish oil encapsulated in oleogel-based β-cyclodextrins complex, further coated with whey protein isolate, effectively protected the functionality of omega-3 FAs (Lee et al., 2018). Protein-based cryo-oleogels composed of whey protein isolate and fish gelatin crosslinked with tannic acid resulted in high oil-holding capacity (96.80 ± 0.69%), low peroxide value, and controlled release profile in gastrointestinal conditions (Purba et al., 2025). Fish oil entrapped in large yellow croaker roe protein hydrolysates and tannic acid conjugate showed improved oxidative stability, resulting in higher omega-3 FA and reduced formation of undesirable volatile compounds such as

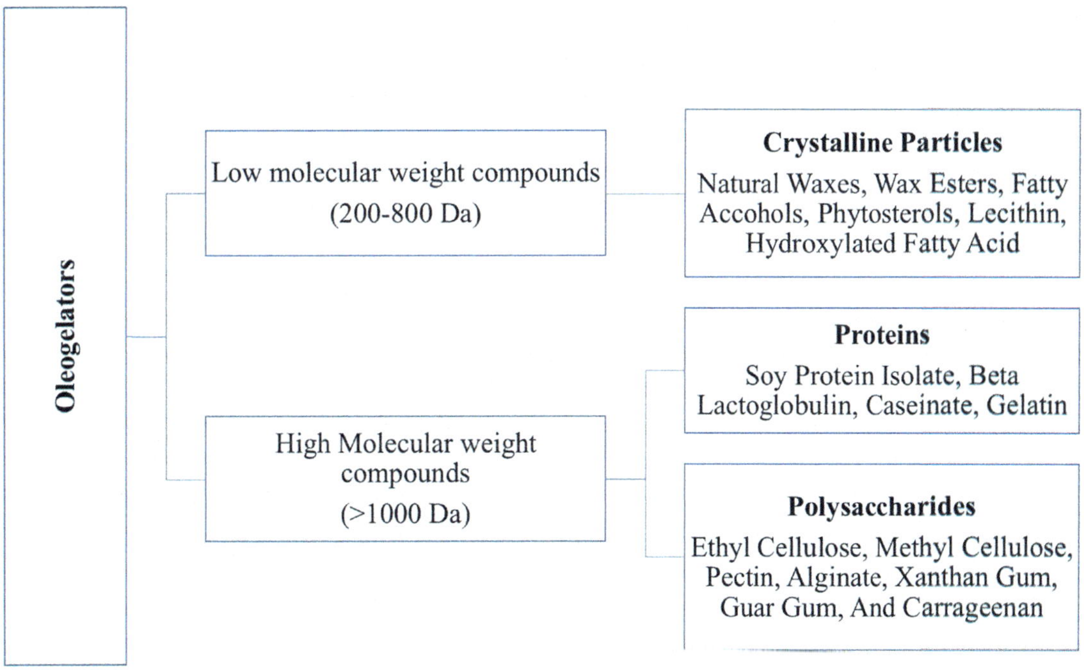

FIGURE 16.7 Classification of oleogelators (O'Sullivan et al., 2016).
Source: From O'Sullivan, C.M., Barbut, S., & Marangoni, A.G. (2016). Edible oleogels for the oral delivery of lipid soluble molecules: Composition and structural design considerations. Trends in Food Science & Technology, 57(5), 59–73https://doi.org/10.1016/j.tifs.2016.08.018; Sivakanthan, S., Fawzia, S., Madhujith, T., & Karim, A. (2022). Synergistic effects of oleogelators in tailoring the properties of oleogels: A review. Comprehensive Reviews in Food Science and Food Safety, 21(4), 3507–3539. https://doi.org/10.1111/1541-4337.12966.

hexanal and octen-3-ol, indicating the enhanced stability of the developed oleogel (Zhang et al., 2025). Wax-based oleogel delivery system utilizes plant-derived (rice bran, carnauba, candelilla, sunflower, and sugarcane) and animal-derived (shellac, bees, and propolis) waxes (1–4 wt.% concentration) to immobilize the oil (Soleimanian et al., 2020). The gelation behavior is influenced by the components present in the wax, including aldehydes. Oleogel microstructure depends on the viscosity of the oil, which in turn depends on the composition of unsaturated FAs. Firmness of gel is inversely proportional to viscosity of the oil, which is influenced by the degree of unsaturation of FA molecules.

A novel oleogel system for the codelivery of omega-3 FAs and polyphenols has been developed using algal oil and polyphenol-enriched whey protein microgels as gelling agents. This system exhibited high loading efficiency and improved oxidative stability, highlighting its potential for delivering multiple bioactive nutrients simultaneously (Wang et al., 2022). In addition, ethylcellulose oleogels prepared from PUFA-rich linseed and chia oils have demonstrated their potential as fat substitutes, retaining high PUFA contents (64.28 and 73.02 g/100 g, respectively) without producing trans FAs. Although chia oil oleogels initially showed lower oxidative stability, the addition of antioxidants like BHT effectively managed peroxide values, confirming the potential of these matrices for stabilizing PUFA-rich oils in food formulations (Millao et al., 2023).

To improve the oleogel strength, water-holding capacity, and thermal stability in food applications (Abou-Elsoud et al., 2026), utilized multiple biopolymers, such as pectin and egg yolk low-density lipoprotein. Breads made with this multipolymer oleogel exhibited superior softness and elasticity, indicating that it is a promising alternative for the development of gluten-free bakery products without alteration in the FA profile. Furthermore, soy wax and bee wax (5 wt. %) oleogelators melted at 65°C and mixed with oil blends of flaxseed oil and palm olein (40:60) at 500 rpm for 15 min at 60°C, followed by overnight refrigeration for gelation. The hardness of soy (4.3 N) and bee (2.2 N) wax oleogels is lower than that of butter. Cookies made with developed oleogel resulted in an enriched nutritional profile, higher spread ratio, lower hardness, and fracturability (Chand et al., 2026). Chickpea (*Cicer arietinum L.*) oil-based oleogel developed using rice bran wax as gelator (wax-to-oil ratio 3:7) resulted 96% oil binding capacity, firmness retention (4.8 N), and improved oxidative stability (peroxide value 1.8 meq O_2/kg) while retaining the bioactivity of unsaturated FAs such as linoleic and oleic acids. Also, chickpea oil and rice bran wax oleogel exhibited good DPPH inhibition (39.82%). A lower wax-to-oil ratio (1:9) resulted in higher antimicrobial activity against food-borne pathogens *E. coli* and *Staphylococcus aureus* compared with a 3:7 ratio, indicating that the increased wax content may limit the diffusion of active compounds to inhibit pathogens. However, significant antimicrobial potential was observed overall (Awlqadr et al., 2026).

16.8 Quality and shelf-life assessment

16.8.1 Oxidative stability

High levels of unsaturation make omega-3 FAs highly susceptible to oxidative degradation, which often leads to undesirable sensory attributes and reduced shelf life of fortified foods. Lipid oxidation occurs by free-radical mechanism, producing both primary oxidation products (hydroperoxides) and secondary products like aldehydes and ketones. These oxidative reactions deteriorate the nutritional quality and flavor of the food, thereby reducing the shelf life of PUFA-incorporated food products (Islam et al., 2023; Zhang, Freund, et al., 2020). The oxidative stability of emulsions is confirmed by measuring both primary (peroxide value, tocopherol content) and secondary (thiobarbituric acid reactive substances) lipid oxidation products, which are typically assessed using p-anisidine value or total oxidation (TOTOX) index (Ghelichi et al., 2026; Lakhlifi El Idrissi et al., 2024).

Essential factors that affect oxidative stability are oxygen exposure, light intensity, temperature, presence of trace metals (e.g., iron, copper), water activity, and absence or presence of natural and synthetic antioxidants (e.g., tocopherols, rosemary extract, TBHQ). The retardation of oxidation by encapsulation, emulsification, and the encapsulation of lipid-soluble antioxidants within the core or at the oil-water interface limits oxygen diffusion and quenches free radicals. On the practical scale in formulation methods, nitrogen blanketing, light-blocking packaging and storage at low-temperatures, and use of metal chelators such as citric acid or EDTA at levels which are permitted by regulations are important (Zhang et al., 2019). In a conventional colloidal system, surfactants are used to stabilize the oil droplets dispersed in the aqueous phase and to minimize the flocculation, coalescence, and creaming (Karthik et al., 2018). However, the protection offered by the surfactants is limited by environmental factors such as temperature, pH, and ionic strength of the emulsion. The presence of natural antioxidants in the PUFA-rich oil source or the addition of synthetic or natural antioxidants during the emulsification step reduced lipid oxidation during storage (He et al., 2025). To improve the oxidative stability, emulsions are stabilized with dense interfacial layers, formed by proteins or polysaccharides, to provide a more effective physical barrier against pro-oxidants compared to surfactant-based emulsion systems (Alijani et al., 2026; Ghelichi et al., 2026; Hu et al., 2019).

16.8.2 Accelerated storage stability

Accelerated stability testing is commonly applied to determine PUFA-enriched products' shelf life by controlled accelerated temperature (e.g., 40°C–65°C), and the change in indices of oxidation, FA profile, and sensory characteristics are monitored. The typical protocol involves storing the product under constant temperature and humidity conditions and periodically measuring peroxide value (PV), anisidine value, conjugated dienes, and free fatty acids at different time intervals. In some cases, these analyses are supplemented with gas chromatography to evaluate FA profiles and volatile compounds.

Physiochemical quality characteristics of dried microcapsules can be evaluated by different parameters such as microencapsulation yield, encapsulation efficiency, moisture content and water activity, wettability and solubility, hygroscopicity, bulk density, particle density, flowability, porosity, color, particle size, crystallinity, particle morphology, and oxidative stability in accelerated storage (Hussain et al., 2025). The data collected from accelerated studies are then correlated with consumer-acceptable sensory threshold values or with chemical limit values determined by Codex and regional standards, to estimate the actual shelf life at ambient conditions. Care must be taken to make sure that the heat generated during the studies has not created nonoxidative changes (e.g., protein denaturation, starch retrogradation, or separation of emulsion layers) that would influence the forecast. Together with models (Arrhenius-type models or empirical kinetic models), the accelerated data may be very useful to estimate a "best before date" and storage conditions on commercially available PUFA-enriched foods (Islam et al., 2023). Most of the studies focused on the preparation, oxidative stability, and physicochemical characteristics of encapsulates for fortification in food products. Despite these advancements, recent research works are increasingly focusing on targeted delivery mechanisms to improve the bioavailability and therapeutic potential of omega-3 FAs (Zhu et al., 2025).

16.9 Emerging trends and future perspectives

The demand for foods enriched with functional nutrients has increased significantly. Incorporation of encapsulated omega-3 FAs into staple foods enhances their functional and nutritional profiles. An efficient delivery system of omega-3 FAs must ensure a high level of physicochemical stability along with acceptable sensory attributes. Moreover, controlled release of functional components is often preferred in the nutraceutical field, as it can enhance the bioavailability and efficacy (Kumar et al., 2024; Vera et al., 2026). Over the last two decades, various emulsion stabilization and encapsulation techniques and formulations have been developed to make the omega-3 PUFAs more accessible and acceptable. These techniques are carefully designed to incorporate the essential PUFAs into food matrices with improved gastrointestinal stability and bioavailability. Recent research has increasingly focused on improving the bioaccessibility of functional PUFAs. For instance, studies on examining the relationship between the degree of unsaturation and bioaccessibility of encapsulated oils, through the evaluation of free oxylipins in digested samples, provide insights for designing the digestion-driven delivery system for PUFAs (Auñon-Lopez et al., 2025).

Furthermore, the increasing importance of food-grade wall materials for PUFA encapsulation and subsequent fortification. Although the nanoscale delivery system has demonstrated promising results, its application in food systems is subject to rigorous safety evaluations. Another challenge is scalability, as encapsulation techniques that perform well at laboratory scale often face limitations during industrial-scale level implementation due to the process complexities in maintaining consistency. In addition, production cost is another critical factor influencing the choice of encapsulation technique, and achieving a balance between the cost of production and functional performance remains a key consideration (Karthik & Anandharamakrishnan, 2016b; Kumar et al., 2024; Vijaykrishnaraj et al., 2024).

16.10 Conclusion

Health benefits of PUFAs, particularly omega-3 and omega-6 FAs, have been extensively demonstrated by various researchers. Flaxseed and chia seeds are rich sources of essential fatty acid ALA, whereas fatty fish and microalgae are important direct natural sources of omega-3 FAs such as EPA and DHA. However, the recommended daily dietary intake is often not met due to changing dietary patterns and limited distribution of these constituents in commonly consumed foods. The incorporation of functional lipids into food systems is limited by their hydrophobic nature, unacceptable flavor, and low oxidative stability during storage. To address these challenges, various encapsulation techniques and delivery systems have been developed to improve stability, mask the off-flavors, and enhance bioavailability in the gastrointestinal tract. Recent advances in targeted delivery systems like micro- and nanoemulsions, gelled emulsions, and dried micro- and nanocapsules have improved their bioavailability and enable the provision of customized nutrition and meet the diverse demands of the public population. Further research is required to explore alternative and sustainable sources such as microalgae, bacteria, and fungi, and to develop effective fortification strategies for stable, widely consumed food products to meet the daily nutritional requirements and promote overall health.

References

Abdel-Razek, A. G., Hassanein, M. M., Ozçelik, B., Baranenko, D. A., & El-Messery, T. M. (2022). Omega fatty acid-balanced oil formula and enhancing its oxidative stability by encapsulation with whey protein concentrate. *Food Bioscience, 50*, 101975. https://doi.org/10.1016/J.FBIO.2022.101975.

Abdelhafez, A., Khabir, Z., Garcia-Bennett, A., Prestidge, C. A., Camponovo, F. F., & Joyce, P. (2026). Omega-3 PUFA concentration and emulsification govern lipid digestion, micellar vesicle formation, and oral bioavailability of fish oil concentrates. *Food Bioscience, 79*(4), 108574. https://doi.org/10.1016/j.fbio.2026.108574.

Abou-Elsoud, M., Khoder, R. M., Salama, M., Wang, S., Khalifa, I., Cai, Z., Ahn, D. U., & Huang, X. (2026). Novel pectin-low-density lipoprotein oleogels as techno-functional ingredients improved the structural and textural characteristics of gluten-free bread. *Food Chemistry, 509*, 148617. https://doi.org/10.1016/j.foodchem.2026.148617.

Akhtar, G., Masoodi, F. A., Rather, Z. U. K., & Wani, T. A. (2022). Exploiting encapsulated Himalayan walnut oil as a vivid source of essential fatty acids for the development of novel functional bread. *International Journal of Food Science and Technology, 57*(7), 4129–4137. https://doi.org/10.1111/ijfs.15729.

Al-Madhagy, S., Ashmawy, N. S., Mamdouh, A., Eldahshan, O. A., & Farag, M. A. (2023). A comprehensive review of the health benefits of flaxseed oil in relation to its chemical composition and comparison with other omega-3-rich oils. *European Journal of Medical Research, 28*(1), 240. https://doi.org/10.1186/s40001-023-01203-6 *2023 28:1*.

Ali, K., Niaz, N., Haq, F. U., Waseem, M., Ashraf, W., Guoxun, C., & Wu, M. (2026). Electrospinning of food-grade polysaccharides and proteins: Materials, challenges, and applications. *Carbohydrate Polymers, 380*, 125070. https://doi.org/10.1016/j.carbpol.2026.125070.

Alijani, S., Hahn, A., Harris, W. S., & Schuchardt, J. P. (2025). Bioavailability of EPA and DHA in humans – A comprehensive review. *Progress in Lipid Research, 97*, 101318. https://doi.org/10.1016/j.plipres.2024.101318.

Alijani, S., Hahn, A., Harris, W. S., & Schuchardt, J. P. (2026). Omega-3 microalgal oil-in-water nanoemulsions stabilized by red seaweed extracts: Physical and oxidative stability. *Algal Research, 93*, 104461. https://doi.org/10.1016/j.plipres.2024.101318.

Anand, V., Ksh, V., Kar, A., Varghese, E., Vasudev, S., & Kaur, C. (2024). Encapsulation efficiency and fatty acid analysis of chia seed oil microencapsulated by freeze-drying using combinations of wall material. *Food Chemistry, 430*, 136960. https://doi.org/10.1016/J.FOODCHEM.2023.136960.

Anwar, S. H., & Kunz, B. (2011). The influence of drying methods on the stabilization of fish oil microcapsules: Comparison of spray granulation, spray drying, and freeze drying. *Journal of Food Engineering, 105*(2), 367–378. https://doi.org/10.1016/j.jfoodeng.2011.02.047.

Areekal, N. N., Chakkaravarthi, A., & Debnath, S. (2024). Effect of microencapsulation on physical properties of powder developed from blended oils rich in PUFA. *Journal of Food Science and Technology, 61*(12), 2275–2286. https://doi.org/10.1007/s13197-024-05992-4.

Arnoldussen, I. A. C., & Kiliaan, A. J. (2014). Impact of DHA on metabolic diseases from womb to tomb. *Marine Drugs, 12*(12), 6190. https://doi.org/10.3390/md12126190.

Attri, N., Arora, D., Saini, R., Chandel, M., Suthar, P., & Dhiman, A. (2024). Health promoting benefits of krill oil: Mechanisms, bioactive combinations, and advanced encapsulation technologies. *Food Science and Biotechnology, 34*(6), 1285–1308. https://doi.org/10.1007/s10068-024-01737-3.

Auñon-Lopez, A., Alberdi-Cedeño, J., Martinez-Yusta, A., Aichner, M., Suwattanasophon, C., & Pignitter, M. (2025). Understanding the bioaccessibility of lipidic compounds and the formation of free oxylipins of encapsulated omega-3-rich marine oils during in vitro digestion. *LWT, 234*(22), 118574. https://doi.org/10.1016/j.lwt.2025.118574.

Awlqadr, F. H., Mohammed, O. A., Qadir, S. A., Qadir, A. M., Faraj, A. M., & Arab, K. (2026). Characterization of chickpea seed oil and its structuring into oleogels using rice bran wax: A study on the physicochemical, thermal, textural, and antioxidant properties for potential use in health-conscious and sustainable food products. *Food Science and Nutrition, 14*(2), e71511. https://doi.org/10.1002/fsn3.71511.

Bisinotto, M. S., Castro, I. A., Guadix, E. M., & García-Moreno, P. J. (2026). Encapsulation of echium oil by electrospraying and mono- or coaxial spray-drying using plant protein hydrolysates as emulsifiers. *Food Chemistry, 512*, 148893. https://doi.org/10.1016/j.foodchem.2026.148893.

Castejón, N., Luna, P., & Señoráns, F. J. (2021). Microencapsulation by spray drying of omega-3 lipids extracted from oilseeds and microalgae: Effect on polyunsaturated fatty acid composition. *LWT, 148*, 111789. https://doi.org/10.1016/j.lwt.2021.111789.

Chand, M., Chopra, R., Dhiman, A., & Singh, D. K. (2026). Development of omega-3 rich oleogels using blended flaxseed oil and their application as a fat replacer in cookies. *Discover Food, 6*(1), 90. https://doi.org/10.1007/s44187-025-00764-1.

Chang, C., & Nickerson, M. T. (2018). Encapsulation of omega 3-6-9 fatty acids-rich oils using protein-based emulsions with spray drying. *Journal of Food Science and Technology, 55*(8), 2850–2861. https://doi.org/10.1007/s13197-018-3257-0.

Chen, Q., Zhao, C., Ma, X., Yan, W., & Wang, F. (2025). Preparation and characterization of walnut oil microcapsules by complex coacervation with sodium alginate and chitosan. *LWT, 222*(2), 117630. https://doi.org/10.1016/j.lwt.2025.117630.

Cholewski, M., Tomczykowa, M., & Tomczyk, M. (2018). A comprehensive review of chemistry, sources and bioavailability of omega-3 fatty acids. *Nutrients, 10*(11), 1662. https://doi.org/10.3390/nu10111662.

Cui, Y., Chen, K., Chen, K., Li, Y., & Jiang, L. (2025). The complex coacervation of gum Arabic and krill protein isolate and their application for Antarctic krill oil encapsulation. *Carbohydrate Polymers, 348*, 122831. https://doi.org/10.1016/j.carbpol.2024.122831.

Da Rosa, J., Marin, D. R., Vieira da Silva, A. M., De Souza, E. M. G., Rech, E. L., Nepomuceno, A. L., & Mertz-Henning, L. M. (2025). Biotechnological advances in enhancing soybean oil quality for human health and food industry applications. *Frontiers in Food Science and Technology, 5*, 1658589. https://doi.org/10.3389/frfst.2025.1658589.

Dabiri Movahed, M., Sahari, M. A., & Barzegar, M. (2024). Microencapsulation of flaxseed oil by complex coacervation of with apricot tree (*Prunus armeniaca* L.) gum and low molecular chitosan: Formation and structural characterization. *Applied Food Research, 4*(2), 100519. https://doi.org/10.1016/j.afres.2024.100519.

Edel, A. L., Patenaude, A. F., Richard, M. N., Dibrov, E., Austria, J. A., Aukema, H. M., Pierce, G. N., & Aliani, M. (2015). The effect of flaxseed dose on circulating concentrations of alpha-linolenic acid and secoisolariciresinol diglucoside derived enterolignans in young, healthy adults. *European Journal of Nutrition, 55*(2), 651–663. https://doi.org/10.1007/s00394-015-0885-2.

Eghbal, N., & Choudhary, R. (2018). Complex coacervation: Encapsulation and controlled release of active agents in food systems. *LWT, 90*, 254–264. https://doi.org/10.1016/j.lwt.2017.12.036.

Elik, A., Koçak Yanık, D., & Göğüş, F. (2021). A comparative study of encapsulation of carotenoid enriched-flaxseed oil and flaxseed oil by spray freeze-drying and spray drying techniques. *LWT, 143*, 111153. https://doi.org/10.1016/j.lwt.2021.111153.

Ezhilarasi, P. N., Karthik, P., Chhanwal, N., & Anandharamakrishnan, C. (2012). Nanoencapsulation techniques for food bioactive components: A review. *Food and Bioprocess Technology, 6*(3), 628–647. https://doi.org/10.1007/s11947-012-0944-0.

Gammone, M. A., Riccioni, G., Parrinello, G., & D'orazio, N. (2018). Omega-3 polyunsaturated fatty acids: Benefits and endpoints in sport. *Nutrients, 11*(1), 46. https://doi.org/10.3390/NU11010046 *2019, Vol. 11, Page 46*.

Ganesan, B., Brothersen, C., & McMahon, D. J. (2014). Fortification of foods with omega-3 polyunsaturated fatty acids. *Critical Reviews in Food Science and Nutrition, 54*(1), 98–114. https://doi.org/10.1080/10408398.2011.578221.

Gharsallaoui, A., Roudaut, G., Chambin, O., Voilley, A., & Saurel, R. (2007). Applications of spray-drying in microencapsulation of food ingredients: An overview. *Food Research International, 40*(9), 1107–1121. https://doi.org/10.1016/j.foodres.2007.07.004.

Ghelichi, S., Hajfathalian, M., García-Moreno, P. J., Yesiltas, B., Moltke-Sørensen, A.-D., & Jacobsen, C. (2021). Food enrichment with omega-3 polyunsaturated fatty acids. *Omega-3 Delivery Systems*, 395–425. https://doi.org/10.1016/b978-0-12-821391-9.00020-x.

Ghelichi, S., McClements, D. J., Sørensen, A. D. M., & Jacobsen, C. (2026). Omega-3 microalgal oil-in-water nanoemulsions stabilized by red seaweed extracts: Physical and oxidative stability. *Algal Research, 93*, 104461. https://doi.org/10.1016/j.algal.2025.104461.

Gill, I., & Valivety, R. (1997). Polyunsaturated fatty acids, part 1: Occurrence, biological activities and applications. *Trends in Biotechnology, 15*(10), 401–409. https://doi.org/10.1016/S0167-7799(97)01076-7.

Glomm, W. R., Molesworth, P. P., Yesiltas, B., Jacobsen, C., & Johnsen, H. (2023). Encapsulation of salmon oil using complex coacervation: Probing the effect of gum acacia on interfacial tension, coacervation and oxidative stability. *Food Hydrocolloids, 140*(2), 108598. https://doi.org/10.1016/j.foodhyd.2023.108598.

Gu, C. Y., Shao, J. Q., Liu, X. L., Wei, J. T., Huang, G. Q., & Xiao, J. X. (2024). Spray drying the Pickering emulsions stabilized by chitosan/ovalbumin polyelectrolyte complexes for the production of oxidation stable tuna oil microcapsules. *International Journal of Biological Macromolecules, 273*, 133139. https://doi.org/10.1016/j.ijbiomac.2024.133139.

Guan, L., Zhu, L., Zhang, X., Han, Y., Wang, K., Ji, N., Yao, X., Zhou, Y., Li, B., Chen, Q., Fan, J., Sha, D., & Lu, S. (2024). Perilla seed oil and protein: Composition, health benefits, and potential applications in functional foods. *Molecules (Basel, Switzerland), 29*(22), 5258. https://doi.org/10.3390/molecules29225258 *2024, Vol. 29, Page 5258*.

Halliwell, B., & Chirico, S. (1993). Lipid peroxidation: Its mechanism, measurement, and significance. *American Journal of Clinical Nutrition, 57*(SUPPL. 5), 715S–725S. https://doi.org/10.1093/ajcn/57.5.715s.

Hashim, N. A., Mohd Norzi, M. F. A., Mohd Arshad, Z. I., Mohd Azman, N. A., & Abdul Mudalip, S. K. (2023). Effect of spray drying parameters on the physicochemical properties and oxidative stability of oil from menhaden (*Brevoortia* spp.) and Asian swamp eel (*Monopterus albus*) oil extract microcapsules. *Food Chemistry Advances, 3*, 100392. https://doi.org/10.1016/j.focha.2023.100392.

He, R., Liu, Y., Zhou, M., Wei, C., Liu, W., Ma, Y., & Luo, P. (2025). Comparison of co-pressing and separate pressing on the oxidative stability and lipidomic signature of ω-6/ω-3 balanced flaxseed-peanut blended oils. *Journal of Food Composition and Analysis, 148*, 108356. https://doi.org/10.1016/j.jfca.2025.108356.

Heinzelmann, K., Franke, K., Jensen, B., & Haahr, A. (2000). Protection of fish oil from oxidation by microencapsulation using freeze-drying techniques. *European Journal of Lipid Science and Technology*. https://doi.org/10.1002/(SICI)1438-9312(200002)102:2.

Ho, T. M., Lehtonen, M., Räikkönen, H., Halahlah, A., & Mikkonen, K. S. (2025). Storage stability of spray-dried flaxseed oil powders protected by wood hemicelluloses – Part 1: Physical properties and initial stage oxidation. *Future Foods, 12*, 100744. https://doi.org/10.1016/j.fufo.2025.100744.

Hu, X., Karthik, P., & Chen, J. (2019). Manipulating oral behaviour of food emulsions using different emulsifiers. *International Journal of Food Science and Technology, 54*(7), 2408–2415. https://doi.org/10.1111/ijfs.14152.

Hussain, M., Bisht, A., Khan, I., Chaudhary, M. N., Kanwal, N., Khalid, M. U., Yiasmin, M. N., Hussain, A., & Zou, X. (2025). Enhanced stability of n-3 PUFAs rich structured lipids via spray-dried microencapsulation with tailored wall materials. *Sustainable Food Technology, 3*(5), 1492–1504. https://doi.org/10.1039/d5fb00185d.

Islam, F., Imran, A., Nosheen, F., Fatima, M., Arshad, M. U., Afzaal, M., Ijaz, N., Noreen, R., Mehta, S., Biswas, S., Rasool, I. F. U., Aslam, M. A., Usman, I., Zahra, S. M., Segueni, N., & Amer Ali, Y. (2023). Functional roles and novel tools for improving-oxidative stability of polyunsaturated fatty acids: A comprehensive review. *Food Science and Nutrition, 11*(6), 2471–2482. https://doi.org/10.1002/fsn3.3272.

Jacobsen, C., & Let, M. B. (2006). Using polyunsaturated fatty acids (PUFAs) as functional ingredients. *Improving the Fat Content of Foods*, 428–453. https://doi.org/10.1533/9781845691073.3.428.

Kapoor, B., Kapoor, D., Gautam, S., Singh, R., & Bhardwaj, S. (2021). Dietary polyunsaturated fatty acids (PUFAs): Uses and potential health benefits. *Current Nutrition Reports, 10*(3), 232–242. https://doi.org/10.1007/s13668-021-00363-3.

Karthik, P., & Anandharamakrishnan, C. (2012). Microencapsulation of docosahexaenoic acid by spray-freeze-drying method and comparison of its stability with spray-drying and freeze-drying methods. *Food and Bioprocess Technology, 6*(10), 2780–2790. https://doi.org/10.1007/s11947-012-1024-1.

Karthik, P., & Anandharamakrishnan, C. (2016a). Fabrication of a nutrient delivery system of docosahexaenoic acid nanoemulsions via high energy techniques. *RSC Advances, 6*(5), 3501–3513. https://doi.org/10.1039/c5ra12876e.

Karthik, P., & Anandharamakrishnan, C. (2016b). Enhancing omega-3 fatty acids nanoemulsion stability and in-vitro digestibility through emulsifiers. *Journal of Food Engineering, 187*, 92–105. https://doi.org/10.1016/j.jfoodeng.2016.05.003.

Karthik, P., S., P. I., & Anandharamakrishnan, C. (2018). Droplet coalescence as a potential marker for physicochemical fate of nanoemulsions during in-vitro small intestine digestion. *Colloids and Surfaces A: Physicochemical and Engineering Aspects, 553*, 278–287. https://doi.org/10.1016/j.colsurfa.2018.05.066.

Kavya, M., Udayarajan, C., Fabra, M. J., López-Rubio, A., & Nisha, P. (2024). Edible oleogels based on high molecular weight oleogelators and its prospects in food applications. *Critical Reviews in Food Science and Nutrition, 64*(13), 4432–4455. https://doi.org/10.1080/10408398.2022.2142195.

Keshmiri, N., Najmi, P., Milani, A. S., & Arjmand, M. (2025). Electrospinning for electromagnetic interference shielding: Principles, challenges, and future directions. *Carbon, 245*(3), 120831. https://doi.org/10.1016/j.carbon.2025.120831.

Koo, H. W., Kim, S. H., & Lee, J. H. (2023). Comparison of physicochemical properties and oxidative stability of microencapsulated perilla oil powder prepared by freeze-drying and spray-drying. *Food Science and Biotechnology, 32*(13), 1831. https://doi.org/10.1007/s10068-023-01299-w.

Kumar, A., Singh, U., Jaiswal, S. G., Dave, J., Wei, S., & Hailu, G. G. (2024). Recent trends in the encapsulation of functional lipids: Comprehensive review. *Sustainable Food Technology, 2*(6), 1610–1630. https://doi.org/10.1039/d4fb00205a.

Lakhlifi El Idrissi, Z., El Guezzane, C., Boujemaa, I., El Bernoussi, S., Sifou, A., El Moudden, H., Ullah, R., Bari, A., Goh, K. W., Goh, B. H., Bouyahya, A., Harhar, H., & Tabyaoui, M. (2024). Blending cold-pressed peanut oil with omega-3 fatty acids from walnut oil: Analytical profiling and prediction of nutritive attributes and oxidative stability. *Food Chemistry: X, 22*(3), 101453. https://doi.org/10.1016/j.fochx.2024.101453.

Lazăr, A. R., Pușcaș, A., Tanislav, A. E., & Mureșan, V. (2024). Bioactive compounds delivery and bioavailability in structured edible oils systems. *Comprehensive Reviews in Food Science and Food Safety, 23*(6), e70020. https://doi.org/10.1111/1541-4337.70020.

Lee, M. C., Jiang, X., Brenna, J. T., & Abbaspourrad, A. (2018). Oleogel-structured composite for the stabilization of ω3 fatty acids in fish oil. *Food & Function, 9*(11), 5598–5606. https://doi.org/10.1039/c8fo01446a.

Liu, Y., Ren, X., Fan, C., Wu, W., Zhang, W., & Wang, Y. (2022). Health Benefits, Food Applications, And Sustainability Of Microalgae-derived N-3 PUFA. *Foods, 11*(13), 1883. https://doi.org/10.3390/foods11131883 *2022, Vol. 11, Page 1883*.

Liu, Y., Shen, N., Xin, H., Yu, L., Xu, Q., & Cui, Y. (2023). Unsaturated fatty acids in natural edible resources, a systematic review of classification, resources, biosynthesis, biological activities and application. *Food Bioscience, 53*, 102790. https://doi.org/10.1016/j.fbio.2023.102790.

Lopes, P. A., Alfaia, C. M., Pestana, J. M., & Prates, J. A. M. (2023). Structured lipids engineering for health: Novel formulations enriched in n-3 long-chain polyunsaturated fatty acids with potential nutritional benefits. *Metabolites, 13*(10), 1060. https://doi.org/10.3390/metabo13101060 *2023, Vol. 13, Page 1060*.

Mehany, T., Zannou, O., Oussou, K. F., Chabi, I. B., & Tahergorabi, R. (2025). Innovative oleogels: Developing sustainable bioactive delivery systems for healthier foods production. *Food Chemistry: X, 29*, 102768. https://doi.org/10.1016/j.fochx.2025.102768.

Millao, S., Iturra, N., Contardo, I., Morales, E., Quilaqueo, M., & Rubilar, M. (2023). Structuring of oils with high PUFA content: Evaluation of the formulation conditions on the oxidative stability and structural properties of ethylcellulose oleogels. *Food Chemistry, 405*, 134772. https://doi.org/10.1016/j.foodchem.2022.134772.

Mondor, M., & Hernández-Álvarez, A. J. (2022). *Camelina sativa* composition, attributes, and applications: A review. *European Journal of Lipid Science and Technology, 124*(3), 2100035. https://doi.org/10.1002/ejlt.202100035.

Mu, H., Song, Z., Wang, X., Wang, D., Zheng, X., & Li, X. (2022). Microencapsulation of algae oil by complex coacervation of chitosan and modified starch: Characterization and oxidative stability. *International Journal of Biological Macromolecules, 194*, 66–73. https://doi.org/10.1016/J.IJBIOMAC.2021.11.168.

Natsia, A., Papadaki, A., Manikas, A. C., Pastore Carbone, M. G., Dracopoulos, V., & Kopsahelis, N. (2026). Electrosprayed hempseed protein/oilbody emulsions for encapsulation and oxidative stabilization of PUFA-rich oils. *Food Hydrocolloids, 175*, 112436. https://doi.org/10.1016/j.foodhyd.2026.112436.

Nyström, L., Mira, I., Benjamins, J. W., Gopaul, S., Granfeldt, A., Abrahamsson, B., von Corswant, C., & Abrahmsén-Alami, S. (2023). In vitro and in vivo performance of pickering emulsion-based powders of omega-3 polyunsaturated fatty acids. *Molecular Pharmaceutics, 21*(2), 677–687. https://doi.org/10.1021/acs.molpharmaceut.3c00804.

Ortiz Sánchez, C. A., Zavaleta, E. B., García, G. R. U., Solano, G. L., & Díaz, M. P. R. (2021). Krill oil microencapsulation: Antioxidant activity, astaxanthin retention, encapsulation efficiency, fatty acids profile, in vitro bioaccessibility and storage stability. *LWT, 147*, 111476. https://doi.org/10.1016/j.lwt.2021.111476.

O'Sullivan, C. M., Barbut, S., & Marangoni, A. G. (2016). Edible oleogels for the oral delivery of lipid soluble molecules: Composition and structural design considerations. *Trends in Food Science & Technology, 57*(5), 59–73. https://doi.org/10.1016/j.tifs.2016.08.018.

Pattnaik, M., & Mishra, H. N. (2022). Amelioration of the stability of polyunsaturated fatty acids and bioactive enriched vegetable oil: Blending, encapsulation, and its application. *Critical Reviews in Food Science and Nutrition, 62*(23), 6253–6276. https://doi.org/10.1080/10408398.2021.1899127.

Pires, J. B., Santos, F. N.dos, Costa, I. H.de L., Kringel, D. H., Zavareze, E.da R., & Dias, A. R. G. (2023). Essential oil encapsulation by electrospinning and electrospraying using food proteins: A review. *Food Research International, 170*, 112970. https://doi.org/10.1016/j.foodres.2023.112970.

Presa-Lombardi, J., García, F., Gutierrez-Barrutia, M. B., & Cozzano, S. (2023). Hemp seed's (*Cannabis sativa* L) nutritional potential for the development of snack functional foods. *OCL, 30*, 24. https://doi.org/10.1051/ocl/2023025.

Purba, D. T., Dave, J., & Somboon, P. (2025). Sustainable oleogel encapsulation of tilapia fish oil using protein-based cryogels: Fabrication, characterization, and digestion behavior. *Sustainable Food Technology, 3*(5), 1480–1491. https://doi.org/10.1039/d5fb00322a.

Rojas, V. M., Marconi, L. F.da C. B., Guimarães-Inácio, A., Leimann, F. V., Tanamati, A., Gozzo, Â. M., Fuchs, R. H. B., Barreiro, M. F., Barros, L., Ferreira, I. C. F. R., Tanamati, A. A. C., & Gonçalves, O. H. (2019). Formulation of mayonnaises containing PUFAs by the addition of microencapsulated chia seeds, pumpkin seeds and baru oils. *Food Chemistry, 274*, 220–227. https://doi.org/10.1016/j.foodchem.2018.09.015.

Ruiz-López, N., Sayanova, O., Napier, J. A., & Haslam, R. P. (2012). Metabolic engineering of the omega-3 long chain polyunsaturated fatty acid biosynthetic pathway into transgenic plants. *Journal of Experimental Botany, 63*(7), 2397–2410. https://doi.org/10.1093/jxb/err454.

Saini, R. K., & Keum, Y. S. (2018). Omega-3 and omega-6 polyunsaturated fatty acids: Dietary sources, metabolism, and significance — A review. *Life Sciences, 203*, 255–267. https://doi.org/10.1016/j.lfs.2018.04.049.

Semenoglou, I., Katsouli, M., Giannakourou, M., & Taoukis, P. (2025). Effect of high-pressure homogenization and wall material composition on the encapsulation of polyunsaturated fatty acids from fish processing. *Molecules (Basel, Switzerland), 30*(7). https://doi.org/10.3390/molecules30071434.

Shahid, M. Z., Imran, M., Khan, M. K., Ahmad, M. H., Nadeem, M., Muhammad, N., & Yasmin, A. (2020). OMEGA-3 fatty acids retention, oxidative quality, and sensoric acceptability of spray-dried flaxseed oil. *Journal of Food Quality, 2020*. https://doi.org/10.1155/2020/7286034.

Shahidi, F., & Hossain, A. (2022). Role of lipids in food flavor generation. *Molecules (Basel, Switzerland), 27*(15), 5014. https://doi.org/10.3390/molecules27155014 *2022, Vol. 27, Page 5014*.

Sivakanthan, S., Fawzia, S., Madhujith, T., & Karim, A. (2022). Synergistic effects of oleogelators in tailoring the properties of oleogels: A review. *Comprehensive Reviews in Food Science and Food Safety, 21*(4), 3507–3539. https://doi.org/10.1111/1541-4337.12966.

Soleimanian, Y., Goli, S. A. H., Shirvani, A., Elmizadeh, A., & Marangoni, A. G. (2020). Wax-based delivery systems: Preparation, characterization, and food applications. *Comprehensive Reviews in Food Science and Food Safety, 19*(6), 2994–3030. https://doi.org/10.1111/1541-4337.12614.

Swetha, N., & Mathanghi, S. K. (2024). Towards sustainable omega-3 fatty acids production – A comprehensive review on extraction methods, oxidative stability and bio-availability enhancement. *Food Chemistry Advances, 4*, 100603. https://doi.org/10.1016/J.FOCHA.2023.100603.

Tak, Y., Kaur, M., Kumar, R., Gautam, C., Singh, P., Kaur, H., Kaur, A., Bhatia, S., Jha, N. K., Gupta, P. K., & Amarowicz, R. (2022). Repurposing chia seed oil: A versatile novel functional food. *Journal of Food Science, 87*(7), 2798–2819. https://doi.org/10.1111/1750-3841.16211.

Timilsena, Y. P., Wang, B., Adhikari, R., & Adhikari, B. (2017). Advances in microencapsulation of polyunsaturated fatty acids (PUFAs)-rich plant oils using complex coacervation: A review. *Food Hydrocolloids, 69*, 369–381. https://doi.org/10.1016/j.foodhyd.2017.03.007.

Turp, G. Y., & Ozuesen, S. (2025). Health benefits of fish oil and the application of encapsulated fish oil in meat and dairy products. *Marine Science and Technology Bulletin, 14*(1), 41–55. https://doi.org/10.33714/masteb.1635847.

Vera, W., Muñoz-More, H. D., Ruiz-Flores, L. A., Nole-Jaramillo, J. M., Nolazco-Cama, D. M., & Espinoza-Espinoza, L. A. (2026). Trends and viability of omega-3 fatty acid microencapsulation: A bibliometric and critical analysis. *Applied Food Research, 6*(1), 101685. https://doi.org/10.1016/j.afres.2026.101685.

Vijaykrishnaraj, M., Kiran Kumar, P., & Karthik, P. (2024). Polyunsaturated fatty acid fortification. *Food Fortification: Trends and Technologies*, 329–354. https://doi.org/10.1201/9781003160663-18.

Villamil, R. A., Cortés, L. Y., & Gutiérrez, L. F. (2024). Technological strategies to enhance yogurt's fatty acid profile and its health-related effects. *Food Reviews International, 40*(2), 771–791. https://doi.org/10.1080/87559129.2023.2197994.

Visioli, F., Alfredo Martínez, J., & Tomé-Carneiro, J. (2026). Genetic modulation of omega-3 and omega-6 polyunsaturated fatty acid metabolism and health outcomes: A systematic review. *Food & Function, 17*(5), 2176–2191. https://doi.org/10.1039/d5fo04964d.

Walker, R., Decker, E. A., & McClements, D. J. (2015). Development of food-grade nanoemulsions and emulsions for delivery of omega-3 fatty acids: Opportunities and obstacles in the food industry. *Food & Function, 6*(1), 41–54. https://doi.org/10.1039/c4fo00723a.

Wang, C., Sun, C., Lu, W., Gul, K., Mata, A., & Fang, Y. (2020). Emulsion structure design for improving the oxidative stability of polyunsaturated fatty acids. *Comprehensive Reviews in Food Science and Food Safety, 19*(6), 2955–2971. https://doi.org/10.1111/1541-4337.12621.

Wang, G. S., Chen, H. Y., Feng, G. X., Yuan, Y., Wan, Z. L., Guo, J., Wang, J. M., & Yang, X. Q. (2022). Polyphenol-enriched protein oleogels as potential delivery systems of omega-3 fatty acids. *Journal of Agricultural and Food Chemistry, 71*(1), 749–759. https://doi.org/10.1021/acs.jafc.2c06348.

Wang, Y., Wu, G., Wang, Y., Rehman, A., Yu, L., Zhang, H., Jin, Q., Suleria, H. A. R., & Wang, X. (2025). Recent developments, challenges, and prospects of dietary omega-3 PUFA-fortified foods: Focusing on their effects on cardiovascular diseases. *Food Chemistry, 470*, 142498. https://doi.org/10.1016/J.FOODCHEM.2024.142498.

Wangsuntornpakdee, P., Sae-tan, S., Iwamoto, S., & Peanparkdee, M. (2023). Optimisation of soybean oil enriched with lipophilic antioxidants from Thai rice germs and their nanoparticles developed using complex coacervation. *Food Bioscience, 54*, 102888. https://doi.org/10.1016/j.fbio.2023.102888.

Wei, W., Cheng, Z., Wang, X., Chang, M., Xie, D., Sun, C., Guo, X., & Li, B. (2025). The potential of marine oils as functional foods: Nutritional composition, health benefits, applications, and future perspectives. *Food Reviews International*. https://doi.org/10.1080/87559129.2025.2528083.

Yang, H., Feng, H., Chen, Q., Xu, C., Song, M., Hou, J., & Chang, Y. (2025). Fabrication and characterization of Idesia polycarpa-derived conjugated linoleic acid microcapsules by spray drying: In vitro digestion and release kinetics. *Food Chemistry: X, 33*, 103420. https://doi.org/10.1016/j.fochx.2025.103420.

Yang, M., Li, L., Zhu, X., Liang, L., Chen, J., Cao, W., Liu, W., Duan, X., Ren, G., & Liu, Z. (2024). Microencapsulation of fish oil by spray drying, spray freeze-drying, freeze-drying, and microwave freeze-drying: Microcapsule characterization and storage stability. *Journal of Food Science, 89*(6), 3276–3289. https://doi.org/10.1111/1750-3841.17098.

Yashodhara, B. M., Umakanth, S., Pappachan, J. M., Bhat, S. K., Kamath, R., & Choo, B. H. (2009). Omega-3 fatty acids: A comprehensive review of their role in health and disease. *Postgraduate Medical Journal, 85*(1000), 84–90. https://doi.org/10.1136/pgmj.2008.073338.

Yuan, Q., Xie, F., Huang, W., Hu, M., Yan, Q., Chen, Z., Zheng, Y., & Liu, L. (2022). The review of alpha-linolenic acid: Sources, metabolism, and pharmacology. *Phytotherapy Research : PTR, 36*(1), 164–188. https://doi.org/10.1002/ptr.7295.

Zakaria, M. F., Mat Zaidi, F. N. A., Ahmad Kamal, A. H., Aleng, N. A., Abd Wahid, M. E., Katayama, T., & Jusoh, M. (2025). PUFA from microalgae: Challenges, factors affecting high production and industrial application. *Aquaculture and Fisheries, 10*(4), 545–555. https://doi.org/10.1016/j.aaf.2025.01.004.

Zhang, H., Yang, Q., Zheng, B., & Liang, P. (2025). Improvement of flavor and gel properties of sea bass surimi gel by fish oil oleogel combined with antioxidants. *Journal of Aquatic Food Product Technology, 34*(5), 261–279. https://doi.org/10.1080/10498850.2025.2526654.

Zhang, J., Freund, M. A., Culler, M. D., Yang, R., Chen, P. B., Park, Y., Decker, E. A., & Zhang, G. (2020). How to stabilize ω-3 polyunsaturated fatty acids (PUFAs) in an animal feeding study?—Effects of the temperature, oxygen level, and antioxidant on oxidative stability of ω-3 PUFAs in a mouse diet. *Journal of Agricultural and Food Chemistry, 68*(46), 13146–13153. https://doi.org/10.1021/acs.jafc.9b08298.

Zhang, Y., Pang, X., Zhang, S., Liu, L., Ma, C., Lu, J., & Lyu, J. (2020). Buttermilk as a wall material for microencapsulation of omega-3 oils by spray drying. *LWT, 127*, 109320. https://doi.org/10.1016/j.lwt.2020.109320.

Zhang, Z.shan, Zhang, L.xia, Xie, Q.fang, & Che, L.ming (2019). Effect of accelerated storage on fatty acids, thermal properties and bioactive compounds of kenaf seed oil. *Journal of Food Science, 84*(8), 2121–2127. https://doi.org/10.1111/1750-3841.14653.

Zhu, P., Li, J., Zhou, Y., Li, J., & Yu, Q. (2025). Precision targeted delivery based on PUFAs: Overview, strategies and applications. *Food Chemistry, 493*, 145800. https://doi.org/10.1016/j.foodchem.2025.145800.

Chapter 17

Packaging innovations for enhancing polyunsaturated fatty acid stability and shelf life

Aditya Madan[1] and Ajay Kumar Swarnakar[2]

[1]*Department of Food Technology, Parul Institute of Applied Sciences, Parul University, Vadodara, Gujarat, India,* [2]*Department of Agricultural Engineering, Triguna Sen School of Technology, Assam University Silchar, Assam, India*

17.1 Introduction

The functional food sector has been gaining traction over the past decade, reflecting increased consumer awareness of the connection between diet and healthy living. Consumers are now looking for foods that provide benefits beyond basic nutrition. Functional foods are designed by incorporating bioactive components, and polyunsaturated fatty acids (PUFAs) form one such group of components. To be specific, omega-3 and omega-6 fatty acids (FAs) offer numerous health benefits and fall under the category of essential FAs, meaning these cannot be synthesized efficiently by the human body. Therefore, these need to be included in the diet. There is an ample amount of scientific evidence claiming a wide range of health benefits, including cardiovascular, neurological, and immunological system (Gill et al., 2024; Patted et al., 2024; Shahidi & Ambigaipalan, 2018a, 2018b). On the contrary, the higher amount of unsaturation renders them more sensitive to oxidation and rancidity, which in turn affects their shelf-life and poses serious formulation challenges (Dyall et al., 2022).

Omega-3 FAs include eicosapentaenoic acid (EPA; 20:5 n-3), docosahexaenoic acid (DHA; 22:6 n-3), and α-linolenic acid (ALA; 18:3 n-3). These are associated with improved brain development and cognitive function, reduced cardiovascular disease risk, neuroprotection in neurodegenerative conditions, and antiinflammatory activity (Gill et al., 2024; Wysoczański et al., 2016). Omega-6 FAs, specifically, linoleic acid (18:2 n-6) and arachidonic acid (20:4 n-6), modulate cardiovascular and immune function. The evidence also supports reduced type 2 diabetes incidence at higher intakes (Hooper et al., 2018; Visioli & Poli, 2025). Moving on to the sources, fish, fish oil, and algae supply EPA and DHA. Flax, chia, perilla, and hemp oils supply ALA. Fermentation can produce DHA without using marine sources (Moi et al., 2018; Rizzo et al., 2023; Saini et al., 2021). In foods, PUFAs affect texture and emulsion stability. They are added to a wide range of food products, namely bakery, dairy, infant formula, and meat products for added nutrition (Fu et al., 2021; Islam et al., 2023).

The chemical structure of PUFAs is a primary determinant of the oxidative stability of oils; each additional double bond substantially increases susceptibility to oxidation, with the relative autoxidation rate of oleic, linoleic, and linolenic acids reported as 1:40 to 50:100 based on oxygen uptake (Choe & Min, 2006). Oxidative deterioration proceeds through enzymatic and nonenzymatic pathways, producing lipid peroxides and secondary by-products that impair sensory and nutritional quality (Dyall et al., 2022; Lee-Okada et al., 2024). External factors such as temperature, Ultraviolet A radiation, and catalytic metal ions further accelerate degradation (Dyall et al., 2022). Consequently, PUFA-rich foods, particularly fish oils and fortified products, may develop off-flavors within days or weeks if inadequately protected (Jacobsen, 2015; Kolanowski et al., 2007). Moisture also acts as a critical factor influencing the oxidative stability of oils (Aberkane et al., 2013; Frankel et al., 2002). Hence, the desirable properties of packaging material must meet criteria to restrict oxygen, light, and moisture. Sometimes, the addition of antioxidants, which either act as chain breakers or radical scavengers, also comes in handy (Hennebelle et al., 2024).

Omega-3 and Omega-6 Polyunsaturated Fatty Acids in Food Systems. DOI: https://doi.org/10.1016/B978-0-443-43810-3.00014-2

For PUFA-rich foods, packaging solutions matter just as much as formulation for nutrient protection. This chapter examines packaging innovations that keep PUFA-rich foods fresh longer. These include strong plastic barriers, oxygen removers, special gas mixes, and freshness tags. Sections 17.2 and 17.3 cover oxidation mechanisms, the market today, and the materials and barriers that work best. Sections 17.4 and 17.5 cover packaging innovations, how to test packaging, and measure shelf life. Section 17.6 reviews applications in edible oils, emulsions, marine, meat, and dairy-based food products. Sections 17.7 and 17.8 look ahead to next-generation materials, sustainability, and research priorities before concluding remarks.

17.2 Background and current scenario

Owing to the presence of double bonds in their chemical structure, PUFAs are highly vulnerable to oxidative degradation. Even though these offer significant nutritional and physiological benefits, this susceptibility is highly concerning and remains a critical challenge for the global market. To address this, it requires an understanding of various oxidation mechanisms, overcoming traditional packaging limitations, and advanced packaging strategies. From the consumer's perspective, clean-label and safe food products are gaining traction in the PUFA-rich product segment.

17.2.1 Mechanistic basis of polyunsaturated fatty acid oxidation

The oxidation process involves multiple interconnected mechanisms that create unstable primary oxidation products and a variety of secondary compounds that contribute to rancidity and deterioration in quality (Shahidi & Zhong, 2010a, 2010b). Therefore, a thorough understanding of these degradation mechanisms is crucial for creating effective packaging solutions that can reduce oxidative reactions in real-world scenarios (Islam et al., 2023).

Autoxidation is the primary mechanism responsible for the degradation of PUFAs in oils and food products, occurring through a self-sustaining free-radical chain reaction involving initiation, propagation, and termination (Choe & Min, 2006; Geng et al., 2023) (see Fig. 17.1).

The process begins with hydrogen removal from allylic or bis-allylic positions, followed by rapid interaction of lipid radicals with oxygen to form peroxyl radicals (Shahidi & Zhong, 2010a, 2010b). Oxidation rates increase with higher unsaturation levels and may initiate at interfacial regions in heterogeneous systems (Hennebelle et al., 2024). Primary hydroperoxides decompose into aldehydes, ketones, malonaldehyde, and hydroxyalkenals (4-HHE, 4-Hydroxy-2-nonenal [4-HNE]), causing rancidity and nutritional degradation (Esterbauer et al., 1991). Photo-induced oxidation occurs when photosensitizers absorb UV or visible light and transfer energy to oxygen, generating singlet oxygen ($^1O_2$) that reacts directly with double bonds via nonradical mechanisms (Bacellar & Baptista, 2019; Choe & Min, 2009), producing distinct hydroperoxides (Choe & Min, 2006). Additionally, transition metals such as iron and copper catalyze oxidation by decomposing hydroperoxides into reactive radicals, accelerating chain reactions even at low concentrations (Elias et al., 2008; Choe & Min, 2006), highlighting the importance of protective packaging strategies (Ahmed et al., 2017; Shao et al., 2023).

Secondary oxidation products—including volatile aldehydes, ketones, and malonaldehyde—are directly responsible for the sensory defects and nutritional losses that define oxidative rancidity in PUFA-rich products (Domínguez et al., 2019).

17.2.2 Conventional packaging limitations and recent advances

PUFA-rich foods are often packaged in traditional packaging materials such as glass bottles, metal cans, aluminium foil laminates, and polymeric films such as LDPE, Polypropylene (PP), and even polyethene terephthalate (PET). Each of

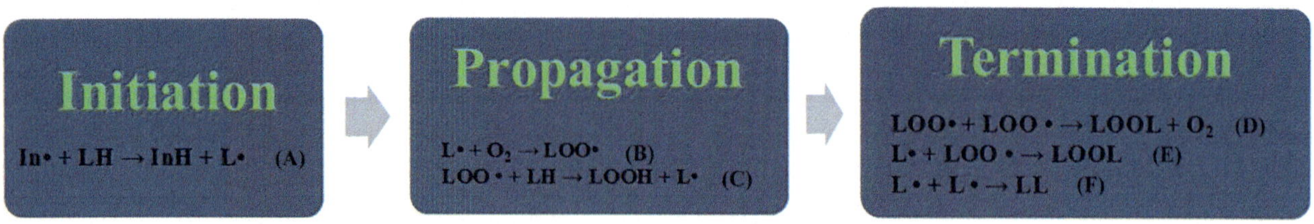

FIGURE 17.1 Lipid auto-oxidation mechanism in food. (A) is the initiation period, (B–C) is the propagation period, and (D–F) is the termination period of lipid oxidation. ln: the free radicals; LH: the unsaturated fatty acid molecules; LOO: the lipid peroxyl radical; L: the lipid free radicals; O_2: oxygen; LOOH: the lipid hydroperoxides; LOOL, LL: the lipid polymers.

Source: Geng, L., Liu, K., & Zhang, H. (2023). Lipid oxidation in foods and its implications on proteins. Frontiers in Nutrition, 10, 1192199. https://doi.org/10.3389/fnut.2023.1192199.

these materials provides distinct barrier properties. Standard single-layer polymers exhibit oxygen transmission rates (OTR) of 50–200 $cm^3/m^2/day/atm$, exceeding the <1–5 $cm^3/m^2/day/atm$ threshold required for PUFA-sensitive products (Siracusa, 2012). Aluminium cans exhibit excellent barrier performance but limit recyclability and visibility properties. On the other hand, glass permits light transmission unless pigmented and has negligible oxygen permeability (Han et al., 2018; Siracusa, 2012). As compared to monolayer materials, multilayer and coated structures enhance barrier performance. Composite films employing ethylene vinyl alcohol (EVOH) or polyvinylidene chloride (PVDC) reduce OTR by 95%–99% as compared to monolayers. Also, metallized or SiOx/AlOx-coated PET structures deliver near-glass-equivalent barrier performance in flexible formats (Han et al., 2018; Siracusa, 2012).

Nevertheless, even the slightest headspace oxygen can initiate oxidation (Jacobsen, 2015). Other factors that can contribute to accelerated degradation include temperature fluctuations, light exposure, and moisture (Durand et al., 2025). However, passive barrier improvements alone cannot eliminate entrapped oxygen, necessitating complementary active packaging approaches (Gupta, 2024; Shao et al., 2023).

Recent trends include the usage of nanocomposite coatings employing graphene oxide, nanocellulose, and montmorillonite nanoclay, which reduce oxygen permeability by 60%–80% through the tortuous diffusion path effect (Lopez de Dicastillo et al., 2020; Vilela et al., 2018). Another advancement includes reducing headspace oxygen below 0.01% by using iron-based or ascorbate-based oxygen scavengers. These components are deployed in the form of sachets, integrated film labels, or direct polymer matrix additives. (Dey & Neogi, 2019; Gupta, 2024). As a part of active packaging, antioxidant-releasing packaging films are also gaining popularity in the research world (Gomez-Estaca et al., 2014; Vilela et al., 2018). Eco-friendly botanicals and biopolymeric matrices are also in demand as consumers look for natural preservation (Hussain et al., 2024; Kozik-Kołodziej, 2026).

17.2.3 Market trends and regulatory challenges

Consumers are expecting clean-label, natural, and eco-friendly packaged products. Additionally, they expect extended shelf life and higher nutritional quality. The global market is therefore influenced and shaped by these demands. Apart from consumer preferences, stringent safety standards and complex regulatory frameworks also contributors to shaping the evolving market. Around the world, manufacturers must comply with food safety regulations. Health claims, oxidation limits, labeling accuracy, and material interaction and safety in the packaging system are some of the important considerations in PUFA-rich products undertaken by regulatory bodies. For any country, these factors, backed up with scientific evidence, form the basis for product and packaging innovations, and commercialization strategies. However, the scattered nature of current scientific data and the inadequate regulatory frameworks for nonmigratory systems continue to hamper innovation, particularly in markets with more restrictive legal constraints (Tian et al., 2013). Table 17.1 reflects the regulatory landscape for PUFA-rich products across nations/regions.

17.3 Packaging materials and barrier requirements

Careful and evidence-based evaluation of three interdependent environmental parameters, namely oxygen ingress, light exposure, and moisture transfer, plays a vital role in the selection of appropriate packaging materials for PUFA-rich food products. Effective barrier performance can prevent lipid degradation during storage and retain product quality. This section discusses barrier requirements, selection of high-performance polymers and multilayer structures, as well as material suitability for various applications. Moreover, it also addresses food packaging interactions that may influence overall product stability and safety.

17.3.1 Control of oxygen, light, and moisture

17.3.1.1 Oxygen permeability

Oxygen permeability is a crucial factor for PUFA-rich foods. Oxygen is a strong oxidizing agent for PUFAs. PUFAs contain bis-allylic methylene groups, which increase oxidation rates by lowering the activation energy for hydrogen abstraction (Jacobsen, 2015). Therefore, even a low level of oxygen can also cause significant oxidative rancidity in PUFAs. Low oxygen permeability packaging materials are essential for long shelf life. These materials can suppress initiation and lower lipid oxidation rate. However, oxygen permeability depends on several factors, including film thickness, polymer type, degree of crystallinity, relative humidity, oxygen partial pressure, and temperature. High-barrier polymer materials such as PVDC, EVOH, and aluminium-based laminated materials are commonly used for PUFA. These packaging materials significantly reduce oxygen permeability. Oxygen permeability follows Fickian behavior of mass

TABLE 17.1 Regulatory frameworks for polyunsaturated fatty acids (PUFAs)-rich food products and packaging across nations/regions.

Region/nation	Regulatory framework	Key requirements	References
European Union	Commission regulation (EU) no 10/2011 and regulation (EC) no 1935/2004	• Migration testing with food simulants: D2 (olive oil) for PUFA-rich fatty foods • Overall migration limit (OML) ≤ 10 mg/dm² (60 mg/kg food) • Alternative simulants: D2e (95% ethanol) or D2i (isooctane) when D2 not feasible • Temperature control: ≤ 60°C for D2e and D2i • Specific migration limits for restricted substances: PFAS, BPA prohibited • Bioactive compound preservation requirements (Article 3)	European Commission (2011)
United States (Federal)	Food and Drug Administration (FDA) food contact notification (FCN) program; PFAS phase-out (2024–25)	• Voluntary market phase-out: PFAS-containing grease-proofing agents no longer sold (announced February 2024, completed by January 2025) • 35 FCNs for PFAS declared no longer effective as of January 6, 2025 • Compliance deadline: June 30, 2025 for existing paper packaging stocks • FDA monitoring: screening method for PFAS detection in paper/paperboard packaging • No federal mandate for PUFA-specific oxidation standards; gap in harmonized testing	FDA (2024), FDA (2025)
United States (State-Level)	California AB 1,200, New York, Oregon, Rhode Island PFAS Bans (2025–26)	• California AB 1,200: prohibition of intentionally added PFAS in food packaging (plant-fiber and other materials) • 100 ppm total organic fluorine threshold for plant-fiber packaging • Oregon and Rhode Island: PFAS bans effective January 1, 2025 • Maine: phase-out by May 25, 2026; broader ban by 2032 • State-level enforcement creates market fragmentation; hinders innovation uniformity	Bryan Cave Leighton Paisner LLP (2025), This Element (2025)
India	FSSAI Food Safety and Standards (Packaging) Regulations, 2018	• Migration testing aligned with EU/US standards: food simulants A (10% ethanol), B (3% acetic acid), D2 (olive oil) • Exact migration thresholds per IS 9835 (Indian Standard) • OML: ≤ 10 mg/dm² (or 60 mg/kg food) • Acceptable material lists for food contact • Nonintentionally added substances (NIAS) risk assessment • Protection of bioactive compounds during packaging and storage	FSSAI (2018)

(Continued)

TABLE 17.1 (Continued)

Region/nation	Regulatory framework	Key requirements	References
Global Industry Standard	GOED (Global Organization for EPA and DHA Omega-3s) voluntary monograph	• Peroxide value (PV) ≤ 5 meq O_2/kg (primary oxidation) • Para-anisidine value ≤ 20 (secondary oxidation) • TOTOX (total oxidation) ≤ 26 (combined oxidation: TOTOX=2×PV + AV) • Testing methods: AOCS methods for oxidation assessment • Oxidation preservation during storage and transportation • Product labeling must reflect oxidation status and EPA/DHA content claims • No regulatory mandate; voluntary industry standard with regulatory advocacy ongoing	Global Organization for EPA and DHA Omega-3s (2022)

transfer. The effective diffusivity of oxygen depends on factors that affect the concentration and partial pressure gradients, as well as those that influence the resistance to mass transfer.

17.3.1.2 Light protection requirements

Food containing photosensitizers, such as chlorophylls, riboflavin, and hem pigments, accelerates PUFA oxidation through a photo-oxidative mechanism upon exposure to light. In photo-oxidation, singlet oxygen reacts directly with unsaturated FAs at a rate much higher than the triplet oxygen-mediated pathway. Therefore, packaging must provide protection against ultraviolet and visible light. Plastic materials such as PET provide insufficient protection until they are modified with a light barrier or light-absorbing coating. Metallized films, aluminium foils, and pigmented polymers can effectively reduce light transmission. It reduces the formation of hydroperoxides and aldehydes in PUFA-rich systems (Lee et al., 2008). In any packaging material, light barrier properties depend on absorption, reflection, and scattering. So, incorporating such a material can improve light barrier properties. For example, titanium dioxide can reduce photon penetration significantly without compromising mechanical integrity. This type of packaging is important for edible oils, omega-3-rich FAs, functional foods, and dairy products.

17.3.1.3 Moisture management

Maintaining a desirable moisture level inside the packet stabilizes oxygen permeability, interfacial reactions, and physical stability. Higher moisture can increase water activity, which can affect lipid oxidation rates by altering reactant mobility, metal ion solubility, and antioxidant efficacy. Poorly permeable packaging materials allow moisture to migrate into the packet and accelerate oxidation due to increased oxygen permeability in hydrophilic polymer. Therefore, water vapor transmission is a key factor in PUFA-rich food items. It needs to be considered during the selection or design of packaging. Polyethene and PP provide effective moisture barrier properties due to their semicrystalline structures. Paper packaging may be used after the coating or lamination (Siracusa et al., 2008). Moisture diffusion is also governed by transport phenomena theory and depends upon material permeability, moisture concentration, and vapor pressure (Siracusa, 2012).

17.3.2 High-barrier polymers and multilayer structures

17.3.2.1 Polymer selection criteria

Polymer packaging is popular for PUFA-rich food. In this context, the barrier properties of the polymer, along with its mechanical and chemical resistance, become important. The primary criterion for PUFA-rich food polymer packaging is to restrict oxygen, light, and moisture while maintaining structural integrity for storage and processing. Semicrystalline polymers like PET, PP, and high-density polyethene have sufficient mechanical and barrier properties; on the other hand, amorphous polymers such as ethylene vinyl alcohol show good barrier properties against oxygen but suffer from moisture migration. Therefore, the selection process must consider morphology, glass transition temperature, and permeability. If a polymer is laminated or used in a multilayer configuration, its compatibility needs to be examined. Polymer should also be chemically inert toward lipid. The choice of polymer also depends on the food that is to be packed, particularly for active and coated systems. For the manufacturing of polymer-based packaging material, thermoformability and processability are often considered. All criteria are important for the selection of polymer-based packaging in PUFA-rich food (Robertson, 2016).

17.3.2.2 Multilayer design strategies

Single-layer packaging is sometimes insufficient to perform multiple functions for protecting PUFA-rich foods. To overcome this problem, a multilayer packaging structure is used. Multilayer packaging material comprises multiple materials, providing multifunctional properties. In general, for PUFA-rich foods, the outer layer acts as a moisture barrier, and the other layers act as oxygen barriers, providing mechanical robustness and sealing. Common configurations for multilayer packaging in PUFA-rich foods include PET/EVOH/PE and paperboard/aluminium/PE laminates. From an engineering perspective, multilayer barrier properties depend on thickness optimization, adhesion, and interfacial diffusion resistance. The resultant permeability also depends on the layer sequence, with each layer acting as a resistance to mass transfer. As required, the thicknesses of the different layers can be adjusted. This strategy also allows us to reduction in the thickness of some layers. Multilayer packaging systems also pose environmental challenges, such as recyclability and sustainability. Accept these problems, multilayer packaging is still a good option for stabilized PUFA-rich food (Marsh & Bugusu, 2007).

17.3.2.3 Functional coating systems

Functional coating approach is used to enhance the barrier and protective properties of the packaging without increasing material thickness. Protective coatings, such as biopolymers and organic or inorganic materials, can reduce oxygen and moisture migration (Ahmad et al., 2025; Jahangiri et al., 2024; Kunam et al., 2022). For PUFA-rich food packaging, ceramic coating can be applied via plasma-enhanced chemical vapor deposition. It can reduce the oxygen transmission rate near aluminium foil while maintaining transparency. These coatings also serve as carriers of antioxidants, UV absorbers, or oxygen scavengers, enabling multifunctional protection (Mahmud et al., 2024). The performance of the coating depends on its uniformity, adhesion strength, and resistance to mechanical cracking. Therefore, coating packaging materials requires precise control to ensure their quality. An optimized coated packaging material offers high-performance, lightweight packaging for PUFA-rich foods (Siracusa, 2012).

17.3.3 Packaging material types for polyunsaturated fatty acid-rich foods

17.3.3.1 Paper-based materials

Paper-based packaging materials are well accepted and popular due to their renewability and biodegradability. However, paper has a hydrophilic nature, which limits its direct use in PUFA-rich foods. Uncoated paper allows oxygen and moisture to migrate, which can trigger or accelerate lipid oxidation. Paper packaging is commonly used for PUFA-rich foods after lamination with other materials, such as metal or polymer film. As already discussed, these materials have good barrier properties against moisture, light, and oxygen. Multilayer paper-based structures are widely used for dried PUFA-rich food. Still in a high-moisture environment, lipid migration in paper fiber packaging can cause it to lose its integrity. Therefore, optimization of layer thickness and adhesion becomes important for ensuring oxidative stability in these types of packaging (Marsh & Bugusu, 2007).

17.3.3.2 Plastic packaging systems

Plastic packaging for PUFA-rich foods is widely used in the food processing industry. As we already discussed in previous sections. Polyolefins like PE, PP, and PET offer excellent barrier properties with structure integration as required. These properties can be modified through copolymerization or blending. Plastic packaging also provides an opportunity to integrate active components, antioxidants, or antibacterial agents (Robertson, 2016).

17.3.3.3 Glass and metal containers

Glass and metal containers do not allow oxygen, moisture, or light to enter, as these packaging materials provide excellent barriers. Glass is chemically inert but allows light to pass. It is necessary to take light-protective measures, such as using amber-colored glass. Metal packaging offers excellent mechanical strength along with these barrier properties. Glass and metal are popular options for packaging lipid-based foods, although their cost and weight are higher than those of polymer- and paper-based packaging (Lee et al., 2008).

17.3.4 Food-packaging interactions

17.3.4.1 Migration phenomena

Stability of packed PUFA-rich food depends upon migration phenomena. It involves the transfer of a low-molecular-weight compound between the food and the packaging material. Lipid migration into polymer matrices can lead to plasticization and swelling. Simultaneously, monomers may migrate into the food, enabling oxidation or affecting sensory quality (Arvanitoyannis & Bosnea, 2004). Migration depends on the diffusion coefficient, concentration gradient, temperature, and time. Therefore, understanding the kinetics becomes essential for designing or selecting packaging materials (Robertson, 2016).

17.3.4.2 Surface and interfacial effects

Food's shelf life in the packaging system depends upon the interaction of the food and the packaging system. Surface and interfacial phenomena play a crucial role in stabilizing packaging system for PUFA-rich foods. Often, oxidation is initiated at the lipid-water or lipid-solid interface where metal ions or oxygen molecules accumulate. This accumulation depends upon packaging surface properties, such as roughness, polarity, and chemical functionality (Laguerre et al., 2007). These properties influence interfacial reaction and the adsorption of reactive species. Therefore, modifying the surface chemistry by applying coatings or treatments can reduce catalytic activity and oxygen availability. Table 17.2 shows some packaging materials used for PUFA-rich food and key findings. Also, depicts barrier properties, applications, and key findings for different packaging materials for PUFA-rich foods.

17.4 Packaging innovation: principles and methods

17.4.1 Active packaging systems

17.4.1.1 Antioxidant-based systems

Antioxidant-based active packaging helps retard lipid oxidation by interrupting the propagation of free radicals or by reducing the free radicals responsible for oxidation in PUFA-rich foods. These antioxidants are incorporated by various methods (Gomez-Estaca et al., 2014) (see Fig. 17.2). Tocopherols, ascorbic acid derivatives, plant polyphenols, and synthetic compounds like butylated hydroxytoluene are common antioxidants used for the purpose. The effectiveness of an antioxidant-based active packaging system depends upon antioxidant polarity, migration kinetics, and spatial localization. Controlled release of antioxidants from packaging systems is important to protect food for long storage and sensorial perspectives (Laguerre et al., 2007; Shahidi & Zhong, 2015). Controlled release of antioxidants from active packaging is illustrated in Fig. 17.3.

17.4.1.2 Oxygen-scavenging technologies

Oxygen-scavenging packaging systems significantly reduce oxygen levels in the packaging headspace, thereby reducing autoxidative reactions in PUFA-rich foods. For the purpose of the iron-based oxidation reaction, ascorbate chemistry or enzymatic systems can be embedded in a polymer packaging system. Oxygen-scavenging systems reduce oxygen levels, unlike barriers to oxygen diffusion or antioxidant-based active packaging that reduce oxidation rates. Therefore, low-oxygen concentrations below the critical threshold are required for lipid radical propagation. Scavengers can be kept in sachets, labels, or polymer layers that can be activated by moisture or heat. Polymer-integrated scavengers can be a good choice for safety and eliminate the need for sachets (Brody et al., 2008).

17.4.2 Smart packaging of polyunsaturated fatty acid-rich foods

Smart packaging plays an essential role in food supply chain management around the globe. It enables continuous monitoring of product conditions during storage, transportation, and distribution. The real-time information helps improve quality control, traceability, and inventory management across the supply chain.

PUFA-rich foods, such as seafood, spoilage is often indicated by the release of total volatile basic nitrogen, biogenic amines (e.g., putrescine, cadaverine), and secondary lipid oxidation products (Arulkumar et al., 2023; Hidalgo et al., 2013). Colorimetric indicators detect these spoilage metabolites and provide real-time freshness of

TABLE 17.2 Packaging materials for polyunsaturated fatty acids (PUFAs)-rich foods: barrier properties, applications, and key findings.

Packaging material	Type/structure	Key barrier property	Light barrier	PUFA application	Key findings from source	Limitation	Reference
Ethylene vinyl alcohol (EVOH) multilayer (PET/EVOH/PE)	Synthetic multilayer coextrusion	Excellent O_2 barrier; low OTR	None	Fish oil pouches; omega-3 sachets	Widely used for PUFA-rich products requiring extended shelf life; combines the processability of PE with the O_2 barrier of EVOH	Nonrecyclable in most current streams; EVOH degrades at high RH	Ranjit et al. (2024)
Aluminium foil laminate	Metallic laminate (Al/PET/PE)	Near-zero OTR and WVTR; total barrier	Complete UV+VIS	Supplements; sachets; retort pouches	Provides complete exclusion of O_2 and light; standard for premium omega-3 supplements and shelf-stable pouches	Not microwave-safe; nontransparent; sustainability concerns	Ranjit et al. (2024)
PLA-based biopolymer film	Bioplastic from lactic acid fermentation	Moderate barrier; improves with nanofillers	Partial UV	Sustainable flexible packaging for PUFA-enriched foods	PLA and PHA are identified as primary sustainable alternatives to synthetic plastics; nanomaterials are needed to match barrier properties	Lower barrier than conventional EVOH; brittle at low temperatures	Nibret (2025)
Chitosan-based edible film	Biopolymer from chitin deacetylation	Good gas and UV barrier (dry); WVTR high	Partial UV	Edible coatings for omega-3 enriched foods	Good gas/UV barrier; high WVTR; suitable only in low-humidity environments; SWOT shows limited water resistance	Poor barrier at high RH; limited scalability	Perera et al. (2023)
Zein-based packaging film	Corn prolamin protein biopolymer	Good O_2 barrier; low WVTR	Partial	Coatings for omega-3 fortified foods	Zein shows good O_2 barrier and excellent moisture resistance; SWOT analysis confirms antioxidant potential and superior water barrier properties	Poor processability; high cost of zein extraction	Perera et al. (2023)
Starch-based film	Biopolymer from cereal/tuber starch	Low WVTR; poor water resistance	None	Composite packaging for dry PUFA products	Starch shows low WVTR but poor water resistance; often blended with other biopolymers or nanoclay to improve properties	Very poor water resistance; degrades on contact with moisture	Perera et al. (2023)

Biopolymer-nanocomposite (PLA + nanoclay)	Bioplastic with montmorillonite nanofiller	Improved O_2 and moisture barrier vs neat PLA	None	Sustainable flexible PUFA packaging	Functionalisation via blending and edible coatings enables sustainable packaging; nanosensors integrated for quality monitoring	Lower barrier than EVOH; limited food contact clearances in the EU	Sharma et al. (2025)
UV-absorbing packaging (light barrier)	Inorganic/organic UV absorbers in polymer	Blocks critical degradation wavelengths	High (absorbs 200–450 nm; 640–670 nm for oils)	Retail PUFA oils; fish oil transparent containers	Vegetable oils degrade at 200–450 nm and 640–670 nm; specific UV-blocking packaging suppresses photo-oxidation initiation	UV stabilizer leaching concerns; cost of specialized films	Kwon et al. (2018)
Active antioxidant film (tocopherol-loaded)	LDPE compounded with alpha-tocopherol	Moderate O_2 barrier; active O_2 scavenging within package	None	PUFA-enriched food contact applications	Alpha-tocopherol is identified as a key active packaging agent for antioxidant migration; butylated hydroxytoluene is also used to delay oxidation in the headspace	Antioxidant depletion over shelf life; regulatory approval needed for novel combinations	Ranjit et al. (2024)
O_2 scavenger sachets (iron-based)	Electrochemical O_2 removal sachet	Removes residual O_2 to less than 0.01%	N/A	Fish oil supplements; omega-3 capsule bottles	Iron-based sachets (e.g., ageless; freshpax) are widely cited for headspace O_2 reduction; ascorbate and glucose oxidase variants are also reviewed	Single-use; cost per pack; not suitable for liquid products	Ranjit et al. (2024)
Biopolymer-based edible coating (WPI)	Whey protein isolate (WPI) edible film	Excellent gas barrier when dry (1–5 cc/m^2/day)	None	Edible coatings for PUFA emulsions and fortified foods	WPI highlighted for shielding PUFAs from oxidation; used in conjunction with lecithin for fish oil encapsulation	Very moisture sensitive; fragile; short functional life on the food surface	Kassem et al. (2025)
Intelligent modified atmosphere (MAP)	Gas flushing + colorimetric sensor label	Displaces O_2; monitors CO_2/O_2 real-time	None	Fresh omega-3 fish; seafood products	Smart MAP combines O_2 displacement with sensor labels (pH indicators for TMA/amine detection) to monitor freshness in fish	Gas distribution uniformity challenges require hermetic sealing	Lokuge (2025)

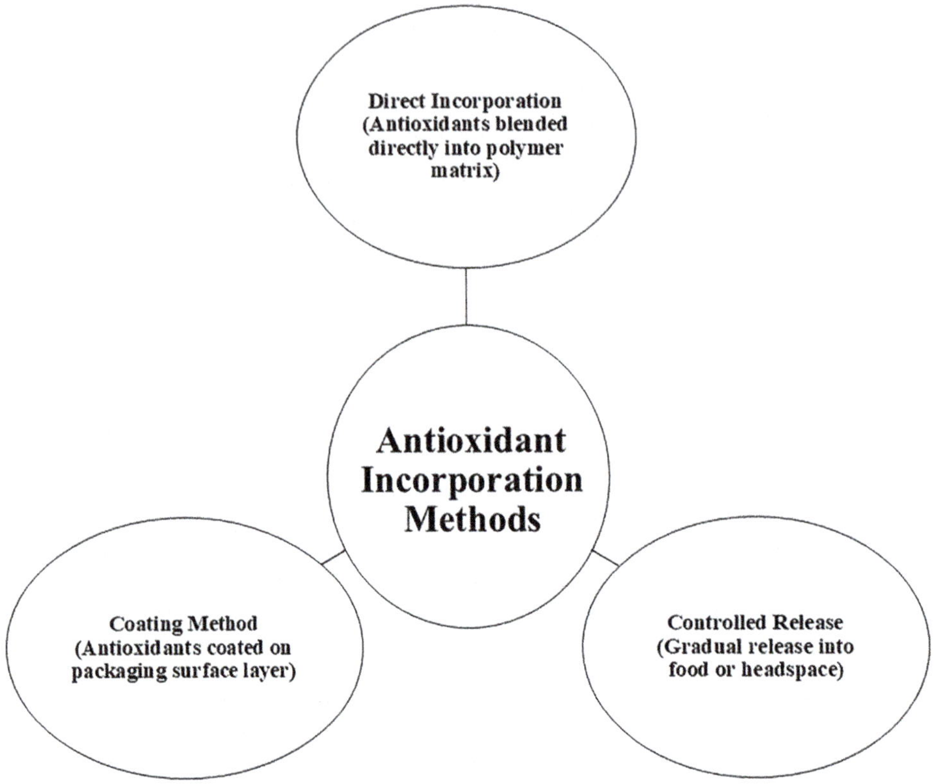

FIGURE 17.2 Methods of incorporating antioxidants.
Source: Gomez-Estaca, J., Lopez-de-Dicastillo, C., Hernandez-Munoz, P., Catala, R., & Gavara, R. (2014). Advances in antioxidant active food packaging. Trends in Food Science & Technology, 35(1), 42–51. https://doi.org/10.1016/j.tifs.2013.10.008.

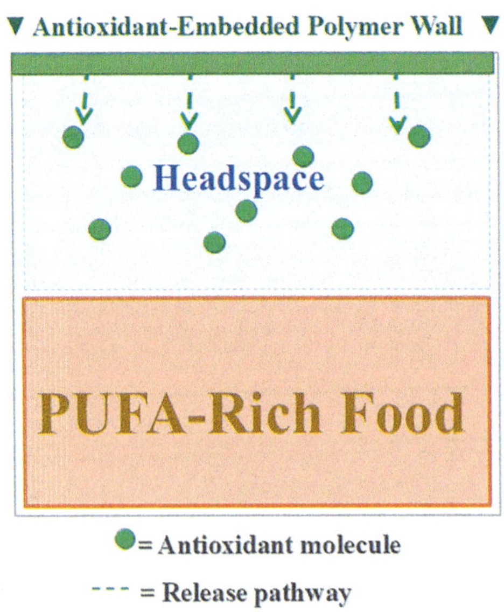

FIGURE 17.3 Controlled release of antioxidants from active packaging for lipid oxidation inhibition in polyunsaturated fatty acids (PUFAs)-rich foods (Kuai et al., 2021).
Source: Kuai, L., Liu, F., Chiou, B.-S., Avena-Bustillos, R.J., McHugh, T.H., & Zhong, F. (2021). Controlled release of antioxidants from active food packaging: A review. Food Hydrocolloids, 120, 106992. https://doi.org/10.1016/j.foodhyd.2021.106992.

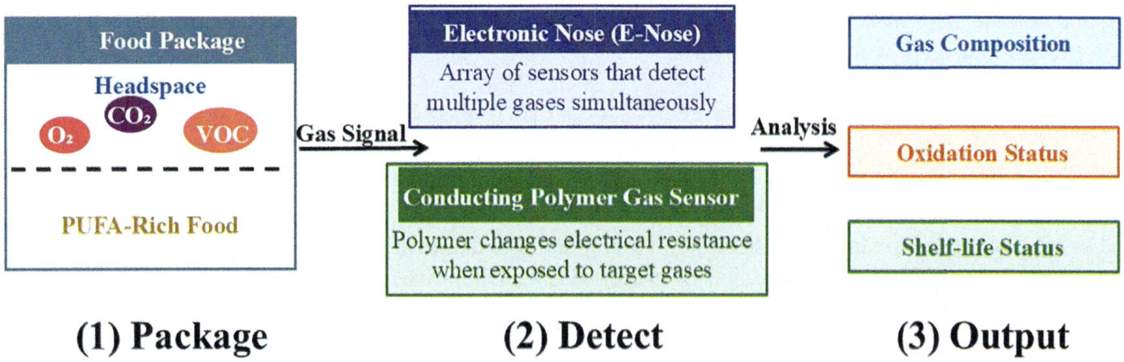

FIGURE 17.4 Advanced smart packaging for nondestructive detection of headspace gas composition in polyunsaturated fatty acid (PUFA)-rich foods. Source: Sohail, M., Sun, D.W., & Zhu, Z. (2018). Recent developments in intelligent packaging for enhancing food quality and safety. Critical Reviews in Food Science and Nutrition, 58(15), 2650–2662. https://doi.org/10.1080/10408398.2018.1449731, https://www.tandfonline.com/loi/bfsn2.

seafood (Zhai et al., 2025). Modified atmosphere packaging (MAP), active antioxidant packaging films, chitosan coatings, oxygen absorbers, and smart freshness indicators represent some of the promising approaches currently employed for the protection of PUFA oxidation (Baptista et al., 2020; Kontominas et al., 2021).

Advanced smart packaging goes one step further and offers a nondestructive way to detect headspace gas composition by incorporating electronic nose (e-nose) arrays and conducting polymer gas sensors (Sohail et al., 2018) (see Fig. 17.4). Time temperature integrators complement these sensors by gathering thermal exposure data to predict remaining PUFA product shelf life along the cold chain (Tsironi et al., 2016). RFID-enabled smart labels wirelessly relay real-time quality data to retailers and consumers. This ensures complete traceability from production to point of use (Ghaani et al., 2016).

17.4.3 Modified atmosphere packaging of polyunsaturated fatty acid-rich foods

Foods rich in PUFAs are highly susceptible to lipid oxidation. Rancid off-flavors and degradation of nutritional value are outcomes of the same (McManus et al., 2011). MAP addresses this problem and can be employed for the preservation of PUFA-rich foods. The headspace oxygen is replaced with precise gas combinations. Most common combinations employ CO_2 (40%–60%) and N_2 (40%–60%), with or without trace O_2 (<5%). This low-oxygen or anaerobic microenvironment retards aerobic microbial growth and protects vulnerable PUFA double bonds from oxidative chain reactions (Stamatis & Arkoudelos, 2007).

Few studies on the MAP of PUFA-rich foods have confirmed the retention of key quality parameters and extended shelf life. PUFA-enriched fish fillets showed a significant reduction in peroxide value (PV) and thiobarbituric acid reactive substances (TBARS) compared with aerobic packaging, thereby extending shelf life by 6–10 days (Duan et al., 2010). Antioxidant surface coatings (e.g., chitosan-krill oil) enhance preservation when combined with MAP (Duan et al., 2010; Messina et al., 2015). High-oxygen MAP with vitamin E supplementation maintained greater PUFA compositional integrity in PUFA-enriched lamb than refrigerated storage. (Alvarez et al., 2009). Omega-3-enriched lamb muscle also confirmed superior oxidative stability when packed in vacuum packaging as compared to air-packaged controls (Ponnampalam et al., 2001). Protective matrices are used for omega-3 supplements during encapsulation. However, when combined with packaging, they further reduce the formation of peroxides and preserve sensory properties (Yenipazar & Şahin-Yeşilçubuk, 2023). Optimal microbial stability for fatty fish such as sea bass has been confirmed by predictive modeling of MAP gas compositions (Tsironi et al., 2019).

17.5 Shelf-life evaluation

17.5.1 Oxidative stability assessment methods

Oxidative stability in PUFA-rich foods is evaluated using chemical, instrumental, and sensorial methods. Primary oxidation is expressed with the PV. Conjugated diene formation and hydroperoxide concentration show initiation of the early stage of the oxidation process. Afterwards, peroxides accumulate in the system, typically following an induction period, and then undergo a rapid increase reflecting autocatalytic kinetics. During secondary oxidation, anisidine value,

TBARS, and volatile aldehydes are assessed and are strongly correlated with sensory value degradation. Primary oxidation follows a pseudo-first-order reaction (Eq. 17.1).

$$\frac{d\,[\mathrm{PV}]}{dt} = k\,[\mathrm{PUFA}] \tag{17.1}$$

Where k - rate constant.

Value of k depends upon oxygen availability and temperature. Chemical changes affect sensory properties, which are captured as off-flavors due to rancidity. Therefore, it is important to define the product's shelf life. Assessment of different packaging with varying oxygen transmission characteristics can improve predictive accuracy (Laguerre et al., 2007; Robertson, 2016).

17.5.2 Accelerated shelf-life testing and modeling

Accelerated shelf-life estimation is a commonly used tool to predict the stability of PUFA-rich food. This estimation is carried out under controlled conditions such as elevated temperature, oxygen concentration, and light exposure. Rate of change is modeled by using Arrhenius Eq. (17.2).

$$k = k_0 \exp\left(-\frac{E_a}{RT}\right) \tag{17.2}$$

Where k - oxidation rate constant, E_a - activation energy, R - gas constant, T - absolute temperature.

High E_a values show greater resistance to oxidation and efficient packaging. Zero- and first-order reaction kinetics models are frequently used to describe oxygen-dependent kinetics, whereas moisture is generally expressed as water activity. These kinetic constants are used to predict shelf life in real storage conditions. Models are valuable for comparing the packaging system capabilities and design (Robertson, 2016).

17.5.3 Comparative evaluation of packaging systems

Comparative shelf-life evaluation is useful for selecting the packaging system. For PUFA-rich foods, we assess oxidation by benchmarking kinetic parameters, quality indices, and sensory acceptability. Comparison can be carried out on the basis of the oxidation rate constant (k), extension induction period, and time required to reach critical limits of PV and AV (Calligaris et al., 2016; Shahidi & Zhong, 2015). A packaging system having a lower oxygen transmission rate shows a lower oxidation rate, which also reflects the mass transfer and reaction kinetics relationship (Frojan et al., 2023). Shelf life reflects failure or reaching the parameter beyond the desirable limit for the product under any packaging system. Therefore, shelf-life extension can be compared under identical storage conditions. For quality retention comparison, sensory parameters such as color, flavor, taste, smell, and textural values can be compared depending on the food. Statistical tools are helpful in analyzing and comparing for the selection of packaging material by establishing correlation with material properties, kinetic behavior, sensory quality, and consumer acceptability (Frojan et al., 2023).

17.6 Applications in polyunsaturated fatty acid-rich food systems

PUFAs are widely introduced into diverse food systems to enhance their nutritional profile. This section highlights the practical application of packaging and stability strategies essential for preserving PUFA integrity in edible oils and emulsions, marine, meat, and dairy PUFA products. It further delves into how the product matrix characteristics affect oxidative behavior and packaging requirements, examining active and intelligent packaging systems, antioxidant integration, microencapsulation strategies, and material selection frameworks tailored to specific PUFA sensitivity and distribution conditions.

17.6.1 Edible oils and emulsions

The preservation of polyunsaturated fatty acid (PUFA)-rich foods presents a significant scientific and industrial challenge due to the inherent chemical instability of PUFAs (Zende et al., 2024). For bulk edible oils, the primary strategy involves creating an effective barrier against oxygen and light through active and intelligent packaging systems. Natural antioxidants like α-tocopherol (vitamin E) or rosemary extract can be used in polylactic acid (PLA) films, which function in the form of controlled-release manner to scavenge free radicals within the oil (Wang et al., 2024). Oxidation can also be effectively slowed down using multilayered biodegradable structures (Glicerina et al., 2023). For refined sunflower oil stored for 12 months, Tetra Brick packaging provided the best protection against oxidation (Romanić et al., 2009).

In the case of emulsified systems, the oil-water interface acts as a critical site for oxidation (Hennebelle et al., 2024). Flaxseed oil emulsions have reportedly shown enhanced oxidative stability as complexes are formed between plant proteins like pea protein and polyphenols such as tannic acid, providing a robust antioxidant shield at the droplet surface (Li et al., 2020). Localization of sesamol at the interface of whey protein isolate (WPI)-stabilized fish oil emulsions has been shown to be an effective strategy for protecting PUFAs from oxidation (Gao et al., 2023). A significant improvement in physical and oxidative stability was observed when double emulsions encapsulating fish oil within structured systems were stabilized with whey protein hydrolysate (Padial-Domínguez et al., 2023). Increased homogenization pressures of oil-in-water emulsions have been shown to improve oxidative stability (Horn et al., 2013).

17.6.2 Marine, meat, and dairy polyunsaturated fatty acid products

Marine-based PUFA products are extremely perishable due to their high content of long-chain omega-3 PUFAs (EPA and DHA). Their preservation requires combining MAP with active components. Antimicrobial films employed alongside MAP have demonstrated shelf-life extension in packaged fish, while incorporating UV-blocking or antimicrobial nanoparticles in nanotechnology-based biodegradable films provided enhanced protection (Cicek & Ozogul, 2022). Real-time quality monitoring has become possible due to intelligent packaging systems integrating freshness indicators, including pH-sensitive smart packaging films for detecting spoilage (Alizadeh-Sani et al., 2020; Alizadeh Sani et al., 2024).

For PUFA-enriched meat and dairy products, a dominant strategy to prevent oxidation and sensory deterioration in formulations such as NaCl-reduced burgers is microencapsulation (Rios-Mera et al., 2021). In dairy systems, emulsion-based fortification boosts bioavailability while maintaining quality attributes (Gumus & Gharibzahedi, 2021). Microencapsulation with omega-3 FAs using fish oil showed a protective effect against lipid oxidation of frozen chicken nuggets, especially during the first month of storage (Jiménez-Martín et al., 2016). Omega-3 UHT milk, fortified yogurt tends to retain >90% DHA after 9 months in Tetra Pak cartons; nitrogen-flushed PE/EVOH yogurt cups significantly reduce fishy off-flavor versus standard PP equivalents (Han et al., 2018). Omega-3 softgel supplements in HDPE bottles flushed with nitrogen and oxygen scavenger achieve 24–36 months ambient shelf life with PV <5 meq O_2/kg, versus >20 meq O_2/kg without active headspace control (Kolanowski, 2010).

17.7 Future perspectives

Future developments in packaging for PUFA-rich food products are expected to move toward integrated, adaptive, and sustainable systems. Advances in nanotechnology, materials science, and digital sensing are allowing packaging to not only provide basic barrier protection but also actively monitor product quality.

17.7.1 Next-generation materials and multifunctional packaging

The next-generation packaging materials will integrate multiple protective functions within a single system, including coextruded or nanocomposite film structures, eliminating reliance on separate sachet inserts or externally attached indicators (Lopez de Dicastillo et al., 2020; Vilela et al., 2018). Biopolymer and biobased systems reinforced with nanocellulose or organoclay are progressively narrowing the performance gap with petroleum-derived multilayer films, thereby supporting biodegradable or compostable end-of-life pathways (Asgher et al., 2020; Lopez de Dicastillo et al., 2020; Mahmud et al., 2024). Additive manufacturing allows packaging structures to act as precision localized active compound release depots, which would otherwise not be achievable by conventional film extrusion (Han et al., 2018).

17.7.2 Sustainability and research priorities

While innovations in packaging are encouraged, sustainability and recyclability should not be given less attention. The use of recyclable and biodegradable materials, due to either regulatory pressure or environmental concerns, is gaining importance. At the same time, smart packaging systems with sensors and indicators can help monitor product quality and improve supply chain management, highlighting the need for continued research that balances performance, sustainability, and cost-effectiveness. It is worth mentioning here that, alone, sensors cannot be relied upon; a combination of sensors and sensory analysis is crucial for judging the quality of PUFA-rich foods, which can provide deeper insights into the oxidation process and shelf-life extension (Clarke et al., 2021).

Some of the critical research gaps include standardized PUFA protection efficacy testing protocols, molecular-level understanding of nanomaterial lipid interactions, standardized, predictive shelf-life models that integrate multiscale variables right from packaging material properties to internal lipid composition and external environmental stressors, inadequate assessment of migration safety and regulatory compliance for emerging biopolymer-nanocomposite systems.

17.8 Conclusion

Polyunsaturated FAs are used in functional foods, nutraceuticals, and fortified food products due to their rich nutritional value. However, it contains double bonds, which are susceptible to oxidation, leading to the formation of hydroperoxides and volatile secondary compounds that affect nutritional and sensorial acceptance. These negative effects on quality ultimately reduce the shelf-life of products. Therefore, PUFA-rich foods require protection against oxidative reactions through a well-designed packaging system that serves as a barrier to light, moisture, and oxygen. Advanced packaging techniques can significantly help us to fulfill these objectives by stabilizing PUFA-containing foods. High-barrier polymers, a multilayer structure, and active packaging can be helpful. Shelf-life prediction using oxidation indices under accelerated storage and kinetics modeling can also help predict quality parameter levels. Future packaging for PUFA is likely to focus on multifunctional, sustainable, and smart technologies to enhance oxidation stability while minimizing environmental impact.

References

Aberkane, L., Roudaut, G., & Saurel, R. (2013). Encapsulation and oxidative stability of PUFA-rich oil microencapsulated by spray drying using pea protein and pectin. *Food and Bioprocess Technology, 7*(5), 1505–1517. https://doi.org/10.1007/s11947-013-1202-9.

Ahmad, K., Ahmad, R., Faizan, M., Farah, Ali, F., Yousaf, M. M., Ali, F., Niaz, W., Khan, T. U., Khan, S., Ali, S., Ahmed, I., & Hassan, H. (2025). A review of nanotechnology in food industry with implication for viable outlook and safety issues. *Hybrid Advances, 10*, 100487. https://doi.org/10.1016/j.hybadv.2025.100487, https://www.sciencedirect.com/journal/hybrid-advances.

Ahmed, I., Lin, H., Zou, L., Brody, A. L., Li, Z., Qazi, I. M., Pavase, T. R., & Lv, L. (2017). A comprehensive review on the application of active packaging technologies to muscle foods. *Food Control, 156*, 109726. https://doi.org/10.1016/j.foodcont.2023.109726.

Alizadeh Sani, M., Zhang, W., Abedini, A., Khezerlou, A., Shariatifar, N., Assadpour, E., Zhang, F., & Jafari, S. M. (2024). Intelligent packaging systems for the quality and safety monitoring of meat products: From lab scale to industrialization. *Food Control, 160*, 110359. https://doi.org/10.1016/j.foodcont.2024.110359.

Alizadeh-Sani, M., Mohammadian, E., Rhim, J. W., & Jafari, S. M. (2020). pH-sensitive (halochromic) smart packaging films based on natural food colorants for the monitoring of food quality and safety. *Trends in Food Science and Technology, 105*, 93–144. https://doi.org/10.1016/j.tifs.2020.08.014, http://www.elsevier.com/wps/find/journaldescription.cws_home/601278/description#description.

Alvarez, I., De La Fuente, J., Caneque, V., Lauzurica, S., Perez, C., & Diaz, M. T. (2009). Changes in the fatty acid composition of M. longissimus dorsi of lamb during storage in a high-oxygen modified atmosphere at different levels of dietary vitamin E supplementation. *Journal of Agricultural and Food Chemistry, 57*(1), 140–146. https://doi.org/10.1021/jf801940c.

Arulkumar, A., Paramithiotis, S., & Paramasivam, S. (2023). Biogenic amines in fresh fish and fishery products and emerging control. *Aquaculture and Fisheries, 8*(4), 431–450. https://doi.org/10.1016/j.aaf.2021.02.001.

Arvanitoyannis, I. S., & Bosnea, L. (2004). Migration of substances from food packaging materials to foods. *Critical Reviews in Food Science and Nutrition, 44*(2), 63–76. https://doi.org/10.1080/10408690490424621.

Asgher, M., Qamar, S. A., Bilal, M., & Iqbal, H. M. N. (2020). Bio-based active food packaging materials: Sustainable alternative to conventional petrochemical-based packaging materials. *Food Research International, 137*, 109625. https://doi.org/10.1016/j.foodres.2020.109625, www.elsevier.com/inca/publications/store/4/2/2/9/7/0.

Bacellar, I. O. L., & Baptista, M. S. (2019). Mechanisms of photosensitized lipid oxidation and membrane permeabilization. *ACS Omega, 4*(26), 21636–21646. https://doi.org/10.1021/acsomega.9b03244, pubs.acs.org/journal/acsodf.

Baptista, R. C., Horita, C. N., & Sant'Ana, A. S. (2020). Natural products with preservative properties for enhancing the microbiological safety and extending the shelf-life of seafood: A review. *Food Research International, 127*, 108762. https://doi.org/10.1016/j.foodres.2019.108762, www.elsevier.com/inca/publications/store/4/2/2/9/7/0.

Brody, A. L., Bugusu, B., Han, J. H., Sand, C. K., & McHugh, T. H. (2008). Scientific status summary. Innovative food packaging solutions. *Journal of Food Science, 73*(8), R107–R116. https://doi.org/10.1111/j.1750-3841.2008.00933.x.

Bryan Cave Leighton Paisner LLP. (2025, December). PFAS in food packaging: State-by-state regulations. Retrieved from https://www.bclplaw.com/en-US/events-insights-news/pfas-in-food-packaging-state-by-state-regulations.html.

Calligaris, S., Manzocco, L., Anese, M., & Nicoli, M. C. (2016). Shelf-life assessment of food undergoing oxidation–A review. *Critical Reviews in Food Science and Nutrition, 56*(11), 1903–1912. https://doi.org/10.1080/10408398.2013.807222, www.tandf.co.uk/journals/titles/10408398.asp.

Choe, E., & Min, D. B. (2006). Mechanisms and factors for edible oil oxidation. *Comprehensive Reviews in Food Science and Food Safety, 5*(4), 169–186. https://doi.org/10.1111/j.1541-4337.2006.00009.x, http://www.blackwell-synergy.com/doi/pdf/10.1111/j.1541-4337.2006.00009.x.

Choe, E., & Min, D. B. (2009). Mechanisms of antioxidants in the oxidation of foods. *Comprehensive Reviews in Food Science and Food Safety, 8*(4), 345–358. https://doi.org/10.1111/j.1541-4337.2009.00085.x.

Cicek, S., & Ozogul, F. (2022). Nanotechnology-based preservation approaches for aquatic food products: A review with the current knowledge. *Critical Reviews in Food Science and Nutrition, 63*(19), 3255–3278. https://doi.org/10.1080/10408398.2022.2096563.

Clarke, H. J., McCarthy, W. P., O'sullivan, M. G., Kerry, J. P., & Kilcawley, K. N. (2021). Oxidative quality of dairy powders: Influencing factors and analysis. *Foods, 10*(10), 2315. https://doi.org/10.3390/foods10102315, https://www.mdpi.com/2304-8158/10/10/2315/pdf.

Dey, A., & Neogi, S. (2019). Oxygen scavengers for food packaging applications: A review. *Journal of Food Engineering, 247*, 95–106. https://doi.org/10.1016/j.jfoodeng.2018.11.020.

Domínguez, R., Pateiro, M., Gagaoua, M., Barba, F. J., Zhang, W., & Lorenzo, J. M. (2019). A comprehensive review on lipid oxidation in meat and meat products. *Antioxidants, 8*(10), 429. https://doi.org/10.3390/antiox8100429, https://www.mdpi.com/2076-3921/8/10/429/pdf.

Duan, J., Jiang, Y., Cherian, G., & Zhao, Y. (2010). Effect of combined chitosan-krill oil coating and modified atmosphere packaging on the storability of cold-stored lingcod (*Ophiodon elongates*) fillets. *Food Chemistry, 122*(4), 1035–1042. https://doi.org/10.1016/j.foodchem.2010.03.065.

Durand, E., Laguerre, M., Bourlieu-Lacanal, C., Lecomte, J., & Villeneuve, P. (2025). Navigating the complexity of lipid oxidation and antioxidation: A review of evaluation methods and emerging approaches. *Progress in Lipid Research, 97*, 101317. https://doi.org/10.1016/j.plipres.2024.101317.

Dyall, S. C., Balas, L., Bazan, N. G., Brenna, J. T., Chiang, N., da Costa Souza, F., Dalli, J., Durand, T., Galano, J. M., Lein, P. J., Serhan, C. N., & Taha, A. Y. (2022). Polyunsaturated fatty acids and fatty acid-derived lipid mediators: Recent advances in the understanding of their biosynthesis, structures, and functions. *Progress in Lipid Research, 86*, 101165. https://doi.org/10.1016/j.plipres.2022.101165, www.elsevier.com/locate/plipres.

Elias, R. J., Kellerby, S. S., & Decker, E. A. (2008). Antioxidant activity of proteins and peptides. *Critical Reviews in Food Science and Nutrition, 48*(5), 430–441. https://doi.org/10.1080/10408390701425615.

Esterbauer, H., Schaur, R. J., & Zollner, H. (1991). Chemistry and biochemistry of 4-hydroxynonenal, malonaldehyde and related aldehydes. *Free Radical Biology and Medicine, 11*(1), 81–128. https://doi.org/10.1016/0891-5849(91)90192-6.

European Commission (2011). Commission regulation (EU) No 10/2011 of 14 January 2011 on plastic materials and articles intended to come into contact with food. *Official Journal of the European Union*, 1–89. L 12 https://eur-lex.europa.eu/eli/reg/2011/10/oj/eng.

FDA. (2024, February 28). FDA announces PFAS used in grease-proofing agents for food packaging no longer being sold in the U.S. https://www.fda.gov/food/hfp-constituent-updates/fda-announces-pfas-used-grease-proofing-agents-food-packaging-no-longer-being-sold-us.

FDA. (2025, January 6). FDA determines authorization for 35 food contact notifications related to PFAS are no longer effective. Federal Register Notice. https://www.fda.gov/food/hfp-constituent-updates/fda-determines-authorization-35-food-contact-notifications-related-pfas-are-no-longer-effective.

Food Safety and Standards Authority of India. (2018). Food Safety and Standards (Packaging) Regulations, 2018. Government of India Official Gazette, Notification No. 1-95/Stds/Packaging/SP(L&C/A)/FSSAI-2017, December 24, 2018. Retrieved from https://fssai.gov.in/upload/uploadfiles/files/Compendium_Packaging_01_02_2022.pdf.

Frankel, E. N., Satué-Gracia, T., Meyer, A. S., & German, J. B. (2002). Oxidative stability of fish and algae oils containing long-chain polyunsaturated fatty acids in bulk and in oil-in-water emulsions. *Journal of Agricultural and Food Chemistry, 50*(7), 2094–2099. https://doi.org/10.1021/jf0111458.

Frojan, J., Bisquert, P., Buche, P., Gontard, N., Boone, L., Nhu Thuy, T., Vermeulen, A., Ragaert, P., Dewulf, J., & Guillard, V. (2023). Scoring methodology for comparing the environmental performance of food packaging. *Packaging Technology and Science, 36*(6), 439–463. https://doi.org/10.1002/pts.2720.

Fu, Y., Wang, Y., Gao, H., Li, D. H., Jiang, R. R., Ge, L., Tong, C., Xu, K., & Wu, M. (2021). Associations among dietary omega-3 polyunsaturated fatty acids, the gut microbiota, and intestinal immunity. *Mediators of Inflammation, 2021*(1), 8879227. https://doi.org/10.1155/2021/8879227.

Gao, Z., Ji, Z., Wang, L., Deng, Q., Quek, S. Y., Liu, L., & Dong, X. (2023). Improvement of oxidative stability of fish oil-in-water emulsions through partitioning of sesamol at the interface. *Foods, 12*(6), 1287. https://doi.org/10.3390/foods12061287.

Geng, L., Liu, K., & Zhang, H. (2023). Lipid oxidation in foods and its implications on proteins. *Frontiers in Nutrition, 10*, 1192199. https://doi.org/10.3389/fnut.2023.1192199.

Ghaani, M., Cozzolino, C. A., Castelli, G., & Farris, S. (2016). An overview of the intelligent packaging technologies in the food sector. *Trends in Food Science and Technology, 51*, 1–11. https://doi.org/10.1016/j.tifs.2016.02.008, http://www.elsevier.com/wps/find/journaldescription.cws_home/601278/description#description.

Gill, R., Al-Badr, M., Alghouti, M., Mohamed, N. A., Abou-Saleh, H., & Rahman, M. M. (2024). Revolutionizing cardiovascular health with nano encapsulated omega-3 fatty acids: A nano-solution approach. *Marine Drugs, 22*(6), 256. https://doi.org/10.3390/md22060256, http://www.mdpi.com/journal/marinedrugs.

Glicerina, V., Siroli, L., Gottardi, D., Ticchi, N., Capelli, F., Accorsi, R., Gherardi, M., Minelli, M., Fiorini, M., Andrisano, V., Colombo, V., Manzini, R., Lanciotti, R., & Romani, S. (2023). Influence of an innovative, biodegradable active packaging on the quality of sunflower oil and "pesto" sauce during storage. *Applied Food Research, 3*(2), 100313. https://doi.org/10.1016/j.afres.2023.100313.

Global Organization for EPA and DHA Omega-3s. (2022). GOED voluntary monograph on EPA and DHA omega-3 products (Version 8.1, Issue Date January 6, 2022). Retrieved fromhttps://goedomega3.com/storage/app/media/Monograph/GOED%20Monograph%20-%202022%2001%2006%20-%20FINAL.pdf.

Gomez-Estaca, J., Lopez-de-Dicastillo, C., Hernandez-Munoz, P., Catala, R., & Gavara, R. (2014). Advances in antioxidant active food packaging. *Trends in Food Science & Technology, 35*(1), 42–51. https://doi.org/10.1016/j.tifs.2013.10.008.

Gumus, C. E., & Gharibzahedi, S. M. T. (2021). Yogurts supplemented with lipid emulsions rich in omega-3 fatty acids: New insights into the fortification, microencapsulation, quality properties, and health-promoting effects. *Trends in Food Science and Technology, 110*, 267–279. https://doi.org/10.1016/j.tifs.2021.02.016, http://www.elsevier.com/wps/find/journaldescription.cws_home/601278/description#description.

Gupta, P. (2024). Role of oxygen absorbers in food as packaging material, their characterization and applications. *Journal of Food Science and Technology, 61*(2), 242–252. https://doi.org/10.1007/s13197-023-05681-8.

Han, J. W., Ruiz-Garcia, L., Qian, J. P., & Yang, X. T. (2018). Food packaging: A comprehensive review and future trends. *Comprehensive Reviews in Food Science and Food Safety, 17*(4), 860–877. https://doi.org/10.1111/1541-4337.12343, http://onlinelibrary.wiley.com/journal/10.1111/(ISSN)1541-4337.

Hennebelle, M., Villeneuve, P., Durand, E., Lecomte, J., van Duynhoven, J., Meynier, A., Yesiltas, B., Jacobsen, C., & Berton-Carabin, C. (2024). Lipid oxidation in emulsions: New insights from the past two decades. *Progress in Lipid Research, 94*, 101275. https://doi.org/10.1016/j.plipres.2024.101275.

Hidalgo, F. J., Navarro, J. L., Delgado, R. M., & Zamora, R. (2013). Histamine formation by lipid oxidation products. *Food Research International, 52*(1), 206–213. https://doi.org/10.1016/j.foodres.2013.03.031.

Hooper, L., Al-Khudairy, L., Abdelhamid, A. S., Rees, K., Brainard, J. S., Brown, T. J., Ajabnoor, S. M., O'Brien, A. T., Winstanley, L. E., Donaldson, D. H., Song, F., & Deane, K. H. (2018). Omega-6 fats for the primary and secondary prevention of cardiovascular disease. *Cochrane Database of Systematic Reviews, 11*, CD011094. https://doi.org/10.1002/14651858.CD011094.pub3.

Horn, A. F., Barouh, N., Nielsen, N. S., Baron, C. P., & Jacobsen, C. (2013). Homogenization pressure and temperature affect protein partitioning and oxidative stability of emulsions. *Journal of the American Oil Chemists' Society, 90*(10), 1541–1550. https://doi.org/10.1007/s11746-013-2292-2.

Hussain, S., Akhter, R., & Maktedar, S. S. (2024). Advancements in sustainable food packaging: From eco-friendly materials to innovative technologies. *Sustainable Food Technology, 2*(5), 1297–1364. https://doi.org/10.1039/d4fb00084f, https://www.rsc.org/journals-books-databases/about-journals/sustainable-food-technology/.

Islam, F., Imran, A., Nosheen, F., Fatima, M., Arshad, M. U., Afzaal, M., Ijaz, N., Noreen, R., Mehta, S., Biswas, S., Rasool, I. F. U., Aslam, M. A., Usman, I., Zahra, S. M., Segueni, N., & Amer Ali, Y. (2023). Functional roles and novel tools for improving-oxidative stability of polyunsaturated fatty acids: A comprehensive review. *Food Science and Nutrition, 11*(6), 2471–2482. https://doi.org/10.1002/fsn3.3272, onlinelibrary.wiley.com/journal/10.1002/%28ISSN%292048-7177.

Jacobsen, C. (2015). Some strategies for the stabilization of long chain n-3 PUFA-enriched foods: A review. *European Journal of Lipid Science and Technology, 117*(11), 1853–1866. https://doi.org/10.1002/ejlt.201500137.

Jahangiri, F., Mohanty, A. K., & Misra, M. (2024). Sustainable biodegradable coatings for food packaging: challenges and opportunities. *Green Chemistry, 26*(9), 4934–4974. https://doi.org/10.1039/d3gc02647g, http://pubs.rsc.org/en/journals/journal/gc.

Jiménez-Martín, E., Pérez-Palacios, T., Carrascal, J. R., & Rojas, T. A. (2016). Enrichment of chicken nuggets with microencapsulated omega-3 fish oil: Effect of frozen storage time on oxidative stability and sensory quality. *Food and Bioprocess Technology, 9*(2), 285–297. https://doi.org/10.1007/s11947-015-1621-x, http://www.springer.com/life+sci/food+science/journal/11947.

Kassem, J. M., Abdulqahar, F. W., Zaky, A. A., Boulkrane, M. S., Darwish, A., Farouk, A., Ozçelik, B., Magouz, O., Liu, X., & El-Messery, T. M. (2025). Micro and nanoencapsulation of omega-3 fatty acids: Functional applications and future perspectives in food systems. *Food Safety and Health*. https://doi.org/10.1002/fsh3.70071, https://onlinelibrary.wiley.com/journal/28351096.

Kolanowski, W. (2010). Omega-3 LC PUFA contents and oxidative stability of encapsulated fish oil dietary supplements. *International Journal of Food Properties, 13*(3), 498–511. https://doi.org/10.1080/10942910802652222.

Kolanowski, W., Jaworska, D., & Weißbrodt, J. (2007). Importance of instrumental and sensory analysis in the assessment of oxidative deterioration of omega-3 long-chain polyunsaturated fatty acid-rich foods. *Journal of the Science of Food and Agriculture, 87*(2), 181–191. https://doi.org/10.1002/jsfa.2733.

Kontominas, M. G., Badeka, A. V., Kosma, I. S., & Nathanailides, C. I. (2021). Recent developments in seafood packaging technologies. *Foods, 10*(5), 940. https://doi.org/10.3390/foods10050940, https://www.mdpi.com/2304-8158/10/5/940/pdf.

Kozik-Kołodziej, N. (2026). Consumer attitudes and perceptions toward sustainable packaging: A systematic literature review. *Sustainability, 18*(3), 1235. https://doi.org/10.3390/su18031235.

Kuai, L., Liu, F., Chiou, B.-S., Avena-Bustillos, R. J., McHugh, T. H., & Zhong, F. (2021). Controlled release of antioxidants from active food packaging: A review. *Food Hydrocolloids, 120*, 106992. https://doi.org/10.1016/j.foodhyd.2021.106992.

Kunam, P. K., Ramakanth, D., Akhila, K., & Gaikwad, K. K. (2022). Bio-based materials for barrier coatings on paper packaging. *Biomass Conversion and Biorefinery, 13*, 15399–15419. https://doi.org/10.1007/s13399-022-03241-2.

Kwon, S., Orsuwan, A., Bumbudsanpharoke, N., Yoon, C. S., Choi, J., & Ko, S. (2018). A short review of light barrier materials for food and beverage packaging. *Korean Journal of Packaging Science and Technology, 24*(3), 141–148. https://doi.org/10.20909/kopast.2018.24.3.141.

Laguerre, M., Lecomte, J., & Villeneuve, P. (2007). Evaluation of the ability of antioxidants to counteract lipid oxidation: Existing methods, new trends and challenges. *Progress in Lipid Research, 46*(5), 244–282. https://doi.org/10.1016/j.plipres.2007.05.002.

Lee, D. S., Yam, K. L., & Piergiovanni, L. (2008). *Food packaging science and technology food packaging science and technology*. South Korea: CRC Press, 1–632. https://www.taylorfrancis.com/books/e/9781439894071.

Lee-Okada, H.-C., Xue, C., & Yokomizo, T. (2024). Recent advances on the physiological and pathophysiological roles of polyunsaturated fatty acids and their biosynthetic pathway. *Biochimica et Biophysica Acta (BBA) - Molecular and Cell Biology of Lipids, 1870*(1), 159564. https://doi.org/10.1016/j.bbalip.2024.159564.

Li, R., Dai, T., Tan, Y., Fu, G., Wan, Y., Liu, C., & McClements, D. J. (2020). Fabrication of pea protein-tannic acid complexes: Impact on formation, stability, and digestion of flaxseed oil emulsions. *Food Chemistry, 310*, 125828. https://doi.org/10.1016/j.foodchem.2019.125828.

Lokuge, E. L. (2025). Recent trends in smart packaging. *Journal of Research Technology and Engineering, 6*(3), 176–201.

Lopez de Dicastillo, C., Velasquez, E., Rojas, A., Guarda, A., & Galotto, M. J. (2020). The use of nanoadditives within recycled polymers for food packaging: Properties, recyclability, and safety. *Comprehensive Reviews in Food Science and Food Safety, 19*(4), 1760–1776. https://doi.org/10.1111/1541-4337.12575.

Mahmud, M. Z. A., Mobarak, M. H., & Hossain, N. (2024). Emerging trends in biomaterials for sustainable food packaging: A comprehensive review. *Heliyon, 10*(1), e24122. https://doi.org/10.1016/j.heliyon.2024.e24122.

Marsh, K., & Bugusu, B. (2007). Food packaging - Roles, materials, and environmental issues. *Journal of Food Science, 72*(3), R39–R55. https://doi.org/10.1111/j.1750-3841.2007.00301.x.

McManus, A., Merga, M., & Newton, W. (2011). Omega-3 fatty acids. What consumers need to know. *Appetite, 57*(1), 80–83. https://doi.org/10.1016/j.appet.2011.03.015.

Messina, C. M., Bono, G., Renda, G., La Barbera, L., & Santulli, A. (2015). Effect of natural antioxidants and modified atmosphere packaging in preventing lipid oxidation and increasing the shelf-life of common dolphinfish (Coryphaena hippurus) fillets. *LWT - Food Science and Technology, 62*(1), 271–277. https://doi.org/10.1016/j.lwt.2015.01.029.

Moi, I. M., Leow, A. T. C., Ali, M. S. M., Rahman, R. N. Z. R. A., Salleh, A. B., & Sabri, S. (2018). Polyunsaturated fatty acids in marine bacteria and strategies to enhance their production. *Applied Microbiology and Biotechnology, 102*(14), 5811–5826. https://doi.org/10.1007/s00253-018-9063-9, link.springer.de/link/service/journals/00253/index.htm.

Nibret, A. M. (2025). Emerging trends in biomaterials for sustainable food packaging: A comprehensive review. *International Journal of Food Engineering and Technology, 9*(2), 71–77. https://doi.org/10.11648/j.ijfet.20250902.12.

Padial-Domínguez, M., García-Moreno, P. J., González-Beneded, R., Guadix, A., & Guadix, E. M. (2023). Evaluation of the physical and oxidative stabilities of fish oil-in-water-in-olive oil double emulsions (O1/W/O2) stabilized with whey protein hydrolysate. *Antioxidants, 12*(3), 762. https://doi.org/10.3390/antiox12030762.

Patted, P. G., Masareddy, R. S., Patil, A. S., Kanabargi, R. R., & Bhat, C. T. (2024). Omega-3 fatty acids: A comprehensive scientific review of their sources, functions and health benefits. *Future Journal of Pharmaceutical Sciences, 10*(1), 94. https://doi.org/10.1186/s43094-024-00667-5.

Perera, K. Y., Jaiswal, A. K., & Jaiswal, S. (2023). Biopolymer-based sustainable food packaging materials: Challenges, solutions, and applications. *Foods, 12*(12), 2422. https://doi.org/10.3390/foods12122422, www.mdpi.com/journal/foods.

Ponnampalam, E. N., Trout, G. R., Sinclair, A. J., Egan, A. R., & Leury, B. J. (2001). Comparison of the color stability and lipid oxidative stability of fresh and vacuum packaged lamb muscle containing elevated omega-3 and omega-6 fatty acid levels from dietary manipulation. *Meat Science, 58*(2), 151–161. https://doi.org/10.1016/S0309-1740(00)00143-1.

Ranjit, P., Reddy, K. V., Venkatesh, B. M., Akila, A., Vijay, P. P., Vajran, G. G. D. D. S., Maddela, N. R., & Prasad, R. (2024). Advancements in food packaging strategies with a focus on antimicrobials and sensor technologies: A comprehensive review. *Sustainable Food Technology*. https://doi.org/10.1039/d5fb00303b.

Rios-Mera, J. D., Saldaña, E., Patinho, I., Selani, M. M., & Contreras-Castillo, C. J. (2021). Enrichment of NaCl-reduced burger with long-chain polyunsaturated fatty acids: Effects on physicochemical, technological, nutritional, and sensory characteristics. *Meat Science, 177*, 108497. https://doi.org/10.1016/j.meatsci.2021.108497, http://www.elsevier.com/locate/meatsci.

Rizzo, G., Baroni, L., & Lombardo, M. (2023). Promising sources of plant-derived polyunsaturated fatty acids: A narrative review. *International Journal of Environmental Research and Public Health, 20*(3), 1683. https://doi.org/10.3390/ijerph20031683.

Robertson, G. L. (2016). *Food packaging: Principles and practice* (3rd ed). Australia: CRC Press, 1–688. http://doi.org/10.1201/b21347, http://www.tandfebooks.com/doi/book/9781439862421.

Romanić, R., Dimić, E., Lazić, V., & Vujasinović, V. (2009). Oxidative stability and tocopherol content of refined sunflower oil during long-term storage in different commercial packagings. *Acta Alimentaria, 38*(3), 319–327. https://doi.org/10.1556/aalim.2009.0001.

Saini, R. K., Prasad, P., Sreedhar, R. V., Naidu, K. A., Shang, X., & Keum, Y. S. (2021). Omega−3 polyunsaturated fatty acids (PUFAs): Emerging plant and microbial sources, oxidative stability, bioavailability, and health benefits—A review. *Antioxidants, 10*(10), 1627. https://doi.org/10.3390/antiox10101627, https://www.mdpi.com/2076-3921/10/10/1627/pdf.

Shahidi, F., & Ambigaipalan, P. (2018a). Omega-3 polyunsaturated fatty acids and their health benefits. *Annual Review of Food Science and Technology, 9*(1), 345–381. https://doi.org/10.1146/annurev-food-111317-095850.

Shahidi, F., & Ambigaipalan, P. (2018b). Omega-3 polyunsaturated fatty acids and their health benefits. *Annual Review of Food Science and Technology, 9*, 355–381. https://doi.org/10.1146/annurev-food-052720-112054.

Shahidi, F., & Zhong, Y. (2010a). Lipid oxidation and improving the oxidative stability. *Chemical Society Reviews, 39*(11), 4067. https://doi.org/10.1039/b922183m.

Shahidi, F., & Zhong, Y. (2010b). Lipid oxidation and improving the oxidative stability. *Chemical Society Reviews, 53*(1), 201–262. https://doi.org/10.1039/b922183m.

Shahidi, F., & Zhong, Y. (2015). Measurement of antioxidant activity. *Journal of Functional Foods, 18*, 757–781. https://doi.org/10.1016/j.jff.2015.01.047.

Shao, H., Liu, C., Wen, Y., Zhang, J., & Wang, Y. (2023). Mono-layer films with superior barrier properties and full recyclability: The system of Poly(ethylene terephthalate)/Poly(glycolic acid). *Polymer, 265*, 125594. https://doi.org/10.1016/j.polymer.2022.125315.

Sharma, C., Kundu, S., Singh, S., Saxena, J., Gautam, S., Kumar, A., & Pathak, P. (2025). From concept to shelf: engineering biopolymer-based food packaging for sustainability. *RSC Sustainability, 3*(11), 4992–5026. https://doi.org/10.1039/d5su00483g.

Siracusa, V. (2012). Food packaging permeability behaviour: A report. *International Journal of Polymer Science, 2012*, 1–11. https://doi.org/10.1155/2012/302029. 302029.

Siracusa, V., Rocculi, P., Romani, S., & Rosa, M. D. (2008). Biodegradable polymers for food packaging: A review. *Trends in Food Science and Technology, 19*(12), 634–643. https://doi.org/10.1016/j.tifs.2008.07.003.

Sohail, M., Sun, D. W., & Zhu, Z. (2018). Recent developments in intelligent packaging for enhancing food quality and safety. *Critical Reviews in Food Science and Nutrition, 58*(15), 2650–2662. https://doi.org/10.1080/10408398.2018.1449731, https://www.tandfonline.com/loi/bfsn20.

Stamatis, N., & Arkoudelos, J. (2007). Quality assessment of Scomber colias japonicus under modified atmosphere and vacuum packaging. *Food Control, 18*(4), 292–300. https://doi.org/10.1016/j.foodcont.2005.10.009.

This Element. (2025, September). PFAS-free take-out packaging: A practical state-by-state guide (Updated September 2025). Retrieved from https://this-element.com/blogs/news/pfas-free-take-out-packaging-a-practical-state-by-state-guide-updated-september-2025.

Tian, F., Decker, E. A., & Goddard, J. M. (2013). Controlling lipid oxidation of food by active packaging technologies. *Food and Function, 4*(5), 669–680. https://doi.org/10.1039/c3fo30360h.

Tsironi, T., Giannoglou, M., Platakou, E., & Taoukis, P. (2016). Evaluation of time temperature integrators for shelf-life monitoring of frozen seafood under real cold chain conditions. *Food Packaging and Shelf Life, 10*, 46–53. https://doi.org/10.1016/j.fpsl.2016.09.004.

Tsironi, T., Ntzimani, A., Gogou, E., Tsevdou, M., Semenoglou, I., Dermesonlouoglou, E., & Taoukis, P. (2019). Modeling the effect of active modified atmosphere packaging on the microbial stability and shelf life of gutted sea bass. *Applied Sciences, 9*(23), 5019. https://doi.org/10.3390/app9235019.

Vilela, C., Kurek, M., Hayouka, Z., Röcker, B., Yildirim, S., Antunes, M. D. C., Nilsen-Nygaard, J., Pettersen, M. K., & Freire, C. S. R. (2018). A concise guide to active agents for active food packaging. *Trends in Food Science and Technology, 80*, 212–222. https://doi.org/10.1016/j.tifs.2018.08.006, http://www.elsevier.com/wps/find/journaldescription.cws_home/601278/description#description.

Visioli, F., & Poli, A. (2025). Omega 6 fatty acids: Helpful, harmless or harmful? *Current Opinion in Clinical Nutrition and Metabolic Care, 28*(2), 114–120. https://doi.org/10.1097/MCO.0000000000001096, http://journals.lww.com/co-clinicalnutrition/pages/default.aspx.

Wysoczański, T., Sokoła-Wysoczańska, E., Pękala, J., Lochyński, S., Czyż, K., Bodkowski, R., Herbinger, G., Patkowska-Sokoła, B., & Librowski, T. (2016). Omega-3 fatty acids and their role in central nervous system - A review. *Current Medicinal Chemistry, 23*(8), 816–831. https://doi.org/10.2174/0929867323666160122114439, PMID:26795198.

Yenipazar, H., & Şahin-Yeşilçubuk, N. (2023). Effect of packaging and encapsulation on the oxidative and sensory stability of omega-3 supplements. *Food Science and Nutrition, 11*(3), 1426–1440. https://doi.org/10.1002/fsn3.3182, onlinelibrary.wiley.com/journal/10.1002/%28ISSN%292048-7177.

Zende, R., Ghase, V., & Jamdar, V. (2024). Recent advances in the antimicrobial and antioxidant capabilities of PLA based active food packaging. *Polymer-Plastics Technology and Materials, 64*(4), 439–464. https://doi.org/10.1080/25740881.2024.2409311.

Zhai, X., Xue, Y., Sun, Y., Ma, X., Ban, W., Marappan, G., Tahir, H. E., Huang, X., Wu, K., Chen, Z., Zou, W., Liu, B., Zhang, L., Yang, Z., & Katona, J. (2025). Colorimetric food freshness indicators for intelligent packaging: Progress, shortcomings, and promising solutions. *Foods, 14*(16), 2813. https://doi.org/10.3390/foods14162813.

Chapter 18

Preventing polyunsaturated fatty acid oxidation: technological advancements for food and nutraceuticals

Mintu Martin[1], Namita Patil[1], Shivanand Shirkole[1], Vijaya Raghavan[2], and Gurunath Mote[1]

[1]*Department of Food Technology, School of Engineering and Technology, D. Y. Patil Agriculture and Technical University, Talsande, Maharashtra, India,* [2]*Department of Bioresource Engineering, Sainte-Anne-de-Bellevue, Montreal, McGill University Canada, Montreal, QC, Canada*

18.1 Introduction to polyunsaturated fatty acids

Fatty acids have an important role in human nutrition and have significant functions associated with cellular structure, energy metabolism, and other elements (Calder et al., 2020). Polyunsaturated fatty acids (PUFAs) have garnered significant interest due to their unique chemical structures with multiple double bonds and biological roles. In comparison to other fatty acids, double bonds have an impact on biological function and make them more susceptible to oxidation (Shahidi & Ambigaipalan, 2015). PUFAs are classified into two types: omega-3 (n-3) PUFAs and omega-6 (n-6) PUFAs, depending on the location of the first double bond from the methyl end of the carbon chain (Simopoulos, 2016). These essential PUFAs, particularly alpha-linolenic acid (ALA, n-3) and linoleic acid (LA, n-6), must be part of the diet because the body is unable to produce them and lacks the enzymes necessary for their synthesis (Burdge & Calder, 2005).

Fatty fish, flaxseeds, walnuts, and vegetable oils (sunflower and soybean oils) are rich sources of PUFAs (Kris-Etherton et al., 2000). Several studies conducted over the years have shed light on the nutritional significance of PUFAs in inflammatory control, cardiovascular protection, and cellular membrane structure. Furthermore, PUFAs may be bioactive lipid mediators that contribute to immunological and inflammatory responses, such as resolvins and eicosanoids (Serhan & Levy, 2018). Numerous health advantages, including neuroprotection, support of cardiovascular health, and fostering metabolic health, have also been linked to adequate PUFA intake (Mozaffarian & Wu, 2011). Despite this, there are still discussions on the appropriate dietary levels and whether the omega-3 to omega-6 PUFA ratio matters more; in particular, too much omega-6 may result in a pro-inflammatory state (Simopoulos, 2016).

Despite their health benefits, PUFAs are highly susceptible to oxidative deterioration, owing to their multiple double bonds. Oxidative degradation results in lipid peroxides and volatile compounds that affect flavor, decrease nutritional quality, and produce potentially harmful secondary oxidation lipids (Shahidi & Zhong, 2010). This represents a significant concern for the food and nutraceutical industries, where effective stabilization of PUFAs is warranted. Examples of the strategies evaluated include antioxidant utilization, recent advances in packaging technology, and novel encapsulation techniques to improve PUFA stability and extend its shelf-life (Frankel, 2012). This review discusses these avenues and recent advancements in PUFA oxidation limitation strategies for nutraceuticals and functional foods. The graphical abstract of this chapter is given in Fig. 18.1.

18.1.1 Definition and types of polyunsaturated fatty acids

PUFAs are fatty acids with two or more double bonds in their hydrocarbon chains. These fatty acids are necessary for nutrition and metabolism in humans, as they serve as precursors to bioactive lipid mediators that mediate a multitude of

Omega-3 and Omega-6 Polyunsaturated Fatty Acids in Food Systems. DOI: https://doi.org/10.1016/B978-0-443-43810-3.00010-5

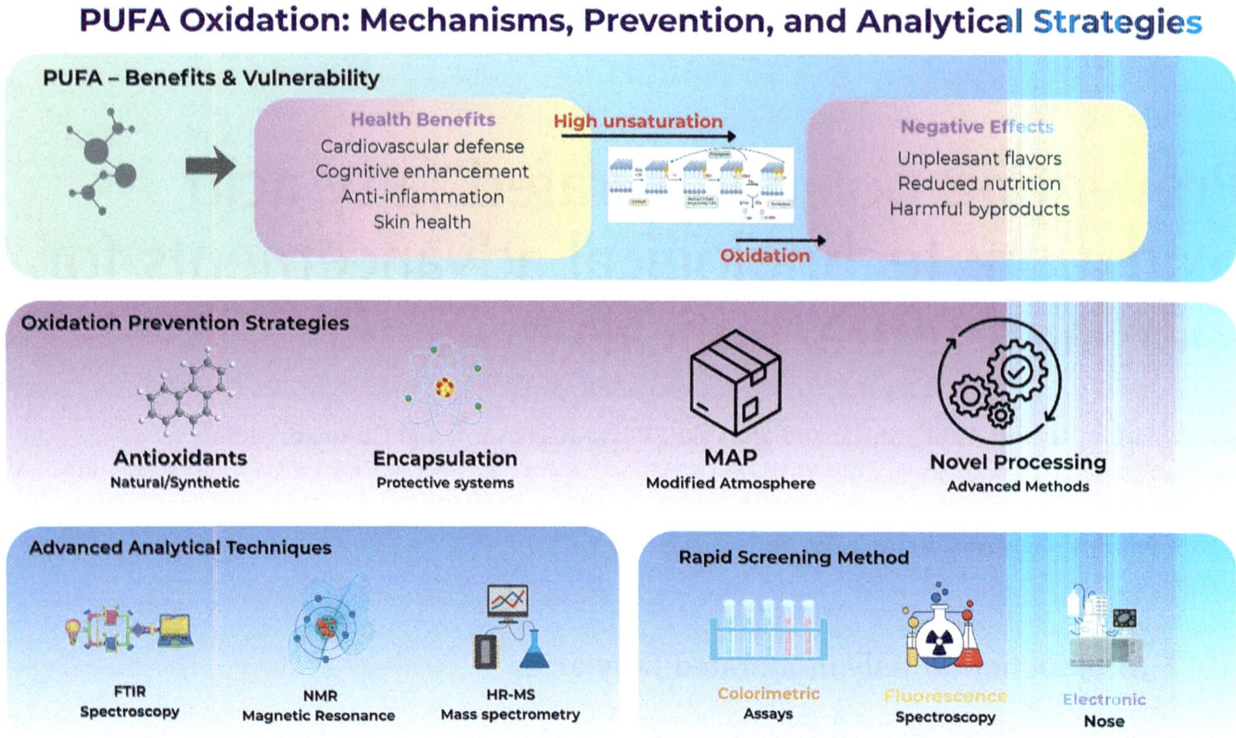

FIGURE 18.1 The graphical abstract on PUFA oxidation, covering benefits, vulnerabilities, prevention strategies and analytical techniques.

physiological functions (Calder, 2005). There are two main classifications of PUFAs, according to where the initial double bond from the carbon chain's methyl terminus is located.

1. Omega-6 (n-6) fatty acids: this classification includes LA (18:2 n-6), which can be converted to arachidonic acid (AA) (20:4 n-6). Omega-6 fatty acids are typically observed in certain plant-derived oils, namely, soybean, corn, and sunflower oil (Calder, 2005).
2. Omega-3 (n-3) fatty acids: this classification contains ALA (18:3 n-3), which can be chemically elongated to form derivatives such as docosahexaenoic acid (DHA, 22:6 n-3) and eicosapentaenoic acid (EPA, 20:5 n-3). Omega-3 fatty acids, like chia seeds and flaxseeds, are found in plant sources and fish oils (Calder, 2005).

Since mammals lack desaturase enzymes to produce ALAs and LA, these PUFAs must come from the diet (Calder, 2005). Maintaining an appropriate ratio of n-3 and n-6 PUFAs is substantial for metabolic homeostasis because they utilize overlapping pathways in metabolic and enzymatic processes. Foods rich in PUFAs are presented in Fig. 18.2 and Table 18.1 summarizes the classification of PUFAs.

18.1.2 Present practices to prevent oxidation of polyunsaturated fatty acid

Currently, preventing the oxidation of PUFAs in foods and nutraceuticals relies on a multipronged approach. A powerful strategy involves the addition of synthetic and natural antioxidants to neutralize free radicals and disrupt the oxidative chain reactions. Modified atmospheric packaging and oxygen scavengers can limit PUFA exposure to oxidative species. Encapsulation techniques (including microencapsulation and nanoencapsulation) can also establish physical barriers to shield PUFAs from environmental conditions. Additionally, controlled storage conditions (such as cold temperatures and light exclusion) can help mitigate the oxidation risk. To address oxidation, recent developments have promoted innovation in the effectiveness and sustainability of these approaches, with attention paid to designing new antioxidant formulations, enhancing packaging barrier properties, and improving encapsulation technologies to support PUFA stability and bioavailability. These new approaches are designed with a greater degree of specificity concerning food matrices for nutraceutical formulations and the multiple challenges posed by product types and intended uses.

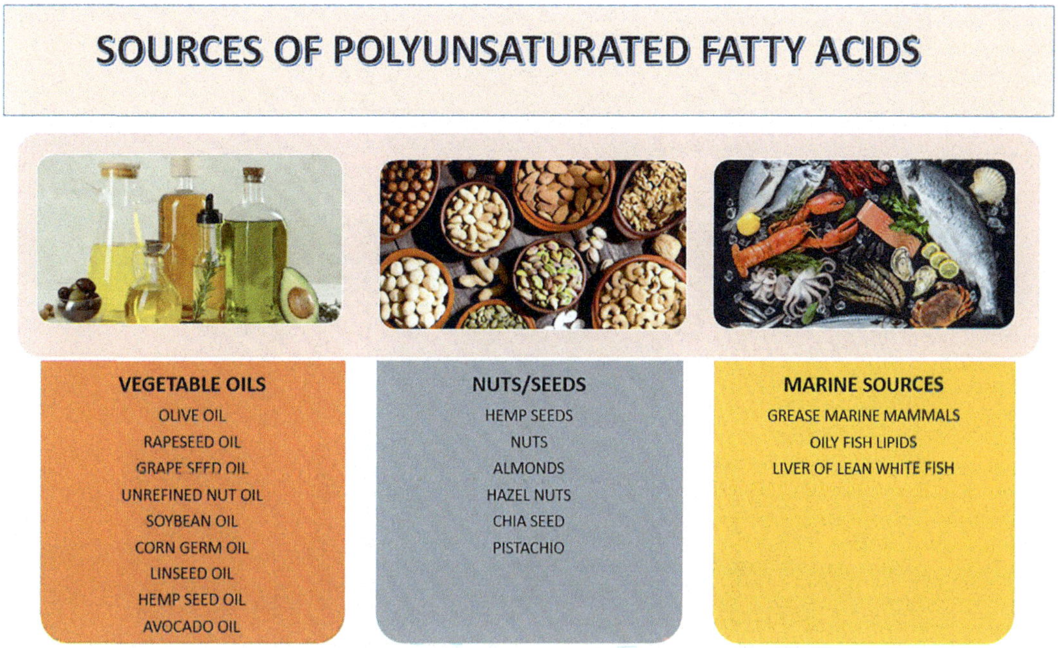

FIGURE 18.2 An infographic listing sources of polyunsaturated fatty acids. (Amjad Khan et al., 2017; Balić et al., 2020; Mititelu et al., 2025; Saini & Keum, 2018).

18.1.3 Challenges in preventing polyunsaturated fatty acid oxidation

Many factors must be considered when developing methods for delaying PUFA oxidation. Existing antioxidant strategies are underwhelming in effectiveness; it is always difficult to provide sufficient protection to PUFA during processing and storage, incorporating protection from oxidation that restricts sensory attributes, regulatory issues are always an issue with synthetic antioxidants, and economic considerations play a role in cost-efficient food systems. The effectiveness of the antioxidants available for the above food formulations is highly dependent on their solubility and concentration, as well as their ability to interact with the food matrix (Shahidi & Zhong, 2010). Second, it can be especially difficult to provide stability to PUFAs because these lipids are susceptible to high heat and exposure to oxygen and light, resulting in their deterioration during food processing and storage (Frankel, 2012). Finally, oxidation can cause off-flavors and rancidity, which can have detrimental effects on sensory attributes and the consumer base. All these attributes must be understood and considered along with PUFA/stability antioxidant strategies, the limitations of regulatory bodies on synthetic antioxidant use, and the current trends for producing clean labels and/or natural ingredients (Shahidi & Zhong, 2010). Moreover, using alternative methods to stabilize PUFA, such as microencapsulation and modified atmosphere packaging (MAP), can increase production costs and should be considered if the goal is to produce economically efficient foods and food systems.

18.2 Health benefits of polyunsaturated fatty acid and mechanisms of polyunsaturated fatty acid oxidation

PUFAs are vital components of a balanced diet, imparting numerous health advantages. Their importance extends to cardiovascular health, brain function, inflammation regulation, ocular health, skin integrity, fetal development, and weight control.

18.2.1 Health benefits of polyunsaturated fatty acid

PUFAs, specifically omega-6 and omega-3 fatty acids, have numerous prominent health effects on various body systems. Omega-3 PUFAs, such as DHA and EPA, are known for their cardiovascular-protective effects. They reduce triglyceride levels, enhance endothelial function, lower blood pressure, and decrease the chances of atherosclerosis by preventing platelet aggregation and systemic inflammation (Mozaffarian & Wu, 2011; Shahidi & Ambigaipalan, 2015). Similarly,

TABLE 18.1 Classification of polyunsaturated fatty acids (PUFAs).

Category	Abbreviation	Fatty acid	Structure	Common sources
Omega-3 (n-3) PUFAs	ALA	α-linolenic acid	18:3 n-3	flaxseeds, walnuts, canola oil, soybean oil, and chia seeds
	EPA	Eicosapentaenoic acid	20:5 n-3	Fish oil and fatty fish (mackerel, sardines, tuna, salmon)
	DPA	Docosapentaenoic acid	22:5 n-3	Fish, seal oil, grass-fed meat
	DHA	Docosahexaenoic acid	22:6 n-3	Fatty fish, breast milk, fish oil, and algae oil
Omega-6 (n-6) PUFAs	LA	Linoleic acid	18:2 n-6	Vegetable oils (soybean, corn, sunflower, safflower), nuts, seeds
	GLA	γ-linolenic acid	18:3 n-6	Evening primrose oil, borage oil, black currant seed oil
	Dihomo-γ-linolenic acid	DGLA	20:3 n-6	Small amounts in human milk, animal fats
	Arachidonic acid	AA	20:4 n-6	Meat, dairy, fish, poultry, eggs
Omega-9 (n-9) PUFAs (nonessential)	Mead acid	MA	20:3 n-9	Synthesized in the body when essential fatty acids are deficient
Other less common PUFAs	Eicosadienoic acid	-	20:2 n-6	Certain vegetable oils

Source: Data elaborated from Amjad Khan et al. (2017); Balić et al. (2020); Calder (2015); Mariamenatu and Abdu (2021); and Saini and Keum (2018).

omega-6 PUFAs like LA are associated with cardiovascular health because of their low levels of low-density lipoprotein cholesterol, which reduces the risk of coronary artery disease (Harris et al., 2009).

DHA serves as an integral structural element in the brain and retina, in areas of neurodevelopment and cognitive health. DHA is crucial for synaptic functions, learning, and memory. While there is suggestive evidence linking perinatal and early childhood DHA intake with cognitive performance and lower neurodegenerative disease risk (Bazinet & Layé, 2014; Joffre et al., 2019), it is unclear whether DHA intake translates into improved cognitive health later in life. Omega-3 PUFAs have positive effects on depression and mood disorders by ameliorating inflammatory processes in the brain (Layé et al., 2018). EPA and DHA also have vigorous antiinflammatory effects by modulating cytokine production in the brain and serving as precursors to special pro-resolving mediators, including resolvins and protectins, which are important for immune homeostasis and the resolution of chronic inflammation (Calder, 2017).

The health of the skin and eyes depends on PUFAs. DHA is a crucial structural element of retinal photoreceptor membranes and is particularly crucial for the formation of vision during pregnancy and early infancy (SanGiovanni & Chew, 2005). Age-related macular degeneration is less common in persons who consume more omega-3 fatty acids (Merle et al., 2014). In terms of skin health, both omega-6 and omega-3 fatty acids are essential for maintaining the function of the epidermal barrier, retaining moisture even in the face of external stressors, and promoting antiinflammatory reactions in the skin, which can help manage skin conditions like psoriasis and eczema, as well as improving elastin and signs of aging skin (Boelsma et al., 2001; Fluhr et al., 2001; Pilkington et al., 2011). Lipid supplementation with DHA and AA throughout pregnancy and lactation is essential for the development of the fetal immunological and neurological systems. Research has shown that supplementation during pregnancy is associated with improved cognitive function in infants and a reduced risk of preterm birth (Carlson, 2009; Innis, 2007; Koletzko et al., 2008). Recent research indicates that omega-3 PUFAs may also assist in weight management by increasing fat oxidation, improving insulin sensitivity, influencing appetite-regulating hormones, and improving metabolic health (Buckley & Howe, 2010; Kunesová et al., 2006). The health benefits of fatty acids are presented in Fig. 18.3.

18.2.2 Mechanisms of polyunsaturated fatty acid oxidation

Lipid hydroperoxides (LOOH) and a variety of secondary degradation products are produced by the autocatalytic process of PUFA oxidation, which takes place through a free radical chain reaction mechanism (Frankel, 2012). The oxidation pathways and biological outcomes of long-chain PUFAs are represented in Fig. 18.4.

There are three stages to the reaction: initiation, propagation, and termination. A lipid radical (L•), a precursor for radical reactions, is created during the initiation phase when external stimuli like heat, metal ions, or light extract a hydrogen atom from the methylene group next to the double bond in the PUFA chain (Shahidi & Zhong, 2010).

The L• quickly reacts with molecular oxygen during the propagation phase to produce a peroxyl radical (LOO•), which then takes a hydrogen atom from another PUFA molecule to produce LOOH and L•. Lipid oxidation continues to propagate as a result of this chain reaction (Mcclements & Decker, 2000). The termination of the reaction happens when two radicals bond to generate stable, nonradical products, or antioxidants donate electrons to the radicals to neutralize

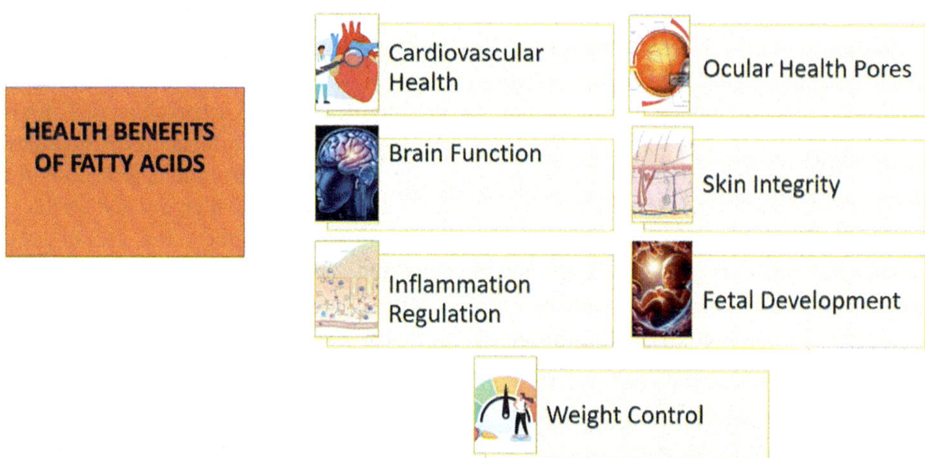

FIGURE 18.3 An infographic listing the health benefits of polyunsaturated fatty acids. (Akbar et al., 2021; Kapoor et al., 2021; Mititelu et al., 2025).

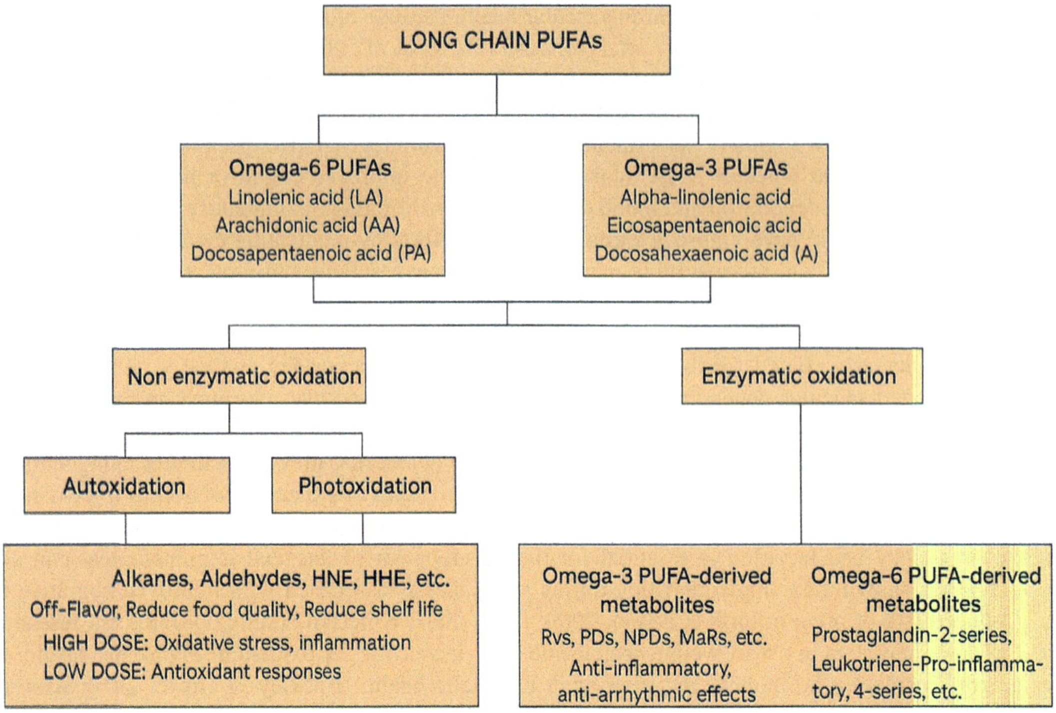

FIGURE 18.4 A Flowchart of oxidation pathways and outcomes of long-chain polyunsaturated fatty acids (PUFAs). (Baral et al., 2022; Sokoła-Wysoczańska et al., 2018; Tao, 2015).

them and prevent the oxidative chain reaction. In PUFA-rich foods, the main primary oxidation products, hydroperoxides, are unstable substances that break down into secondary oxidation products, such as alcohols, ketones, and aldehydes, which cause rancidity, off-taste, and losses in nutritional quality (Laguerre et al., 2017).

18.2.3 Factors that impact polyunsaturated fatty acid oxidation rates

The rate at which PUFAs oxidize is influenced by both intrinsic characteristics of fatty acids and extrinsic environmental factors. The degree of unsaturation is crucial; fatty acids with more double bonds, including DHA (22:6 n-3) and EPA (20:5 n-3), are more susceptible to oxidation because they have more reactive sites (Shahidi & Ambigaipalan, 2015). The presence of oxygen in the environment accelerates oxidation, particularly during the lipid peroxidation propagation stage when oxygen reacts with lipid radicals to form LOO• (Johnson & Decker, 2015). Temperature also plays a crucial role, as higher temperatures increase the kinetic energy of molecules and shorten both the initiation and propagation stages of lipid oxidation (Choe & Min, 2006). Similarly, exposure to light, particularly in the visible and ultraviolet wavelength ranges, produces radicals and begins oxidation, which is an issue for transparent packaging materials (McClements, 2004).

Iron, copper, and other catalytic metal ions also play important roles in PUFA oxidation via redox cycling, which converts LOOH into highly reactive free radicals. The water activity (aw) has two effects on lipid oxidation. Very low-aw enhances the number of pro-oxidant elements, whereas very high-aw promotes hydrolytic degradation of lipids, eventually leading to oxidative degradation of lipids (Shahidi & Zhong, 2010). These effects, which depend on the presence of water, support the need for controlled humidity during the storage of PUFA-rich food products. It is also essential to consider the presence of antioxidants, such as natural (e.g., polyphenols and tocopherols) and/or synthetic (e.g., butylated hydroxytoluene (BHT) and butylated hydroxyanisole [BHA]) antioxidants, to reduce oxidation rates. Antioxidants act through various mechanisms, including chelating pro-oxidant metals, scavenging free radicals, and reducing LOOH to more stable nonreactive species. The food matrix itself also affects oxidation kinetics. In emulsion systems, characteristics such as droplet size, type of emulsifier, and interfacial properties of the droplets alter the rate and pathway of oxidation. Storage conditions, including temperature, light exposure, and packaging atmosphere, also affect oxidative stability. Therefore integrated formulation and packaging must be considered to maximize shelf life and maintain PUFA integrity. Effects of PUFAs oxidation products on health and food quality are given in Fig. 18.5.

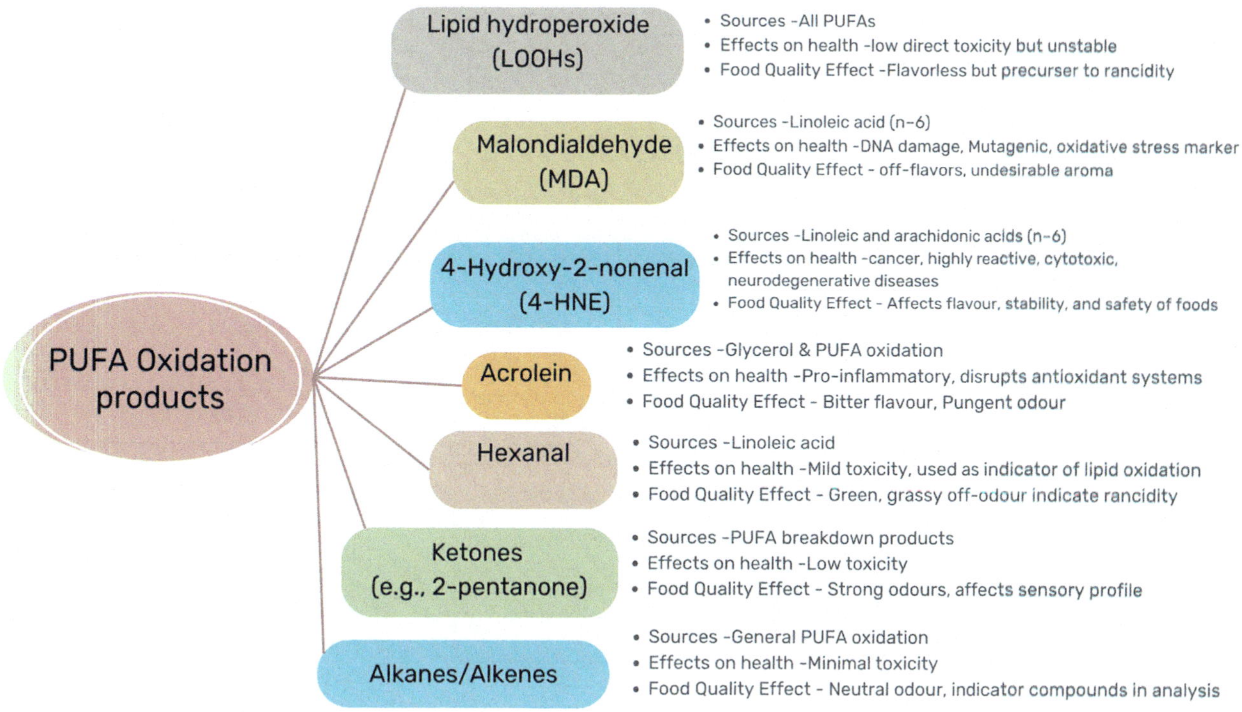

FIGURE 18.5 An infographic summarizing PUFA oxidation products and their effects on health and food quality.

18.3 Methods and technological advancements for preventing polyunsaturated fatty acid oxidation

18.3.1 Antioxidant additives

Antioxidants are one of the easiest methods to stop PUFA from oxidizing. Antioxidants can be divided into two categories: natural and synthetic. Natural antioxidants include compounds from both phytochemical and animal sources, such as carotenoids, ascorbic acid (vitamin C), flavonoids, tocopherols (vitamin E), and polyphenols. Natural antioxidants are Generally Recognized as Safe and meet consumer trends for clean label products. Synthetic antioxidants, such as BHA, BHT, tertiary butyl hydroquinone (TBHQ), and propyl gallate, are inexpensive, readily available, easy to prepare, and very stable at low concentrations against oxidation. However, their use is restricted or banned in some markets owing to possible safety concerns. According to Ayoka et al. (2022), synthetic phenolic antioxidants like BHA and BHT have been found to be carcinogenic and cytotoxic. Additionally, Xu et al. (2017) note that there are regulatory challenges associated with their use, which differ depending on the country and food category. Antioxidants delay oxidative degradation through a range of mechanisms, including free radical scavenging, chain propagation prevention, and metal ion chelation (Shahidi & Zhong, 2010). Free radical scavenging is a well-known and well-studied mechanism, similar to tocopherols (vitamin E), which are capable of scavenging free radicals for hydrogen atoms and, therefore promote the dissociation of chain reactions in lipid oxidation (Shahidi & Ambigaipalan, 2015).

Metal chelation is another way to slow oxidation degradation through a chelating agent (EDTA and citric acid), thereby preventing metal-catalyzed oxidation reactions. The propensity of these metals to oxidize and catalyze oxidizing reactions makes their removal from any system an ideal approach for increasing the oxidative stability. Antioxidants neutralize radicals and chelate metals; however, they also deplete singlet oxygen, an extremely reactive form of oxygen associated with PUFA degradation. Carotenoids are particularly effective because they absorb excess oxidative energy, thereby preventing the damage caused by singlet oxygen. Notably, several antioxidants act synergistically in this process. Ascorbic acid (vitamin C) can reduce oxidized tocopherols to their antioxidant form, or at the very least maximize antioxidant activity in lipid systems (Shahidi & Ambigaipalan, 2015). Overall, this combination of bioregulatory functions makes antioxidant strategies particularly effective for preserving PUFA-rich food quality and nutrition. Packaging together with antioxidant(s) provides even higher protection against PUFA onset, based on complementary functions against PUFA-oxidized species; tocopherol reacts with lipid radicals, and ascorbic acid can restore oxidized tocopherols,

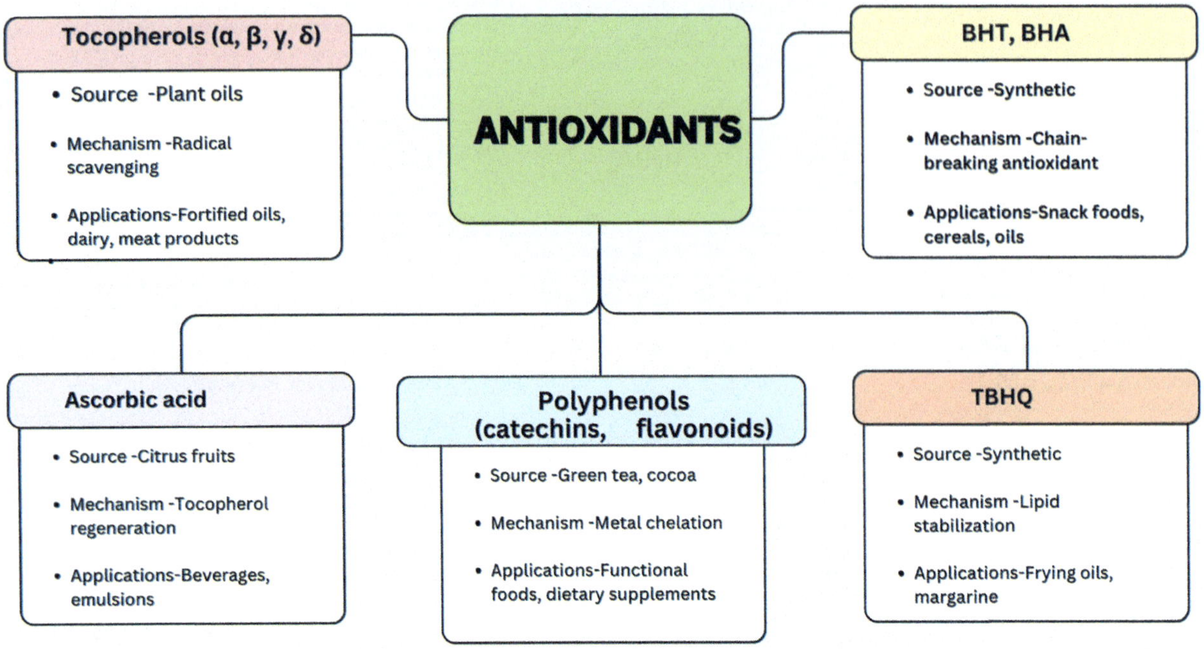

FIGURE 18.6 A flowchart detailing the sources, mechanisms and applications of various antioxidant additives.

or green tea polyphenols can enhance the activities of other antioxidants by generating radical scavenging and metal chelation activities (Shahidi & Ambigaipalan, 2015). The mechanism, source, and various applications of antioxidant additives are given in Fig. 18.6.

The FDA and EFSA provide recommended upper limits for synthetic antioxidants, but as consumers increasingly prefer natural, clean labels, and sustainably derived products, there has been a shift toward plant-based sources of antioxidants, as well as food waste (Shahidi & Zhong, 2010). Despite their positive attributes, antioxidants still have limitations in terms of solubility (especially lipophilic antioxidants), thermal instability, and, in some cases, pro-oxidant activity in some reaction systems with metal components. Newer forms, such as nanoemulsions, liposomal encapsulation, and antioxidant-loaded edible films, allow for the design of processes using antioxidants to enhance their delivery and improve their stability. Effectiveness can also be influenced by the food matrix; for example, tocopherols and rosemary extracts improve the stability of antioxidants in processed meats (Walpurgis et al., 2020), vitamins C and E prolong the stabilization of dairy products enriched with PUFA, and TBHQ can prolong the shelf life of fried oil, especially for oils containing PUFA. Microencapsulation is another common method for encapsulating omega-3 oils in nutraceuticals. Future directions will include sustainability issues and new explorations of bio-based antioxidants, intelligent encapsulation to induce targeted release profiles, enzymatic antioxidants (SOD and catalase), and combined techniques integrating current antioxidants with other food technologies, such as MAP, to provide optimized protection against PUFA oxidation.

18.3.2 Encapsulation techniques

Encapsulation is a physical barrier that shields PUFAs from environmental threats, including heat, oxygen, or light. It is an essential technique in food and nutraceuticals that improves the stability, bioavailability, and precisely controlled release of PUFAs. Encapsulation involves both microencapsulation and nanoencapsulation. Microencapsulation refers to the envelopment of PUFAs in microscale carriers (1–1000 μm) that creates a barrier to both chemical and physical oxidation. Spray drying is a widely employed method for microencapsulation. In this method, an aqueous emulsion containing PUFA is sprayed into a heated chamber under conditions that enable rapid evaporation to produce a powder that provides protection to PUFA. Spray drying offers a cost-effective and uniformly scalable method for microencapsulation; however, the high-temperature nature of the formulation process can denature any compounds that are heat-sensitive, thus affecting the extent of encapsulation. Another method of microencapsulation is complex coacervation, which is based on the electrostatic attraction between two biopolymers that have opposite charge (e.g., gelatin and gum Arabic), which spontaneously coacervate to form a shell around the PUFA to "trap" it. Complex coacervation offers significant encapsulation efficiency and release; nevertheless, it is influenced by environmental factors, including ionic strength and pH, which may impact stability. The third method of microencapsulation is extrusion technology, which uses pressure to push the emulsified PUFA through a small opening and then solidifies the capsule with either calcium ions or at cooler temperatures (Risch & Reineccius, 1995).

Nanoencapsulation is the use of delivery carriers at the nanoscale size (1–1000 nm) to encapsulate PUFA, which has been shown to dramatically improve PUFA solubility, stability, and bioavailability (Walker et al., 2015). Liposome technology, a commonly used nanoencapsulation method, involves a phospholipid-based vesicle that encapsulates PUFA within its bilayer membranes and protects PUFA from oxidative degradation (Fathi et al., 2012). Although liposomes demonstrate good biocompatibility and acceptability, leading to increased PUFA delivery, they are sensitive to oxidation potential, complicated to produce, and tend to be relatively expensive (Walker et al., 2015). Another method is used more often than the nanoencapsulation of liposomes into nanoemulsions. Oil-in-water (or water-in-oil) emulsions with droplet or particle sizes measured in the nano range are known as nanoemulsions, most of which can be understood through surfactant stabilization. They can also increase PUFA solubility, improve oxidative stability, and control release from nanoemulsions. However, they generally require high-energy emulsification techniques, as is required for liposomes, which can increase the production costs (McClements & Rao, 2011). Another technique for encapsulating PUFAs is polymeric nanoparticles, which are stable, nanoscale particles made of biodegradable polymers like polylactic acid and chitin. The most effective PUFA delivery techniques are polymeric nanoparticles because of their strong oxidative protection and controlled-release characteristics. However, there are still issues with the safety and regulatory approval of polymeric materials for food applications (Fathi et al., 2012). Encapsulation strategies have notable advantages in preventing PUFA oxidation; however, they have significant limitations. Microencapsulation approaches (e.g., extrusion, complex coacervation, and spray drying) are popular means of encapsulation because they are easily scalable and cost-efficient; however, they may have limitations associated with oxidative stability in extreme processing environments. Nanoencapsulation enablers (liposomes, nanoemulsions, and polymeric nanoparticles) provide benefits in terms of biocompatibility and oxidative stability, yet their increased industrialized production costs and socioeconomic/administrative realm limitations may prevent and hinder equal adoption by individual producers and consumers.

18.3.3 Modified atmosphere packaging

A popular technique for extending the shelf life of PUFA is MAP, which contains food items by lowering their exposure to oxygen, the most common oxidizing agent (Robertson, 2016). MAP is implemented in multiple formats, including inert gas flushing, oxygen scavengers, and vacuum packaging, and can aid in optimizing oxidative stability while preserving the nutritional value (Kirtil et al., 2016). Inert gas flushing involves displacing oxygen in packaging with an inert gas such as nitrogen. Nitrogen is commonly used because it is inert and effective in protecting lipid-based foods such as fish and nuts from the effects of oxidation. CO_2 has antimicrobial properties and is useful in seafood and meat applications. Flushing inert gases does not completely displace oxygen; therefore high-barrier materials are still typically used in conjunction with MAP to provide long-term protection from oxidation (Robertson, 2016). Oxygen scavengers, such as ascorbic acid and iron-based compounds, as well as enzymatic agents, such as glucose oxidase, can actively remove residual oxygen and limit the damage associated with the oxidation of PUFA, especially when combined with flushing techniques (Miltz & Perry, 2005; Vermeiren et al., 2000). In addition, to oxygen scavengers, the success of flushing procedures as an intervention is dependent on the oxygen permeability of the material used for packaging and the initial amount of oxygen inside the product at the start of the intervention (Robertson, 2016).

Vacuum packaging, which involves complete air removal before sealing, is another method that can delay lipid oxidation and the spoilage of vegetable oils, fatty fish, and nuts. Nonetheless, vacuum packaging can negatively affect the appearance and texture of delicate foods and has no impact on the growth of anaerobic bacteria. Overall, MAP technology will continue to be an important intervention for prolonging PUFA's shelf life, and the intervention can be elevated from effectiveness with multiple interventions.

18.3.4 Novel processing methods

The growing need for foods and nutraceuticals rich in PUFAs has sparked research on modern mild and nonthermal processing methods that can limit oxidation and maintain nutritional quality. The induction of PUFA breakdown has been linked to the thermal processing of food, which is one of the reasons why the use of low-and-high-pressure processing (HPP), ultrasound, cold plasma, ohmic heating, pulsed electric field processing (PEF), and supercritical fluid extraction techniques has been studied in place of thermal processes. They act by reducing oxidative stress, inactivating pro-oxidant enzymes, and modifying food matrices for PUFA stability. Ultrasound processing (20–100 kHz) inactivates oxidative enzymes and increases the emulsion stability. However, high-intensity ultrasound has been shown to cause cavitation, which generates free radicals that decrease its protective effect. Consequently, ultrasound applications may require optimization (Al-Sharify et al., 2025). HPP relies on hydrostatic pressure (100–600 MPa) to inactivate spoilage microorganisms and lipoxygenases to extend the shelf life of PUFA-rich foods, such as fish and omega-3 fortified dairy. Ohmic heating is a slightly different technique in that it is a liquid food method that provides a uniform heat distribution, resulting in lower localized hot spots and reduced oxidation risk. PEF technology uses high-voltage electric pulses to effectively inactivate oxidative enzymes in liquid products (e.g., omega-3-enriched juices) without causing heat damage.

Cold plasma treatment, which relies on ionized gases to create reactive species, has been considered for microbial and oxidative enzyme inactivation, while maintaining PUFA functionality in oils and emulsions. Similarly, SFE, specifically CO_2 SFE, has been used for the extraction and purification of omega-3 fatty acids from algae and fish oil without exposing PUFA to heat or oxygen, thereby lowering the possibility of oxidative degradation. While these approaches yield advantages, processes such as SFE and HPP are limited owing, in part, to the high cost of operation and investment in equipment. However, these novel processes can be advantageous when coupled with traditional preservation methods, such as the antioxidant fortification of oils, PUFA encapsulation, and MAP designs, to create a multihurdle system for preserving PUFA. Future research should focus on optimizing processing parameters, creating economic viability, and gaining consumer acceptance. Additionally, sustainable and environmentally friendly processes deserve attention with respect to energy consumption and waste if these methods are to gain competitiveness for widespread industrial use.

18.4 Functional roles of polyunsaturated fatty acids in food and nutraceuticals

18.4.1 Nutritional benefits

Omega-6 (n-6) and omega-3 (n-3) fatty acids, in particular, are PUFAs, which are vital dietary components with a variety of health benefits. Cardioprotective omega-3 fatty acids, like ALA, DHA, and EPA, reduce triglycerides, improve endothelial function, and lessen the incidence of arrhythmias and coronary heart disease (Mozaffarian & Wu, 2011). High levels in the brain and retina are necessary for neuroprotection, cognitive development, and visual function during pregnancy and infancy (SanGiovanni & Chew, 2005). Furthermore, omega-3 PUFAs have numerous therapeutic advantages in chronic inflammatory disorders such as rheumatoid arthritis and inflammatory bowel disease, and they alter inflammatory responses through the production of resolvin and protectin (Calder, 2017).In addition, to cardiovascular and cognitive health, PUFAs assist skin health, hormonal regulation, and metabolism. Omega-3s promote skin hydration and improve elasticity, while providing a protective effect against photoaging and inflammatory skin conditions such as psoriasis. They enhance insulin sensitivity and support normal leptin production, highlighting omega-3s as a potential approach for tackling obesity and metabolic syndrome. Pregnancy-related DHA intake has been linked to better fetal brain development and neonatal outcomes (Koletzko et al., 2008). Despite the documented benefits, owing to oxidative instability and imbalanced dietary sources, it can be difficult to optimize PUFA consumption, especially in terms of delivery systems, personalized nutrition, and sustainable PUFA sources, which should be further examined (Akbar et al., 2021).

18.4.2 Sensory properties

Sensory qualities of food, such as appearance, flavor, texture, aroma, and mouth feel, are significantly impacted by PUFAs. These biologically important lipids possess a high degree of unsaturation, which lowers the melting point and facilitates fat crystallization, ultimately improving or facilitating smooth, creamy, or spreadable textures in emulsified and lipid-rich food products such as margarines, dressings, and dairy alternatives (Duan et al., 2023). In particular, PUFAs lower the melting point of fats and lead to desirable textures in plant-based butters and soft candy; however, they often require structuring, such as oleogelation, to maintain consistency in the final product. As PUFAs are also reactive and oxidatively unstable, they may degrade lipids via polymerization or other oxidation reactions, resulting in unpleasant graininess and/or discoloration and alterations in viscosity.

Flavor and aroma susceptibilities to PUFA oxidation were also significant. Fresh PUFAs contribute mild, nutty, and buttery flavor to foods, whereas oxidation produces an unpleasant odor and flavor because of the development of aldehydes, ketones, and other volatile compounds, leading to rancid, rotten fish, or cardboard attributes. Sensory degradation can lead to consumer rejection of omega-3-enriched products due to off-flavor or staleness. PUFAs also affect emulsion stability and the desirable flavors formed during cooking (controlled oxidation and Maillard reactions); however, excess thermal exposure can lead to burnt or bitter flavors (Choe & Min, 2006). To maintain sensory acceptability, food formulators utilize microencapsulation, antioxidant fortification, gas flushing, or MAP. The future of food science lies in the discovery of innovative methods for PUFA stabilization, safe avenues for antioxidant delivery, and the improvement of packaging technologies to prolong the shelf life of items high in PUFAs while maintaining optimal sensory quality.

18.4.3 Shelf-life extension

PUFAs are easily oxidized, which causes a reduction in the sensory characteristics, nutritional value, and shelf life of foods and nutraceuticals. Oxidation can produce off-flavors, rancidity, color changes, and changes in textural properties, all of which contribute to consumer rejection (McClements & Decker, 2000). Although some derivatives of PUFAs, such as conjugated linoleic acid, have antioxidant properties, their endogenous effects are not strong enough to prevent autoxidation. Therefore several strategies have been developed to preserve PUFAs, such as the use of natural (e.g., rosemary extract and tocopherols) or synthetic (e.g., BHA, TBHQ, and BHT) methods, refrigeration, flushing with nitrogen prior to packaging, and more sophisticated techniques, such as MAP, to reduce oxidation and/or prolong shelf life (Choe & Min, 2006; Frankel, 2012).

Encapsulation methods, including microencapsulation, nanoemulsions, and liposomes, are crucial for ensuring the stability of PUFA because they physically separate PUFA from pro-oxidizing elements, such as heat, light, oxygen, and moisture. By incorporating PUFA within these systems, the PUFA content and bioactivity are preserved during the storage of dairy products, baked goods, or functional foods. The oxidation of PUFA has also been associated with textural challenges and color instability of PUFAs in processed meat, dairy, and seafood, mainly owing to pigment degradation and lipid polymerization. Synergistic strategies, such as the encapsulation of antioxidants and lipid structuring strategies (i.e., oleogelation) with emulsions, have shown improved protection of sensory characteristics and prevention of lipid rancidity in food systems.

Although PUFAs do not have a strong antimicrobial effect, some oxidation products (hydroperoxides) may play a role in inhibiting microorganisms by disrupting their cell membranes. However, these products exhibit conditions that promote spoilage and contamination. Thus novel preservation strategies such as cold plasma treatment, active packaging, and enzymatic stabilization are being studied. Future research should seek to provide clean-label antioxidant systems, facilitate violet nanoencapsulation for bioavailability, and develop environmentally friendly packaging propositions to accommodate consumer perceptions about having what they consider safe, stable, and desirable PUFA-enriched food products.

18.5 Novel tools for assessing polyunsaturated fatty acid oxidation

Accurate assessment of PUFA oxidation is key to ensuring the nutritional quality of food, shelf life, and nutraceutical products. The most common traditional methods are the anisidine value, thiobarbituric acid reactive substances (TBARS), and peroxide value. However, these methods tend to be both sensitive and specific. However, advances in both analytical and rapid screening methods have markedly improved our ability to detect, quantify, and measure lipid oxidation in real-time. The advanced analytical techniques for assessing PUFA oxidation are presented in Fig. 18.7.

18.5.1 Advanced analytical techniques

When attempting to decipher the complexities of metabolic pathways and degradation products of PUFA oxidative metabolism, there is a need for advanced analytical methods that can detect minor chemical transformations. High-resolution analytical methods not only allow for detailed analysis of oxidation products but also assist in creating products for targeted stabilization of PUFA foods and nutraceuticals.

1. High-resolution mass spectrometry (HRMS) is an advanced technique that measures oxidation-derived compounds, specifically hydroperoxides, aldehydes, and ketones, with high accuracy and precision. The high accuracy and resolution of HRMS allow for effective differentiation, even for structurally similar oxidation product isomers. HRMS has been extensively used to investigate the degradation pathways of PUFAs in functional foods and marine oils (Kang & Yeo, 2024). Although HRMS is highly specific and sensitive, its use can be impractical because of the complex instrumentation and sample processing required.
2. Fourier transform infrared (FTIR) spectroscopy is commonly used to determine functional group changes in oxidized lipids by identifying alterations in carbonyl and hydroxyl functional groups, which provides a fast instrument for nondestructive analysis of lipid oxidation. FTIR is useful for real-time monitoring and assessment of the quality of edible oils and fortified PUFA emulsions (Li et al., 2019; Vlachos et al., 2006). Although FTIR is not as specific as chromatographic analyses, it is helpful for preliminary screening of oxidative changes in complex food products.

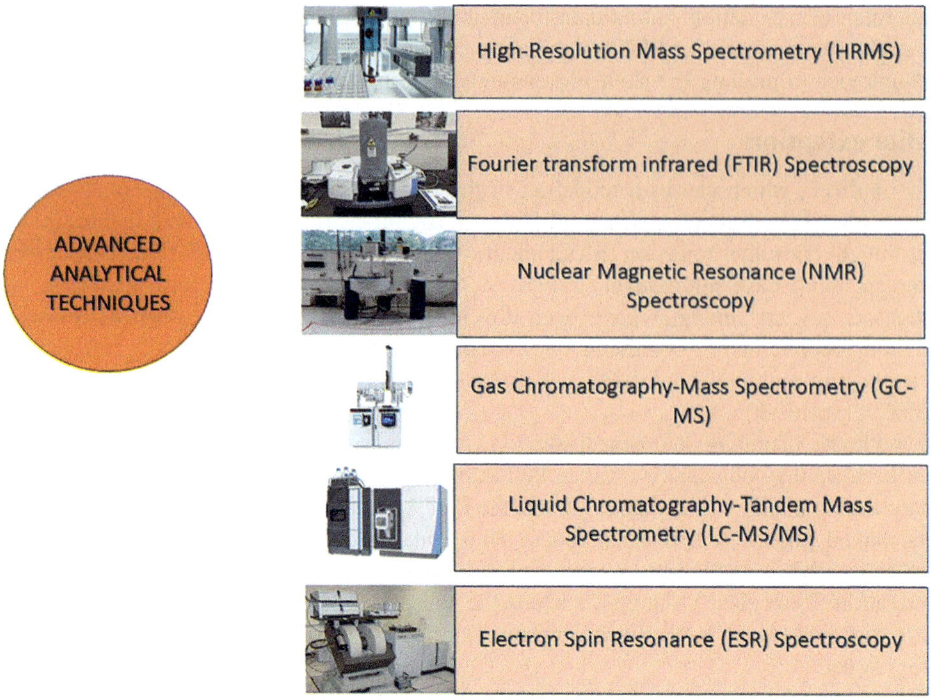

FIGURE 18.7 A diagram listing advanced analytical techniques for assessing PUFA oxidation

3. Nuclear magnetic resonance (NMR) spectroscopy can be used nondestructively for assessing lipid oxidation (Alexandri et al., 2017; Hwang, 2015; Shahidi & Zhong, 2010). By examining chemical shifts and coupling patterns, NMR gives information about the chemical micro-environment of PUFA molecules and provides important data on the type and extent of lipid oxidation. Use of 2-dimensional (2D) NMR and chemometric integrative models has further enhanced the resolution and interpretation of NMR, making it a valuable tool for monitoring the oxidation of vegetable oils and omega-3 supplements.
4. Gas chromatography-mass spectrometry (GC-MS) is the standard method for classifying volatile secondary oxidation byproducts (aldehydes, alcohols, and ketones). GC-MS has been specifically used for determining the rancidity of PUFA-rich foods, including those derived from fish oils, dairy, and meat products (Frankel, 2012). GC-MS is very sensitive and produces reliable results, but is often limited to volatile compounds and extensive sample preparation.
5. Liquid chromatography-tandem mass spectrometry (LC-MS/MS) has complementary advantages that allow non-volatile-based primary oxidation, including hydroperoxides and oxidized phospholipids. Oxidation of PUFAs by free radicals has been linked with various human diseases, such as atherosclerosis and neurodegenerative conditions. This process results in the formation of hydroperoxides and cyclic peroxides, which are subsequently reduced to lipid alcohols such as hydroxyeicosatetraenoic acid (HETEs) and isoprostanes (IsoPs), respectively. Ito et al. (2017) present a protocol for studying HETEs and F2-IsoPs utilizing a triple quadrupole mass spectrometer combined with reverse phase liquid chromatography. This highly selective method allows for the simultaneous analysis of multiple oxidation products, such as HETEs and F2-IsoPs. This LC-MS method can be used to assess the effects of oxidative stress in fluids and biological tissues and to study the process of free radical oxidation in vitro.
6. Electron spin resonance (ESR) spectroscopy was used to directly confirm the presence of free radical vectors in lipid peroxidation. It provides crucial real-time information regarding the onset, propagation, and mechanism of oxidation to identify the oxidation potential, providing specific critical information that is particularly useful in the assessment of functional and nutraceutical foods. The assessment of radical formation using two distinct ESR spectroscopy methods has been conducted to gather objective analytical data on the oxidative vulnerability of fish oils under mild oxidation conditions (Falch et al., 2005). Similarly, chemiluminescent techniques (Rolewski et al., 2009) are widely used because of their high sensitivity to the presence of oxidative and peroxidative products, which assess the light produced by oxidative reactions. These assays are useful for determining the oxidation in emulsified lipid systems and PUFA-enriched formulations.

Moreover, the advancement of hyphenated techniques that involve the combination of several multiplexing analytical platforms to obtain a comprehensive oxidation profile is particularly novel in the field. GC-MS, in addition, to FTIR, enables comprehensive characterization of volatile oxidation products, whereas LC-MS/MS in combination with NMR allows quantification of the PUFA oxidation mechanism, including detailed structures. These techniques offer the best analytical platforms, combining the dimensionality of characterization and accuracy for the overall management of oxidation in food and nutraceuticals.

18.5.2 Rapid screening methods

There is a need for a rapid and cost-effective screening method to evaluate the lipid oxidation levels in PUFA-rich foods and nutraceuticals. Colorimetric assays, such as ferric reducing antioxidant power assays (Gulcin, 2020) and TBARS assays (Zeb & Ullah, 2016), can be used routinely for quality control because of their simplicity, cost, and low bias in assessing the extent of oxidative damage (Abeyrathne et al., 2021). These assays provide a rapid way to estimate secondary oxidation products and malondialdehyde (MDA) in food, but may lack specificity as food matrices become more complex. Fluorescence spectroscopy can improve sensitivity by capturing fluorescence changes in lipids altered by oxidation and may be particularly useful in emulsions and encapsulated PUFA systems. Additionally, the advancement of portable spectrophotometers can greatly assist in in-field monitoring of oxidation levels in oils and supplements in food production and storage environments.

Innovative technologies, such as electrochemical sensors and electronic nose (E-nose) devices, are changing the landscape for in situ, and real-time measurements of both volatile oxidized and nonvolatilized markers (Karami et al., 2020). Electrochemical sensors, including cutting-edge graphene-based devices, have shown excellent sensitivity in the detection of redox-active compounds in oxidized lipids. E-noses have also proven useful in measuring and testing the rancidity and oxidation stability of edible oil (Xu et al., 2016). Immunoassays, such as ELISA, targeting specific biomarkers, including 4-hydroxynonenal and MDA, exhibit excellent specificity and the ability to measure low levels of oxidation of nutraceuticals. Microfluidic devices, or lab-on-a-chip systems, which measure lipid oxidation in food matrices and are emerging as platforms for high-throughput analysis with miniaturization, quick testing, and minimal reagent use, have also attracted attention in the field. Future research will likely connect AI prediction models for oxidation, smart packaging, and/or enzyme-based biosensors to develop a more intelligent and sustainable approach for monitoring PUFA oxidation.

18.6 Future perspectives and challenges

Future strategies to overcome the oxidation of PUFAs should focus on the development of more effective, sustainable, and consumer-friendly technologies. Anticipated advancements include the formulation of novel antioxidants that leverage the synergistic or combined use of naturally-derived oxidant substances to enhance the oxidative stability of PUFAs. Additionally, microencapsulation and nano-delivery systems present promising solutions for the targeted, controlled release of PUFAs and antioxidants, thereby improving their bioavailability and oxidative functionality. Innovations in food processing and active packaging designs, which have the potential to prevent oxidation throughout the supply chain and within the food product, are also essential. Moreover, the employment of more sensitive and rapid analytical techniques to monitor real-time oxidative markers can support the development of artificial intelligence and predictive modeling to optimize PUFA stability and protect it from the complexities of the food matrix. Nonetheless, challenges persist, such as identifying cost-effective options and creating a "clean label" that protects PUFA oxidation while being economically viable in terms of scalability and potentially aligning with all international regulatory requirements. Other challenges include the long-term safety profiles (metabolically) of new antioxidants, packaging systems, and compounds. Addressing these significant challenges will clearly necessitate a multidisciplinary approach that integrates food science, nanotechnology, toxicology, and data analytics to advance the next phase of PUFA stabilization technology.

18.7 Conclusion

This review has emphasized that preventing PUFA oxidation is vital to ensure nutritional value, safety, and quality of foods and nutraceutical products high in PUFA. While the health benefits of PUFAs have been well-established, the food industry is cursed by a number of issues associated with the rapid oxidation of PUFAs. To address these issues, the industry has implemented various alternatives, including innovative new antioxidant formulations and microencapsulation methods, MAP, and advanced processing technologies such as high-pressure processing, cold plasma, etc. that utilize free radical scavenging, create physical or chemical barriers, adapt environmental conditions, and inactivate pro-oxidant enzymes to improve stability and product shelf life. Moreover, new analytical tools have enhanced the detection and target quantification of oxidation products for more accurate monitoring and control. Nevertheless, issues with scale, cost-effectiveness, and food regulatory compliance still exist, particularly when trying to accommodate consumers' preferences for natural, clean-label products. Future research needs to focus on optimizing antioxidant synergy from natural sources, developing efficient and targeted encapsulation methods, improving active and intelligent packaging solutions, and advancing rapid, nondestructive analytical methods. It will also be vital to develop novel processing methods that deliver food-grade PUFA while meeting safety standards. Addressing these challenges may require a multidisciplinary approach and the harmonization. Over time, as new innovations are generated, the food sector will have the capacity to create adaptive solutions that can preserve the stability of health-promoting PUFA-enriched food that can also meet the changing needs and demands of consumers.

References

Abeyrathne, E. D. N. S., Nam, K., & Ahn, D. U. (2021). Analytical methods for lipid oxidation and antioxidant capacity in food systems. *Antioxidants, 10*(10). https://doi.org/10.3390/antiox10101587, https://www.mdpi.com/2076-3921/10/10/1587/pdf.

Akbar, S., Bhatti, M. Z., Saeed, R. F., & Qazi, A. S. (2021). Polyunsaturated fatty acids: Impact on health and disease status. *Life and Science, 2*(2), 12. https://doi.org/10.37185/lns.1.1.85.

Alexandri, E., Ahmed, R., Siddiqui, H., Choudhary, M. I., Tsiafoulis, C. G., & Gerothanassis, I. P. (2017). High resolution NMR spectroscopy as a structural and analytical tool for unsaturated lipids in solution. *Molecules (Basel, Switzerland), 22*(10), 1663. https://doi.org/10.3390/molecules22101663.

Al-Sharify, Z. T., Al-Najjar, S. Z., Anumudu, C. K., Hart, A., Miri, T., & Onyeaka, H. (2025). Non-thermal technologies in food processing: Implications for food quality and rheology. *Applied Sciences, 15*(6), 3049. https://doi.org/10.3390/app15063049.

Amjad Khan, W., Chun-Mei, H., Khan, N., Iqbal, A., Lyu, S.-W., & Shah, F. (2017). Bioengineered plants can be a useful source of omega-3 fatty acids. *BioMed Research International,* 7348919. https://doi.org/10.1155/2017/7348919.

Ayoka, T. O., Nwachukwu, N., Ene, A. C., Igwe, C. U., Ogara, A. L., & Nnadi, C. O. (2022). In-vitro antioxidant activity and acute toxicity of the alkaloidal constituents of Zanthoxylum zanthoxyloides leaves. *Tropical Journal of Natural Product Research, 6*(2), 276–280. https://doi.org/10.26538/tjnpr/v6i2.17, https://www.tjnpr.org/img/manuscript_2202_17-TJNPR-2022-M018%20Galley%20Proof%20C.pdf.

Balić, A., Vlašić, D., Žužul, K., Marinović, B., & Bukvić Mokos, Z. (2020). Omega-3 versus omega-6 polyunsaturated fatty acids in the prevention and treatment of inflammatory skin diseases. *International Journal of Molecular Sciences, 21*(3), 741. https://doi.org/10.3390/ijms21030741.

Baral, P. K., Amin, M. T., Rashid, M. M. O., & Hossain, S. M. (2022). Assessment of polyunsaturated fatty acids on COVID-19-associated risk reduction. *Revista Brasileira de Farmacognosia, 32*(1), 50–64. https://doi.org/10.1007/s43450-021-00213-x.

Bazinet, R. P., & Layé, S. (2014). Polyunsaturated fatty acids and their metabolites in brain function and disease. *Nature Reviews. Neuroscience, 15*(12), 771–785. https://doi.org/10.1038/nrn3820.

Boelsma, E., Hendriks, H. F. J., & Roza, L. (2001). Nutritional skin care: Health effects of micronutrients and fatty acids. *The American Journal of Clinical Nutrition, 73*(5), 853–864. https://doi.org/10.1093/ajcn/73.5.853.

Buckley, J. D., & Howe, P. R. C. (2010). Long-chain omega-3 polyunsaturated fatty acids may be beneficial for reducing obesity-A review. *Nutrients, 2*(12), 1212–1230. https://doi.org/10.3390/nu2121212, http://www.mdpi.com/2072-6643/2/12/1212/pdf.

Burdge, G. C., & Calder, P. C. (2005). Dietary α-linolenic acid and health-related outcomes: A metabolic perspective. *Proceedings of the Nutrition Society, 64*(3), 327–333. https://doi.org/10.1079/PNS2005447.

Calder, P., Carr, A., Gombart, A., & Eggersdorfer, M. (2020). Optimal nutritional status for a well-functioning immune system is an important factor to protect against viral infections. *Nutrients, 12*(4), 1181. https://doi.org/10.3390/nu12041181.

Calder, P. C. (2005). Dietary fatty acids and immune function. *Nutrition Reviews, 63*(6 Pt 2), S150–S160. https://doi.org/10.1111/j.1753-4887.2005.tb00154.x.

Calder, P. C. (2015). Functional roles of fatty acids and their effects on human health. *Journal of Parenteral and Enteral Nutrition, 39*(1_suppl), 18S–32S. https://doi.org/10.1177/0148607115595980.

Calder, P. C. (2017). Omega-3 fatty acids and inflammatory processes: From molecules to man. *Biochemical Society Transactions, 45*(5), 1105–1115. https://doi.org/10.1042/BST20160474, http://www.biochemsoctrans.org/content/45/5/1105.full-text.pdf.

Carlson, S. E. (2009). Docosahexaenoic acid supplementation in pregnancy and lactation. *The American Journal of Clinical Nutrition, 89*(2), 678S. https://doi.org/10.3945/ajcn.2008.26811e.

Choe, E., & Min, D. B. (2006). Mechanisms and factors for edible oil oxidation. *Comprehensive Reviews in Food Science and Food Safety, 5*(4), 169–186. https://doi.org/10.1111/j.1541-4337.2006.00009.x.

Duan, H., Song, W., Zhao, J., & Yan, W. (2023). Polyunsaturated fatty acids (PUFAs): Sources, digestion, absorption, application and their potential adjunctive effects on visual fatigue. *Nutrients, 15*(11), 2633. https://doi.org/10.3390/nu15112633.

Falch, E., Velasco, J., Aursand, M., & Andersen, M. L. (2005). Detection of radical development by ESR spectroscopy techniques for assessment of oxidative susceptibility of fish oils. *European Food Research and Technology, 221*(5), 667–674. https://doi.org/10.1007/s00217-005-0009-y.

Fathi, M., Mozafari, M. R., & Mohebbi, M. (2012). Nanoencapsulation of food ingredients using lipid based delivery systems. *Trends in Food Science & Technology, 23*(1), 13–27. https://doi.org/10.1016/j.tifs.2011.08.003.

Fluhr, J. W., Kao, J., Jain, M., Ahn, S. K., Feingold, K. R., & Elias, P. M. (2001). Generation of free fatty acids from phospholipids regulates stratum corneum acidification and integrity. *Journal of Investigative Dermatology, 117*(1), 44–51. https://doi.org/10.1046/j.0022-202X.2001.01399.x.

Frankel, E. N. (2012). Lipid oxidation: Mechanisms, inhibition, and analysis. *Lipid Technology, 24*(11), 247–250. https://doi.org/10.1002/lite.20120025.

Gulcin, İ. (2020). Antioxidants and antioxidant methods: An updated overview. *Archives of Toxicology, 94*(3), 651–715. https://doi.org/10.1007/s00204-020-02689-3.

Harris, W. S., Mozaffarian, D., Rimm, E., Kris-Etherton, P., Rudel, L. L., Appel, L. J., Engler, M. M., Engler, M. B., & Sacks, F. (2009). Omega-6 fatty acids and risk for cardiovascular disease: A science advisory from the American Heart Association Nutrition Subcommittee. *Circulation, 119*(6), 902–907. https://doi.org/10.1161/CIRCULATIONAHA.108.191627.

Hwang, H.-S. (2015). NMR spectroscopy for assessing lipid oxidation. *Lipid Technology, 27*(8), 187–189. https://doi.org/10.1002/lite.201500037.

Innis, S. M. (2007). Dietary omega-3 fatty acids and the developing brain. *Brain Research, 1237*, 35–43.

Ito, J., Shimizu, N., Kobayashi, E., Hanzawa, Y., Otoki, Y., Kato, S., Hirokawa, T., Kuwahara, S., Miyazawa, T., & Nakagawa, K. (2017). A novel chiral stationary phase LC-MS/MS method to evaluate oxidation mechanisms of edible oils. *Scientific Reports, 7*(1). https://doi.org/10.1038/s41598-017-10536-2, www.nature.com/srep/index.html.

Joffre, C., Rey, C., & Layé, S. (2019). N-3 polyunsaturated fatty acids and the resolution of neuroinflammation. *Frontiers in Pharmacology, 10*. https://doi.org/10.3389/fphar.2019.01022.

Johnson, D. R., & Decker, E. A. (2015). The role of oxygen in lipid oxidation reactions: A review. *Annual Review of Food Science and Technology, 6*, 171–190. https://doi.org/10.1146/annurev-food-022814-015532, http://www.annualreviews.org/journal/food.

Kang, J., & Yeo, J. (2024). Critical overview of mass spectrometry-based lipidomics approach for evaluating lipid oxidation in foods. *Food Science and Biotechnology, 34*, 837–849. https://doi.org/10.1007/s10068-024-01726-6.

Kapoor, B., Kapoor, D., Gautam, S., Singh, R., & Bhardwaj, S. (2021). Dietary polyunsaturated fatty acids (PUFAs): Uses and potential health benefits. *Current Nutrition Reports, 10*(3), 232–242. https://doi.org/10.1007/s13668-021-00363-3.

Karami, H., Rasekh, M., & Mirzaee-Ghaleh, E. (2020). Application of the E-nose machine system to detect adulterations in mixed edible oils using chemometrics methods. *Journal of Food Processing and Preservation, 44*(9). https://doi.org/10.1111/jfpp.14696.

Kirtil, E., Kilercioğlu, M., & Oztop, M. H. (2016). Modified atmosphere packaging of foods. In *Reference module in food science*. Elsevier, 1–6. https://doi.org/10.1016/B978-0-08-100596-5.03218-2.

Koletzko, B., Cetin, I., & Brenna, J. T. (2008). Dietary fat intakes for pregnant and lactating women. *British Journal of Nutrition, 100*(3), 473–479. https://doi.org/10.1017/S0007114507764747.

Kris-Etherton, P. M., Taylor, D. S., Yu-Poth, S., Huth, P., Moriarty, K., Fishell, V., Hargrove, R. L., Zhao, G., & Etherton, T. D. (2000). Polyunsaturated fatty acids in the food chain in the United States. *American Journal of Clinical Nutrition, 71*(1 Suppl), 179S–188S. https://doi.org/10.1093/ajcn/71.1.179s.

Kunesová, M., Braunerová, R., Hlavatý, P., Tvrzická, E., Stanková, B., Skrha, J., Hilgertová, J., Hill, M., Kopecký, J., Wagenknecht, M., Hainer, V., Matoulek, M., Parízková, J., Zák, A., & Svacina, S. (2006). The influence of n-3 polyunsaturated fatty acids and very low calorie diet during a short-term weight reducing regimen on weight loss and serum fatty acid composition in severely obese women. *Physiological Research, 55*(1), 63–72. https://doi.org/10.33549/physiolres.930770.

Laguerre, M., Lecomte, J., & Villeneuve, P. (2017). Lipid oxidation in food emulsions: Impact of physical and chemical properties on chemical pathways and kinetics. *Critical Reviews in Food Science and Nutrition, 57*(4), 697–715. https://doi.org/10.1080/10408398.2014.972091.

Layé, S., Nadjar, A., Joffre, C., & Bazinet, R. (2018). Anti-inflammatory effects of omega-3 fatty acids in the brain: Physiological mechanisms and relevance to pharmacology. *Pharmacological Reviews, 70*(1), 12–38.

Li, Q., Chen, J., Huyan, Z., Kou, Y., Xu, L., Yu, X., & Gao, J. M. (2019). Application of Fourier transform infrared spectroscopy for the quality and safety analysis of fats and oils: A review. *Critical Reviews in Food Science and Nutrition, 59*(22), 3597–3611. https://doi.org/10.1080/10408398.2018.1500441, https://www.tandfonline.com/loi/bfsn20.

Mariamenatu, A. H., & Abdu, E. M. (2021). Overconsumption of omega-6 polyunsaturated fatty acids (PUFAs) versus deficiency of omega-3 PUFAs in modern-day diets: The disturbing factor for their "Balanced Antagonistic Metabolic Functions" in the human body. *Journal of Lipids, 2021*, 8848161. https://doi.org/10.1155/2021/8848161.

Mcclements, D. J., & Decker, E. A. (2000). Lipid oxidation in oil-in-water emulsions: impact of molecular environment on chemical reactions in heterogeneous food systems. *Journal of Food Science, 65*(8), 1270–1282. https://doi.org/10.1111/j.1365-2621.2000.tb10596.x.

McClements, D. J., & Rao, J. (2011). Food-Grade nanoemulsions: Formulation, fabrication, properties, performance, biological fate, and potential toxicity. *Critical Reviews in Food Science and Nutrition, 51*(4), 285–330. https://doi.org/10.1080/10408398.2011.559558.

McClements, D. J. (2004). *Food emulsions: Principles, practices, and techniques* (2th ed.). CRC Press.

Merle, B. M. J., Benlian, P., Puche, N., Bassols, A., Delcourt, C., Souied, E. H., Allaire, C., Bassols, A., Belabbas, K., Brault, D., Brouquet, Y., Castagnet, S., Crié, A., Gaudino, I., Gawrilow, P., Lablache-Combier, M., Leveziel, N., Mechai, N., Morineau, G., ... Turquois, I. (2014). Circulating omega-3 fatty acids and neovascular age-related macular degeneration. *Investigative Ophthalmology and Visual Science, 55*(3), 2010–2019. https://doi.org/10.1167/iovs.14-13916, http://www.iovs.org/content/55/3/2010.full.pdf.

Miltz, J., & Perry, M. (2005). Evaluation of the performance of iron-based oxygen scavengers, with comments on their optimal applications. *Packaging Technology and Science, 18*(1), 21–27. https://doi.org/10.1002/pts.671.

Mititelu, M., Lupuliasa, D., Neacşu, S. M., Olteanu, G., Busnatu, Ş. S., Mihai, A., Popovici, V., Măru, N., Boroghină, S. C., Mihai, S., Ioniţă-Mîndrican, C. B., & Scafa-Udrişte, A. (2025). Polyunsaturated fatty acids and human health: A key to modern nutritional balance in association with polyphenolic compounds from food sources. *Foods, 14*(1). https://doi.org/10.3390/foods14010046, www.mdpi.com/journal/foods.

Mozaffarian, D., & Wu, J. H. Y. (2011). Omega-3 fatty acids and cardiovascular disease: Effects on risk factors, molecular pathways, and clinical events. *Journal of the American College of Cardiology, 58*(20), 2047–2067. https://doi.org/10.1016/j.jacc.2011.06.063, www.elsevier.com/locate/jacc.

Pilkington, S. M., Watson, R. E. B., Nicolaou, A., & Rhodes, L. E. (2011). Omega-3 polyunsaturated fatty acids: Photoprotective macronutrients. *Experimental Dermatology, 20*(7), 537–543. https://doi.org/10.1111/j.1600-0625.2011.01294.x.

Risch, S.J., & Reineccius, G.A. (Eds.). (1995). Encapsulation and controlled release of food ingredients (ACS symposium series no. 590). American Chemical Society. https://doi.org/10.1021/bk-1995-0590.

Robertson, G. L. (2016). *Food packaging: Principles and practice* (3rd ed.). CRC Press. https://doi.org/10.1201/b21347.

Rolewski, P., Siger, A., Nogala-Kałucka, M., & Polewski, K. (2009). Chemiluminescent assay of lipid hydroperoxides quantification in emulsions of fatty acids and oils. *Food Research International, 42*(1), 165–170. https://doi.org/10.1016/j.foodres.2008.09.010.

Saini, R. K., & Keum, Y. S. (2018). Omega-3 and omega-6 polyunsaturated fatty acids: Dietary sources, metabolism, and significance — A review. *Life Sciences, 203*, 255–267. https://doi.org/10.1016/j.lfs.2018.04.049, www.elsevier.com/locate/lifescie.

SanGiovanni, J. P., & Chew, E. Y. (2005). The role of omega-3 long-chain polyunsaturated fatty acids in health and disease of the retina. *Progress in Retinal and Eye Research, 24*(1), 87–138. https://doi.org/10.1016/j.preteyeres.2004.06.002.

Serhan, C. N., & Levy, B. D. (2018). Resolvins in inflammation: Emergence of the pro-resolving superfamily of mediators. *Journal of Clinical Investigation, 128*(7), 2657–2669. https://doi.org/10.1172/JCI97943, https://www.jci.org/articles/view/97943/pdf.

Shahidi, F., & Zhong, Y. (2010). Lipid oxidation and improving the oxidative stability of foods. *Chemical Society Reviews, 39*(11), 4067–4079. https://doi.org/10.1039/B922183M.

Shahidi, F., & Ambigaipalan, P. (2015). Phenolics and polyphenolics in foods, beverages and spices: Antioxidant activity and health effects – A review. *Journal of Functional Foods, 18*, 820–897. https://doi.org/10.1016/j.jff.2015.06.018.

Simopoulos, A. P. (2016). An increase in the Omega-6/Omega-3 fatty acid ratio increases the risk for obesity. *Nutrients, 8*(3). https://doi.org/10.3390/nu8030128, http://www.mdpi.com/2072-6643/8/3/128/pdf.

Sokoła-Wysoczańska, E., Wysoczański, T., Pękala, J., Czyż, K., Bodkowski, R., Lochyński, S., & Patkowska-Sokoła, B. (2018). Polyunsaturated fatty acids and their potential therapeutic role in cardiovascular system disorders: A review. *Nutrients, 10*(10), 1561.

Tao, L. (2015). Oxidation of polyunsaturated fatty acids and its impact on food quality and human health. *Advances in Food Technology and Nutritional Sciences, 1*(6), 135–137. https://doi.org/10.17140/AFTNSOJ-1-123.

Vermeiren, L., Devlieghere, F., VanBeen, M., De Kruijf, N., & Debevere, J. (2000). Development in the active packaging of foods. *Journal of Food Technology in Africa, 5*(1). https://doi.org/10.4314/jfta.v5i1.19249.

Vlachos, N., Skopelitis, Y., Psaroudaki, M., Konstantinidou, V., Chatzilazarou, A., & Tegou, E. (2006). Applications of Fourier transform-infrared spectroscopy to edible oils. *Analytica Chimica Acta, 573-574*, 459–465. https://doi.org/10.1016/j.aca.2006.05.034.

Walker, R., Decker, E. A., & McClements, D. J. (2015). Development of food-grade nanoemulsions and emulsions for delivery of omega-3 fatty acids: Opportunities and obstacles in the food industry. *Food and Function, 6*(1), 42–55. https://doi.org/10.1039/c4fo00723a, http://www.rsc.org/Publishing/Journals/FO/about.asp.

Walpurgis, K., Thomas, A., Geyer, H., Mareck, U., & Thevis, M. (2020). Dietary supplement and food contaminations and their implications for doping controls. *Foods, 9*(8), 1012. https://doi.org/10.3390/foods9081012.

Xu, D. P., Li, Y., Meng, X., Zhou, T., Zhou, Y., Zheng, J., Zhang, J. J., & Li, H. B. (2017). Natural antioxidants in foods and medicinal plants: Extraction, assessment and resources. *International Journal of Molecular Sciences, 18*(1). https://doi.org/10.3390/ijms18010096, http://www.mdpi.com/1422-0067/18/1/96/pdf.

Xu, L., Yu, X., Liu, L., & Zhang, R. (2016). A novel method for qualitative analysis of edible oil oxidation using an electronic nose. *Food Chemistry, 202*, 225–231. https://doi.org/10.1016/j.foodchem.2016.01.144.

Zeb, A., & Ullah, F. (2016). A simple spectrophotometric method for the determination of thiobarbituric acid reactive substances in fried fast foods. *Journal of Analytical Methods in Chemistry, 2016*, 9412767. https://doi.org/10.1155/2016/9412767.

Chapter 19

Novel packaging strategies for polyunsaturated fatty acid-enriched food products

Khaoula Elhadef[1], Bouthaina Ben Hadj Hmida[2], Sarra Akermi[1], Moufida Chaari[1], Fakhreddine Ben Amara[1], and Slim Smaoui[1]

[1]*Laboratory of Microbial Biotechnology, Enzymatic and Biomolecules, Centre of Biotechnology of Sfax, Sfax, Tunisia,* [2]*Laboratory of Biochemistry and Enzymatic Engineering of Lipases, National Engineering School of Sfax, University of Sfax, Sfax, Tunisia*

19.1 Introduction

Owing to the existence of multiple unsaturations in their structure, polyunsaturated fatty acids (PUFAs) are considered highly valuable dietary components in terms of nutritional value and health benefits. This class may include diverse components such as arachidonic acid, eicosapentaenoic acid (EPA), and docosahexaenoic acid (DHA), which are significant long-chain fatty acids (Kus-Yamashita et al., 2016). Over time, researchers have demonstrated the benefits of PUFAs in modulating inflammation, cognitive activity, and metabolism of cholesterol (Fig. 19.1) (Palacios et al., 2022). On the other side, several studies have associated PUFAs with cardiovascular illnesses (CVDs). However, their metabolic effect is still very controversial and unclear, despite their advantageous health benefits. The effect of plasma levels of omega-3 and omega-6 PUFA on the risk of CVDs was investigated by Borges et al. (2022) using Mendelian randomization. Due to oxidative degradation caused by the high quantities of monounsaturated fatty acids (MUFA) and PUFA, groundnut, fish, and sunflower oils develop rancid smells (Peter et al., 2022). According to a WHO report, noncommunicable illnesses alone were responsible for almost 41 million deaths in 2018. Both inflammation and oxidative stress play an important role in the development of the risk of noncommunicable chronic illnesses. Both the inflammatory and antioxidant signaling pathways are impacted by PUFAs (Djuricic & Calder, 2021). In addition, PUFAs play a role as antioxidants by changing the inflammatory process and regulating the antioxidant signaling pathway (Calder, 2020). The three stages of lipid oxidation are the following: initiation, development, and termination. The most important free radicals in the mentioned process are the fatty acid radicals, including LOO-, LO-, and L- (Li et al., 2022). PUFAs' propensity to undergo oxidation is crucial for preserving the integrity of cellular membranes and foods high in lipids (Dessì et al., 2002). Omega-3, including DHA and EPA, is advantageous for providing defense against many metabolic diseases (Saini et al., 2021). By decreasing the risk of cancer, cardiovascular disease, and inflammation, omega-3 PUFAs could enhance health. According to the literature, improving the amount of unsaturation increases the fraction of lipid oxidation. Hence, omega-3 PUFAs are more vulnerable to oxidation because of the double bonds they contain (Zhang et al., 2020). Likewise, due to its unsaturated link, which generates a range of metabolites and reactive oxygen species (ROS), PUFAs are especially susceptible to oxidation. Oxidation levels and metabolites might have a positive or negative effect on PUFA efficiency. Because PUFA has a large number of unsaturated bonds, it is more vulnerable to oxidation, which can be further grouped into two types: nonenzymatic oxidation and enzymatic oxidation. Other subtypes of nonenzymatic oxidation include autoxidation, which is mediated by free radicals, and photo-oxidation (Tao, 2015). When handling, cooking, and storing edible oils, lipid oxidation causes deterioration processes. Any loss of oil quality, such as a deterioration in the oil's nutritional quality or the development of unwanted off-flavors that make the oil less appealing to customers, is caused by the oxidation mechanism. Furthermore, lipid oxidation typically produces dangerous byproducts, which may lead to the creation of novel lipid peroxidation end products that could be fatal to human wellness. Lipid oxidation is controlled by temperature, oxygen consumption, and antioxidants. High temperatures and the degree of lipid unsaturation could cause chain reactions to proceed more quickly, which could

Omega-3 and Omega-6 Polyunsaturated Fatty Acids in Food Systems. DOI: https://doi.org/10.1016/B978-0-443-43810-3.00018-X

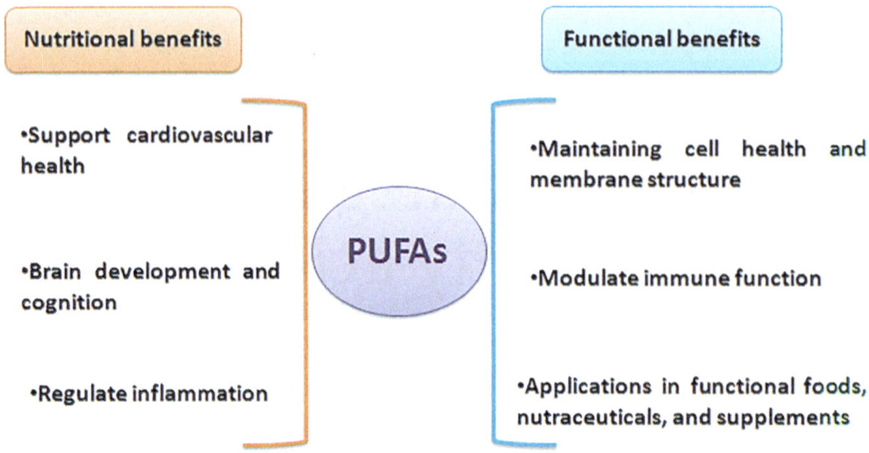

FIGURE 19.1 Benefits of polyunsaturated fatty acids (PUFAs) for nutrition and function.

increase the interaction of oils with oxygen (Fadda et al., 2022). This chapter provides a detailed overview of packaging innovations aimed at enhancing the stability of PUFAs. It looks into the main factors affecting PUFA stability as well as how innovative packaging may prolong product shelf life and lessen deterioration. This chapter looks at a number of packing techniques, evaluates the usefulness of different materials, and emphasizes how they protect PUFA-rich foods from oxidative and environmental challenges. Researchers wishing to optimize PUFA stability with cutting-edge packaging alternatives may find useful information about how packaging techniques impact the overall safety and quality of food goods.

19.2 Challenges in polyunsaturated fatty acid stability

Oxidation, hydrolysis, and environmental factors are the major stability challenges that PUFAs may face owing to the presence of unsaturations in their structure. These compounds are highly reactive, and lipid peroxidation may cause the deterioration of their nutritional value and the formation of undesirable flavors (Machado et al., 2023). In fact, the exposure to various factors, including oxygen, light, heat, and moisture, can accelerate their degradation, raising concerns towards storage and processing processes (Jurić et al., 2022).

19.2.1 Chemical instability

Oxidation of PUFAs can be defined as a complex biochemical process that begins with the initiation phase and ends with the termination (Islam et al., 2023). At the beginning, a hydrogen atom from a PUFA is oxidized by ROS promoting the production of an unstable radical (Juan and Pérez de la Lastra, 2021). Moreover, the oxidation process continues to propagate by reacting with lipid radicals, resulting in the formation of lipid peroxyl radicals and hydroperoxides (Aureliano et al., 2023). Eventually, the oxidized PUFA is transformed into secondary products, derived from hydroperoxides, including aldehydes, ketones, and short-chain fatty acids (Machado et al., 2023). Toxic forms of aldehydes can contribute to oxidative stress and membrane destabilization by reacting with cellular components. On the other side, PUFA oxidation is considered a major factor in multiple pathological factors such as neurodegenerative and cardiovascular problems (Cordiano et al., 2023). In food products, rancidity, deterioration in nutritional value, and undesirable flavors are tightly linked to the oxidative degradation of PUFAs (Gengatharan, 2025). Therefore controlling PUFA oxidation can be realized via various antioxidant mechanisms, including enzymatic defenses (including superoxide dismutase and glutathione peroxidase) and nonenzymatic antioxidants (such as polyphenols and vitamin E) in order to neutralize free radicals and stabilize lipid membranes (Gouvêa et al., 2023). Understanding the different steps of the oxidative process can ameliorate human health and preserve the safety and stability of food products (Fig. 19.2).

19.2.2 The factors destabilizing polyunsaturated fatty acids

PUFAs are essential components of biological structures and play a crucial role in contributing to human well-being. Nevertheless, their instability can be a challenging matter, especially in the food and pharmaceutical industries. Different factors, including oxygen exposure, light, heat, and moisture, can facilitate the deterioration of these products, making the use of proper storage and stabilization methods indispensable (Fig. 19.3).

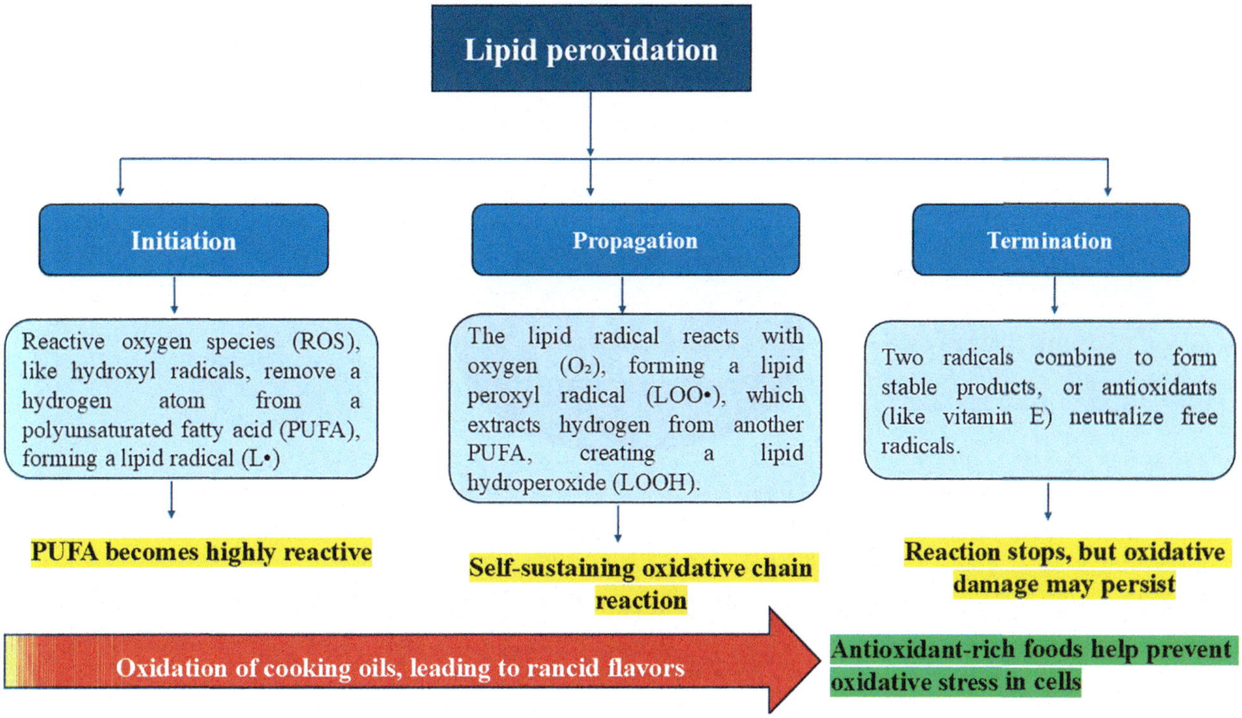

FIGURE 19.2 The process of lipid peroxidation.

19.2.2.1 Oxygen exposure

The existence of catalysts, including metal ions and the continuous exposure to oxygen, can accelerate the oxidation of (PUFAs) (Musakhanian et al., 2022). It is important to mention that PUFA degradation is the result of exposure to different forms and concentrations of oxygen, which highly influence the oxidation rate. For example, lipid peroxidation in biological and food systems can occur when the amount of absorbed oxygen by PUFAs is affected by the presence of a partial pressure. Moreover, under ambient conditions, oxidative damage can be initiated when PUFA-rich membranes absorb an amount of oxygen (Machado et al., 2023). On the other side, during harsh conditions, including high temperatures and UV light exposure, the increasing of pressure and the amount of dissolved oxygen may intensify the oxidation. At high temperatures, the decrease of oxygen solubility in lipid structures can be explained by the reduction of oxidation dependence on dissolved oxygen.

19.2.2.2 Light

The oxidation of (PUFAs) can be accelerated via permanent exposure to UV light, resulting in their degradation and the loss of their valuable nutritional benefits (Lopes & Courrol, 2023). In this sense, lipid peroxidation can be initiated when ROS, such as hydroxyl radicals, singlet oxygen, and superoxide, are produced by the UV-B radiation, leading to the alteration of PUFAs' structural integrity (Pathak et al., 2019). In addition, fatty acids such as EPA and DHA, involved in brain development and cardiovascular health, were noticed to rapidly degrade when exposed to UV light (Mora et al., 2022). Literature reports demonstrated that the reduction of the production of these fatty acids in marine organisms, caused by excessive exposure to UV, can significantly affect the food chain and human nutrition (Conceição et al., 2020; Kannan et al., 2021). Additionally, further research has shown that the oxidation of PUFAs present in skin sebum can contribute to premature aging and skin inflammation (Gruber et al., 2021). On the other side, the shelf life and sensory qualities of PUFA-rich oils, such as flaxseed, fish oil, and sunflower oil, known to bear large amounts of omega-6 and omega-3 fatty acids, can diminish due to UV light exposure (Pattnaik & Mishra, 2022; Saini et al., 2021).

19.2.2.3 Moisture

Moisture is among the main factors that can significantly destabilize PUFAs by increasing hydrolytic rancidity and oxidative degradation (Melgosa et al., 2019). This usually happens when PUFAs are exposed to water, converting

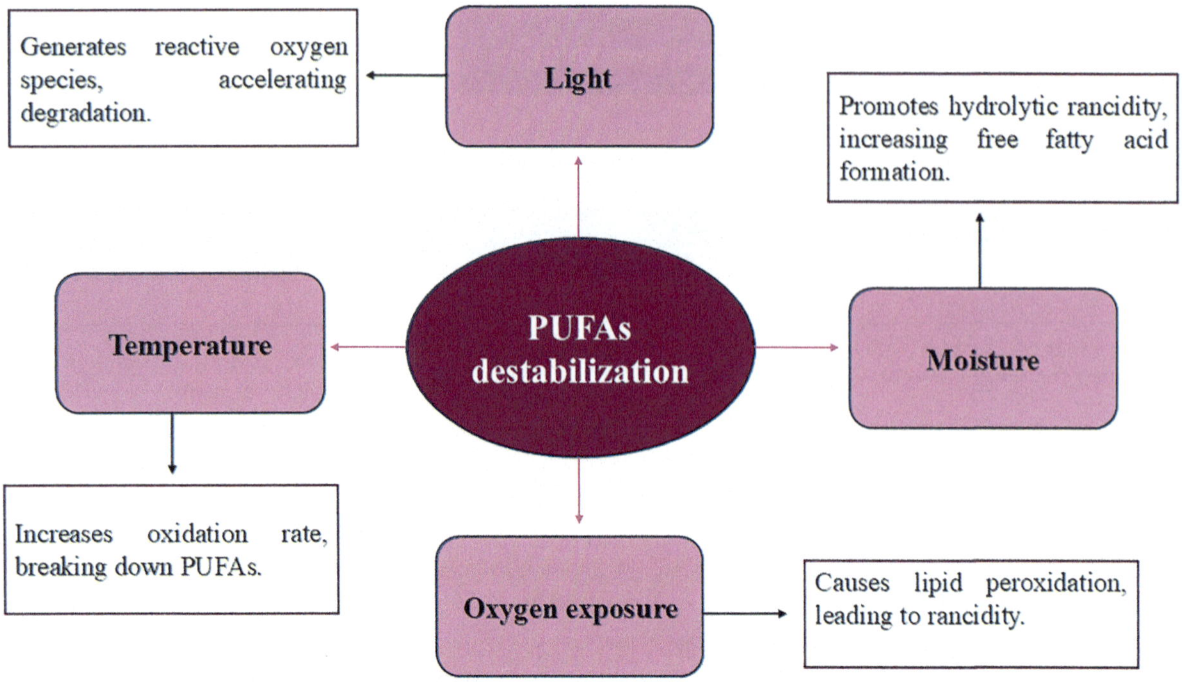

FIGURE 19.3 The different factors influencing the polyunsaturated fatty acids (PUFAs) stability.

triglycerides into free fatty acids. This process can cause heavy losses in the food industry, especially during the storage process, as high levels of humidity can deteriorate PUFA-rich oils. Furthermore, this factor can facilitate microbial growth and proliferation, leading to lipid degradation of the food products through enzymatic activity. It can also damage the membrane integrity by influencing PUFA functionality in cell signaling pathways (Das, 2021). It can intensify lipid oxidation by boosting the interaction between PUFAs and oxygen, resulting in the production of ROS that degrade fatty acids (Islam et al., 2023).

To resolve the problem of PUFA degradation by moisture, various preservation techniques were suggested to be used to maintain their stability and nutritional value. In this context, silica gel and calcium chloride were employed to absorb the excess moisture from different food matrices in order to inhibit microbial proliferation and growth (Kaushani et al., 2022). In addition, vacuum-sealed packaging was used especially in fish oil capsules and nut conservation to reduce oxygen and moisture exposure (Nagarajarao, 2016). Freeze-drying is another technique that was applied to remove water through sublimation. It enhanced PUFA shelf life by converting them from liquid to powder (Islam et al., 2018). Finally, vitamin E and polyphenols, which serve as powerful antioxidant agents, can protect PUFAs through free radical scavenging and the reduction of oxidative stress.

19.2.2.4 Temperature

It was found that the formation of toxic oxidation products, including malondialdehyde and 4-Hydroxy-2 (E)-nonenal, is generally caused by lipid peroxidation induced by high temperatures. This degradation can give rise to several problems, particularly in cooking oils, resulting in their reduced effectiveness in supporting cardiovascular and neurological health. However, low temperatures (refrigeration) can be used to preserve PUFA stability in food storage by slowing and limiting lipid oxidation. A previous study has shown that cold storage significantly reduces oxidative degradation in PUFA-rich products, including fish and vegetable oils (Méndez et al., 2022). However, extreme cold can also impact PUFA bioavailability by altering their crystalline structure, potentially affecting absorption in biological systems (Delmas & Aires, 2025).

19.3 Innovative packaging for enhancing polyunsaturated fatty acid stability

19.3.1 Stabilization of polyunsaturated fatty acid-containing foods with antioxidants

Lipid oxidation causes foods to lose their nutritional value and develop unappealing characteristics for consumers. Moreover, conditions such as cancer and atherosclerosis can be brought on by oxidation. Antioxidants are therefore necessary for foods to retain their safety and quality (Poljsak et al., 2021). Interest in utilizing biological antioxidants has grown owing to the toxicological hazards of synthetic ones and customer demand for natural products (Uzombah, 2022). Anthocyanins, flavonoids, carotenoids, vitamin E, and phenolic compounds are among the elements of natural goods that are known to act as oxidation process scavengers (Abeyrathne et al., 2022). Metal chelation, oxygen scavenging, and radical scavenging are the three primary antioxidative mechanisms required to prevent food systems from oxidizing. Numerous possible ways of action can be attributed to specific antioxidants. Furthermore, an antioxidant's polarity and solubility dictate where it is placed in a certain food matrix, which also affects how powerful the antioxidant is (Parcheta et al., 2021).

19.3.1.1 Tocopherol

Tocopherols are a type of fat-soluble antioxidant that assist in reducing oxidative stress by efficiently neutralizing lipid peroxyl radicals. Because tocopherols can reverse the harm that free radicals have caused, they may also help lower the risk of neurological diseases such as Alzheimer's, and some types of cancer, in addition to cardiovascular health (Abdelqader et al., 2023). The majority of dietary tocopherols come from plant-based sources, such as seed oils (safflower, corn, and soybean), almonds, whole grains, sunflower seeds, and wheat germ. On the other hand, meals originating from animals usually include very little of this vitamin. Due to the fact that vitamin E is fat-soluble, proper digestion and absorption of dietary fat are required for its absorption (Andrès et al., 2024). In α-tocopherol, the highest level of biological activity is observed. It breaks chains and is the best lipid-soluble antioxidant. The physical state bulk phase or emulsion, concentration, temperature, and lipid composition all influence whether α-tocopherol in food has an antioxidant, pro-oxidant, or neutral effect. Serfert et al. (2009) used α-tocopherol as a stabilizer of chemicals during the time of homogenization, microencapsulation, and storage of oils that contained long-chain PUFAs. After storing fish oil-enriched energy bars at room temperature for 10 weeks, Horn et al. (2009) demonstrated the effects of ascorbyl palmitate, γ-tocopherol, and caffeic acid on preventing lipid oxidation.

19.3.1.2 Polyphenols

The antioxidative, anticarcinogenic, antiinflammatory, and angiogenesis-inhibiting properties of bioactive compounds, especially polyphenols, naturally occurring in vegetables, herbs, and fruits, have been demonstrated to have potential health effects (Mitropoulou et al., 2023; Pan et al., 2021; Samtiya et al., 2021). Fruits, vegetables, and a variety of aromatic and medicinal plants all contain flavonols, a subgroup of flavonoids (Carpena et al., 2021). Additionally, in different in vitro models (the oxygen radical absorbance capacity [ORAC]), a well-known flavonol (quercetin) has shown effectiveness as a potent antioxidant agent (Pozo-Martínez et al., 2022). It showed an inhibitory activity against lipid oxidation in many foodstuffs fortified with PUFAs and marine oils (Liu et al., 2021). Rupasinghe et al. (2010) stipulated that EPA and fish oil have antioxidant potential to prevent oxidation by the addition of polyphenolic-enriched apple skin extract. Moreover, Huber et al. (2009) indicated that quercetin glycosides can limit the peroxidation of omega-3 PUFAs and fish oil lipids.

19.3.2 Applying innovative methods to reduce oxidation

To prevent PUFA oxidation, it is important to design an interfacial structure. To alter the covalent and noncovalent molecules of those interfacial layers, many physical, enzymatic, and chemical methods are employed. A previous study reported that the encapsulation of PUFAs in microcapsules to enhance Maillard reaction products reduced surface oil, resulting in enhanced oxidation-protection efficiency (Wang et al., 2025). Furthermore, the process of free radical linking is employed to produce polysaccharide polyphenol or protein–polyphenol pairings. It permits the creation of free radicals by facilitating the interaction of residues on the polysaccharide or protein chain with hydroxyl radicals, resulting in the formation of conjugates (Liu et al., 2016). The rise in the number of phenolic hydroxyl content in conjugates has shown an improvement in their capacity to neutralize and reduce free radicals (Zhang et al., 2023). In addition, enzymatic crosslinking was used to reinforce intramolecular and intermolecular interactions between biopolymers (Zeeb et al., 2017). This method may enhance PUFA stability in emulsions and limit the lipid oxidation process. The microfluidic-jet spray-drying is another method that ensures the creation of microcapsules with potent particles to ameliorate the uniformity of omega-3 fatty acid emulsions. Additionally, the electrospray method is generally based on the electrohydrodynamic principle of the systems and solvent media. It guarantees the production of omega-3 PUFA microcapsules at low temperatures to reduce the effect of heated airflow on these molecules. Nevertheless, several studies discussed the use of mixtures derived from both plants and animals. It was reported that those extracts have efficient and powerful antioxidant biomolecules that may work together, when mixed, to avoid omega-3 oxidation. A previous study of Islam et al. (2023)

stated that the mixture of phlobatannins, tannins, and flavonoids from the coconut's carapace can limit the oxidative alterations. Another research suggested that the addition of 200 mg/L of coconut shell extract to shrimp oil emulsion can delay lipid degradation up to 12 days under refrigerated conditions at 30°C. This finding can be explained by the extract, which created hydrophobicity in saponifiable molecules and regenerated antioxidant compounds through hydrophobic ring topologies. The same study has demonstrated that the refining processes, including neutralization, bleaching, and deodorization, had a considerable effect on the oil composition, stability kinetics, and quality indices (Gharby et al., 2021).

19.3.2.1 Encapsulation

The efficacy of the encapsulation of omega-3 oil and the maintenance of its stability during storage are crucial factors in developing effective delivery systems. In this sense, the choice of encapsulating material, processing conditions, and formulation strategy are the major factors that should be taken into consideration (Habib et al., 2022).

The use of milk proteins, dextrins, modified cellulose, gelatin, plant gums, and modified starches, as encapsulants, can preserve delicate PUFAs and extend their shelf life. When selecting a coating material, it is necessary to guarantee oxidative stability, food application compatibility, and regulatory approval (Rodríguez Cortina, 2022). Although it only offers a small selection of wall materials, spray-drying is the widely known and economical encapsulation technique available (Díaz-Montes, 2023). Other options include double-coating methods, ultrasonic spray nozzles, and freeze-drying (Legako & Dunford, 2010a, 2010b). Legako and Dunford discovered that, at comparable core-to-wall ratios, ultrasonic two-channel nozzles generated more homogeneous microcapsules, but their encapsulation efficiency was lower than that of freeze-dried systems.

Numerous substances, such as complex coacervates of gelatin and sugar beet and gum arabic, pectin, and glucose sirup, have been studied for microencapsulation (Fig. 19.4) (Ghorchi et al., 2025). However, spray-drying's need for high temperatures, which, when paired with oxygen exposure, might hasten PUFA oxidation, is still an obstacle. Thus at lower processing temperatures, freeze-drying has become a viable substitute for preserving oil stability (Anwar & Kunz, 2011).

19.3.2.2 Modified atmosphere packaging

Modified Atmosphere Packaging is a widely utilized protection method for maintaining the quality and increasing the storage stability of perishable items, including meat products, fruits, fish, and fresh vegetables. This technique slows down oxidative reactions and microbiological growth by changing the makeup of internal packing gases. Game meat is particularly vulnerable to oxidation because it contains high levels of PUFAs, proteins, and myoglobin, which are pro-oxidant substances that enhance the meat's vulnerability to oxidative deterioration (Chaijan, 2008).

Bak et al. (1999) looked into how modified atmosphere packaging (MAP) affected the oxidative changes that occurred in cold-water shrimp that were kept in frozen storage. Their research looked at the effects of temperature changes, light exposure, and packaging conditions on shell-on shrimp during a 12-month period in terms of frost formation, lipid oxidation, discolouration, and textural alterations (i.e., meat toughness). In comparison to traditional packaging, the results showed that MAP produced better preservation results by drastically lowering color fading, rancidity, and hardness. However, lipid oxidation and discolouration were made worse by light exposure, and frost formation inside the packing was significantly influenced by temperature changes.

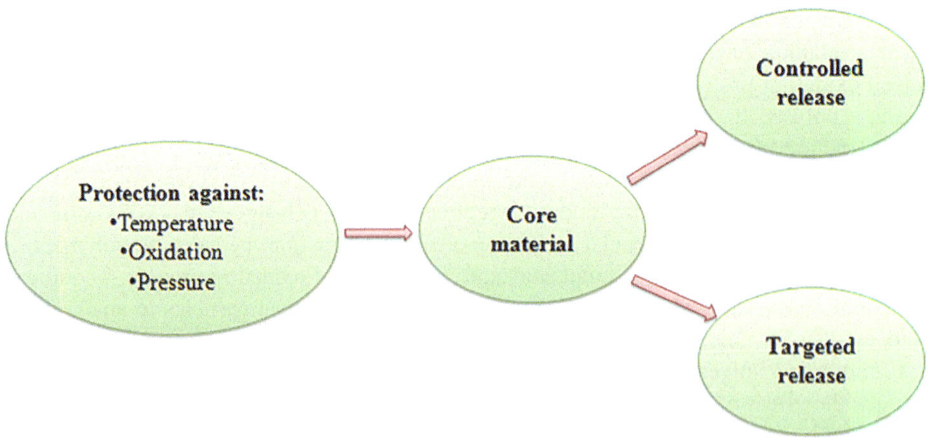

FIGURE 19.4 Fundamental idea of bioactive chemical microencapsulation.

In addition to shrimp, MAP has been shown to effectively enhance the storage stability of other seafood elements. As an illustration of MAP's wider usefulness in protecting seafood quality during storage, investigations by Yesudhason et al. (2010) verified its efficacy in keeping seer fish (*Scomberomorus commerson*), while Kykkidou et al. (2009) found similar benefits for Mediterranean fish.

19.4 Packaging materials and their role

Packaging materials are highly relevant to the final product quality. The production of different packaging materials has been made from various sources. The packaging material quality was the link between the consumers and the producer, that encouraging them to believe in the product (Pal et al., 2019). The selection of these materials for packaging influences its appearance and guarantees its protection. Many types of packaging materials were developed depending on the application area (cosmetics, food, meat, pharmaceuticals, etc.)

19.4.1 Material types

19.4.1.1 Petroleum-based plastic materials

Even though petroleum-based plastic materials allow easy handling and have good physical and functional properties, they are poorly degradable and inefficient (Mendes & Pedersen, 2021). Polypropylene (PP), polyethylene (PE), polyurethane, polystyrene (PS), poly(ethylene terephthalate) (PET), expanded PS, polyvinyl chloride, and polyamides are polymers applied in food packaging (Luzi et al., 2019). Plastic-based materials remain the greatest material used, with 26% of the total polymers (Mendes & Pedersen, 2021). Over the next 20 years, the consumption of plastics is predicted to increase twofold, as they rapidly substitute for other materials used for packaging. The main reasons for this are their good barrier properties, light weight, and reduced cost (MacArthur et al., 2016).

19.4.1.2 Biobased packaging materials

These polymers are produced by microorganisms or plants by metabolic methods and from sustainable resources such as polysaccharides, wood, agricultural waste, or lignocellulosic materials (Menon & Rao, 2012). The main advantages of these materials were related to their biodegradability and biocompatibility, which make them an ideal candidate for food applications. Bio-based materials can be classified into several categories, such as microorganism-derived polymers (e.g., xanthan, alginate, and polysaccharides), protein-based polymers, and wood-derived polymers. Biobased packaging materials such as chitin and cellulose can be transformed into nanomolecules (Agarwal et al., 2023; Vähä-Nissi et al., 2017). The use of cellulose as an intelligent agent with biobased nanomaterials enhances its bioactivity as an antioxidant, antibacterial, and freshness sensor.

19.4.1.3 Wood based polymers

Wood-derived polymers containing approximately 25% lignin, 50% cellulose, 30% hemicellulose, and originate from lignocellulosic polysaccharides. Exceptionally, these materials were mainly used for nonwoven products, paper products, etc. (Sakr et al., 2021).

19.4.2 Functional additives

The integration of natural additives into packaging was assessed due to their high antioxidant activities. Different components were used, such as rosemary essential oil, green tea leaf extracts, cinnamon essential oil, flaxseed and flaxseed essential oil, grape extracts, etc. (Elgadir & Mariod, 2025). These compounds were especially used to protect various types of meat food. Table 19.1 summarizes the advantages of these components in meat preservation.

19.5 Impact of packaging on food shelf life

The protection of food products rich in PUFAs, which are susceptible to oxidative spoilage, heavily depends on the type of packaging used. Different studies mentioned that both the material and its barrier properties significantly impact how quickly oxidation occurs. For example, glass containers reduce oxygen transmission, making them more effective than plastic ones in dark settings. Additionally, encapsulation is essential for enhancing stability. For instance, compared to sirups, which showed significant deterioration (PV = 44.6 meq/kg oil) due to increased oxygen interaction, omega-3 capsules had much lower peroxide (7.62 meq/kg oil) and TOTOX values (30.44) after storage (Yenipazar & Şahin-Yeşilçubuk, 2023). In another study,

TABLE 19.1 Natural additives in meat preservation.

Food ingredient	Meat used	Active compound	Role	References
Green tea leaf extracts	Beef, chicken	Catechins	Extend shelf life	Elgadir and Mariod (2025), Gallego et al. (2015)
Rosemary extract	Chicken	Carnosol	Enhance shelf life and meat quality	AL-hijazeen and AL-rawashdeh (2019)
Cinnamon essential oil	Beef, chicken	Cinnamaldehyde	Enhance storage stability by inhibition of microbial proliferation and lipid oxidation	Diniz do Nascimento et al. (2020)
Grape extracts	Beef, chicken	Syringic acid	Enhance the shelf life of chicken and chicken patties, beef and beef patties.	Horbańczuk et al. (2019)
Flaxseed and flaxseed essential oil	Beef	α-linolenic acid	Improve the meat with total polyunsaturated fatty acid and omega-3 with higher nutritional values and sensory profiles	Raole and Raole (2022), Reyes-Padilla et al. (2018)

the quality of liquid whole egg can be preserved through the use of PE terephthalate, high-density PE, and Tetra Rex (Kocetkovs et al., 2022). Among these, PET packaging proved most efficient in preserving PUFAs over 35 days, presenting only a 2.1% reduction in amino acid content, which surpassed the performance of HDPE. In contrast, packaging types such as Tetra Rex® led to moisture loss, likely due to the delamination of their layered structure, which in turn sped up the changes in the composition of fatty acids (Kocetkovs et al., 2022).

Different studies in sustainable packaging have targeted enhancing the quality of fish and fish products, particularly salmon, using bio-based and active materials. In the study of Nilsuwan et al. (2021), packaging was formulated using fish gelatin-based films, combined with emulsified gelatin or polylactic acid layers. These types of packaging limited fat oxidation in fried salmon skin and preserved its freshness during storage (Nilsuwan et al., 2021). Another study used a mixture of chitosan and rice protein hydrolysates, which helps delay the oxidation in fresh salmon. This combination was reported to maintain the product's shelf life by 7 days in comparison with control samples (Yan et al., 2022). Additionally, Azizi-Lalabadi et al. (2020) used PP-based nanocomposites enhanced with ZnO nanoparticles, green tea extract, and zeolite 4A. This packaging composition stated a functional effect by improving the storage stability and safety of salmon (Azizi-Lalabadi et al., 2020). A comparable development was detected with a nanocomposite made of methoxyl pectin and gelatin, enriched with curcumin, which maintained the shelf life of salmon fillets up to 6 days (Candra et al., 2023). Essential oils and plant extracts have also been integrated into active packaging. For instance, a protein-based film incorporating ginger, garlic, and cinnamon essential oils demonstrated high antioxidant effects. In fact, cinnamon essential oil contributed to limiting oxidative changes in salmon over a 9-day refrigeration period. These compounds led to a significant reduction in peroxide value in salmon (Cheng et al., 2024). Similarly, packaging developed with pectin and blueberry extract helped maintain a lower pH level and slowed spoilage during storage (Romero et al., 2022). In addition, *Otolithes ruber* fillets stored in sage seed gum films, including *Zataria multiflora* essential oil, showed low levels of spoilage indicators such as biogenic amines, which leads to extended freshness due to the film's antimicrobial and antioxidant activity (Mohammadi et al., 2023). Furthermore, rainbow trout fillets treated with a gelatin film enriched with propolis extract experienced reduced rates of lipid oxidation and microbial growth indicators. These results effectively prolong the shelf life of rainbow trout fillets and maintain sensory quality (Ucak et al., 2020). Pérez-Córdoba et al. (2022) developed a gelatin and chitosan active packaging system with a nanoemulsion of garlic essential oil and α-tocopherol. This film presents a protective layer for refrigerated slices of omega-3-enriched mortadella. After 5 days of storage, the film extended the shelf life of refrigerated slices of omega-3-enriched mortadella by inhibiting the growth of pathogenic bacteria and decreasing lipid oxidation processes (Pérez-Córdoba et al., 2022). In the study of Dantas et al. (2022), who investigated the long-term stability of omega-3-fortified milk powder stored at 25°C and 75% relative humidity over a period of 360 days. The product was sealed in four types of packaging: BOPP/PP (biaxially oriented PP with PP),

TABLE 19.2 Packaging application for polyunsaturated fatty acid-rich food products.

Food matrix	Packaging	Main results	References
Omega-3-fortified milk powder	Metallized polyethylene (PE) terephthalate with low-density PE, BOPP/PP, metal cans, and composite cans	- Milk powders stored in these three packaging systems retained sufficient omega-3 levels even after 12 months of storage	Dantas et al. (2022)
Slices of omega-3-enriched mortadella	Gelatin–chitosan-based + nanoemulsified garlic essential oil and α-tocopherol	- Slowing down lipid oxidation processes, effectively maintaining the quality of the meat for 5 days during cold storage	Pérez-Córdoba et al. (2022)
Fried salmon	Fish gelatin/poly(lactic) acid	- EF/E-GF packaging decreases oxidation in salmon	Nilsuwan et al. (2021)
Fresh salmon	Rice protein hydrolysateS(RPH) -+ chitosan	- RPH/CS packaging prolongs the shelf life of salmon for 7 days.	Yan et al. (2022)
Salmon	Polypropylene (PP) nanocomposites containing green tea extract, 4A zeolite, and ZnO nanoparticles	- PP, ZnO NPs/4A Z/GTE, increase the shelf life of salmon.	Azizi-Lalabadi et al. (2020)
Fresh salmon fillets	Methoxyl pectin/gelatin/TiO_2/curcumin nanocomposite	- Prolongation of fresh salmon fillets' shelf life for 6 days	Candra et al. (2023)
Salmon	Protein isolate-EO emulsions (garlic, ginger, and cinnamon)	- Inhibition of lipid oxidation.	Cheng et al. (2024)
Salmon	Pectin-blueberries extract	- Low values of pH	Romero et al. (2022)
Otolithes ruber fillets	Sage seed gum +essential oil of *Zataria multiflora*	- Decrease biogenic amines. - Prolong the fish shelf life	Mohammadi et al. (2023)
Rainbow trout fillet	Propolis extract (PE) + gelatin	- Delay the lipid oxidation in trout fillets - Delay microbial deterioration in trout fillets	Ucak et al. (2020)

PETmet/LDPE (metallized PE terephthalate with low-density PE), composite cans, and metal cans. All samples were stored under normal atmospheric conditions with 21% oxygen. During the storage period, measurements were noted for headspace oxygen levels and omega-3 fatty acid content (specifically EPA + DHA). Among the tested packaging types, the BOPP/PP film performed the poorest, displaying a notable decline in EPA + DHA levels (from 390.2 to 352.0 mg/100 g). This deterioration was due to the material's permeability to water vapor and oxygen. In contrast, the PETmet/LDPE film, composite cans, and metal cans provided better protection, with minimal changes observed across all quality parameters. Their superior barrier properties helped maintain the product's chemical and physical integrity over time. As a result, milk powders stored in these three packaging systems preserved sufficient omega-3 levels even after 12 months of storage (Table 19.2) (Dantas et al., 2022).

19.6 Conclusion

PUFAs are crucial elements in a balanced diet; nevertheless, their susceptibility to degradation and oxidation restricts their application in food industries. Conventional packaging approaches often fall short of addressing the complicated issues related to preserving PUFA quality throughout storage and distribution processes. Novel advances in packaging techniques have enabled innovative results, such as active packaging methods with natural components, including intelligent materials that can regularly authenticate the quality. Additionally, to ameliorate the shelf life of food, these improvements increase the nutrient retention, client safety, and marketability of food products with PUFAs. Then, packaging improvements are an essential plan for enhancing the stability, safety, and quality of food products with PUFAs, encouraging consumer health.

References

Abdelqader, A., Obeidat, M. D., Al-Rawashdeh, M. S., & Alrazak, A. A. (2023). The role of vitamin E as an antioxidant and preventing damage caused by free radicals. *Journal of Life Science and Applied Research, 4*(2), 88–95.

Abeyrathne, E. D. N. S., Nam, K., Huang, X., & Ahn, D. U. (2022). Plant-and animal-based antioxidants' structure, efficacy, mechanisms, and applications: A review. *Antioxidants, 11*(5). https://doi.org/10.3390/antiox11051025, https://www.mdpi.com/2076-3921/11/5/1025/pdf?version=1653297413.

Agarwal, A., Shaida, B., Rastogi, M., & Singh, N. B. (2023). Food packaging materials with special reference to biopolymers-properties and applications. *Chemistry Africa, 6*(1), 117–144. https://doi.org/10.1007/s42250-022-00446-w, https://www.springer.com/journal/42250.

AL-hijazeen, M., & AL-rawashdeh, M. (2019). Preservative effects ofrosemary extract (Rosmarinus officinalis L.) on quality andstorage stability of chicken meat patties. Food Science and Technology, *39*(1), 27–34.

Andrès, E., Lorenzo-Villalba, N., Terrade, J.-E., & Méndez-Bailon, M. (2024). Fat-soluble vitamins A, D, E, and K: Review of the literature and points of interest for the clinician. *Journal of Clinical Medicine, 13*(13), 3641. https://doi.org/10.3390/jcm13133641.

Anwar, S. H., & Kunz, B. (2011). The influence of drying methods on the stabilization of fish oil microcapsules: Comparison of spray granulation, spray drying, and freeze drying. *Journal of Food Engineering, 105*(2), 367–378.

Aureliano, M., De Sousa-Coelho, A. L., Dolan, C. C., Roess, D. A., & Crans, D. C. (2023). Biological consequences of vanadium effects on formation of reactive oxygen species and lipid peroxidation. *International Journal of Molecular Sciences, 24*(6), 5382. https://doi.org/10.3390/ijms24065382.

Azizi-Lalabadi, M., Rafiei, L., Divband, B., & Ehsani, A. (2020). Active packaging for Salmon stored at refrigerator with polypropylene nanocomposites containing 4A zeolite, ZnO nanoparticles, and green tea extract. *Food Science & Nutrition, 8*(12), 6445–6456. https://doi.org/10.1002/fsn3.1934.

Bak, L. S., Andersen, A. B., Andersen, E. M., & Bertelsen, G. (1999). Effect of modified atmosphere packaging on oxidative changes in frozen stored cold water shrimp (Pandalus borealis). *Food Chemistry, 64*(2), 169–175. https://doi.org/10.1016/s0308-8146(98)00152-6.

Borges, M. C., Haycock, P. C., Zheng, J., Hemani, G., Holmes, M. V., Davey Smith, G., Hingorani, A. D., & Lawlor, D. A. (2022). Role of circulating polyunsaturated fatty acids on cardiovascular diseases risk: Analysis using Mendelian randomization and fatty acid genetic association data from over 114,000 UK Biobank participants. *BMC Medicine, 20*(1). https://doi.org/10.1186/s12916-022-02399-w, http://www.biomedcentral.com/bmcmed/.

Calder, P. C. (2020). N-3 PUFA and inflammation: From membrane to nucleus and from bench to bedside. *Proceedings of the Nutrition Society, 79*(4), 404–416. https://doi.org/10.1017/S0029665120007077, http://journals.cambridge.org/PNS.

Candra, A., Tsai, H. C., Saragi, I. R., Hu, C. C., Yu, W. T., Krishnamoorthi, R., Hong, Z. X., & Lai, J. Y. (2023). Fabrication and characterization of hybrid eco-friendly high methoxyl pectin/gelatin/TiO2/curcumin (PGTC) nanocomposite biofilms for salmon fillet packaging. *International Journal of Biological Macromolecules, 232*. https://doi.org/10.1016/j.ijbiomac.2023.123423, www.elsevier.com/locate/ijbiomac.

Carpena, M., Caleja, C., Nuñez-Estevez, B., Pereira, E., Fraga-Corral, M., Reis, F.S., & Barros, L. (2021). Flavonoids: A group of potential food additives with beneficial health effects.

Chaijan, M. (2008). Lipid and myoglobin oxidations in muscle foods. *Songklanakarin Journal of Science & Technology, 30*(1).

Cheng, J., Kandula, N., Cortes, V. E., Choi, H., Singh, P., & Cui, L. (2024). Pea protein isolate-based active films for salmon preservation: The role of different essential oils in film properties, antioxidant, and antibacterial activities. *Current Research in Food Science, 9*, 100936. https://doi.org/10.1016/j.crfs.2024.100936.

Conceição, D., Lopes, R. G., Derner, R. B., Cella, H., do Carmo, A. P. B., Montes D'Oca, M. G., Petersen, R., Passos, M. F., Vargas, J. V. C., Galli-Terasawa, L. V., & Kava, V. (2020). The effect of light intensity on the production and accumulation of pigments and fatty acids in Phaeodactylum tricornutum. *Journal of Applied Phycology, 32*(2), 1017–1025. https://doi.org/10.1007/s10811-019-02001-6.

Cordiano, R., Di Gioacchino, M., Mangifesta, R., Panzera, C., Gangemi, S., & Minciullo, P. L. (2023). Malondialdehyde as a potential oxidative stress marker for allergy-oriented diseases: An update. *Molecules, 28*(16), 5979. https://doi.org/10.3390/molecules28165979.

Dantas, F. B. H., Alvim, I. D., Miguel, A. M. R.de O., Alves, R. M. V., & Marangoni Júnior, L. (2022). Influence of different packaging materials on the stability of omega-3-enriched milk powder during storage. *Journal of Packaging Technology and Research, 6*(3), 225–233. https://doi.org/10.1007/s41783-022-00143-6.

Das, U. N. (2021). "Cell membrane theory of senescence" and the role of bioactive lipids in aging, and aging associated diseases and their therapeutic implications. *Biomolecules, 11*(2), 241. https://doi.org/10.3390/biom11020241.

Delmas, D., & Aires, V. (2025). Polyunsaturated fatty acids: New molecular mechanisms and nutritional therapeutic challenges. *Nutrients, 17*(3), 588. https://doi.org/10.3390/nu17030588.

Dessì, M. A., Deiana, M., Day, B. W., Rosa, A., Banni, S., & Corongiu, F. P. (2002). Oxidative stability of polyunsaturated fatty acids: Effect of squalene. *European Journal of Lipid Science and Technology, 104*(8), 506–512. https://doi.org/10.1002/1438-9312(200208)104:8<506::AID-EJLT506>3.0.CO;2-1.

Diniz do Nascimento, L., de Moraes, A. A. B., Costa, K. S.da, Pereira Galúcio, J. M., Taube, P. S., Costa, C. M. L., Neves Cruz, J., de Aguiar Andrade, E. H., & de Faria, L. J. G. (2020). Bioactive natural compounds and antioxidant activity of essential oils from spice plants: New findings and potential applications. *Biomolecules, 10*(7), 988. https://doi.org/10.3390/biom10070988.

Djuricic, I., & Calder, P. C. (2021). Beneficial outcomes of omega-6 and omega-3 polyunsaturated fatty acids on human health: An update for 2021. *Nutrients, 13*(7), 2421. https://doi.org/10.3390/nu13072421.

Díaz-Montes, E. (2023). Wall materials for encapsulating bioactive compounds via spray-drying: A review. *Polymers, 15*(12), 2659.

Elgadir, M., & Mariod, A. (2025). Effect of selected food additives on quality of meat and meat products, recent advances. *Agriculture and Food Bioactive Compounds, 2*(4), 76–85. https://doi.org/10.31989/afbc.v2i4.1615.

Fadda, A., Sanna, D., Sakar, E. H., Gharby, S., Mulas, M., Medda, S., Yesilcubuk, N. S., Karaca, A. C., Gozukirmizi, C. K., Lucarini, M., Lombardi-Boccia, G., Diaconeasa, Z., & Durazzo, A. (2022). Innovative and sustainable technologies to enhance the oxidative stability of vegetable oils. *Sustainability, 14*(2), 849. https://doi.org/10.3390/su14020849.

Gallego, M., Gordon, M., Segovia, F., & Almajano, M. (2015). Caesalpinia decapetala extracts as inhibitors of lipid oxidation in beef patties. *Molecules, 20*(8), 13913–13926. https://doi.org/10.3390/molecules200813913.

Gengatharan, A. (2025). Chapter 18 - Degradation of lipids during food processing. In Brijesh K. Tiwari, & Mysore Lokesh Bhavya (Eds.). *Chemistry of thermal and non-thermal food processing technologies* (pp. 429–460). Academic Press. https://doi.org/10.1016/B978-0-443-22182-8.00019-X.

Gharby, S., Hajib, A., Ibourki, M., Sakar, E. H., Nounah, I., Moudden, H. E., Elibrahimi, M., & Harhar, H. (2021). Induced changes in olive oil subjected to various chemical refining steps: A comparative study of quality indices, fatty acids, bioactive minor components, and oxidation stability kinetic parameters. *Chemical Data Collections, 33*. https://doi.org/10.1016/j.cdc.2021.100702, http://www.journals.elsevier.com/chemical-data-collections/.

Ghorchi, A., Arianfar, A., Hakimzadeh, V., & Naji-Tabasi, S. (2025). Nano-encapsulation of red beetroot extract based on betalain using of complex coacervation in gummy candies. *Iranian Food Science and Technology Research Journal, 21*(2), 147–164. https://doi.org/10.22067/ifstrj.2024.88135.1333, https://ifstrj.um.ac.ir/article_46647_405db51938e86f2b5be1a8f078c45b3a.pdf.

Gouvêa, F.de J., de Oliveira, V. S., Mariano, B. J., Takenaka, N. A. R., Gamallo, O. D., da Silva Ferreira, M., & Saldanha, T. (2023). Natural antioxidants as strategy to minimize the presence of lipid oxidation products in canned fish: Research progress, current trends and future perspectives. *Food Research International, 173*(November), 113314. https://doi.org/10.1016/j.foodres.2023.113314.

Gruber, F., Marchetti-Deschmann, M., Kremslehner, C., & Schosserer, M. (2021). The skin epilipidome in stress, aging, and inflammation. *Frontiers in Endocrinology, 11*. https://doi.org/10.3389/fendo.2020.607076.

Habib, M., Jan, K., & Bashir, K. (2022). Fortification of bioactive components for the development of functional foods. In *Bioactive components: A sustainable system for good health and well-being*. Singapore: Springer Nature Singapore, 381–401.

Horbańczuk, O., Kurek, M., Atanasov, A., Brncic, M., Rimac, S., & Brncic (2019). The effect of natural antioxidants on quality and shelflife of beef and beef products. *Food Technology and Biotechnology, 57*(4), 439–447.

Horn, A. F., Nielsen, N. S., & Jacobsen, C. (2009). Additions of caffeic acid, ascorbyl palmitate or γ-tocopherol to fish oil-enriched energy bars affect lipid oxidation differently. *Food Chemistry, 112*(2), 412–420. https://doi.org/10.1016/j.foodchem.2008.05.094.

Huber, G. M., Vasantha Rupasinghe, H. P., & Shahidi, F. (2009). Inhibition of oxidation of omega-3 polyunsaturated fatty acids and fish oil by quercetin glycosides. *Food Chemistry, 117*(2), 290–295. https://doi.org/10.1016/j.foodchem.2009.04.007.

Islam, F., Imran, A., Nosheen, F., Fatima, M., Arshad, M. U., Afzaal, M., Ijaz, N., et al. (2023). Functional roles and novel tools for improving-oxidative stability of polyunsaturated fatty acids: A comprehensive review. *Food Science & Nutrition, 11*(6), 2471–2482. https://doi.org/10.1002/fsn3.3272.

Islam, M., Mahmud, N., Nawas, T., Yang, F., & Xia, W. (2018). Health benefits and spray drying microencapsulation process of fish oil (omega-3).

Juan, C. A., Pérez de la Lastra, J. M., Plou, F. J., & Pérez-Lebeña, E. (2021). The chemistry of reactive oxygen species (ROS) revisited: Outlining their role in biological macromolecules (DNA, lipids and proteins) and induced pathologies. *International Journal of Molecular Sciences, 22*(9), 4642. https://doi.org/10.3390/ijms22094642.

Jurić, S., Jurić, M., Siddique, M. A. B., & Fathi, M. (2022). Vegetable oils rich in polyunsaturated fatty acids: Nanoencapsulation methods and stability enhancement. *Food Reviews International, 38*(1), 32–69. https://doi.org/10.1080/87559129.2020.1717524.

Kannan, N., Rao, A. S., & Nair, A. (2021). Microbial production of omega-3 fatty acids: An overview. *Journal of Applied Microbiology, 131*(5), 2114–2130. https://doi.org/10.1111/jam.15034.

Kaushani, K. G., Rathnasinghe, N. L., Katuwawila, N., Jayasinghe, R. A., Nilmini, A. H. L. R., & Priyadarshana, G. (2022). Trends in smart packaging technologies for sustainable monitoring of food quality and safety. *International Journal of Research and Innovation in Applied Science, 07*(07), 07–30. https://doi.org/10.51584/ijrias.2022.7702.

Kocetkovs, V., Radenkovs, V., Juhnevica-Radenkova, K., & Muizniece-Brasava, S. (2022). Variation in the fatty acid and amino acid profiles of pasteurized liquid whole hen egg products stored in four types of packaging. *Animals (Basel), 12*(21), 2990. https://doi.org/10.3390/ani12212990.

Kus-Yamashita, M. M. M., Mcdonald, B., Ravacci, G., Rogero, M. M., Santos, R. D., Waitzberg, D., & Lajolo, F. M. (2016). Polyunsaturated fatty acids: Health impacts. European Journal of Nutrition and Food Safety, *6*(3), 111–131.

Kykkidou, S., Giatrakou, V., Papavergou, A., Kontominas, M. G., & Savvaidis, I. N. (2009). Effect of thyme essential oil and packaging treatments on fresh Mediterranean swordfish fillets during storage at 4°C. *Food Chemistry, 115*(1), 169–175. https://doi.org/10.1016/j.foodchem.2008.11.083.

Legako, J., & Dunford, N. T. (2010a). Effect of spray nozzle design on fish oil–whey protein microcapsule properties. *Journal of Food Science, 75*(6), E394–E400.

Legako, J., & Dunford, N. T. (2010b). Effect of spray nozzle design on fish oil-whey protein microcapsule properties. *Journal of Food Science, 75*(6), E394. https://doi.org/10.1111/j.1750-3841.2010.01708.x.

Li, H., Chen, Y., Peng, Q., Tan, X., Chen, G., Zhou, H., & Yan, R. (2022). Flavonoids from bamboo leaves improve the stability of unsaturated fatty acids in the lipids of walnut emulsions. *Industrial Crops and Products, 178*, 114609. https://doi.org/10.1016/j.indcrop.2022.114609.

Liu, C., Ge, S., Yang, J., Xu, Y., Zhao, M., Xiong, L., & Sun, Q. (2016). Adsorption mechanism of polyphenols onto starch nanoparticles and enhanced antioxidant activity under adverse conditions. *Journal of Functional Foods, 26*, 632–644.

Liu, S., Zhu, Y., Liu, N., Fan, D., Wang, M., & Zhao, Y. (2021). Antioxidative properties and chemical changes of quercetin in fish oil: Quercetin reacts with free fatty acids to form its ester derivatives. *Journal of Agricultural and Food Chemistry, 69*(3), 1057–1067.

Lopes, C. R. B., & Courrol, L. C. (2023). Evaluation of steady-state and time-resolved fluorescence spectroscopy as a method for assessing the impact of photo-oxidation on refined soybean oils. *Foods, 12*(9), 1862. https://doi.org/10.3390/foods12091862.

Luzi, F., Torre, L., Kenny, J. M., & Puglia, D. (2019). Bio-and fossil-based polymeric blends and nanocomposites for packaging: Structure–property relationship. *Materials, 12*(3), 471.

MacArthur, E., Waughray, D., & Stuchtey, M. (2016). Rethinking Plastics, starting with packaging. In Cologny World Economic Forum (pp. 1-206).

Machado, M., Rodriguez-Alcalá, L. M., Gomes, A. M., & Pintado, M. (2023). Vegetable oils oxidation: Mechanisms, consequences and protective strategies. *Food Reviews International, 39*(7), 4180–4197. https://doi.org/10.1080/87559129.2022.2026378.

Melgosa, R., Benito-Román, Ó., Sanz, M. T., de Paz, E., & Beltrán, S. (2019). Omega–3 Encapsulation by PGSS-drying and conventional drying methods. Particle characterization and oxidative stability. *Food Chemistry, 270*(January), 138–148. https://doi.org/10.1016/j.foodchem.2018.07.082.

Mendes, A. C., & Pedersen, G. A. (2021). Perspectives on sustainable food packaging:– Is bio-based plastics a solution? *Trends in Food Science and Technology, 112*, 839–846. https://doi.org/10.1016/j.tifs.2021.03.049, http://www.elsevier.com/wps/find/journaldescription.cws_home/601278/description#description.

Méndez, L., Sacchi, R., Medina, I., & Aubourg, S. P. (2022). Nutritional and preservative properties of polyphenol-rich olive oil: Effect on seafood processing and storage. In C. Bravo-Diaz (Ed.). *Lipid oxidation in food and biological systems: A physical chemistry perspective* (pp. 455–477). Cham: Springer International Publishing. https://doi.org/10.1007/978-3-030-87222-9_20.

Menon, V., & Rao, M. (2012). Trends in bioconversion of lignocellulose: Biofuels, platform chemicals & biorefinery concept. *Progress in Energy and Combustion Science, 38*(4), 522–550. https://doi.org/10.1016/j.pecs.2012.02.002.

Mitropoulou, G., Stavropoulou, E., Vaou, N., Tsakris, Z., Voidarou, C., Tsiotsias, A., Tsigalou, C., Taban, B. M., Kourkoutas, Y., & Bezirtzoglou, E. (2023). Insights into antimicrobial and anti-inflammatory applications of plant bioactive compounds. *Microorganisms, 11*(5), 1156. https://doi.org/10.3390/microorganisms11051156.

Mohammadi, M., Hosseini, H., Shahraz, F., Hosseini, S. M., Alizadeh, A. M., Taghizadeh, M., Mohammadi, A., & Shojaee-Aliabadi, S. (2023). Effect of sage seed gum film incorporating Zataria multiflora Boiss essential oil on the storage quality and biogenic amine content of refrigerated Otolithes ruber fillets. *International Journal of Biological Macromolecules, 238*, 123711. https://doi.org/10.1016/j.ijbiomac.2023.123711.

Mora, I., Arola, L., Caimari, A., Escoté, X., & Puiggròs, F. (2022). Structured long-chain omega-3 fatty acids for improvement of cognitive function during aging. *International Journal of Molecular Sciences, 23*(7), 3472. https://doi.org/10.3390/ijms23073472.

Musakhanian, J., Rodier, J.-D., & Dave, M. (2022). Oxidative stability in lipid formulations: A review of the mechanisms, drivers, and inhibitors of oxidation. *AAPS PharmSciTech, 23*(5), 151. https://doi.org/10.1208/s12249-022-02282-0.

Nagarajarao, R. C. (2016). Recent advances in processing and packaging of fishery products: A review. Aquatic Procedia, 2nd international symposium on aquatic products processing and health, ISAPPROSH 2015, 7(August), 201–213. https://doi.org/10.1016/j.aqpro.2016.07.028.

Nilsuwan, K., Guerrero, P., Caba, K.de la, Benjakul, S., & Prodpran, T. (2021). Fish gelatin films laminated with emulsified gelatin film or poly(lactic) acid film: Properties and their use as bags for storage of fried salmon skin. *Food Hydrocolloids, 111*, 106199. https://doi.org/10.1016/j.foodhyd.2020.106199.

Pal, M., Devrani, M., & Hadush, A. (2019). Recent developments in food packaging technologies. *Beverage Food World, 46*(1), 21–25.

Palacios, D., Busto, M. D., Albillos, S. M., & Ortega, N. (2022). Synthesis and oxidative stability of monoacylglycerols containing polyunsaturated fatty acids by enzymatic glycerolysis in a solvent-free system. *LWT, 154*. https://doi.org/10.1016/j.lwt.2021.112600, https://www.journals.elsevier.com/lwt.

Pan, D., Gong, X., Wang, X., & Li, M. (2021). Role of active components of medicinal food in the regulation of angiogenesis. *Frontiers in Pharmacology, 11*. https://doi.org/10.3389/fphar.2020.594050.

Parcheta, M., Świsłocka, R., Orzechowska, S., Akimowicz, M., Choińska, R., & Lewandowski, W. (2021). Recent developments in effective antioxidants: The structure and antioxidant properties. *Materials, 14*(8), 1984. https://doi.org/10.3390/ma14081984.

Pathak, J., Rajneesh, Ahmed, H., Singh, D. K., Singh, P. R., Kumar, D., Kannaujiya, V. K., Singh, S. P., & Sinha, R. P. (2019). Oxidative stress and antioxidant defense in plants exposed to ultraviolet radiation. In *Reactive oxygen, nitrogen and sulfur species in plants*. John Wiley & Sons, Ltd, 371–420. https://doi.org/10.1002/9781119468677.ch16.

Pattnaik, M., & Mishra, H. N. (2022). Amelioration of the stability of polyunsaturated fatty acids and bioactive enriched vegetable oil: Blending, encapsulation, and its application. *Critical Reviews in Food Science and Nutrition, 62*(23), 6253–6276. https://doi.org/10.1080/10408398.2021.1899127, https://www.tandfonline.com/loi/bfsn20.

Pérez-Córdoba, L. J., Pinheiro, A. C., de Núñez de Villavicencio-Ferrer, M., Trindade, M. A., & Sobral, P. J. A. (2022). Applying gelatine:chitosan film loaded with nanoemulsified garlic essential oil/α-tocopherol as active packaging of sliced Omega-3-rich mortadella. *International Journal of Food Science and Technology, 57*(10), 6378–6388. https://doi.org/10.1111/ijfs.15938, http://onlinelibrary.wiley.com/journal/10.1111/(ISSN)1365-2621.

Peter, M. J., Lalithapriya, U., Venkatachalapathy, R., & Sukumar, M. (2022). Characterization of an effective drug carrier system for improved oxidative and thermal stability of essential fatty acids: A review. *International Journal of Food Properties, 25*(1), 1753–1772.

Poljsak, B., Kovač, V., & Milisav, I. (2021). Antioxidants, food processing and health. *Antioxidants, 10*(3), 433. https://doi.org/10.3390/antiox10030433.

Pozo-Martínez, J., Vázquez-Rodríguez, S., Olea-Azar, C., & Moncada-Basualto, M. (2022). Evaluation of ORAC methodologies in determination of antioxidant capacity of binary combinations of quercetin and 3-(3,4,5-trihydroxybenzoyl) coumarin derivatives. *Arabian Journal of Chemistry, 15*(11), 104298. https://doi.org/10.1016/j.arabjc.2022.104298.

Raole, V. M., & Raole, V. V. (2022). Flaxseed and seed oil: Functional food and dietary support for health. *EAS Journal of Nutrition and Food Sciences, 4*(2), 68–77. https://doi.org/10.36349/easjnfs.2022.v04i02.007.

Reyes-Padilla, E., Valenzuela-Melendres, M., Camou, J. P., Sebranek, J. G., Alemán-Mateo, H., Dávila-Ramírez, J. L., Cumplido-Barbeitia, G., & González-Ríos, H. (2018). Quality evaluation of low fat bologna-type meat product with a nutritional profile designed for the elderly. *Meat Science, 135*, 115–122. https://doi.org/10.1016/j.meatsci.2017.09.007, http://www.elsevier.com/locate/meatsci.

Rodríguez Cortina, A. (2022). Sacha Inchi seed oil encapsulation as a strategy for the development of new functional foods.

Romero, J., Cruz, R. M. S., Díez-Méndez, A., & Albertos, I. (2022). Valorization of berries' agro-industrial waste in the development of biodegradable pectin-based films for fresh salmon (*Salmo salar*) shelf-life monitoring. *International Journal of Molecular Sciences, 23*(16), 8970. https://doi.org/10.3390/ijms23168970.

Rupasinghe, H. V., Erkan, N., & Yasmin, A. (2010). Antioxidant protection of eicosapentaenoic acid and fish oil oxidation by polyphenolic-enriched apple skin extract. *Journal of Agricultural and Food Chemistry, 58*(2), 1233–1239.

Saini, R. K., Prasad, P., Sreedhar, R. V., Akhilender Naidu, K., Shang, X., & Keum, Y. S. (2021). Omega- 3 polyunsaturated fatty acids (PUFAs): Emerging plant and microbial sources, oxidative stability, bioavailability, and health benefits—A review. *Antioxidants, 10*(10), 1627.

Sakr, E. A. E., Massoud, M. I., & Ragaee, S. (2021). Food wastes as natural sources of lactic acid bacterial exopolysaccharides for the functional food industry: A review. *International Journal of Biological Macromolecules, 189*, 232–241. https://doi.org/10.1016/j.ijbiomac.2021.08.135, www.elsevier.com/locate/ijbiomac.

Samtiya, M., Aluko, R. E., Dhewa, T., & Moreno-Rojas, J. M. (2021). Potential health benefits of plant food-derived bioactive components: An overview. *Foods, 10*(4). https://doi.org/10.3390/foods10040839, https://www.mdpi.com/2304-8158/10/4/839/pdf.

Serfert, Y., Drusch, S., & Schwarz, K. (2009). Chemical stabilisation of oils rich in long-chain polyunsaturated fatty acids during homogenisation, microencapsulation and storage. *Food Chemistry, 113*(4), 1106–1112. https://doi.org/10.1016/j.foodchem.2008.08.079.

Tao, L. (2015). Oxidation of polyunsaturated fatty acids and its impact on food quality and human health. *Advances in Food Technology and Nutritional Sciences - Open Journal, 1*(6), 135–142. https://doi.org/10.17140/AFTNSOJ-1-123.

Ucak, I., Khalily, R., Carrillo, C., Tomasevic, I., & Barba, F. J. (2020). Potential of propolis extract as a natural antioxidant and antimicrobial in gelatin films applied to rainbow trout (*Oncorhynchus mykiss*) fillets. *Foods, 9*(11), 1584. https://doi.org/10.3390/foods9111584.

Uzombah, T. A. (2022). The implications of replacing synthetic antioxidants with natural ones in the food systems. In *Natural food additives*. IntechOpen.

Vähä-Nissi, M., Koivula, H. M., Räisänen, H. M., Vartiainen, J., Ragni, P., Kenttä, E., & Harlin, A. (2017). Cellulose nanofibrils in biobased multilayer films for food packaging. *Journal of Applied Polymer Science, 134*(19).

Wang, K. L., Yu, B. K., Zhao, H. F., Liu, Y. X., Wu, C. Y., Zhang, Y. H., & Mu, Z. S. (2025). Preparation and characterization of microcapsules for tuna oil by maillard reaction products of whey protein isolate and Arabic gum via complex coacervation. *Food Chemistry, 475*. https://doi.org/10.1016/j.foodchem.2025.143269, https://www.sciencedirect.com/science/journal/03088146.

Yan, Q., Wang, L., Sun, X., Fan, F., Ding, J., Li, P., Zhu, Y., Xu, T., & Fang, Y. (2022). Improvement in the storage quality of fresh salmon (*Salmo salar*) using a powerful composite film of rice protein hydrolysates and chitosan. *Food Control, 142*, 109211. https://doi.org/10.1016/j.foodcont.2022.109211.

Yenipazar, H., & Şahin-Yeşilçubuk, N. (2023). Effect of packaging and encapsulation on the oxidative and sensory stability of omega-3 supplements. *Food Science & Nutrition, 11*(3), 1426–1440. https://doi.org/10.1002/fsn3.3182.

Yesudhason, P., Gopal, T. K. S., Ravishankar, C. N., Lalitha, K. V., & Kumar, A. (2010). Effect of potassium sorbate and modified atmosphere packaging on the shelf-life extension of seer fish (Scomberomorus Commerson) steaks during iced storage. *Journal of Food Biochemistry, 34*(2), 399–424. https://doi.org/10.1111/j.1745-4514.2009.00288.x.

Zeeb, B., McClements, D. J., & Weiss, J. (2017). Enzyme-based strategies for structuring foods for improved functionality. *Annual Review of Food Science and Technology, 8*, 21–34. https://doi.org/10.1146/annurev-food-030216-025753, http://www.annualreviews.org/journal/food.

Zhang, J., Freund, M. A., Culler, M. D., Yang, R., Chen, P. B., Park, Y., & Zhang, G. (2020). How to stabilize ω-3 polyunsaturated fatty acids (PUFAs) in an animal feeding study?—effects of the temperature, oxygen level, and antioxidant on oxidative stability of ω-3 PUFAs in a mouse diet. *Journal of Agricultural and Food Chemistry, 68*(46), 13146–13153.

Zhang, W., Sun, J., Li, Q., Liu, C., Niu, F., Yue, R., & Deng, S. (2023). Free radical-mediated grafting of natural polysaccharides such as chitosan, starch, inulin, and pectin with some polyphenols: Synthesis, structural characterization, bioactivities, and applications—A review. *Foods, 12*(19), 3688.

Chapter 20

Quality control measures for ensuring polyunsaturated fatty acid product integrity

Tendai Abgirl Makore, Brighton Marimanzi Mvumi, and Tonderayi Mathew Matsungo
University of Zimbabwe, Harare, Zimbabwe

20.1 Introduction

20.1.1 Background and importance of polyunsaturated fatty acid

Omega-3 and omega-6 are integral components of polyunsaturated fatty acids (PUFAs) that are essential nutrients with well-established roles in supporting cardiovascular, neurological, and metabolic health (Petersen et al., 2024; Saini et al., 2021; Venugopalan et al., 2021). The human body cannot produce the essential fatty acids, therefore it must be acquired from dietary sources, making their inclusion in functional foods a public health priority (Tocher et al., 2019). Food systems have responded by fortifying a diversity of products such as milk based alternatives, baked goods, beverages, and infant formulas with PUFAs to enhance their nutritional profile. Eicosapentaenoic acid (EPA) and docosahexaenoic acid (DHA) are specifically recognized omega-3s, that are involved in reducing blood triglycerides, regulating heart rhythm, and supporting cognitive functions (Ristic-Medic et al., 2013; Wani et al., 2023). Ensuring the quality, potency, and safety of PUFAs in functional foods through robust quality control (QC) is essential for maximizing health benefits and maintaining consumer confidence.

20.1.2 Challenges in maintaining polyunsaturated fatty acid integrity in post harvest handling and storage

The incorporation of PUFAs into food products poses various complexities owing to their inherent tendency toward oxidation, isomerization, and polymerization during processing and storage of these products. Various exposures of PUFAs to heat, photochemical, oxidative, and trace metals may trigger lipid peroxidation, resulting in the development of unacceptable compounds that affect product quality in terms of taste, safety, and nutritional value (Geng et al., 2023; Ma et al., 2019; Repetto et al., 2012). Additionally, as integral components of the structural composition of a phospholipid bilayers, PUFAs endow food emulsions and delivery matrices with functional integrity (Islam, Imran, et al., 2023). Consequently, the chemical and functional stability of PUFAs, which is essential for the maintenance of quality in these characteristics, requires the use of sophisticated instrumental techniques and specific formulation techniques at all stages of food processing and packaging. Such control is especially important in functional foods, where chemical degradation of PUFAs can affect efficacy and also trigger regulatory issues.

20.1.3 Scope and rationale of the chapter

The current chapter offers a critical analysis of QC interventions helpful in the maintenance of stability and functionality in the context of PUFAs in food-based delivery systems. Within the context of functional food product development and formulation, the current chapter seeks to address issues related to the use of state-of-the-art technology in the determination of PUFAs, encapsulation techniques and strategies, processing techniques and strategies, and packaging technologies in the mitigation of oxidative stability in the context of PUFAs. The chapter provides a practical interface

Omega-3 and Omega-6 Polyunsaturated Fatty Acids in Food Systems. DOI: https://doi.org/10.1016/B978-0-443-43810-3.00021-X

between the biochemistry of PUFAs and food processing technology. The overall goal is to contribute to the overarching goal of improving the safety and bioavailability of PUFAs in functional food systems.

20.2 Literature review

20.2.1 Current market dynamics of polyunsaturated fatty acid products

The market for PUFAs has witnessed significant growth in recent times due to the awareness among consumers regarding the potential impact of the products on their health. The market for packaged foods containing n-3 PUFAs, such as infant formula, was valued at $34.7 billion in 2016. The market is expected to grow at a compound annual growth rate of 9.1% from 2016 to 2030. This is a result of the growing interest among consumers to take active steps to maintain their health (Essential Oils Market Size & Share I Industry Report, 2030 [Internet], n.d.; Kolanowski, 2010a; Petersen et al., 2024; Saini et al., 2021). The availability of PUFA products in various forms, such as fish oil capsules, algal-based supplements, and omega-3 PUFA-fortified food products, caters for various consumer requirements and dietary preferences. Major market participants, including Koninklijke DSM N.V. (Royal DSM), BASF, and Aker BioMarine, are engaged in research and development efforts aimed at improving the efficacy, bioavailability, and sustainability of PUFA ingredients (Insights for Polyunsaturated fatty acids supplement ingredients, n.d.; Bhat et al., 2024; Tańska et al., 2016; Tulimaa, 2022). The market's rapidly changing dynamics highlight how important it is to ensure the products' quality and purity in order to maintain consumer trust and deliver the desired health benefits (Tańska et al., 2016; Tulimaa, 2022). The large size of the market, coupled with ongoing growth, underscores the extensive consumer base that depends on the quality of PUFA products for healthy living. This high demand highlights how crucial it is to have strict QC procedures in place to guarantee customer trust and product efficacy.

20.2.2 Lipid oxidation mechanism

Oxidation of lipids is a significant factor contributing to food spoilage. It is the slow oxidation of unsaturated fatty acids present in fats upon exposure to atmospheric oxygen, ultraviolet (UV), and pro-oxidant metal ions (Ghelichi et al., 2023). Auto-oxidation, photo-oxidation, and enzymatic oxidation are all forms of lipid oxidation (Geng et al., 2023; Ma et al., 2019; Repetto et al., 2012). Among these, auto-oxidation is a chain reaction of free radicals that is started when oxygen and unsaturated fatty acids interact (Repetto et al., 2012) (Fig. 20.1). When oil molecules are exposed to heat, light, or transition metal catalysts during initiation, free radicals are created. Following this, radicals undergo propagation, in which they react to create more radicals, and termination, in which they unite to create stable, nonradical products, which puts an end to the chain reaction.

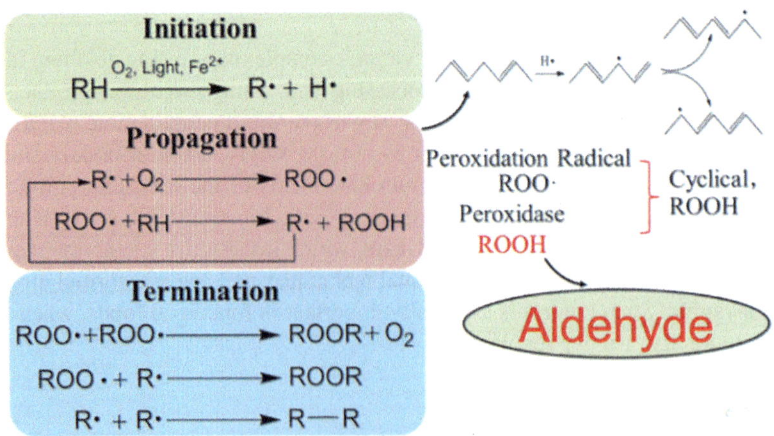

FIGURE 20.1 Mechanism of lipid oxidation from initiation to termination.
Adapted from Geng, L., Liu, K., & Zhang, H. (2023). Lipid oxidation in foods and its implications on proteins. Frontiers Nutrition, 10, 1192199. https://doi.org/10.3389/fnut.2023.1192199.

Rancidity occurs when lipid auto-oxidation reaches a specific threshold. Further, it can be responsible for producing aromatic molecules due to a large number of carbonyls, which play a significant role in determining food products rich in (PUFAs) (Ayala et al., 2014; Islam, Imran, et al., 2023; Repetto et al., 2012).

Hydroperoxides represent the primary products resulting from the auto-oxidation of lipids, with the oxidation of various fatty acids potentially yielding multiple hydroperoxides (Ayala et al., 2014). The generation of hydroperoxides occurs due to the influence of free radicals, specifically through the abstraction of a hydrogen atom from the α-methylene group linked to the double

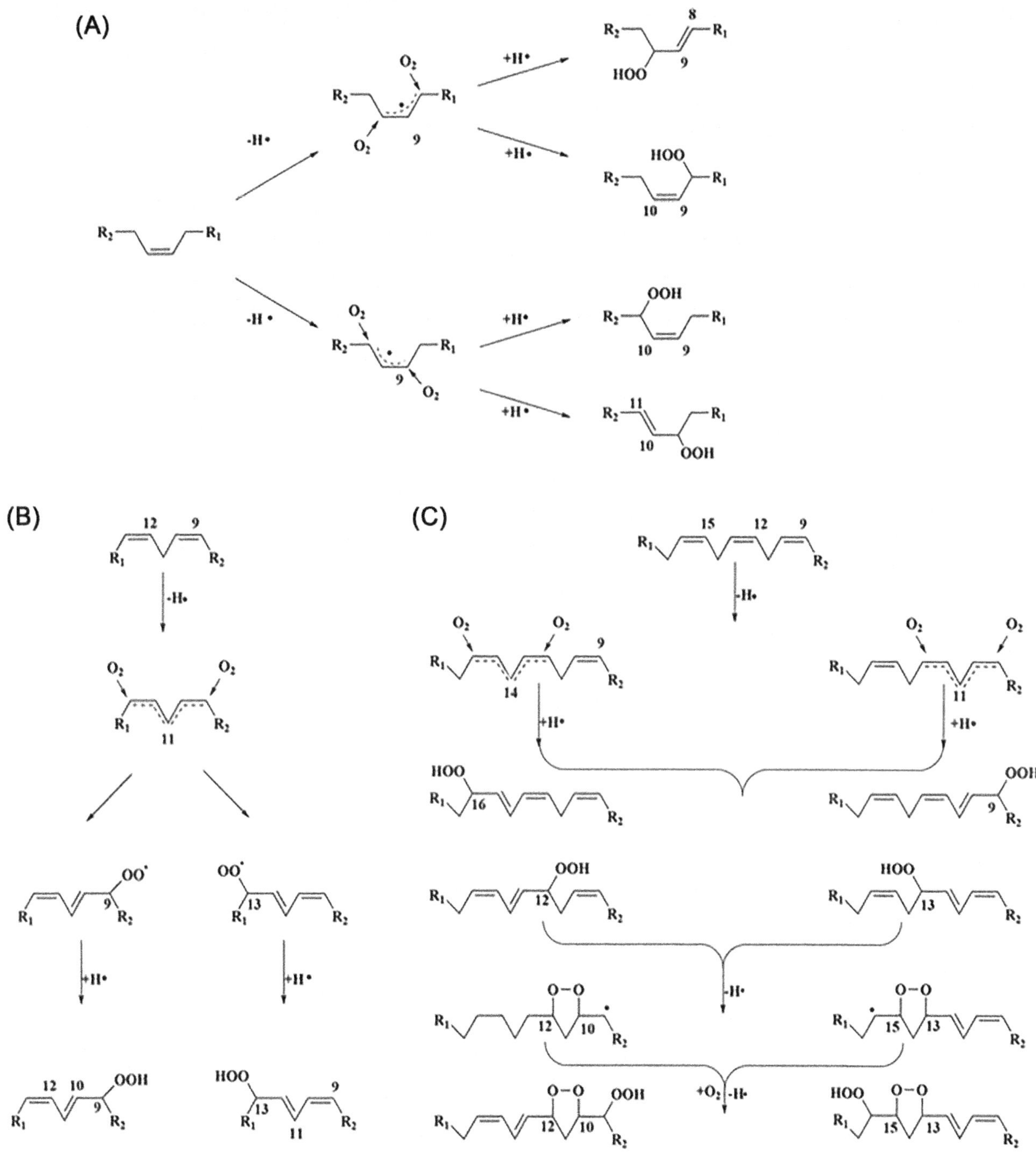

FIGURE 20.2 Classic mechanism for auto-oxidation: (A) Oleic acid; (B) Linoleic acid; and (C) α-Linoleic acid.
Adapted from Geng, L., Liu, K., & Zhang, H. (2023). Lipid oxidation in foods and its implications on proteins. Frontiers Nutrition, 10, 1192199. https://doi.org/10.3389/fnut.2023.1192199.

bond present in lipids. This process subsequently results in the creation of allyl radicals (Ayala et al., 2014; Mostafa Abd El-Aal, 2012; Resende et al., 2021). Allyl radicals possess electrons that are capable of delocalizing across three carbon atoms, as demonstrated in the case of oleic acid, or across five carbon atoms, as observed in linoleic acid (Fig. 20.2).

The departure of hydrogen from C8 and C11 penta-dienyl may lead to the structuring of two allylic radicals (Repetto et al., 2012). Furthermore, reactivity of intermediates with oxygen could result in the production of 8-, 9-, 10-, and 11-allyl hydroperoxides (Mendonça et al., 2017; Repetto et al., 2012). The auto-oxidation of linoleic acid entails a doubly reactive process, during which penta-dienyl radicals may be produced by the allyl groups of C11 (Kolanowski, 2010a; Saini et al., 2021; Tao, Department of Animal Science, Cornell University, Ithaca, NY, USA, 2015). The hydroperoxides of conjugated 9- and 13-dienes may be generated through the interaction of intermediates with oxygen.

Linolenic acid has the potential to produce two penta-dienyl radicals by the abstraction of hydrogen from the methylene groups located at C11 and C14 (Domijan et al., 2015; Geng et al., 2023; Kolanowski, 2010a; Repetto et al., 2012). Furthermore, unsaturated fatty acids interact with singlet oxygen, potentially leading to an increase in the number of double bonds and resulting in instability within the food system (Ayala et al., 2014; Benatti et al., 2004). The breakdown products of hydroperoxides are influenced by factors such as temperature, pressure, and the concentration of oxygen. The cleavage of hydroperoxides can lead to the formation of a range of volatile aromas and nonvolatile compounds. Certain degradation products consistently impact the aroma and odor of meat products that are either cooked or stored (Geng et al., 2023). The degradation of hydroperoxide may lead to the formation of alkoxy and hydroxyl radicals as a result of the homogeneous cleavage of OOH.

The alkoxy radicals undergo cleavage at the C-C bond, resulting in the production of aldehydes and vinyl radicals, or alternatively, unsaturated aldehydes and alkyl radicals. This process subsequently yields volatile organic compounds, including aldehydes, alkenes, and alcohols (Fig. 20.3).

Among the compounds produced through the cleavage of alkoxy radicals, aldehydes represent the crucial aroma substances (Pizzimenti et al., 2013; Repetto et al., 2012). The outcomes of the cleavage reaction are influenced by the stability of fatty acids present in food and the degradation products resulting from hydroperoxide isomers.

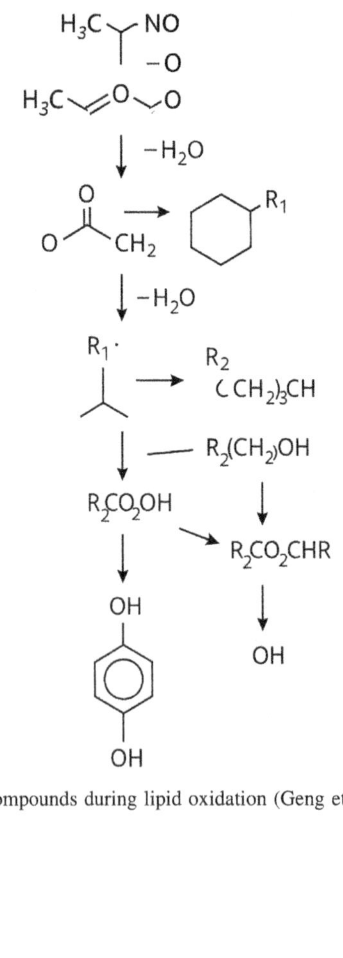

FIGURE 20.3 Mechanism of formation of aroma compounds during lipid oxidation (Geng et al., 2023).

20.2.3 Quality control analytical methods to detect lipid oxidation

Lipid oxidation is crucial for the stability and quality of functional foods rich in (PUFAs) (Robert, n.d.). Given that foods with high PUFA content are particularly susceptible to oxidative degradation, it is essential to employ sensitive analytical techniques to identify early-stage and advanced oxidation byproducts, including, hydroperoxides to aldehydes (Ayala et al., 2014; Bhat et al., 2024; Islam, Imran, et al., 2023; Kolanowski, 2010a; Repetto et al., 2012; Rudy et al., 2016). Common analytical techniques include spectrophotometric assays, chromatographic methods, and spectroscopic tools for accurate monitoring and QC (Table 20.1).

20.2.3.1 Chemical methods

The assessment of oxidative stability has great significance for ensuring the functional integrity of foods that are polyunsaturated with fatty acids (PUFAs). Chemical indices of oxidation enable a rapid quantification of the initial and subsequent oxidation-derived compounds of lipids for effective QC of functional foods. Table 20.2 illustrates the most significant chemical techniques for the assessment of PUFAs that have applications in functional foods, indicating sensitivity, applicability, and significance.

20.2.3.2 Instrumental methods

Sophisticated analytical techniques, including spectrophotometric analyses, chromatographic analyses, and spectroscopy, are being more widely used for the selective, sensitive, and comprehensive analysis of the oxidation level of PUFA in functional foods (Table 20.3). This has significantly helped in carrying out the quality analysis in functional food systems.

20.2.3.3 Sensory evaluation in polyunsaturated fatty acid product for product integrity

Organoleptic assessment, by trained descriptive panels (with intensity scales) and untrained panels (tested hedonic and just about right scales using descriptive statistics), provides valuable information on perceived quality of oxidized PUFA-enriched foods (Cheseto et al., 2020; Ghelichi et al., 2023; Kolanowski, 2010a). Untrained panels provide a direct measure of consumer acceptability, while trained panels provide quantitative, detailed profiles of each off-flavor. These sensory perceptions are the human response to a complex mixture of volatile molecules developed during lipid oxidation (Adámek et al., 2018; Cheseto et al., 2020; Murage et al., 2021).

In order to establish the chemical basis of these sensory attributes, instrumental methods such as gas chromatography-mass spectrometry (GC-MS) and bioassays for primary and secondary oxidation products are employed to give quantitative data on individual volatiles and total oxidation levels. Descriptive statistics are required to summarize these chemical measurements (Adámek et al., 2018). Principal Component Analysis (PCA) is a handy way for decreasing the dimensionality of sensory and chemical datasets in such a way that it becomes easier to visualize correlations between the presence of specific volatile compounds and certain sensory descriptors. For instance, a PCA biplot may reveal how increased concentrations of some aldehydes are associated with increased "rancid" or "fishy" scores by the trained panel (Murage et al., 2021).

Furthermore, analysis of variance (ANOVA) is crucial for ascertaining if there are statistically significant differences in sensory qualities (as assessed by expert panels) and in chemical markers among various treatment categories (e.g.,

TABLE 20.1 Oxidation substrates, initiators, catalysts, intermediaries, and byproducts (Ayala et al., 2014; Domínguez et al., 2019; Ghelichi et al., 2023; Robert, n.d.).

Substrates	Intiators, catalysts	Primary byproducts	Intermediaries	Secondary species
Oxyethylene bond RH	Light	Hydroperoxide ROOH	Alkoxyl radical RO*	Water
Allylic bonds	Triplet oxygen	Peroxide ROOR	Hydroxyl radical HO*	Small organic acids, carbonyl compounds (ketones, aldehydes) Volatiles
Antioxidant AH	Transition metal Antioxidant radical	Free radical R. Transition metal	Peroxyl radical ROO. Hydroperoxide ROOH	

TABLE 20.2 Analytical chemical methods for polyunsaturated fatty acid oxidation analysis.

Method	Principle	Sample preparation	Valuation stage	Oxidation stage detected	Representative compounds	Cost impact	Permissible levels	Detection sensitivity	References
Peroxide value	Iodometric titration quantifies hydroperoxides by reacting with iodide under acidic conditions.	Lipid extracted, treated with KI in acetic acid, and titrated with $Na_2S_2O_3$.	Processing, early storage, and packaging QC.	Primary oxidation	Lipid hydroperoxides (e.g., 13-HPODE, 9-HPODE)	Low; inexpensive reagents and equipment (routine lab use).	≤5 meq/kg (ISO 3960:2017)	Moderate (≥1 meq/kg)	Saini et al. (2021), Kolanowski (2010b), Tulimaa (2022), Quality Control Management of Nutraceuticals and Dietary Supplements [Internet] (n.d)
p-Anisidine value	Aromatic aldehydes react with p-anisidine to form chromophores measured at 350 nm.	Fat dissolved in iso-octane reacted with p-anisidine.	Shelf life testing, oxidative degra-dation.	Secondary oxidation	2-alkenals (e.g., 2-octenal), 2,4-dienals	Low to moderate; requires specific reagents but is still cost-effective for routine tests.	≤20 (ISO 6885:2016)	Moderate (~1 μmol/g)	Islam, Kaczmarek, et al. (2023), Pizzimenti et al. (2013), Nielsen (2010), Hocquette et al. (2005)
Thiobarbituric acid reactive substances	MDA reacts with thiobarbituric acid to form a pink chromogen at 532 nm.	Homogenization in TCA, heating with TBA, and centrifugation.	Late-stage rancidity assessment.	Secondary to terminal oxidation	Malondialdehyde (MDA), lipid aldehydes	Low; standard lab equipment, relatively low-cost reagents.	≤1.0 mg MDA/kg	High (0.1 μmol/kg)	Geng et al. (2023), Repetto et al. (2012)

TABLE 20.3 Instrumental methods for polyunsaturated fatty acid (PUFA) oxidation analysis.

Method	Principle	Sample preparation	Application stage	Oxidation stage detected	Representative compounds	Cost impact	Permissible levels	Sensitivity	References
Gas chromatography (GC-FID/MS)	FAMEs are separated and quantified via volatility and retention times using FID or MS.	Transesterification of extracted lipids into FAMEs.	Raw materials, formulation, baseline profiling.	Full spectrum	EPA, DHA, LA, ALA, AA (as FAMEs), hexanal, nonanal, pentanal, volatile alcohols	High GC system is expensive, and MS or FID detectors further increase costs.	<1% degradation for PUFA-rich oils	Very high (ppb–ppm)	Benatti et al. (2004), Nielsen (2010)
Fourier transform infrared spectroscopy (FTIR)	Detects vibrational changes due to new functional groups (carbonyls, hydroxyls).	Minimal prep (direct film or ATR analysis).	Real-time QC, in-line oxidation monitoring.	Primary and secondary oxidation	C=O (~1740/cm), OH, CH deformation	Moderate; FTIR equipment is costly but requires minimal sample preparation.	ΔAbs > 0.05 AU indicates oxidation	High	Repetto et al. (2012), Islam, Imran, et al. (2023), van de Voort et al. (1994)
Differential scanning calorimetry (DSC)	Measures thermal transitions affected by structural oxidation (melting, enthalpy loss).	Lipid samples were sealed in aluminum pans.	Processing, encapsulation stability.	Structural impact of oxidation	Crystalline loss, oxidized triacylglycerols	Moderate to high; DSC equipment is specialized, though reusable for various analyses.	ΔH loss >2%–5% signals oxidation	Moderate	Belayneh et al. (2017), Giuffrida et al. (2007), Islam, Kaczmarek et al. (2023)
High-performance liquid chromatography (HPLC)	Separates and quantifies polar oxidized lipids and antioxidants.	Filtration: mobile phases based on polarity.	Antioxidant evaluation, degradation kinetics.	Secondary and terminal oxidation	Oxidized sterols, tocopherol degradation products. Malondialdehyde, 4-HNE, hydroxyl fatty acids	High; HPLC systems and specific detectors (e.g., UV, fluorescence) are costly.	Ox. sterols >1 mg/kg indicate damage	High	Mendonça et al. (2017), Domijan et al. (2015)

(*Continued*)

TABLE 20.3 (Continued)

Method	Principle	Sample preparation	Application stage	Oxidation stage detected	Representative compounds	Cost impact	Permissible levels	Sensitivity	References
Nuclear magnetic resonance (^{1}H-, ^{13}C-NMR)	Elucidates molecular environments and changes in proton or carbon signals.	Dissolved in deuterated solvents ($CDCl_3$, DMSO-d_6).	Research, product validation, and structural studies.	All stages	Allylic protons, hydroperoxides, aldehyde resonances	Very high; NMR equipment is very expensive and requires skilled operation.	Hydroperoxides >5% total intensity=-concern	Very high	Resende et al. (2021)
Dielectric spectroscopy	Measures dielectric constant and conductivity changes due to molecular structure alterations.	Minimal to none	Real-time/inline monitoring.	Primary and secondary oxidation	Polar lipids, hydroperoxides	Low–moderate	Requires model calibration	Moderate (μS/cm, dielectric loss)	Saini et al. (2021), Venugopalan et al. (2021)
UV-Vis spectrophotometry	Measures absorbance of conjugated dienes (232 nm) and TBARS (532 nm).	Minimal (dilution or solvent extraction)	Laboratory, routine testing.	Primary and secondary oxidation	Conjugated dienes, MDA	Low	AOCS/ISO reference thresholds	Moderate (μmol/L)	Stoffel et al. (2020)

antioxidant levels, packaging materials, or storage conditions). Subsequently, post hoc tests such as Tukey's HSD test can then be used for further comparisons among groups to identify which specific groups differ significantly from each other. By comparing the important sensory differences generated by ANOVA in combination with the respective significant variances in chemical markers, one can obtain a complete overview of the chemical causes behind changes in sensory quality (Schroën & Berton-Carabin, 2022). This integrated approach, leveraging the insights from both human sensory panels and objective chemical analyses, is enhanced by the dimensionality reduction capabilities of PCA and the comparative power of ANOVA. Therefore the implementation of effective measures to retain the quality characteristics of PUFA-enriched formulation products is critically important (Tulimaa, 2022).

20.3 Regulatory standards, guidelines and quality management systems

The emergence of regulations and guidelines by both government and professional bodies has played a crucial role in ensuring the safety of PUFA products (Resende et al., 2021; Rudy et al., 2016). These instruments often set limits for various quality parameters, including oxidation markers and limits of contaminant levels, and requirements for labeling and nutrient content.

20.3.1 Global organization for eicosapentaenoic acid and docosahexaenoic acid omega-3s

The Global organization for EPA and DHA omega-3s (GOED) has established a voluntary monograph that serves as a benchmark for the quality of omega-3 oils. The members are required to adhere to the monograph as a condition of membership. This monograph specifies stringent limits for oxidative markers: a peroxide value (PV) of ≤5 meq O_2/kg, an anisidine value (AV) of ≤20, and a total oxidation value (TOTOX) of ≤26 (Bannenberg et al., 2020). Furthermore, GOED requires that EPA and DHA make up at least 60% of the oil's total fatty acid composition (GOED | The Global Organization for EPA and DHA Omega-3s [Internet], n.d.). The purpose of these guidelines is to guarantee the efficacy, safety, and sensory quality of omega-3 products. GOED also provides technical guidance on acceptable levels of contaminants such as heavy metals and dioxins, aligning with international safety benchmarks (Kolanowski, 2010a; GOED | The Global Organization for EPA and DHA Omega-3s [Internet], n.d.).

20.3.2 European food safety authority

In Europe, the European food safety authority establishes, oversees, and regulates nutraceuticals, which encompasses PUFA supplements, and categorizes them as food supplements. These supplements are concentrated nutrient sources designed to enhance the standard diet and offer nutritional or physiological advantages. The regulations set forth by the EU delineate the substances permissible in food supplements and the allowable concentrations, as detailed in Directive 2002/46/EC (Knutsen et al., 2017). The European Commission has also established rules on nutraceutical ascertains through Regulation (EC) No 1924/2006, ensuring that any statements on food labels are precise, unambiguous, and supported by scientific data (Bhat et al., 2024; Knutsen et al., 2017). Furthermore, as stated in the Food information to consumers regulation, the EU has standards pertaining to food labeling requiring information including the item's name, ingredients list, nutrition statement, and date marking (Knutsen et al., 2017). Enforcing food laws and keeping an eye on food firms' compliance at every stage of production, processing, and distribution are the responsibilities of member states (Islam, Imran, et al., 2023; Mititelu et al., 2025).

20.3.3 Food and Drug Administration

The United States Food and Drug Administration (FDA) regulates dietary supplements, including omega-3 fatty acid supplements, under the Dietary Supplement Health and Education Act (DSHEA) of 1994 (FDA Releases Small Entity Compliance Guide on Omega-3 Fatty Acids Final Rule | FDA [Internet], n.d.; FDA Updates "Healthy" Claim, Providing a Refreshed Tool for Consumers | FDA [Internet], n.d.). While the FDA does not have specific mandatory quality standards for all dietary supplements, it has established current good manufacturing practice guidelines for dietary supplement production, packaging, labeling, and storage. The purpose of these rules is to guarantee the purity and quality of dietary supplements. For infant formula, which often contains added PUFAs, the FDA has more stringent regulations, including requirements for nutrient levels, lack of contaminants, and comprehensive QC procedures. The FDA also oversees food labeling, requiring accurate information about nutrient content, including fats and fatty acids (FDA Releases Small Entity Compliance Guide on Omega-3 Fatty Acids Final Rule | FDA [Internet], n.d.; FDA Updates "Healthy" Claim, Providing a Refreshed Tool for Consumers | FDA [Internet], n.d.).

TABLE 20.4 Oxidative stability parameters for polyunsaturated fatty acid-enriched oils.

Organization	Peroxide value (PV, meq O_2/kg)	Anisidine value	TOTOX value (2 × PV + AV)	EPA + DHA%	References
Codex Alimentarius	≤10 (refined oils); ≤15 (virgin oils)	Not specified	Not specified	Not specified	Guidelines I CODEXALIMENTARIUS FAO-WHO [Internet] (n.d.)
GOED	≤5	≤20	≤26	≥60%	GOED I The Global Organization for EPA and DHA Omega-3s [Internet] (n.d.)
EFSA	Not specified	Not specified	Not specified	Safe upper limit: 5 g/day	Rudy et al. (2016), GOED I The Global Organization for EPA and DHA Omega-3s [Internet] (n.d.)
FDA	Not specified	Not specified	Not specified	Max: 3 g/day (2 g from supplements)	FDA Updates "Healthy" Claim, Providing a Refreshed Tool for Consumers I FDA [Internet] (n.d.), FDA Releases Small Entity Compliance Guide on Omega-3 Fatty Acids Final Rule I FDA [Internet] (n.d.)

20.3.4 Codex alimentarius commission

The Codex alimentarius commission is a widely acknowledged resource that provides guidelines on food safety and quality, including those directly relevant to PUFA-supplemented foods (Guidelines | CODEXALIMENTARIUS FAO-WHO [Internet], n.d.). The Standard for named vegetable oils (CODEX STAN 210–1999) contains rules that may be directly applied to PUFA-supplemented compounds, notwithstanding the lack of particular PUFA monographs. These guidelines highlight important elements involved in establishing the quality and shelf life of edible oils (Codex Alimentarius Approves New Food Standards [Internet], n.d.). For example, it can be noted that according to regulations, refined oils' PV should not exceed 10 milliequivalents active oxygen per kilogram of oil, while cold-pressed and virgin oils' value should not surpass 15 milliequivalents per kilogram (Table 20.4). Because omega-3 oils are particularly susceptible to hydroperoxide formation, these values are essential for monitoring initial oxidation (Kolanowski, 2010a; Saini et al., 2021).

The CODEX standard emphasizes the need for PV and AV, where the latter measures secondary oxidation products that may be present in the product, including aldehydes that affect product safety and flavor. The industry also follows other complementary standards, including those of GOED, which recommend that the AV be ≤20, whereas TOTOX, calculated as 2 x PV + AV, be ≤26 for fish oils and algal oils, even though no specific limits are recommended by CODEX STAN 210–1999 for AV. These parameters offer a detailed analysis of both primary and secondary oxidation products in PUFA-enriched products (Ghelichi et al., 2023; Quality Control Management of Nutraceuticals and Dietary Supplements [Internet], n.d).

Moreover, the general standard for food additives (CODEX STAN 192–1995) allows antioxidants, including tocopherols, to be used in oils that are high in PUFAs, but this should be done within specified limits that ensure safety and increase stability (Mureşan et al., 2020). The General standard for the labeling of prepackaged foods (CODEX STAN 1–1985) requires that information on nutrient content be provided correctly. The label indicating the omega-3 or omega-6 fatty acid content should be an accurate reflection of the composition within specified limits of tolerance. These standards ensure that products containing PUFAs are of high quality, safe, and transparent throughout their production and consumption process (Bhat et al., 2024).

20.4 Applications of quality control measures across the polyunsaturated fatty acid product life cycle

The need for quality and authenticity of PUFA-containing products requires the implementation of QC measures that cover all stages of the product's life cycle, including raw material sourcing, storage, and distribution. The delivery of quality PUFA-enriched functional foods relies on the implementation of good manufacturing practices (GMP) (Mureşan et al., 2020), (hazard analysis and critical control points, HACCP) (HACCP Principles & Application Guidelines | FDA [Internet], n.d.), and (food safety system certification, FSSC 22000 (FSSC 22000 - Delivering trust and impact for global food safety [Internet], n.d.) for all stages of product manufacture (Fig. 20.4).

20.4.1 Quality control in raw material sourcing

The production of quality PUFA-based products depends on the careful selection of raw materials, which is a crucial step to ensure that the end product meets the quality requirements for the content of PUFAs, and the quality of its freshness and purity. The raw materials should, therefore, be procured from reliable sources that meet the quality requirements, which can only be achieved through a supplier qualification system. The supplier qualification system should, therefore, be robust, as a reliable supply chain is a major contributor to quality (Hocquette et al., 2005).

After procuring the raw materials, the quality of the raw materials is verified through verification tests to ensure the quality, purity, and freshness of the raw materials. The quality assessments for the raw materials are carried out through quality profiling, which involves the use of gas chromatography (GC) for the identification of PUFAs, and the use of GC for the quantification of EPA, DHA, and α-Linoleic acid. The raw materials are also tested for oxidation, which involves the use of the PV, acid value (AV), and the use of the TOTOX for the assessment of the raw materials' freshness. The raw materials are also tested for the presence of heavy metals and for the presence of persistent organic pollutants for the marine oils, and for the presence of pesticide residues for the plant-based oils. The raw materials are then stored under cool, dry, and oxygen-free conditions to prevent (Bhat et al., 2024; Kolanowski, 2010a; Resende et al., 2021; Saini et al., 2021).

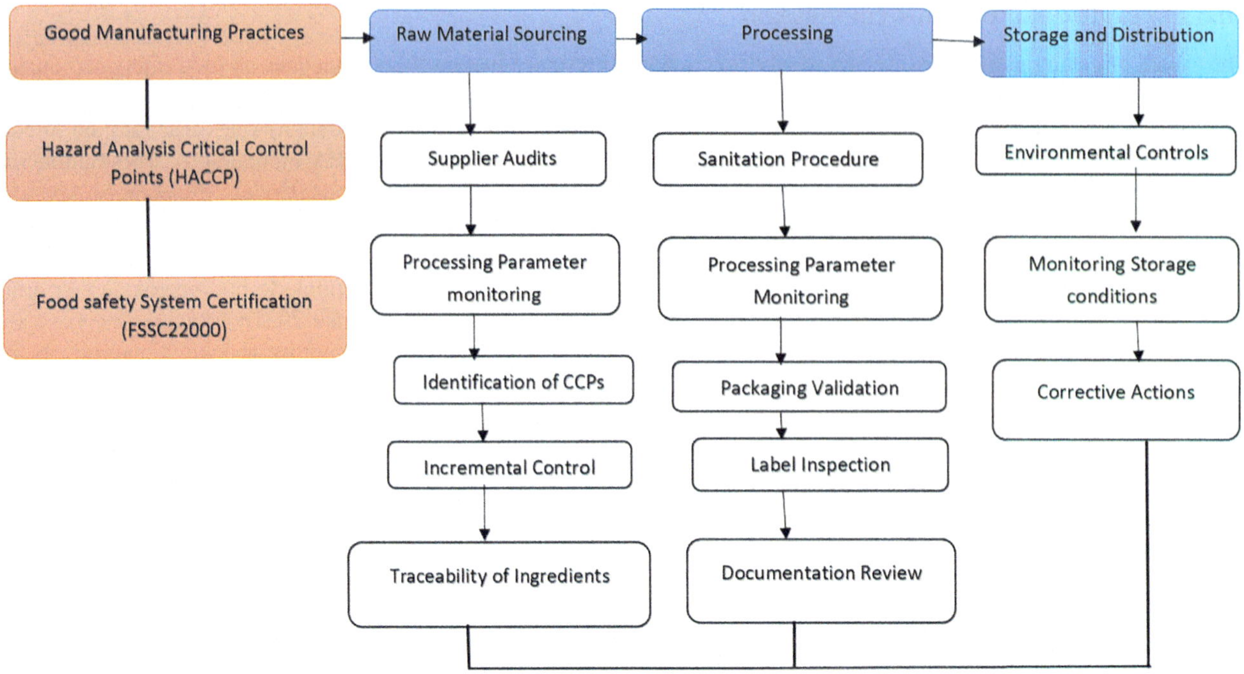

FIGURE 20.4 Value chain quality control measures.

20.4.2 Quality control during processing and manufacturing

In the production phase, the QC focuses on the minimization of oxidation and contaminants. The mild processing procedures, such as supercritical fluid extraction and enzymatic processing, are increasingly being adopted to maintain the integrity of the PUFAs under mild processing conditions (Đorđević et al., 2015; Geng et al., 2023; Kolanowski, 2010a). The early use of antioxidants such as tocopherols and rosemary is essential to prevent the formation of free radicals that initiate the oxidation reaction (Mostafa Abd El-Aal, 2012). The processing conditions are strictly controlled to ensure that the product is subjected to minimum heat, light, and oxygen. The implementation of GMP is essential to maintain a clean manufacturing environment. This includes training the staff and ensuring the cleanliness of the facilities. Cross-contamination is also prevented. The in-process testing of the product for the presence of oxidation products and the PUFAs is done to ensure that the product is of the desired quality (FSSC 22000 - Delivering trust and impact for global food safety [Internet], n.d.).

In the case of PUFAs in supplement form, such as soft gels, the QC of the encapsulation process is strictly implemented to prevent the entry of oxygen. The materials for the capsule should be inert and nonreactive with the oil (Du et al., 2022; FSSC 22000 - Delivering trust and impact for global food safety [Internet], n.d.). Purification procedures such as molecular distillation are implemented to remove the contaminants without affecting the fatty acid composition. This is a precise procedure that should be strictly controlled to prevent further oxidation (Ghelichi et al., 2023).

The implementation of GMP (Pirsa & Asadi, 2021; Teixeira-Costa & Andrade, 2022; Tian et al., 2013) is essential to ensure the standardization and cleanliness of the entire manufacturing process. This includes the training of the staff and the cleanliness of the facilities. The HACCP (HACCP Principles & Application Guidelines | FDA [Internet], n.d.) is a system that identifies the hazards that may be encountered in the facilities. This may include the presence of oxidizing factors such as heat, metal ions, and light. HACCP helps to define the critical control points during the entire manufacturing process. The FSSC 22000 is a standard that combines the ISO 22000 standard with the industry-specific requirements. The FSSC is essential to ensure the implementation of the HACCP and the GMP principles. The traceability and the monitoring of the entire manufacturing process are critical (FSSC 22000 - Delivering trust and impact for global food safety [Internet], n.d.).

20.4.3 Quality control in storage and distribution

The quality assurance process in postmanufacturing activities includes careful management of storage and distribution. The quality assurance process in postmanufacturing activities for PUFAs includes careful management of storage and distribution. The products are highly prone to oxidation in an uncontrolled environment. Therefore low temperatures and low humidity, along with protection from light during storage, are important factors (Pirsa & Asadi, 2021; Tian et al., 2013). Refrigeration or freezing can also be done for a longer shelf life. The packaging material should have low oxygen permeability. The packaging should be opaque for protection against photo-oxidation (Pirsa & Asadi, 2021). The transportation should also be carried out in a controlled environment. The shelf life is determined by carrying out stability studies under different conditions. The factors taken into consideration include the quality of oil, antioxidant content, and packaging. The storage should ensure that there is no product degradation and that quality is maintained (Ghelichi et al., 2023; Tian et al., 2013).

20.4.4 Role of packaging in preventing oxidation

It is noteworthy that packaging is a critical factor in the prevention of PUFAs from oxidation. The use of suitable packaging that can effectively inhibit the entry of oxygen into the package is important. Multilayer plastics, glass, and metallic packaging can effectively inhibit the entry of oxygen (Tian et al., 2013). The use of opaque packaging or material resistant to UV light can effectively inhibit light-induced oxidation. The use of active packaging technology provides effective protection against oxidation. The active packaging technology can be in the form of oxygen scavengers and antioxidant-releasing packaging. The active packaging technology can effectively inhibit the oxidation process by incorporating active substances in the packaging matrix that can effectively inhibit the oxidation process in the PUFAs product. The packaging should be inert and meet regulatory requirements to avoid leaching of active substances. The use of effective packaging can also help in building consumer confidence and enhancing product appeal (Pirsa & Asadi, 2021; Teixeira-Costa & Andrade, 2022).

20.5 Advancements in analytical techniques

The area of PUFA quality measurement is increasingly incorporating innovative technology such as high-resolution instruments, analytics, and automation. This technology also shows promise not only to offer better analytical accuracy but to provide faster and cheaper QCs on a real-time basis throughout the PUFA product chain. Examples of some technologies available to measure PUFA integrity are summarized in Table 20.5.

20.5.1 Raman spectroscopy for lipid and polyunsaturated fatty acid integrity analysis

Raman spectroscopy is a noninvasive, powerful optical method applied in the molecular characterization of lipids by investigating their vibrational modes via the inelastic scattering of monochromatic light, most commonly derived from a laser with an operating wavelength ranging from 405 to 1064 nm (Chen et al., 2018). In a standard arrangement, a confocal Raman microscope illuminates the sample with the laser beam through an objective lens, which results in the generation of Rayleigh (elastic) and Raman (inelastic) scattered photons (Hong et al., 2025; Uematsu & Shimizu, 2021). The Stokes Raman-scattered photons are subsequently separated by a spectrograph according to their wavelengths, producing a Raman spectrum that plots Raman shift (in per cm) against photon intensity (Baeten, 2010; Chen et al., 2018). The resultant spectral data yield highly detailed molecular fingerprints of tremendous usefulness for lipid characterization (Higgins et al., 2022; Hong et al., 2025).

Prominent Raman bands characteristic of lipids are the symmetric (2851/cm) and asymmetric (2881/cm) stretching modes of CH_2, ester carbonyl stretch at 1740/cm, and unsaturation bands like C=C–H stretching at 3010/cm and C=C deformation at 1262/cm (Baeten, 2010; Higgins et al., 2022). Raman spectroscopy is particularly well adapted to analyzing PUFA integrity as it can identify structural information like levels of unsaturation and fatty acid esterification without labels or advanced sample preparation (Hong et al., 2025). Raman spectroscopy has been applied to measure lipid oxidation, differentiate between types of oils, and monitor fat content in meat. Its low water interference is a major advantage, making it especially suitable for biological and food matrices. (Wrona et al., 2023). In addition, the ratiometric analysis of Raman peak intensities has allowed the measurement of lipid unsaturation and the monitoring of the composition of lipid droplets in cells (Higgins et al., 2022; Uematsu & Shimizu, 2021).

Still, traditional Raman spectroscopy may suffer from its comparably high detection limits and low sensitivity. SERS is a solution to this problem (Drabik et al., 2023). SERS was developed as a supporting method that drastically increases the

TABLE 20.5 Advanced technologies for PUFA integrity quality control.

Technology	Principle	Application mode	Analyte/target	Advantages	Limitations	Applications / references
Raman spectroscopy	Inelastic scattering of light to identify molecular vibrations	Nondestructive, point scan	C=C bonds, lipid oxidation markers	Rapid, solvent-free, portable	Fluorescence interference, complex spectra	Used for assessing vegetable oils (Baeten, 2010; Chen et al., 2018; Higgins et al., 2022; Hong et al., 2025; Uematsu and Shimizu, 2021; Wrona et al., 2023)
NIR spectroscopy	Absorption of near-infrared radiation by molecular bonds	Nondestructive, inline	Fatty acid profile, oxidation status	Fast, in-line compatible, requires minimal prep	Lower specificity, needs chemometric calibration	Applied in edible oil and meat industry oxidation (Fernández-Cabanás et al., 2011; Jayaselan et al., 2017)
Hyperspectral imaging (HSI)	Combines spectroscopy and imaging for spatial-spectral mapping	Surface imaging	Oxidative degradation patterns, lipid mapping	High resolution, visualization capability	High data volume, computationally intense	Used in meat products and fish oil oxidation detection (Aqeel et al., 2024; Bhargava et al., 2024)
GC-MS/LC-MS	Separation and identification of oxidation compounds	Lab-based, quantitative	Aldehydes, hydroxy acids, epoxides	High sensitivity and specificity	High cost, time-consuming	Gold standard in PUFA oxidation studies. (Hewavitharana et al., 2020)
AI/machine learning	Data-driven models for prediction/classification	Embedded in software	Spectral/chromatographic profiles, oxidation level	Predictive power, automation	Requires large training datasets	Used in real-time edible oil quality prediction and sorting (Ali et al., 2025; Aqeel et al., 2024)
Chemometrics	Multivariate statistical analysis of complex data	Data interpretation	Spectral data, quality indices	Enhances data utility, enables real-time decisions	Requires expert setup	Applied with NIR and HSI in PUFA quality classification (El Orche et al., 2020; Maggio et al., 2012; Muzolf-Panek et al., 2020)
Biosensors	Biochemical detection via enzymes/antibodies	Portable or in situ	Peroxides, aldehydes, free radicals	Rapid, field-usable, specific	Limited shelf life, calibration issues	Used in fish oil and packaged meat oxidation monitoring (Daci et al., 2024)

intensity of the Raman signal by using substrates covered with roughened noble metals such as silver, gold, or copper (Chen et al., 2018). Up to 10^{11} enhancement factors have been demonstrated, enabling ultra-sensitive detection of trace-level analytes. While SERS has been explored in lipid analysis, SERS application to detect lipid oxidation in meat products is underdeveloped and is one interesting research frontier to be pursued in the future (Hong et al., 2025; Surmacki et al., 2022). In general, Raman spectroscopy, particularly when enhanced by SERS, offers a selective, rapid, and versatile analytical method for qualitative and quantitative analysis of PUFA oxidation and food lipid quality (Hong et al., 2025; Wang et al., 2022; Zhou et al., 2019).

20.5.2 Near-infrared spectroscopy for polyunsaturated fatty acid quality and oxidation analysis

Near-Infrared (NIR) spectroscopy is now a very powerful analytical technique for the quick, nondestructive evaluation of PUFA quality and oil loss control in foods and lipid-based systems. Operating between the electromagnetic spectrum of approximately 800 to 2500 nm (Fernández-Cabanás et al., 2011), combination vibrations and molecular overtones of bonds like C–H, N–H, and O–H functional groups that are frequently found in fatty acids and lipids are highly sensitive to NIR spectroscopy (Fernández-Cabanás et al., 2011). Provided these functional groups are at concentrations above approximately 0.1%, NIR provides consistent and reproducible results and is therefore very well suited to high-throughput screening of PUFA-rich samples (Fernández-Cabanás et al., 2011). The fundamental principle of NIR spectroscopy is the absorption of radiation due to molecular vibration. However, unlike in mid-infrared spectroscopy, the absorption bands for the NIR range are combination and overtone bands, which are broader and more complex in nature. Therefore spectral features overlap each other considerably, and interpretation is not feasible directly. In addressing this challenge, modern NIR spectroscopy primarily relies on multivariate statistical techniques, where chemometrics play a fundamental role in interpreting complex spectral information and obtaining valuable information. In this regard, a set of reference samples is normally used to establish a calibration model based on multivariate regression techniques, such as PCA and partial least squares (PLS). Subsequently, these models are normally used in assessing fatty acid composition, oxidation levels, and water activity in lipids in newly presented samples (Jayaselan et al., 2017; Murage et al., 2021).

In terms of its components, a NIR spectrometer normally includes a light source, such as a quartz tungsten halogen lamp or an incandescent lamp, and optical components like a prism or a diffraction grating for light dispersion (Beć et al., 2020). In addition, a silicon charge-coupled device is normally used as a detector, especially for lower near-infrared ranges, or a more sensitive detector like indium gallium arsenide (InGaAs) and lead sulfide (PbS), especially for a broader near-infrared range. In more sophisticated spectrometers, fourier transform near-infrared interferometers are normally used in obtaining high-resolution spectral information with high signal-to-noise ratios, especially for ranges above 1000 nm (Alamu et al., 2021).

The main advantage of NIR spectroscopy is that it requires minimal sample handling and can perform fast analysis. Such characteristics make NIR spectroscopy highly suitable for process monitoring and QC in food products. The capability to examine bulk samples in a nondestructive manner allows for the continuous monitoring of oil quality and the rate of oxidation and degradation of PUFAs. Recent advances in NIR spectroscopy have shown that it can be effectively applied to monitoring and assessment of the loss of palm oil (Beć et al., 2020) and other vegetable oils. It has been successfully applied in the food industry for QC in dairy products, meat products, and processed foodstuffs. Despite the advantages of NIR spectroscopy, there are some disadvantages that can be encountered. The complex nature of NIR spectra makes it difficult to interpret results. The specificity of NIR spectroscopy can also be low in comparison to other techniques that can be applied. Despite these disadvantages, NIR spectroscopy can be an effective and environmentally friendly method for ensuring the quality and stability of PUFAs in different food products (Murage et al., 2021).

20.5.3 Hyperspectral imaging

Hyperspectral imaging (HSI) is an important analytical tool that combines the principles of spectroscopy and imaging to provide spatially resolved information on the chemistry of a material. HSI technology has found significant application as a nondestructive tool for QC in the food industry, including the assessment of the quality of PUFAs (Bhargava et al., 2024). HSI technology provides information on the entire spectrum of the material under study, including the visible region (400–700 nm) (Aqeel et al., 2024), the NIR region (700–1000 nm), and the short-wave infrared region (SWIR) (1000–2500 nm) (Aqeel et al., 2024). This information is provided as a three-dimensional data-set known as a "hypercube," where the two spatial dimensions are correlated to the one spectral dimension. This allows the identification of the spatial distribution of the chemical signals (Bhargava et al., 2024).

In the case of PUFAs in foods such as meat products, fish products, dairy products, and edible oils, the occurrence of oxidation can cause significant alterations to the chemistry of the material. However, such alterations are not visible to the naked eye. HSI technology can provide the tools to identify the alterations to the chemistry of the material. This can be achieved by the identification of the molecular features associated with the products of lipid oxidation, such as hydroperoxides, aldehydes, and the levels of unsaturation. Alterations in the features associated with the C–H, O–H, and C=O bonds can be correlated to the primary and secondary levels of lipid oxidation. HSI technology can provide information on the spatial distribution of the oil, the distribution of the lipids, and the spatial distribution of the degradation of the PUFAs (Aqeel et al., 2024; Bhargava et al., 2024).

The instrumental setup generally consists of a broad-spectrum light source (e.g., quartz-halogen lamp), a spectrograph/imaging filter, and a detector that can cover a specific spectral range (e.g., InGaAs detector for NIR and SWIR regions). The scanning process can be carried out using a line-scan or an area-scan approach. Sophisticated analytical techniques such as PCA, PLS regression, and machine learning (ML) algorithms can be applied for classification and prediction purposes due to the high dimensionality associated with the HSI data (Aqeel et al., 2024).

The potential of HSI technology has been explored in the detection of lipid oxidation in fish fillet products (Du et al., 2022), quality grading of beef products based on fat content and distribution, and oxidative rancidity in food oils. The potential use of this technology in QC and traceability in both laboratory and industrial environments is evident. Despite the advantages offered by this technology, the use of HSI technology requires high computational capabilities for data acquisition and analysis. Calibration of the model can also vary from sample to sample. Nevertheless, the use of HSI technology in combination with chemometric and AI techniques has shown increased potential for the technology in terms of predictive capability and efficiency for overall PUFA quality monitoring in food matrices (Aqeel et al., 2024; Bhargava et al., 2024).

20.5.4 Chromatographic techniques

The major analytical tools for the detailed characterization of PUFAs and their oxidized derivatives are GC and liquid chromatography (LC), particularly in combination with mass spectrometry (MS). These chromatographic techniques allow for the high-resolution separation of complex mixtures of fatty compounds, facilitating the qualitative and quantitative analysis of PUFAs and a wide range of secondary products of their oxidative degradation (Domijan et al., 2015; Goldring et al., 1993; Hewavitharana et al., 2020). Aldehydes, ketones, and hydrocarbons are volatile or semivolatile secondary products of the oxidative degradation of PUFAs that can be detected with the help of GC-MS and GC tandem mass spectrometry (GC-MS/MS) (Hewavitharana et al., 2020). The formation of these compounds is a result of primary and secondary lipid oxidation. The derivatives of these compounds are significant secondary products of the degradation of PUFAs. The derivatives may be formed with the help of methylation of fatty acids to form fatty acid methyl esters, which is a common practice to enhance the GC analysis of nonvolatile substances. The trace-level quantification of the individual fatty acids and the secondary products of the degradation of PUFAs is also possible in complex food products due to the exceptional sensitivity of MS/MS detection (Hewavitharana et al., 2020).

On the other hand, complementary techniques can be provided by high-performance liquid chromatography (HPLC), especially when coupled with high-resolution mass spectrometry (HRMS). HPLC-HRMS techniques are particularly useful for the analysis of nonvolatile, polar oxidation products, including hydroperoxides, oxylipins, and conjugated dienes (CD) (Domijan et al., 2015; Mendonça et al., 2017). The techniques can be used without derivatization, with the additional advantage of ambient-temperature separations. The use of ultra-high-performance liquid chromatography systems can increase the analysis speed, making the technique advantageous for the QC of food products containing PUFAs, emulsions, and functional foodstuffs (Domijan et al., 2015). The current generation of chromatographic techniques can now incorporate sampling systems, ultra-fast column technology, and integrated data analysis tools that utilize artificial intelligence (AI) and chemometrics, which can significantly improve the analysis speed, and the reproducibility, sensitivity, and reliability of the results (Fernández-Cabanás et al., 2011). Two-dimensional chromatography techniques, including 2D-LC/GC, are increasingly being used for the comprehensive analysis of the lipidome and for the separation of coeluting oxidation products, which can only be identified as a single peak with conventional one-dimensional techniques (Mendonça et al., 2017).

The applications of the techniques are varied, covering the entire food production cycle, from the analysis of food ingredients to the prediction of shelf life, and the analysis of foodstuffs for regulatory purposes (Ghelichi et al., 2023). For instance, GC-MS was used to analyze the oxidation of PUFAs, as indicated by the production of hexanal and nonanal, while HPLC-HRMS was used for the analysis of the oxidation of linoleic acid, as indicated by the production of OXLAMs, in infant formula and dietary supplements (Mendonça et al., 2017).

Although the techniques are more time-consuming, the advantages of the techniques are undeniable, making them essential tools for the analysis of PUFAs and for the analysis of the oxidation of PUFAs. The techniques can now be used with real-time tools, including NIR, Raman spectroscopy, and biosensors, making them a robust technique for the comprehensive analysis of foodstuffs for QC, and for the confirmation of results, as indicated by the use of the techniques for the analysis of the quality and the shelf life of foodstuffs, as indicated by the use of the techniques for the analysis of foodstuffs containing PUFAs, emulsions, and functional foodstuffs (Domijan et al., 2015).

20.5.5 Integration of data-driven artificial intelligence and machine learning

The monitoring of PUFA integrity and oxidation state is a QC measure in food systems in transition, driven by advances in AI and ML technologies (Fernández-Cabanás et al., 2011). These technologies are particularly useful for handling the large and complex datasets generated by spectroscopic, chromatographic, and physicochemical analyses used in food quality assessment (El Orche et al., 2020). In order for AI systems to correctly predict different attributes of food samples, such as oxidation state, shelf life, and levels of adulteration, they should be able to recognize different patterns and relationships in complex, high-dimensional datasets.

To perform these tasks, different ML algorithms, such as artificial neural networks (ANN), random forest classifiers, and convolutional neural networks (CNN), are used for classifying oil samples according to their oxidation levels, predicting PVs, and distinguishing authentic sources of PUFA from adulterated ones (Cao et al., 2014). For example, CNNs have been effectively applied in predicting the oxidation status of fish and meat samples using their hyperspectral images, while ANNs have been applied in modeling different parameters, such as peroxide and AVs from Fourier transform infrared spectroscopy and Raman spectra with high accuracy levels (Ayala et al., 2014).

In addition, reinforcement learning and ensemble approaches are being incorporated into different control systems for decision-making purposes in order to optimize different parameters in food processing, particularly in optimizing PUFA processing parameters in order to maintain their oxidative stability in food systems in transition, leading to the creation of smart factories with continuously optimized parameters in food processing (Ghelichi et al., 2023; Jackowski et al., 2015; Tao, Department of Animal Science, Cornell University, Ithaca, NY, USA, 2015). In addition, cloud-based AI systems are able to facilitate different aspects of food traceability (Fernández-Cabanás et al., 2011). In spite of different challenges in implementing these technologies, their integration in food systems in transition is promising for predicting, scaling, and automating PUFA QC in food systems in transition.

20.5.6 Chemometrics as a decision-support tool

Indicates that chemometrics is of critical value in converting complex data obtained during analysis into valuable information that can be used in decision-making processes, especially when considering the oxidation of PUFAs, where several factors affect their stability and degradation (Muzolf-Panek et al., 2020). By applying statistical and mathematical calculations on data obtained through Raman spectroscopy, NIR spectroscopy, GC-MS, HPLC, and HSI, chemometrics improves data interpretability, accuracy, and usefulness of analysis data (Maggio et al., 2012).

To reduce dimensionality, highlight relevant information in datasets, and create accurate calibration models, chemometrics uses statistical methods such as PCA, PLS regression, discriminant analysis, and support vector machines (El Orche et al., 2020). These models enable accurate predictions of oxidation indices of lipids without requiring direct chemical analysis of datasets, offering timely predictions of CD concentrations, thiobarbituric acid reactive substances, and PV levels (Ghelichi et al., 2023).

Chemometrics is also of critical value in monitoring multivariate processes, where chemometrics helps in identifying abnormalities in lipid oxidation patterns during production processes. This is of critical value, especially in real-time applications where chemometrics is used in monitoring systems in edible oil refining processes or in manufacturing processes involving PUFAs (El Orche et al., 2020; Maggio et al., 2012; Muzolf-Panek et al., 2020). In addition, chemometric models can be integrated into digital twin technology, where product performance under different environmental conditions is simulated, offering valuable information on product formulation and storage strategies. By improving the accuracy, rate, and efficiency of PUFA analysis, chemometrics is of critical value in modern QC processes, bridging the gap between analysis data obtained through laboratory-grade analysis and industrial processes (El Orche et al., 2020; Maggio et al., 2012; Muzolf-Panek et al., 2020).

20.5.7 Emerging role of biosensors

Biosensors offer an innovative and increasingly viable method for in situ and real-time assessment of PUFA oxidation, especially in a decentralized environment (Signal and Information Processing for Sensing Systems - Institute for Bioengineering of Catalonia- Santiago Marco Colás [Internet], n.d.). Biosensors use a physicochemical detector and a biological recognition component that produce a measurable signal in the presence of a specific analyte (Daci et al., 2024). Biosensors that use enzymes and electrochemical detection have been developed for detecting PUFA degradation products such as hydroperoxides, malondialdehyde , and 4-hydroxynonenal. These biomarkers are strong indicators of oxidative stress in lipid-enriched meals and tissues (Daci et al., 2024).

Significant advances in technology have greatly improved the performance and capabilities of biosensors. The use of nanomaterials such as gold nanoparticles, graphene, and metal-organic frameworks has greatly improved the performance and amplification capabilities of biosensors. Label-free optical biosensors, such as surface plasmon resonance and interferometry, offer real-time and rapid quantification capabilities (Daci et al., 2024). The miniaturization of biosensors and their integration with smartphone technology offer exciting possibilities for the use of biosensors in the assessment

TABLE 20.6 Quality control parameters for polyunsaturated fatty acid (PUFA) integrity in developed and developing countries.

Quality control parameter	Developed countries	Developing countries	References
Regulatory framework	Harmonized regulations (e.g., EFSA, FDA); mandatory labeling of omega-3s	Often limited or fragmented; donor-supported frameworks dominate	Regulation - 1924/2006 - EN - EUR-Lex [Internet] (n.d.), Robert (n.d.), FDA Updates "Healthy" Claim, Providing a Refreshed Tool for Consumers I FDA [Internet] (n.d.), Program (2025)
Analytical capabilities	Use of GC-MS, LC-MS/MS, Fourier transform infrared spectroscopy, NIR, Raman spectroscopy for PUFA profiling	Reliance on classical methods: peroxide, TBARS; limited access to high-end instruments	Hewavitharana et al. (2020), Li et al. (2014)
Monitoring of oxidation products	Monitors hydroperoxides, MDA, 4-HNE, and anisidine values	Primarily peroxide values; MDA analysis limited	Ghelichi et al. (2023), Bannenberg et al. (2020), Du et al. (2022), Cao et al. (2014)
Use of AI/ML in QC	AI models (ANN, CNN, RF) used for oxidation prediction and classification	Largely absent or limited to pilot studies	Aqeel et al. (2024), Ali et al. (2025), El Orche et al. (2020)
Biosensor application	Enzyme/electrochemical biosensors, SPR, nanomaterial-enhanced systems	Few biosensor applications; mostly donor-supported labs	Daci et al. (2024), Smart et al. (2023)
Personnel expertise	Multidisciplinary staff with expertise in lipidomics, analytical chemistry	Lack of training and limited continuous professional development	Saini et al. (2021), Tao, Department of Animal Science, Cornell University, Ithaca, NY, USA (2015), The State of Food Security and Nutrition in the World (2022)
Traceability and documentation	Blockchain and LIMS used in supply chains	Predominantly paper-based or semiautomated systems	Knutsen et al. (2017), Mititelu et al. (2025)
Shelf life prediction models	Machine learning models, Rancimat, Arrhenius kinetics	Historical or empirical models only	Islam, Kaczmarek, et al. (2023), Du et al. (2022)
Labeling of EPA/DHA content	Standardized with approved health claims (e.g., heart health)	Often lacking; no mandatory EPA/DHA disclosure	Bannenberg et al. (2020), PDF.pdf [Internat] (n.d.), Federal Register: Food Labeling: Nutrient Content Claims; Alpha-Linolenic Acid, Eicosapentaenoic Acid, and Docosahexaenoic Acid Omega-3 Fatty Acids [Internet] (n.d.)
Innovation and R&D	Active investment by companies like DSM, Badische Anilin- und Soda-Fabrik, and Aker BioMarine	Limited domestic research; mostly driven by NGOs or collaborations	Hong et al. (2025), Uematsu and Shimizu (2021), Daci et al. (2024)

and monitoring of PUFAs in the field. Such miniaturization offers potential for the use of biosensors by producers, regulators, and consumers for assessing the quality of PUFAs in foodstuffs such as oil, meat, and dairy products, and in functional food products (Tao, Department of Animal Science, Cornell University, Ithaca, NY, USA, 2015).

Despite the relatively limited capabilities of biosensors in detecting and analyzing PUFAs and their oxidation products compared to other techniques such as chromatography and spectroscopy, biosensors offer a viable alternative for assessing and detecting PUFAs in a decentralized environment. The relatively low costs associated with biosensors make them a viable alternative for detecting and assessing PUFAs in a QC environment (Jackowski et al., 2015; Signal and Information Processing for Sensing Systems - Institute for Bioengineering of Catalonia- Santiago Marco Colás [Internet], n.d.).

20.6 Comparative analysis of quality control parameters for polyunsaturated fatty acid integrity in developed and developing countries

Table 20.6 shows a comparative analysis of the factors critically involved in monitoring and sustaining the quality of PUFAs in both developed and developing countries. Interestingly, the analysis reveals trends that are different for each country with regard to analytical ability, regulatory practices, and technological trends concerning the quality of PUFA. The factors presented in Table 20.6 offer perspectives on gaps within capacities and their implications on PUFA utilization within industrial, nutritional, and commercial applications.

20.7 Conclusions

It is imperative that PUFA products are ensured of integrity, given their substantial positive impact on human health and their increasing demand as a result of their health benefits. This chapter sought to highlight the complexity of QC in the PUFA industry, further emphasizing the importance of a holistic approach in ensuring product integrity, that is, an entire product life cycle or entire value chain.

Prevention of oxidation remains a fundamental concept in ensuring PUFA product integrity. This is in light of the PUFA inherent tendency toward oxidation, which demands that these products are strictly controlled in terms of their exposure to oxygen, temperature, and light throughout their entire value chain. Strategic utilization of antioxidants, and packaging materials with low oxygen and light transmission, are integral in preventing oxidation and, consequently, extending their shelf life. Adherence to regulatory policies and guidelines, as set by organizations such as GOED and national food safety authorities, remains a fundamental concept in ensuring a minimum level of quality and safety in PUFA products, which is necessary for entry into and for building trust among consumers in their quality and reliability.

The future trend in the QC of PUFA is expected to be greatly influenced by the latest advances in analytical and processing techniques. The latest advances in rapid and nondestructive techniques such as Raman and NIR spectroscopy have shown potential for more efficient quality assessment. The development and implementation of green processing techniques cannot only benefit the environment but also contribute to the QC of PUFA by avoiding harsh conditions that can trigger degradation. The diversification trend in the sources of PUFA, including algae and genetically modified plants, poses opportunities and challenges for QC. New strategies will be required to address the unique characteristics and risks associated with these new sources in order to maintain a consistent supply of premium quality PUFA products and meet the increasing demand globally. The advancement in this field is important to further improve QC measures and ensure that the consumer can confidently benefit from the health merits associated with PUFA products.

References

Adámek, M., Adámková, A., Jiří Mlček, Borkovcová, M., & Bednářová, M. (2018). Acceptability and sensory evaluation of energy bars and protein bars enriched with edible insect. *Potravinarstvo Slovak Journal of Food Sciences, 12*(1), 431–437. https://doi.org/10.5219/925.

Alamu, E. O., Nuwamanya, E., Cornet, D., Meghar, K., Adesokan, M., Tran, T., Belalcazar, J., Desfontaines, L., & Davrieux, F. (2021). Near-infrared spectroscopy applications for high-throughput phenotyping for cassava and yam: A review. *International Journal of Food Science & Technology, 56*(3), 1491–1501. https://doi.org/10.1111/ijfs.14773.

Ali, M., Benfante, V., Basirinia, G., Alongi, P., Sperandeo, A., Quattrocchi, A., et al. (2025). Applications of artificial intelligence, deep learning, and machine learning to support the analysis of microscopic images of cells and tissues. *Journal of Imaging, 11*(2), 59. https://doi.org/10.3390/jimaging11020059.

Aqeel, M., Sohaib, A., Iqbal, M., Rehman, H. U., & Rustam, F. (2024). Hyperspectral identification of oil adulteration using machine learning techniques. *Current Research in Food Science, 8*, 100773. https://doi.org/10.1016/j.crfs.2024.100773.

Ayala, A., Muñoz, M. F., & Argüelles, S. (2014). Lipid peroxidation: Production, metabolism, and signaling mechanisms of malondialdehyde and 4-hydroxy-2-nonenal. *Oxidative Medicine and Cellular Longevity, 2014*, 360438. https://doi.org/10.1155/2014/360438, http://www.landesbioscience.com/journals/oximed.

Baeten, V. (2010). Raman spectroscopy in lipid analysis. *Lipid Technology, 22*(2), 36–38. https://doi.org/10.1002/lite.200900082.

Bannenberg, G., Rice, H. B., Bernasconi, A., Ferrari, A., Mallon, C., Navarrete, L., Hughes, R., Igarashi, J., Persons, K., Latynski, L., Phung, A., Wang, S., & Ismail, A. (2020). Ingredient label claim compliance and oxidative quality of EPA/DHA omega-3 retail products in the U.S. *Journal of Food Composition and Analysis, 88*, 103435. https://doi.org/10.1016/j.jfca.2020.103435.

Beć, K. B., Grabska, J., & Huck, C. W. (2020). Near-infrared spectroscopy in bio-applications. *Molecules (Basel, Switzerland), 25*(12), 2948. https://doi.org/10.3390/molecules25122948.

Belayneh, H. D., Wehling, R. L., Cahoon, E. B., & Ciftci, O. N. (2017). Effect of extraction method on the oxidative stability of camelina seed oil studied by differential scanning calorimetry. *Journal of Food Science, 82*(3), 632–637. https://doi.org/10.1111/1750-3841.13652, http://www3.interscience.wiley.com/journal/118509799/issueyear?year=2008.

Benatti, P., Peluso, G., Nicolai, R., & Calvani, M. (2004). Polyunsaturated fatty acids: Biochemical, nutritional and epigenetic properties. *Journal of the American College of Nutrition, 23*(4), 281–302. https://doi.org/10.1080/07315724.2004.10719371.

Bhargava, A., Sachdeva, A., Sharma, K., Alsharif, M. H., Uthansakul, P., & Uthansakul, M. (2024). Hyperspectral imaging and its applications: A review. *Heliyon, 10*(12), e33208. https://doi.org/10.1016/j.heliyon.2024.e33208.

Bhat, R. S., Alsuhaibani, A. S., Albugami, F. S., & Aldawsari, F. S. (2024). Omega 3 fatty acid as a health supplement: An overview of its manufacture and regulatory aspects. *Current Research in Nutrition and Food Science, 12*(1), 70–90. https://doi.org/10.12944/CRNFSJ.12.1.06, https://www.foodandnutritionjournal.org/download/19688.

Cao, J., Deng, L., Zhu, X.-M., Fan, Y., Hu, J.-N., Li, J., et al. (2014). Novel Approach To Evaluate The Oxidation State Of Vegetable Oils Using Characteristic Oxidation Indicators. *Journal of Agricultural and Food Chemistry, 62*(52), 12545–12552. https://doi.org/10.1021/jf5047656, http://pubs.acs.org/journal/jafcau.

Chen, Q., Xie, Y., Xi, J., Guo, Y., Qian, H., Cheng, Y., Chen, Y., & Yao, W. (2018). Characterization of lipid oxidation process of beef during repeated freeze-thaw by electron spin resonance technology and Raman spectroscopy. *Food Chemistry, 243*, 58–64. https://doi.org/10.1016/j.foodchem.2017.09.115.

Cheseto, X., Baleba, S. B. S., Tanga, C. M., Kelemu, S., & Torto, B. (2020). Chemistry and sensory characterization of a bakery product prepared with oils from African edible insects. *Foods, 9*(6). https://doi.org/10.3390/foods9060800, https://www.mdpi.com/2304-8158/9/6/800.

Codex Alimentarius Approves New Food Standards [Internet]. (n.d.). Retrieved May 10, 2025 from https://natlawreview.com/article/codex-alimentarius-main-outcome-47th-session-cac47?utm_source=chatgpt.com.

Daci, M., Berisha, L., Mercatante, D., Rodriguez-Estrada, M. T., Jin, Z., Huang, Y., & Amorati, R. (2024). Advancements in biosensors for lipid peroxidation and antioxidant protection in food: A critical review. *Antioxidants, 13*(12), 1484. https://doi.org/10.3390/antiox13121484.

Domijan, A., Ralić, J., Radić Brkanac, S., Rumora, L., & Žanić-Grubišić, T. (2015). Quantification of malondialdehyde by HPLC-FL – application to various biological samples. *Biomedical Chromatography, 29*(1), 41–46. https://doi.org/10.1002/bmc.3361.

Domínguez, R., Pateiro, M., Gagaoua, M., Barba, F. J., Zhang, W., & Lorenzo, J. M. (2019). A comprehensive review on lipid oxidation in meat and meat products. *Antioxidants, 8*(10), 429. https://doi.org/10.3390/antiox8100429.

Đorđević, V., Balanč, B., Belščak-Cvitanović, A., Lević, S., Trifković, K., Kalušević, A., et al. (2015). Trends in encapsulation technologies for delivery of food bioactive compounds. *Food Engineering Reviews, 7*(4), 452–490. https://doi.org/10.1007/s12393-014-9106-7.

Drabik, J., Kaźmierczak, B., Kozdrach, R., & Rogoś, E. (2023). The use of Raman spectroscopy to monitor changes in the intensity of ratio of integral unsaturated bands in bio-greases. *Molecules (Basel, Switzerland), 28*(7), 3033. https://doi.org/10.3390/molecules28073033.

Du, Q., Zhou, L., Li, M., Lyu, F., Liu, J., & Ding, Y. (2022). Omega-3 polyunsaturated fatty acid encapsulation system: Physical and oxidative stability, and medical applications. *Food Frontiers, 3*(2), 239–255. https://doi.org/10.1002/fft2.134.

El Orche, A., Bouatia, M., & Mbarki, M. (2020). Rapid analytical method to characterize the freshness of olive oils using fluorescence spectroscopy and chemometric algorithms. *Journal of Analytical Methods in Chemistry, 2020*, 1–9. https://doi.org/10.1155/2020/8860161.

Essential Oils Market Size & Share | Industry Report, 2030 [Internet]. (n.d.). Retrieved March 03, 2025 from https://www.grandviewresearch.com/industry-analysis/essential-oils-market.

FDA Releases Small Entity Compliance Guide on Omega-3 Fatty Acids Final Rule | FDA [Internet]. (n.d.). Retrieved May 10, 2025, from https://www.fda.gov/food/hfp-constituent-updates/fda-releases-small-entity-compliance-guide-omega-3-fatty-acids-final-rule.

FDA Updates "Healthy" Claim, Providing a Refreshed Tool for Consumers | FDA [Internet]. (n.d.). Retrieved May 10, 2025, from https://www.fda.gov/news-events/press-announcements/fda-updates-healthy-claim-providing-refreshed-tool-consumers.

Federal Register: Food Labeling: Nutrient Content Claims; Alpha-Linolenic Acid, Eicosapentaenoic Acid, and Docosahexaenoic Acid Omega-3 Fatty Acids [Internet]. (n.d.). Retrieved May 10, 2025, from https://www.federalregister.gov/documents/2014/04/28/2014-09492/food-labeling-nutrient-content-claims-alpha-linolenic-acid-eicosapentaenoic-acid-and-docosahexaenoic.

Fernández-Cabanás, V. M., Polvillo, O., Rodríguez-Acuña, R., Botella, B., & Horcada, A. (2011). Rapid determination of the fatty acid profile in pork dry-cured sausages by NIR spectroscopy. *Food Chemistry, 124*(1), 373–378. https://doi.org/10.1016/j.foodchem.2010.06.031.

FSSC 22000 - Delivering trust and impact for global food safety [Internet]. (n.d.). Retrieved May 10, 2025, from https://www.fssc.com/fssc-22000/.

Geng, L., Liu, K., & Zhang, H. (2023). Lipid oxidation in foods and its implications on proteins. *Frontiers Nutrition, 10*, 1192199. https://doi.org/10.3389/fnut.2023.1192199.

Ghelichi, S., Hajfathalian, M., Yesiltas, B., Sørensen, A. D. M., García-Moreno, P. J., & Jacobsen, C. (2023). Oxidation and oxidative stability in emulsions. *Comprehensive Reviews in Food Science and Food Safety, 22*(3), 1864–1901. https://doi.org/10.1111/1541-4337.13134, http://onlinelibrary.wiley.com/journal/10.1111/(ISSN)1541-4337.

Giuffrida, F., Destaillats, F., Egart, M. H., Hug, B., Golay, P. A., Skibsted, L. H., & Dionisi, F. (2007). Activity and thermal stability of antioxidants by differential scanning calorimetry and electron spin resonance spectroscopy. *Food Chemistry, 101*(3), 1108–1114. https://doi.org/10.1016/j.foodchem.2006.03.010, www.elsevier.com/locate/foodchem.

GOED I The Global Organization for EPA and DHA Omega-3s [Internet]. (n.d.). Retrieved May 10, 2025, from https://goedomega3.com/.

Goldring, C., Casini, A. F., Maellaro, E., Del Bello, B., & Comporti, M. (1993). Determination of 4-hydroxynonenal by high-performance liquid chromatography with electrochemical detection. *Lipids, 28*(2), 141–145. https://doi.org/10.1007/BF02535778.

Guidelines I CODEXALIMENTARIUS FAO-WHO [Internet]. (n.d.). Retrieved May 10, 2025, from https://www.fao.org/fao-who-codexalimentarius/codex-texts/guidelines/en/?utm.

HACCP Principles & Application Guidelines I FDA [Internet]. (n.d.). Retrieved May 10, 2025, from https://www.fda.gov/food/hazard-analysis-critical-control-point-haccp/haccp-principles-application-guidelines.

Hewavitharana, G. G., Perera, D. N., Navaratne, S. B., & Wickramasinghe, I. (2020). Extraction methods of fat from food samples and preparation of fatty acid methyl esters for gas chromatography: A review. *Arabian Journal of Chemistry, 13*(8), 6865–6875. ScienceDirect. https://doi.org/10.1016/j.arabjc.2020.06.039, http://colleges.ksu.edu.sa/Arabic%20Colleges/CollegeOfScience/ChemicalDept/AJC/default.aspx, http://www.sciencedirect.com/science/journal/18785352.

Higgins, S., Biswas, S., Goff, N. K., Septiningsih, E. M., & Kurouski, D. (2022). Raman spectroscopy enables non-invasive and confirmatory diagnostics of aluminum and iron toxicities in rice. *Frontiers in Plant Science, 13*. https://doi.org/10.3389/fpls.2022.754735, https://www.frontiersin.org/journals/plant-science.

Hocquette, J. F., Richardson, R. I., Prache, S., Medale, F., Duffy, G., & Scollan, N. D. (2005). The future trends for research on quality and safety of animal products. *Italian Journal of Animal Science, 4*(3), 49–72. https://doi.org/10.4081/ijas.2005.3s.49, http://www.aspajournal.it/atti_aspa/Session%20II.pdf.

Hong, C., Shi, M., Wang, S., Yang, Y., & Pu, Z. (2025). Novel analysis based on Raman spectroscopy in nutrition science. *Analytical Methods, 17*(9), 1977–1996. https://doi.org/10.1039/d4ay02129k.

Insights for Polyunsaturated fatty acids supplement ingredients. (n.d.). Retrieved May 09, from https://www.datainsightsmarket.com/reports/polyunsaturated-fatty-acid-supplement-ingredient-307891.

Islam, F., Imran, A., Nosheen, F., Fatima, M., Arshad, M. U., Afzaal, M., Ijaz, N., Noreen, R., Mehta, S., Biswas, S., Rasool, I. F. U., Aslam, M. A., Usman, I., Zahra, S. M., Segueni, N., & Amer Ali, Y. (2023). Functional roles and novel tools for improving-oxidative stability of polyunsaturated fatty acids: A comprehensive review. *Food Science & Nutrition, 11*(6), 2471–2482. https://doi.org/10.1002/fsn3.3272.

Islam, M., Kaczmarek, A., & Tomaszewska-Gras, J. (2023). Differential scanning calorimetry as a tool to assess the oxidation state of cold-pressed oils during shelf-life. *Journal of Food Measurement and Characterization, 17*(6), 6639–6651. https://doi.org/10.1007/s11694-023-02152-8.

Jackowski, S. A., Alvi, A. Z., Mirajkar, A., Imani, Z., Gamalevych, Y., Shaikh, N. A., & Jackowski, G. (2015). Oxidation levels of North American over-the-counter n-3 (omega-3) supplements and the influence of supplement formulation and delivery form on evaluating oxidative safety. *Journal of Nutritional Science, 4*, e30. https://doi.org/10.1017/jns.2015.21, http://journals.cambridge.org/action/displayJournal?jid=JNS.

Jayaselan, H., Nawi, N., Ismail, W., Shariff, A., Rajah, V., & Arulandoo, X. (2017). Application of spectroscopy for nutrient prediction of oil palm. *Journal of Experimental Agriculture International, 15*(3), 1–9. https://doi.org/10.9734/jeai/2017/31502.

Knutsen, H. K., Alexander, J., Barregård, L., Bignami, M., Brüschweiler, B., Ceccatelli, S., Cottrill, B., Dinovi, M., Edler, L., Grasl-Kraupp, B., Hoogenboom, L., Nebbia, C. S., Oswald, I. P., Petersen, A., Rose, M., Roudot, A. C., Schwerdtle, T., Vleminckx, C., Vollmer, G., ... Hogstrand, C. (2017). Assessment of a decontamination process for dioxins and dioxin-like PCBs in fish oil by physical filtration with activated carbon. *EFSA Journal, 15*(7). https://doi.org/10.2903/j.efsa.2017.4961, efsa.onlinelibrary.wiley.com/journal/18314732/.

Kolanowski, W. (2010a). Omega-3 LC PUFA Contents and Oxidative Stability of Encapsulated Fish Oil Dietary Supplements, [Internet].

Kolanowski, W. (2010b). Omega-3 LC PUFA contents and oxidative stability of encapsulated fish oil dietary supplements. *International Journal of Food Properties, 13*(3), 498–511. https://doi.org/10.1080/10942910802652222.

Li, Y., Ghasemi Naghdi, F., Garg, S., Adarme-Vega, T., Thurecht, K. J., Ghafor, W., Tannock, S., & Schenk, P. M. (2014). A comparative study: The impact of different lipid extraction methods on current microalgal lipid research. *Microbial Cell Factories, 13*(1), 14. https://doi.org/10.1186/1475-2859-13-14.

Ma, L., Liu, G., & Liu, X. (2019). Malondialdehyde, 4-hydroxy-2-hexenal, and 4-hydroxy-2-nonenal in vegetable oils: Formation kinetics and application as oxidation indicators. *European Journal of Lipid Science and Technology, 121*(7), 1900040. https://doi.org/10.1002/ejlt.201900040.

Maggio, R. M., Cerretani, L., Barnaba, C., & Chiavaro, E. (2012). Application of Differential Scanning Calorimetry-Chemometric Coupled Procedure to the Evaluation of Thermo-Oxidation on Extra Virgin Olive Oil. *Food Biophysics, 7*(2), 114–123. https://doi.org/10.1007/s11483-012-9248-1.

Mendonça, R., Gning, O., Di Cesaré, C., Lachat, L., Bennett, N. C., Helfenstein, F., & Glauser, G. (2017). Sensitive and selective quantifcation of free and total malondialdehyde in plasma using UHPLC-HRMS. *Journal of Lipid Research, 58*(9), 1924–1931. https://doi.org/10.1194/jlr.D076661, http://www.jlr.org/content/58/9/1924.full.pdf.

Mititelu, M., Lupuliasa, D., Neacşu, S. M., Olteanu, G., Busnatu, Ştefan S., Mihai, A., Popovici, V., Măru, N., Boroghină, S.ţa. C.ţa, Mihai, S., Ioniţă-Mîndrican, C.-B., & Scafa-Udrişte, A. (2025). Polyunsaturated fatty acids and human health: A key to modern nutritional balance in association with polyphenolic compounds from food sources. *Foods, 14*(1), 46. https://doi.org/10.3390/foods14010046.

Mostafa Abd El-Aal, H. A. H. (2012). Lipid peroxidation end-products as a key of oxidative stress: Effect of antioxidant on their production and transfer of free radicals. In A. Catala (Ed.). *Lipid peroxidation*. InTech. https://doi.org/10.5772/45944.

Murage, M. W., Muge, E. K., Mbatia, B. N., & Mwaniki, M. W. (2021). Development and sensory evaluation of omega-3-rich nile perch fish oil-fortified yogurt. *International Journal of Food Science, 2021*, 1–7. https://doi.org/10.1155/2021/8838043, http://www.hindawi.com/journals/ijfs/.

Mureşan, C. C., Marc, R. A. V., Jimborean, M., Rusu, I., Mureşan, A., Nistor, A., Cozma, A., & Suharoschi, R. (2020). Food safety system (HACCP) as quality checkpoints in a spin-off small-scale yogurt processing plant. *Sustainability, 12*(22), 9472. https://doi.org/10.3390/su12229472.

Muzolf-Panek, M., Kaczmarek, A., Tomaszewska-Gras, J., Cegielska-Radziejewska, R., Szablewski, T., Majcher, M., et al. (2020). A chemometric approach to oxidative stability and physicochemical quality of raw ground chicken meat affected by black seed and other spice extracts. *Antioxidants, 9*(9), 903. https://doi.org/10.3390/antiox9090903.

Nielsen, S. S. (Ed.). (2010). *Food analysis [Internet]*Boston, MA: Springer US.

Petersen, K. S., Maki, K. C., Calder, P. C., Belury, M. A., Messina, M., Kirkpatrick, C. F., & Harris, W. S. (2024). Perspective on the health effects of unsaturated fatty acids and commonly consumed plant oils high in unsaturated fat. *British Journal of Nutrition, 132*(8), 1039–1050. https://doi.org/10.1017/S0007114524002459, https://www.cambridge.org/core/journals/british-journal-of-nutrition/issue/D14C123362887C2EE9A7DB9363C7E6A6.

Pirsa, S., & Asadi, S. (2021). Innovative smart and biodegradable packaging for margarine based on a nano composite polylactic acid/lycopene film. *Food Additives & Contaminants: Part A, 38*(5), 856–869. https://doi.org/10.1080/19440049.2021.1891299.

Pizzimenti, S., Ciamporcero, E., Daga, M., Pettazzoni, P., Arcaro, A., Cetrangolo, G., et al. (2013). Interaction of aldehydes derived from lipid peroxidation and membrane proteins. Frontiers in Physiology, *4*. https://doi.org/10.3389/fphys.2013.00242.

Program H.F. (2025). FDA's Nutrition Initiatives. FDA.

Quality Control Management of Nutraceuticals and Dietary Supplements [Internet]. bioMérieux Website. (n.d.). Retrieved May 02, 2025, from https://www.biomerieux.com/us/en/education/resource-hub/scientific-library/food-safety-library/quality-control-management-of-nutraceuticals-and-dietary-supplements.html.

Regulation - 1924/2006 - EN - EUR-Lex [Internet]. Retrieved June 15, 2025, from https://eur-lex.europa.eu/eli/reg/2006/1924/oj/eng.

Repetto, M., Semprine, J., & Boveris, A. (2012). Lipid peroxidation: Chemical mechanism, biological implications and analytical determination. In A. Catala (Ed.). *Lipid peroxidation*. InTech. https://doi.org/10.5772/45943.

Resende, M. T., Osheter, T., Linder, C., & Wiesman, Z. (2021). Proton low Field NMR relaxation time domain sensor for monitoring of oxidation stability of PUFA-rich oils and emulsion products. *Foods, 10*(6), 1385. https://doi.org/10.3390/foods10061385.

Ristic-Medic, D., Vucic, V., Takic, M., Karadzic, I., & Glibetic, M. (2013). Polyunsaturated fatty acids in health and disease. *Journal of the Serbian Chemical Society, 78*(9), 1269–1289. https://doi.org/10.2298/jsc130402040r.

Robert G.S. (n.d.). Mechanisms of lipid oxidation [Internet]. Mechanisms of lipid oxidative fragmentation. Retrieved May 09, 2025, from https://case.edu/artsci/chem/faculty/salomon/Mechanisms.htm.

Rudy, M. D., Kainz, M. J., Graeve, M., Colombo, S. M., & Arts, M. T. (2016). Handling and storage procedures have variable effects on fatty acid content in fishes with different lipid quantities. Soengas JL, editor. *PLoS One, 11*(8), e0160497. https://doi.org/10.1371/journal.pone.0160497.

Saini, R. K., Prasad, P., Sreedhar, R. V., Akhilender Naidu, K., Shang, X., & Keum, Y.-S. (2021). Omega−3 polyunsaturated fatty acids (PUFAs): Emerging plant and microbial sources, oxidative stability, bioavailability, and health benefits—A review. *Antioxidants, 10*(10), 1627. https://doi.org/10.3390/antiox10101627.

Schroën, K., & Berton-Carabin, C. C. (2022). A unifying approach to lipid oxidation in emulsions: Modelling and experimental validation. *Food Research International, 160*, 111621. https://doi.org/10.1016/j.foodres.2022.111621.

Signal and Information Processing for Sensing Systems - Institute for Bioengineering of Catalonia- Santiago Marco Colás [Internet]. (n.d.). Retrieved May 10, 2025, from https://ibecbarcelona.eu/ca/sensingsys.

Smart, A., Crew, A., Doran, O., & Hart, J. P. (2023). Development of a novel dual-enzyme screen-printed amperometric biosensor for the analysis of esterified fatty acids. *Journal of Food Composition and Analysis, 122*, 105488. https://doi.org/10.1016/j.jfca.2023.105488.

Stoffel, W., Schmidt-Soltau, I., Binczek, E., Thomas, A., Thevis, M., & Wegner, I. (2020). Dietary ω3-and ω6-Polyunsaturated fatty acids reconstitute fertility of Juvenile and adult Fads2-Deficient mice. *Molecular Metabolism, 36*, 100974. https://doi.org/10.1016/j.molmet.2020.100974.

Surmacki, J. M., Quiros-Gonzalez, I., & Bohndiek, S. E. (2022). Evaluation of label-free confocal Raman microspectroscopy for monitoring oxidative stress in vitro in live human cancer cells. *Antioxidants, 11*(3), 573. https://doi.org/10.3390/antiox11030573.

Tańska, M., Roszkowska, B., Skrajda, M., & Dąbrowski, G. (2016). Commercial cold pressed flaxseed oils quality and oxidative stability at the beginning and the end of their shelf life. *Journal of Oleo Science, 65*(2), 111–121. https://doi.org/10.5650/jos.ess15243.

Tao, L. Department of Animal Science, Cornell University, Ithaca, NY, USA. (2015). Oxidation of polyunsaturated fatty acids and its impact on food quality and human health. *Advances in Food Technology and Nutritional Sciences – Open Journal, 1*(6), 135–142. https://doi.org/10.17140/AFTNSOJ-1-123.

Teixeira-Costa, B. E., & Andrade, C. T. (2022). Natural polymers used in edible food packaging—History, function and application trends as a sustainable alternative to synthetic plastic. *Polysaccharides, 3*(1), 32–58. https://doi.org/10.3390/polysaccharides3010002, https://www.mdpi.com/journal/polysaccharides.

The State of Food Security and Nutrition in the World FAO. (2022). https://doi.org/10.4060/cc0639en.

Tian, F., Decker, E. A., & Goddard, J. M. (2013). Controlling lipid oxidation of food by active packaging technologies. *Food & Function, 4*(5), 669. https://doi.org/10.1039/c3fo30360h.

Tocher, D. R., Betancor, M. B., Sprague, M., Olsen, R. E., & Napier, J. A. (2019). Omega-3 long-chain polyunsaturated fatty acids, EPA and DHA: Bridging the gap between supply and demand. *Nutrients, 11*(1), 89. https://doi.org/10.3390/nu11010089, https://www.mdpi.com/2072-6643/11/1/89/pdf.

Tulimaa, T. (2022). *Product quality management in the procurement of italian olive oil*. South Eastern Finland University of Applied Sciences, 1–45.

Uematsu, M., & Shimizu, T. (2021). Raman microscopy-based quantification of the physical properties of intracellular lipids. *Communications Biology, 4*(1), 1176. https://doi.org/10.1038/s42003-021-02679-w.

van de Voort, F. R., Ismail, A. A., Sedman, J., & Emo, G. (1994). Monitoring the oxidation of edible oils by Fourier transform infrared spectroscopy. *Journal of the American Oil Chemists' Society, 71*(3), 243–253. https://doi.org/10.1007/BF02638049.

Venugopalan, V. K., Gopakumar, L. R., Kumaran, A. K., Chatterjee, N. S., Soman, V., Peeralil, S., Mathew, S., McClements, D. J., & Nagarajarao, R. C. (2021). Encapsulation and protection of omega-3-rich fish oils using food-grade delivery systems. *Foods, 10*(7). https://doi.org/10.3390/foods10071566, https://www.mdpi.com/2304-8158/10/7/1566/pdf.

Wang, P., Huang, J., Sun, J., Liu, R., Jiang, T., & Sun, G. (2022). Evaluating the nutritional properties of food: A scoping review. *Nutrients, 14*(11), 2352. https://doi.org/10.3390/nu14112352.

Wani, S. A., Elshikh, M. S., Al-Wahaibi, M. S., & Naik, H. R. (2023). *Functional foods: Technological challenges and advancement in health promotion functional foods: Technological challenges and advancement in health promotion*. India: CRC Press, 1–339. http://doi.org/10.1201/9781003315100, https://www.taylorfrancis.com/books/edit/10.1201/9781003315100/functional-foods-sajad-ahmad-wani-mohamed-elshikh-mona-al-wahaibi-haroon-rashid-naik?context=ubx&refId=54d5528e-c8f5-4478-8ef6-fa243e1cab6a.

Wrona, M., Lours, J., Salafranca, J., Joly, C., & Nerín, C. (2023). Innovative surface-enhanced raman spectroscopy method as a fast tool to assess the oxidation of lipids in ground pork. *Applied Sciences, 13*(9), 5533. https://doi.org/10.3390/app13095533.

Zhou, Q., Jia, X., Deng, Q., Chen, H., Tang, H., & Huang, F. (2019). Quality evaluation of rapeseed oil in Chinese traditional stir-frying. *Food Science & Nutrition, 7*(11), 3731–3741. https://doi.org/10.1002/fsn3.1232.

Chapter 21

Market trends and opportunities in the polyunsaturated fatty acid food industry

Devanampriyan Rajan[1], Sankari Rajan[1], Kalaivani Sundaravadivelu[1], and Rakesh Kumar Gupta[2]

[1]*Department of Food Technology, Kongu Engineering College, Erode, Tamil Nadu, India,* [2]*Agricultural and Food Engineering Department, Indian Institute of Technology, Kharagpur, West Bengal, India*

21.1 Introduction and overview of polyunsaturated fatty acid food systems

Polyunsaturated fatty acids (PUFAs) were considered to be the vital dietary source essential for overall health, distinguishing themselves from saturated fats by their involvement in several fundamental biological processes. Essential fats have been incorporated into the phospholipids inside the cell membranes, where they influence fluidity flow, and functionality of the embedded proteins. Furthermore, PUFAs are crucial for physiological regulation, contributing significantly to blood pressure control and coagulation with are responsible for the functioning of the human nervous system, including being critical for infant brain and nervous system development (e.g., docosahexaenoic acid [DHA]). Since it cannot be synthesized by our human body, which are classified as the essential fatty acids (EFAs), as omega-3 and omega-6, being alpha-linolenic acid (ALA), eicosapentaenoic acid (EPA), and DHA (Mititelu et al., 2025). PUFAs were crucial for the overall well-being by actively contributing to the maintenance and protection of major organ systems, including the brain, nerves, and eyes. Furthermore, their benefits support several chronic conditions, such as cardiovascular fat reduction, neurodegenerative disorders, as well as various inflammatory diseases (Mukherjee et al., 2024). These adverse conditions span multiple organ systems and include dermatitis, renal hypertension, and mitochondrial dysfunction. Furthermore, this deficiency can elevate the risk of Type II diabetes. The lack of these essential fats also severely impacts neurological and immunological health, leading to impaired brain development, arthritis, depression, and reduced immune resistance to infections (Mukherjee et al., 2024). A review on plant-based sources of PUFA states that the sources of PUFAs include flaxseeds (high in ALA, 39%–64% of total fat) and soybean oil. Promising novel sources for long-chain omega-3 PUFAs are algae, microorganisms, stearidonic acid (SDA)-rich plants, and genetically modified (GM) plants (Rizzo et al., 2023). The PUFAs were produced from waste sources by cultivating the microorganism *Aurantiochytrium* sp. strain L3W, a thraustochytrid which obtained from eight different sources, such as sake lees, Japanese mustard spinach leaves, lemon peels, Hiroshimana old pickle, soy sauce residue, crown daisy, orange peel, and grape skin, as well as liquid wastes from udon-type noodle boiling waste water on top layer and pickle seasoning liquid type waste were separated (Rizzo et al., 2023). Generally, in the food industry, PUFA-based functional foods and nutraceuticals were major market products with high commercial value. Furthermore, it extends to applications such as animal feed and aquaculture applications.

This chapter covers the commercial realities of the PUFA landscape, beginning with a detailed market overview that identifies key industry players and the dynamic competitive environment. This analysis will set the stage for exploring the common driving factors, such as consumer health awareness, the urgent need for sustainable sourcing methods, and continuous technological advancements. Furthermore, this chapter examines emerging trends and innovations, highlighting the shift toward plant-based sources like algae, the role of nanoencapsulation in enhancing product quality, and the expansion of applications in functional foods and customized fortification. Finally, providing a comprehensive look at sophisticated processing technologies, including novel delivery systems and stability enhancements that underpin product development, culminating in a strategic SWOT analysis and a forward-looking perspective on the future direction of PUFA food systems.

Omega-3 and Omega-6 Polyunsaturated Fatty Acids in Food Systems. DOI: https://doi.org/10.1016/B978-0-443-43810-3.00009-9

21.2 Market overview, industry players, and landscape

The global PUFAs market has emerged as a dynamic segment within the broader functional food, nutrition, and health supplement industry (Toopcham et al., 2021). It can be increased starting from USD 3824.9 million in 2025, close to USD 6913.8 million by 2035 at a compound annual growth rate of 6.1%. This growth mainly increases the consumer demand for omega-fortified nutrition products, robust clinical validation of the EFAs such as EPA, DHA, ALA, linoleic acid (LA), and arachidonic acid (AA), and incorporation of PUFAs in functional foods, dietary supplements, and algal/marine oil production processes (Future Market Insights, 2025; Kumar & Sharma, 2023). Omega-3 fatty acids currently dominate the market with approximately 79.3% share, led by DHA and EPA, which are key ingredients in infant formulas, cardiovascular supplements, and fortified food products (Simopoulos, 2022). Omega-6 fatty acids constitute the remaining 20.7%, supported by growing applications of LA and AA, especially in infant nutrition (Calder, 2020). Marine-derived sources constitute about 37.2% of the market supply, with plant sources contributing the majority share (62.8%) (Toopcham et al., 2021). The supplement and functional food sectors represent the largest application segments, accounting for 37.3% of PUFA demand, followed by pet animal feed and infant nutrition segments (Future Market Insights, 2025).

It has a diverse portfolio of multinational corporations alongside regionally important players. Leading global manufacturers include BASF, DSM-Firmenich, Cargill, Archer Daniels Midland, Epax AS, Omega Protein Corporation, and Aker BioMarine, each investing heavily in product innovation, sustainability certifications, and advanced refining technologies (Kumar & Sharma, 2023). These entities primarily focus on marine-derived sources of omega-3 fatty acids such as EPA and DHA, refining fish oil (FO) and algal oil through fermentation to sustain supply and premium positioning (Simopoulos, 2022). Concurrently, Indian companies such as Gangwal Healthcare, Ennature Biopharma, Arjuna Natural, and Blue Line Foods are strengthening local supply chains and expanding capacity for both marine- and plant-based PUFA products (Future Market Insights, 2025). This segment remains fragmented, with varied specialization in formulation stability, purity optimization, and value-added PUFA derivatives. Within this competitive landscape, companies are differentiating through proprietary extraction and encapsulation technologies, sustainability certifications (e.g., MSC, IFFO-RS), and targeting growth in pharmaceutical, infant nutrition, and clinical nutrition segments to capture higher-margin opportunities (Calder, 2020).

Geographically, North America and Europe lead adoption due to mature markets and regulatory frameworks, while East Asia and South Asia Pacific emerge as the fastest-growing regions, fueled by demographic trends and expanding infant formula markets (Kumar & Sharma, 2023; Toopcham et al., 2021). The increasing focus on sustainability, clean-label products, and infant nutrition regulations continues to favor premium, high-purity PUFA concentrates, including algal-derived omega-3 oils and biotech-enabled plant oils (Simopoulos, 2022). For example, East Asia prioritizes infant formula fortification and marine algal oil adoption, while India focuses on accessible plant-based PUFA formulations to meet rising cardiovascular health awareness (Future Market Insights, 2025). Major challenges like raw material pricing volatility, stringent regulatory frameworks, and high processing costs were dominant in the food industry. Sustainability considerations drive a shift toward traceable and carbon-neutral sourcing, underpinning long-term competitive advantages in the evolving PUFA marketplace (Calder, 2020). Table 21.1 shows the market players with their special grades.

21.3 Common driving factors in the polyunsaturated fatty acid industry

The primary driver for the PUFA industry is the well-established protective health benefits of omega-3s (EPA and DHA) against metabolic and chronic diseases, which, coupled with the rising global incidence of these conditions, fuels massive consumer demand. This high nutritional and commercial importance necessitates the continuous exploration and exploitation of **diverse, sustainable production sources,** including plants, microalgae, macroalgae, and thraustochytrids (Saini et al., 2021).

21.3.1 Consumer health awareness and demand

Driven by the persistent and increasing prevalence of diet-related chronic illnesses and associated comorbidities globally, consumers are exhibiting a marked shift toward proactive health management. This involves a deliberate prioritization of healthy lifestyles, particularly emphasizing the crucial and recognized role of nutritional intake ((Gutierres et al., 2025). The growing awareness of the a crucial role of PUFAs in maintaining human health contrasts with the established effects associated with the saturated fat intake still common in modern food systems. Dietary intakes to increase PUFA consumption are often recommended and found in synergy with polyphenols in traditional food sources (Mititelu et al., 2024).

TABLE 21.1 Market overview of industry players with their specialty grades.

Company	Category	Primary PUFA types	Key sources	Specialty grade PUFA	Refrences
BASF (Germany)	Global	Omega-3 (EPA, DHA)	Marine (fish/algal), plant	High-purity concentrates, sustainability certifications (MSC), pharma-grade	Kumar and Sharma (2023)
DSM-Firmenich (Netherlands)	Global	Omega-3 (EPA, DHA), omega-6 (LA)	Marine, plant (canola/sunflower)	Marine refining, algal fermentation, infant nutrition blends	Toopcham et al. (2021)
Cargill (USA)	Global	Omega-3 (EPA, DHA), omega-6 (LA, ALA)	Marine, plant (canola, sunflower)	Bulk supply for supplements/functional foods, plant oil refining	Kumar and Sharma (2023)
ADM (USA)	Global	Omega-6 (LA), omega-3 (ALA)	Plant-dominant (canola, sunflower, flaxseed)	Plant-based oils, fortified foods, cooking oils	Kumar and Sharma (2023)
Epax AS (Norway)	Global	Omega-3 (EPA, DHA)	Marine (fish oil [FO])	High-concentration marine EPA/DHA, cardiovascular supplements	Simopoulos (2022)
Omega Protein Corp. (USA)	Global	Omega-3 (EPA, DHA)	Marine (FO)	FO refining, pet feed, functional foods	Calder (2020)
Aker BioMarine (Norway)	Global	Omega-3 (EPA, DHA)	Marine (krill oil)	Krill phospholipids, enhanced absorption supplements	Rizzo et al. (2023)
Golden Omega (Chile)	Global	Omega-3 (EPA, DHA)	Marine (FO)	South American FO, sustainability-focused	Oliver et al. (2020)
Zhoushan Sinomega (China)	Global	Omega-3 (EPA, DHA)	Marine (fish/algal)	East Asia marine production, infant formulas	Lenihan-Geels et al. (2013)
Cellana Inc. (USA)	Global	Omega-3 (DHA)	Algal	Vegan algal DHA, infant nutrition	Adeyomoye et al. (2023)
Arista Industries (USA)	Global	Omega-3 (EPA, DHA), omega-6	Marine, plant	Blends for supplements, oxidative stability	Future Market Insights (2025)
Gangwal Healthcare	Indian	Omega-3 (EPA, DHA), omega-6 (LA)	Marine, plant	Nutraceuticals, distribution partnerships	Saini et al. (2021)
Ennature Biopharma	Indian	Omega-3 (DHA), algal oils	Algal, marine	Biotech algal fermentation, vegan products	Lenihan-Geels et al. (2013)
Arjuna Natural	Indian	Omega-3 (ALA), omega-6 (LA)	Plant (flaxseed, others)	Herbal extracts, plant-based supplements	Rizzo et al. (2023)
Blue Line Foods	Indian	Omega-3 (EPA, DHA)	Marine (FO)	Fishmeal/oil, pet feed, industrial	Oliver et al. (2020)
Mukka Proteins	Indian	Omega-3 (EPA, DHA)	Marine (FO)	FO processing, regional supply	Calder (2020)

Global demand for PUFAs has intensified significantly, driven by their widely recognized role in promoting diet and human health. This escalating awareness and the diverse essential applications of PUFAs—spanning aquafeed, superfoods, and therapeutic medical formulations targeting diseases like cancer, cardiovascular disease, and diabetes—have created an immense need for a reliable supply. Consequently, interest has surged in microbial cell biotechnologies as a critical and sustainable solution capable of producing the necessary quantities of PUFAs to meet this burgeoning global demand (Adeyomoye et al., 2023). Demand is driven by long-chain polyunsaturated fatty acids (LC-PUFAs), which are key components for nutritional and pharmacological applications (Saikia & Diganta, 2023).

However, challenges such as declining natural fish catches, and climatic changes threaten the PUFA supply chain, highlighting the demand for sustainable substitute sources such as zoospore microorganisms, to meet the increasing market demand effectively (Saikia & Diganta, 2023). Traditional sources such as fish and FO have been directly used for supplying these EFAs (which humans cannot synthesize), as they are now insufficient to meet global needs and are severely threatened by overexploitation. This crisis in supply is driving the urgent exploration of novel and sustainable alternatives (Demets & Foubert, 2021).

21.3.2 Advances in sustainable sourcing

The omega-3 fatty acids, such as EPA and DHA have led to research focusing on three main nonfish alternatives: microalgae and other microorganisms, GM plants, and SDA-rich plants. Microalgae (like *Schizochytrium*) and microbes (like engineered yeasts) are cultivated in bioreactors with high yields, and GM crops (like engineered *Camelina sativa*) produce omega-3-rich oil in their seeds using genes from these microbes, offering a scalable agricultural solution. Finally, SDA-rich plants (like Ahiflower) provide a precursor that is more efficiently converted to EPA by the body than the standard precursor, bypassing a key metabolic limitation. Microalgae, which are photosynthetic single-celled organisms, were increasingly a primary source of PUFA. They are cultivated in the bioreactors for scalable and high-yield production (20%–50% dry weight total fat), and species like *Schizochytrium* and *Crypthecodinium* are already commercially used to fortify foods, including infant formula. Furthermore, algal oil is considered a safer alternative to FO due to a lower risk of pollutant contamination (Rizzo et al., 2023). SDA, a promising plant-based alternative, is found in oils like *Buglossoides arvensis* (Ahiflower). SDA is efficiently converted to EPA within the body, suggesting it can deliver comparable health benefits across immunity, brain function, and intestinal microbial health. This makes SDA-rich oils an eco-friendly, sustainable, and dependable omega-3 supplementation option for clinicians and health-conscious consumers (Baker et al., 2025). Research on developing and deregulating genetically engineered oilseed crops to serve as a renewable, terrestrial source for obtaining omega-3 LC-PUFAs was complex, requiring two decades of work to introduce biosynthetic pathways that produce FO equivalent profiles with nutrient content and an optimal omega-3/omega-6 ratio. Despite regulatory challenges associated with these novel traits, some engineered crops approved for large-scale cultivation and incorporation into food and feed have positioned these crops as a safe, cost-efficient, and scalable solution capable of meeting rising demands in aquaculture and human nutrition with favorable health, economic, and environmental impacts (Zhou et al., 2023).

A study identifies crop-derived PUFAs as an environmentally sustainable solution to meet the rising worldwide demands of essential lipids. The core sustainable strategy detailed is the use of genetic engineering in crop development in biotechnology, which leverages the advancement and application of genetic engineering techniques within genomics and molecular biology to understand and manipulate the complex biochemical pathways of lipid metabolism in plants. This knowledge allows researchers to engineer transgenic oil crops with improved or tailored fatty acid compositions, specifically engineering plants to produce nutritionally improved oils characterized by significantly increased PUFA levels (ALA, gamma-linolenic acid) that are beneficial for human health. This approach aims to create new, improved varieties of oil crops that offer unique qualities for both food production and industrial applications, thereby providing a plant-based, sustainable alternative (Assefa et al., 2025).

21.3.3 Technological innovations in extraction and delivery systems

21.3.3.1 Supercritical fluid extraction

The study highlights supercritical CO_2 ($scCO_2$) processing as a compelling alternative technology for extracting n-3 PUFAs, especially in the context of valorizing fish by-products. The key advantages of using $scCO_2$ over conventional methods are that it allows the replacement of toxic organic solvents, operates under milder processing conditions (which helps preserve the quality of the delicate lipids), and creates an inert atmosphere that significantly reduces the risk of oxidation of the easily degradable omega-3 PUFAs. Commercial omega-3 concentrates frequently exhibit limitations in purity and bioavailability and are highly susceptible to oxidation. These persistent quality issues are the primary factors driving the industry's search for more efficient and advanced extraction methods, concentration, and final formulation of the target compounds (Melgosa et al., 2021).

The supercritical fluid extraction (SFE) of microalgae, such as *Nannochloropsis* sp., utilizes supercritical CO_2 ($scCO_2$). While $scCO_2$ has low polarity, adding cosolvents like n-hexane significantly increases its solvating power for a broader range of extraction. This combined method, in studies on *N. oculata* successfully doubled the EPA yield and nearly doubled the total PUFA content relative to saturated fatty acids (SFAs). Furthermore, the SFE process can be precisely tailored to isolate specific omega-3 fatty acids: higher pressures and temperatures (550 bar, 75°C) maximize EPA yield, while milder conditions (400 bar, 50°C) are optimal for DHA recovery (Sousa et al., 2023).

21.3.3.2 Ultrasound-assisted extraction

Ultrasound-assisted extraction (UAE) disrupts cell walls through cavitation, a process where ultrasound waves create and collapse vacuum bubbles, generating intense shearing forces and liquid jets that mechanically break cell structures. This mechanism improves extraction yields by reducing particle size, increasing solvent-compound contact, and enhancing mass transfer, ultimately leading to reduced solvent usage and shorter extraction times at lower temperatures (Sousa et al., 2023). UAE demonstrates significant superiority over conventional methods like Soxhlet extraction for the production of omega-3 PUFAs from traditional sources, including fish waste. Under optimized conditions, UAE achieved a high oil extraction yield of 45.11% (g/g freeze-dried fish waste). The quality of the extracted FO was markedly improved, featuring 39.41% omega-3 fatty acids and 45.21% total PUFA content (g/g extracted oil). Compared with the Soxhlet extraction, UAE showed a remarkable 90.50% efficiency in oil extraction, leading to enhanced omega-3 and total PUFA while significantly decreasing SFA content ($p < 0.05$). Furthermore, the oil obtained via UAE exhibited enhanced oxidative stability, confirmed by better values for onset time, acidity, peroxide, p-anisidine, and total oxidation, signifying an overall improved oil quality (Ciftci & Çavdar, 2025). When ultrasound applied to microalgae like *Nannochloropsis* sp., UAE often operates at frequencies like 20 or 37 kHz. Combining UAE with switchable hydrophilicity solvents significantly damages cell walls, achieving high lipid extraction efficiency (up to 98.2%) and increasing EPA content. Furthermore, UAE enhances enzymatic extraction by increasing total lipid yields and specifically improving the content of polar lipids; for example, using an ultrasound probe with ethanol on *N. oceanica* enhanced the recovery of total PUFA and EPA by 47% and 35%, respectively, compared to ethanol alone (Sousa et al., 2023). See Fig. 21.1 shows the ultrasound extraction process.

21.3.3.3 Microwave-assisted extraction

Microwave-assisted extraction (MAE) was initially employed in experiments to evaluate its effectiveness for recovering DHA and other PUFAs from *Crypthecodinium cohnii* biomass, utilizing various solvents, including organic and food-grade options like n-hexane, 2-butanol, and an n-hexane:isopropanol (2:3) mixture. However, in comparison with other tested methods, MAE did not prove to be the most efficient technique; instead, UAE, particularly when using n-hexane:isopropanol (2:3) and 2-butanol, delivered higher extraction rates, leading the researchers to select and further optimize UAE rather than MAE in subsequent experiments (Stramarkou et al., 2021). The application of low temperature microwave-ultrasound-assisted extraction significantly improved the obtainment of PUFAs from tomato seed oil, resulting in a 30.91% increase in PUFA content, notably LA, compared to the conventional Soxhlet method. This combined

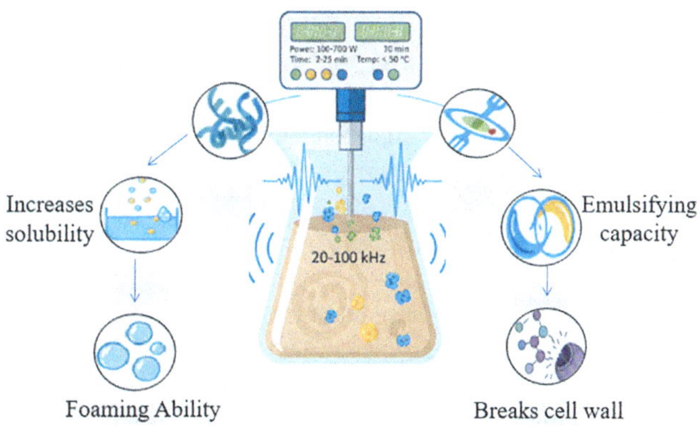

FIGURE 21.1 Ultrasound extraction methods processing (pictures were self-made).

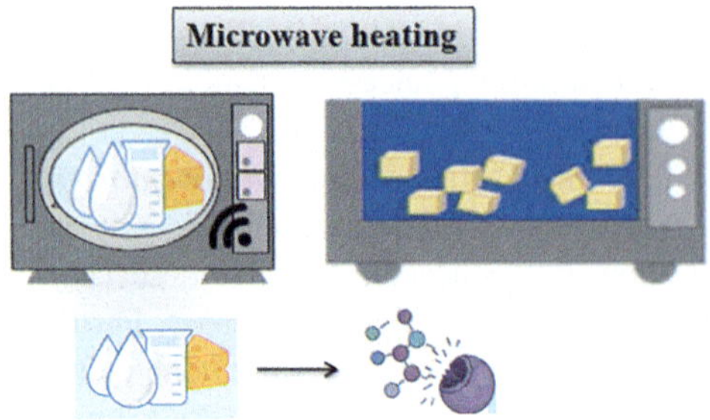

FIGURE 21.2 Microwave extraction methods and processing.

technique also successfully enhanced both the overall oil quality and yield (Kumar et al., 2023). The MAE-brine method leverages the high polarity of water, with salt present in the 10% brine medium, to significantly absorb microwave energy. This process improves the dielectric loss, which efficiently converts microwave energy into heat, leading to increased microalgae cell disruption. This enhanced cell wall breakdown is crucial because it promotes the release of PUFAs, which are regarded as the primary constituents of microalgal polar lipids, including glycolipids and phospholipids. Furthermore, minimal extraction time in MAE is advantageous, as it helps preserve thermolabile (Zghaibi et al., 2019). See Fig. 21.2 shows the microwave extraction methods and processing.

21.3.3.4 Enzyme-assisted extraction

The green technology of enzyme-assisted extraction (EAE) is utilized to break the cell walls of microalgae like *Nannochloropsis* sp., promoting the release of PUFAs by breaking down complex polysaccharides using enzymes such as cellulase, laccase, hemicellulase, papain, pectinase, and mannase. The efficacy of EAE is heavily reliant on the optimization of parameters like enzyme ratio, pH, temperature, and reaction time. Successful implementation has been demonstrated, with cellulase alone achieving a high lipid yield of 88.70% and an extracted oil composition containing 19.91% PUFA. Additionally, combining cellulase and mannanase resulted in 73% total lipid recovery, although the released lipids usually require a subsequent extraction step using solvents such as ethanol or n-hexane:2-propanol for full recovery (Sousa et al., 2023).

A study reveals that characterization of Nile tilapia waste, which was found to have a significant 30.3% lipid content, confirming its suitability for oil recovery and subsequent PUFA enrichment. The enrichment of PUFAs was achieved using lipases sourced from *Pseudomonas fluorescens* and *Thermomyces lanuginosa*. Enzymatic concentration significantly improved the oil's nutritional profile, yielding a high final PUFA percentage of 59.0% and a beneficial n-6/n-3 fatty acid ratio of 1.2, while the concentrated Nile tilapia waste oil (TWO) maintained acceptable peroxide and acid values for human consumption. Specifically, the optimization focused on enriching EPA and DHA; the increased accumulation of EPA + DHA (6.0%) was achieved using 0.1 g of immobilized *T. lanuginosa* lipase per 2 g of oil after an 18-hour reaction process duration, outperforming the 4.0% content obtained under similar conditions with *P. fluorescens* lipase (Sangkharak et al., 2020).

21.3.3.5 Delivery systems in polyunsaturated fatty acid

Delivery systems for omega-3 PUFA are vital because PUFAs readily undergo lipid oxidation, compromising their nutritional value, creating off-flavors, and generating toxic aldehydes during processing and digestion. The controlled-release systems discussed include both low-fat and high-fat emulsions, whose oxidative stability can be influenced by the choice of emulsifiers. Additionally, the technique of microencapsulation is employed to protect FO; this is achieved through various encapsulation techniques like spray drying and electro spraying, where the choice of encapsulating materials is crucial for controlling the oxidative stability of the final delivery system (Jacobsen et al., 2022). The novel delivery system for essential long-chain n-3 PUFAs (like EPA and DHA) from FO is built upon Complexes formed by sodium caseinate (SC) and phosphatidylcholine (PC) liposomes carrying FO, delivering n-3 and n-6 PUFAs in equal mass amounts. This system, which can optionally include the plant antioxidant clove bud essential oil for enhanced protection, is characterized by nanosized and spherical-shaped particles. These complexes exhibit complete solubility in an aqueous environment (pH 7.0, 0.001 M ionic strength), substantial encapsulation capacity (SC retaining up to 70% of liposomes), and strong antioxidant protection, preventing up to 96% of lipid oxidation throughout 20 days of light-exposed storage at ambient temperature (Semenova et al., 2022).

An advanced move toward precision delivery is described through three main types of carrier systems. Nanoencapsulation and nanoliposomes rely on lipid-based structures that resemble natural cell membranes, enabling PUFAs to pass efficiently through the gastrointestinal barrier. To provide stronger protection against harsh digestive conditions, Pickering emulsions use solid particles, such as cellulose nanocrystals, to form a protective barrier that withstands stomach acid and preserves the active compounds until they reach the small intestine for regulated release. In addition, chitosan-based nanoparticles are presented as a targeted approach for colon delivery. these systems are designed to stay intact in the upper digestive tract and degrade only in response to specific gut microbiota, making them especially suitable for treating inflammatory bowel conditions (Zhu et al., 2025).

The nanoencapsulation of omega-3 PUFAs utilizes hexosomes that were formulated using omega-3 PUFA monoglycerides. These hexosomal nanocarriers, which belong to a class of nano-self-assemblies known for their well-defined nanostructures and lower viscosity compared to bulk liquid crystalline phases, are considered highly promising delivery systems due to the known health benefits of omega-3 lipids. They are versatile, capable of delivering omega-3 PUFAs as a standalone ingredient or in combination with other nutritional compounds, owing to their high capacity to solubilize various food additives (hydrophilic, amphiphilic, and hydrophobic molecules) and their capacity to provide sustained release of these nutritional compounds (Yaghmur, 2019). Future research into drug delivery systems (DDS) for omega-3 PUFAs is fundamental. The focus must be on overcoming current challenges like low bioavailability and high oxidation susceptibility while simultaneously maximizing therapeutic benefits. This goal requires the development and optimization of advanced encapsulation techniques, with a particular emphasis on utilizing metal-organic framework nanoparticles (Gill et al., 2024).

21.3.4 Regulatory support and health claims

Global health organizations, including the WHO, recommend a daily dietary intake of n-3 PUFAs, specifically EPA and DHA, generally ranging from 250 to 1000 mg, with 500 mg/day being the most common recommended dose. Supporting the expansion of these nutrients, microalgae-derived DHA and arachidonic acid (ARA) oils received and recognized as Generally Recognized As Safe by the US Food and Drug Administration (FDA) in 2001, allowing their use in infant formulae and marking the first commercially successful food product fortified with microalgae-derived n-3 PUFAs; furthermore, supplements from species like *Schizochytrium* sp. have been granted FDA approval for use in humans. Despite these regulatory successes and widespread interest, the scientific literature presents inconsistencies in the dose-dependent contribution of EPA and DHA to inflammatory regulation and cardiovascular health and in establishing optimal dosages for diverse population groups (Liu et al., 2022).

The deregulation of transgenic crops with novel nutritional characteristics, such as omega-3 LC-PUFAs, faces significant regulatory challenges. Crucially, despite these hurdles, some oilseed crops engineered for the production of omega-3 LC-PUFAs have already achieved successful regulatory approval for large-scale cultivation and are cleared and suitable for incorporation into animal feed as well as human food, confirming that viable regulatory pathways for these innovative agricultural products exist and have been successfully navigated. The study also suggests that these issues could be better addressed through the adoption of a more trait-based regulatory approach (Zhou et al., 2023).

PUFAs, including omega-3 fatty acids, DHA, and EPA, are subject to specific regulatory permissions for nutrition claims. General nutrition content claims permitted include being products can be labelled as *"high in polyunsaturated fats"* or as a *"source of omega-3 fatty acids."* In the European Union, certain health claims are permitted. For example, EFAs can be claimed to support normal growth in children. DHA has additional allowed claims, such as supporting normal visual and brain development in infants, and benefiting maternal intake during pregnancy and breastfeeding. Both DHA and EPA can be linked to the maintenance of normal heart function, often in association with omega-3 claims on fish and fish products (Harland & Sanders, 2024). An authorized EU health claim supports that the substituting SFAs with unsaturated fatty acids, including PUFAs, supports the maintenance of normal blood cholesterol, a conclusion based on metaanalytic evidence. However, future efforts in both practical implementation and the development of new claims are expected to shift focus toward more stable cardiovascular health markers beyond just cholesterol (Livingstone, 2014).

21.4 Emerging trends and innovations

The shift toward algal-based vegan DHA/EPA growing demand for sustainable, allergen-free, and vegan nutrition is accelerating the shift toward algal-derived DHA and EPA. Algal fermentation provides consistent, high-purity omega-3 concentrates without reliance on marine ecosystems, enabling formulators to meet clean-label expectations and environmental commitments (Oliver et al., 2020). Rising adoption of plant-forward diets across Europe, North America, and Asia is strengthening interest in vegan DHA for fortified beverages, infant formulas, cognitive-health supplements, and premixes. Algal oils offer superior stability, controlled fatty acid profiles, and easier regulatory management for infant and clinical nutrition products. As consumers increasingly prioritize sustainability, traceability, and ethical sourcing, algal-based omega-3s are rapidly emerging as premium alternatives to fish and krill oils across global markets (Lenihan-Geels et al., 2013).

The adoption of microencapsulated PUFA formats is increasing across functional foods, beverages, and nutritional supplements by improving oxidative stability, flavor neutrality, and shelf life (Venugopalan et al., 2021). Encapsulated EPA, DHA, ALA, and LA provide superior protection against heat, moisture, and oxidation, enabling seamless incorporation into RTD beverages, bakery products, dairy alternatives, bars, powdered mixes, and infant nutrition formulations (Anwar, 2011). Manufacturers are adopting spray-drying, complex coacervation, liposomal systems, and starch- or protein-based encapsulation to enhance bioavailability while preventing off-flavors typically associated with marine oils. This technology is enabling PUFA inclusion in clean-label applications and broadening use beyond traditional softgels (Muhoza et al., 2023). As demand for convenient, fortified, and taste-optimized nutrition grows, encapsulated PUFAs are becoming a core innovation driver for both food and supplement manufacturers (Venugopalan et al., 2021).

The rise of personalized PUFA-based nutrition and diets is increasingly integrating omega-3 and omega-6 profiling into tailored health solutions targeting cardiometabolic wellness, cognitive function, inflammation management, and hormone balance (Nilsson et al., 2012). At-home blood testing, genetic screening, and AI-driven diet analysis are enabling brands to deliver individualized EPA/DHA ratios, ALA/LA recommendations, and customized PUFA blends. Brands are also developing subscription-based PUFA supplement programs for seniors, athletes, women's health, and individuals with specific dietary patterns (Pokushalov et al., 2024; Smith et al., 2015). With rising consumer interest in quantifiable health outcomes and precision nutrition, PUFA suppliers are collaborating with digital-health companies, D2C wellness brands, and clinical nutrition platforms to deliver differentiated, evidence-backed offerings. This trend reinforces the shift from generic PUFA supplements to science-guided, personalized lipid solutions (Blomquist et al., 2025).

Manufacturers are increasingly producing high-concentration PUFA blends formulated for targeted health outcomes, such as heart health, prenatal care, cognitive support, and antiinflammatory benefits (Nicholls and Lincoff, 2020). These blends combine optimized ratios of EPA, DHA, ALA, LA, and AA to meet the needs of specialized segments across infant nutrition, clinical care, sports nutrition, and aging populations (Troesch et al., 2020). Advances in molecular distillation, enzymatic concentration, and fermentation technologies allow suppliers to deliver precise fatty acid profiles while maintaining purity and stability. This shift toward outcome-specific PUFA blends is strengthening product differentiation and elevating the functional value of PUFA-enriched products (Swetha & Mathanghi, 2024).

21.5 Processing technologies and product development

Biomass particles are extracted using the solvents, which make the oil more consistent. Extraction of the oil process involves cold pressing, blending, pulverization, defatting and extraction. The most widely used solvents include chloroform, methanol, propanol and multicomponent solvent system. Green solvent technologies have been widely utilized for the extraction due to the nature of solvent chemistry. Terpenes have been widely used for the extraction of biomaterials from pine trees and other algal species (Sati et al., 2019). The supercritical extraction method is an advanced and secure technology that can serve for the extraction and refinement of PUFAs from microbial and algal biomass under the maintained temperature and pressure conditions (Li et al., 2019).

21.5.1 Stability and bioavailability enhancements

Adding vegan, PUFA-rich seed oils to foods can help our bodies absorb these fats and make them more stable against oxidation. Oils like olive, corn, safflower, and sunflower are especially rich PUFAs. This makes them more stable during cooking and storage, giving them good resistance to heat and oxidation (Zuk et al., 2015). It is hard to produce foods enriched with DHA and EPA, because these n-3 fatty acids breakdown easily when exposed to oxidation (Colombo et al., 2020). It can reduce the nutritional value of foods by destroying important fatty acids and fat-soluble vitamins like A, D, E, and K, and it can also lower the overall calorie content. Oxidation causes rancidity, which leads to unpleasant flavors and strong odors (Shahidi & Hossain, 2022). Sunflower contains a lot of PUFAs, which can easily oxidize and cause rancidity (Wang, Fan, et al., 2018). Different methods have been used to control the oxidation of PUFAs, which involves the addition of antioxidants (Wang, Zhu, et al., 2018), encapsulation, and forming into a stable emulsion (Miyashita et al., 2018). Harmful aldehydes produced during oxidation, such as malondialdehyde and 4-hydroxy-2-nonenal (4-HNE), can damage the body by cross-linking proteins and binding to the nucleic acids (Zhang et al., 2021). Stability is typically improved by incorporating natural and synthetic antioxidants, which are used as additives (Yui et al., 2016). Lately, people prefer natural ingredients instead of synthetic ones. Because of this, researchers have been testing natural antioxidants from plants, such as polyphenols, carotenoids, and tocopherols. One example is rosemary extract, which shields n-3 PUFAs in flaxseed oil better than α-tocopherols or butylated hydroxytoluene (Wang, Fu, et al., 2018). The n-3 index is usually seen as a wide measure of the extended availability of very long-chain PUFAs like EPA and DHA in the body (Schuchardt & Hahn, 2013). Many research show that plant-based oils or algae-obtained PUFAs can effectively raise concentration in bloods of EPA + DHA. In a trial of placebo-controlled study, pregnant women who took 400 mg of algal DHA daily from mid-pregnancy until six months after giving birth had much higher DHA levels in their red blood cell phospholipids (1.94% of fatty acids) at delivery compared to the placebo group (0.84%) (Khandelwal et al., 2020). In a 14-week study involving 93 adults with high triglycerides, taking 2.4 g/day of algal oil (rich in DHA and EPA at a 2.7:1 ratio) lowered triglycerides by about 18.9%, while the FO group (2.0 g/day, ratio 0.7:1) showed a 22.9% decrease (Ryan & Symington, 2015). Choosing the right encapsulation method can make omega-3 oils much more stable, easier to mix in water, and easier for our body to absorb (Xiong et al., 2021).

21.5.2 Novel delivery systems for polyunsaturated fatty acid supplements

Liposomes offer an excellent means to deliver EFAs in a targeted and efficient way, especially for individuals with special healthcare needs, particularly those suffering from malnutrition, inflammatory conditions, neurological disorders, and cardiovascular disease. Nano liposomes have been studied as efficient carriers for orally delivering n-3 FA, and they may also improve intestinal absorption and influence on inflammation-related markers (Shabana et al., 2024). Solid lipid nanoparticles (SLN) and nanostructured lipid carriers (NLCs) are novel lipid delivery techniques. These particles are very small (typically between 40 and 1000 nm in diameter), and the lipids used remain solid at both room temperature (25°C to 37°C). SLNs are grouped into three basic types based on the drug (bioactive compound) that is encapsulated inside the solid lipid matrix. In Type I, the compound is blended evenly throughout the lipid; in Type II, the compound ends up concentrated in an outer shell; and in Type III, the compound forms the inner core, surrounded by solid lipid (Gordillo-Galeano & Mora-Huertas, 2018). NLCs come in three structural types. Type I, the "imperfect" matrix, has a disordered lipid core created by mixing solid and liquid lipids, which leaves extra space for higher loading capacity. Type II, the "amorphous" type, forms a noncrystalline, structureless core to reduce drug loss during storage, while Type III, the "multiple-compartment" type, contains tiny oil droplets inside a solid lipid matrix, allowing controlled release systems designed for the coencapsulation of diverse compounds (Garg et al., 2022). Emulsion-based DDS have increased encapsulation yield (43%–87%) and provide controlled release and penetration compared to tablets and capsules (Hosny et al., 2021). Hybrid emulsions are done by mixing materials like natural polymers, structured lipids, and solid nanoparticles, that offers a new way to overcome traditional limitations of nanoemulsions. They provide greater stability, controlled release, and in some cases, targeted delivery of bioactive compounds, along with better protection against oxidation (Zhou et al., 2024). An innovative self-micro-emulsifying delivery system (SMEDS) for concentrated omega-3 fatty acids, when exposed to the gut's watery environment, quickly forms microdroplets, improving the absorption. In two studies, total absorption of EPA + DHA from the SMEDS formulation PRF-021 was 6.4 times (low dose) and 11.5 times (high dose) higher than from standard formulations, demonstrating more effective omega-3 absorption from the supplement (West et al., 2018).

21.5.3 Microencapsulation and liposomal technologies

Encapsulation is a well-established way to improve the oxidative stability and overall functionality of PUFAs such as n-3 fatty acids. Microencapsulating garden cress helped to protect it from oxidation (Umesha et al., 2013). Microencapsulation can help oils last longer by wrapping them in protective materials like milk proteins, dextrin, modified cellulose, gelatin, plant gums, or modified starch and keeps the oils stability, thereby extending shelf life (Castejón et al., 2021). There are many techniques for the microencapsulation process, which include spray drying, freeze drying, and spray nozzle coating for encapsulating the end product (Pattnaik & Mishra, 2020). Research has also explored that encapsulating oils includes long-chain PUFA-rich systems (e.g., FO) coated with SC, dextrins, highly branched cyclic dextrins, and modified cellulose (Bratovcic & Suljagic, 2019). Liposomal technology involves layers of phospholipids united together. Generally consists of many phospholipids arranged together to get a ring like structure and ingested into the polar and nonpolar matrix, enhances the microencapsulation of lipophilic and lipophobic materials (Amoabediny et al., 2018). Many methods, including thin layer hydration, reverse phase evaporation, microfluid microencapsulation, and ethanol injection, can also be used (Tsai & Rizvi, 2016). Nano liposomal encapsulation has a diameter of 50–200 nm and has an increased stability against oxidation compared to the encapsulation done with increased size of liposomes ($d > 200$ nm) (Rasti et al., 2012). Encapsulating the shrimp oil using the liposomal technologies has an increased in the encapsulation yield and has a higher stability against oxidation (McClements, 2012). The thin-film hydration (Bangham) method is a conventional way to make liposomes. Phospholipids are mixed with organic solvents like chloroform or methanol, and these solvents are evaporated, leaving a thin lipid film on the flask. When a water-based solution is added and mixed, usually by vortexing or sonication process, where it has a lower the encapsulation efficiency (Trier et al., 2011). Reverse-phase evaporation vesicles (REVs) are liposomes made by first dissolving phospholipids in a volatile organic solvent and then mixing in an aqueous solution enabled water-in-oil emulsion formation. As the solvent is evaporated under vacuum, this emulsion gradually flips into a water-based double emulsion, creating liposomes with relatively high encapsulation efficiency, but the removal of solvent will be quite difficult (Yokoyama et al., 2003). Three frequencies (43, 133, and 480 kHz) and two power levels (8 and 18 W) of liposomal encapsulation are treated under ultrasonication. The findings showed that lower frequencies shrink liposomes faster than higher ones, and that short, high-power sonication is more effective than longer, low-power treatments. Under these conditions, the liposomes reached a size of about 50–70 nm (Yamaguchi et al., 2009). Microfluidic encapsulation is made by fitting a small round glass tube inside a square glass tube, with a tapered tube inserted from the other side. The inner water-based fluid with tiny microspheres and the middle oil-based fluid with lipids were pumped through the tubes, mixing at the tip to form liposomes. An outer water layer helped shape the final droplets. By adjusting flow rates and tube sizes, uniform liposomes between 20 and 150 μm are formed. This method has a reduced usage of organic solvents(Shum et al., 2008). Supercritical Reverse Phase Evaporation is a liposomal microencapsulation technique that is similar to REV method, but uses SC-CO_2 instead of organic solvents. Soy lecithin was pressurized with SC-CO_2 at 12–30 MPa and 60°C, and then a glucose dissolved in water was added in a controlled, gradual manner, followed by rapid depressurization to form liposomes. High-PC lecithin produced large unilamellar vesicles (0.2–1.2 μm), while low-PC lecithin formed smaller multilamellar liposomes (0.1–0.25 μm); adding ethanol improved phospholipid solubility and encapsulation efficiency. Liposome size was also influenced by pressure, with droplets larger below 20 MPa than above (Imura et al., 2003). Supercritical microencapsulation has gained significant attention because the usage of hazard-free solvents and the encapsulation efficiency is higher (Tsai & Rizvi, 2016). Fig. 21.3 shows the liposomal preparation methods for the PUFA processing conditions. See Table 21.2 shows the encapsulation techniques for the different PUFA products with benefits.

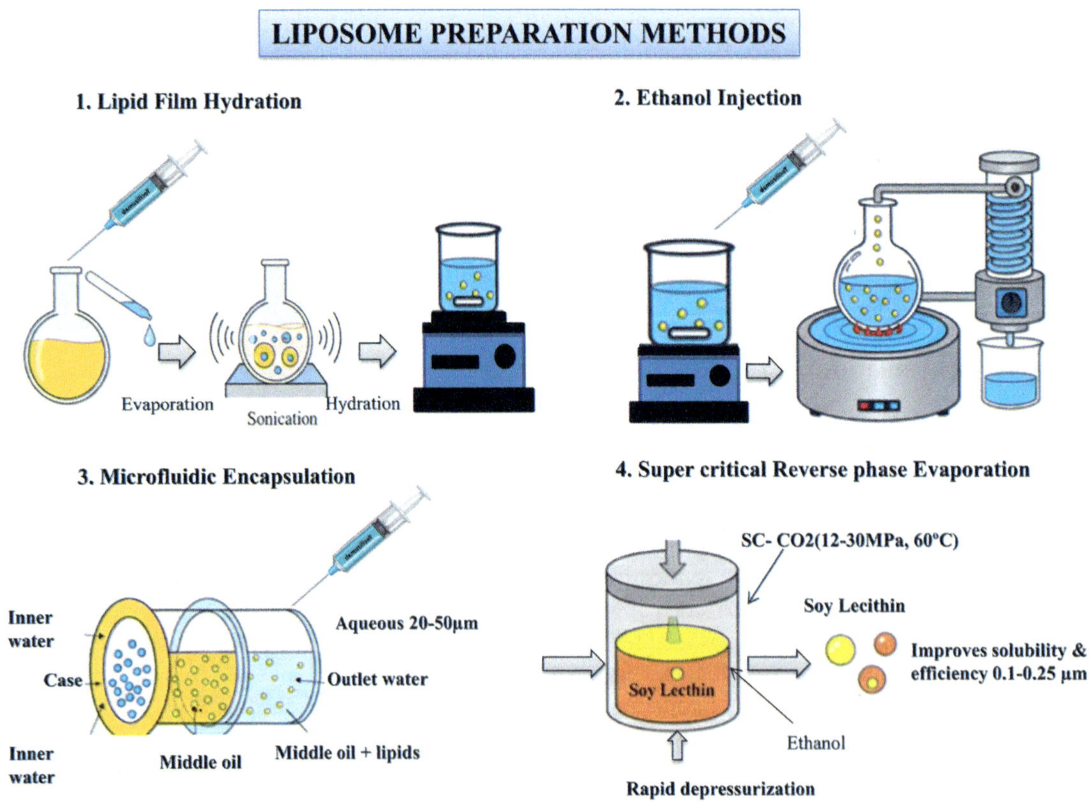

FIGURE 21.3 Liposomal encapsulation methods processing (pictures were self-made).

TABLE 21.2 Encapsulation of polyunsaturated fatty acids from different sources.

Source of PUFAs	Encapsulation composition	Production method	Size of encapsulation	Encapsulation benefits	References
Plant oil	Polymers protein solution + aqueous solution + Oil	Complex coacervation	10:1–20:1 Ratio	Highest encapsulation efficiency and yield, delays oxidation	Timilsena et al. (2017)
Chia seeds, echium seeds, camelina seeds, algal biomass of *Nannochloropsis gaditana*	Sodium caseinate and Lactose	Spray drying	1.5 to 30 μm	7.0 to 76.9% High encapsulation efficiency, high payload (142 mg/g)	Castejón et al. (2021)
Fish oil (FO)	Sodium alginate.3%, 1.0%, and 2.0% concentration Glucose sirup	Needle drop method	17–33 μm (0.3%), 10–18 μm (1.0%), and 5–10 μm (2.0%)	Increased intestinal availability of EPA and DHA,	Olloqui and Castañeda-Ovando, 2018
FO	Lecithin, polyethylene glycol, propylene glycol ester, and polysorbate	Self microencapsulating delivery systems and liposomal encapsulation, soft gel preparation method	100–300 nm	Enhanced bioavailability and prevents oxidation	Ahmad et al. (2025)
Shrimp lipid extract, FO, and fish protein hydrolysate	Soya lecithin, chitosan and whey protein concentrate (WPC)	Ultrasonication	38.12 to 100.02 nm	Increased solubility (28.83 mg/100 g), encapsulation efficiency (97.67%), and oxidative stability	Amiri et al. (2024)
Chia oil	Hydroxyl propyl β-cyclodextrin + lipoic acid, chia oil	Nanoliposomal encapsulation + inclusion complex	52.19 ± 7.00 nm	Increased encapsulation efficiency 80.24 ± 0.49%	Choudhary et al. (2022)
Pistachio oil	Pistachio oil + soya Lecithin	Ultrasonication + liposomal method	100–250 nm	Decrease in inflammation, Increase in the EPA and DHA	Hassanshahi et al. (2022)
Tuna eyeball oil	soy phosphatidylcholine lecithin + Tuna oil	Nanoliposomal encapsulation + ultrasonication	31.6–67.2 nm	Highest encapsulation yield of 98% and Increased in the PUFAs content with enhanced stability	Kurniawan et al. (2024)
Soybean-and-walnut oil	Xanthan gum + sodium azide + inulin	High-pressure homogenization	138 nm	Increased viscoelastic property and gel strength	Alfaro-Rodríguez et al. (2022)
Fish and linseed oil	Tween 80 + transcutol-P	High-pressure homogenization	Less than 130 nm	Helps in the improved treatment of psoriasis	Mittal et al. (2021)
Omega-6/omega-3 fatty acids	WPC + maltodextrin + gum arabic	ultrasonic or micro fluidizer, freeze drying and spray drying	198.5 nm, 201.3 nm, 824.9 nm, 714.2 nm	High encapsulation efficiency, emulsion and oxidative stability	Abdel-Razek et al. (2022)

21.5.4 Innovations in fortification techniques

For biscuits fortified with 10%, 20%, and 30% flax fiber, the total PUFAs rise markedly from 10.50% to 20.50%, while SFAs declined from 48.22% to 40.20%. This indicates a substantial increase in omega-3 levels compared to biscuits without flaxseed, accompanied by a major reduction in the omega-6/omega-3 ratiofrom 8.50 down to 1.00 (Elshehy et al., 2018). Cheese quality after adding flaxseed oil at different points in production (homogenization, coagulation, and salting) has been assessed. After 30 days of storage at 8°C, the homogenization stage produced the most favorable results, although it was accompanied by higher levels of lipid oxidation (Calligaris et al., 2015). Fortification of Turkish white cheese with corn oil is a live result which shows the rise in the PUFA content in the cheese and provide scientific proof which decreases the bad cholesterol. Overall, it has a higher sensory acceptance than the control cheese (Arslan et al., 2014). Cereals and bars offer practical options for PUFA fortification. However, because omega-3 PUFAs are inefficiently incorporated into membrane phospholipids and provide limited benefits to plasma omega-3 levels, it remains unclear whether fortification of human milk can supply infants with sufficient amounts of omega-3 PUFAs. Milk can be enriched through two main approaches: (1) direct addition of oil or an omega-3 PUFA carrier, or (2) dietary supplementation of animals with omega-3-rich ingredients so that their milk becomes naturally enriched, as mammary glands naturally produce milk with higher levels of these fatty acids (Lock & Bauman, 2004). The low levels of omega-3 PUFAs in most meats indicate that fortification is needed to help people reach the recommended intake of 0.5 g per day (Maia et al., 2007). Bread recipes use various fats depending on the style of bread, making it simple to include n-3 PUFAs during dough mixing. Likewise, baked goods include bakery and confectionery products that contain other components, so using n-3 fortified eggs or dairy offers an effective way to improve their health benefits (Yep et al., 2002). Methods which include microencapsulation or emulsification, which trap PUFAs can improve fortified yogurt quality. They help boost water-holding capacity and have the refine texture, which reduces the rate of oxidation (Gumus & Gharibzahedi, 2021). A well-designed capsule system needs to trap a sizable amount of oil rich in fatty acids inside a food-grade coating material. This approach helps in several ways: it protects the oils from chemical degradation, enables the nutrients to be released at the right place and time depending on conditions, allows the enriched ingredient to mix smoothly with the surrounding food without changing its look or texture, and ensures the final product remains appealing to consumers (Chang & Nickerson, 2018). Nanoliposome are made by using a mixture of PC, ethanol, glycerol, and water. These were made up and dried by freeze-drying or spray-drying using carboxymethyl cellulose as the encapsulating wall material and fumed silica to prevent clumping. The dried nano liposomes help hide the fishy odor and protect the shrimp oil from oxidizing, making the oil more stable and better suited for use in foods (Gulzar & Benjakul, 2020). Many PUFA supplements we can find in the market come in the form of fish-derived oils, which are usually packaged as soft-gel capsules (Hegde et al., 2025). Aquatic oil, which has long-chain PUFAs, was coated with a wall material of glucose sirup and gelatin matrix. Splash encapsulation allows different liquid channels that allow the wall material and core material to mix right at the point where the droplets are formed. Sonic energy can also be used to create the droplets (Selim et al., 2021).

21.5.5 SWOT analysis

The major strength is the growing demand for omega-fortified nutrition. The rising global shift toward preventive health, functional nutrition, and evidence-backed dietary supplementation has emerged as one of the strongest demand drivers for PUFAs. Consumers across key markets are increasingly incorporating omega-3 and omega-6 ingredients into daily nutrition, driven by their validated roles in cardiovascular health, cognitive performance, inflammation control, and infant development. Simultaneously, ALA- and LA-rich plant sources such as flaxseed, canola, sunflower, and safflower oils are witnessing expanded utilization in bakery, dairy, snacking, and ready-to-drink nutritional formulations, enabling manufacturers to create clean-label and plant-forward products (Kiefer & Pantuso, 2012).

In infant nutrition, the continued requirement for DHA and AA fortification has strengthened PUFA integration across premium formula launches, particularly in Asia Pacific and Europe. As global consumers increasingly prioritize heart health, metabolism, mental well-being, and immunity, demand for omega-fortified functional foods, nutraceuticals, and clinical nutrition products continues to accelerate across both developed and emerging markets. The stronger clinical backing of the EPA/DHA, the expanding body of clinical and nutritional science continues to reinforce the PUFAs—EPA, DHA, ALA, LA, and AA—in cardiometabolic health, cognitive development, inflammatory regulation, and immune function. Growing evidence from randomized clinical trials, large-scale epidemiological studies, and infant-nutrition research has elevated the significance of marine-derived EPA/DHA and plant-derived ALA/LA in preventing chronic lifestyle disorders. DHA and AA, in particular, remain foundational components in global infant nutrition standards in retinal and neurological improvement, driving sustained adoption across premium formula categories (Einerhand et al., 2023). Within adult and senior populations, clinical validation around triglyceride reduction, endothelial function, mood balance, and neuroprotective benefits has strengthened demand for high-purity EPA/DHA concentrates, increasingly sourced from aquatic oils. PUFA sources including flaxseed, canola, sunflower, and safflower oils, continue to gain traction as clean-label options for functional food fortification and personalized nutrition programs. As evidence-based health management becomes central to consumer decision-making, clinically supported PUFA formulations remain positioned as essential lipids across supplements, pharmaceuticals, infant nutrition, and functional food applications (Wei et al., 2025).

The rising use of functional foods and supplements and the accelerating shift toward functional nutrition has significantly increased the incorporation of PUFAs across mainstream food and supplement categories. Consumers seeking convenient, evidence-backed solutions for heart health, cognitive function, inflammatory balance, and overall wellness are driving ingredients in daily nutrition. Manufacturers of functional beverages, fortified dairy, bakery products, snack bars, and ready-to-mix powders are increasingly utilizing EPA- and DHA-rich marine oils. Technological improvements in microencapsulation and deodorization have enhanced stability and taste neutrality, allowing PUFAs to be blended into wider product matrices without oxidative concerns. Supplements continue to remain a major demand center, with high-concentration EPA/DHA softgels, gummies, powders, and vegan algal DHA gaining notable traction. As functional foods and wellness-driven supplementation rise globally, PUFA-enriched formulations remain central to growth across developed and emerging markets (Yeşilçubuk et al., 2021).

The expansion of marine and algal oil production has become a critical enabler of sustained growth in the global PUFA market. Rising demand for high-purity EPA and DHA across supplements, pharmaceuticals, infant formulas, and fortified foods is accelerating investment in advanced extraction, fermentation, and purification technologies. Marine sources—particularly FO and krill oil—continue to dominate EPA and DHA supply, supported by improved fisheries management, upgraded refining capacity, and enhanced sustainability certifications that strengthen their acceptance in regulated applications. Parallelly, algal oil production is scaling rapidly as consumers and formulators seek vegan, allergen-free, and environmentally resilient alternatives to marine oils. Algal fermentation allows consistent output, controlled fatty acid profiles, and suitability for infant nutrition, where DHA purity and regulatory compliance are essential. Vegan oils, such as canola, sunflower, and safflower continue to support ALA and LA availability, but the strongest capacity expansion is occurring in microbial and marine segments. As global PUFA demand diversifies across end-use sectors, scalable algal and marine oil production remains fundamental to ensuring stability, quality, and long-term industry competitiveness (Yan et al., 2024).

The constraints is that volatility in marine raw material prices remains one of the most persistent restraints affecting the global PUFA market. EPA- and DHA-rich oils sourced from fish, krill, and marine microorganisms are highly sensitive to fluctuations in seasonal catch volumes, environmental disruptions, and long-term sustainability pressures on wild fisheries. Variability in anchovy, sardine, and tuna stocks—key feedstock species for FO—directly influences crude oil availability and pricing, with ripple effects across refining, concentration, and downstream PUFA ingredient costs. Marine-derived inputs also face tightening regulatory controls, rising quotas, and increased competition from aquaculture and animal-feed industries, further intensifying pricing instability. Krill oil production is especially affected by geopolitical conditions in Antarctic harvesting zones, while algal fermentation, though stable, remains costlier at scale. These fluctuations challenge manufacturers producing EPA/DHA concentrates for supplements, fortified foods, infant nutrition, and pharmaceutical-grade formulations. In contrast, ALA- and LA-rich plant oils from canola, flaxseed, sunflower, and safflower offer more stable supply, yet cannot fully offset marine dependency. Overall, raw material price volatility continues to constrain cost predictability and margin stability for marine PUFA producers (Hoang et al., 2024; Wei et al., 2025).

Regulatory complexities surrounding PUFA labeling, health claims, purity requirements, and oxidative stability continue to act as a major restraint across global markets. Authorities in North America, Europe, and Asia enforce stringent controls on EPA, DHA, ALA, LA, and AA content declarations, contaminant limits, and permissible nutritional or therapeutic claims, particularly for products positioned in supplements, fortified foods, and infant formulas. Manufacturers sourcing marine-based oils must comply with rigorous standards for heavy metals, dioxins, PCBs, and oxidation indices, often increasing testing, refining, and documentation costs. Infant nutrition regulations are even more demanding, requiring precise DHA/AA ratios, validated sourcing, and strict adherence to Codex and region-specific guidelines. For plant-derived oils including canola, flaxseed, sunflower, and safflower, clean-label positioning demands additional scrutiny around processing aids, stability enhancers, and allergen declarations. The growing need to substantiate structure–function claims, meet country-specific PUFA fortification rules, and navigate varying global regulatory frameworks delays product approvals and elevates compliance burdens for both established and emerging PUFA manufacturers (Fuentes et al., 2024).

The opportunities is that the global shift toward plant-based nutrition, clean-label ingredients, and sustainable sourcing models is driving a significant rise in demand for plant-derived PUFAs. Oils rich in ALA and LA, particularly flaxseed, canola, sunflower, and safflower, are gaining strong traction across functional foods, dietary supplements, dairy alternatives, and ready-to-eat nutrition formats due to their favorable fatty acid profiles, mild sensory attributes, and broad regulatory acceptance. As consumers increasingly seek vegan, allergen-free, and environmentally responsible alternatives to marine-derived EPA and DHA sources, plant PUFAs are emerging as preferred ingredients for both mainstream and premium product lines. Advances in refining, cold pressing, and deodorization technologies have further improved purity, oxidative stability, and application versatility, enabling plant oils to be incorporated into bakery products, beverages, spreads, bars, and microencapsulated supplement formats. Their compatibility with fortification systems makes them particularly suitable for clean-label functional food innovation. Growing adoption in infant nutrition blends, clinical nutrition, and pet health formulations also expands long-term demand. Overall, the surge in plant-based PUFA consumption represents a high-value opportunity for manufacturers across both developed and emerging markets. PUFA use in the rising emphasis on companion animal health, functional pet food formulations, and preventive veterinary nutrition is driving strong growth in PUFA adoption across pet and livestock categories. Marine-based oils are increasingly incorporated into premium dog and cat food products to support skin and coat health, immune function, joint mobility, and cognitive development. Algal DHA is gaining traction due to its sustainability, purity, and favorable regulatory acceptance, particularly in formulations targeting senior pets and developmental nutrition (Rizzo et al., 2023; Saini et al., 2021).

Plant-derived ALA- and LA-rich oils from flaxseed, canola, sunflower, and safflower are also widely used to enhance overall fatty acid balance, support metabolic health, and improve feed efficiency in both companion animals and livestock. Their clean-label positioning and cost-effectiveness make them suitable for mainstream and economy feed segments. As pet humanization accelerates and veterinary recommendations shift toward evidence-based functional diets, PUFA-enriched formulations across marine and plant sources represent a strategic opportunity for manufacturers supplying pet food, animal feed, and targeted veterinary nutrition products (Monnard & Dulloo, 2021). Fig. 21.4 shows the SWOT analysis of PUFA-based system.

21.5.6 Emerging innovations trends, and future perspectives

Microorganisms offer a powerful and versatile platform for advancing lipid production. Over millions of years, they have evolved a wide range of metabolic pathways capable of synthesizing many different lipids, making them an efficient and cost-effective source for industrial applications. Modern "omics" technologies are playing a key role in this progress. Tools such as next-generation sequencing, transcriptomics, proteomics, and advanced mass spectrometry are helping researchers map the missing links in single-cell lipid biosynthesis. Insights gained from these approaches will support the design and scale-up of more efficient production processes. Fatty acid profiles of oils derived from microorganisms can

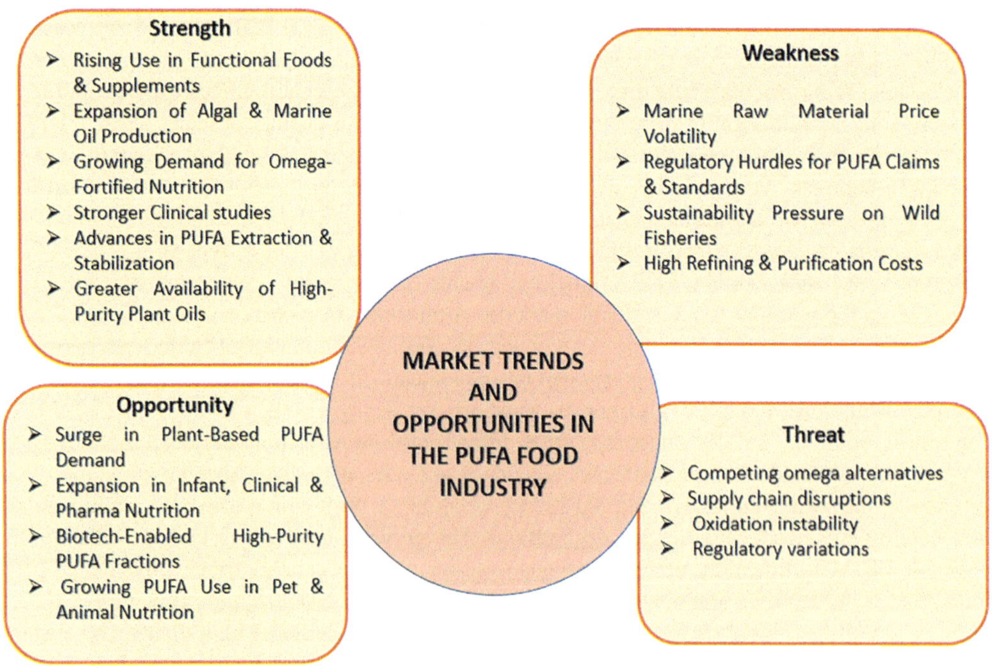

FIGURE 21.4 SWOT analysis of polyunsaturated fatty acid (PUFA)-based products.

also be tailored, such as increasing PUFA content by introducing specific enzymes into the host organisms. Better regulation of PUFA-related pathways will greatly streamline the final production steps (Swetha & Mathanghi, 2024). Microencapsulation offers an effective approach to protect PUFAs from oxidative degradation caused by environmental factors, dramatically improving their stability. Still, encapsulating PUFA-rich oils into powder changes their original liquid form, which can limit how those oils are used. An alternative approach is to naturally enrich oil-seed crops with antioxidants such as tocols (tocopherols), so the extracted oils are more resistant to oxidation without needing encapsulation. Academic. Going forward, research should look into metabolic-engineering strategies for oilseed crops. This could raise their internal antioxidant levels, helping oils stay fresher, more stable, and shelf-ready (Saini et al., 2021). European Food Safety Authority recommends boosting dietary DHA to maintain healthy levels 250 mg of EPA + DHA daily for adults and 100 mg of DHA for infants and children less than 2 years (EFSA Panel on Dietetic Products, N., & Allergies, 2010). Marine nutraceuticals are gaining significant interest as marine organisms provide a plentiful source of biologically active molecules used in promoting health and treating disease (Suleria et al., 2015). Marine-derived foods supply proteins, peptides, polysaccharides, PUFAs, vitamins, minerals, and many other beneficial nutrients, thus it gains a potential market insights and future growth towards innovative supplements and products.

21.6 Summary

This chapter comprehensively analyzes the PUFA food industry's market dynamics, featuring global leaders and Indian players with the competitive landscapes of the industry, navigating marine-to-plant source shifts amid regional growth patterns with different extraction techniques and emerging trends in the processing conditions. Furthermore, this chapter examines driving factors including consumer health awareness for chronic disease prevention, sustainable sourcing via microalgae, thraustochytrids, and GM crops, alongside extraction innovations techniques like supercritical CO_2, ultrasound, microwave, enzyme-assisted and nanoencapsulation delivery systems enabling PUFA integration into functional foods, beverages, bakery, dairy, and infant nutrition while overcoming oxidation challenges. Emerging trends highlight the algal vegan DHA/EPA, microencapsulated formats, personalized AI-driven nutrition, and high-concentration blends for targeted cardiometabolic, cognitive, and immune outcomes.

21.7 Conclusion

The PUFA industry represents the convergence of nutritional science, sustainability, and delivery innovation, transitioning from marine dependency to scalable algal and microbial platforms that position PUFAs as cornerstone functional ingredients across fortified foods and precision nutrition. Food technologists must prioritize hybrid extraction technologies, advanced nanoencapsulation, and AI-guided personalization to mainstream clean-label applications, while industry leaders address volatility through traceability, sustainability certifications, and harmonized health claims. This evolution establishes PUFAs as foundational preventive nutrition solutions, bridging consumer demand for evidence-based cardiovascular, cognitive, and immune health benefits with global functional food expansion.

Acknowledgments

The authors would like to thank the staff of the Department of Food Technology, Kongu Engineering College, for their extensive technical support, and all coauthors for their assistance with this chapter.

Conflict of interest

The authors declare no conflicts of interest relevant to the content of this chapter.

References

Abdel-Razek, A. G., Hassanein, M. M., Ozçelik, B., Baranenko, D. A., & El-Messery, T. M. (2022). Omega fatty acid-balanced oil formula and enhancing its oxidative stability by encapsulation with whey protein concentrate. *Food Bioscience, 50*. https://doi.org/10.1016/j.fbio.2022.101975, http://www.journals.elsevier.com/food-bioscience/.

Adeyomoye, O., Olaniyan, O. T., & Adetunji, C. O. (2023). Production of polyunsaturated fatty acids (PUFAs) and their biomedical application. In *Next-Generation algae: Volume II: Applications in medicine and the pharmaceutical industry*. Nigeria: wiley, 125–137. https://doi.org/10.1002/9781119857860.ch5, https://onlinelibrary.wiley.com/doi/book/10.1002/9781119857860.

Ahmad, I., Dogra, A., Nagpal, T., Sharma, C., Singh, S., Shaiva, N., Saini, G., & Luhach, K. (2025). Liposome-like encapsulation of fish oil-based self-nano emulsifying formulation for improved bioavailability. *Applied Food Research, 5*(1), 100745. https://doi.org/10.1016/j.afres.2025.100745.

Alfaro-Rodríguez, M.-C., Prieto, P., García, M. C., Martín-Piñero, M. J., & Muñoz, J. (2022). Influence of nanoemulsion/gum ratio on droplet size distribution, rheology and physical stability of nanoemulgels containing inulin and omega-3 fatty acids. *Journal of the Science of Food and Agriculture, 102*(14), 6397–6403. https://doi.org/10.1002/jsfa.12005.

Amiri, H., Shabanpour, B., Pourashouri, P., & kashiri, M. (2024). Preparation of functional supplement powder using nanoliposome-containing marine bioactive compounds. *Journal of Food Science, 89*(12), 8658–8672. https://doi.org/10.1111/1750-3841.17543.

Amoabediny, G., Haghiralsadat, F., Naderinezhad, S., Helder, M. N., Akhoundi Kharanaghi, E., Mohammadnejad Arough, J., & Zandieh-Doulabi, B. (2018). Overview of preparation methods of polymeric and lipid-based (niosome, solid lipid, liposome) nanoparticles: A comprehensive review. *International Journal of Polymeric Materials and Polymeric Biomaterials, 67*(6), 383–400. https://doi.org/10.1080/00914037.2017.1332623, www.tandf.co.uk/journals/titles/00914037.asp.

Anwar, S. H. (2011). Microencapsulation of omega-3 fatty acids: What it is, how it's made, and challenges in food technology. *Life Science, 39*.

Arslan, S., Topcu, A., Saldamli, I., & Koksal, G. (2014). Use of corn oil in the production of Turkish white cheese. *Journal of Food Science and Technology, 51*(10), 2382–2392. https://doi.org/10.1007/s13197-012-0752-6.

Assefa, M., Zhao, Y., Zhou, C., Song, Y., & Zhao, X. (2025). Advancements in crop PUFAs biosynthesis and genetic engineering: A systematic and mixed review system. *International Journal of Molecular Sciences, 26*(8), 3462. https://doi.org/10.3390/ijms26083462.

Baker, E. J., Cumberford, G., & Hanaway, P. (2025). Recognizing the health benefits of plant-sourced omega-3 stearidonic acid: Exploring its complementary role to preformed EPA/DHA. *Lipids, 60*(6), 435–442. https://doi.org/10.1002/lipd.12452, http://www.springerlink.com/content/0024-4201.

Blomquist, S. A., Albrecht, J. H., Hallmark, B., Klimentidis, Y. C., Garcia, L. A., Mandarino, L. J., Coletta, D. K., & Chilton, F. H. (2025). The influence of FADS genetic variation and omega-3 fatty acid deficiency on cardiometabolic disease risk in a Mexican American population. *Frontiers in Nutrition, 12*. https://doi.org/10.3389/fnut.2025.1538505, journal.frontiersin.org/journal/nutrition.

Bratovcic, A., & Suljagic, J. (2019). Micro-and nano-encapsulation in food industry. *Croatian Journal of Food Science and Technology, 11*(1), 113–121.

Calder, P. C. (2020). Omega-3 fatty acids and inflammatory processes: From molecules to man. *Biochemical Society Transactions, 48*(2), 1–15. https://doi.org/10.1042/BST20200467.

Calligaris, S., Ignat, A., Biasutti, M., Innocente, N., & Nicoli, M. C. (2015). Cheese fortification using saturated monoglyceride self-assembly structures as carrier of omega-3 fatty acids. *International Journal of Food Science and Technology, 50*(9), 2129–2134. https://doi.org/10.1111/ijfs.12877, http://onlinelibrary.wiley.com/journal/10.1111/(ISSN)1365-2621.

Castejón, N., Luna, P., & Señoráns, F. J. (2021). Microencapsulation by spray drying of omega-3 lipids extracted from oilseeds and microalgae: Effect on polyunsaturated fatty acid composition. *LWT, 148*, 111789. https://doi.org/10.1016/j.lwt.2021.111789.

Chang, C., & Nickerson, M. T. (2018). Encapsulation of omega 3-6-9 fatty acids-rich oils using protein-based emulsions with spray drying. *Journal of Food Science and Technology, 55*(8), 2850–2861. https://doi.org/10.1007/s13197-018-3257-0, http://www.springerlink.com/content/121580/.

Choudhary, P., Dutta, S., Moses, J. A., & Anandharamakrishnan, C. (2022). Liposomal encapsulation of omega-3 fatty acid and α-lipoic acid conjugate for cow milk fortification. *Journal of Food Processing and Preservation, 46*(9). https://doi.org/10.1111/jfpp.16082.

Ciftci, O. N., & Çavdar, H. K. (2025). Ultrasound-assisted extraction improved the extraction rate, omega-3, and polyunsaturated fatty acid content of fish oil from Atlantic bonito waste. *European Journal of Lipid Science and Technology*.

Colombo, S. M., Rodgers, T. F. M., Diamond, M. L., Bazinet, R. P., & Arts, M. T. (2020). Projected declines in global DHA availability for human consumption as a result of global warming. *Ambio, 49*(4), 865–880. https://doi.org/10.1007/s13280-019-01234-6, http://www.bioone.org/loi/ambi.

Demets, R., & Foubert, I. (2021). Traditional and novel sources of long-chain omega-3 fatty acids. In P. J. García-Moreno, C. Jacobsen, & A.-D. Moltke Sørensen (Eds.)

EFSA Panel on Dietetic Products, N., & Allergies (2010). Scientific opinion on dietary reference values for fats, including saturated fatty acids, polyunsaturated fatty acids, monounsaturated fatty acids, trans fatty acids, and cholesterol. *Efsa Journal, 8*(3), 1461.

Einerhand, A. W. C., Mi, W., Haandrikman, A., Sheng, X. Y., & Calder, P. C. (2023). The impact of linoleic acid on infant health in the absence or presence of DHA in infant formulas. *Nutrients, 15*(9). https://doi.org/10.3390/nu15092187, http://www.mdpi.com/journal/nutrients/.

Elshehy, H., Agamy, N., & Ismail, H. (2018). Effect of fortification of biscuits with flaxseed on omega 3 and calcium content of the products. *Journal of High Institute of Public Health, 48*(2), 58–66. https://doi.org/10.21608/jhiph.2018.19901.

Fuentes, J. B., Beara, I., & Torović, L. (2024). Regulatory compliance of health claims on omega-3 fatty acid food supplements. *Foods, 14*(1), 67.

Future Market Insights (2025). *Global polyunsaturated fatty acids market: Global industry analysis 2020-2024 and opportunity assessment 2025-2035*. Future Market Insights.

Garg, J., Pathania, K., Sah, S. P., & Pawar, S. V. (2022). Nanostructured lipid carriers: A promising drug carrier for targeting brain tumours. *Future Journal of Pharmaceutical Sciences, 8*(1). https://doi.org/10.1186/s43094-022-00414-8.

Gill, R. W., Al-Badr, M., Al-Ghouti, M. A., Mohamed, N. A., Abou-Saleh, H., & Rahman, M. M. (2024). Revolutionizing cardiovascular health with nano-encapsulated omega-3 fatty acids: A nano-solution approach. https://doi.org/10.20944/preprints202404.1839.v1

Gordillo-Galeano, A., & Mora-Huertas, C. E. (2018). Solid lipid nanoparticles and nanostructured lipid carriers: A review emphasizing on particle structure and drug release. *European Journal of Pharmaceutics and Biopharmaceutics, 133*, 285–308. https://doi.org/10.1016/j.ejpb.2018.10.017, www.elsevier.com/locate/ejphabio.

Gulzar, S., & Benjakul, S. (2020). Nanoliposome powder containing shrimp oil increases free flowing behavior and storage stability. *European Journal of Lipid Science and Technology, 122*(6). https://doi.org/10.1002/ejlt.202000049.

Gumus, C. E., & Gharibzahedi, S. M. T. (2021). Yogurts supplemented with lipid emulsions rich in omega-3 fatty acids: New insights into the fortification, microencapsulation, quality properties, and health-promoting effects. *Trends in Food Science and Technology, 110*, 267–279. https://doi.org/10.1016/j.tifs.2021.02.016, http://www.elsevier.com/wps/find/journaldescription.cws_home/601278/description#description.

Gutierres, D., Pacheco, R., & Reis, C.P. (2025). We are what we eat: The role of omega-3 and omega-6 polyunsaturated fatty acids in human health.

Harland, J.I., & Sanders, T.A.B. (2024). 12 - Regulatory issues, Editor(s): Thomas A.B. Sanders, in Woodhead Publishing Series in Food Science, Technology and Nutrition. In Functional dietary lipids (second edition). Woodhead Publishing, pp. 261–294). ISBN 9780443153273.

Hassanshahi, G., Karimabad, M. N., & Jebali, A. (2022). The therapeutic effect of PEGlated nanoliposome of pistachio unsaturated oils and its efficacy to attenuate inflammation in multiple sclerosis: A randomized, double-blind, placebo-controlled clinical trial phase I. *Journal of Neuroimmunology, 362*, 577768. https://doi.org/10.1016/j.jneuroim.2021.577768.

Hegde, M. V., Zanwar, A. A., & Adekar, S. P. (2025). Nutrition, Life, Disease, and Death. In *Omega-3 fatty acids: Keys to nutritional health and disease*. India: Springer Science+Business Media, 1–11. https://doi.org/10.1007/978-3-031-84200-9_1.

Hoang, T. V., Tran, T. T., Mafruhah, O. R., Pham, T. T. L., Hsieh, M. T., & Ha, H. A. (2024). Comparison of Omega-3 polyunsaturated fatty acids bioavailability in fish oil and krill oil: Network meta-analyses. *Food Chemistry: X, 24*, 101880.

Hosny, K. M., Sindi, A. M., Alkhalidi, H. M., Kurakula, M., Hassan, A. H., Bakhaidar, R. B., Abualsunun, W. A., Almehmady, A. M., Khames, A., Rizg, W. Y., Khallaf, R. A., Alruwaili, N. K., & Alhakamy, N. A. (2021). Development of omega-3 loxoprofen-loaded nanoemulsion to limit the side effect associated with NSAIDs in treatment of tooth pain. *Drug Delivery, 28*(1), 741–751. https://doi.org/10.1080/10717544.2021.1909179, https://www.tandfonline.com/loi/idrd20.

Imura, T., Gotoh, T., Otake, K., Yoda, S., Takebayashi, Y., Yokoyama, S., Takebayashi, H., Sakai, H., Yuasa, M., & Abe, M. (2003). Control of physicochemical properties of liposomes using a supercritical reverse phase evaporation method. *Langmuir: The ACS Journal of Surfaces and Colloids, 19*(6), 2021–2025. https://doi.org/10.1021/la020589a.

Jacobsen, C., Sørensen, A.-D.M., &Yesiltas, B. (2022). Delivery systems for omega-3 oils. Proceedings of 2022 AOCS Annual Meeting & Expo. https://doi.org/10.21748/sedt7727.

Khandelwal, S., Kondal, D., Chaudhry, M., Patil, K., Swamy, M. K., Metgud, D., Jogalekar, S., Kamate, M., Divan, G., Gupta, R., Prabhakaran, D., Tandon, N., Ramakrishnan, U., & Stein, A. D. (2020). Effect of maternal docosahexaenoic acid (DHA) supplementation on offspring neurodevelopment at 12 months in India: A randomized controlled trial. *Nutrients, 12*(10), 3041. https://doi.org/10.3390/nu12103041.

Kiefer, & Pantuso (2012). Omega-3 fatty acids: An update emphasizing clinical use. *Agro Food Industry Hi-Technology, 23*(4).

Kumar, A., & Sharma, R. (2023). Polyunsaturated fatty acids market trends: Focus on omega-3 and omega-6 in functional foods and nutraceuticals. *Journal of Food Science and Technology, 60*(8), 2456–2468. https://doi.org/10.1007/s13197-023-05789-2.

Kumar, S., Nirmal Thirunavookarasu, S., Sunil, C. K., Vignesh, S., Venkatachalapathy, N., & Rawson, A. (2023). Mass transfer kinetics and quality evaluation of tomato seed oil extracted using emerging technologies. *Innovative Food Science & Emerging Technologies, 83*, 103203 ISSN 1466-8564.

Kurniawan, M. O., Mittal, A., Benjakul, S., & Singh, A. (2024). Ultrasonicated omega-3-enriched skipjack tuna eyeball oil nanoliposome: Preparation, characterisation, and fortification in milk. *International Journal of Food Science and Technology, 59*(10), 6975–6986. https://doi.org/10.1111/ijfs.17405, http://onlinelibrary.wiley.com/journal/10.1111/(ISSN)1365-2621.

Lenihan-Geels, G., Bishop, K. S., & Ferguson, L. R. (2013). Alternative sources of omega-3 fats: Can we find a sustainable substitute for fish? *Nutrients, 5*(4), 1301–1315. https://doi.org/10.3390/nu5041301, http://www.mdpi.com/2072-6643/5/4/1301/pdf171301-1315.

Li, X., Liu, J., Chen, G., Zhang, J., Wang, C., & Liu, B. (2019). Extraction and purification of eicosapentaenoic acid and docosahexaenoic acid from microalgae: A critical review. *Algal Research, 43*, 101619. https://doi.org/10.1016/j.algal.2019.101619.

Liu, Y., Ren, X., Fan, C., Wu, W., Zhang, W., & Wang, Y. (2022). Health benefits, food applications, and sustainability of microalgae-derived N-3 PUFA. *Foods, 11*(13), 1883. https://doi.org/10.3390/foods11131883.

Livingstone, K. M. (2014). 14 - Authorised EU health claims for the replacement of saturated fats. In M. J. Sadler (Ed.). *Woodhead publishing series in food science, technology and nutrition, foods, nutrients and food ingredients with authorised EU health claims* (pp. 298–317). Woodhead Publishing. https://doi.org/10.1533/9780857098481.4.298 ISBN 9780857098429.

Lock, A. L., & Bauman, D. E. (2004). Modifying milk fat composition of dairy cows to enhance fatty acids beneficial to human health. *Lipids, 39*(12), 1197–1206. https://doi.org/10.1007/s11745-004-1348-6.

Maia, M. R. G., Chaudhary, L. C., Figueres, L., & Wallace, R. J. (2007). Metabolism of polyunsaturated fatty acids and their toxicity to the microflora of the rumen. *Antonie Van Leeuwenhoek, 91*(4), 303–314. https://doi.org/10.1007/s10482-006-9118-2.

McClements, D. J. (2012). Nanoemulsions versus microemulsions: Terminology, differences, and similarities. *Soft Matterial, 8*(6), 1719–1729. https://doi.org/10.1039/c2sm06903b.

Melgosa, R., Sanz, M. T., & Beltrán, S. (2021). Supercritical CO_2 processing of omega-3 polyunsaturated fatty acids – towards a biorefinery for fish waste valorization. *The Journal of Supercritical Fluids, 169*, 105121 ISSN 0896-8446.

Mititelu, M., Lupuliasa, D., Neacşu, S. M., Olteanu, G., Busnatu, Ş. S., Mihai, A., Popovici, V., Măru, N., Boroghină, S. C., Mihai, S., Ioniţă-Mîndrican, C. B., & Scafa-Udrişte, A. (2025). Polyunsaturated fatty acids and human health: A key to modern nutritional balance in association with polyphenolic compounds from food sources. *Foods, 14*(1). https://doi.org/10.3390/foods14010046, www.mdpi.com/journal/foods.

Mititelu, M., Lupuliasa, D., Neacşu, S. M., Olteanu, G., Busnatu, Ş. S., Mihai, A., & Scafa-Udrişte, A. (2024). Polyunsaturated fatty acids and human health: A key to modern nutritional balance in association with polyphenolic compounds from food sources. *Foods, 14*(1), 46.

Mittal, S., Ali, J., & Baboota, S. (2021). Enhanced anti-psoriatic activity of tacrolimus loaded nanoemulsion gel via omega 3 - fatty acid (EPA and DHA) rich oils-fish oil and linseed oil. *Journal of Drug Delivery Science and Technology, 63*, 102458. https://doi.org/10.1016/j.jddst.2021.102458.

Miyashita, K., Uemura, M., & Hosokawa, M. (2018). Effective prevention of oxidative deterioration of fish oil: focus on flavor deterioration. *Annual Review of Food Science and Technology, 9*(1), 209–226. https://doi.org/10.1146/annurev-food-030117-012320.

Monnard, C. R., & Dulloo, A. G. (2021). Polyunsaturated fatty acids as modulators of fat mass and lean mass in human body composition regulation and cardiometabolic health. *Obesity Reviews, 22*, e13197.

Muhoza, B., Yuyang, H., Uriho, A., Harindintwali, J. D., Liu, Q., & Li, Y. (2023). Spray-and freeze-drying of microcapsules prepared by complex coacervation method: A review. *Food Hydrocolloids, 140*, 108650.

Mukherjee, S., Mohanty, A. K., Rao, U., & Poddar, A. (2024). Microbial polyunsaturated fatty acids (PUFAs) for human health: A comprehensive review of evidence from in vivo preclinical models. *Discover Applied Sciences, 6*(10). https://doi.org/10.1007/s42452-024-06238-w, https://link.springer.com/journal/42452.

Nicholls, S. J., Lincoff, A. M., Garcia, M., Bash, D., Ballantyne, C. M., Barter, P. J., Davidson, M. H., Kastelein, J. J. P., Koenig, W., McGuire, D. K., Mozaffarian, D., Ridker, P. M., Ray, K. K., Katona, B. G., Himmelmann, A., Loss, L. E., Rensfeldt, M., Lundström, T., & Agrawal, S. E. (2020). Effect of high-dose omega-3 fatty acids vs corn oil on major adverse cardiovascular events in patients at high cardiovascular risk: The STRENGTH randomized clinical trial. *JAMA - Journal of the American Medical Association, 324*(22), 2268–2280. http://jama.jamanetwork.com/journal.aspx.

Nilsson, A., Radeborg, K., Salo, I., & Björck, I. (2012). Effects of supplementation with n-3 polyunsaturated fatty acids on cognitive performance and cardiometabolic risk markers in healthy 51 to 72 years old subjects: A randomized controlled cross-over study. *Nutrition Journal, 11*(1). https://doi.org/10.1186/1475-2891-11-99.

Oliver, L., Dietrich, T., Marañón, I., Villarán, M. C., & Barrio, R. J. (2020). Producing omega-3 polyunsaturated fatty acids: A review of sustainable sources and future trends for the EPA and DHA market. *Resources, 9*(12), 1–15. https://doi.org/10.3390/resources9120148, https://www.mdpi.com/2079-9276/9/12/148.

Olloqui, E. J., Castañeda-Ovando, A., Contreras-López, E., Hernandez-Sanchez, D., Tapia-Maruri, D., Piloni-Martini, J., & Añorve-Morga, J. (2018). Encapsulation of fish oil into low-cost alginate beads and EPA-DHA release in a rumino-intestinal in vitro digestion model. *European Journal of Lipid Science and Technology, 120*(9). https://doi.org/10.1002/ejlt.201800036, http://onlinelibrary.wiley.com/journal/10.1002/(ISSN)1438-9312.

Pattnaik, M., & Mishra, H. N. (2020). Effect of microwave treatment on preparation of stable PUFA enriched vegetable oil powder and its influence on quality parameters. *Journal of Food Processing and Preservation, 44*(4). https://doi.org/10.1111/jfpp.14374, http://onlinelibrary.wiley.com/journal/10.1111/(ISSN)1745-4549.

Pokushalov, E., Ponomarenko, A., Shrainer, E., Kudlay, D., & Miller, R. (2024). Biomarker-guided dietary supplementation: A narrative review of precision in personalized nutrition. *Nutrients, 16*(23), 4033. https://doi.org/10.3390/nu16234033.

Rasti, B., Jinap, S., Mozafari, M. R., & Yazid, A. M. (2012). Comparative study of the oxidative and physical stability of liposomal and nanoliposomal polyunsaturated fatty acids prepared with conventional and Mozafari methods. *Food Chemistry, 135*(4), 2761–2770. https://doi.org/10.1016/j.foodchem.2012.07.016.

Rizzo, G., Baroni, L., & Lombardo, M. (2023). Promising sources of plant-derived polyunsaturated fatty acids: A narrative review. *International Journal of Environmental Research and Public Health, 20*(3), 1683. https://doi.org/10.3390/ijerph20031683.

Ryan, L., & Symington, A. M. (2015). Algal-oil supplements are a viable alternative to fish-oil supplements in terms of docosahexaenoic acid (22:6n-3; DHA). *Journal of Functional Foods, 19*, 852–858. https://doi.org/10.1016/j.jff.2014.06.023, http://www.elsevier.com/wps/find/journaldescription.cws_home/717426/description#description.

Saikia, & Diganta (2023). A review of polyunsaturated fatty acids (PUFA) of marine zoosporic microorganisms and their commercialization. *Botanica Marina, 66*. https://doi.org/10.1515/bot-2022-0073.

Saini, Prasad, Sreedhar, Akhilender Naidu, Shang, & Keum (2021). Omega-3 polyunsaturated fatty acids (PUFAs): Emerging plant and microbial sources, oxidative stability, bioavailability, and health benefits-a review. *Antioxidants (Basel, Switzerland), 10*(10).

Sangkharak, K., Paichid, N., Yunu, T., & Klomklao, S. (2020). Improvement of extraction and concentration method for polyunsaturated fatty acid production from *Nile tilapia* processing waste. *Biomass Conversion and Biorefinery*, 1–13.

Sati, H., Mitra, M., Mishra, S., & Baredar, P. (2019). Microalgal lipid extraction strategies for biodiesel production: A review. *Algal Research, 38*, 101413. https://doi.org/10.1016/j.algal.2019.101413.

Schuchardt, J. P., & Hahn, A. (2013). Bioavailability of long-chain omega-3 fatty acids. *Prostaglandins, Leukotrienes, and Essential Fatty Acids, 89*(1), 1–8. https://doi.org/10.1016/j.plefa.2013.03.010.

Selim, K. A., Alharthi, S. S., Abu El-Hassan, A. M., Elneairy, N. A., Rabee, L. A., & Abdel-Razek, A. G. (2021). The effect of wall material type on the encapsulation efficiency and oxidative stability of fish oils. *Molecules (Basel, Switzerland), 26*(20). https://doi.org/10.3390/molecules26206109, https://www.mdpi.com/1420-3049/26/20/6109/pdf.

Semenova, M. G., Antipova, A. S., Martirosova, E. I., Chebotarev, S. A., Palmina, N. P., Bogdanova, N. G., Krikunova, N. I., Zelikina, D. V., Anokhina, M. S., & Kasparov, V. V. (2022). The relationship between the structure and functionality of essential PUFA delivery systems based on sodium caseinate with phosphatidylcholine liposomes without and with a plant antioxidant: An in vitro and in vivo study. *Food and Function, 13*(4), 2354–2371. https://doi.org/10.1039/d1fo03336k, http://pubs.rsc.org/en/journals/journal/fo.

Shabana, S., Hamouda, H. I., Hamadou, A. H., Ahmed, B., Chi, Z., & Liu, C. (2024). Marine phospholipid nanoliposomes: A promising therapeutic approach for inflammatory bowel disease: Preparation, safety, and efficacy evaluation. *Colloids and Surfaces B: Biointerfaces, 234*. https://doi.org/10.1016/j.colsurfb.2023.113702, https://www.sciencedirect.com/science/journal/09277765.

Shahidi, F., & Hossain, A. (2022). Role of lipids in food flavor generation. *Molecules (Basel, Switzerland), 27*(15), 5014. https://doi.org/10.3390/molecules27155014.

Shum, H. C., Lee, D., Yoon, I., Kodger, T., & Weitz, D. A. (2008). Double emulsion templated monodisperse phospholipid vesicles. *Langmuir: The ACS Journal of Surfaces and Colloids, 24*(15), 7651–7653. https://doi.org/10.1021/la801833a.

Simopoulos, A. P. (2022). The importance of the omega-6/omega-3 fatty acid ratio in cardiovascular disease and other chronic diseases. *Experimental Biology and Medicine, 247*(5), 456–472.

Smith, C. E., Follis, J. L., Nettleton, J. A., Foy, M., Wu, J. H. Y., Ma, Y., Tanaka, T., Manichakul, A. W., Wu, H., Chu, A. Y., Steffen, L. M., Fornage, M., Mozaffarian, D., Kabagambe, E. K., Ferruci, L., Chen, Y. D. I., Rich, S. S., Djoussé, L., Ridker, P. M., ... Lemaitre, R. N. (2015). Dietary fatty acids modulate associations between genetic variants and circulating fatty acids in plasma and erythrocyte membranes: Meta-analysis of nine studies in the CHARGE consortium. *Molecular Nutrition and Food Research, 59*(7), 1373–1383. https://doi.org/10.1002/mnfr.201400734, http://onlinelibrary.wiley.com/journal/10.1002/(ISSN)1613-4133.

Sousa, S. C., Freitas, A. C., Gomes, A. M., & Carvalho, A. P. (2023). Extraction of nannochloropsis fatty acids using different green technologies: The current path. *Marine Drugs, 21*(6). https://doi.org/10.3390/md21060365, http://www.mdpi.com/journal/marinedrugs.

Stramarkou, M., Oikonomopoulou, V., Chalima, A., Boukouvalas, C., Topakas, E., & Krokida, M. (2021). Optimization of green extractions for the recovery of docosahexaenoic acid (DHA) from Crypthecodinium cohnii. *Algal Research, 58*, 102374. https://doi.org/10.1016/j.algal.2021.102374.

Suleria, H. A. R., Osborne, S., Masci, P., & Gobe, G. (2015). Marine-based nutraceuticals: An innovative trend in the food and supplement industries. *Marine Drugs, 13*(10), 6336–6351. https://doi.org/10.3390/md13106336, http://www.mdpi.com/1660-3397/13/10/6336/pdf.

Swetha, N., & Mathanghi, S. K. (2024). Towards sustainable omega-3 fatty acids production – A comprehensive review on extraction methods, oxidative stability and bio-availability enhancement. *Food Chemistry Advances, 4*, 100603. https://doi.org/10.1016/j.focha.2023.100603.

Timilsena, Y. P., Wang, B., Adhikari, R., & Adhikari, B. (2017). Advances in microencapsulation of polyunsaturated fatty acids (PUFAs)-rich plant oils using complex coacervation: A review. *Food Hydrocolloids, 69*, 369–381. https://doi.org/10.1016/j.foodhyd.2017.03.007, https://www.journals.elsevier.com/food-hydrocolloids.

Toopcham, T., Roytrakul, S., & Roytrakul, S. (2021). Marine and plant-derived polyunsaturated fatty acids: Sources, health benefits, and market dynamics. *Trends in Food Science & Technology, 115*, 102–115.

Trier, S., Henriksen, J. R., & Andresen, T. L. (2011). Membrane fusion of pH-sensitive liposomes - A quantitative study using giant unilamellar vesicles. *Soft Matter, 7*(19), 9027–9034. https://doi.org/10.1039/c1sm05818e.

Troesch, B., Eggersdorfer, M., Laviano, A., Rolland, Y., Smith, A. D., Warnke, I., Weimann, A., & Calder, P. C. (2020). Expert opinion on benefits of long-chain omega-3 fatty acids (DHA and EPA) in aging and clinical nutrition. *Nutrients, 12*(9), 1–25. https://doi.org/10.3390/nu12092555, https://www.mdpi.com/2072-6643/12/9/2555/pdf.

Tsai, W. C., & Rizvi, S. S. H. (2016). Liposomal microencapsulation using the conventional methods and novel supercritical fluid processes. *Trends in Food Science and Technology, 55*, 61–71. https://doi.org/10.1016/j.tifs.2016.06.012, http://www.elsevier.com/wps/find/journaldescription.cws_home/601278/description#description.

Umesha, S. S., Monahar, B., & Naidu, K. A. (2013). Microencapsulation of α-linolenic acid-rich garden cress seed oil: Physical characteristics and oxidative stability. *European Journal of Lipid Science and Technology, 115*(12), 1474–1482. https://doi.org/10.1002/ejlt.201300181.

Venugopalan, V. K., Gopakumar, L. R., Kumaran, A. K., Chatterjee, N. S., Soman, V., Peeralil, S., Mathew, S., McClements, D. J., & Nagarajarao, R. C. (2021). Encapsulation and protection of omega-3-rich fish oils using food-grade delivery systems. *Foods, 10*(7). https://doi.org/10.3390/foods10071566, https://www.mdpi.com/2304-8158/10/7/1566/pdf.

Wang, D., Fan, W., Guan, Y., Huang, H., Yi, T., & Ji, J. (2018). Oxidative stability of sunflower oil flavored by essential oil from *Coriandrum sativum* L. during accelerated storage. *LWT, 98*, 268–275.

Wang, X., Zhu, C., Peng, T., Zhang, W., Zhang, J., Liu, H., ... Wu, C. (2018). Enhanced stability of an emulsion enriched in unsaturated fatty acids by dual natural antioxidants fortified in both the aqueous and oil phases. *Food Hydrocolloids, 82*, 322–328.

Wang, Y. Z., Fu, S. G., Wang, S. Y., Yang, D. J., Wu, Y. H. S., & Chen, Y. C. (2018). Effects of a natural antioxidant, polyphenol-rich rosemary (*Rosmarinus officinalis* L.) extract, on lipid stability of plant-derived omega-3 fatty-acid rich oil. *LWT, 89*, 210–216. https://doi.org/10.1016/j.lwt.2017.10.055, https://www.journals.elsevier.com/lwt.

Wei, W., Cheng, Z., Wang, X., Chang, M., Xie, D., Sun, C., & Li, B. (2025). The potential of marine oils as functional foods: Nutritional composition, health benefits, applications, and future perspectives. In *Food reviews international*1–32 (Mititelu *et al.*, 2025).

West, A. L., Kindberg, G. M., Hustvedt, S. O., & Calder, P. C. (2018). A novel self-micro-emulsifying delivery system enhances enrichment of eicosapentaenoic acid and docosahexaenoic acid after single and repeated dosing in healthy adults in a randomized trial. *Journal of Nutrition, 148*(11), 1704–1715. https://doi.org/10.1093/jn/nxy127, http://jn.nutrition.org.

Xiong, X., Zhang, S., Fu, N., Lei, H., Wu, W. D., & Chen, X. D. (2021). Effects of particle formation behavior on the properties of fish oil microcapsules fabricated using a micro-fluidic jet spray dryer. *International Journal of Food Engineering, 17*(1), 27–36. https://doi.org/10.1515/ijfe-2019-0162, www.degruyter.com/view/j/ijfe.

Yaghmur, A. (2019). *Nanoencapsulation of food ingredients by cubosomes and hexosomes*. Elsevier BV, 483–522. https://doi.org/10.1016/b978-0-12-815673-5.00012-x.

Yamaguchi, T., Nomura, M., Matsuoka, T., & Koda, S. (2009). Effects of frequency and power of ultrasound on the size reduction of liposome. *Chemistry and Physics of Lipids, 160*(1), 58–62. https://doi.org/10.1016/j.chemphyslip.2009.04.002.

Yan, K., Guo, F., Kainz, M. J., Li, F., Gao, W., Bunn, S. E., & Zhang, Y. (2024). The importance of omega-3 polyunsaturated fatty acids as high-quality food in freshwater ecosystems with implications of global change. *Biological Reviews, 99*(1), 200–218. https://doi.org/10.1111/brv.13017, http://onlinelibrary.wiley.com/journal/10.1111/(ISSN)1469-185X.

Yep, Y. L., Li, D., Mann, N. J., Bode, O., & Sinclair, A. J. (2002). Bread enriched with microencapsulated tuna oil increases plasma docosahexaenoic acid and total omega-3 fatty acids in humans. *Asia Pacific Journal of Clinical Nutrition, 11*(4), 285–291. https://doi.org/10.1046/j.1440-6047.2002.00309.x.

Yeşilçubuk, N.Ş., Demirel, B., & Bilsel, A. Y. (2021). Attitudes and preferences of consumers towards functional foods enriched with Omega-3 fatty acids. *AvrupaBilimveTeknolojiDergisi,* (25), 485–492.

Yokoyama, S., Takeda, T., & Abe, M. (2003). Preparation of ganglioside GM3 liposomes and their membrane properties. *Colloids and Surfaces B: Biointerfaces, 27*(2-3), 181–187. https://doi.org/10.1016/s0927-7765(02)00071-1.

Yui, Y., Miyazaki, S., Ma, Y., Ohira, M., Fiehn, O., Ikegami, T., McCalley, D. V., & Tanaka, N. (2016). Distinction of synthetic dl-α-tocopherol from natural vitamin E (d-α-tocopherol) by reversed-phase liquid chromatography. Enhanced selectivity of a polymeric C18 stationary phase at low temperature and/or at high pressure. *Journal of Chromatography. A, 1450*, 45–52. https://doi.org/10.1016/j.chroma.2016.04.076.

Zghaibi, N., Omar, R., Kamal, S. M. M., Biak, D. R. A., & Harun, R. (2019). Microwave-assisted brine extraction for enhancement of the quantity and quality of lipid production from microalgae *Nannochloropsis* sp. *Molecules (Basel, Switzerland), 24*(19), 3581. https://doi.org/10.3390/molecules24193581.

Zhang, N., Li, Y., Wen, S., Sun, Y., Chen, J., Gao, Y., Sagymbek, A., & Yu, X. (2021). Analytical methods for determining the peroxide value of edible oils: A mini-review. *Food Chemistry, 358*, 129834. https://doi.org/10.1016/j.foodchem.2021.129834.

Zhou, Q., Lane, K. E., & Li, W. (2024). Evaluating the stability and digestibility of long-chain omega-3 algal oil nanoemulsions prepared with lecithin and Tween 40 emulsifiers using an in vitro digestion model. *Foods, 13*(15). https://doi.org/10.3390/foods13152407, www.mdpi.com/journal/foods.

Zhou, X.-R., Yao, Z. J., Benedicto, K., Nichols, P. D., Green, A., & Singh, S. (2023). New sustainable oil seed sources of omega-3 long-chain polyunsaturated fatty acids: A journey from the ocean to the field. *Sustainability, 15*(14), 11327. https://doi.org/10.3390/su151411327.

Zhu, P., Li, J., Zhou, Y., Li, J., & Yu, Q. (2025). Precision targeted delivery based on PUFAs: Overview, strategies and applications. *Food Chemistry, 493*(Pt 2), 145800. https://doi.org/10.1016/j.foodchem.2025.145800.

Zuk, M., Richter, D., Matuła, J., & Szopa, J. (2015). Linseed, the multipurpose plant. *Industrial Crops and Products, 75*, 165–177. https://doi.org/10.1016/j.indcrop.2015.05.005.

Chapter 22

Regulatory landscape of polyunsaturated fatty acids in food products: labeling and claims

Vignaesh Dhanabalan[1], Masilan Karunanithi[2], Bharathipriya Rajasekaran[3], Sarojini Andiappan[1], and Mohammed Javith[4]

[1]*Paraprofessional Institute of Fisheries Technology, Tamil Nadu Dr. J. Jayalalithaa Fisheries University, Madhavaram Campus, Chennai, Tamil Nadu, India,* [2]*Department of Fish Processing Technology, TNJFU – Fisheries College and Research Institute, Tamil Nadu Dr. J. Jayalalithaa Fisheries University, Ponneri, Tamil Nadu, India,* [3]*Institute of Food Science and Technology, National Taiwan University, Taipei, Taiwan,* [4]*Directorate of Extension Education, Tamil Nadu Dr. J. Jayalalithaa Fisheries University, Nagapattinam, Tamil Nadu, India*

22.1 Introduction to polyunsaturated fatty acids in the modern diet

22.1.1 Definition and classification

Polyunsaturated fatty acids (PUFAs) are essential fatty acids with two or more double bonds in the hydrocarbon structure. These essential fatty acids can be obtained from the diet and cannot be synthesized by the human body. PUFAs are classified into omega-3 and omega-6 fatty acids. The main sources of omega-3 fatty acids include fish oil, flaxseed oil, chia seeds, walnuts, soyabeans, and canola oil, whereas soybean oil, sunflower oil, corn oil, cottonseed oil, safflower oil, and grapeseed oil are the key sources of omega-6 fatty acids (Mititelu et al., 2025). One of the omega-3 fatty acids, α-linolenic acid (ALA), acts as a precursor for the synthesis of eicosapentaenoic acid (EPA) and docosahexaenoic acid (DHA). Similarly, an omega-6 fatty acid is linoleic acid, which acts as a precursor for the synthesis of gamma-linolenic acid and arachidonic acid (Islam et al., 2023; Kapoor et al., 2021). These PUFAs are also important in the synthesis of eicosanoids and docosanoids, which serve as signaling molecules for maintaining optimal health (Papandreou, 2014a,b).

22.1.1.1 Classification

PUFAs are classified into two types based on the position of the double bond in the hydrocarbon structure. Table 22.1 shows the application of different categories of lipids (Gunstone and Herslof, 1992; Gunstone et al., 2007; Zhang and Xu, 2025).

22.1.1.1.1 Omega-3 fatty acids

This mainly includes ALA (18:3 n-3) that acts as a precursor for long-chain derivatives such as EPA and DHA.

22.1.1.1.2 Omega-6 fatty acids

The primary member is linoleic acid (LA). LA serves as the precursor for arachidonic acid (AA or ARA), which is vital for the structural integrity of skeletal muscle and the functioning of the immune and neurological systems. Fig. 22.1 presents the oxidation of PUFA.

22.1.1.2 Dietary food sources

The primary sources of PUFAs are plant sources, algal sources, and marine/aquatic sources.

Omega-3 and Omega-6 Polyunsaturated Fatty Acids in Food Systems. DOI: https://doi.org/10.1016/B978-0-443-43810-3.00011-7

TABLE 22.1 Applications of different categories of lipids.

S. no.	Categories	Definition	Types of applications
	Nutritional lipids	Lipids essential for human metabolism and health, including fatty acids, phospholipids, sterols, etc.	Heart-healthy oils, weight management, antiinflammatory diets
	Healthy lipids	Lipids promoting health and preventing disease (e.g., monounsaturated fatty acids, polyunsaturated fatty acids, Medium chain Triglycerides MCTs); often overlap with nutritional lipids	Infant formula, dietary supplements, fortified oils, daily nutrition
	Functional lipids	Lipids providing physiological benefits beyond basic nutrition (e.g., omega-3s, structured lipids, Fatty acid esters of hydroxy fatty acids FAHFAs)	Functional foods, nutraceuticals, metabolic therapy (e.g., Diacylglycerol DAG, omega-3s, phytosterols)
	Bioactive lipids	Lipids with direct biological activity (e.g., DHA, tocopherols, FAHFAs, odd-chain fatty acids).	Precision nutrition, metabolic disease therapy (e.g., obesity), neurological/immune support
	Bio-medical lipids	Lipids specifically designed or applied for medical purposes (e.g., enteral/parenteral emulsions, immune-support lipids)	Enteral/parenteral nutrition, malnutrition treatment, metabolic disorders

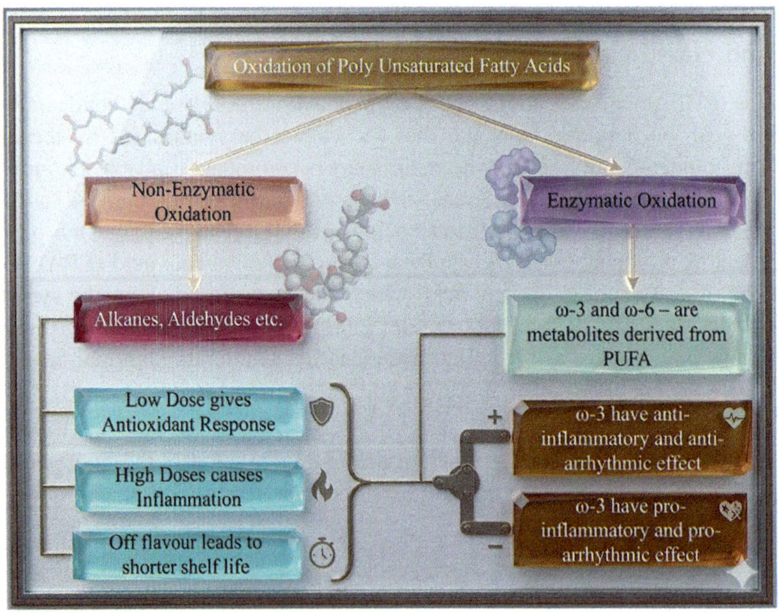

FIGURE 22.1 Polyunsaturated fatty acids (PUFA)—oxidation.

22.1.1.2.1 Omega-3 sources

- Plant sources: plant seeds such as flaxseeds (linseeds), chia seeds, perilla seeds, green leafy vegetables, cereals, and walnuts.
- Aquatic/marine sources: fatty fishes such as salmon and tuna. Marine algal polysaccharides and krill are also significant sources.

22.1.1.2.2 Omega-6 sources

Vegetable oils, including soybean, sunflower, corn, safflower, and canola oils, are the chief sources of LA. AA is found in peanut oil, eggs, and various dairy products.

*22.1.1.3 Health benefits of **polyunsaturated fatty acids***

The inclusion of PUFAs in a balanced diet is linked to the prevention and management of several chronic conditions.

22.1.1.3.1 Cardiovascular health

PUFAs are a recognized therapeutic tool for cardioprotection. They contribute to heart health by:

- regulating blood pressure and improving cholesterol metabolism;
- exhibiting antiarrhythmic effects by altering sodium, potassium, and calcium channels in heart cells, reducing their excitability and slowing atrioventricular conduction;
- reducing the risk of myocardial infarction and sudden cardiac death (Narayan et al., 2006).

22.1.1.3.2 Brain and neurological function

- PUFAs are fundamental for the central nervous system.
- DHA is a structural lipid in the brain and retina, accounting for nearly 90% of the n-3 PUFAs in the brain and 10-20% of its total lipid content. They are essential for fetal brain development and visual maturation during pregnancy. Higher intake is associated with a reduced risk of cognitive decline, dementia, and Alzheimer's disease (Weiser et al., 2016).

22.1.1.3.3 Inflammation and autoimmune disorders

EPA and DHA produce metabolites with potent antiinflammatory properties. Supplementation can benefit patients with asthma by inhibiting bronchial inflammation and mitigating exercise-induced bronchoconstriction (Miyata & arita., 2015).

22.1.1.3.4 Autoimmune conditions

Symptoms of multiple sclerosis (MS), rheumatoid arthritis, and psoriasis may be altered or improved through the modulation of pro-inflammatory cytokines.

22.1.1.3.5 Metabolic health and obesity

The omega–3 PUFAs are crucial in body weight management by (Chacińska et al., 2019):

- Enhancing β-oxidation of fatty acids in adipose tissues and decreasing lipogenic enzyme activity;
- improving insulin resistance by stimulating the release of adiponectin.

22.1.1.3.6 Cancer prevention

- Epidemiological studies suggest that PUFAs may protect against certain malignancies, including colorectal, breast, and prostate cancers.
- For cancer patients, omega–3 fatty acids can help maintain lean body mass and boost appetite (D'Eliseo & Velotti, 2016).

22.1.2 Physiological importance

PUFAs ensure the fluidity and structural stability of all cellular membranes. These fatty acids also act as primary substrates for the synthesis of eicosanoids, which are bioactive mediators that regulate immune activity, vascular pressure, and inflammatory pathways. Particularly, EPA and DHA play essential roles in maintaining heart health, facilitating normal visual good vision, and supporting neurological development (Parasannanavar et al., 2021). Table 22.2 presents the sources and benefits of different fatty acids (Gunstone & Herslof, 1992; Gunstone et al., 2007; Zhang & Xu, 2025).

22.1.2.1 Novel foods and new polyunsaturated fatty acid sources

The Novel Food Regulation (EU) 2015/2283 applies to many innovative PUFA sources, which ensures safety through rigorous scientific review. Examples of authorized novel sources include algal oil from *Ulkenia* sp. (high in DHA), Antarctic krill oil (rich in phospholipids), and chia oil (*Salvia hispanica*). Interestingly, ethyl esters of fish oil are

TABLE 22.2 Source and benefits of different fatty acids.

S. no.	Types of fatty acids	Sources	Beneficial properties
1.	Oleic acid (C18:1 n-9)	Olive oil, avocado oil	Improves lipid profile; supports heart health
2.	Nervonic acid (C24:1 n-9)	Fish, seed oils, human brain tissue	Very long chain fatty acids; important in nerve cell membranes
3.	Linoleic acid (C18:2 n-6)	Sunflower oil, corn oil, soybean oil	Essential fatty acid (EFA); supports skin, inflammation modulation
4.	CLA	Ruminant fats (beef, dairy), grass-fed animal products	Anticarcinogenic, antiinflammatory; potential in weight management
5.	Alpha-linolenic acid (C18:3 n-3)	Flaxseed, chia seeds, walnuts	EFA; supports heart and brain function
6.	Arachidonic acid (C20:4 n-6)	Meat, eggs, organ meats	Precursor to eicosanoids; pro-inflammatory in excess
7.	Eicosapentaenoic acid (C20:5 n-3)	Fatty fish, fish oil, algae oil	Antiinflammatory; supports cardiovascular and brain health
8.	Docosapentaenoic acid (C22:5 n-3)	Fish oil, marine sources	Intermediate omega-3; supports DHA synthesis
9.	Docosahexaenoic acid (DHA) (C22:6 n-3)	Fatty fish, fish oil, breast milk	Crucial for brain and eye development; antiinflammatory
10.	Branched chain fatty acids	Dairy, ruminant fat, some fermented foods	Influence gut microbiota and metabolic health
11.	Fatty acid esters of hydroxy fatty acids	Adipose tissue, fermented foods, milk, rice bran oil	Antiinflammatory, glucose-regulating. Potential therapeutic lipokines

authorized for use only in food supplements, as they are considered unauthorized novel foods in conventional food categories. Fig. 22.2 shows the sources of PUFA.

22.1.3 The nutritional imbalance challenge

The variation in modern nutritional diets among developed countries is typically characterized by saturated lipids and a lesser availability of omega-3s. Consequently, global health guidelines increasingly support a diet that increases the consumption of unsaturated fatty acids over saturated and trans-fat components (Turck et al., 2022).

22.2 Labeling and health claims of polyunsaturated fatty acids in foods

Labeling is an important tool for increasing consumer awareness and trust. Labels should be precise and transparent. Labelling ensures that the that information relevant to dietary decisions adheres to established legal frameworks. As oxidative stability is a challenge for the packaging and labeling of products supplemented with PUFAs, protective packaging is essential. Therefore labeling regulations and elements are necessary for preserving the actual nutritional profile mentioned and delivered to the consumer.

22.2.1 Agencies maintaining mandatory global regulations

Major Global agencies, which include USFDA, EFSA (European Food Safety Authority), and FSSAI, establish guidelines and regulations for labeling to prevent false or misleading information.

22.2.1.1 Ingredient statements

All labels should include common names of all fats and oils in the packaging label in descending order by weight. For example, specific names such as "sunflower oil" or "flax seed" oil must be used on the ingredients list in the packaging label instead of using non-specific names such as "vegetable oil."

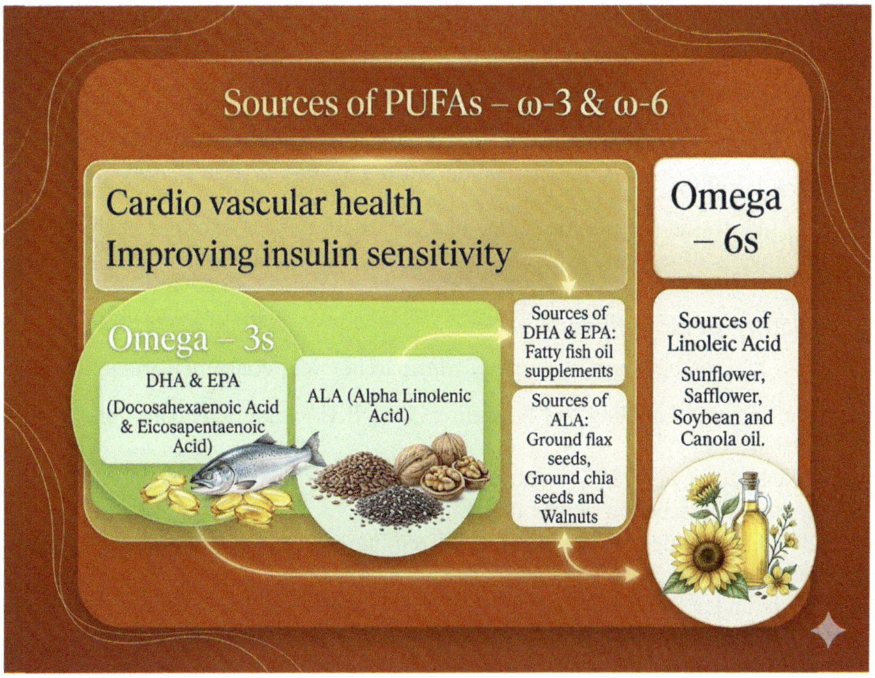
Sources of PUFAs – ω-3 & ω-6
Cardio vascular health
Improving insulin sensitivity
Omega – 6s
Omega – 3s
DHA & EPA
(Docosahexaenoic Acid & Eicosapentaenoic Acid)
ALA (Alpha Linolenic Acid)
Sources of DHA & EPA: Fatty fish oil supplements
Sources of ALA: Ground flax seeds, Ground chia seeds and Walnuts
Sources of Linoleic Acid
Sunflower, Safflower, Soybean and Canola oil.

FIGURE 22.2 Sources of polyunsaturated fatty acid.

22.2.1.2 *Nutrition facts panels*

The tables mentioned on the label should be properly quantified, such as saturated, unsaturated, and trans fats. Several labels should also be required to separate the fatty acids into constituent types such as n-3, n-6, fat-soluble vitamins (A, D, E, and K), and their composition. These constituents must also be validated through laboratory testing for ensuring its accuracy.

22.2.1.3 *Nutrition and health claims*

According to the USFDA regulation, the nutrients are classified as:

- **Class I:** nutrients that are fortified in foods and must be at 100% of the declared value on the label;
- **Class II:** nutrients that are native or indigenous to the food itself and must be present at least at 80% of the declared value on the label.

22.2.1.4 *Nutrient content claims*

Nutrient content claims describe the level of a nutrient in a food. These may be absolute claims (e.g., 'High in DHA or EPA'), indicating that a product meets a minimum specified content threshold, or relative claims, which compare nutrient content to that of another food.

22.2.1.5 *Health claims*

This was related to the food components and treatment of disease by maintaining the normal physiological function. For example, products claiming EPA and DHA support cardiac health and brain development require scientific evidence. Also, in the United States, these claims must meet the "significant scientific agreement" standard. Whereas, European Union countries mandate authorization by the European Food Safety Authority (EFSA) (EFSA Panel on Nutrition, Novel Foods and Food Allergens NDA, 2022).

22.2.1.6 *Nutrient profiling and front-of-pack labelling*

Nutrient profiling is the evaluation of foods based on their nutritional composition to make a healthier choice and reduce the risk of diet-related diseases.

22.2.1.6.1 Restricting claims

A primary goal of nutrient profiling is to restrict the use of nutrition and health claims on foods that are high in fat, sugar, or salt. This ensures consumers aren't misled by products that may be rich in PUFAs yet still high in sodium or added sugars.

22.2.1.6.2 Front-of-pack labelling

Front-of-pack (FOP) tools like traffic-light colors or Nutri-Score help consumers spot healthier options at a glance. In Europe, nutrient-profiling models often emphasize replacing saturated fatty acids with PUFAs to support heart health.

22.2.1.7 Global regulatory perspectives

Labeling rules differ across regions but share the aim of transparency and consumer protection.

- **United States:** under the Nutrition Labeling and Education Act (NLEA), the FDA bans generic oil names and mandates fat breakdowns on the labels.
- **European Union:** EU Regulation 1169/2011 requires nutrition declarations per 100 g or 100 mL. The "Farm to Fork" strategy seeks to harmonize FOP labeling across the Union.
- **China:** labels must follow Codex rules, including standardized ingredient labeling and stringent checks on health claims related to children's growth.
- **Japan:** food labeling falls under the Food Sanitation Act; any health claims require approval from the Secretary of Health, Labor and Welfare based on systematic evidence reviews.
- India: the FSSAI mandates symbols for vegetarian/nonvegetarian status and requires extensive scientific dossiers for health claim approval.

22.2.1.8 Compliance and accuracy

The reliability of label claims is a critical concern for consumer safety. A study of omega-3 supplements in the French market found that while most products were compliant, approximately 2.5% failed to meet their label claims for EPA or DHA content. Such discrepancies highlight the need for continuous market surveillance and rigorous adherence to manufacturing standards (Pasini et al., 2022).

22.2.1.9 Advanced metabolism and bioavailability

The human diet primarily depends on the PUFAs, but the capacity to transform the plant-derived precursor fatty acid, such as ALA, to the omega-3 fatty acids is limited. Research has shown that a "bottleneck" effect exists in the transformation of precursors to omega fatty acids. About 10%–20% of ALA is only converted to EPA, and as little as 1%–9% of ALA is only transformed to DHA. Therefore the efficiency of this fatty acid conversion is largely determined by bioavailability, which is defined as the extent of their entrance into the systemic circulation of specific organs. After ingestion, the PUFAs are found in both free-state or bound to glycerol, such as mono, di, or triacylglycerols, which ultimately build the cell membrane phospholipids (Wood et al., 2015).

22.2.1.10 Detailed physiological mechanisms

PUFAs exert protective effects on the cardiovascular system through sophisticated molecular strategies. They provide cardio-protection by modulating ion channels—specifically potassium, sodium, and calcium channels—which makes heart cells "less impulsive" and significantly reduces the risk of dangerous heart rhythm intervals, such as a prolonged QT interval (Marcus and Link, 2024). In terms of physical performance, PUFAs possess potent antioxidative and antiinflammatory properties that help manage the enhanced generation of reactive oxygen species in individuals performing strenuous physical activities.

22.2.1.11 Oxidative stability and food science technologies

The chemical structure of PUFAs, characterized by multiple double bonds, renders them highly susceptible to lipid oxidation, which proceeds through three sequential stages: initiation, propagation, and termination. Factors such as temperature, pH, light, and ionic strength can weaken food emulsions and lead to the formation of hazardous by-products, such as reactive carbonyl compounds. To mitigate these risks, the following innovative preservative strategies are employed (Islam et al., 2023).

- **Encapsulation:** micro and nanoencapsulation protect PUFAs from the environment, mask off-flavours such as "fishy" odors, and improve distribution to target cells.
- **Advanced emulsions:** technologies such as pickering emulsions, which use solid particles for stabilization, and bilayer emulsions, which create a thicker physical barrier, significantly reduce the rate of oxidation.
- **Maillard reaction products:** these can be used to capture volatile chemicals that cause flavor deterioration, particularly in fish oils.

22.2.1.12 Quality assessment in supplements

Ensuring the safety of omega-3 supplements involves monitoring their oxidative status through standardized metrics.

- **Peroxide value (PV):** a marker for the first stage of oxidation; guidelines typically require a PV of less than 5 mEq. $O_2\,kg^{-1}$.
- **p-Anisidine value (AV):** used as a marker for the secondary stage of oxidation.
- **Totox value:** a consolidated score calculated as $(2 \times PV) + AV$ to represent total oxidation; a maximum limit of 26 is standard for fish oils. Additionally, supplements often contain tocols (tocopherols and tocotrienols), which act as essential antioxidants to maintain the shelf life of sensitive oils (Bannenberg et al., 2017).

22.2.1.13 Emerging trends in labeling and packaging

Modern consumer preferences are driving shifts in how PUFA-rich foods are marketed and protected.

- **Clean labelling:** clean labeling makes clear whether the product is minimally processed and free from artificial additives, ensuring transparency for consumers.
- **Sustainability claims:** today, labels highlight certifications for responsible practises such as sustainable, organic, and fair trade.
- **Technology enhancements:** packages now use QR codes to give consumers instant access to details such as storage conditions and preparation steps on their mobile devices.
- **Active packaging:** advanced packaging uses smart sensors to track freshness in real time and release antioxidants to maintain the quality of the product during storage.

22.3 The global framework: Codex Alimentarius and international standardization

22.3.1 Role of the Codex Alimentarius

Codex Alimentarius sets food-labeling standards to protect consumer health and ensure fair practices. The WTO's SPS and TBT Agreements recognise Codex standards as international benchmarks for resolving trade disputes (Codex Alimentarius Commission, 1985).

22.3.1.1 General principles for labeling

Codex's core principle is that food labels must not mislead consumers; prepackaged labels should avoid a false impression of a product's nature (Codex Alimentarius Commission, 1985).

22.3.1.2 Codex guidelines for polyunsaturated fatty acid labeling

Specific guidelines regarding nutrition labeling recommend that it remain voluntary unless a nutrition claim is made. When a claim is made regarding fatty acids, Codex mandates the listing of saturated, monounsaturated, and PUFAs, as well as cholesterol (Codex Alimentarius Commission, 1985).

22.3.1.3 International harmonization

Differences in national regulations can act as trade barriers, requiring exporters to modify labels for different markets. Regional entities such as ASEAN and MERCOSUR work toward harmonizing these regulations to facilitate the free movement of food products while maintaining consumer protection (Codex Alimentarius Commission, 1985).

22.3.2 The American regulatory landscape: FDA oversight

22.3.2.1 Statutory framework

In the United States, food labeling and health claims come under the Nutrition Labeling and Education Act of 1990 (NLEA), codified in 21 CFR and enforced by the FDA (Hoadley, 2017a,b).

22.3.2.2 Nutrient classification and compliance

For label compliance, the FDA classifies nutrients: Class I (added) must meet or exceed 100% of the declared value, while Class II (natural) must reach at least 80%. Because EPA and DHA exist in nature, they are often treated as Class II nutrients by industry practice (Hoadley, 2017a,b) (Bannenberg et al., 2020).

22.3.2.3 Types of claims

The United States allows three categories of claims: nutrient content claims, structure/function claims, and health claims. Health claims are further divided into authorized health claims—which require significant scientific agreement (SSA)—and qualified health claims (QHCs), which are supported by emerging evidence and must include a disclaimer to prevent consumer deception (Bannenberg et al., 2020).

22.3.2.4 Categories of permitted claims

The FDA recognizes three main categories of health-related messages:

- **Nutrient content claims:** these describe the level of a nutrient, such as "low fat" or "high in Omega-3."
- **Structure/function claims:** these describe the role of a nutrient in affecting the normal structure or function of the body (e.g., "DHA supports brain health") without referencing a disease.
- **Health claims:** these link a food component to the reduced risk of a disease or health condition.

22.3.2.5 Significant scientific agreement versus qualified claims

Authorized health claims must be supported by SSA among qualified experts. However, the FDA also permits QHCs, which are based on emerging scientific evidence and must include a disclaimer to prevent consumer deception. For example, the QHC for walnuts and heart disease states that the research is "supportive but not conclusive."

22.3.2.6 Nutrient profiling: the "Jelly Bean Rule"

To prevent unhealthy foods from bearing health claims, the FDA employs nutrient profiling. Products are disqualified if they exceed set limits for "negative" nutrients, such as saturated fat, cholesterol, or sodium.

22.4 The European approach: European Food Safety Authority and regulation (EC) 1924/2006

22.4.1 Harmonized EU legislation

In the European Union, Regulation (EC) No 1924/2006 provides a comprehensive framework for nutrition and health claims. This regulation ensures that any claim displayed on labeling or advertising is clear, reliable, and substantiated by scientific evidence (European Union, 2006).

22.4.1.1 Authorization process

All nutrition and health claims must be authorized by the European Commission following a scientific assessment by the EFSA. To be approved, claims must demonstrate a cause-and-effect relationship between the food/constituent and the claimed health benefit, often requiring gold-standard human intervention trials (European Union, 2006).

22.4.1.2 Authorized polyunsaturated fatty acid claims

Remarkable numbers of health claims have been authorized for n-3 and n-6 fatty acids based on their essentiality. For example, ALA and LA maintain the normal blood cholesterol levels. EPA and DHA are authorized for claims related to normal heart function, while DHA specifically is linked to brain and vision maintenance (European Union, 2006). Table 22.3 shows the health-beneficial properties of PUFA (Islam et al., 2023; Ali et al., 2024).

TABLE 22.3 Health-beneficial properties of polyunsaturated fatty acid (PUFA).

S. no.	PUFA	Health benefits	References
Omega-3 fatty acids			
1.	Alpha-linolenic acid	Promotes cardiovascular functioning, blood pressure regulation, and neurological problems; antiinflammatory and antiarrhythmic characteristics	Blondeau et al. (2015) and Gogna et al. (2023)
2.	Eicosapentaenoic acid	Antiinflammatory qualities, fewer serious coronary incidents, and better antiplatelet actions increase cardiovascular performance. Protects against severe brain damage	Narayan et al. (2006) Swanson et al. (2012)
3.	Docosahexaenoic acid		
Omega-6 fatty acids			
4.	Arachidonic acid	The neurological system (cognitive and brain processes), skeletal muscle, and immune processes all require it for proper growth and functioning	Tallima and El Ridi (2018)
5.	Linoleic acid	Decrease body fat with increasing lean body mass, and modify immunological and/or inflammatory reactions to decrease the formation of atherosclerosis	Kim et al. (2016)

22.4.1.3 Nutrient profiling

The EU is developing nutrient profiles—criteria that foods must respect to bear claims—to prevent products high in fat, sugar, or salt from using health messages to appear "healthy" (Turck et al., 2022).

22.4.2 The role of the European Food Safety Authority

New health claims undergo a rigorous assessment by EFSA, which evaluates the "highest possible scientific standard" of evidence, primarily relying on human intervention studies. EFSA maintains the "EU Register of nutrition and health claims," which contains all permitted and rejected claims (Turck et al., 2022).

22.4.3 Specific authorized polyunsaturated fatty acid claims

The EU has authorized several claims related to lipids and PUFAs, including:

- **Replacement claims:** "Replacing saturated fats with unsaturated fats in the diet has been shown to lower/reduce blood cholesterol."
- **Essential fatty acids** claims**:** claims for ALA in relation to sustaining normal blood cholesterol levels.

22.5 Regulatory landscapes in Asia and evolving markets

22.5.1 Japan: the pioneer of functional foods

In 1991, Japan pioneered the introduction of a regulatory framework for functional foods, known as food for specified health use (FOSHU). FOSHU products are evaluated for both safety and effectiveness and are authorized to indicate health-related physiological benefits (Government of Japan, 1991).

22.5.2 Japan's food with nutrient function claims

Unlike FOSHU, food with nutrient function claims products do not require premarketing approval if they contain standardized amounts of specific vitamins or minerals. Japan permits the use of QHCs with scientific evidence (Government of Japan, 1991).

22.5.3 Indian context

FSSAI oversees the regulation of PUFA in India, which directs the fortification initiatives to develop functional foods and sets labeling standards to combat national nutritional deficiencies.

22.5.3.1 Dietary guidelines and requirements

The 2024 ICMR-NIN, 2024 Dietary Guidelines for Indians highlight the importance of PUFA for overall health and development. Special attention is given to DHA, which contributes to the growth of an infant's brain and retina. To meet the needs, guidelines recommend that n-6 PUFA provides at least 3% of daily energy, while n-3 PUFA should contribute between 0.6% and 1.2%. On a standard 2000 Kcal diet, this translates into about 6.6 g of n-6 PUFA and 2.2 g of n-3 PUFA each day.

22.5.3.1.1 Multisource edible oils

FSSAI encourages the use of multisource edible oils, which are admixtures of two vegetable oils where neither is less than 20% by weight. These blends are regulated to ensure they do not exceed 33% saturated fatty acids and are often promoted for supporting the n-6 to n-3 ratio, typically between 1:5 and 1:10. Mandatory FOP declarations must state "MULTI-SOURCE EDIBLE OIL" in bold capital letters along with the constituent oils and their percentages.

22.5.3.2 Fortification and labeling regulations

India's approach to PUFA fortification is currently in an evolving stage:

- **Voluntary fortification:** nutrients such as vitamins A and D, iron, iodine, n-3, etc. require fortification in food products.
- **Multisource edible oils:** FSSAI has given special standards for multisource edible oils. These oil products are produced by blending two different vegetable oils. To safeguard consumer health, the regulations also limit saturated fatty acids to not more than 33% (IVPA, 2022).
- **Ratio claims:** to support the claim about the "ideal ratio" of n-3 to n-6, which is typically 1:5 to 1:10, FSSAI permits the manufacturers to add up to 5% of a third oil, such as Chia oil or flaxseed/linseed oil, to obtain this balance (IVPA, 2022).
- **Compliance and misbranding:** under the Prevention of Food Adulteration Act and current FSSAI norms, products that carry misleading or false claims are classified as misbranded and prohibited. In India, implied nutritional and health claims are permitted. The FSSAI oversees the fortification landscape. While fortification with iodine and vitamins A and D is often mandatory for certain oils, omega-3 fortification remains voluntary. Manufacturers must comply with FSSAI guidelines to ensure safety and accurate labeling, particularly regarding the n-3 to n-6 ratio (targeted at 1:5 to 1:10) (IVPA, 2022). Fig. 22.3 illustrates the regulatory landscape of PUFA in food products.

22.5.3.3 Public health challenges and the Indian diet

The regulatory landscape is shaped by specific dietary patterns and health data in the region:

- **Low omega-3 intake:** research on Indian school children (ages 7–13) reveals an average omega-3 PUFA intake of only 55.46 mg day^{-1}, which is significantly lower than recommended levels.
- **Omega-6 imbalance:** modern Indian diets have an excess of n-6 fatty acids, which inhibit the ALA conversion into more bioactive forms, such as EPA and DHA.
- **Trans-fat concerns:** in South Asia, the high consumption of partially hydrogenated oils (vanaspati ghee) remains a major regulatory challenge, as these are the prominent source of industrial trans fats linked to heart disease and diabetes (Meier et al., 2021).

22.5.3.4 Labeling for special uses

India mandates nutrition labeling for foods with special dietary uses. If a nutrition claim is made, the label must verify the nutrient's presence. Broader mandatory labeling of prepackaged foods is largely driven by public health concerns over noncommunicable diseases (Banović Fuentes et al., 2025).

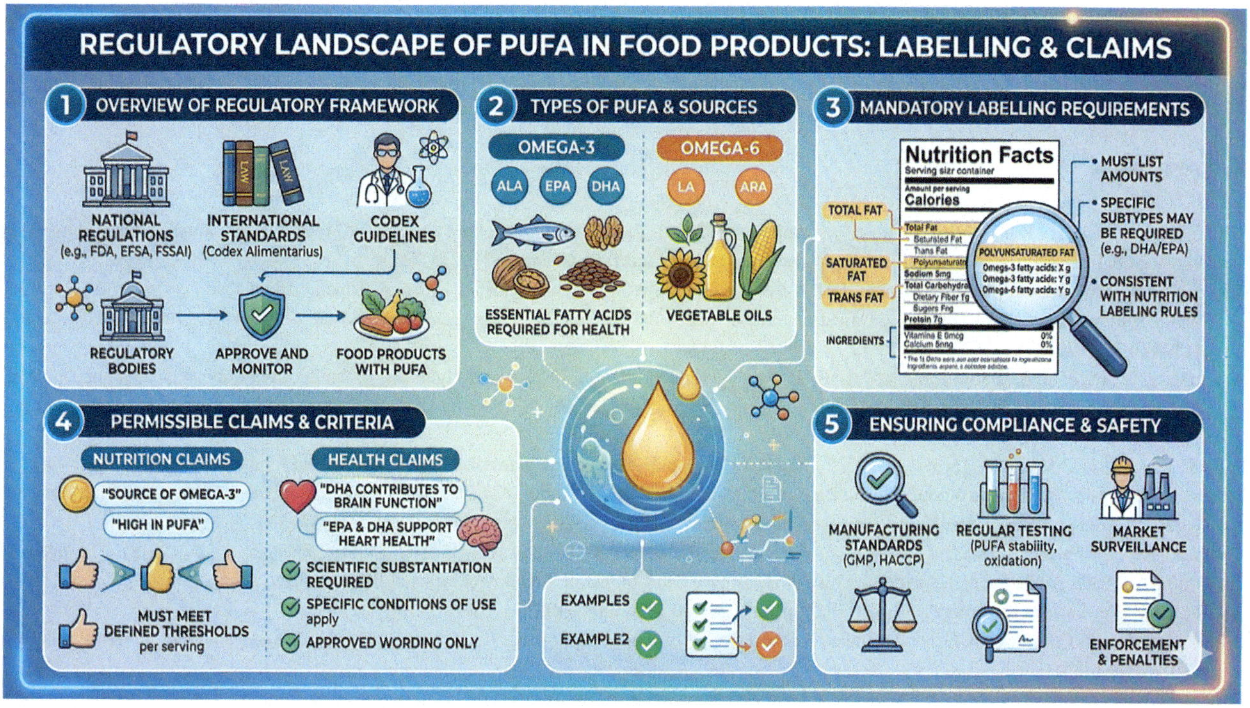

FIGURE 22.3 Regulatory landscape of polyunsaturated fatty acid (PUFA) in food products.

22.5.4 Emerging standards in other regions

In Australia and New Zealand, regulations ensure that products have a minimum 92% of the claimed omega-3 content to maintain consumer trust. In Brazil, mandatory labeling for trans fatty acids was implemented to assist in reducing cardiovascular risk (Domínguez Díaz et al., 2020).

22.6 Implementation challenges and future directions

22.6.1 The controversy of trans-fat labeling

Globally, the labeling of trans fat is an ongoing debate and controversy. Trans-fat labeling is mandated in the USFDA and Canada due to its link to heart disease, while the Codex Committee placed responsibility on the national government, citing the lack of worldwide agreement on definitions and risk levels (Hawkes, 2004).

22.6.2 Consumer understanding and format

Regulators face challenges to keep the food label simple and easy for consumers to understand. Several reports showed that consumers struggle to interpret numbers, quantities, and fat types. To simply the comparison, labels often use %DV (daily value) or per 100 g or per mL format (Miró-Colmenárez et al., 2024).

22.6.3 Trade and regulatory barriers

Strict preauthorization rules are often seen as barriers to trade. For food companies, particularly small and medium enterprises, the challenge is even greater, as limited financial resources make the claim approval difficult (Miró-Colmenárez et al. 2024).

22.7 Conclusion

The PUFA regulation in food products requires a balance between ensuring safety, applying nutrition science, and safeguarding consumer interests. The EU's centralized and restricted systems make regulatory approval of health claims more stringent. In contrast, the United States provides greater flexibility through qualified claims while developing countries such as India emphasize the strategic blending of oils as a public health approach. The key takeaways for future regulation include harmonization of standards, standardization of oxidative quality metrices, nutrient profiling, and personalized nutrition.

References

Ali, F., Ilyas, A., Ali, H., Kalaiselvan, V., Ali, V., & Anjum, V. (2024). Packaging and labelling policies for bioactive constituents from edible oils and fats: A global perspective. In Bioactive compounds of edible oils and fats (Chapter 17). CRC Press.

Bannenberg, Gerard, Mallon, Craig, Edwards, Holly, Yeadon, Derek, Yan, Kevin, Johnson, Holly, & Ismail, Adam (2017). Omega-3 Long-Chain Polyunsaturated Fatty Acid Content and Oxidation State of Fish Oil Supplements in New Zealand. *Scientific Reports, 7*(1). https://doi.org/10.1038/s41598-017-01470-4.

Bannenberg, G., Rice, H. B., Bernasconi, A., Ferrari, A., Mallon, C., Navarrete, L., Hughes, R., Igarashi, J., Persons, K., Latynski, L., Phung, A., Wang, S., & Ismail, A. (2020). Ingredient label claim compliance and oxidative quality of EPA/DHA omega-3 retail products in the U.S. *Journal of Food Composition and Analysis, 88*, 103435.

Banović Fuentes, J., Beara, I., & Torović, L. (2025). Regulatory compliance of health claims on omega-3 fatty acid food supplements. *Foods, 14*(1), 67.

Blondeau, N., Lipsky, R. H., Bourourou, M., Duncan, M. W., Gorelick, P. B., & Marini, A. M. (2015). Alpha-linolenic acid: An omega-3 fatty acid with neuroprotective properties—Ready for use in the stroke clinic? *BioMed Research International, 2015*(1), 519830.

Chacińska, M., Zabielski, P., Książek, M., Szałaj, P., Jarząbek, K., Kojta, I., Chabowski, A., & Błachnio-Zabielska, A. U. (2019). The Impact of OMEGA-3 Fatty Acids Supplementation on Insulin Resistance and Content of Adipocytokines and Biologically Active Lipids in Adipose Tissue of High-Fat Diet Fed Rats. *Nutrients, 11*(4), 835. https://doi.org/10.3390/nu11040835.

Codex Alimentarius Commission. General standard for the labeling of prepackaged foods (CODEX STAN 1-1985) and guidelines on nutrition labeling (CAC/GL 2-1985).

D'Eliseo, D., & Velotti, F. (2016). Omega-3 Fatty Acids and Cancer Cell Cytotoxicity: Implications for Multi-Targeted Cancer Therapy. *Journal of Clinical Medicine, 5*(2), 15. https://doi.org/10.3390/jcm5020015.

EFSA Panel on Nutrition, Novel Foods and Food Allergens (NDA). (2022). Scientific advice related to nutrient profiling for the development of harmonised mandatory front-of-pack nutrition labelling and the setting of nutrient profiles for restricting nutrition and health claims on foods. EFSA Journal, 20(4), 7259.

European Union. Regulation (EC) No 1924/ 2006 on nutrition and health claims made on foods.

Gogna, S., Kaur, J., Sharma, K., Bhadariya, V., Singh, J., Kumar, V., Rasane, P., & Vipasha, V. (2022). A systematic review on the role of alpha linolenic acid (ALA) in combating non-communicable diseases (NCDs). *Nutrition & Food Science, 53*(2), 221–233. https://doi.org/10.1108/nfs-01-2022-0023.

Government of Japan. (1991). Health Promotion Act (Act No. 103 of 2002) and Food for Specified Health Use (FOSHU) system regulations.

Domínguez Díaz, L., Fernández-Ruiz, V., & Cámara, M. (2020). An international regulatory review of food health-related claims in functional food products labeling. *Journal of Functional Foods, 68*, 103896.

Gunstone, F. D., & Herslof, B. G. (1992). *A lipid glossary*. London: The Oily Press.

Gunstone, F. D., Harwood, J. L., & Dijkstra, A. J. (2007). *The lipid handbook with CD-ROM*. CRC press.

Hawkes, C. (2004). Nutrition labels and health claims: The global regulatory environment. Geneva: World Health Organization. ISBN 92 4 159171.

Hoadley, J. E. (2017a). US regulation of food label claims. In *Developing new functional food and nutraceutical products*. Academic Press, 291–308.

Hoadley, J. E. (2017b). *US regulation of food label claims developing new functional food and nutraceutical products*. United States: Elsevier Inc, 291–308. http://www.sciencedirect.com/science/book/9780128027806, https://doi.org/10.1016/B978-0-12-802780-6.00016-X.

ICMR-NIN. (2024). Dietary guidelines for Indians.

Islam, F., Imran, A., Nosheen, F., Fatima, M., Arshad, M. U., Afzaal, M., Ijaz, N., Noreen, R., Mehta, S., Biswas, S., Rasool, I. F. U., Aslam, M. A., Usman, I., Zahra, S. M., Segueni, N., & Amer Ali, Y. (2023). Functional roles and novel tools for improving-oxidative stability of polyunsaturated fatty acids: A comprehensive review. *Food Science & Nutrition, 11*(6), 2471–2482. https://doi.org/10.1002/fsn3.3272.

IVPA. (2022). Evolving regulatory landscape of edible oils and fats in India. In IVPA Souvenir 2022.

Kapoor, B., Kapoor, D., Gautam, S., Singh, R., & Bhardwaj, S. (2021). Dietary polyunsaturated fatty acids (PUFAs): Uses and potential health benefits. *Current Nutrition Reports, 10*(3), 232–242. https://doi.org/10.1007/s13668-021-00363-3.

Kim, J. H., Kim, Y., Kim, Y. J., & Park, Y. (2016). Conjugated linoleic acid: Potential health benefits as a functional food ingredient. *Annual Review of Food Science and Technology, 7*, 221–244. https://doi.org/10.1146/annurev-food-041715-033028, http://www.annualreviews.org/journal/food.

Marcus, M. D., & Link, M. S. (2024). Omega-3 Fatty Acids and Arrhythmias. *Circulation, 150*(6), 488–503. https://doi.org/10.1161/circulationaha.123.065769.

Meier, C., Harms, E., Früh, B., Stoffers, H., Bee, G., Hugelshofer, D. H., Quander-Stoll, N., & Stolz, H. (2021). The effect of polyunsaturated fatty acids (PUFA) and organic labeling on Swiss consumers' acceptance of pork salami. *Organic Agriculture, 11*(4), 519–537. https://doi.org/10.1007/s13165-021-00369-9, www.springer.com/life+sciences/agriculture/journal/13165.

Miró-Colmenárez, P. J., Illán-Marcos, E., Díaz-Cruces, E., Rocasolano, M. M., Martínez-Hernandez, J. M., Zamora-Ledezma, E., & Zamora-Ledezma, C. (2024). Current insights into industrial trans fatty acids legal frameworks and health challenges in the European Union and Spain. *Foods, 13*(23), 3845.

Mititelu, M., Lupuliasa, D., Neacşu, S. M., Olteanu, G., Busnatu, Ş. S., Mihai, A., Popovici, V., Măru, N., Boroghină, S. C., Mihai, S., Ioniţă-Mîndrican, C. B., & Scafa-Udrişte, A. (2025). Polyunsaturated fatty acids and human health: A key to modern nutritional balance in association with polyphenolic compounds from food sources. *Foods, 14*(1). https://doi.org/10.3390/foods14010046, www.mdpi.com/journal/foods.

Miyata, J., & Arita, M. (2015). Role of omega-3 fatty acids and their metabolites in asthma and allergic diseases. *Allergology International, 64*(1), 27–34. https://doi.org/10.1016/j.alit.2014.08.003.

Narayan, B., Miyashita, K., & Hosakawa, M. (2006). Physiological effects of eicosapentaenoic acid (EPA) and docosahexaenoic acid (DHA) - A review. *Food Reviews International, 22*(3), 291–307. https://doi.org/10.1080/87559120600694622.

Papandreou, C. (2014a). Polyunsaturated fatty acids in relation to sleep quality and depression in obstructive sleep apnea hypopnea syndrome. In *Omega-3 fatty acids in brain and neurological health*. Academic Press, 337–347.

Papandreou, C. (2014b). *Polyunsaturated fatty acids in relation to sleep quality and depression in obstructive sleep apnea hypopnea syndrome omega-3 fatty acids in brain and neurological health*. Greece: Elsevier, 337–347. https://www.sciencedirect.com/book/9780124105270, https://doi.org/10.1016/B978-0-12-410527-0.00027-2.

Parasannanavar, D., Gaddam, I., Bukya, T., Ibrahim S, A., Reddy K, S., Banjara, S. K., Salvadi, B. P. P., Kumar B, N., Rao, S. F., Geddam, J. J. B., & Rajkumar, H. (2021). Omega-3 polyunsaturated fatty acid intake and plasma fatty acids of school going Indian children - a cross-sectional study. *Prostaglandins, Leukotrienes, and Essential Fatty Acids, 170*. https://doi.org/10.1016/j.plefa.2021.102294, http://www.elsevier-international.com/journals/plef/.

Pasini, F., Gómez-Caravaca, A. M., Blasco, T., Cvejić, J., Caboni, M. F., & Verardo, V. (2022). Assessment of lipid quality in commercial omega-3 supplements sold in the French market. *Biomolecules, 12*(10), 1361.

Swanson, D., Block, R., & Mousa, S. A. (2012). Omega-3 Fatty Acids EPA and DHA: Health Benefits Throughout Life. *Advances in Nutrition, 3*(1), 1–7. https://doi.org/10.3945/an.111.000893.

Tallima, H., & El Ridi, R. (2018). Arachidonic acid: Physiological roles and potential health benefits–A review. *Journal of Advanced Research, 11*, 33–41.

Turck, D., Bohn, T., Castenmiller, J., de Henauw, S., Hirsch-Ernst, K. I., Knutsen, H. K., Maciuk, A., Mangelsdorf, I., McArdle, H. J., Naska, A., Peláez, C., Pentieva, K., Thies, F., Tsabouri, S., Vinceti, M., Bresson, J. L., & Siani, A. (2022). Scientific advice related to nutrient profiling for the development of harmonised mandatory front-of-pack nutrition labelling and the setting of nutrient profiles for restricting nutrition and health claims on foods. *EFSA Journal, 20*(4). https://doi.org/10.2903/j.efsa.2022.7259, efsa.onlinelibrary.wiley.com/journal/18314732/.

Weiser, M., Butt, C., & Mohajeri, M. (2016). Docosahexaenoic Acid and Cognition throughout the Lifespan. *Nutrients, 8*(2), 99. https://doi.org/10.3390/nu8020099.

Wood, K. E., Mantzioris, E., Gibson, R. A., Ramsden, C. E., & Muhlhausler, B. S. (2015). The effect of modifying dietary LA and ALA intakes on omega-3 long chain polyunsaturated fatty acid (n-3 LCPUFA) status in human adults: A systematic review and commentary. *Prostaglandins, Leukotrienes and Essential Fatty Acids, 95*, 47–55. https://doi.org/10.1016/j.plefa.2015.01.001.

Zhang, H., & Xu, X. (2025). Nutritional lipids: An overview of nutritional progress and market trends. *Journal of Food Bioactives*, 8–30. https://doi.org/10.26599/jfb.2025.95031418.

Chapter 23

Sensory evaluation and consumer acceptance of polyunsaturated fatty acid-enriched foods

Jagan Karthik Sugumar, K.S. Krithiga, Dhivya Pandiyan, Saranya Venkatajalam, and Pothiyappan Karthik
Department of Food Technology, Faculty of Engineering, Karpagam Academy of Higher Education, Coimbatore, Tamil Nadu, India

23.1 Introduction

The essential macronutrients from dietary fats have a fundamental role in human health, which promote a concentrated source of energy for structural integrity of cell membranes, and act as precursors for a wide range of bioactive lipid mediators (Calder, 2015). Among different classes of dietary lipids, polyunsaturated fatty acids (PUFAs) have gained particular attention for their physiological and functional benefits. Particularly in PUFAs, omega-3 (n-3) and omega- 6 (n-6) fatty acids are connected with biological processes including inflammation regulation, lipid metabolism, immune function, and neural development (Shahidi & Ambigaipalan, 2018). Eicosapentaenoic acid (EPA) and docosahexaenoic acid (DHA), two long-chain n-3 PUFAs, have been shown to protect against cardiovascular diseases, metabolic problems, and neurological conditions (Swanson et al., 2012). Dietary reference consumption suggested by the European Food Safety Authority also highlights the adequate consumption of EPA and DHA across different age groups to support optimal health outcomes(EFSA Panel on Dietetic Products, Nutrition, and Allergies (NDA), 2010). In reaction to the instruction of the food industry has increasingly focused on the evolution of PUFA—enriched functional foods, including dairy products, bakery items, meat products, spreads, and ready-to-eat food. The PUFAs incorporated in food matrices have significant technological challenges. The food fortification and reformulation approach mainly aims to highlight the nutritional quality of commonly consumed products without requiring necessary changes from the consumers. On account of a high degree of unsaturation, PUFAs are highly prone to oxidative deterioration, which leads to constitution of volatile organic compounds triggering off-flavours, rancid odors, discoloration, and textural defects. (Jacobsen, 2015). These oxidative reaction with harmful consequences to product quality, shelf-life, and consumer perception. A number of studies have reported that PUFA-enriched food can significantly alter the sensory characteristics of foods, particularly aroma and flavor, which are mainly a consumer preference (Mehta, 2015). In animal-derived foods, dietary influence approach for supplementing feed with fish oil (FO) or linseed oil has been shown to alter the fatty acid composition but may also initiate unwanted sensory notes. For example, enrichment of pork with n-3 fatty acids has been associated with changes in volatile flavor compounds, including susceptibility to oxidation-derived odors (Hui et al., 2025). Homogeneously sensory challenges have been reported in PUFA-enriched milk, eggs, and meat products (Rymer & Givens, 2005). Perceptual attributes such as taste, aroma, texture, and appearance play a leading role in consumer preference in food choices, frequently outweighing nutritional considerations during procurement decisions. Even when consumers are apprised of the health benefits associated with PUFA-enriched foods, Negative sensory impressions have the potential to drastically lower acceptability and willingness to buy such goods. (Verbeke, 2005). Consequently, one of the important obstacle's effective commercializations of PUFA—fortified foods is customer acceptance. To overcome these hurdles, various approaches, including microencapsulation, use of antioxidants, emulsification technologies, and formulation optimization, have been investigated to enhance the quality of sensation and stability in oxidation (Jacobsen et al., 2008). Nevertheless, the effectiveness of this method must be analyzed not only through physicochemical and nutritional evaluation but also

Omega-3 and Omega-6 Polyunsaturated Fatty Acids in Food Systems. DOI: https://doi.org/10.1016/B978-0-443-43810-3.00013-0

through systematic sensory evaluation and consumer studies. In addition, consumer acceptance plays an essential role in understanding the perception, preference, willingness to purchase, and influence of health information on the food choices of consumers. Integrating the sensory data with the consumer research enables the food developers to produce the design PUFA-enriched products that optimize the optimal balance between nutritional enhancement and sensory quality. The evolution of consumer acceptance is necessary for the successful development and commercialization of PUFA-enriched foods. The present chapter focuses on the sensory evaluation and consumer acceptance of PUFA-enriched foods, discussing the impact of PUFA incorporation on sensory attributes, the methodologies used for sensory and consumer testing, and the challenges and opportunities associated with developing sensorially acceptable PUFA-fortified products.

23.2 Polyunsaturated fatty acid sources and their application in various foods

23.2.1 Classification of polyunsaturated fatty acids sources

PUFAs are fatty acids characterized by having more than one double bond in their carbon backbone. They are highly abundant in cell membranes, where they are primarily incorporated into membrane phospholipids (Torres-Vanegas et al., 2025). PUFAs are generally classified as either omega-3 or omega-6 based on the position of the first double bond in the long-chain fatty acid. The first double bond between the sixth and seventh carbon atoms from the terminal methyl group is found in all members of the omega-6 family, whereas the omega-3 family members have their initial double bond between the third and fourth carbon atoms. Fig. 23.1 shows the contents of omega-3 and omega-6 PUFA sources in plant and animal foods.

These fatty acids serve as essential precursors to eicosanoids, a group of hormone-like inflammatory mediators (Lovegrove, 2025).

23.2.2 Sources of polyunsaturated fatty acid

The sources of PUFA are widespread and have varied sources ranging from microalgal to marine sources. Based on the members of omega-3 and omega-6 fatty acids, the selected dietary sources are classified below.

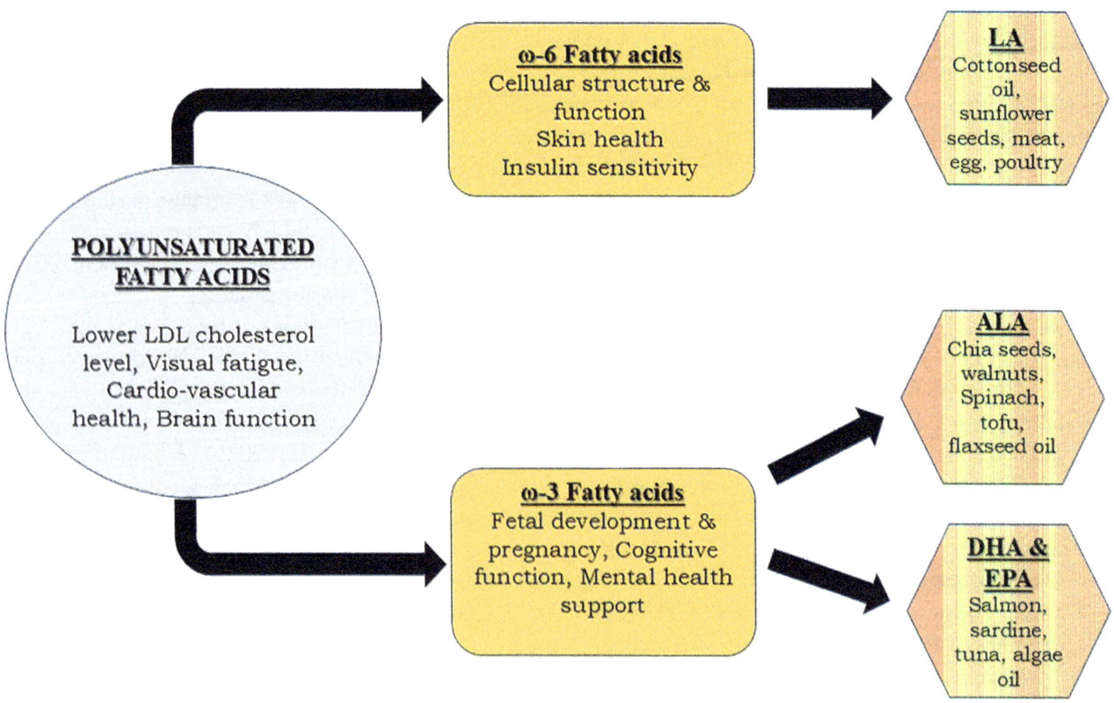

FIGURE 23.1 Omega-3 and omega-6 polyunsaturated fatty acids (PUFAs) sources in plant and animal foods.

TABLE 23.1 The most common sources of polyunsaturated fatty acids are found within marine food products.

Fish	Scientific name	Eicosapentaenoic acid (% of total fatty acids)	Docosahexaenoic acid (% of total fatty acids)	References
Blue fish	*Pomatomus saltatrix*	0.323	0.991	Ianora et al. (2003)
Carp	*Cyprinus carpio*	0.305	0.146	Ianora et al. (2003)
Cat fish	*Silurus glanis*	0.100	0.137	Waldron et al. (1998)
Dolphin	*Delphinus delphis*	0.026	0.113	Gill et al. (2003)
Shark	*Carcharodon carcharias*	0.316	0.527	Rangel et al. (2022)

23.2.2.1 Marine sources

Marine organisms such as fish and krill, store fat in their skin, which are present in low-temperature, high-pressure, and anoxic environments, produce long-chain PUFAs by the anaerobic pathway (Tian et al., 2024). The major source of PUFAs has been found in FO, particularly EPA and DHA, which are preferred for their substantial health benefits, such as enhancing mental health and developmental outcomes (Mukherjee et al., 2024). Table 23.1 shows the most common sources of PUFAs found within marine food products. Marine foods, such as fish and krill, are primarily found in omega-3 PUFAs. The derived food products from fish and krill, such as FO and krill oil (KO), represent high-level dietary content of omega-3 PUFAs. These FO and KO consist of both EPA and DHA in various molecular structures (Pham et al., 2024a, 2024b).

23.2.2.2 Plant sources

Plants serve as essential plant-derived sources of PUFAs, that offers effectual alternatives to conventional meat and marine sources. According to the researchers, nuts and seeds contain major amounts of PUFA content. Soybean, oil palm, rapeseed, and sunflower are the four substantial crops derived from plant oils. Although genetic research aims to increase fatty acid profile, and such procedures are mostly relevant to soybeans and rapeseed. On the other hand, *Camelina sativa* has surfaced as a nidus point for genetic engineering due to its simplicity of modification, excellent stress resilience, and exceptionally high PUFA content (Chen et al., 2020; Yang et al., 2025).

23.2.2.3 Microbial sources

Microbes are generally known for their ability to generate PUFAs (MANZOOR et al., 2022). Omega-3 and omega-6 fatty acids can be synthesized from various microalgae, bacteria, fungi, and yeasts (Ramachandran et al., 2024). The two main sources of microalgae include *Schizochytrium and Nannochloropsis*, which can accumulate up to 5% (w/w) of EPA, and 15%–20% (w/w) of DHA (Navalho et al., 2025). Consequently, these microalgae are being used to partially replace FO in human and animal diets (Sandoval et al., 2023).

Yeast represents another significant microbial source. As a genetically traceable organism, it naturally produces fatty acids such as oleic and palmitic acid, though typically at levels below 5% of total fatty acids (Kumari et al., 2025). However, recent advancements in engineered strains of oleaginous yeasts have enabled the production of arachidonic acid and linoleic acid (LA) (Sharma et al., 2025).

Animal sources such as beef, lamb, pork, poultry, milk, and eggs contain fatty acids, and these sources are influenced by the impact of diet composition and the digestive system of the animals (Eaton et al., 1998; Pusceddu et al., 2015). Eggs are a good source of PUFAs, especially DHA (Bavelaar & Beynen, 2004). Egg yolk contains 0.1% EPA, 6%–7% DHA, and 0.8% α-linoleic acid (ALA) (Huang et al., 2008). ALA and the long-chain n-3 PUFA, such as EPA, docosapentaenoic acid, and DHA, are found in meat and meat products, which play a crucial role in the human diet (Givens et al., 2006). Additionally, milk and dairy products play an essential role in providing fatty acids to the human diet (Crawford et al., 1976). The total PUFA in cow milk is approximately $3.6 \pm 0.57\%$ (Aleksandra et al., 2009).

23.2.3 Applications of polyunsaturated fatty acid

23.2.3.1 Functional foods

PUFAs are linked to numerous health benefits; for instance, a high proportion of PUFAs is known to be associated with a lower risk of cardiovascular diseases (Sekikawa et al., 2019). The addition of one or more of PUFAs from natural sources to foods is the main focus of the current methodologies being developed to develop PUFA functional foods (Cardoso et al., 2025).

23.2.3.2 Bakery and cereal-based products

The modification of the fatty acids, such as interesterification and microencapsulation, helps in developing PUFA-rich bakery fatty acids. In addition, cereal is also modified to PUFA-containing food products. For example, numerous cereal substrates can be transformed by lower filamentous fungi into products containing various n-6 and n-3 PUFAs (White et al., 2025).

23.2.3.3 Beverages and ready-to-drink

The fortification of beverages with omega-3 fatty acids has many potential applications, including lowering the risk of cardiovascular diseases. In recent years, the fortification of PUFAs in beverages and drinks has grown tremendously (Shahidi & Ambigaipalan, 2016).

23.2.3.4 Meat and processed foods

Seafood is one of the most important dietary sources of n-3 PUFA, which are vital for human health. It is significant in human health due to the presence of various volatile compounds that are produced by a variety of volatile compounds in meat products, such as aldehydes, alcohols, ketones, and hydrocarbons (Hui et al., 2025; Yang et al., 2025).

23.2.3.5 Confectionery and snacks

The mean fat intake from snacks was 34.5 g/day, covering nearly 47% of the recommended daily intake (Haque Akanda et al., 2020). The partially hydrogenated fat items, such as cakes, cookies, donuts, and potato chips, were substantially lower in EPA and contained relatively greater levels of trans-PUFAs (Haque Akanda et al., 2020).

23.2.3.6 Cooking oils and spreads

PUFAs in vegetable oils are pressed from the plants and undergo processing and refinement to produce premium oils. It serves as the main source of naturally occurring plant sterols in the diet (Jandacek, 2017).

23.3 Why is consumer acceptance needed for enriched foods?

Consumer acceptance is a key determinant of successful formulation, commercialization, and long-term consumption of enriched foods, particularly those fortified with omega-3 PUFAs. The enriched food is formulated with nutritional value beyond basic dietary requirements to promote the health benefits, such as improved cardiovascular function, enhanced cognitive function, and overall well-being. The nutritional superiority alone is not sufficient to ensure success. Without consumer approval and regular consumption, even scientifically proven products cannot achieve a meaningful public health impact or commercial sustainability. The main acceptance of consumers is crucial for translating the health claims into real-world benefits, influencing sensory satisfaction, market success, and dietary behavior change.

The fundamental determinant for market success is consumer acceptance, that are successful development and commercialization of food innovations. Consumer preference toward enriched foods is strongly influenced by purchase intention, repeat consumption, and long-term market sustainability, as well as the willingness to buy the premium for incorporated functional benefits (Nazzaro et al., 2024). In the failure of consumer acceptance, the fortified foods remain confined to a niche market or remain absent to achieve widespread adoption. Food manufacturers, retailers, and product developers invest substantial resources in research and development, processing technologies, quality control, and marketing strategies. The enriched product does not fulfill the expectations in terms of sensory attributes such as taste, texture, and overall perceived value; they face a higher risk of market failure, resulting in financial losses and reduced confidence among the industry stakeholders.

Sensory quality frequently appears as one of the most significant factors for consumer acceptance. Overall, enriched food items' taste, texture, aroma, and appearance are considered the health claims in developing consumer preference (Carrillo et al., 2012). This is mainly relevant to PUFA-enriched foods, as omega-3 fatty acids are major amount in off-flavours and undesirable aromas, leading to oxidation and textural changes (Ganesan et al., 2014). The formulation control in omega-3 enriched eggs with flaxseed oil or FO, compared to conventional egg have optimized carefully while maintaining the acceptance. The consumer accepts more on formulation, ingredient form, and storage conditions than on the enriched food (Scheideler et al., 1997).

Consumer acceptance of lipid-modified foods in dairy products has been shown to vary by product type. Monounsaturated fatty acid-enriched milk that had been lowered in SFA showed acceptance levels that were similar to control samples, but modified cheese products frequently scored worse on liking tests because of their textural constraints (Markey et al., 2017). Consumer acceptance is not only influenced by intrinsic sensory attributes but also by the extrinsic factors and health communication. The conjugated linoleic acid (CLA)-enriched dairy products maintain that consumer awareness of health benefits alone does not ensure acceptance; attitude, trust in functional claims, and perceived relevance strongly influence purchasing decisions (Peng et al., 2006).

The choice of experiments conducted among Italian consumers they performed and show the willingness to pay for functional attributes, mainly in long-chain omega-3 fatty acids, in products that include olive oil, and in pasta. Factors affecting consumer utility, the presence of functional ingredients significantly influences the acceptance of food categories, and also supports the economic sustainability of enriched strategies (Nazzaro et al., 2024). These help in acceptance in translating nutritional innovation into market success. The lipid-modified foods are significantly consumer acceptance dairy by product type. Modified cheese products have low performance in consumer preference due to the textural limitations, while SFA-reduced monounsaturated fatty acid-enriched milk demonstrated the acceptance levels compared to control samples (Markey et al., 2017). Consumer awareness of health benefits fails to ensure the acceptance, rather than attitude, trust in functional claims, and perceived relevance are majorly influenced by the purchasing mindset and decisions in the CLA-enriched dairy products (Peng et al., 2006). The experiments performed among the consumers in Italy they out show the willingness to buy for functional attributes such as long-chain omega-3 fatty acids in products including olive oil and pasta. The presence of functional ingredients enhances the acceptance of food categories, and price influences the consumer utility, and favors the economic sustainability of enrichment strategies that are reflected in the market success. Unfamiliar ingredients or novel technology of enriched food of fortified or biofortified food that represent the unfamiliar sensory characteristics or perceived artificiality, which can reduce the acceptance due to a lack of clear information and trust-building strategies (Razzaq et al., 2021). Optimizing the technology plays a main role in oxidative degradation of PUFA-enriched lipid-based nutrition supplements. The sensory factors such as color, taste, and flavor strongly influence the consumer acceptance, while European consumers commonly agree that microalgae are acceptable food ingredients, by the sensory factors. Minimal consumer refuse because of vivid green colouration and marine off-flavors; they need careful incorporation and sensory control (Olsen et al., 2024). In animal-derived foods, formulated PUFA enrichment does not rely on consumer acceptance. Sensory evaluations of PUFA-enriched pork salami with high PUFA levels within a defined range did not reduce overall liking, although higher PUFA products were frequently perceived as softer or greasier. Majorly, the acceptance is high in level when the product is named as organic, which displays the influence of extrinsic cues and information on consumer perception (Meier et al., 2021). As a whole, these studies identify that overpowering enrichment may negatively affect sensory quality, oxidative stability, and palatability, even when nutritional value is higher in amount (Betti et al., 2009). The consumer acceptance is essential for enriched food because it determines market adoption, sustained consumption, public health impact, and industry investment. PUFA-enriched food products from scientific innovation to dietary norm, consumer acceptance must be addressed throughout product development and implementation.

23.4 Types of sensory analyses used in the evaluation of consumer acceptance

PUFAs are now incorporated into new products that are commonly consumed, and this shows the trends in public health policies and new innovations. The essential fatty acids, mainly omega-3 and omega-6 fatty acids, maintain heart health, support neural development, and regulate inflammatory responses. This was highlighted by the international experts convened by the World Health Organization and the Food and Agriculture Organization (Calder, 2015). So the modern food industry develops many PUFA-enriched food products, which include milk, yogurt, cheese spreads, infant formula, bakery products, meat products, margarine, and ready-to-drink beverages (Kolanowski & Laufenberg, 2006). But not only fortification but also consumer acceptance is also important to achieve the success of the PUFA-enriched products in food markets. The consumer perception of taste, aroma, texture, and overall acceptability determines the product acceptance and market purchasing by consumers repeatedly (Verbeke, 2006). Therefore, sensory analysis plays an important role in the marketing and development of PUFA-enriched foods (Granato et al., 2010). The sensory characteristics of PUFA-enriched foods depend on the chemical instability of highly unsaturated fatty acids (Choe & Min, 2006). PUFAs are sensitive to oxidation reactions that can lead to secondary compounds such as hexanal, propanal, and other aldehydes, giving rancid and fishy odors due to the presence of multiple double bonds Shahidi and Zhong, 2020. But consumers may detect slight changes in aroma or flavor, which can reduce overall acceptability even when oxidation levels are below regulatory limits (Kolanowski et al., 2004). This issue points out the importance of integrating sensory analysis with instrumental analysis, such as peroxide value and thiobarbituric acid reactive substances (TBARS) values (Gray et al., 1996). If any slight oxidative changes are detected in spite of acceptable chemical stability in PUFA-enriched dairy beverages and spreads, it will reduce flavor acceptance scores (Jacobsen et al., 2013).

The sensory methods are important for evaluating consumer acceptance (Bareen et al., 2025). The sensory tests involve people who can represent the consumer market and aim to measure liking and preference rather than explaining product characteristics (Baker et al., 2022). David Peryam and Herbert Pilgrim developed a 9-point hedonic scale, which remains as basic of acceptance testing of sensory characteristics (Lim, 2011). In sensory testing, people express their liking for attributes such as appearance, aroma, flavor, texture, and overall acceptability on a scale. In the case of omega-3 enriched with milk or yogurt, flavor is the primary factor in overall acceptance in hedonic scaling (Granato et al., 2010). When oxidative flavor is detectable, overall liking scores may decline significantly, even among the health-conscious people (Kolanowski et al., 2004). Preference testing can further explain the understanding of consumer choice characteristics. In these tests, consumers give priority to their preferred sample among the sample alternatives (Bareen et al., 2025). This test was employed for comparing the PUFA enriched with free FO and microencapsulated oil. Microencapsulation has been shown to enhance the sensory score by suppressing the contact between PUFAs and the food matrix so that the oxidation and oxidative flavor were limited (Drusch & Mannino, 2009). When the bakery items incorporated with flaxseed oil or FO microcapsules are tested for preference testing, they often show higher sensory acceptance for encapsulated trials than in direct addition of oils (Kolanowski & Laufenberg, 2006).

While affective tests measure liking among the consumers in the market, discriminative tests detect whether sensory differences exist between samples (Bareen et al., 2025). These types of testing are important during the storage and shelf-life studies of PUFA-enriched food products. The triangle test involves panelists with three identified samples, two identical and one different, and asks them to find the different one. This method is sensitive to small sensory alterations, and this method is widely applied in assessing whether fortification of PUFA changes the flavor of a control product (Kolanowski et al., 2004). In omega-3-enriched milk powders or spreads, the panelists cannot differentiate the enriched sample from controls, so that masking strategies were confirmed (Jacobsen et al., 2008).

The duo-trio test is another discriminative method in sensory testing. In DHA-enriched infant formula, it is essential that the sensory profile closely resembles the reference product to maintain people's trust and infant acceptance. Paired comparison difference tests may also be employed to detect if one product gives a fishy smell or rancid aroma than another sample, mainly during accelerated shelf-life studies (Gray et al., 1996). Descriptive sensory analysis results in deeper insight into the specific attributes responsible for acceptance or rejection (Bareen et al., 2025). Quantitative descriptive analysis (QDA) involves trained panelists who develop a shared vocabulary and rate attribute intensities using structured scales (Murray et al., 2001). The indicators, such as oxidized aroma, metallic taste, creaminess, mouthfeel, bitterness, and color changes, are included in PUFA-enriched foods (Domínguez et al., 2019). These detailed profiles help the researchers to relate sensory testing with chemical indicators of oxidation in the food product (Kolanowski et al., 2004). For example, sensory rancidity scores were correlated with TBARS values in PUFA-fortified meat systems. Flavor profile analysis involves the identification of flavor sequence over a period of time (Pineau et al., 2009).

The understanding of sensory attributes can be further enhanced by dynamic sensory methods, such as time-intensity analysis (Pineau et al., 2009). In PUFA-enriched beverages or emulsions, this analysis method has been useful to detect delayed fishy tastes that may not be felt during initial testing (Drusch & Mannino, 2009). Apart from sensory attributes, consumer acceptance of these products can be influenced by extrinsic factors such as labeling, health claims, and knowledge about nutraceuticals (Verbeke, 2005). The market studies indicate that sensory experience determines repeat purchase, although the health information can initiate expectations and liking of a product (Ares & Deliza, 2010). Thus, sensory analysis must be analyzed in a broader manner that integrates nutritional information and consumer psychology (Baker et al., 2022). Consequently, the sensory evaluation of PUFA-enriched foods includes affective, discriminative, and dynamic technologies. Each method offers deep insight into how nutritional enhancement interacts with sensory perception. This type of sensory analysis becomes unavoidable as they are essential to ensure that they achieve both health benefits and consumer acceptance, as PUFA are highly sensitive to oxidation (Choe & Min, 2006).

23.5 Preparation of panel members and training

When it comes to organoleptic acceptance and analysis of sensory data of any formulated and fortified product, the panel members who represent, take part in the analysis, and contribute to the measurement of sensory responses play a vital role and are to follow standards laid out under ISO – 13300. The sensory panel members act as the sample representation of the market target, and thus the selection and screening of panel members for specific sensory analyses is key to gaining insight into the probable market preference for any formulated product as per ISO standard – 5492:2008. The choice of panel members is dependent on several influencing factors and demographic criteria, as the panel would function similarly to the target market. The panel members may be required to undergo learning, training, and screening for the respective type of sensory evaluation and the level of knowledge required for the evaluation. These are designed as necessary selection criteria, as further elucidated below.

23.5.1 Selection criteria for sensory panel

The sensory evaluation process is usually preceded by a sensory panel leader who curates and organizes the evaluation procedure and who selects and trains panel members. The panel leader is supposed to be unbiased and is required to have knowledge of how and why the sensory evaluation is to be conducted. They are also responsible for conveying essential information to the panel members and avoiding any form of influence or bias between the panel members, and avoiding any presumptions on the product to be evaluated. The sensory assessors/panel members are selected for the evaluation based on age, health, personal habits, personality, and experience (depending upon the type of sensory evaluation), and their ability to take in information and carry out the task of evaluating the product (Carpenter et al., 2000). The panel members should be volunteers for the sensory analysis, or if public/external members are involved, they can be compensated monetarily, but making sure there is no bias among the panel members towards a positive evaluation (Ojeh, 2021). It is the duty of the panel leader to identify potential assessors for that particular sensory evaluation study based on the needs and ideal requirements for the evaluation (International Organization for Standardization, 2012). The selection of the sensory assessors is based on criteria such as attitude, communication, willingness, health, ability to understand and identify, and ascertain properties. Psychological criteria, such as interest and decision-making, also influence selection. The preliminary screening of the recruited panel members is carried out by performing a threshold screening study.

23.5.2 Threshold tests and screening of panelists

Threshold refers to the least concentration of a sample/sensory perception of an attribute required for the detection, identification, and differentiation of the sensation of the sample. These threshold tests are done to identify potentially sensitive assessors for the evaluation. The threshold tests are carried out by preparing samples for evaluating the sensory perception of smell, flavor, and taste. Color, appearance and textural perceptions are tested with simple questionnaire and using specific standard solutions for identification (International Organization for Standardization, 2012) based on ISO standard – 8586 based on ISO standard – 8586. For odor, flavor, and taste thresholds, test samples are prepared for sensing particular flavor/taste in increasing concentrations, ranging from not detectable range to very predominant concentrations to be sensed and recognized.

For example, sourness is evaluated using increasing concentrations of citric acid solution, where usually the detection threshold is at 1 g/L for an average assessor. For odor thresholds, essential oils of spices and condiments are used. These tests not only help us identify panel members with similar threshold/ sensory acuity levels for perception but also help identify supertasters and a-tasters; Therefore, they can be excluded from the sensory panel. The panel members are also evaluated for their ability to differentiate thresholds between two tastes/flavors, and usually, panel members with low or average concentrations for detection, recognition, and difference are preferred as panel members.

23.5.3 Standards for sensory panel members

The screening and selection of panel members are technically regulated and assessed based on ISO (8586:2023) standards and guidelines provided by the American Society for Testing and Materials (ASTM) manual. The standards are essential in identifying the sensory assessors based on their acuity in sensory perception, ability to discriminate different flavors, odors, and tastes, and rank them, and also provide reliable and repeatable measurements of sensory data. These standards are utilized to filter out the possible sensorially impaired assessors as they could affect the scores in a sensory evaluation or could end up confusing/misinterpreting sensory descriptors. These standards are also used for carrying out the sensory assessment in a standard test manner to prevent irregularities in the evaluation part and avoid any bias. Some standard methods adopted from ASTM-based standards are E1885 for the triangle test method, E3041 for establishing necessary sensory scales for the respective assessment process, and MNL14 for using sensory analysis as a quality control tool. Certain ISO standards, such as ISO 3972:2011, help in other aspects, such as describing the methods for evaluating the sensitivity of certain tastes. These standards help in not only selecting the right assessor for the sensory evaluation but also help train them for specific tests, especially the descriptive sensory analyses.

23.5.4 Educating and training the sensory panel

The process of educating and training panel members is carried out as part of the sensory evaluation process. But not all sensory evaluation studies require education and training, for example acceptance tests such as hedonic scale testing which is usually done using a 9-point scale does not require any essential training of panel members as this type of acceptance test is a representation of common/general population identical to the average consumer (Contador et al., 2014; Deliza et al., 2005; Labbe et al., 2004). Even if training is not required, education of panel members is carried out in order to identify the product parameters and interpret the scales, and also understand the sensory evaluation sheet and the scoring/ scale system used in the study. Other sensory evaluations, such as preference and discrimination tests, require minimal training of the panel members in order to ensure that the attributes are represented correctly and evaluated with a better understanding of the products. These include paired and ranked preference tests, duo-trio test, triangle test, and tests such as just-about-right analysis and survey-like evaluations, such as check all that apply studies.

The representation of the general population/consumers is referred to as untrained panel members, and those who receive minor training for carrying out the evaluation are referred to as semitrained panel members. Typically, the training period of semitrained panel members is in the range of 5–8 hours. The panel members who are recruited and trained for descriptive sensory analyses are referred to as trained panel members or expert assessors. Typically, the training of expert assessors is rigorous and requires a training period of 80–150 hours, depending upon the type of descriptive analysis, and is carried out for short-term and long-term sensory memory for the product (Contador et al., 2014; Elgaard et al., 2019; Monteiro & Vasconcelos, 2024; Purriños et al., 2022).

Studies such as flavor and texture profile analysis and time-intensity studies require the longest training time, usually ranging from 60–100 hours and in case of assessors for QDA require a training period of 50–80 hours but for long-term sensory memory and building expertise on specific recognition of attributes may take from 2 to 5 years, depending upon the food product (Kemp et al., 2018). This level of training is required to ensure the repeatability and reproducibility of sensory responses consistently.

23.5.5 Number of panel members

The number of sensory assessors is decided based on the type and requirements of the sensory evaluation process. Usually, when representing the general population/consumers in acceptance, discrimination, and preference tests, untrained panel members are used. The number of untrained panel members typically ranges from 50–70 members, and in certain cases, for hedonic tests done for consumer acceptability, may even have close to 300 panel members. Some discrimination tests, such as duo-trio and triangle test, and hedonic test handling very similar samples, may require semitrained panel members, and in that case, 35–50 panel members with 5–8 hours of training is sufficient. In the case of descriptive sensory analysis requires 6–15 expertly trained assessors to carry out the evaluation. The different types of sensory analyses, types of panel members, and number of panel members used in various sensory studies involving PUFA-enriched foods are listed in Table 23.2.

23.5.6 Participation and sensory assessment

The sensory evaluations involving hedonic tests carried out with untrained panel members usually consider the entire dataset produced by the sensory panel. The discrimination/difference tests and affirmative/preference test data undergo screening, and among 30–50 assessor data, only 12–20 assessor data are considered (Carpenter et al., 2000; Pecore, 1993), and this screening is done based on assessor acuity to sensory perception, which is measured by using ANOVA (International Organization for Standardization, 2016). For descriptive sensory analysis, the data assessment is primarily done by MANOVA, factor analysis, or two-way ANOVA (for QDA) and is interpreted accordingly. These assessment of sensory data helps in making informed decisions in the identification of key attributes and understanding the sensory quality attributes that affect overall sensory acceptance and help create a qualitative sensory fingerprint for foods based on using descriptive analysis data (Brockhoff et al., 1996; Heymann & Noble, 1989; Moskowitz & Meiselman, 1977; Schlich, 2017).

There are some descriptive analyses such as spectrum analysis and free choice profiling, require basic statistical studies, such as measurements of descriptive statistics, and in certain cases, one-way ANOVA is used. For paired comparison and ranking test, statistical significance between samples is evaluated using Student's—t-test, Tukey's (HSD) test, least significant difference test, and Duncan's multiple range test, provided the means are more leaned towards alternate hypothesis. The use of statistical tools helps discriminate and make informed decisions, as sensory data is primarily considered psychometric data.

23.6 Sensory descriptors used for polyunsaturated fatty acid-enriched foods

23.6.1 Attributes and descriptors

The sensory attributes are characteristics that determine or influence the overall acceptability/ preferability of the evaluated food sample. In PUFA-enriched foods, the set of attributes evaluated is mostly common amongst each other. A descriptor refers to the standard sensory adjective for a particular sensory attribute, which describes the nature of the food on sensory perception. In general, the sensory attributes are classified into (1) appearance and color, (2) odor, (3) flavor, (4) taste, and (5) texture and mouthfeel. We evaluated 325 research articles via Scopus pertaining to PUFA-enriched foods

TABLE 23.2 Type and number of sensory panel members for various polyunsaturated fatty acid-enriched foods.

S.no.	Food product category	Product	Sensory evaluation used	Panel type	Panel size	References
1.	Meat and poultry	Chicken nuggets with encapsulated fish oil (FO)	Triangle test	Untrained	48	Pérez-Palacios et al. (2018)
			Quantitative descriptive analysis (QDA)	Trained	15	
			Hedonic scale test (5-point scale)	untrained	48	
		Pork with linseed oil	Taste activity value	Trained	8	Hui et al. (2025)
		Cooked sausages with encapsulated FO, dry-cured sausages	QDA	Trained	14	Solomando et al. (2021)
			Temporal dominance of sensation	Trained	14	
			Hedonic scale test and purchase intent	Untrained	154	
		Raw meat, cooked ham, and dry-cured shoulder meat enriched with DHA	QDA	Trained	6	Sárraga et al. (2007)
		Dry-cured ham	QDA	Trained	12	Mairesse et al. (2011)
		Dry fermented sausages n-3 fatty acid (FA) enriched	QDA	Trained	10	Valencia et al. (2006)
		Surimi franks enriched with n-3 FA	Hedonic scale test (9-point scale)	Untrained	79	Sell (2012)
2.	Egg	Hard-boiled eggs and scrambled eggs	Descriptive analysis (unstructured)	Trained	8	Lawlor et al. (2010)
		n-3 FA-enriched eggs	Triangle test	Untrained	20	Tserveni-Gousi et al. (2006)
		Hard-boiled eggs, scrambled eggs, madeira cake	QDA (7-point scale)	Semitrained	30	Parpinello et al. (2006)
			Hedonic scale test	Untrained	24	
3.	Milk and milk products	Microalgal extract fortified yogurt	Hedonic scale test	Untrained	20	Robertson et al. (2016)
		Yogurt fortified with flaxseed powder	Hedonic scale test (7-point scale)	Semitrained	30	Ardabilchi Marand et al. (2020)
		Yogurt, soft cheese, cream, butter, processed cheese, fortified with FO	Scaling method	trained	16	Kolanowski and Weißbrodt (2007)

4.	Bakery and pasta	Croissants, muffins	Triangle test	Untrained (habitual consumer)	30	Quílez et al. (2006)
		Cookies, pasta	Hedonic scale test	Untrained	54	Babuskin et al. (2014)
		Dry pasta	Hedonic scale test	Untrained	71	Rodríguez De Marco et al. (2018)
			Check all that apply	Untrained	71	
5.	Other foods	Instant foods (concentrates): mushroom soup, tomato soup, pudding, rice cereal, milk-rice cereal, jelly, cocoa, potato purée	Duo-trio test	Trained	12–16	Kolanowski et al. (1999), Kolanowski, Jaworska and Weißbrodt (2007), Kolanowski, Jaworska, Laufenberg, et al. (2007)
			Hedonic scale test	Untrained	20	
			Palatability test	Trained	20	
			Intensity test (graphic scale test)	Trained	8–12	

with keywords encompassing sensory analysis and various sensory attributes and performed a cooccurrence study to map potential attributes and descriptors used in those articles using VOSviewer (Ver. 1.6.20). The mapped descriptors/attributes are given in Fig. 23.2. Each of the attributes is explored for various PUFA-enriched foods and is studied in detail.

23.6.2 Commonly used sensory descriptors

The common sensory descriptors for fat-rich PUFA-enriched foods are discussed with respect to each sensory attribute accordingly. These sensory descriptors act as terminologies signifying the sensory characteristics of the food products. The sensory attributes and indicators used in PUFA-enriched foods are shown in Table 23.3.

23.6.2.1 Color/appearance

The most common descriptors for color refer to redness and pinkness, which are usually indicators for fresh or cured meat products. For sausages, the descriptors used are homogeneity, so as to indicate the structural distribution of meat and fat. In certain foods, marbling is also used as a visual descriptor for the appearance attribute (Pérez-Palacios et al., 2018; Solomando et al., 2021). In dairy-based products, the color attribute uses descriptors such as oily, glossy, creamy, and homogenous, which are predominantly used. In a few product descriptors such as colored, smooth, and shiny were used.

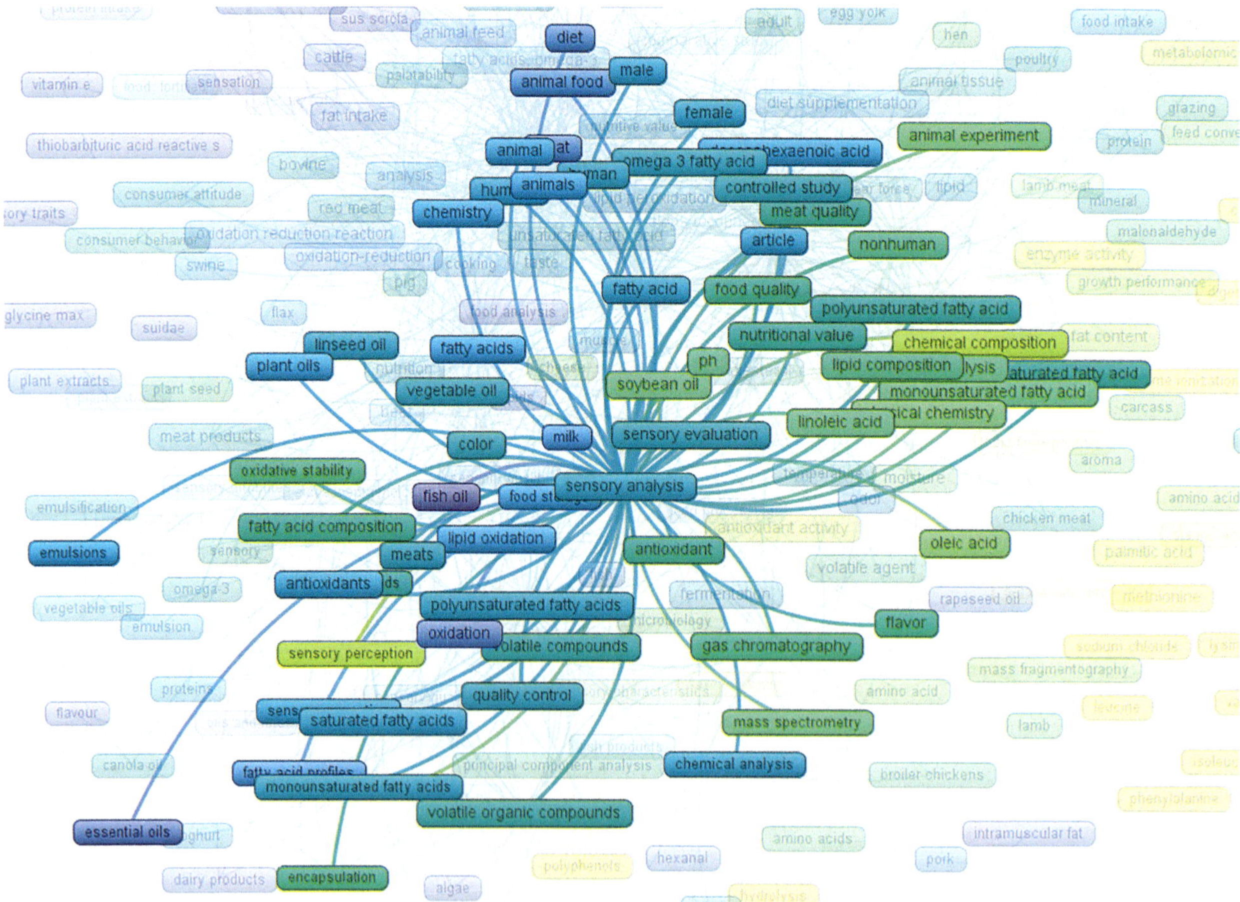

FIGURE 23.2 Mapping of keyword co-occurrences for sensory analysis to identify attributes and descriptors.

TABLE 23.3 Sensory attributes and indicators used in polyunsaturated fatty acid-enriched foods.

S.no.	Product evaluated	Sensory attribute	Sensory descriptor	References
1.	Ready to cook meat	Appearance	Homogeneous color, structure	Pérez-Palacios et al. (2018)
		Odor	Fried, fishy, rancid	
		Texture	Crustiness, oiliness, juiciness, firmness	
		Taste and flavor	Intensity, meaty, oily, salty, spicy, rancid, and fishy	
2.	Pork	Odor	Aromatic, sulfurous, and alcoholic	Hui et al. (2025)
		Taste	Sourness, saltiness, sweetness, and bitterness	
3.	Cooked sausages and dry-cured sausages	Appearance	Homogeneous, bright, and color intensity	Solomando et al. (2021)
		Odor	Spicy, smoky, and rancid	
		Taste/Flavor	Saltiness, smoky, and rancid flavor	
		Texture	Hardness, chewiness, juiciness, elasticity, granularity, and oiliness	
		Dynamic sensory perception (temporal dominance of sensation)	Saltiness, smoky, rancid, meaty, tender, juicy, oily, and fishy	
4.	Raw meat, dry-cured shoulder meat	Odour	Metallic odor	Sárraga et al. (2007)
		Flavor	Metallic, saltiness, mustiness, sweetness, piquantness, bitterness, cured flavor, aged flavor, and fishy	
		Texture	Adhesiveness, hardness, crumbliness, pastiness, fibrousness, and fat-meltiness	
5.	Dry-cured ham	Color	Fat color, muscle color, marbling, and surface shininess	Mairesse et al. (2011)
		Odor	Abnormal odor	
		Flavor	Salty, peppery, rancid, spicy, moldy, and herby	
		Texture	Tenderness	
6.	Dry fermented sausages	Color	Saturation	Valencia et al. (2006)
		Odor	Typical odor	

(Continued)

TABLE 23.3 (Continued)

S.no.	Product evaluated	Sensory attribute	Sensory descriptor	References
		Flavor	Fishy	
		Texture	Tender, chewy, and juiciness	
7.	Hard-boiled eggs	Odor	Buttery, off-odor, and sulfurous	Lawlor et al. (2010)
		Flavor	Aftertaste, astringent, buttery, salty, and sweet	
		Taste	Intensity	Parpinello et al. (2006), Tserveni-Gousi et al. (2006)
		Aroma	Off-odor, and sulfurous	
		Color	Yolk color, whiteness, and yellowness	
8.	Yogurt	Appearance	Color, whiteness, and yellowness	Ardabilchi Marand et al. (2020), Kolanowski and Weißbrodt (2007), Robertson et al. (2016)
		Odor/flavor	Aromatic, off-odor, and fishy	
		Texture	Thickness	
		Taste	Acidic, and rancid	
9.	Bakery and pasta	Appearance	Visual appeal	Babuskin et al. (2014), Quílez et al. (2006), Rodríguez De Marco et al. (2018)
		Texture	Firmness, and hardness	
		Odor	Unpleasant, and pleasant	
		Flavor	Fishy	
10.	Other instant foods and beverages	Odor/flavor	Buttery, fishy, smoky, and herby	Kolanowski et al. (1999, 2004), Kolanowski, Jaworska, and Weißbrodt (2007), Kolanowski, Jaworska, Laufenberg et al. (2007)
		Texture	Springiness, pastiness, and gumminess,	
		Taste	Meaty, oily, spicy, smoky, astringent, salty, grassy, moldy, bitter, and nutty	

23.6.2.2 Odor

Odor is considered the most critical and challenging attribute for PUFA-enriched foods, as fatty volatile compounds are the first indicators to signal lipid degradation to the consumer and suggest the quality of the food.

1. Fishy odor: This is the most common negative descriptor associated with omega-3-enriched foods, particularly when FO or algal oil is used (Babuskin et al., 2014; Drusch & Mannino, 2009; Lawlor et al., 2010). It arises from volatile compounds present in foods, such as fatty acid volatiles, which have extremely low odor thresholds. This note is generally considered a negative attribute as an off-odor unless the product is inherently seafood-based.
2. Earthy: Plant-based PUFA-enriched foods are common products containing LA oxidation. Similarly, some studies have shown that controlled enrichment can sometimes suppress these specific volatiles in meat, though they remain a key marker of oxidative processes. In certain foods, a metallic odor is also reported in foods enriched with PUFA.
3. Rancid/fried/oily/pungent: As oxidation progresses in fatty foods, the generation of short-chain aldehydes produces sharp, pungent, or "oily/rancid" notes reminiscent of old cooking oil or stale nuts. This is the hallmark of sensory rejection. As n-3 fatty acids are unstable and prone to oxidation easily, and for degradation products, which is typically a characteristic of PUFA-rich foods (Mairesse et al., 2011; Sárraga et al., 2007).
4. Grassy: Some volatiles derived from PUFA degradation (such as hexanal at lower concentrations) can present as green or grassy notes. While not always negative, they indicate a departure from the expected neutral or "fresh" aroma of the base product.

23.6.2.3 Flavor

PUFA-rich foods have a characteristic flavor that is indicative of oily/rancidness, which refers to the quality of the product. In foods such as dried/cured meat products, descriptors such as meaty, fried, smoky, salty, and intense are used (Domínguez et al., 2019; Gray et al., 1996; Mairesse et al., 2011; Sárraga et al., 2007; Solomando et al., 2021; Domínguez et al., 2019). Off-flavor descriptors such as bitterness and astringency are also predominant in PUFA-rich foods.

23.6.2.4 Taste

Common descriptors indicative of taste attributes are mustiness, fishy, rancid, soapy, sweet, and meaty in products such as fried/cured meat, dried and fresh sausages, and are indicators of quality, which mostly imply undesirable qualities. Herby, earthy, moldy, and acidic descriptors are used in foods such as dairy, cheese, spreads, concentrates, and soups, which indicate the freshness of the food samples.

23.6.2.5 Texture

Texture-based descriptors are more common with respect to the type of food used, and the most common descriptors are juiciness, firmness, hardness, springiness, crustiness, smoothness, chewiness, and smoothness in meat and meat-based products. Dairy and instant foods have other descriptors such as creaminess, oily, buttery, slimy, thick, gumminess, and pastiness (Kolanowski et al., 1999, 2004; Kolanowski, Jaworska, Laufenberg et al., 2007; Kolanowski & Weißbrodt, 2007). Textural descriptors are also predominant indicators of food quality. Off-texture descriptors used are ropiness, stringy, rubbery, and dry in meat-based products enriched with PUFA (Kolanowski et al., 2004).

23.7 Indicators of sensory quality for polyunsaturated fatty acid-enriched foods

The incorporation of nutraceuticals, such as PUFA, in food products has evolved as a new trend in modern food development techniques (Granato et al., 2010). While the nutritional significance of PUFA is well known, it is a challenge for maintaining a preferable sensory quality (Kolanowski & Laufenberg, 2006). The consumers may be willing to choose nutritional food products, but they hardly ought to compromise on taste, aroma, or texture (Verbeke, 2006). So, it is necessary to identify the indicators to test for sensory quality in PUFA-enriched foods for successful commercialization (Baker et al., 2022). The sensory indicators for PUFA-enriched foods include oxidative stability, absence of rancid aroma, flavor, and stable texture and color, hedonic scale ratings, shelf-life, and storage quality (Kolanowski & Laufenberg, 2006). Integrating physical, chemical, and sensory tests gives the most reliable result for ensuring consumer satisfaction. As the functional food fortification is emerging in new product development techniques, maintaining sensory quality with nutritional stability continues to be important for consumer acceptance (Calder, 2015). One of the most important indicators is the oxidative stability of PUFA (Choe & Min, 2006). PUFAs are sensitive to oxidation as they contain more double bonds, which lead to the formation of aldehydes and ketones that give rancid, fishy smells (Shahidi & Zhong,

2005). The chemical indicators, such as peroxide value and TBARS values, serve as indirect indicators of sensory quality as they can be inferred with oxidative stability. While these are chemical analyses rather than sensory tests, they correlate strongly with the sensory view of rancidity (Kolanowski et al., 2004). In PUFA-enriched meat products or dairy systems, an increase in TBARS values often relates to sensory score with oxidized flavor (Domínguez et al., 2019). Thus, the combined results of sensory evaluation with chemical indicators provide a more detailed understanding of quality.

Aroma is an essential indicator of sensory quality in PUFA-enriched foods. Aroma compounds generated during oxidative rancidity can significantly interrupt consumer perception. In products enhanced with marine FOs, volatile compounds such as trimethylamine may cause fishy notes if formulation and development are inefficient (Shahidi & Zhong, 2005). Flavor is an equally important attribute as aroma in sensory tests (Pineau et al., 2009). A fishy taste in omega-3 fortified beverages reduces consumer satisfaction even when the initial taste profile is neutral (Kolanowski & Laufenberg, 2006). Encapsulation technologies have been declared to reduce flavor release and improve sensory quality by decreasing the chances for lipid exposure to oxygen (Drusch & Mannino, 2009). Texture and mouthfeel also act as another important indicator of sensory quality in food products (Bareen et al., 2025). The incorporation of PUFA in emulsified products such as yogurt and mayonnaise may alter viscosity, creaminess, and stability (MCCLEMENTS & DECKER, 2000). The consumers will accept the emulsions with a stable and homogeneous texture without any phase separation. Oil separation in emulsion indicates poor formulation, and that can negatively affect quality (Kolanowski & Laufenberg, 2006).

Color stability is an influential indicator in sensory analysis. In meat products enriched with omega-3 fatty acids, lipid oxidation may lead to degradation of pigments and also browning reactions (Gray et al., 1996). People often relate discoloration to spoilage, even when the product is microbially safe (Ares & Deliza, 2010). Maintaining color similar to conventional products helps to improve positive views on sensory quality (Baker et al., 2022). PUFA-enriched products may give acceptable results at the time of testing, but the product can spoil during spoilage, so the shelf-life is also an indicator of sensory quality (Kolanowski et al., 2004). The sensory quality can be maintained by effective antioxidants, efficient packaging, and storage conditions until the product is consumed (Choe & Min, 2006). Advanced technologies such as encapsulation help to protect PUFA from oxidation, which increases the shelf-life. They reduce the chances for oxidation so that the absence of rancid smell can give positive effects in sensory evaluation (Kolanowski & Laufenberg, 2006). Consumers cannot distinguish enriched products from conventional products in discriminative tests when the encapsulation technologies are optimized .

23.8 Conclusion and future prospects

The PUFA-enriched food presents a significant scientific leap in the field of functional food products, which is pushed forward by prominent evidence of their prospective health benefits in preventing cardiovascular diseases, regulating neuro-muscular development and inflammatory responses. However, the success of any nutritionally innovative product is that consumers can actually buy these products and consume them, which depends on consumer acceptance of the enriched product, and this primarily is dependent on the sensory quality of the enriched food product. The important takeaway from this chapter is that while the health consciousness for PUFA-enrichment in food is sound, the practical hurdles posed by quality issues, such as oxidative instability, decolouration, and textural changes on processing and storage, create a very difficult sensory obstacle that cannot be underestimated. PUFAs, especially the long-chain omega-3 varieties, readily undergo oxidation and generate volatile compounds that produce rancid, fishy, and metallic off-flavors. The consumers will be able to detect these off-flavors, and when detected, rejection is the evidentnt way to report them.

The sensory evaluation methods discussed in this chapter offer tools for assessing and improving a product's organoleptic quality. From preference and acceptance tests such as hedonic scale testing, captures how the general uninformed consumers would respond to PUFA-enriched products, to discriminative methods such as triangle test, that reveals if consumer can differentiate between enriched and conventional foods and finally, through descriptive analyses such as QDA, temporal dominance of sensation and intensity studies, where trained expert panel members provide detailed profiles of specific attributes or create product specific organoleptic fingerprint, each method contributes significant and valuable insights into food product quality. It is critical to carefully identify, select, train, and screen panel members, using international standards as a guide, to help ensure that sensory data obtained from the analyses are reliable and meaningful. Identifying the right sensory descriptors for expressing different attributes, such as appearance, aroma, flavor, taste, and texture, allows food producers and assessors to identify and pinpoint where exactly the problem lies, while indicators such as oxidative stability, aroma profile, flavor balance, texture integrity, and color consistency serve as practical, measurable markers of food quality. Thus, there is a clear need for an integrated approach for PUFA-enriched food products and sensory acceptance. Sensory evaluation works alongside chemical analysis, processing technologies such as encapsulation, antioxidant content measurements, and genuine consumer surveys and research, providing the most reliable data to develop PUFA-enriched foods that deliver both nutritional benefits and organoleptic acceptance. As the market for functional foods continues to grow, the methods and guidelines covered in this chapter will remain a critical tool to make sure that health-conscious products actually find sensory acceptance with the respective target consumers.

References

Aleksandra, A., Niveska, P., Vesna, V., Jasna, T., Tamara, P., Vrvic, M., & Marija, G. (2009). Milk in human nutrition: Comparison of fatty acid profiles. *Acta Veterinaria, 59*(5-6), 569–578. https://doi.org/10.2298/AVB0906569A.

Ardabilchi Marand, M., Amjadi, S., Ardabilchi Marand, M., Roufegarinejad, L., & Jafari, S. M. (2020). Fortification of yogurt with flaxseed powder and evaluation of its fatty acid profile, physicochemical, antioxidant, and sensory properties. *Powder Technology, 359*, 76–84. https://doi.org/10.1016/j.powtec.2019.09.082, www.elsevier.com/locate/powtec.

Ares, G., & Deliza, R. (2010). Studying the influence of package shape and colour on consumer expectations of milk desserts using word association and conjoint analysis. *Food Quality and Preference, 21*(8), 930–937. https://doi.org/10.1016/j.foodqual.2010.03.006.

Babuskin, S., Krishnan, K. R., Babu, P. A. S., Sivarajan, M., & Sukumar, M. (2014). Functional foods enriched with marine microalga *Nannochloropsis oculata* as a source of ω-3 fatty acids. *Food Technology and Biotechnology, 52*(3), 292–299. http://www.ftb.com.hr/images/pdfarticles/2014/July-September/ftb_52-3_292-299.pdf.

Baker, M. T., Lu, P., Parrella, J. A., & Leggette, H. R. (2022). Consumer acceptance toward functional foods: A scoping review. *International Journal of Environmental Research and Public Health, 19*(3). https://doi.org/10.3390/ijerph19031217, https://www.mdpi.com/1660-4601/19/3/1217/pdf.

Bareen, M. A., Prasannakumaran, K. M., & Sahu, J. K. (2025). *Recent developments in sensory assessment and consumer preference techniques* (pp. 369–402). https://doi.org/10.1007/978-3-031-75834-8_14.

Bavelaar, F. J., & Beynen, A. C. (2004). Relationships between the intake of n-3 polyunsaturated fatty acids by hens and the fatty acid composition of their eggs. *International Journal of Poultry Science, 3*(11), 690–696. https://doi.org/10.3923/ijps.2004.690.696, http://www.pjbs.org/ijps/fin274.pdf.

Betti, M., Schneider, B. L., Wismer, W. V., Carney, V. L., Zuidhof, M. J., & Renema, R. A. (2009). Omega-3-enriched broiler meat: 2. Functional properties, oxidative stability, and consumer acceptance. *Poultry Science, 88*(5), 1085–1095. https://doi.org/10.3382/ps.2008-00158.

Brockhoff, P. M., Hirst, D., & Ns, T. (1996). Analysing individual profiles by three-way factor analysis. *Data Handling in Science and Technology, 16*(C), 307–342. https://doi.org/10.1016/S0922-3487(96)80034-7.

Calder, P. C. (2015). Functional roles of fatty acids and their effects on human health. *Journal of Parenteral and Enteral Nutrition, 39*(1S). https://doi.org/10.1177/0148607115595980.

Cardoso, C. L., Gomes, R., Matos, J., Lopes, P. A., Bandarra, N. M., & Afonso, C. M. (2025). A comparison of alternative oil supplements as a source of bioaccessible key fatty acids. *International Journal of Food Science and Technology, 60*(2). https://doi.org/10.1093/ijfood/vvaf224, https://academic.oup.com/ijfst/issue.

Carpenter, R. P., Lyon, D. H., & Hasdell, T. A. (2000). *Guidelines for sensory analysis in food product development and quality control*. Springer US. https://doi.org/10.1007/978-1-4615-4447-0.

Carrillo, E., Varela, P., & Fiszman, S. (2012). Effects of food package information and sensory characteristics on the perception of healthiness and the acceptability of enriched biscuits. *Food Research International, 48*(1), 209–216. https://doi.org/10.1016/j.foodres.2012.03.016.

Chen, C. G., Wang, P., Zhang, Z. Q., Ye, Y. B., Zhuo, S. Y., Zhou, Q., Chen, Y. M., Su, Y. X., & Zhang, B. (2020). Effects of plant oils with different fatty acid composition on cardiovascular risk factors in moderately hypercholesteremic Chinese adults: A randomized, double-blinded, parallel-designed trial. *Food and Function, 11*(8), 7164–7174. https://doi.org/10.1039/d0fo00875c, http://pubs.rsc.org/en/journals/journal/fo.

Choe, E., & Min, D. B. (2006). Mechanisms and factors for edible oil oxidation. *Comprehensive Reviews in Food Science and Food Safety, 5*(4), 169–186. https://doi.org/10.1111/j.1541-4337.2006.00009.x, http://www.blackwell-synergy.com/doi/pdf/10.1111/j.1541-4337.2006.00009.x.

Contador, L., Shinya, P., Bunger, A., Sáenz, C., & Infante, R. (2014). Training a sensory panel for describing texture in peach and nectarines. *Journal of Food, Agr and Environment, 12*(3–4), 65–70. https://www.scopus.com/inward/record.uri?eid=2-s2.0-84908116811&partnerID=40&md5=1db561360af72980d89e8bb4e039d46f.

Crawford, M. A., Hall, B., Laurance, B. M., & Munhambo, A. (1976). Milk lipids and their variability. *Current Medical Research and Opinion, 4*(1), 33–43. https://doi.org/10.1185/03007997609109350.

Deliza, R., MacFie, H., & Hedderley, D. (2005). The consumer sensory perception of passion-fruit juice using free-choice profiling. *Journal of Sensory Studies, 20*(1), 17–27. https://doi.org/10.1111/j.1745-459X.2005.050604.x.

Domínguez, R., Pateiro, M., Gagaoua, M., Barba, F. J., Zhang, W., & Lorenzo, J. M. (2019). A comprehensive review on lipid oxidation in meat and meat products. *Antioxidants, 8*(10), 429. https://doi.org/10.3390/antiox8100429.

Drusch, S., & Mannino, S. (2009). Patent-based review on industrial approaches for the microencapsulation of oils rich in polyunsaturated fatty acids. *Trends in Food Science & Technology, 20*(6-7), 237–244. https://doi.org/10.1016/j.tifs.2009.03.007.

Eaton, S. B., Eaton III, S. B., Sinclair, A. J., Cordain, L., & Mann, N. J. (1998). Dietary intake of long-chain polyunsaturated fatty acids during the paleolithic. In *The return of w3 fatty acids into the food supply*. KARGER, 12–23. https://doi.org/10.1159/000059672.

EFSA Panel on Dietetic Products, Nutrition, and Allergies (NDA). (2010). Scientific Opinion on Dietary Reference Values for fats, including saturated fatty acids, polyunsaturated fatty acids, monounsaturated fatty acids, trans fatty acids, and cholesterol. *EFSA Journal, 8*(3). https://doi.org/10.2903/j.efsa.2010.1461.

Elgaard, L., Jensen, S., Mielby, L. A., & Byrne, D. V. (2019). Performance of beer sensory panels: A comparison of experience level, product knowledge, and responsiveness to feedback calibration. *Journal of Sensory Studies, 34*(6). https://doi.org/10.1111/joss.12540, http://onlinelibrary.wiley.com/journal/10.1111/(ISSN)1745-459X.

Ganesan, B., Brothersen, C., & McMahon, D. J. (2014). Fortification of foods with omega-3 polyunsaturated fatty acids. *Critical Reviews in Food Science and Nutrition, 54*(1), 98–114. https://doi.org/10.1080/10408398.2011.578221.

Gill, J. M. R., Brown, J. C., Caslake, M. J., Wright, D. M., Cooney, J., Bedford, D., Hughes, D. A., Stanley, J. C., & Packard, C. J. (2003). Effects of dietary monounsaturated fatty acids on lipoprotein concentrations, compositions, and subfraction distributions and on VLDL apolipoprotein B kinetics: Dose-dependent effects on LDL. *American Journal of Clinical Nutrition, 78*(1), 47–56. https://doi.org/10.1093/ajcn/78.1.47, http://www.ajcn.org/contents-by-date.2005.shtml.

Givens, D. I., Kliem, K. E., & Gibbs, R. A. (2006). The role of meat as a source of n−3 polyunsaturated fatty acids in the human diet. *Meat Science, 74*(1), 209–218. https://doi.org/10.1016/j.meatsci.2006.04.008.

Granato, D., Branco, G. F., Cruz, A. G., Faria, J.de A. F., & Shah, N. P. (2010). Probiotic dairy products as functional foods. *Comprehensive Reviews in Food Science and Food Safety, 9*(5), 455–470. https://doi.org/10.1111/j.1541-4337.2010.00120.x.

Gray, J. I., Gomaa, E. A., & Buckley, D. J. (1996). Oxidative quality and shelf-life of meats. *Meat Science, 43*, 111–123. https://doi.org/10.1016/0309-1740(96)00059-9.

Haque Akanda, M. J., M.R., N., F.S., A., Shaarani, S., Mamat, H., Lee, J. S., J., N., A.H., M., Selamat, J., Khan, F., Matanjun, P., & Islam Sarker, M. Z. (2020). Hard fats improve the physicochemical and thermal properties of seed fats for applications in confectionery products. *Food Reviews International, 36*(6), 601–625. https://doi.org/10.1080/87559129.2019.1657443.

Heymann, H., & Noble, A. C. (1989). Comparison of canonical variate and principal component analyses of wine descriptive analysis data. *Journal of Food Science, 54*(5), 1355–1358. https://doi.org/10.1111/j.1365-2621.1989.tb05991.x.

Huang, J. H., Jiang, S. G., Lin, H. Z., Zhou, F. L., & Ye, L. (2008). Effects of dietary highly unsaturated fatty acids and astaxanthin on the fecundity and lipid content of pond-reared Penaeus monodon (Fabricius) broodstock. *Aquaculture Research, 39*(3), 240–251. https://doi.org/10.1111/j.1365-2109.2007.01868.x.

Hui, T., Li, Q., Fang, Z., Li, R., Sun, Y., Li, J., & Yang, Y. (2025). Sensory qualities markers of n-3 PUFA enriched fresh pork meat fattened by linseed oil and selenium methionine. *Food Chemistry, 464*(Pt 3), 141832. https://doi.org/10.1016/j.foodchem.2024.141832.

Ianora, A., Poulet, S. A., & Miralto, A. (2003). The effects of diatoms on copepod reproduction: a review. *Phycologia, 42*(4), 351–363. https://doi.org/10.2216/i0031-8884-42-4-351.1.

International Organization for Standardization. (2012). *Sensory analysis - General guidelines for the selection, training and monitoring of selected assessors and expert sensory assessors (ISO standard No.8586:2012(E)).*

International Organization for Standardization. (2016). *Sensory analysis-Methodology-General guidance for establishing a sensory profile (ISO standard - 13299).* www.iso.org.

Jacobsen, C. (2015). Some strategies for the stabilization of long chain n-3 PUFA-enriched foods: A review. *European Journal of Lipid Science and Technology, 117*(11), 1853–1866. https://doi.org/10.1002/ejlt.201500137, http://www3.interscience.wiley.com/journal/69502350/home.

Jacobsen, C., Let, M. B., Nielsen, N. S., & Meyer, A. S. (2008). Antioxidant strategies for preventing oxidative flavour deterioration of foods enriched with n-3 polyunsaturated lipids: a comparative evaluation. *Trends in Food Science and Technology, 19*(2), 76–93. https://doi.org/10.1016/j.tifs.2007.08.001.

Jacobsen, C., Sørensen, A.-D. M., & Nielsen, N. S. (2013). Stabilization of omega-3 oils and enriched foods using antioxidants. In *Food enrichment with omega-3 fatty acids*. Elsevier, 130–149. https://doi.org/10.1533/9780857098863.2.130.

Jandacek, R. J. (2017). Linoleic acid: A nutritional quandary. *Healthcare, 5*(2), 25. https://doi.org/10.3390/healthcare5020025.

Kemp, S. E., Hort, J., & Hollowood, T. (2018). Setting up and training a descriptive analysis panel. In *Descriptive analysis in sensory evaluation*. Wiley, 81–112. http://doi.org/10.1002/9781118991657.ch3.

Kolanowski, W., Jaworska, D., Laufenberg, G., & Weißbrodt, J. (2007). Evaluation of sensory quality of instant foods fortified with omega-3 PUFA by addition of fish oil powder. *European Food Research and Technology, 225*(5–6), 715–721. https://doi.org/10.1007/s00217-006-0474-y.

Kolanowski, W., Jaworska, D., & Weißbrodt, J. (2007). Importance of instrumental and sensory analysis in the assessment of oxidative deterioration of omega-3 long-chain polyunsaturated fatty acid-rich foods. *Journal of the Science of Food and Agriculture, 87*(2), 181–191. https://doi.org/10.1002/jsfa.2733.

Kolanowski, W., Swiderski, F., Jaworska, D., & Berger, S. (2004). Stability, sensory quality, texture properties and nutritional value of fish oil-enriched spreadable fat. *Journal of the Science of Food and Agriculture, 84*(15), 2135–2141. https://doi.org/10.1002/jsfa.1770.

Kolanowski, W., Swiderski, F.Â., & Aw Berger, S. (1999). Possibilities of fish oil application for food products enrichment with v-3 PUFA. *International Journal of Food Sciences and Nutrition, 50*.

Kolanowski, W., & Laufenberg, G. (2006). Enrichment of food products with polyunsaturated fatty acids by fish oil addition. *European Food Research and Technology, 222*(3-4), 472–477. https://doi.org/10.1007/s00217-005-0089-8.

Kolanowski, W., Swiderski, F., Jaworska, D., & Berger, S. (2004). Stability, sensory quality, texture properties and nutritional value of fish oil-enriched spreadable fat. *Journal of the Science of Food and Agriculture, 84*(15), 2135–2141. https://doi.org/10.1002/jsfa.1770.

Kolanowski, W., & Weißbrodt, J. (2007). Sensory quality of dairy products fortified with fish oil. *International Dairy Journal, 17*(10), 1248–1253. https://doi.org/10.1016/j.idairyj.2007.04.005.

Kumari, P., Sharma, J., & Khare, P. (2025). Recent advancements and strategies for omega-3 fatty acid production in yeast. *Journal of Basic Microbiology, 65*(3). https://doi.org/10.1002/jobm.202400491.

Labbe, D., Rytz, A., & Hugi, A. (2004). Training is a critical step to obtain reliable product profiles in a real food industry context. *Food Quality and Preference, 15*(4), 341–348. https://doi.org/10.1016/S0950-3293(03)00081-8.

Lawlor, J. B., Gaudette, N., Dickson, T., & House, J. D. (2010). Fatty acid profile and sensory characteristics of table eggs from laying hens fed diets containing microencapsulated fish oil. *Animal Feed Science and Technology, 156*(3-4), 97–103. https://doi.org/10.1016/j.anifeedsci.2010.01.003.

Lim, J. (2011). Hedonic scaling: A review of methods and theory. *Food Quality and Preference, 22*(8). https://doi.org/10.1016/j.foodqual.2011.05.008.

Lovegrove, J. A. (2025). Dietary fats and cardiometabolic health—from public health to personalised nutrition: 'One for all' and 'all for one' *Nutrition Bulletin, 50*(1), 132–141. https://doi.org/10.1111/nbu.12722, http://onlinelibrary.wiley.com/journal/10.1111/(ISSN)1467-3010.

Mairesse, G., Benet, M., Méteau, K., Juin, H., Durand, D., & Mourot, J. (2011). Effect of plant antioxidant in n-3 polyunsaturated fatty acid-enriched diet on fatty acid composition and sensorial attributes of dry-cured ham. *International Journal of Food Science & Technology, 46*(12), 2656–2662. https://doi.org/10.1111/j.1365-2621.2011.02797.x.

MANZOOR, M. F., SHABBIR, U., GILANI, S. M., SAMEEN, A., AHMAD, N., SIDDIQUE, R., AHMED, Z., QAYYUM, A., & REHMAN, A. (2022). Characterization of bioactive fatty acids and oxidative stability of microwave vacuum dried fish powder supplemented extruded product. *Food Science and Technology, 42*. https://doi.org/10.1590/fst.22720.

Markey, O., Souroullas, K., Fagan, C. C., Kliem, K. E., Vasilopoulou, D., Jackson, K. G., Humphries, D. J., Grandison, A. S., Givens, D. I., Lovegrove, J. A., & Methven, L. (2017). Consumer acceptance of dairy products with a saturated fatty acid–reduced, monounsaturated fatty acid–enriched content. *Journal of Dairy Science, 100*(10), 7953–7966. https://doi.org/10.3168/jds.2016-12057, http://www.elsevier.com/wps/find/journaldescription.cws_home/721317/description#description.

MCCLEMENTS, D. J., & DECKER, E. A. (2000). Lipid oxidation in oil-in-water emulsions: Impact of molecular environment on chemical reactions in heterogeneous food systems. *Journal of Food Science, 65*(8), 1270–1282. https://doi.org/10.1111/j.1365-2621.2000.tb10596.x.

Mehta, B. M. (2015). Lipid oxidation (2005), 2nd edn, edited by E.N.Frankel, Woodhead Publishing Ltd., Sawston, Cambridge, UK. ISBN-13: 978-0-9531949-8-8. *International Journal of Dairy Technology, 68*(1), 148–149. https://doi.org/10.1111/1471-0307.12128.

Meier, C., Harms, E., Früh, B., Stoffers, H., Bee, G., Hugelshofer, D. H., Quander-Stoll, N., & Stolz, H. (2021). The effect of polyunsaturated fatty acids (PUFA) and organic labeling on Swiss consumers' acceptance of pork salami. *Organic Agriculture, 11*(4), 519–537. https://doi.org/10.1007/s13165-021-00369-9, www.springer.com/life+sciences/agriculture/journal/13165.

Monteiro, B., & Vasconcelos, S. (2024). Sensory panel training: Developing hospitality students analytical and research skills. In A. I. Azevedo (Ed.), *Proceedings of the European conference on research methods in business and management studies* (Vol. 23, Number 1, pp. 153–160). Academic Conferences and Publishing International Limited. https://doi.org/10.34190/ecrm.23.1.2514

Moskowitz, H. R., & Meiselman, H. L. (1977). Psychophysical and psychometric approaches to sensory evaluation. *C R C Critical Reviews in Food Science and Nutrition, 9*(1), 41–79. https://doi.org/10.1080/10408397709527230.

Mukherjee, S., Mohanty, A. K., Rao, U., & Poddar, A. (2024). Microbial polyunsaturated fatty acids (PUFAs) for human health: A comprehensive review of evidence from in vivo preclinical models. *Discover Applied Sciences, 6*(10). https://doi.org/10.1007/s42452-024-06238-w, https://link.springer.com/journal/42452.

Murray, J. M., Delahunty, C. M., & Baxter, I. A. (2001). Descriptive sensory analysis: Past, present and future. *Food Research International, 34*(6), 461–471. https://doi.org/10.1016/S0963-9969(01)00070-9.

Navalho, S., Ferrer-Ledo, N., Barbosa, M. J., & Varela, J. (2025). Nannochloropsis lipids and polyunsaturated fatty acids: Potential applications and strain improvement. *Marine Drugs, 23*(3). https://doi.org/10.3390/md23030128, http://www.mdpi.com/journal/marinedrugs.

Nazzaro, C., Stanco, M., Uliano, A., & Marotta, G. (2024). Consumers' acceptance and willingness to pay for enriched foods: Evidence from a choice experiment in Italy. *Future Foods, 10*, 100405. https://doi.org/10.1016/j.fufo.2024.100405.

Ojeh, S. (2021). The role of sensory analysis in quality controlIn *The role of sensory analysis in quality control* (2nd Edition). ASTM International. https://doi.org/10.1520/mnl14-2nd-eb.

Olsen, M. L., Olsen, K., & Jensen, P. E. (2024). Consumer acceptance of microalgae as a novel food - Where are we now? And how to get further. *Physiologia Plantarum, 176*(3). https://doi.org/10.1111/ppl.14337.

Parpinello, G. P., Meluzzi, A., Sirri, F., Tallarico, N., & Versari, A. (2006). Sensory evaluation of egg products and eggs laid from hens fed diets with different fatty acid composition and supplemented with antioxidants. *Food Research International, 39*(1), 47–52. https://doi.org/10.1016/j.foodres.2005.05.010.

Pecore, D. S. (1993). Guidelines for sensory analysis in food product development and quality control. *Trends in Food Science & Technology, 4*(6), 200. https://doi.org/10.1016/0924-2244(93)90132-T.

Peng, Y., West, G. E., & Wang, C. (2006). Consumer attitudes and acceptance of CLA-enriched dairy products. *Canadian Journal of Agricultural Economics/Revue Canadienne d'agroeconomie, 54*(4), 663–684. https://doi.org/10.1111/j.1744-7976.2006.00072.x.

Pham, T. P. T., Hoang, T. V., Le, T. T. D., Cao, P. T. N., Ho, V. T. N., Vu, T. M. H., Le, T. H. T., Pham, H. T. X., Ratna Mafruhah, O., Pham, T. T. L., Hsieh, M. T., & Ha, H. A. (2024a). Comparing the cardiovascular risk-reducing effects of polyunsaturated fatty acids in fish oil and krill oil: A network meta analysis. *Journal of Functional Foods, 120*. https://doi.org/10.1016/j.jff.2024.106379, https://www.sciencedirect.com/science/journal/17564646.

Pham, T.-P.-T., Le, T.-T.-D., Cao, P.-T.-N., Ho, V.-T.-N., Vu, T.-M.-H., Le, T.-H.-T., Pham, H.-T.-X., Mafruhah, O.R., Pham, T.-T.-L., Hsieh, M.-T., Ha, H.-A., & Hoang, T.-V. (2024b). Comparing the cardiovascular risk-reducing effects of polyunsaturated fatty acids in fish oil and krill oil: A network meta-analysis. https://doi.org/10.20944/preprints202405.0128.v1

Pineau, N., Schlich, P., Cordelle, S., Mathonnière, C., Issanchou, S., Imbert, A., Rogeaux, M., Etiévant, P., & Köster, E. (2009). Temporal dominance of sensations: Construction of the TDS curves and comparison with time–intensity. *Food Quality and Preference, 20*(6), 450–455. https://doi.org/10.1016/j.foodqual.2009.04.005.

Purriños, L., Pateiro, M., Rosmini, M., Domínguez-Valencia, R., Teixeira, A., Sichetti Munekata, P. E. S., Campagnol, P. C. B., & Lorenzo, J. M. (2022). Descriptive sensory analysis as an analytical tool for the sensory characterization of meat products: Fundaments, panel training, and descriptors of meat products. In *Sensory analysis for the development of meat products: Methodological aspects and practical applications*. Elsevier, 51–76. https://doi.org/10.1016/B978-0-12-822832-6.00003-5.

Pusceddu, M. M., El Aidy, S., Crispie, F., O'Sullivan, O., Cotter, P., Stanton, C., Kelly, P., Cryan, J. F., & Dinan, T. G. (2015). N-3 polyunsaturated fatty acids (PUFAs) reverse the impact of early-life stress on the gut microbiota. *PLoS ONE, 10*(10). https://doi.org/10.1371/journal.pone.0139721, http://www.plosone.org/article/fetchObject.action?uri=info:doi/10.1371/journal.pone.0139721&representation=PDF.

Pérez-Palacios, T., Ruiz-Carrascal, J., Jiménez-Martín, E., Solomando, J. C., & Antequera, T. (2018). Improving the lipid profile of ready-to-cook meat products by addition of omega-3 microcapsules: effect on oxidation and sensory analysis. *Journal of the Science of Food and Agriculture, 98*(14), 5302–5312. https://doi.org/10.1002/jsfa.9069, http://onlinelibrary.wiley.com/journal/10.1002/(ISSN)1097-0010.

Quílez, J., Ruiz, J. A., Brufau, G., & Rafecas, M. (2006). Bakery products enriched with phytosterols, α-tocopherol and β-carotene. Sensory evaluation and chemical comparison with market products. *Food Chemistry, 94*(3), 399–405. https://doi.org/10.1016/j.foodchem.2004.11.029.

Ramachandran, V., Gopakumar, S. T., Ramachandra, K. S. S., Chandrasekar, S., Tejpal, C. S., Nair, A. V., Pootholathil, S., Sreenath, K. R., Nithyashree, J. K., & Achamveetil, G. (2024). Insights into the methodological perspectives for screening polyunsaturated fatty acids-containing bacteria. *Archives of Microbiology, 206*(11). https://doi.org/10.1007/s00203-024-04155-5, https://www.springer.com/journal/203.

Rangel, B. S., Hammerschlag, N., Martinelli, L. A., & Moreira, R. G. (2022). Effects of urbanization on the nutritional ecology of a highly active coastal shark: Preliminary insights from trophic markers and body condition. *Science of the Total Environment, 826*. https://doi.org/10.1016/j.scitotenv.2022.154082, www.elsevier.com/locate/scitotenv.

Razzaq, A., Tang, Y., & Qing, P. (2021). Towards sustainable diets: Understanding the cognitive mechanism of consumer acceptance of biofortified foods and the role of nutrition information. *International Journal of Environmental Research and Public Health, 18*(3), 1175. https://doi.org/10.3390/ijerph18031175.

Robertson, R. C., Gracia Mateo, M. R., O'Grady, M. N., Guihéneuf, F., Stengel, D. B., Ross, R. P., Fitzgerald, G. F., Kerry, J. P., & Stanton, C. (2016). An assessment of the techno-functional and sensory properties of yoghurt fortified with a lipid extract from the microalga Pavlova lutheri. *Innovative Food Science and Emerging Technologies, 37*, 237–246. https://doi.org/10.1016/j.ifset.2016.03.017.

Rodríguez De Marco, E., Steffolani, M. E., Martínez, M., & León, A. E. (2018). The use of Nannochloropsis sp. as a source of omega-3 fatty acids in dry pasta: chemical, technological and sensory evaluation. *International Journal of Food Science and Technology, 53*(2), 499–507. https://doi.org/10.1111/ijfs.13609.

Rymer, C., & Givens, D. I. (2005). n−3 fatty acid enrichment of edible tissue of poultry: A review. *Lipids, 40*(2), 121–130. https://doi.org/10.1007/s11745-005-1366-4.

Sandoval, C., Nahuelqueo, K., Mella, L., Recabarren, B., Souza-Mello, V., & Farías, J. (2023). Role of long-chain polyunsaturated fatty acids, eicosapentaenoic and docosahexaenoic, in the regulation of gene expression during the development of obesity: a systematic review. *Frontiers in Nutrition, 10*. https://doi.org/10.3389/fnut.2023.1288804.

Sárraga, C., Guàrdia, M. D., Díaz, I., Guerrero, L., García Regueiro, J. A., & Arnau, J. (2007). Nutritional and sensory quality of porcine raw meat, cooked ham and dry-cured shoulder as affected by dietary enrichment with docosahexaenoic acid (DHA) and α-tocopheryl acetate. *Meat Science, 76*(2), 377–384. https://doi.org/10.1016/j.meatsci.2006.12.007.

Scheideler, S. E., Froning, G., & Cuppett, S. (1997). Studies of consumer acceptance of high omega-3 fatty acid-enriched eggs. *Journal of Applied Poultry Research, 6*(2), 137–146. https://doi.org/10.1093/japr/6.2.137.

Schlich, P. (2017). Temporal Dominance Of Sensations (TDS): A new deal for temporal sensory analysis. *Current Opinion in Food Science, 15*, 38–42. https://doi.org/10.1016/j.cofs.2017.05.003.

Sekikawa, A., Ihara, M., Lopez, O., Kakuta, C., Lopresti, B., Higashiyama, A., Aizenstein, H., Chang, Y. F., Mathis, C., Miyamoto, Y., Kuller, L., & Cui, C. (2019). Effect of S-equol and soy isoflavones on heart and brain. *Current Cardiology Reviews, 15*(2), 114–135. https://doi.org/10.2174/1573403X15666181205104717.

Sell, C. R. (2012). Sensory characteristics and storage quality indicators of Surimi franks nutritionally enhanced with omega-3 rich flaxseed oil and Salmon oil [West Virginia University]. https://researchrepository.wvu.edu/etd/4917

Shahidi, F, & Zhong, H. J. (2020). Methods for Measuring Lipid Oxidation. In *Bailey's Industrial Oil and Fat Products*1–27. https://doi.org/10.1002/047167849X.bio050.pub2.

Shahidi, F., & Ambigaipalan, P. (2016). *Beverages fortified with omega-3 fatty acids, dietary fiber, minerals, and vitamins*. Informa UK Limited, 801–813. http://doi.org/10.1201/b19490-69.

Shahidi, F., & Ambigaipalan, P. (2018). Omega-3 polyunsaturated fatty acids and their health benefits. *Annual Review of Food Science and Technology, 9*(1), 345–381. https://doi.org/10.1146/annurev-food-111317-095850.

Shahidi, F., & Zhong, Y. (2005). Lipid oxidation: Measurement methods. In *Bailey's industrial oil and fat products*. Wiley. https://doi.org/10.1002/047167849X.bio050.

Sharma, N., Sharma, S. G., Kocher, G. S., & Dhir, A. (2025). Microalgae: A treasure house for polyunsaturated fatty acid (PUFA) production. *National Academy Science Letters*. https://doi.org/10.1007/s40009-025-01867-0, https://www.springer.com/journal/40009.

Solomando, J. C., Antequera, T., Ventanas, S., & Perez-Palacios, T. (2021). Sensory profile and consumer perception of meat products enriched with EPA and DHA using fish oil microcapsules. *International Journal of Food Science and Technology, 56*(6), 2926–2937. https://doi.org/10.1111/ijfs.14932, http://onlinelibrary.wiley.com/journal/10.1111/(ISSN)1365-2621.

Swanson, D., Block, R., & Mousa, S. A. (2012). Omega-3 fatty acids EPA and DHA: Health benefits throughout life. *Advances in Nutrition, 3*(1), 1–7. https://doi.org/10.3945/an.111.000893.

Tian, L., Chi, G., Lin, S., Ling, X., & He, N. (2024). Marine microorganisms: natural factories for polyunsaturated fatty acid production. *Blue Biotechnology, 1*(1), 15. https://doi.org/10.1186/s44315-024-00012-8.

Torres-Vanegas, J., Rodríguez-Echevarría, R., Campos-Pérez, W., Rodríguez-Reyes, S. C., Reyes-Pérez, S. D., Pérez-Robles, M., & Martínez-López, E. (2025). Effect of a diet supplemented with marine omega-3 fatty acids on inflammatory markers in subjects with obesity: A Randomized active placebo-controlled trial. *Healthcare, 13*(2), 103. https://doi.org/10.3390/healthcare13020103.

Tserveni-Gousi, A., Yannakopoulos, A., Botsoglou, N., Christaki, E., Florou-Paneri, P., & Yannakakis, E. (2006). *Sensory evaluation and oxidative stability of n-3 fatty acid enriched eggs in Greece Sensorische Bewertung und Oxidationsstabilität von mit n-3 Fettsäuren angereicherten Eiern in Griechenland* (Number 5).

Valencia, I., Ansorena, D., & Astiasarán, I. (2006). Nutritional and sensory properties of dry fermented sausages enriched with n - 3 PUFAs. *Meat Science, 72*(4), 727–733. https://doi.org/10.1016/j.meatsci.2005.09.022.

Verbeke, W. (2005). Consumer acceptance of functional foods: Socio-demographic, cognitive and attitudinal determinants. *Food Quality and Preference, 16*(1), 45–57. https://doi.org/10.1016/j.foodqual.2004.01.001.

Verbeke, W. (2006). Functional foods: Consumer willingness to compromise on taste for health? *Food Quality and Preference, 17*(1–2), 126–131. https://doi.org/10.1016/j.foodqual.2005.03.003.

Waldron, M. K., Spencer, A. L., & Bauer, J. E. (1998). Role of long-chain polyunsaturated n-3 fatty acids in the development of the nervous system of dogs and cats. *Journal of the American Veterinary Medical Association, 213*(5), 619–622. https://doi.org/10.2460/javma.1998.213.05.619.

White, M. R., Gibbs, R. L., Grijalva, P. C., Hicks, Z. M., Beer, H. N., Marks-Nelson, E. S., & Yates, D. T. (2025). Reducing systemic inflammation in IUGR-born neonatal lambs via daily oral ω-3 PUFA supplement improved skeletal muscle glucose metabolism, glucose-stimulated insulin secretion, and blood pressure. *Metabolites, 15*(6). https://doi.org/10.3390/metabo15060346, http://www.mdpi.com/journal/metabolites.

Yang, Z., Chen, Y., Ma, S., Zhang, M., Tang, T., & Du, C. (2025). Bioengineering of long-chain polyunsaturated fatty acids in oilseed crops. *Progress in Lipid Research, 99*, 101333. https://doi.org/10.1016/j.plipres.2025.101333.

Chapter 24

Food matrix interactions: enhancing bioavailability and functionality of polyunsaturated fatty acids

H.E. Shweatha[1], Netravati Hiremath[1], Arfa[1], Prashanth Kotthapalli[2], and Sumana Kumar[2]

[1]*Department of Nutrition & Dietetics, JSS Academy of Higher Education and Research, Mysuru, Karnataka, India,* [2]*Department of Microbiology, JSS Academy of Higher Education and Research, Mysuru, Karnataka, India*

24.1 Introduction

24.1.1 Insights on chemical structure of polyunsaturated fatty acids and food matrices

Polyunsaturated fatty acids (PUFAs) are essential dietary lipids characterized by the presence of two or more cis double bonds within their hydrocarbon chains. Omega-6 fatty acids, such as linoleic acid (LA) and arachidonic acid, and omega-3 fatty acids (n-3s), including α-linolenic acid (ALA), eicosapentaenoic acid (EPA), and docosahexaenoic acid (DHA), are essential dietary PUFAs. They function as integral components of cell membranes, precursors to bioactive lipid mediators, and regulators of gene expression and metabolism. These fatty acids are integral to cell membrane composition and play critical roles in the regulation of inflammation, cardiovascular health, neurodevelopment, and metabolic balance. The chemical composition of PUFAs is characterized by long aliphatic carbon chains with several cis-configured double bonds that are separated by methylene groups. The bis-allylic position has relatively weak C–H bonds, which makes PUFAs extremely prone to oxidation. The greater the unsaturation, the greater the susceptibility to oxidation; DHA is much less stable than EPA or LA because of the number of double bonds (Dyall et al., 2022; Harwood, 2023; Mititelu et al., 2025).

Due to this inherent instability, the physical form of PUFAs in food systems—such as the degree of emulsification, interface, and encapsulation—is critically important in preventing oxidative damage during processing, storage, and transit through the gastrointestinal tract. The PUFAs can be unstable due to various factors, such as the level of unsaturation, temperature, oxygen exposure, light exposure, pH levels, enzymatic activity, and interactions with other food components (Szpicer et al., 2025; Zazula et al., 2025). Alterations in the chemical composition of PUFAs, such as oxidation, hydrolysis, isomerization, and polymerization, can impact the sensory, nutritional, and functional properties of lipid-based foods, thereby affecting their bioavailability and associated health benefits. Particle size, texture, degree of processing, and specific processing technique applied during the formulation of food or supplement also determine the interaction and bioavailability of biomolecules in the human body system (Asif et al., 2026; Rahim et al., 2025). The relationship between the food matrix and the bioavailability of PUFAs has garnered significant attention due to the increasing demand for omega-3-rich foods and their associated health benefits. The food matrix is crucial in the release and absorption of nutrients by the human body, with the magnitude and proportion of food components such as proteins, carbohydrates, and dietary fiber influencing the bioavailability of PUFAs. In various food formulations, multiple factors impact the digestion, absorption, and bioavailability of PUFAs (Alijani et al., 2025; Cholewski et al., 2018).

24.1.2 Physical encapsulation and its impact on bioavailability

Lipids are present in natural foods either as components attached to the food matrix, such as proteins, or encapsulated within cells. EPA and DHA are physically encapsulated as triglycerides within the muscle cell membranes of oily fish. In oilseeds, the encapsulation of ALA occurs in the form of oleosomes, which are bound by a protein and membrane matrix. The ability to determine the accessibility of digestive enzymes to lipids is contingent upon the efficiency of the matrix

Omega-3 and Omega-6 Polyunsaturated Fatty Acids in Food Systems. DOI: https://doi.org/10.1016/B978-0-443-43810-3.00032-4

(Oscarsson & Hurt-Camejo, 2017; Song et al., 2023). Although the release of fatty acids from the matrix may be slower, it can also serve as a pathway through which lipids become accessible to digestive enzymes, potentially enhancing the bioavailability of the lipids. The surface area of matrices is increased by mechanical disruption techniques, such as mincing or homogenization, modifying the dynamics of digestion rates. Additionally, the emulsification process facilitates the formation of mixed micelles, which is important for the transport of PUFAs through the unstirred water layer of the mucosa. The incorporation of PUFAs, such as EPA and DHA, into emulsified or micellar structures within the food matrix enhances the dispersion of these PUFAs and their accessibility by digestive enzymes. This enhances the effective production of mixed micelles in the colon, which is essential for fat digestion and absorption. Therefore the stability, digestion, and bioavailability of PUFAs such as EPA and DHA can be improved by the food matrix (Mondal et al., 2024; Parada & Aguilera, 2007; Preeti et al., 2023).

24.1.3 Oxidative status and matrix protection

The food matrix influences the oxidative stability of PUFA in predigestion and at the time of digestion. Lipid oxidation is catalyzed by reactive oxygen species or metal ions, resulting in the formation of lipid radicals, hydroperoxides, and secondary oxidation products such as aldehydes and ketones, which are known to negatively impact the nutritional quality, sensory properties, and safety of food products, as well as the absorption process. Antioxidants, such as phenolic compounds and tocopherols, may assist PUFA in maintaining their structural integrity. PUFAs interact through self-assembly mechanisms, interfacial phenomena, and molecular packing effects to impact oxidative behavior, texture, and structural stability. Multiple cis double bonds provide greater structural flexibility and lower packing density in PUFAs than saturated fatty acids and have a direct impact on the behavior of the lipid phase and physicochemical functioning (Abeyrathne et al., 2021; Geng et al., 2023; Hennebelle et al., 2024).

24.2 Physicochemical interactions

24.2.1 Lipid–polyunsaturated fatty acids interactions: emulsions, micelles, and liposome encapsulation

In complex food systems (solid, semisolid, or liquid), PUFAs are structured and interact with other lipids and amphiphilic compounds to form structured assemblies such as lipid domains, self-assembled micellar structures during digestion, and phospholipid-based liposomes for fortification. The molecular structure of PUFAs in these lipid systems determines their susceptibility to oxygen, light, and pro-oxidative compounds (metal ions), which are the primary oxidative stresses. PUFAs can be produced in lipid systems or enclosed in phospholipid bilayers to improve oxidative stability by decreasing their mobility and reactivity. Additionally, released PUFAs are encapsulated in mixed micelles of bile salts and lipid digestion products during gastrointestinal digestion. This is a crucial step in determining the intestinal absorption and bioavailability of PUFAs (Table 24.1). In this regard, lipid structuring and encapsulation in food systems regulate both the chemical stability of PUFAs and their bioavailability based on microenvironmental exposure and digestive release conditions (Acevedo-Fani et al., 2020; Kupikowska-Stobba et al., 2025).

24.2.1.1 Protein–polyunsaturated fatty acid binding

PUFAs primarily interact with proteins in food systems through noncovalent interactions, such as hydrogen bonding, hydrophobic interactions, and occasionally electrostatic bonding. The presence of multiple cis double bonds in PUFAs predisposes them to interact with nonpolar amino acids, including leucine, isoleucine, and phenylalanine. These interactions can affect oxidation, aggregation, thermal stability, and protein structure within food systems (Islam et al., 2023; Oruch et al., 2010).

24.2.1.2 Casein protein–polyunsaturated fatty acid interactions

Caseins, characterized as elastic and amphiphilic phosphoproteins, assemble into micelles that inherently bind and solubilize hydrophobic substances. The absence of a defined tertiary structure allows caseins to partially envelop lipid molecules within their hydrophobic domains, thereby stabilizing protein–lipid complexes in solution (Parc et al., 2014; Sadiq et al., 2021). While the presence of unsaturated fatty acids and protein-bound metal ions, such as iron, could potentially lead to lipid oxidation, in dairy milk fortified with PUFAs, these interactions may enhance the stability of the dispersion and prevent phase separation. Additionally, the interaction with PUFAs may induce slight conformational modifications in casein micelles, which can subsequently alter the rheological characteristics of cheese and yogurt (Bao & Pignitter, 2023; Cengiz et al., 2019; Cengiz et al., 2021; Xu et al., 2025).

TABLE 24.1 Food matrix factors associated with polyunsaturated fatty acids bioavailability in foods.

Matrix system	Effect on droplet size and stability	Influence on lipase	Influence on micelle formation	Effect on bioavailability
Casein-based emulsion	Small, Stable droplets	Digested gradually	Favorable after proteolysis	Often increases or maintaines
Whey protein at the interface	Highly stable	Delay if rigid	Neutral	Dependent on context
Whey protein gels	Immobilizes droplets	Diffusion restricted	Slight delay	Rate decrease
Plant protein emulsions	Good stability	Hindered	Neutral	Slightly decrease or little change
Soluble fiber	Indirect stabilization	Slower transport of enzymes	May reduce bile availability	Rate decrease
Insoluble fiber	Droplets attach to particles	Restricted	Reduced	Decrease
Starch gel matrix	Restricts mobility	Controlled	Maintained	Tunable
Hydrogel encapsulation	High stability	Depends on the release	Variable	Tunable/targeted

24.2.1.3 Whey protein–polyunsaturated fatty acid interactions

Whey proteins, such as β-lactoglobulin (β-LG), have been known to possess a tertiary structure with hydrophobic binding sites inside that bind fatty acids, including PUFAs. The calyx-like hydrophobic binding pocket of β-LG can bind long-chain fatty acids via hydrophobic interactions and hydrogen bonding at specific binding sites. The binding of PUFAs can either stabilize or destabilize protein structure based on pH, temperature, and ionic strength, which may affect denaturation and aggregation properties during heat treatment (Corfield et al., 2023; Le Maux et al., 2014; Tai et al., 2016). Protein–PUFA complexes may potentially enhance oxidative stability by physically hindering the diffusion and accessibility of PUFAs to pro-oxidants; although, in some instances, protein oxidation and lipid oxidation may occur synergistically through radical transfer mechanisms (Liu et al., 2005). Therefore the interaction of whey proteins with PUFAs has vast potential in modulating functional properties such as foaming, gelation, and heat stability in protein-fortified beverages and protein-based foods (Keramat et al., 2023; Peter et al., 2022).

24.2.1.4 Plant proteins–polyunsaturated fatty acid interaction

Plant storage proteins have a lower fatty acid-binding capacity. Additional nonpolar amino acids may be accessible due to heat or high-pressure treatment, which can increase the affinity of lipid binding but also lead to protein aggregation. Protein–PUFA complexes in plant-based foods can influence emulsifying and gelling abilities, as well as lipid oxidation rates. The binding of PUFAs to plant proteins may lessen oxygen diffusion and the production of radicals, even if oxidation products may also form covalent connections with amino acid side chains, decreasing nutritional value. These interactions are essential for the creation of texture and the distribution of lipids in plant-based dairy and meat alternatives (Aruchunan et al., 2025; Hülsebusch et al., 2025; Paramita et al., 2020; Zhu et al., 2018).

24.2.2 Carbohydrate matrices: fiber, starch gels, and hydrogel entrapment

24.2.2.1 Dietary fiber–polyunsaturated fatty acid interactions

Dietary fibers, such as β-glucans, pectin, cellulose, and arabinoxylans, form viscous or gel-like materials that entrap free fatty acids or lipid droplets in a three-dimensional network. Pectin and β-glucans may slow down the diffusion of pro-oxidants and oxygen by increasing viscosity and steric hindrance, which may indirectly improve the oxidative stability of PUFAs. In structured systems, such as bakery or fiber-enriched spreads, the fiber matrices could potentially affect lipid distribution and retention, hence affecting texture, mouthfeel, and lipid release properties (He et al., 2021; Kivelä et al., 2011; Shuaibu et al., 2026).

24.2.2.2 Starch gels–polyunsaturated fatty acid interactions

Amylose–lipid complexes, or V-type complexes, occur when amylose molecules aggregate with unsaturated fatty acids. Amylose–lipid complexes formed during functional food production with amylose encapsulation help in the stabilization of PUFAs by protecting them from oxidation. Amylose or any starch-based encapsulation creates resistance to enzymatic digestion. In this complex, amylose forms a single left-handed helix around the fatty acids in their aliphatic tail, which induces a stable structure (Lee et al., 2024; Lv et al., 2019; Photinam et al., 2024). By trapping fatty acid molecules with van der Waals and hydrophobic forces, the nonpolar core of the single-helix amylose molecules in these inclusion complexes can stabilize the starch matrix. The stability of this complex depends on the degree of unsaturation. Long-chain fatty acids can be incorporated into amylose helices, but their packing efficiency may be hampered by their high disorder compared to saturated lipids (Cavdar Dincturk et al., 2026; Liu et al., 2023).

24.2.2.3 Hydrogel entrapment–polyunsaturated fatty acid interactions

Hydrogels based on polysaccharides, such as alginate, carrageenan, and xanthan, can establish three-dimensional networks with the ability to immobilize lipids via mechanical entrapment. The size of the network pores defines the degree of entrapment and protection of lipids. Because PUFAs are reactive molecules, they could potentially have lower oxidation rates when encapsulated in hydrogels due to reduced oxygen transport and molecular mobility, especially in more dense or ionically cross-linked hydrogels. Additionally, the system may become more stable because of electrostatic interactions between lipid–protein complexes and charged polysaccharides (Lin et al., 2022; Lin et al., 2022; Lupu et al., 2023; 2023; Nair & Sujith, 2026). Bigels (hydrogel-organogel hybrids) enable dual-phase coencapsulation, with hydrogel–organogel ratios tuning phase distribution (Table 24.2). Organogels outperform for pure PUFA oils, whereas hydrogels are more suitable for emulsion-fortified foods, such as frankfurters (Kasparaviciene et al., 2024; Shakeel et al., 2021).

TABLE 24.2 Comparative overview of hydrogels and organogels as advanced food delivery systems: composition, properties, and applications.

Aspect	Hydrogels	Organogels	Comparison to other systems (liposomes, microcapsules, nanoemulsions)	Quantitative metrics (hydrogels)	Quantitative metrics (organogels)
Base Composition	Hydrophilic polymers: alginate (seaweed-derived), chitosan (crustacean shells), gelatin (collagen hydrolysate), pectin (fruit peels), carrageenan, starch, PVA.	Lipophilic structurants in oils: monoglycerides (MAG/DAG), phytosterols/sterols (plant sources), ethylcellulose (cellulose derivative), waxes (rice bran, sunflower), lecithin, sorbitan esters.	Liposomes: phospholipids (soy lecithin); microcapsules: gelatin/alginate shells; nanoemulsions: surfactants (Tween 80) + oils.	Swelling ratio: 10–100x; water content: 90%–99%.	Oil-binding capacity: 95%–99%; gelator concentration: 1%–10% w/w.
Solvent	Water, buffers (pH 4–8), fruit juices; ionic crosslinkers (Ca^{2+}, Fe^{3+}).	Edible oils (sunflower, canola, olive), fats (palm olein, anhydrous milk fat).	Liposomes/nanoemulsions: aqueous continuous phase; microcapsules: solvent evaporation.	Pore size: 1–100 mm.	Fiber diameter: 50 nm–5 mm.
Structure and formation	3D crosslinked hydrophilic network via ionic (alginate-Ca^{2+}), covalent (genipin), or physical (H-bonds) gelation; extrusion/bead methods.	Self-assembled fibrillar/ crystalline network via cooling/ supercooling; high-shear mixing.	Liposomes: hydration/ sonication (vesicles 50–500 nm); microcapsules: coacervation/spray-drying; nanoemulsions: high-pressure homogenization.	Gel strength: 0.1–10 kPa; Mesh size: 5–50 nm.	Gel strength: 5–50 kPa; critical gelling concentration: 2%–5%.
Key properties	High biocompatibility, shear-thinning (viscosity drop >90% under shear), stimuli-responsive (pH 2–7, 37°C–60°C, enzymes); transparent.	Thermoreversible (melt >50°C), spreadable texture ($G' > G''$), oxidation-resistant; opaque/ white.	Nanoemulsions: low viscosity (<10 mPas), transparent; liposomes: fragile (rupture <40°C).	Viscosity: 10^2–10^5 μmPas.	Solid fat content mimics: 20%–80%.
Food applications	Probiotic encapsulation (yogurt, beverages), vitamin C/E delivery, flavor/oil-in-water emulsions, synbiotic gels, texture modifiers (low-fat dairy).	Trans-fat replacers (margarine, shortenings), w-3/b-carotene carriers, chocolate fillings, meat analogs, bakery emulsions.	Microcapsules: powdered flavors/probiotics; nanoemulsions: clear drinks.	Loading capacity: 10%–40% w/w (hydrophilic).	Loading capacity: 90%–98% oil phase (lipophilic).
Release mechanism	Fickian diffusion/swelling (Higuchi model), surface erosion; responsive to gastric pH (2.0), intestinal enzymes (amylase, lipase).	Partition-controlled diffusion, melting-triggered; sustained in the small intestine (bile salts).	Liposomes: pH/fusion burst; nanoemulsions: dilution-induced (creaming).	Release rate: 20%–80% per 24 h (pH-responsive).	Release rate: 10%–50% per 24 h (sustained).
Stability metrics	Thermal: stable 4°C–60°C; GI simulation: 70%–95% retention (pepsin/pancreatin); storage: 4–8 weeks (4°C, syneresis <5%).	Thermal: 20°C–80°C (no melt); GI: 85%–98% (lipase-resistant); storage: 12–24 weeks (25°C, oxidation <10%).	Nanoemulsions: poor long-term (Ostwald ripening); liposomes: low shear stability.	Viability loss: <1 log CFU g^{-1} (28 days).	Bioactive retention: 85%–95% (90 days).

24.3 Digestion and release mechanisms

The digestion, release, and absorption of PUFAs is a multistep process that involves both mechanical and chemical digestion. Mechanical digestion begins with chewing that happens in the mouth, leading to the breakdown of the food matrix into smaller particles, followed by emulsification, chemical digestion by the action of enzymes, micelle formation, followed by intestinal uptake in the later part of the gastrointestinal tract (Fig. 24.1). PUFAs are triacyl glycerol with unsaturated fatty acids and are usually found in esterified form rather than free fatty acids. As with other nutrients and phytochemicals, PUFAs, being part of the food matrix, interact and exert influence on each other, thus modulating PUFAs accessibility for digestion and thereby influencing absorption efficiency, that is, during digestion, PUFA release may be impeded or facilitated by intact plant cell walls, dense protein–lipid assemblies, and emulsified fat globules (Dehelean et al., 2025; Miao et al., 2022; van Eijnatten et al., 2024).

24.3.1 Gastric phase

Mechanical digestion of the food matrix starts in the mouth, that is, mastication with the help of teeth in this case, PUFAs, from either plant (intact cell walls) or animal (muscle) source, which helps in increasing the surface area of the food matrix for enzymatic breakdown. Lingual lipase secreted by lingual serous glands in the oral cavity plays an important role in initiating lipid hydrolysis, which is crucial in early life stages (infancy) and those with compromised pancreatic function. Therefore compromised oral health and not enough mastication can hinder further digestion (Clemente-Suárez et al., 2025; Swackhamer & Hayes, 2026). The gastric phase of digestion involves the enzyme gastric lipase, secreted by

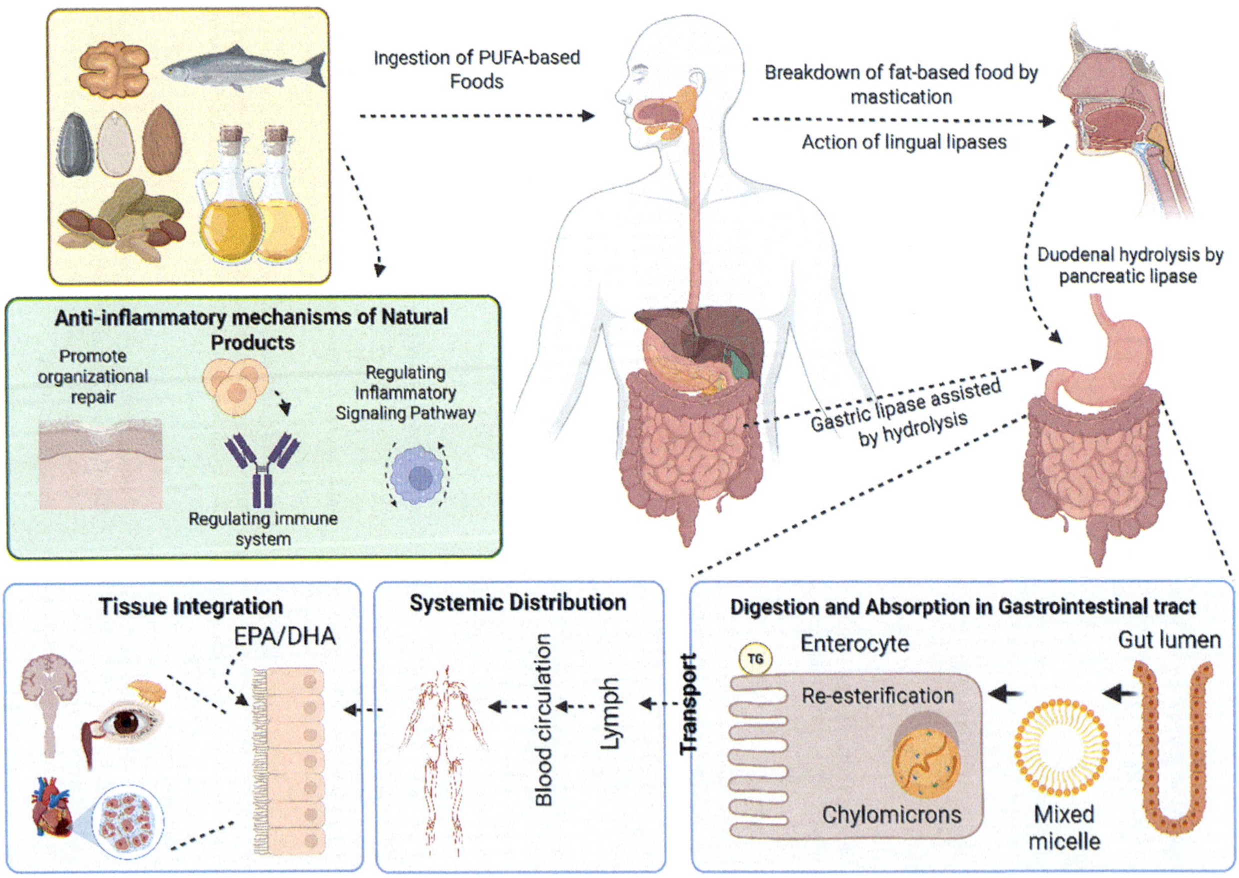

FIGURE 24.1 Schematic of dietary polyunsaturated fatty acids (PUFAs) from ingestion to physiological outcomes. This flowchart illustrates the sequential journey of PUFAs from PUFA-rich foods. Key steps include oral/gastric lipolysis, duodenal hydrolysis by pancreatic lipase into micelles, enterocyte absorption, and chylomicron formation for lymphatic/blood delivery, tissue incorporation into phospholipids or conversion to eicosanoids, and ultimate effects like antiinflammatory signaling and membrane fluidity enhancement; arrows indicate directional flow.

chief cells, that hydrolyzes TAGs, which acts as an important preparatory and regulatory role, It involves cleaving of ester bonds in TAGs, that is, fatty acids from the n-3 position are removed, resulting in only partial hydrolysis resulting in diacyl glycerol, which enters the duodenum for further emulsification (Table 24.3). Food matrices, for example, protein-rich animal sources, such as egg, fish, milk, and milk products, contain lipid present in them that can influence gastric emptying rate and lipid droplet stability, and the degree of protein hydrolysis by pepsin in the stomach influences fat hydrolysis (Dong et al., 2026; Hajfathalian et al., 2025; Pineda-Vadillo et al., 2021).

24.3.2 Intestinal phase

The duodenum, a segment of the small intestine, serves as the primary site for lipid digestion. This process involves the emulsification and subsequent breakdown of lipids by pancreatic lipase, resulting in the formation of free fatty acids, monoacylglycerols, PUFAs, and the breakdown of phospholipid-bound PUFAs by phospholipase, which is particularly significant in the context of marine-derived omega-3 fatty acids (Hussain, 2014; Iqbal & Hussain, 2009). The emulsification of fats by bile salts, which are synthesized by the liver and concentrated, stored, and released from the gallbladder, plays a crucial role in determining the extent of fat digestion. Bile salts facilitate the emulsification of dietary fats and promote the formation of mixed micelles, which comprise cholesterol, free fatty acids, 2-monoacylglycerol, fat-soluble vitamins, bile salts, and other by-products of lipid digestion, including PUFAs (di Gregorio et al., 2021; Monte et al., 2009).

24.3.2.1 Polyphenols and antioxidants

Polyphenolic compounds are said to have both anti and pro-digestive effects on PUFAs. Certain polyphenols impede pancreatic lipase activity and attach to bile acids, reducing the extent of lipid digestion. In turn, their antioxidant properties protect PUFAs from oxidative degradation during digestion, hence retaining their structure and biological activity (Krawczyk et al., 2023; Martinez-Gonzalez et al., 2017).

24.3.2.2 Mineral–lipid interactions

Minerals, such as calcium and magnesium, can combine with free fatty acids, especially with long-chain PUFAs, to form an indigestible phenomenon. This phenomenon is more evident in individuals of those consuming large amounts of calcium supplements or fortified foods, which may influence the availability of PUFAs in some groups (Peñalver et al., 2024; Roth-Walter et al., 2024; Swetha & Mathanghi, 2024).

24.4 Emerging applications and functionality

At present, the usage and applications of beneficial PUFAs, in various sectors in different forms and sources have gained major importance. Due to their multifunctional physiological role and therapeutic importance, the market value has increased for PUFA-based products. PUFAs, specifically omega-3 fatty acids such as ALA, EPA, DHA, and a lower ratio of omega-6 to omega-3 appear to play a major role in various physiological functions. Most of the studies understood that

TABLE 24.3 Gastrointestinal processing of dietary polyunsaturated fatty acids (PUFAs).

Digestive stage	Mechanism	Key factors influencing PUFA release
Oral phase (mouth)	Food is mechanically broken down through chewing, and initial lipid digestion begins.	Lingual lipase activity and the structural integrity of the food matrix determine early PUFA release.
Gastric phase (stomach)	Partial breakdown of triglycerides occurs, mainly at the sn-3 position.	Gastric lipase efficiency and protein–lipid interactions influence the extent of hydrolysis.
Intestinal phase (duodenum)	Lipids are emulsified, micelles are formed, and complete digestion of triglycerides takes place.	Bile salts, pancreatic lipase, and phospholipases play critical roles in facilitating PUFA bioaccessibility.
Absorption (enterocytes)	Fatty acids are re-esterified and incorporated into chylomicrons for systemic transport.	Fatty acid transport proteins, CD36 receptors, and the molecular structure of PUFAs affect absorption efficiency.

supplementation with omega-3 fatty acids with a lower ratio of omega-6 to omega-3 fatty acids aids in inflammation reduction, where low-grade inflammation is known to be related to the risk of cardiovascular diseases, cancer, diabetes mellitus, and most autoimmune disorders. Omega-3 fatty acids such as ALA, EPA, and DHA are essential fatty acids with enormous health benefits. It is well established that omega-3 fatty acids supplementation is directly associated with cognitive function enhancement and immune-related functionality improvement (Das et al., 2024; Zivkovic et al., 2011). Emerging applications are majorly focused on areas of precision nutrition, neuroprotection, cardiometabolic health management, nutrition in oncology, and the area of adjunct therapies emerged with a specific target, along with nanomedicine-based drug delivery systems (Table 24.4). Beyond the traditional cardiovascular, PUFAs are also being explored around innovative delivery systems, such as nanoemulsions and functional biological aids to enhance bioavailability to gain therapeutic benefits in a precise way. However, major applications are integrated in pharmaceuticals and functional foods development, including dietary supplements.

24.4.1 Functional foods: enrichment and fortification

PUFAs are obtained from different food sources of animal and plant origin. Most foods are sourced with omega-3 fatty acids, which are entailed with ALA mainly found in vegetable oils such as soybean oil, nut sources such as walnut, butternut, and other plant sources like flaxseed, canola oil, etc., additional key types of omega-3 fatty acids *viz*., DHA and EPA are primarily obtained from fatty fish and other seafoods (Table 24.5). Studies have also shown that certain microorganisms, such as microalgae, also contain high levels of DHA, as well as EPA. However, it is a crucial task to utilize these sources in functional food formulations in an acceptable way. Increasing awareness about the importance of omega-3 fatty acids in cognitive function, immune-related functionality, and inflammation and inflammation-associated health problems has driven demand for functional foods formulation by enrichment or fortification (Oliver et al., 2020).

Specifically, fortification and enrichment of foods with n-3s with selective inclusion of omega-3-rich source foods are rising. This is specifically aimed at improving the nutritional quality to gain the health benefits. Awareness and utilization of omega-3 fatty acids are increasingly recognized due to their essential role in various physiological processes. Consequently, ensuring sufficient intake of omega-3 fatty acids, whether through dietary sources, fortification, or enrichment, is of utmost importance. Common emerging applications in the food industry include the fortification of dairy products such as yoghurt, ghee, spreads, and dairy-based beverages with omega-3 sources. Microalgae are being incorporated into pasta, bakery products, condiments, and commonly consumed beverages. Cumulative consideration is being given to the development of widely commercialized food products, like pasta, sauces, and noodles, bakery products like biscuits, bread, and soft drinks, as well as soups. Microalgae-based powders and frozen pastes are increasingly being incorporated into soups, juices, various smoothies, cookies, crackers, and are also utilized in ice creams and nutritional supplements. The Food and Drug Administration has approved microalgae as generally recognized as safe for consumption. Specifically, *Euglena gracilis* is employed in conventional food products such as baked goods, milk and

TABLE 24.4 Delivery strategies to enhance polyunsaturated fatty acids (PUFA) bioavailability.

Delivery strategy	Mechanism of action	Key advantages
Natural food matrices (e.g., fish, dairy)	Promote natural digestion and emulsification during digestion	Improve micelle formation, lipid absorption, and protect PUFA from oxidation
Nanoemulsions	Increase surface area available for enzymatic action	Accelerate soluble digestion and enhance absorption kinetics through smaller droplets
Solid lipid nanoparticles	Provide controlled and sustained lipid release	Improve PUFA stability and bioavailability
Polymeric nanocarriers	Enhance mucoadhesion within the intestine; encapsulate PUFAs for protection against degradation	Increase intestinal retention and uptake; augment overall oral bioavailability compared to conventional forms such as free oils or emulsions
Coingestion with probiotics	Modulates gut microbiota composition	Supports improved lipid metabolism, absorption, and short-chain fatty acid production, aiding PUFA uptake

TABLE 24.5 Commercially available omega-3 food sources and possible applications.

Food sources	Possible applications
Flaxseed and oil	Bakery products, fruits and vegetable juices, dairy product formulation, medicines, dietary supplements, 3D-printed products, emulsifiers and stabilisers
Fish (e.g., salmon, tuna, herring, and mackerel) and fish oil	Bakery products, such as oils and medicines, dietary supplements, 3D-printed products
Chia seed and oil	Bakery products, fruits and vegetable juices, dairy product formulation, medicines
Canola oil	As oil, 3D printed products
Seaweed/microalgae (e.g.,*Euglena gracilis)*	Baked products, juices, dairy products, medicines, supplements, 3D-printed products
Garden cress seed and oil	Salad dressing, 3D-printed products
Soybean oil	As oil, 3D-printed products
Nut sources, *viz.*, walnut, almond, hazelnut	Baked products, fruit juices, dairy products, supplements, 3D printed products
Camelina seed oil	As oil, capsules, supplements, 3D-printed products

dairy products, beverages like fruit juices, as well as in soft candies and soups. PUFA-fortified functional foods are anticipated to remain a significant sector within the global food industry. The formulation of products based on PUFAs significantly benefits from the application of emulsion and nano-emulsion technologies, as well as microencapsulation and other techniques, to maintain product stability. For the encapsulation of essential PUFA sources, whey protein isolates, modified starch, and gum acacia play a beneficial role. Sustained innovation, regulatory compliance, and improved stability of functional foods will drive future advancements in this field. The formulation of functional foods enriched with omega-3 sources, with particular attention to the desirable omega-3 to omega-6 ratio, represents a promising avenue in the food industry to address various health issues. PUFA-enriched functional foods aim to deliver health-promoting fats and fat sources to target cardiovascular health risks, modulate inflammation, support cognitive function, and improve various metabolic diseases associated with inflammation (Ganesan et al., 2014; Pandey et al., 2025).

24.4.2 3D-printed matrices utilization in polyunsaturated fatty acids-based functional foods

Three-dimensional printing is an emerging technology that enables to formulate tailor-made PUFA-rich functional foods. 3D food printing provides a novel manufacturing method that helps in the physical realization of any food formulation with tailored textures, nutritional and phytochemical profiles, and required esthetics. The major methods being used in 3D printing include extrusion-printing, inkjet, binder jet, and selective laser sintering. Extrusion-based printing can be applied for developing the PUFA-based formulations in extruded form. Inkjet printing technique is typically used to improve the flavor or omega-3 PUFA bioactive deposition onto the surface of food. Binder jetting approach can be applied to bind PUFA-sourced oil emulsions with powdered food constituents. Selective laser sintering can be applied to fuse the powdered omega-3-sourced ingredients in a tailored texture. Most printing methods basically rely on edible inks and other materials of plant-based purees, formulations enriched with proteins, hydrocolloid matrices, and even cultured meats (Hodhodi et al., 2025; Zhu et al., 2023). As alternate source of these, any raw material can be replaced with an omega-3 source, if there is a possibility of replacement. Extrusion-based method is widely applied with successful results in a broad range of food matrices with or without thermal energy due to its versatility and feasibility. While integrating the omega-3 fatty acids (EPA and DHA) rich food matrices for 3D food print formulation, oxidative instability needs to be considered. Oxidative stability of PUFA poses a major challenge in sensory acceptance and rancidity in food formulations or supplements. Microencapsulation through spray drying or coacervation of n-3s and incorporation of these in 3D food formulation effectively improves the oxidative stability. For example, n-3s molecules can be encapsulated with cocoa powder matrices that can be incorporated in 3D-printed chocolate (Ehsan et al., 2025; Li, Koirala, et al., 2025; Yi-Wu et al., 2022). The research studies have been done on the development of a 3D printed fish analog. In 3D-printed products, PUFA source can be encapsulated with pea protein and other resistant food sources. Cookies were prepared using 3D-printing technology with the inclusion of omega-3 sourced microalgae such as *A. platensis, C. vulgaris,* and *H. pluvial.* Omega-3 fatty acid inclusion in 3D-printed chocolate is one of the promising products to deliver these bioactives in an efficient way. The development of 3D-printed foods with the inclusion of essential oils with omega-3 sources or extracted omega-3 sources in the formulation helps to meet the requirement. Microencapsulated n-3s extracted from fish oil, flaxseed, or any other sources incorporated into protein or starch-based gels can serve as a sustainable approach. PUFAs or any other bioactives highly susceptible to oxidation need to be formulated with utmost care to enhance oxidative stability. However, ethical and regulatory challenges associated with the lack of standardized safety procedures in 3D-printed foods pose prominent barriers in the clinical field (Lim et al., 2024; Wang et al., 2025).

24.4.3 Gut-microbiome modulation: polyunsaturated fatty acids matrix effects on microbiota

Human gut microbiome is diversified with trillions of microorganisms, which play a vital physiological role in metabolic processes and immunological functions. Gut microbiome is commonly considered the largest immune system of the human body. Alteration in the gut microbiome organization, including its abundance and diversity, exerts a multifaceted effect on the overall immune mechanism. Significant studies have revealed that flaws in gut microbiota are associated with most health issues, such as inflammatory bowel diseases, cardiovascular-related diseases, diabetes mellitus, obesity, and many other health problems. Rejuvenation of the gut microbiome with beneficial microorganisms has been used as a primitive factor in treatment. However, most studies revealed that omega-3 fatty acids supplementation has been shown to improve the gut microbiome with beneficial effects. The beneficial effect of omega-3 fatty acids in behavioral problems is presumed to be associated with the regulation of intestinal microbial composition; however, still more research needs to be done for strong authentication. Healthy individuals' gut microbiota is predominantly abundant with Firmicutes and Bacteroidetes. However, Proteobacteria and Actinobacteria species abundance is also evident. The gut microbiome is generally influenced by various factors, such as lifestyle factors, including dietary pattern, sleeping pattern, stress factors, and exposure to antibiotics and other environmental factors (Afzaal et al., 2022; Sun et al., 2025; Zhang et al., 2024).

Despite the extensive research on the effects of prebiotic sources on the gut microbiome, there remains a notable gap in studies focusing on the role of dietary fats, particularly omega-3 polyunsaturated fatty acids (PUFAs), and the critical balance between omega-3 and omega-6 fatty acids in enhancing gut microbiome diversity. Emerging evidence envisages that omega-3 fatty acids serves as an important source of structural and functional biomolecules that serve a significant role in modulating the composition and function of the gut microbiome and are considered as one of the vital key mediators of host health. Research evidence from human trial suggested that omega-3 PUFA supplementation consistently alters the composition of the gut microbiota. Particularly, this results in faecalis bacterium reduction and an improvement in Bacteroidetes and butyrate-producing bacteria of the *Lachnospiraceae* family (Kumar et al., 2022; Sundaram et al., 2022). Research evidence revealed that omega-3 fatty acids, such as ALA, EPA, and DHA, plays significant role in gut microbiome modulation and are key mediator in the upregulation of host health. Although most of the evidence highlighted the positive impact of omega-3 sourced dietary intervention and supplementation on gut microbiota and its relationship with host interaction through modulation of gut microbiome. This, in turn, helps in metabolite production, and the intestinal mucus barrier protection and immune protection. However, a low ratio of omega-6/omega-3 appears to attain the enormous beneficial effects through beneficial microbial diversity amplification, while a balanced proportion fosters a health-favorable microbiome production (Bodur et al., 2025; Zinkow et al., 2025). It is evidence that omega-3 fatty acids, specifically EPA and DHA, are known to increase the *Bifidobacterium* and *Lactobacillus* spp., and this in turn is involved in the reduction of pro-inflammatory bacteria such as *Deferribacteraceae*, as revealed through in vivo studies on human as well as animal models. In addition, omega-3 fatty acids take part in immune modulation mediated through the microbiome by enhancing the short-chain fatty acids (SCFA), making bacterial strains, which further enhance the SCFA production. These SCFAs play an important role in immune modulation and oxidative stress reduction, in turn reducing the inflammatory environment of the intestine. SCFA-producing bacteria such as *Blautia*, *Bacteroides, Roseburia*, and *Coprococcus* have been reported to increase after the supplementation with omega-3 fatty acids. Some studies also highlighted that treatment with omega-3 fatty acids reduced the pathogenic bacteria species, such as *Ruminococcus, Dorea longicatena, Oscillibacter*, and *Eubacterium hallii* (Costantini et al., 2017; Hutchinson et al., 2020; Watson et al., 2018).

24.4.4 Health endpoints: targeted delivery as antiinflammatory, neuroprotection

PUFAs, specifically n-3s such as EPA and DHA known to possess antiinflammatory potential. Omega-3 bioactive involved in the modulation of inflammatory pathways by altering the microstructure of the cell membrane, which in turn influences the transcriptional regulation of cells, and promotes the antiinflammatory mediator production. Research evidence suggests that PUFAs, particularly omega-3, function as antiinflammatory biomolecules, whereas omega-6

PUFAs, such as arachidonic acid and LA, are regarded as pro-inflammatory. Targeted delivery techniques through advanced carriers such as nano-emulsion and liposomes promise the effective utilization of PUFA in the therapeutic or health promotion field. Advanced encapsulation technologies, such as nanoencapsulation and microencapsulation, nanoemulsions, and liposomes, help to protect and enhance stability while overcoming bioavailability limitations, which enables the optimized therapeutic target. These can be applied in functional food formulations or to develop pharmaceutical products and/or any health supplements (Calder, 2013; De Cillis et al., 2025; Djuricic & Calder, 2021). Cyclo-dextrin, oligosaccharide-based nanosponges have emerged as advanced delivery systems to overcome the solubility and stability of PUFA, while these also enable the targeted and sustained release of these bioactive therapeutic agents. Cyclodextrins, being hydrophilic outside and hydrophobic in the interior cavity, can form inclusion complexes with hydrophobic molecules of omega-3 bioactive compounds. When crosslinked with pyromellitic dianhydride or diphenyl carbonate, they generate three-dimensional porous nanostructures known as nanosponges, which further impart controlled release of biomolecules. Magneto liposomes hybrid nanocarriers offer a promising, specialized delivery system for PUFA. Application of this in supplements and other therapeutic formulations serves as carriers to enhance the stability, bioavailability, and targeted delivery of PUFAs, specifically for treating inflammatory diseases (Bahavarnia et al., 2024; Musuc, 2024; Wehl et al., 2025).

PUFAs are the essential components of neuronal and glial cell membranes. It is observed that PUFA intake from dietary sources helps to regulate both prostaglandin and pro-inflammatory cytokine production. Adequate ratio of dietary n-6 and n-3 fatty acids needs to be emphasized to prevent neuroinflammation. This could provide the authentication of the protective role of omega-3 fatty acids in neurodegenerative diseases, which are linked to aging. PUFAs and their metabolites are known to regulate microglia phenotype and function to exert their anti-inflammatory and resolving activities in the brain (Joffre et al., 2019; Martinat et al., 2021). Human tracer studies using stable isotopes, such as ^{13}C-labeled EPA and DHA, investigate omega-3 fatty acid metabolism, absorption, beta-oxidation, and conversion pathways in vivo. These nonradioactive tracers enable safe tracking in plasma, breath, and tissues over days to weeks (Koletzko et al., 1998). Participants typically receive a single oral dose of uniformly ^{13}C-labeled EPA or DHA, with plasma and breath CO_2 monitored via mass spectrometry for up to 28 days. Apparent retro-conversion of ^{13}D-DHA to ^{13}C-EPA in humans is low, indicating minimal direct reversal but possible slowed EPA metabolism during supplementation. These studies clarify age-related omega-3 handling, informing supplementation for cardiovascular or cognitive function, and extend to retro-conversion debates in n-3 PUFA pathways. Uniform labeling ensures precise tracking without natural isotope overlap issues (Loukil et al., 2025; Plourde et al., 2011).

24.5 Challenges and future directions

PUFAs are acknowledged for their substantial health benefits, which contribute to their industrial demand. Formulation of PUFA-enriched or fortified functional foods with a beneficial fatty acid ratio is one of the promising avenues in the food industry. Despite the challenges such as insignificant availability of the required fatty acid ratio, regulatory concern, sensory acceptance, food matrix interactions with bioavailability, low stability and solubility, skill oriented technological advancements in the agriculture field and processing sector have given the array of hope to meet the requirement. Emerging applications are widely intended towards functional food development with omega-3 fatty acid incorporation. Fortification and enrichment of foods with essential fatty acids are getting popularized in the food production sector. Technologically advanced routes, such as nano-emulsion, microencapsulation, fortification, enrichment, and even biofortification, have enabled the successful commercialization of omega-3 sourced functional foods in the market (Chadare et al., 2019; Kumar et al., 2024; Zazula et al., 2025).

24.5.1 Availability of polyunsaturated fatty acid source for product formulations

Severe supply deficits have induced less affordability due to high cost. Most consumed vegetable oils are rich in omega-6 PUFAs, not in omega-3 sources. However, flaxseed and chia seed oils and walnuts have a considerable amount of omega-3 ALA. Along with these marine sources of fish, terrestrial plant sources are being utilized as the major PUFA source for commercialization. While terrestrial plant-derived PUFAs are limited by poor yields and high land needs, overfishing and conflicting demands for other advantages, such as protein sources, threaten the sustainability of the PUFA supply from marine fish. Due to their enormous accumulation capacity, ease of cultivation, and independence from freshwater or arable land, microalgae have thus become a prospective alternative source of PUFAs. Photosynthetic microalgae, such as *Phaeodactylum tricornutum* and *Nannochloropsis oceanica*, are being utilized for commercial purposes. However, these microalgae screening will be tedious and time-consuming (Khozin-Goldberg et al., 2011; Mariamenatu et al., 2021).

24.5.2 Oxidation stability of polyunsaturated fatty acids in complex matrices

Lipid components are highly susceptible to oxidation, especially the oxidation of PUFA lead to the formation of unsaturated carbonyl, harmful compounds which induce the undesirable flavor and rancidity during the extraction process, storage, as well as in food formulations. It is reported that PUFAs are more vulnerable to chemical changes, such as metal-catalyzed autoxidation and hydrogenation, due to the multiple C=C bonds known to be susceptible to electrophilic attack. Increased consumer preference for natural preservatives, validation studies on natural sources like polyphenol-rich rosemary extracts, efficiency in stabilization of the n-3 PUFA in flaxseed oil have been reported. Similarly, catechin from green tea extracts has also shown DHA-rich oil stabilization. The phytochemicals, such as carotenoid, tocopherol, and polyphenol extracts from edible flower sources, have also been shown to impart oxidative protection of cold-pressed linseed and chia seed oils (Briceño et al., 2025; Li, Tang, et al., 2025; Rahim et al., 2024). The oxidation stability of PUFAs in complex matrices (e.g., emulsions, dairy, meats, microcapsules) is primarily hindered by their high degree of unsaturation, making them sensitive to oxygen, light, heat, and pro-oxidants. Due to their multiple double bonds, PUFAs are also highly prone to oxidation, which poses formulation challenges in food matrices. In complex food systems, oxidation typically starts at the interface between oil and water, and the stability of PUFAs is heavily influenced by the interfacial structure, pH, ionic strength, and the presence of natural antioxidants (Singh et al., 2018; Wu et al., 2022). Microencapsulation and nanoencapsulation techniques are known to protect PUFA-based food sources or any formulations from environmental factors like oxygen, light, and transition metals. This, in turn, is known to play a role in preserving oxidative stability and bioactivity. To improve the shelf life of omega-3-rich foods, spray and freeze-drying encapsulation are commonly applied in the food industry. Liposomal encapsulation and coacervation techniques are also used to develop and to improve the stability of PUFA-based functional foods. For the encapsulation of essential PUFA sources, whey protein isolates, modified starch, and gum acacia can serve a beneficial role (Homroy et al., 2024; Xu et al., 2024).

24.5.3 Regulatory and sensory hurdles in product design

Regulatory compliance hurdles associated with the product design of PUFAs, particularly long-chain omega-3s (EPA/DHA), include their susceptibility to oxidation. However, strict nutritional labeling requirements and the need to prove safety for health claims are additional critical tasks. Regulatory standards divergence in different regions poses another hurdle. In any functional food formulations or any product preparation, compliance with regulatory standards related to purity and food source is a major concern. For example, fish oil is a source of omega-3 fatty acids; the purity and safety compliance of the fish source is a critical task. Labeling this source and marketing with reliable standards is also considered as a critical aspect. Extending the shelf life of fish oil or any other sources and its fortification in foods also pose a challenge. Although all challenges may not be solved regarding optimal formulations of such products, studies such as this are needed to help succeed in implementing such new food concepts (Fuentes et al., 2025; Gutierres et al., 2025; Hajfathalian et al., 2025).

24.5.4 Precision nutrition: tailored matrices and artificial intelligence modeling

Precision nutrition focuses on the individual's genetic, metabolic, and microbiome characteristics to develop personalized dietary strategies. Tailor-made food matrices targeting inflammation in specific conditions, along with artificial intelligence (AI) applications, represent a sustainable approach. Custom functional formulations incorporating beneficial PUFAs, especially omega-3 fatty acids, can be employed to target inflammation in any disease condition or to promote well-being. AI can be utilized as a transformative technology, serving as an effective tool in integrating the food system with nutrition to achieve scalable, sustainable health solutions through precision nutrition targeting specific conditions (Nourazarain & Vaziri, 2025; Singar et al., 2024). AI techniques, such as machine learning and deep learning applications, facilitate the interpretation of data related to biological parameters and their association with health-delivering components, as well as specific health outcomes. The application of omega-3 fatty acid-based food matrices in inflammatory pathway interpretation through AI modeling signifies a paradigm shift in AI-based dietary science. By integrating genomics, metabolomics, microbiomics, and individualized nutritional matrices, targeted dynamic strategies for modulating inflammation are offered. Rather than following a general diet, the future lies in data-driven, personalized nutrition, harmonizing biology to enhance technology and clinical practice (Al Shareef et al., 2025; Alkalbani et al., 2026; Guo et al., 2025).

24.6 Conclusion

PUFAs are vital nutrients with profound effects on human health, such as reducing inflammation, lowering cardiovascular risk, modulating gut microbiota, and supporting cancer prevention strategies. However, their therapeutic potential is often hindered by susceptibility to oxidation, poor aqueous solubility, and inconsistent gastrointestinal absorption. To address these challenges, strategies have been developed to stabilize PUFAs against degradation, optimize their release profiles, and enhance bioefficacy through matrix-mediated protection and targeted delivery, effectively bridging the gap between dietary intake and physiological impact. Emerging evidence underscores the translational potential of these approaches. For instance, fortified emulsions in functional foods have shown a threefold increase in postprandial EPA/DHA absorption in clinical trials, while nanoencapsulated PUFAs exhibit superior retention in the gut–liver axis, potentially working synergistically with probiotics to combat chemoresistance in oncology. PUFA-enriched matrices are also being investigated in the context of metabolic disorders, neurodegeneration, and microbiota dysbiosis. Ultimately, mastering food matrix interactions not only enhances PUFA utility but also redefines functional foods as proactive allies in preventive medicine and personalized health.

References

Abeyrathne, E. D. N. S., Nam, K., & Ahn, D. U. (2021). Analytical methods for lipid oxidation and antioxidant capacity in food systems. *Antioxidants, 10*(10). https://doi.org/10.3390/antiox10101587, https://www.mdpi.com/2076-3921/10/10/1587/pdf.

Acevedo-Fani, A., Dave, A., & Singh, H. (2020). Nature-Assembled structures for delivery of bioactive compounds and their potential in functional foods. *Frontiers in Chemistry, 8*. https://doi.org/10.3389/fchem.2020.564021.

Afzaal, M., Saeed, F., Shah, Y. A., Hussain, M., Rabail, R., Socol, C. T., Hassoun, A., Pateiro, M., Lorenzo, J. M., Rusu, A. V., & Aadil, R. M. (2022). Human gut microbiota in health and disease: Unveiling the relationship. *Frontiers in Microbiology, 13*. https://doi.org/10.3389/fmicb.2022.999001, https://www.frontiersin.org/journals/microbiology#.

Al Shareef, R., Fathelrahman, E., Osman, R., Gebiso, T., & Platat, C. (2025). Can artificial intelligence uncover the bioactive peptides' benefits for human health and knowledge? A narrative review. *Frontiers in Nutrition, 12*. https://doi.org/10.3389/fnut.2025.1698147.

Alijani, S., Hahn, A., Harris, W. S., & Schuchardt, J. P. (2025). Bioavailability of EPA and DHA in humans – A comprehensive review. *Progress in Lipid Research, 97*. https://doi.org/10.1016/j.plipres.2024.101318, https://www.sciencedirect.com/science/journal/01637827.

Alkalbani, N., Shahin, L., Benzeghiba, H., Obaid, R. S., Osaili, T. M., Cheik Ismail, L., Al qasssimi, G., Rauf, M., Abdulrahim, K., Almashgouni, A., Ashuweihi, F., & AL-Fuqaha, D. (2026). Artificial intelligence in functional food innovation: Bioactive enhancement and formulation optimization: A quasi-systematic review. *Food Chemistry: X, 34*. https://doi.org/10.1016/j.fochx.2026.103628, https://www.sciencedirect.com/science/journal/25901575.

Aruchunan, U., Henry, C. J., & Sim, S. Y. J. (2025). Role of protein-lipid interactions for food and food-based applications. *Food Hydrocolloids, 160*. https://doi.org/10.1016/j.foodhyd.2024.110715, https://www.sciencedirect.com/science/journal/0268005X.

Asif, Z., Prestidge, C. A., & Joyce, P. (2026). Exploring the impact of lipid structure and composition on the digestion of next-generation meat and dairy analogues. *Foods, 15*(4). https://doi.org/10.3390/foods15040772, www.mdpi.com/journal/foods.

Bahavarnia, F., Hasanzadeh, M., Bahavarnia, P., & Shadjou, N. (2024). Advancements in application of chitosan and cyclodextrins in biomedicine and pharmaceutics: Recent progress and future trends. *RSC Advances, 14*(19), 13384–13412. https://doi.org/10.1039/d4ra01370k.

Bao, Y., & Pignitter, M. (2023). Mechanisms of lipid oxidation in water-in-oil emulsions and oxidomics-guided discovery of targeted protective approaches. *Comprehensive Reviews in Food Science and Food Safety, 22*(4), 2678–2705. https://doi.org/10.1111/1541-4337.13158.

Bodur, M., Yilmaz, B., Ağagündüz, D., & Ozogul, Y. (2025). Immunomodulatory effects of omega-3 fatty acids: Mechanistic insights and health implications. *Molecular Nutrition & Food Research, 69*(10). https://doi.org/10.1002/mnfr.202400752.

Briceño, J., Vásquez, C., Guayta, J., Ramírez, C., Altuna, J., & Silva, M. (2025). Study of the oxidative stability of chia oil (*Salvia hispanica* L.) at various concentrations of alpha tocopherol. *Processes, 13*(12), 3887. https://doi.org/10.3390/pr13123887.

Calder, P. C. (2013). Omega-3 polyunsaturated fatty acids and inflammatory processes: Nutrition or pharmacology? *British Journal of Clinical Pharmacology, 75*(3), 645–662. https://doi.org/10.1111/j.1365-2125.2012.04374.x.

Cavdar Dincturk, H., Akkuzu, N., Günal-Köroğlu, D., Can Karaca, A., & Capanoglu, E. (2026). Molecular insights into bioactive interactions within protein- and polysaccharide-based colloids: Implications for stability, functionality, and bioavailability. *Foods, 15*(1), 112. https://doi.org/10.3390/foods15010112.

Cengiz, A., Kahyaoglu, T., Schröen, K., & Berton-Carabin, C. (2019). Oxidative stability of emulsions fortified with iron: The role of liposomal phospholipids. *Journal of the Science of Food and Agriculture, 99*(6), 2957–2965. https://doi.org/10.1002/jsfa.9509.

Cengiz, A., Schroën, K., & Berton-Carabin, C. (2021). Towards oxidatively stable emulsions containing iron-loaded liposomes: The key role of phospholipid-to-iron ratio. *Foods, 10*(6), 1293. https://doi.org/10.3390/foods10061293.

Chadare, F. J., Idohou, R., Nago, E., Affonfere, M., Agossadou, J., Fassinou, T. K., Kénou, C., Honfo, S., Azokpota, P., Linnemann, A. R., & Hounhouigan, D. J. (2019). Conventional and food-to-food fortification: An appraisal of past practices and lessons learned. *Food Science and Nutrition, 7*(9), 2781–2795. https://doi.org/10.1002/fsn3.1133, onlinelibrary.wiley.com/journal/10.1002/%28ISSN%292048-7177.

Cholewski, M., Tomczykowa, M., & Tomczyk, M. (2018). A comprehensive review of chemistry, sources and bioavailability of omega-3 fatty acids. *Nutrients, 10*(11), 1662. https://doi.org/10.3390/nu10111662.

De Cillis, F., Begni, V., Genini, P., Leo, D., Riva, M. A., & Cattaneo, A. (2025). Restoring balance: The role of omega-3 polyunsaturated fatty acids on the gut–brain axis and other interconnected biological pathways to improve depression. *Nutrients, 17*(21). https://doi.org/10.3390/nu17213426, http://www.mdpi.com/journal/nutrients/.

Clemente-Suárez, V. J., Redondo-Flórez, L., Beltrán-Velasco, A. I., Yáñez-Sepúlveda, R., Rubio-Zarapuz, A., Martín-Rodríguez, A., Navarro-Jimenez, E., & Tornero-Aguilera, J. F. (2025). Human digestive physiology and evolutionary diet: A metabolomic perspective on carnivorous and scavenger adaptations. *Metabolites, 15*(7). https://doi.org/10.3390/metabo15070453, http://www.mdpi.com/journal/metabolites.

Corfield, R., Lalou, G., Di Lella, S., Martínez, K. D., Schebor, C., Allievi, M. C., & Pérez, O. E. (2023). Experimental and modeling approaches applied to the whey proteins and vitamin B9 complexes study. *Food Hydrocolloids, 142*. https://doi.org/10.1016/j.foodhyd.2023.108834, https://www.journals.elsevier.com/food-hydrocolloids.

Costantini, L., Molinari, R., Farinon, B., & Merendino, N. (2017). Impact of omega-3 fatty acids on the gut microbiota. *International Journal of Molecular Sciences, 18*(12), 2645. https://doi.org/10.3390/ijms18122645.

Das, P., Dutta, A., Panchali, T., Khatun, A., Kar, R., Das, T. K., Phoujdar, M., Chakrabarti, S., Ghosh, K., & Pradhan, S. (2024). Advances in therapeutic applications of fish oil: A review. *Measurement: Food, 13*, 100142. https://doi.org/10.1016/j.meafoo.2024.100142.

Dehelean, C. A., Boru, C., Macaşoi, I. G., Dumitrel, Ş. I., Trandafirescu, C., & Ersilia, A. (2025). Obtaining and characterization of nutraceuticals based on linoleic acid derivatives obtained by green synthesis and their valorization in the food industry. *Nutrients, 17*(15). https://doi.org/10.3390/nu17152416, http://www.mdpi.com/journal/nutrients/.

Djuricic, I., & Calder, P. C. (2021). Beneficial outcomes of omega-6 and omega-3 polyunsaturated fatty acids on human health: An update for 2021. *Nutrients, 13*(7), 2421. https://doi.org/10.3390/nu13072421.

Dong, X., Wang, Y., Chen, X. D., & Selomulya, C. (2026). Designing protein gels for nutrient delivery: From formulation to digestion. *Comprehensive Reviews in Food Science and Food Safety, 25*(2). https://doi.org/10.1111/1541-4337.70424, http://onlinelibrary.wiley.com/journal/10.1111/(ISSN)1541-4337.

Dyall, S. C., Balas, L., Bazan, N. G., Brenna, J. T., Chiang, N., da Costa Souza, F., Dalli, J., Durand, T., Galano, J. M., Lein, P. J., Serhan, C. N., & Taha, A. Y. (2022). Polyunsaturated fatty acids and fatty acid-derived lipid mediators: Recent advances in the understanding of their biosynthesis, structures, and functions. *Progress in Lipid Research, 86*. https://doi.org/10.1016/j.plipres.2022.101165, www.elsevier.com/locate/plipres.

Ehsan, M., Shankar, A., Chohan, J. S., Rasheed, B., Imran, A., Usman, I., Rasheed, M., Saeed, F., Afzaal, M., Islam, F., & Ndagire, C. T. (2025). Three-dimensional (3D) food printing applications, techniques, and consumer acceptance. *eFood, 6*(6). https://doi.org/10.1002/efd2.70106, onlinelibrary.wiley.com/journal/26663066.

van Eijnatten, E. J. M., Roelofs, J. J. M., Camps, G., Huppertz, T., Lambers, T. T., & Smeets, P. A. M. (2024). Gastric coagulation and postprandial amino acid absorption of milk is affected by mineral composition: A randomized crossover trial. *Food and Function, 15*(6), 3098–3107. https://doi.org/10.1039/d3fo04063a, http://pubs.rsc.org/en/journals/journal/fo.

Fuentes, J. B., Beara, I., & Torović, L. (2025). Regulatory compliance of health claims on omega-3 fatty acid food supplements. *Foods, 14*(1), 67. https://doi.org/10.3390/foods14010067.

Ganesan, B., Brothersen, C., & McMahon, D. J. (2014). Fortification of foods with omega-3 polyunsaturated fatty acids. *Critical Reviews in Food Science and Nutrition, 54*(1), 98–114. https://doi.org/10.1080/10408398.2011.578221.

Geng, L., Liu, K., & Zhang, H. (2023). Lipid oxidation in foods and its implications on proteins. *Frontiers in Nutrition, 10*. https://doi.org/10.3389/fnut.2023.1192199.

di Gregorio, M. C., Cautela, J., & Galantini, L. (2021). Physiology and physical chemistry of bile acids. *International Journal of Molecular Sciences, 22*(4), 1780. https://doi.org/10.3390/ijms22041780.

Guo, B., Lu, X., Jiang, X., Shen, X. L., Wei, Z., & Zhang, Y. (2025). Artificial intelligence in advancing algal bioactive ingredients: Production, characterization, and application. *Foods, 14*(10). https://doi.org/10.3390/foods14101783, www.mdpi.com/journal/foods.

Gutierres, D., Pacheco, R., & Reis, C. P. (2025). The role of omega-3 and omega-6 polyunsaturated fatty acid supplementation in human health. *Foods, 14*(19). https://doi.org/10.3390/foods14193299, www.mdpi.com/journal/foods.

Hajfathalian, M., Ghelichi, S., & Jacobsen, C. (2025). Anti-obesity peptides from food: Production, evaluation, sources, and commercialization. *Comprehensive Reviews in Food Science and Food Safety, 24*(2). https://doi.org/10.1111/1541-4337.70158.

Harwood, J. L. (2023). Polyunsaturated fatty acids: Conversion to lipid mediators, roles in inflammatory diseases and dietary sources. *International Journal of Molecular Sciences, 24*(10). https://doi.org/10.3390/ijms24108838, http://www.mdpi.com/journal/ijms.

Hennebelle, M., Villeneuve, P., Durand, E., Lecomte, J., van Duynhoven, J., Meynier, A., Yesiltas, B., Jacobsen, C., & Berton-Carabin, C. (2024). Lipid oxidation in emulsions: New insights from the past two decades. *Progress in Lipid Research, 94*, 101275. https://doi.org/10.1016/j.plipres.2024.101275.

He, H. J., Qiao, J., Liu, Y., Guo, Q., Ou, X., & Wang, X. (2021). Isolation, structural, functional, and bioactive properties of cereal arabinoxylan—A critical review. *Journal of Agricultural and Food Chemistry, 69*(51), 15437–15457. https://doi.org/10.1021/acs.jafc.1c04506, http://pubs.acs.org/journal/jafcau.

Hodhodi, A., Rahimabadi, E. Z., Simorgh, S., & Safari, P. (2025). 3D food printing: A promising approach to meet food security. In *Climate change, food security, and land management*. Cham: Springer, 1–43. https://doi.org/10.1007/978-3-031-71164-0_52-1.

Homroy, S., Chopra, R., Singh, P. K., Dhiman, A., Chand, M., & Talwar, B. (2024). Role of encapsulation on the bioavailability of omega-3 fatty acids. *Comprehensive Reviews in Food Science and Food Safety, 23*(1), 1–35. https://doi.org/10.1111/1541-4337.13272, http://onlinelibrary.wiley.com/journal/10.1111/(ISSN)1541-4337.

Hussain, M. M. (2014). Intestinal lipid absorption and lipoprotein formation. *Current Opinion in Lipidology, 25*(3), 200–206. https://doi.org/10.1097/MOL.0000000000000084, http://www.co-lipidology.com/.

Hutchinson, A. N., Tingö, L., & Brummer, R. J. (2020). The potential effects of probiotics and ω-3 fatty acids on chronic low-grade inflammation. *Nutrients, 12*(8), 1–15. https://doi.org/10.3390/nu12082402, https://www.mdpi.com/2072-6643/12/8/2402/pdf.

Hülsebusch, L., Heyn, T. R., Amft, J., & Schwarz, K. (2025). Extrusion of plant proteins: A review of lipid and protein oxidation and their impact on functional properties. *Food Chemistry, 470*, 142607. https://doi.org/10.1016/j.foodchem.2024.142607.

Iqbal, J., & Hussain, M. M. (2009). Intestinal lipid absorption. *American Journal of Physiology - Endocrinology and Metabolism, 296*(6), E1183. https://doi.org/10.1152/ajpendo.90899.2008, http://ajpendo.physiology.org/cgi/reprint/296/6/E1183.

Islam, F., Imran, A., Nosheen, F., Fatima, M., Arshad, M. U., Afzaal, M., Ijaz, N., Noreen, R., Mehta, S., Biswas, S., Rasool, I. F. U., Aslam, M. A., Usman, I., Zahra, S. M., Segueni, N., & Amer Ali, Y. (2023). Functional roles and novel tools for improving-oxidative stability of polyunsaturated fatty acids: A comprehensive review. *Food Science and Nutrition, 11*(6), 2471–2482. https://doi.org/10.1002/fsn3.3272, onlinelibrary.wiley.com/journal/10.1002/%28ISSN%292048-7177.

Joffre, C., Rey, C., & Layé, S. (2019). N-3 polyunsaturated fatty acids and the resolution of neuroinflammation. *Frontiers in Pharmacology, 10*. https://doi.org/10.3389/fphar.2019.01022.

Kasparaviciene, G., Maslii, Y., Herbina, N., Kazlauskiene, D., Marksa, M., & Bernatoniene, J. (2024). Development and evaluation of two-phase gel formulations for enhanced delivery of active ingredients: Sodium diclofenac and camphor. *Pharmaceutics, 16*(3), 366. https://doi.org/10.3390/pharmaceutics16030366.

Keramat, M., Ehsandoost, E., & Golmakani, M.-T. (2023). Recent trends in improving the oxidative stability of oil-based food products by inhibiting oxidation at the interfacial region. *Foods, 12*(6), 1191. https://doi.org/10.3390/foods12061191.

Khozin-Goldberg, I., Iskandarov, U., & Cohen, Z. (2011). LC-PUFA from photosynthetic microalgae: Occurrence, biosynthesis, and prospects in biotechnology. *Applied Microbiology and Biotechnology, 91*(4), 905–915. https://doi.org/10.1007/s00253-011-3441-x.

Kivelä, R., Sontag-Strohm, T., Loponen, J., Tuomainen, P., & Nyström, L. (2011). Oxidative and radical mediated cleavage of β-glucan in thermal treatments. *Carbohydrate Polymers, 85*(3), 645–652. https://doi.org/10.1016/j.carbpol.2011.03.026.

Koletzko, B., Demmelmair, H., Hartl, W., Kindermann, A., Koletzko, S., Sauerwald, T., & Szitanyi, P. (1998). The use of stable isotope techniques for nutritional and metabolic research in paediatrics. *Early Human Development, 53*, S77. https://doi.org/10.1016/s0378-3782(98)00067-x.

Krawczyk, M., Burzynska-Pedziwiatr, I., Wozniak, L. A., & Bukowiecka-Matusiak, M. (2023). Impact of polyphenols on inflammatory and oxidative stress factors in diabetes mellitus: Nutritional antioxidants and their application in improving antidiabetic therapy. *Biomolecules, 13*(9). https://doi.org/10.3390/biom13091402, http://www.mdpi.com/journal/biomolecules.

Kumar, H., Guleria, S., Kimta, N., Nepovimova, E., Dhalaria, R., Dhanjal, D. S., Sethi, N., Alomar, S. Y., & Kuca, K. (2024). Selected fruit pomaces: Nutritional profile, health benefits, and applications in functional foods and feeds. *Current Research in Food Science, 9*. https://doi.org/10.1016/j.crfs.2024.100791, https://www.sciencedirect.com/science/journal/26659271.

Kumar, M., Pal, N., Sharma, P., Kumawat, M., Sarma, D. K., Nabi, B., Verma, V., Tiwari, R. R., Shubham, S., Arjmandi, B., & Nagpal, R. (2022). Omega-3 fatty acids and their interaction with the gut microbiome in the prevention and amelioration of type-2 diabetes. *Nutrients, 14*(9). https://doi.org/10.3390/nu14091723, https://www.mdpi.com/2072-6643/14/9/1723/pdf.

Kupikowska-Stobba, B., Niu, H., Klojdová, I., Agregán, R., Lorenzo, J. M., & Kasprzak, M. (2025). Controlled lipid digestion in the development of functional and personalized foods for a tailored delivery of dietary fats. *Food Chemistry, 466*, 142151. https://doi.org/10.1016/j.foodchem.2024.142151.

Lee, S. H., Huang, W. Y., Hwang, J., Yoon, H., Heo, W., Hong, J., Kim, M. J., Kang, C. S., Han, B. K., & Kim, Y. J. (2024). Characteristics of amylose–lipid complex prepared from pullulanase-treated rice and wheat flour. *Food Science and Biotechnology, 33*(5), 1113–1122. https://doi.org/10.1007/s10068-023-01411-0, https://www.springer.com/journal/10068.

Lim, W. S., Lim, N., Park, H. J., & Lee, M. H. (2024). Emulsion gel-based 3D printable fat analogue prepared with pea protein isolate. *Journal of Food Engineering, 364*. https://doi.org/10.1016/j.jfoodeng.2023.111801, http://www.sciencedirect.com/science/journal/02608774.

Lin, J., Jiao, G., & Kermanshahi-pour, A. (2022). Algal polysaccharides-based hydrogels: Extraction, synthesis, characterization, and applications. *Marine Drugs, 20*(5), 306. https://doi.org/10.3390/md20050306.

Liu, W. Y., Hsieh, Y. S., Ko, H. H., & Wu, Y. T. (2023). Formulation approaches to crystalline status modification for carotenoids: Impacts on dissolution, stability, bioavailability, and bioactivities. *Pharmaceutics, 15*(2). https://doi.org/10.3390/pharmaceutics15020485, http://www.mdpi.com/journal/pharmaceutics.

Liu, X., Powers, J. R., Swanson, B. G., Hill, H. H., & Clark, S. (2005). Modification of whey protein concentrate hydrophobicity by high hydrostatic pressure. *Innovative Food Science and Emerging Technologies, 6*(3), 310–317. https://doi.org/10.1016/j.ifset.2005.03.006.

Li, R., Koirala, S., Prakash, S., Xu, Y., & Bhandari, B. (2025). Omega-3 incorporation effects on the structural, rheological, and sensory properties of 3D-printed chocolate. *Sustainable Food Technology, 3*(6), 2134–2143. https://doi.org/10.1039/d5fb00475f.

Li, S., Tang, S., Mo, R., & Yu, P. (2025). Lipid oxidation and lipidomic profiles of raw and thermal-extracted yak fat under hydroxyl radical-induced oxidative stress. *Food Chemistry: X, 26*, 102295. https://doi.org/10.1016/j.fochx.2025.102295.

Loukil, I., Ku, D., Vachon, A., Metherel, A., & Plourde, M. (2025). Omega-3 supplementation increases 13C-EPA but not 13C-DHA kinetics in healthy older adults after 13C-DHA single dose intake: A secondary analysis. *Nutrition (Burbank, Los Angeles County, Calif.), 136*, 112803. https://doi.org/10.1016/j.nut.2025.112803.

Lupu, A., Gradinaru, L. M., Gradinaru, V. R., & Bercea, M. (2023). Diversity of bioinspired hydrogels: From structure to applications. *Gels, 9*(5). https://doi.org/10.3390/gels9050376, www.mdpi.com/journal/gels.

Lv, R., Qi, L., Zou, Y., Zou, J., Luo, Z., Shao, P., & Tamer, T. M. (2019). Preparation and structural properties of amylose complexes with quercetin and their preliminary evaluation in delivery application. *International Journal of Food Properties, 22*(1), 1445–1462. https://doi.org/10.1080/10942912.2019.1651736, https://www.tandfonline.com/loi/ljfp20.

Mariamenatu, A. H., Abdu, E. M., & Kostner, G. M. (2021). Overconsumption of omega-6 polyunsaturated fatty acids (PUFAs) versus deficiency of omega-3 PUFAs in modern-day diets: The disturbing factor for their "balanced antagonistic metabolic functions" in the human body. *Journal of Lipids, 2021*, 1–15. https://doi.org/10.1155/2021/8848161.

Martinat, M., Rossitto, M., Di Miceli, M., & Layé, S. (2021). Perinatal dietary polyunsaturated fatty acids in brain development, role in neurodevelopmental disorders. *Nutrients, 13*(4). https://doi.org/10.3390/nu13041185, https://www.mdpi.com/2072-6643/13/4/1185/pdf.

Martinez-Gonzalez, A. I., Díaz-Sánchez, Á. G., De La Rosa, L. A., Vargas-Requena, C. L., Bustos-Jaimes, I., & Alvarez-Parrilla, E. (2017). Polyphenolic compounds and digestive enzymes: In vitro non-covalent interactions. *Molecules (Basel, Switzerland), 22*(4). https://doi.org/10.3390/molecules22040669, http://www.mdpi.com/1420-3049/22/4/669/pdf.

Le Maux, S., Bouhallab, S., Giblin, L., Brodkorb, A., & Croguennec, T. (2014). Bovine β-lactoglobulin/fatty acid complexes: Binding, structural, and biological properties. *Dairy Science & Technology, 94*(5), 409–426. https://doi.org/10.1007/s13594-014-0160-y.

Miao, R., Jin, F., Wang, Z., Lu, W., Liu, J., Li, X., & Zhang, R. X. (2022). Oral delivery of decanoic acid conjugated plant protein shell incorporating hybrid nanosystem leverage intestinal absorption of polyphenols. *Biomaterials, 281*, 121373. https://doi.org/10.1016/j.biomaterials.2022.121373.

Mititelu, M., Lupuliasa, D., Neacşu, S. M., Olteanu, G., Busnatu, Ş. S., Mihai, A., Popovici, V., Măru, N., Boroghină, S. C., Mihai, S., Ioniță-Mîndrican, C. B., & Scafa-Udriște, A. (2025). Polyunsaturated fatty acids and human health: A key to modern nutritional balance in association with polyphenolic compounds from food sources. *Foods, 14*(1). https://doi.org/10.3390/foods14010046, www.mdpi.com/journal/foods.

Mondal, D., Awana, M., Mandal, S., Pandit, K., Singh, A., Syeunda, C. O., Thandapilly, S. J., & Krishnan, V. (2024). Functional foods with a tailored glycemic response based on food matrix and its interactions: Can it be a reality? *Food Chemistry: X, 22*. https://doi.org/10.1016/j.fochx.2024.101358, https://www.sciencedirect.com/science/journal/25901575.

Monte, M. J., Marin, J. J. G., Antelo, A., & Vazquez-Tato, J. (2009). Bile acids: Chemistry, physiology, and pathophysiology. *World Journal of Gastroenterology, 15*(7), 804–816. https://doi.org/10.3748/wjg.15.804, http://www.wjgnet.com/1007-9327/15/804.pdf.

Musuc, A. M. (2024). Cyclodextrins: Advances in chemistry, toxicology, and multifaceted applications. *Molecules (Basel, Switzerland), 29*(22), 5319. https://doi.org/10.3390/molecules29225319.

Nair, S. N., & Sujith, S. (2026). Hydrogels and organogels as food delivery system. In *Handbook of nutraceuticals*. Cham: Springer, 849–893. https://doi.org/10.1007/978-3-031-98791-5_30.

Nourazarain, A., & Vaziri, Y. (2025). Nutrigenomics meets multi-omics: Integrating genetic, metabolic, and microbiome data for personalized nutrition strategies. *Genes & Nutrition, 20*(1). https://doi.org/10.1186/s12263-025-00790-9.

Oliver, L., Dietrich, T., Marañón, I., Villarán, M. C., & Barrio, R. J. (2020). Producing omega-3 polyunsaturated fatty acids: A review of sustainable sources and future trends for the EPA and DHA market. *Resources, 9*(12), 1–15. https://doi.org/10.3390/resources9120148, https://www.mdpi.com/2079-9276/9/12/148.

Oruch, R., Lund, A., Pryme, I. F., & Holmsen, H. (2010). An intercalation mechanism as a mode of action exerted by psychotropic drugs: Results of altered phospholipids substrate availabilities in membranes? *Journal of Chemical Biology, 3*(2), 67–88. https://doi.org/10.1007/s12154-009-0034-6.

Oscarsson, J., & Hurt-Camejo, E. (2017). Omega-3 fatty acids eicosapentaenoic acid and docosahexaenoic acid and their mechanisms of action on apolipoprotein B-containing lipoproteins in humans: A review. *Lipids in Health and Disease, 16*(1). https://doi.org/10.1186/s12944-017-0541-3.

Pandey, A., Kamran, F., Choudhury, M., Li, L., Rahman, M. S., & Hussain, M. A. (2025). Omega-3 fatty acid fortification of plant-based beverages to enhance their nutritional profile. *Foods, 14*(9). https://doi.org/10.3390/foods14091602, www.mdpi.com/journal/foods.

Parada, J., & Aguilera, J. M. (2007). Food microstructure affects the bioavailability of several nutrients. *Journal of Food Science, 72*(2), R21. https://doi.org/10.1111/j.1750-3841.2007.00274.x.

Paramita, V. D., Panyoyai, N., & Kasapis, S. (2020). Molecular functionality of plant proteins from low-to high-solid systems with ligand and co-solute. *International Journal of Molecular Sciences, 21*(7). https://doi.org/10.3390/ijms21072550, https://www.mdpi.com/1422-0067/21/7/2550/pdf.

Parc, A. L., Houéto, E. H., Pigat, N., Chat, S., Leonil, J., Chanat, E., & Nabi, I. R. (2014). The membrane-associated form of αs1-casein interacts with cholesterol-rich detergent-resistant microdomains. *PLoS One, 9*(12), e115903. https://doi.org/10.1371/journal.pone.0115903.

Peter, M. J., Lalithapriya, U., Venkatachalapathy, R., & Sukumar, M. (2022). Characterization of an effective drug carrier system for improved oxidative and thermal stability of essential fatty acids: A review. *International Journal of Food Properties, 25*(1), 1753–1772. https://doi.org/10.1080/10942912.2022.2105352.

Peñalver, R., Lorenzo, J. M., & Nieto, G. (2024). Bioaccessibility, digestibility and nutritional properties of algae and *Cyanophyceae* as basis of their potential as functional food ingredients. *Applied Food Research, 4*(1). https://doi.org/10.1016/j.afres.2024.100404, https://www.sciencedirect.com/science/journal/27725022.

Photinam, R., Moongngarm, A., Detchewa, P., & Wang, Y. J. (2024). Improvement of amylose–lipid complex and starch digestibility profiles of corn starch added with rice bran oil or linoleic acid using ultrasonic and microwave treatment. *Journal of Food Science and Technology, 61*(12), 2287–2298. https://doi.org/10.1007/s13197-024-05993-3, https://www.springer.com/journal/13197.

Pineda-Vadillo, C., Nau, F., Guérin-Dubiard, C., Bourlieu, C., Capozzi, F., Bordoni, A., & Dupont, D. (2021). In vivo digestion of egg products enriched with DHA: Effect of the food matrix on DHA bioavailability. *Foods, 10*(1), 6. https://doi.org/10.3390/foods10010006.

Plourde, M., Chouinard-Watkins, R., Vandal, M., Zhang, Y., Lawrence, P., Brenna, J. T., & Cunnane, S. C. (2011). Plasma incorporation, apparent retroconversion and β-oxidation of 13C-docosahexaenoic acid in the elderly. *Nutrition & Metabolism, 8*(1), 5. https://doi.org/10.1186/1743-7075-8-5.

Preeti, Sambhakar, S., Saharan, R., Narwal, S., Malik, R., Gahlot, V., Khalid, A., Najmi, A., Zoghebi, K., Halawi, M. A., Albratty, M., & Mohan, S. (2023). Exploring LIPIDs for their potential to improves bioavailability of lipophilic drugs candidates: A review. *Saudi Pharmaceutical Journal, 31*(12), 101870. https://doi.org/10.1016/j.jsps.2023.101870.

Rahim, M. A., Regenstein, J. M., Al-Asmari, F., Imran, M., Ramadan, M. F., Rocha, J. M. F., Hussain, I., & Zongo, E. (2024). Optimized spray-dried conditions' impact on fatty acid profiles and estimation of in vitro digestion of spray-dried chia/fish oil microcapsules. *Scientific Reports, 14*(1). https://doi.org/10.1038/s41598-024-65214-x, https://www.nature.com/srep/.

Rahim, M. A., Uzma, M., Al-Asmari, F., Koraqi, H., Ramadan, M. F., Castro-Muñoz, R., & Zongo, E. (2025). A Comprehensive review on nutritional traits, extraction methods, oxidative stability, encapsulation technologies, food applications and health benefits of omega fatty acids. *Food Science & Nutrition, 13*(10). https://doi.org/10.1002/fsn3.71008.

Roth-Walter, F., Berni Canani, R., O'Mahony, L., Peroni, D., Sokolowska, M., Vassilopoulou, E., & Venter, C. (2024). Nutrition in chronic inflammatory conditions: Bypassing the mucosal block for micronutrients. *Allergy, 79*(2), 353–383. https://doi.org/10.1111/all.15972.

Sadiq, U., Gill, H., & Chandrapala, J. (2021). Casein micelles as an emerging delivery system for bioactive food components. *Foods, 10*(8), 1965. https://doi.org/10.3390/foods10081965.

Shakeel, A., Farooq, U., Gabriele, D., Marangoni, A. G., & Lupi, F. R. (2021). Bigels and multi-component organogels: An overview from rheological perspective. *Food Hydrocolloids, 111*. https://doi.org/10.1016/j.foodhyd.2020.106190, https://www.journals.elsevier.com/food-hydrocolloids.

Shuaibu, A., Juma, N. S., & Bashir, B. H. (2026). Polysaccharides as carriers and protectors of additives and bioactive compounds in food. *Journal of Future Foods*. https://doi.org/10.1016/j.jfutfo.2025.12.031.

Singar, S., Nagpal, R., Arjmandi, B. H., & Akhavan, N. S. (2024). Personalized nutrition: Tailoring dietary recommendations through genetic insights. *Nutrients, 16*(16). https://doi.org/10.3390/nu16162673, http://www.mdpi.com/journal/nutrients/.

Singh, P., Singh, T. P., & Gandhi, N. (2018). Prevention of lipid oxidation in muscle foods by milk proteins and peptides: A review. *Food Reviews International, 34*(3), 226–247. www.tandf.co.uk/journals/titles/87559129.asp, 10.1080/87559129.2016.1261297.

Song, R., Li, W., Deng, S., Zhao, Y., & Tao, N. (2023). Assessment of lipid composition and eicosapentaenoic acid/docosahexaenoic acid bioavailability in fish oil obtained through different enrichment methods. *Frontiers in Nutrition, 10*. https://doi.org/10.3389/fnut.2023.1136490.

Sundaram, T. S., Giromini, C., Rebucci, R., Pistl, J., Bhide, M., & Baldi, A. (2022). Role of omega-3 polyunsaturated fatty acids, citrus pectin, and milk-derived exosomes on intestinal barrier integrity and immunity in animals. *Journal of Animal Science and Biotechnology, 13*(1). https://doi.org/10.1186/s40104-022-00690-7, www.jasbsci.com/.

Sun, C., Zhu, J., Sun, X., Zhang, Z., Sun, Y., Jin, Y., & Wu, T. (2025). Targeting the human gut microbiome: A comparative review of probiotics, prebiotics, synbiotics, and postbiotics. *Journal of Advanced Research*. https://doi.org/10.1016/j.jare.2025.12.032.

Swackhamer, C., & Hayes, A. M. R. (2026). Something to chew on – oral processing simulators should be developed for integration with in vitro digestion workflows. *Food Bioscience, 76*, 108271. https://doi.org/10.1016/j.fbio.2026.108271.

Swetha, N., & Mathanghi, S. K. (2024). Towards sustainable omega-3 fatty acids production – A comprehensive review on extraction methods, oxidative stability and bio-availability enhancement. *Food Chemistry Advances, 4*, 100603. https://doi.org/10.1016/j.focha.2023.100603.

Szpicer, A., Bińkowska, W., Stelmasiak, A., Wojtasik-Kalinowska, I., Czajkowska, A., Mierzejewska, S., Domiszewski, Z., Rydzkowski, T., Piepiórka-Stepuk, J., & Półtorak, A. (2025). Innovative microencapsulation techniques of bioactive compounds: Impact on physicochemical and sensory properties of food products and industrial applications. *Applied Sciences, 15*(22), 11908. https://doi.org/10.3390/app152211908.

Tai, C. S., Chen, Y. Y., & Chen, W. L. (2016). β -Lactoglobulin influences human immunity and promotes cell proliferation. *BioMed Research International, 2016*. https://doi.org/10.1155/2016/7123587, http://www.hindawi.com/journals/biomed/.

Wang, Z., Zhang, M., Mujumdar, A. S., & Lin, J. (2025). Potential of functional factors in foods for 3D printing to manage metabolic syndrome: a comprehensive review. *Food Reviews International*. https://doi.org/10.1080/87559129.2025.2553684, www.tandf.co.uk/journals/titles/87559129.asp.

Watson, H., Mitra, S., Croden, F. C., Taylor, M., Wood, H. M., Perry, S. L., Spencer, J. A., Quirke, P., Toogood, G. J., Lawton, C. L., Dye, L., Loadman, P. M., & Hull, M. A. (2018). A randomised trial of the effect of omega-3 polyunsaturated fatty acid supplements on the human intestinal microbiota. *Gut, 67*(11), 1974–1983. https://doi.org/10.1136/gutjnl-2017-314968, http://gut.bmj.com/content/by/year.

Wehl, L., Muggli, K., Möller, K., Engelke, H., & Bein, T. (2025). Cross-linked cyclodextrin-based nanoparticles as drug delivery vehicles: Synthesis strategy and degradation studies. *ACS Omega, 10*(10), 10352–10365. https://doi.org/10.1021/acsomega.4c10200.

Wu, H., Richards, M. P., & Undeland, I. (2022). Lipid oxidation and antioxidant delivery systems in muscle food. *Comprehensive Reviews in Food Science and Food Safety, 21*(2), 1275–1299. https://doi.org/10.1111/1541-4337.12890, http://onlinelibrary.wiley.com/journal/10.1111/(ISSN)1541-4337.

Xu, R., Molenaar, A. J., Chen, Z., & Yuan, Y. (2025). Mode and mechanism of action of omega-3 and omega-6 unsaturated fatty acids in chronic diseases. *Nutrients, 17*(9). https://doi.org/10.3390/nu17091540, http://www.mdpi.com/journal/nutrients/.

Xu, Y., Yan, X., Zheng, H., Li, J., Wu, X., Xu, J., Zhen, Z., & Du, C. (2024). The application of encapsulation technology in the food Industry: Classifications, recent Advances, and perspectives. *Food Chemistry: X, 21*, 101240. https://doi.org/10.1016/j.fochx.2024.101240.

Yi-Wu, J., Hsieh, C. H., & Lin, Z. Y. (2022). Novel high-speed 3d printing method using selective oil sintering with thermoplastic polyurethane powder printing. *International Journal of Bioprinting, 8*(2), 159–163. https://doi.org/10.18063/ijb.v8i2.521, https://accscience.com/journal/IJB/volumes_and_issues.

Zazula, M. F., Pozzan, R., dos Reis, G. A., Maciel, M., Horlem, T., Banckes, T. N., Pereira, J. L. S., Sales-Campos, C., Fernandes, L. C., Martinez-Burgos, W. J., & Naliwaiko, K. (2025). Advances in oral drug delivery systems for natural polyunsaturated fatty acids: Enhancing bioavailability and therapeutic potential. *Pharmaceutics, 17*(11). https://doi.org/10.3390/pharmaceutics17111377, http://www.mdpi.com/journal/pharmaceutics.

Zhang, Y., Wang, H., Sang, Y., Liu, M., Wang, Q., Yang, H., & Li, X. (2024). Gut microbiota in health and disease: Advances and future prospects. *MedComm, 5*(12). https://doi.org/10.1002/mco2.70012.

Zhu, W., Iskandar, M. M., Baeghbali, V., & Kubow, S. (2023). Three-dimensional printing of foods: A critical review of the present state in healthcare applications, and potential risks and benefits. *Foods, 12*(17), 3287. https://doi.org/10.3390/foods12173287.

Zhu, Z., Zhao, C., Yi, J., Liu, N., Cao, Y., Decker, E. A., & McClements, D. J. (2018). Impact of interfacial composition on lipid and protein co-oxidation in oil-in-water emulsions containing mixed emulisifers. *Journal of Agricultural and Food Chemistry, 66*(17), 4458–4468. https://doi.org/10.1021/acs.jafc.8b00590, http://pubs.acs.org/journal/jafcau.

Zinkow, A., Grodzicki, W., Czerwińska, M., & Dziendzikowska, K. (2025). Molecular mechanisms linking omega-3 fatty acids and the gut–brain axis. *Molecules (Basel, Switzerland), 30*(1). https://doi.org/10.3390/molecules30010071, http://www.mdpi.com/journal/molecules.

Zivkovic, A. M., Telis, N., German, J. B., & Hammock, B. D. (2011). Dietary omega-3 fatty acids aid in the modulation of inflammation and metabolic health. *California Agriculture, 65*(3), 106–111. https://doi.org/10.3733/ca.v065n03p106, http://ucce.ucdavis.edu/files/repositoryfiles/ca6503p106-90309.pdf.

Section V

Sustainable polyunsaturated fatty acids

Chapter 25

Life cycle assessment of polyunsaturated fatty acids production and processing

Abiram Karanam Rathankumar[1], Kongkona Saikia[2], Vinoth Kumar Vaidyanathan[3], Femil Selta Daniel[4], and Maria del Rayo Sanchez-Carbente[5]

[1]*Department of Biotechnology (FoE), Karpagam Academy of Higher Education, Coimbatore, Tamil Nadu, India,* [2]*Department of Biochemistry, FASCM, Karpagam Academy of Higher Education, Coimbatore, Tamil Nadu, India,* [3]*Integrated Bioprocessing Laboratory, School of Bioengineering, SRM Institute of Science and Technology, Kattankulathur, Tamil Nadu, India,* [4]*Department of Biochemistry, Sri Ramakrishna College of Arts and Science for Women, Coimbatore, Tamil Nadu, India,* [5]*Autonomous University of the State of Morelos, Cuernavaca, Mexico*

25.1 Introduction

Polyunsaturated fatty acids (PUFAs), in recent years, have emerged as industrially important bioactive molecules due to their positive impact on human health, prevention of diseases, and providing a sustainable food system. The common PUFAs are mainly of two types: omega-3 and omega-6 fatty acids (Kapoor et al., 2021). Eicosapentaenoic acid (EPA) and docosahexaenoic acid (DHA) are common examples of omega-3 fatty acids, which have a positive role in neurological development, immunity, cardiovascular regulation, etc. (Kapoor et al., 2021). These PUFAs can be found in fatty fishes (e.g., Salmon) (Ziegler & Hilborn, 2023), flax seeds (Stefanova & Borisova, 2021), chia seeds (Liu & Yan, 2021), and certain edible oils (Hernandez et al., 2025). On the other hand, omega-6 PUFAs (arachidonic acid and linoleic acid) are involved in maintaining cellular function, nervous system, and skin health, and the regulation of inflammation. They are also involved in the regulation of antioxidant signaling (Djuricic & Calder, 2021). Plant-based oils, such as sunflower, corn, and soybean oils, are the primary sources of omega-6 fatty acids. Considering PUFA health benefits, there has been a significant increase in the industrial demand for PUFA-enriched foods, nutraceuticals, therapeutic products, and animal-feed formulations. This global trend shift has also significantly increased consumer awareness and alteration toward health-conscious diets, which in turn has expanded the global PUFA market.

Generally, the dominant sources of long-chain omega-3 fatty acids are extracted from marine fish. However, the overexploitation of resources, bycatch, diminishing marine biodiversity, postharvest processing, and the utilization of commercial fishing vessels challenge the sustainability of the overall production process (Lloret et al., 2025). Moreover, the production of plant-based PUFAs from oilseeds, such as sunflower, flax seeds, chia seeds, etc., requires extensive land and water utilization (Cerone & Smith, 2021; Ziegler & Hilborn, 2023). Further, fertilizers used for agricultural processes can also have an impact on the environment (Penuelas et al., 2023). Considering these factors, recently the focus has shifted to the production of PUFAs in an environmentally friendly way from a variety of sources, such as fungi, microalgae, and genetically engineered crops (Qin et al., 2023). Although these platforms have a promising outcome on the production of highly pure PUFAs and reduced environmental impact, they involve a nutrient-intensive fermentation process, high energy utilization, coupled with extensive downstream and purification processes. Thus, it is necessary to understand the overall environmental impact through a scientific and comprehensive framework. In this regard, life cycle assessment (LCA) is an important source to comprehend the environmental performance of production from "cradle-to-gate" or "cradle-to-grave" systems (Zaimes & Khanna, 2015).

LCA allows a systemic assessment of the environmental burdens across the various stages of PUFA production and supply chain (Zaimes & Khanna, 2015). This evaluation includes biomass cultivation and processing, oil extraction and processing, energy demands, emissions, water footprint, packaging, transportation, and end-of-life management. With technological advancement, several strategies have been developed for PUFA production; however, limited LCA studies have made it difficult to understand and identify the sustainable routes. In this regard, variable functional units, integrated

Omega-3 and Omega-6 Polyunsaturated Fatty Acids in Food Systems. DOI: https://doi.org/10.1016/B978-0-443-43810-3.00027-0

biorefineries, various cultivation routes, extraction processes, circular bioeconomy concepts, etc., further complicate the LCA process. Thus, a comprehensive review is required to understand the current production trend, along with methodical gaps and environmental effects, to standardize PUFA production strategies with a minimal ecological impact. Considering these factors, this chapter provides an elucidated overview of the ecological impacts associated with various PUFA production systems. It also establishes a comparative assessment of different LCA studies to understand their sustainability performances. Overall, this chapter aims to provide an understanding of distinguishing an ideal environmentally efficient PUFA production and supply route, which can cater to global health and nutrition.

25.2 Overview of polyunsaturated fatty acid production

The growing global interest in PUFAs due to their wide range of applications has led to an increase in research done to understand the synthesis pathways and production systems for PUFAs. Due to this increased demand, apart from the traditional marine-derived sources, various biotechnological platforms, such as microalgae, fungi, and engineered microbes, are also being explored to make the PUFA production process scalable and sustainable. The various sources of PUFAs are discussed as follows.

25.2.1 Marine sources

Marine sources are the largest supply of commercial PUFAs, such as EPA and DHA, owing to their naturally high concentrations, easy extraction, and broad regulatory acceptance for human application (Sahena et al., 2009; Taşbozan & Gökçe, 2017). The major source of these PUFAs is fish oils obtained from species such as sardine, tuna, salmon, mackerel, etc. Generally, omega-3 fatty acids are primarily produced by marine microalgae and certain protists through polyketide synthase (PKS) or desaturase/elongase pathways. These primary producers are consumed by zooplankton, which then becomes the diet of oily fish, thereby concentrating and accumulating larger quantities of EPA and DHA (Gladyshev et al., 2013). Thus, the oily fish become major reservoirs for PUFA harvest. The processing and extraction of PUFAs from oily fish include cooking, pressing, centrifugation, and molecular distillation or supercritical extraction to concentrate the PUFAs (Sahena et al., 2009). Another growing marine source is krill oil from *Euphausia superba* (krill), which contains phospholipid-bound EPA and DHA (Shahidi & Abad, 2024). *E. superba* also has astaxanthin, a potent antioxidant, which stabilizes the PUFAs. However, the utilization of krill is restricted to limit environmental impacts.

Despite the wide application of marine sources for PUFA production, their commercial use is facing concerns due to a reduction in resource availability, bioaccumulation of contaminants, and seasonal variations, among other issues (Koch & Jensen, 2016). Due to these sustainability challenges, the focus has recently shifted toward various biotechnological approaches for PUFA production.

25.2.2 Microalgal sources

Microalgae can accumulate substantial amounts of fatty acids, making them one of the primary biological sources of PUFAs (Kumar et al., 2019). They synthesize PUFAs through complex biological pathways, such as denaturation and elongation processes. PUFAs production by microalgae is achieved through two main pathways: aerobic and anaerobic, with the former being the most common route. In the aerobic pathway, desaturases introduce double bonds into fatty acid chains, which are then elongated by elongases (Monroig & Kabeya, 2018; Sun et al., 2018). In previous studies, the action of these two enzymes has been shown to improve the production of EPA (Monroig & Kabeya, 2018). The major factors that affect microalgal PUFAs production are nutrient availability, light, temperature, and salinity. Nitrogen and phosphorus directly influence the microalgal growth and, further, lipid accumulation (Yaakob et al., 2021). Thus, cultivation conditions optimization is needed to attain a desired PUFAs yield. Moreover, PUFAs production also depends on the species used.

Microalgal production has various advantages over marine sources, which include controlled production, limited environmental contaminants, and reduced environmental impact (Qin et al., 2023). However, light limitations, harvesting, and processing costs can be major challenges, which can be addressed by directing more research into metabolic engineering, circular bioeconomy, and LCA-guided optimization.

25.2.3 Fungal and yeast sources

Oleaginous fungi and yeasts are another notable platform used for the commercial production of PUFAs, such as EPA, DHA, γ-linolenic acid (GLA), and arachidonic acid (Calarnou et al., 2024). Fungi, majorly belonging to the phylum

Mucoromycota, can store high quantities of PUFAs-rich lipids when cultivated under optimal conditions (Calarnou et al., 2024). These fungi possess desaturase enzymes, which can introduce double bonds in esterified acyl chains. Generally, GLA is produced by fungi such as *Mucor circinelloides* (Zhang et al., 2022), *Umbellopsis ramanniana*, and *Thamnidium elegans* (Latifi et al., 2025), among others. Similarly, arachidonic acid and EPA can be produced by strains like *Mortierella alpina*. However, DHA can be produced only by *Thraustochytrids* (Parrish, 2024), which are fungoid-like marine protists. To improve the fungal production of PUFAs, various strategies have been utilized, such as chemical mutagenesis, direct gene manipulation (to improve desaturase production), enhanced oxygen utilization, etc. On the other hand, yeasts such as *Yarrowia lipolytica* can show substantial lipid accumulation (up to 40%) (Jia et al., 2022). However, under normal conditions, yeasts synthesize fatty acids having more than one double bond. Thus, metabolic engineering of yeasts is generally performed to produce PUFAs of interest owing to the advancement in genetic tools, the ability to metabolize various substrates, etc.

25.2.4 Engineered microbial sources

Although the natural producers of PUFAs have shown promising potential for their production, the major challenge is the low productivity, which is not sufficient to meet the current market demands. To meet this demand, metabolic engineering of microbial sources has shown acceptable yield and productivity of PUFAs. These advances in metabolic engineering have significantly improved PUFAs production, mainly due to the precision control over the metabolic pathways (Hanley, 2025). For example, the production of an important PUFA, EPA, can be improved by various strategies. In one strategy, the acetyl-CoA pool supply is increased by modulating acetyl-CoA synthetase (ACS), ATP citrate lyase, and pyruvate dehydrogenase complex (Russo et al., 2023). Previous works showed that the ACS gene, involved in ACS production, was overexpressed in *Escherichia coli*, which increased its synthesis. Similarly, the heterologous expression of ACS gene from *Thalassiosira pseudonana* in *Saccharomyces cerevisiae* also improved EPA production. One of the commonly engineered yeasts for PUFAs production is *Y. lipolytica*, which has been achieved by manipulating the desaturase/elongase pathway, introducing PKS pathway, etc. Further, in *E. coli*, DHA production was improved by the integration of DHA biosynthetic gene cluster and pfaE gene from *Moritella marina*.

25.3 Life cycle assessment for polyunsaturated fatty acid production

LCA is a systematic and standardized procedure used for quantifying the environmental impacts of a product, its process, or system, from raw material to product end-of-life (Arvanitoyannis, 2008). This process also includes raw material processing, manufacturing, transport, and product disposal after their intended use. LCA follows standards defined under ISO 14040 and ISO 14044, ensuring methodological consistency and transparency (Finkbeiner et al., 2006). Depending on the objectives and the scope of life the cycle covered, LCA can be classified into different types. Two widely accepted classification approaches are:

(a) Classification based on purpose
(b) Classification based on system boundaries.

25.3.1 Life cycle assessment classification based on purpose

Classification based on purpose focuses on the intent of the assessment—whether the study aims to describe existing systems or evaluate the consequences of decisions.

25.3.1.1 Attributional life cycle assessment

It describes the environmental burden which is associated with existing products or systems at a specific point in time within a defined system boundary (Ekvall, 2019). Allocation of the system's overall environmental impact using average data and physical relationships, and distributing among the system outputs, is considered to be a major objective of attributional life cycle assessment. By this approach, the material and energy flow within the system is accounted for and assigns the environmental loads proportionally to a functional unit. This analysis is commonly applied for carbon footprint studies and comparative assessment of similar products. Due to its simple methodology, it is widely adopted for industrial and regulatory applications. It is used to analyze the current flow in a process.

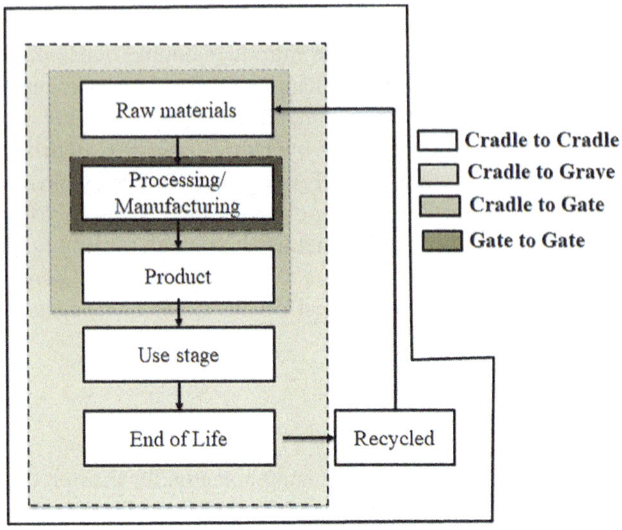

FIGURE 25.1 Classification of life cycle assessment based on system boundaries.

25.3.1.2 Consequential life cycle assessment

Consequential life cycle assessment (CLCA) is designed to analyze the changes in the environmental impact that may arise from changes made in the system (Ekvall, 2019). Instead of studying the existing system, CLCA deals with the changes in the environmental impacts as a result of specific action, such as introducing a new unit operation or modifying the process within a system. By a predictive approach, CLCA uses marginal data by considering system-wide consequences. Due to its high complexity and higher uncertainty, it is often employed for policy analysis and strategic planning. CLCA deals with decision-making and captures the indirect effects of the system.

25.3.2 Life cycle assessment classification based on system boundaries

LCA is also classified based on the system boundaries, which have a direct influence on the scope and completeness of the analysis (Fig. 25.1). One of the common boundary definitions is the "cradle-to-grave" LCA, which includes the environmental impact analysis from raw material extraction to product manufacturing, its utilization till the end-of-life (Zaimes & Khanna, 2015). This assessment does not consider the disposal phase of the products and is particularly utilized for intermediate products, whose downstream applications may vary. On the other hand, in "gate-to-gate" LCA, the boundaries are further narrowed down to only the production stage within the product life cycle. This strategy is typically used while optimizing the process or for developing a cleaning process after a unit operation to assess its environmental performance. The "gate-to-gate" LCA provides valuable information about manipulating the process to reduce the environmental burden on the system. "Cradle-to-cradle" LCA enhances the traditional LCA by incorporating circular economy principles into consideration. In this approach, the end products are recovered and reused to achieve a closed-loop system with effective sustainable material management.

25.4 Major components of life cycle assessment

LCA generally consists of four interlinked phases as outlined by ISO 14040 and ISO 14044 standards. In LCA, (1) goal and scope definition, (2) life cycle inventory (LCI) analysis, (3) life cycle impact assessment (LCIA), and (4) interpretation are the four major components (Fig. 25.2) (Arvanitoyannis, 2008). LCA used for PUFA production assesses from a "cradle-to-gate" or "cradle-to-grave" standpoint. PUFA LCA generally evaluates different stages: extraction of raw materials, PUFA production, processing and purification, and transportation and packaging. LCA is also influenced by various impact categories (climate change, eutrophication, acidification, energy demands).

25.4.1 Goal and scope

As per the ISO standards, the goal and scope definition is to establish the purpose, system boundaries, and functional unit of LCA. Defining a goal and scope is the first and most important step in LCA analysis. In simple terms, it explains "why

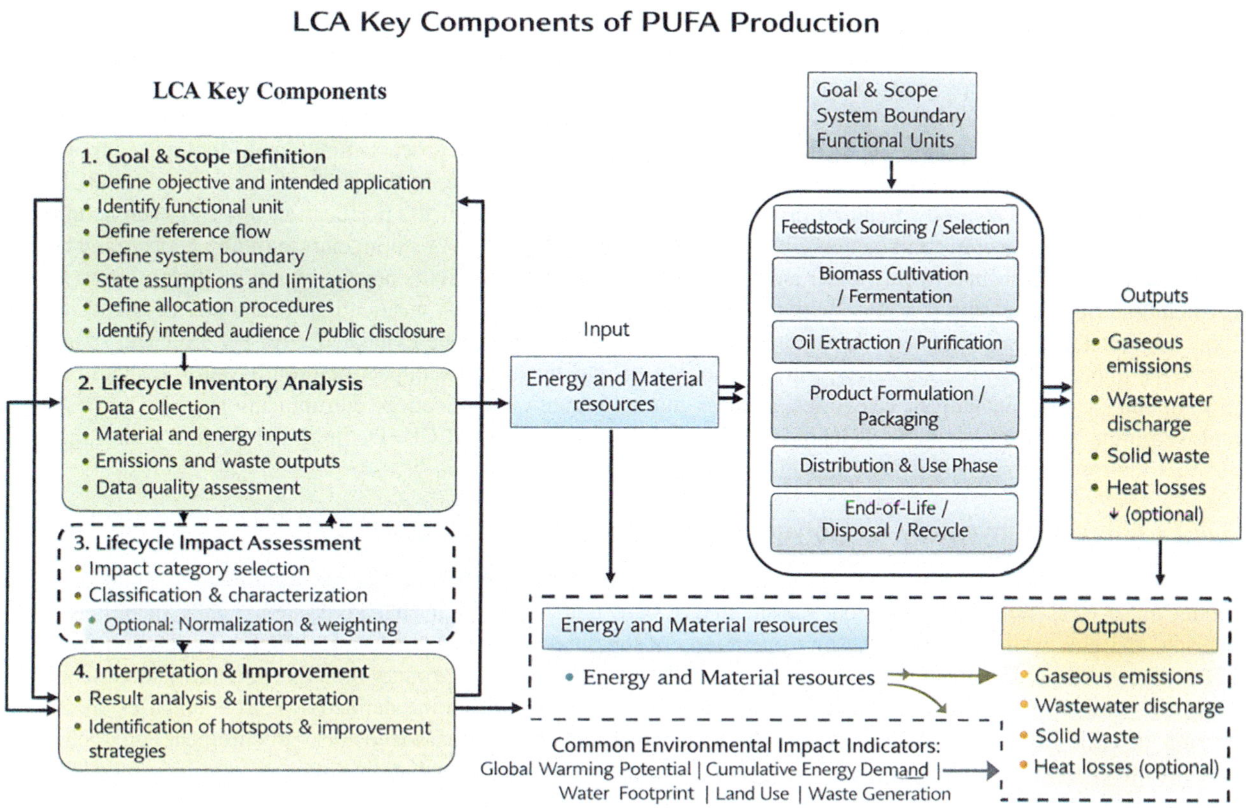

FIGURE 25.2 Life cycle assessment (LCA) key components and system boundary for polyunsaturated fatty acids (PUFAs) production.

the study is done" and "what it covers" respectively, by defining functional units, establishing the system boundaries, and the intended use of the study. As per ISO 14040:2006, Clause 5.1; ISO 14044:2006, Clause 4.2.2, the goal is defined as "the intended application, the reasons for carrying out the study, the intended audience, and whether the results are intended to be used in comparative assertions disclosed to the public" (Standard, 2006; Standardization, 2006). The goal explains the purpose and context of the study, and the application of the results, but it does not include any technical or modeling terms utilized in the process.

On the other hand, the scope of LCA involves establishing the functional units, system boundaries, assumptions, limitations, and other data requirements to describe "how the study will be conducted". From a technical point of view, the scope defines the functional units precisely, which describes the actual service delivered by the system rather than a simple measurement of process variables and raw materials (Arvanitoyannis, 2008). For example, the production of 1 g of 95% pure PUFA from 10 L media via aerobic fermentation rather than stating PUFA production via aerobic fermentation. Further, the reference flow involved is used to represent the amount of product/material or services required to fulfill the functional unit. It acts like a linker between the functional unit and the inventory by defining the input and output required for the defined function (Li et al., 2014). For instance, process water, nutrients, amount of heat, and electricity used to process 10 L of media.

Another major aspect of the scope is to establish the system boundaries, which involves defining the range of the study application, such as "cradle-to-grave" or "cradle-to-cradle" or "cradle-to-gate." The defined system boundary should coincide with the study goal, and all the factors that significantly contribute to the environmental impact have to be included, and omissions, if any, must be justified for the transparency and completeness of the study (Arvanitoyannis, 2008). The scope definition further establishes the system boundaries, level of detail, assumptions, and limitations of the study. System boundaries must be consistent with the stated goal and may range from "cradle-to-gate" to "cradle-to-grave" or "cradle-to-cradle" configurations. ISO standards require the inclusion of all unit processes that significantly contribute to environmental impacts, while permitting exclusions only when they do not compromise the completeness or representativeness of the results (Standardization, 2006). The system boundary includes raw material (feedstock) production, biomass production, extraction and purification, and finally transportation. Some of the feedstock used for PUFA production are sugarcane, marine biomass, food waste substrate, and oilseed. In cases where multifunctional processes occur, allocation procedures must be clearly defined. ISO 14044 recommends avoiding allocation wherever possible by applying system subdivision or system expansion (Standard, 2006). When allocation is unavoidable, it should rely on physical relationships (mass or energy), and the chosen method must be transparently justified.

Once system boundaries are established, the data considered for the study or used for the LCA study has to be specified. Further, in the case of multiple products or functions deriving from a single process, functional input and output can be allocated to the respective products (Zaimes & Khanna, 2015). For example, in the production of PUFA, if PUFA and biomass are considered as product and by-product, the chemicals required for the purification of PUFA can be allocated for only PUFA, rather than in combination with biomass. However, ISO 14044 recommends avoiding allocation whenever possible, and suggests including only under an unavoidable condition based on the physical relation, such as mass, energy, or stoichiometric relationship (e.g.,10% activated carbon used for 67% PUFA purification) (Standard, 2006). Within the scope, the impact assessment methodology specifies "how the impact will be evaluated". As per ISO, the scope must include the impact categories, indicators, and any models that can evaluate the impact before the study. It should identify the midpoint or endpoint impact categories, such as human toxicity, acidification, eutrophication, etc. The commonly employed impact assessment methods include ReCiPe, CML, TRACI, and ILCD. Defining the method within the scope enhances the transparency and avoids bias in the result interpretation.

25.4.2 Life cycle inventory for polyunsaturated fatty acid production

LCI is the second stage, which includes the quantitative specification of inputs and outputs required or associated with the product or services provided throughout the defined system boundaries. LCI analysis systematically quantifies all the materials and energy flows around the unit operations of the smallest elements related to PUFA production within the defined boundaries (Arvanitoyannis, 2008; Li et al., 2014). Considering the primary data that are under direct control of the process and ensuring mass and energy balance across the process within the defined system boundaries are a major criterion in LCI. In case of PUFA, the inventory generally includes biomass/feedstock procurement, production and downstream processing, extraction and purification, transportation and distribution, and waste management (Barr & Landis, 2018). The key inputs of the process are raw materials, energy demands, solvents, and nutrients. The major outputs include PUFAs-enriched oils, coproducts, residual substrates, and other environmental emissions (Davis et al., 2021).

Briefly, the LCI for marine-derived PUFAs is influenced by fuel consumption during fishing and the transportation of marine fish or their by-products to the processing units (Ziegler & Hilborn, 2023; Zlaugotne et al., 2023). Other inputs include the energy consumption, solvents, and water used for extraction and refining processes. In the case of marine PUFAs LCI, fish oil is the major output, along with coproducts such as fishmeal. The emissions that are considered for LCI are mostly the fuel combustion and wastewater discharge from the processing units (Barr & Landis, 2018). Further, the plant-based PUFAs LCI mostly takes agricultural inputs and land-based resources into account. In this LCI, the upstream inputs include fertilizers, irrigation, fuel for farm machinery, and energy used for oil processing and extraction (Al-Mawali et al., 2021). Apart from the PUFAs, oilseed cakes are produced as coproducts that can be upscaled as animal feed (Sarkar et al., 2021; Stefanova & Borisova, 2021). The emissions produced from agricultural source processing, particularly NO_2, are considered one of the major environmental impacts (Zlaugotne et al., 2023).

Similarly, for microalgal PUFAs, the inputs considered are the carbon sources, nutrients, water, and energy demand (used for microalgae growth and process, lipid extraction and processing, and biomass recovery) (Kumar et al., 2019). In the case of microalgae, EPA and DHA of high purity can be attained; however, the production process is greatly influenced by the energy demand of the overall process (Oliver et al., 2020). The LCI of fungal and yeast-based systems is based on heterotrophic fermentation processes (Calarnou et al., 2024). In these systems, the inputs are mainly associated with the fermentation process- carbohydrate sources (glucose, molasses), nitrogen sources, and electricity (sterilization, aeration, agitation, temperature control) (Parsons et al., 2018). The inputs from the downstream processing include lipid extraction and purification, and biomass recovery. The produced PFA-rich microbial oil, along with the residual biomass, constitutes the output of the inventory. Thus, co-product handling and allocation, and utilization of low-impact raw materials can immensely reduce the inventory burdens (Abelleira et al., 2024).

25.4.3 Life cycle impact assessment for polyunsaturated fatty acid production

LCIA is the third stage in LCA and assesses the environmental impact related to all the inputs and outputs quantified in LCI. LCIA relates the raw inventory data to environmental impact indicators that reflect their potential effects (Standard, 2006). In general, LCIA involves the impact categories selection, the assignment or classification of inventory flow, characterization and normalization, and weighting. LCIA links the material and energy flow to different environmental effect categories and evaluates the impact indicators such as global warming potential, acidification, energy demands, land and water utilization, and eutrophication, etc.

Global warming potential is a common impact category considered in PUFA LCIA studies (Standardization, 2006). Energy utilization and fuel consumption in production pathways are the major components that influence global warming potential. In marine-derived PUFAs, it is high owing to the fuel consumption by fishing fleets and refining processes (Ziegler & Hilborn, 2023). Moreover, plant-based PUFA production also contributes to global warming through fertilizer application, NO_2 production, and water consumption (Zlaugotne et al., 2023). On the other hand, microbial and microalgal PUFA production generally involves higher utilization of electricity, which directly influences the global warming potential of the system.

Further, the main inputs for acidification and eutrophication potentials are nutrient emissions and agricultural inputs (Oliver et al., 2020). Acidification impacts are influenced by ammonia volatilization and NO_2 emissions, whereas the eutrophication impacts are mostly the result of fertilizer application and runoff, and nutrient-rich wastewater. Thus, nutrient management and wastewater treatment are crucial to reduce environmental impacts. Another indicator considered during LCIA studies is the land and water usage, which varies greatly across different production pathways. Plant-based PUFAs generally have extensive land usage with high water consumption for irrigation (Zlaugotne et al., 2023). In the case of microalgal systems, although the land utilization is less, these systems have high water and energy demands. Energy demand is another indicator of LCIA, which evaluates the sustainability of the production pathway. The energy profile of marine and plant-based systems is due to fossil fuel consumption for fishing activities and agricultural actions. On the other hand, for microbial and microalgal systems, a high amount of energy is utilized in unit processes, such as sterilization, aeration, agitation, etc. Hence, LCIA can aid in emphasizing the importance of energy balance and suggest tradeoffs across different schemes of energy utilization, thereby reducing overall energy burdens.

25.4.4 Interpretation

It is the final stage, and according to ISO 14044:2006, it is defined as "the phase of LCA in which the results of the inventory analysis and impact assessment are analyzed in relation to the goal and scope, to reach conclusions, explain limitations, and provide recommendations" (Standard, 2006). The primary objective of interpretation is to extract meaningful insights from the LCI and LCIA data, identify environmental hotspots, evaluate uncertainties, and provide scientifically supported recommendations for decision-making. This phase can be divided into three key substeps: significant issue identification, evaluation, and reporting with recommendations. Issue identification involves hotspot analysis and contribution analysis. It identifies the unit operations that contribute most to the environmental burden and are quantified with respect to the functional unit. For example, in PUFA production, the use of solvents during downstream purification may represent a major environmental hotspot (Zlaugotne et al., 2023). Evaluation focuses on completeness, sensitivity, and consistency, ensuring all inputs and outputs are accounted for, assumptions are clearly defined, and methodological choices align with the goal and scope. Sensitivity analysis can evaluate the effect of major parameters such as fermentation yield, energy source, or allocation methods. Finally, the reporting and recommendation stage analyzes the findings to suggest improvements, such as optimizing solvent use, enhancing fermentation efficiency, or integrating renewable energy, which can lower the overall environmental impact of PUFA synthesis.

25.5 Case studies

Being a "cradle-to-grave" approach, LCA provides a unique comparative insight into the production of PUFAs using various strategies (Table 25.1). This analysis also provides insight into the production stage environmental burden, including raw material processing, transport, and production of PUFA, followed by the end-of-life disposal.

25.5.1 Omega-3 fatty acids

A comparative case study using different production pathways, such as marine-based (fish oils), plant-based (alpha-linolenic acid [ALA]-rich oils), and microbial omega-3 fatty acids (algal and bacterial fermentation), provides crucial information on their production strategy preference (Fig. 25.3) (Djuricic & Calder, 2021; Oliver et al., 2020). The omega-3 fatty acids extracted from fatty fish, such as anchovies, sardines, and mackerel, is a prominent strategy due to their high bioavailability in humans (Lloret et al., 2025). However, the environmental impacts associated with marine-based production are significant and multifaceted (Lloret et al., 2025). LCA represented potential environmental concerns, which majorly include overfishing that causes ecological imbalance in marine biodiversity. Further, the logistics involving fish containment, shipping, and processing of the fish increase greenhouse gas emissions due to significant consumption of

TABLE 25.1 Life cycle assessment (LCA) of different polyunsaturated fatty acids production systems.

Source	Goal	Key LCA findings	References
Microalgae	EPA/DHA production from *Schizochytrium* microalgae (heterotrophic cultivation)	Lower GWP and energy use vs. traditional fish oil; cultivation and drying key hotspots	Togarcheti and Padamati (2021)
Algae	EPA production using metabolic engineered *Phaeodactylum tricornutu*	Reduction in energy demand and global warming potential due to metabolism manipulation.	Qin et al. (2023)
Fish	LCA farmed salmon vs wild salmon (fish vs non-fish oil impacts)	Farmed salmon has higher eutrophication and climate impacts; fish oil as diet source	Ziegler and Hilborn (2023)
Fish and algae	Comparative analysis of one metric ton omega-3 fatty acids extraction from fish and algae	Impact was higher in algae-based omega-3 fatty acid extraction than in fish, if filtration was not used	Barr and Landis (2018)
Microbial	Organic feed waste for microbial oil by oleaginous microorganisms	Impact is high due to cell disruption	Abelleira et al. (2024)
Microbial	Hexanoic acid production	MES-based production yields higher carbon dioxide emissions compared with conventional strategies.	Luo et al. (2024)
Plant	Comparison of PUFA extraction by conventional hexane and supercritical extraction	Impact was found to be less while using supercritical extraction	Hernandez et al. (2025)
Plant	Waste date seed for oil extraction	Highest impact was observed during catalyst preparation and reuse	Al-Mawali et al. (2021)
Microalgae	Evaluate environmental impact of PUFAs from heterotrophic algae	Sugar cane cultivation contribute to high impact in all the categories.	Davis et al. (2021)
Microalgae, rapeseed oil, and fish oil	Understand the environmental impact of the sources used	Microalgae contribute to lower environmental impact	Zlaugotne et al. (2023)
Porphyridium purpureum FJ-12	Evaluate the microalgal cultivation in TB-PBRs to obtain high-valued products in a lowcost	TB-PBRs enhanced microalgal growth and bioproduct synthesis.	Guo et al. (2025)

fossil fuels (Ziegler & Hilborn, 2023). On the other hand, the utilization of water needed for refrigeration and large-scale processing, in turn, contributes to the environmental burdens. Although the omega-3 fatty acids extraction has several environmental and sustainability challenges, the high DHA and EPA content make this process a primary source (Lloret et al., 2025).

Another alternative production strategy for the EPA and DHA synthesis is plant-based oils. The ALA content in the oils derived from flax seed, chia, walnuts, and hemp is considered an EPA and DHA precursor, which, by the action of human metabolism, converts into EPA and DHA (Liu & Yan, 2021; Stefanova & Borisova, 2021). Even though the biotransformation reported was lower due to low conversion efficiency, plant-based omega-3 fatty acids are generally a sustainable alternative to the marine-based oils. Further, due to the lower energy requirement for the cultivation and processing of seed, this strategy contributes to a lower carbon footprint compared to marine oil (Zlaugotne et al., 2023). However, this strategy has a significant water footprint, particularly for crops like chia and flaxseed, due to intensive farming. This strategy has low biodiversity and ecosystem risk, as it doesn't involve continuous fishing that significantly disturbs the food chain. While plant-based omega-3 oils offer a more sustainable option in terms of carbon footprint and energy use, issues related to large-scale monoculture farming and pesticide utilization have a negative environmental impact (Zlaugotne et al., 2023).

Further, the microbial-based PUFAs, particularly from algae, are represented as a sustainable alternative, resulting in high EPA and DHA yields through the fermentation process (Abelleira et al., 2024). Minimal use of land and clean water

FUNCTIONAL UNIT

1 kg purified Omega-3 fatty acids (EPA+DHA equivalent), ready for human consumption
(OR)
1 kg formulated Omega-3 product standardized to an equivalent EPA/DHA content

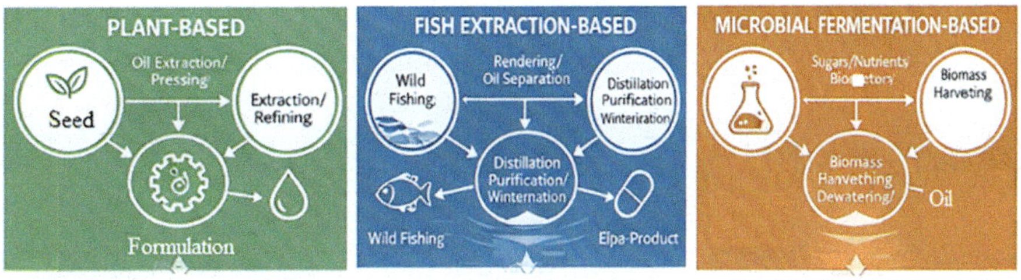

REFERENCE PROCESS
Plant oil required to deliver 1 kg EPA+DHA equivalent

REFERENCE PROCESS
Wild-caught fish oil needed to deliver 1 kg EPA+DHA equivalent

REFERENCE PROCESS
Microbial biomass required to deliver 1 kg EPA+DHA equivalent

Common Inputs
- **Electricity (kWh)**
- **Thermal energy / steam / fuel (MJ)**
- **Process & cooling water (m^3)**
- **Chemicals & processing aids (kg)**
- **Cleaning-in-Place (CIP) chemicals (kg)**
- **Packaging materials (kg)**
- **Transport / logistics**

Common Output
- **Final product**
- **Air emissions**
- **Wastewater**
- **Solid residues**
- **Packaging waste**
- **Waste heat (MJ)**
- **Off-spec material losses (kg)**

Specific Inputs

Plant based	Fish based	Microbial based
• Seeds / algal biomass (kg) • Fertilizers (kg) • Soil amendments (kg) • Irrigation water (m^3) • Herbicides / pesticides (kg a.i.) • Field diesel use (MJ or L) • Solvent for extraction (kg or L) • Steam / heat for oil refining • Energy for winterization / distillation	• Fuel for fishing vessels (L or MJ) • Refrigeration energy at sea (kWh) • Ice / cooling water • Fish raw material (kg wet weight) • Chemicals for purification • Steam / heat for rendering • Electricity for molecular distillation	• Carbon source (kg) • Nitrogen source (kg) • Other nutrients & trace minerals • pH control agents • Aeration (m^3 air or kWh blower energy) • Agitation power (kWh) • Cooling water for fermenters • Dewatering chemicals • Solvents used in oil extraction • Sterilization steam

Specific Outputs

Plant based	Fish based	Microbial based
• Oilseed meal co-product (kg) • Field emissions • Crop residue biomass • Solvent vapour losses	• Fish meal co-product (kg) • Wastewater from rendering • Protein/fat sludge • Vessel exhaust emissions • Discarded by-catch	• Spent fermentation broth • Microbial biomass waste (if not reused) • CO_2 from fermentation • Volatile losses from solvents • Sterilization condensate • Cell debris

FIGURE 25.3 System boundaries, functional unit, and key inputs/outputs for alternative omega-3 polyunsaturated fatty acids production pathways.

TABLE 25.2 Comparative omega-3 fatty acid impact assessment from marine, plant, and microbial sources.

Impact category	Marine source	Plant source	Microbial source
Carbon footprint (kg CO_2eq)	High	Low	Medium
Water use (m^3/kg product)	High	Medium	Low
Land use (m^2/kg product)	Low	High	Low
Energy consumption (MJ)	High	Low	Medium
Biodiversity impact	High (overfishing)	Medium (monoculture)	Low

resources makes this process more sustainable, as it has low land and water usage. In addition, greenhouse gas emissions associated with microbial production are relatively lower compared to the fishing and plant-based production strategies (Table 25.2).

25.6 Future prospective

The key factors that influence environmental integrity across PUFA production and processing are raw materials, energy sources, production processes, and coproduct formation. Although high PUFAs yield is obtained from microalgae, genetically engineered microbes, etc., there are several drawbacks of these methods that can be addressed to attain sustainable PUFAs production. In this regard, photobioreactors can be integrated with urban–industrial symbiosis and renewable energy sources to reduce eutrophication and climate impact. Further, precision fertilization techniques can be applied in plant systems used for PUFAs production. In the case of genetically engineered crops, land and nutrient burden can be reduced. Similarly, to attain a sustainable route of PUFAs production, the microalgae can be grown on waste substrates, which can produce a substantial amount of the product. During the extraction process, green extraction techniques, such as ultrasound-assisted extraction or deep eutectic solvent extraction, can be utilized to reduce the environmental impact. The production sustainability can also be improved by the valorization of the generated waste, which can address environmental impact by integrating the circular economy concept. Future work can be done by emphasizing the LCAs of engineered crops, assessment of extraction techniques, and detailed techno-economic and socio-environmental studies.

25.7 Conclusion

LCA offers a detailed framework to understand the environmental sustainability of PUFAs production and processing. This chapter highlights the variability of PUFAs supply chains and the environmental impacts of different production pathways based on raw material usage, energy demand, water footprint, land usage, emissions, and co-/by-product handling. Across all the production systems, LCAs evaluate the energy demand, nutrient inputs, and extraction processes as the major hotspots of environmental burden while considering functional units, system boundaries, and allocation approaches. Overall, no single production pathway can be considered superior across all impact domains, and thus, future work is required to assess the process sustainability based on circular bioeconomy, renewable energy sources, green extraction, etc.

References

Abelleira, S., Cruz, P. L., & Iribarren, D. (2024). Life cycle sustainability assessment of microbial oil from organic waste. *Cleaner Environmental Systems, 15*. https://doi.org/10.1016/j.cesys.2024.100236, https://www.sciencedirect.com/science/journal/26667894.

Al-Mawali, K. S., Osman, A. I., Al-Muhtaseb, A. H., Mehta, N., Jamil, F., Mjalli, F., Vakili-Nezhaad, G. R., & Rooney, D. W. (2021). Life cycle assessment of biodiesel production utilising waste date seed oil and a novel magnetic catalyst: A circular bioeconomy approach. *Renewable Energy, 170*, 832–846. https://doi.org/10.1016/j.renene.2021.02.027, http://www.journals.elsevier.com/renewable-and-sustainable-energy-reviews/.

Arvanitoyannis, I. S. (2008). ISO 14040: Life Cycle Assessment (LCA) - Principles and guidelines. In *Waste management for the food industries*. Greece: Elsevier Inc, 97–132. http://doi.org/10.1016/B978-012373654-3.50006-7, http://www.sciencedirect.com/science/book/9780123736543.

Barr, W. J., & Landis, A. E. (2018). Comparative life cycle assessment of a commercial algal multiproduct biorefinery and wild caught fishery for small pelagic fish. *International Journal of Life Cycle Assessment, 23*(5), 1141–1150. https://doi.org/10.1007/s11367-017-1395-7, http://www.springerlink.com/content/0948-3349.

Calarnou, L., Vigouroux, E., Thollas, B., Le Grand, F., & Mounier, J. (2024). Screening for the production of polyunsaturated fatty acids and cerebrosides in fungi. *Journal of Applied Microbiology, 135*(2). https://doi.org/10.1093/jambio/lxae030.

Cerone, M., & Smith, T. K. (2021). A brief journey into the history of and future sources and uses of fatty acids. *Frontiers in Nutrition, 8*. https://doi.org/10.3389/fnut.2021.570401, journal.frontiersin.org/journal/nutrition.

Davis, D., Morão, A., Johnson, J. K., & Shen, L. (2021). Life cycle assessment of heterotrophic algae omega-3. *Algal Research, 60*. https://doi.org/10.1016/j.algal.2021.102494, http://www.sciencedirect.com/science/journal/aip/22119264.

Djuricic, I., & Calder, P. C. (2021). Beneficial outcomes of omega-6 and omega-3 polyunsaturated fatty acids on human health: An update for 2021. *Nutrients, 13*(7), 2421. https://doi.org/10.3390/nu13072421.

Ekvall, T. (2019). Attributional and consequential life cycle assessment. *Sustainability Assessment at the 21st Century, 13*.

Finkbeiner, M., Inaba, A., Tan, R. B. H., Christiansen, K., & Klüppel, H. J. (2006). The new international standards for life cycle assessment: ISO 14040 and ISO 14044. *International Journal of Life Cycle Assessment, 11*(2), 80–85. https://doi.org/10.1065/lca2006.02.002, https://www.springer.com/journal/11367.

Gladyshev, M. I., Sushchik, N. N., & Makhutova, O. N. (2013). Production of EPA and DHA in aquatic ecosystems and their transfer to the land. *Prostaglandins and Other Lipid Mediators, 107*, 117–126. https://doi.org/10.1016/j.prostaglandins.2013.03.002.

Guo, S., Xie, D., Xiao, X., Zhou, Y., Yang, Y., Li, L., Wang, M., He, Y., & Chen, B. (2025). *Porphyridium purpureum* cultivation in outdoor pilot-scale: Economic assessment and life cycle assessment of photobioreactor-based cultivation systems. *ACS Sustainable Chemistry & Engineering, 13*(31), 12430–12440. https://doi.org/10.1021/acssuschemeng.5c02921.

Hanley, B. (2025). Genetic manipulation in agriculture. In *Natural and unnatural product chemistry: From molecules to systems*. Springer, 131–153.

Hernandez, C., Kaucz, A. P., Condoret, J.-S., Remigy, J.-C., Azzaro-Pantel, C., & Camy, S. (2025). Life cycle assessment of refined sunflower oil production for food industry: Exploring hexane-free alternative using supercritical CO_2 for processing pressed cake. *The Journal of Supercritical Fluids*, 106735.

Jia, Y. L., Wang, L. R., Zhang, Z. X., Gu, Y., & Sun, X. M. (2022). Recent advances in biotechnological production of polyunsaturated fatty acids by Yarrowia lipolytica. *Critical Reviews in Food Science and Nutrition, 62*(32), 8920–8934. https://doi.org/10.1080/10408398.2021.1937041, https://www.tandfonline.com/loi/bfsn20.

Kapoor, B., Kapoor, D., Gautam, S., Singh, R., & Bhardwaj, S. (2021). Dietary polyunsaturated fatty acids (PUFAs): Uses and potential health benefits. *Current Nutrition Reports, 10*(3), 232–242. https://doi.org/10.1007/s13668-021-00363-3.

Koch, M., & Jensen, M. K. (2016). Limitations of the review and meta-analysis of fish and PUFA intake and mild-to-severe cognitive impairment risks: A dose-response meta-analysis of 21 cohort studies. *American Journal of Clinical Nutrition, 104*(2), 537. https://doi.org/10.3945/ajcn.116.133397, http://ajcn.nutrition.org/content/104/2/537.1.full.pdf.

Kumar, B. R., Deviram, G., Mathimani, T., Duc, P. A., & Pugazhendhi, A. (2019). Microalgae as rich source of polyunsaturated fatty acids. *Biocatalysis and Agricultural Biotechnology, 17*, 583–588. https://doi.org/10.1016/j.bcab.2019.01.017, http://www.journals.elsevier.com/biocatalysis-and-agricultural-biotechnology/.

Latifi, M., Jalali Bidgoli, F., Hajihassani, H., Hassani, D., Ingvarsson, P. K., & Farrokhi, N. (2025). Recent advances and future directions on GLA-producing organisms. *Frontiers in Bioengineering and Biotechnology, 13*. https://doi.org/10.3389/fbioe.2025.1567840.

Li, T., Zhang, H., Liu, Z., Ke, Q., & Alting, L. (2014). A system boundary identification method for life cycle assessment. *The International Journal of Life Cycle Assessment, 19*(3), 646–660. https://doi.org/10.1007/s11367-013-0654-5.

Liu, B., & Yan, W. (2021). Quantitative polyunsaturated fatty acid analysis of chia seed oil by high-performance liquid chromatography. *Journal of Chromatographic Science, 59*(2), 120–127. https://doi.org/10.1093/chromsci/bmaa084.

Lloret, J., Vila-Belmonte, M., Izquierdo, A., San, J., & Biton-Porsmoguer, S. (2025). The unsustainability of the Omega-3 supply from seafood in the Mediterranean under global change. *Food Policy, 136*, 102972. https://doi.org/10.1016/j.foodpol.2025.102972.

Luo, J., Pérez-Fortes, M., Straathof, A. J. J., & Ramirez, A. (2024). Life cycle assessment of hexanoic acid production via microbial electrosynthesis and renewable electricity: Future opportunities. *Journal of Environmental Chemical Engineering, 12*(5), 113924. https://doi.org/10.1016/j.jece.2024.113924.

Monroig, Ó., & Kabeya, N. (2018). Desaturases and elongases involved in polyunsaturated fatty acid biosynthesis in aquatic invertebrates: A comprehensive review. *Fisheries Science, 84*(6), 911–928. https://doi.org/10.1007/s12562-018-1254-x.

Oliver, L., Dietrich, T., Marañón, I., Villarán, M. C., & Barrio, R. J. (2020). Producing omega-3 polyunsaturated fatty acids: A review of sustainable sources and future trends for the EPA and DHA market. *Resources, 9*(12), 1–15. https://doi.org/10.3390/resources9120148, https://www.mdpi.com/2079-9276/9/12/148.

Parrish, C. C. (2024). Thraustochytrids and algae as sustainable sources of long-chain omega-3 fatty acids for aquafeeds. *Sustainability, 16*(21), 9142. https://doi.org/10.3390/su16219142.

Parsons, S., Chuck, C. J., & McManus, M. C. (2018). Microbial lipids: Progress in life cycle assessment (LCA) and future outlook of heterotrophic algae and yeast-derived oils. *Journal of Cleaner Production, 172*, 661–672. https://doi.org/10.1016/j.jclepro.2017.10.014.

Penuelas, J., Coello, F., & Sardans, J. (2023). A better use of fertilizers is needed for global food security and environmental sustainability. *Agriculture & Food Security, 12*(1). https://doi.org/10.1186/s40066-023-00409-5.

Qin, Z. H., Hu, X., Mou, J. H., He, G. H., Ye, G. B., Li, H. Y., Chopra, S. S., Dong, L., Lin, C. S. K., & Wang, X. (2023). Environmental profiling microalgae-based eicosapentaenoic acid production along the technical advancement via life cycle assessment. *Journal of Cleaner Production, 397*. https://doi.org/10.1016/j.jclepro.2023.136477, https://www.journals.elsevier.com/journal-of-cleaner-production.

Russo, M., Pileri, F., & Ghisletti, S. (2023). Novel insights into the role of acetyl-CoA producing enzymes in epigenetic regulation. *Frontiers in Endocrinology, 14*. https://doi.org/10.3389/fendo.2023.1272646.

Sahena, F., Zaidul, I. S. M., Jinap, S., Saari, N., Jahurul, H. A., Abbas, K. A., & Norulaini, N. A. (2009). PUFAs in fish: Extraction, fractionation, importance in health. *Comprehensive Reviews in Food Science and Food Safety, 8*(2), 59–74. https://doi.org/10.1111/j.1541-4337.2009.00069.x.

Sarkar, N., Chakraborty, D., Dutta, R., Agrahari, P., Bharathi, S. D., Singh, A. A., & Jacob, S. (2021). A comprehensive review on oilseed cakes and their potential as a feedstock for integrated biorefinery. *Journal of Advanced Biotechnology and Experimental Therapeutics, 4*(3), 376–387. https://doi.org/10.5455/jabet.2021.d137, https://www.bsmiab.org/jabet/wp-content/uploads/sites/2/2021/08/178-1628068229.pdf.

Shahidi, F., & Abad, A. (2024). Why is Antactic krill (Euphasia superba) oil on the spotlight? A review. *Food Production, Processing and Nutrition, 6*(1). https://doi.org/10.1186/s43014-024-00260-6.

Standard, I. (2006). *Environmental management-Life cycle assessment-Requirements and guidelines*. London: ISO.

Standardization, I. O. F. (2006). *Environmental management: Life cycle assessment; Principles and Framework*. ISO.

Stefanova, I., & Borisova, V. (2021). Using the flax seeds and the flax oil in the production of chopped semi-finished chicken meat products in order to enrich them with polyunsaturated fatty acids. *The International Conference on Advances in Emerging Trends and Technologies*.

Sun, X. M., Geng, L. J., Ren, L. J., Ji, X. J., Hao, N., Chen, K. Q., & Huang, H. (2018). Influence of oxygen on the biosynthesis of polyunsaturated fatty acids in microalgae. *Bioresource Technology, 250*, 868–876. https://doi.org/10.1016/j.biortech.2017.11.005, www.elsevier.com/locate/biortech.

Taşbozan, O., & Gökçe, M. A. (2017). Fatty acids in fish. *Fatty Acids, 1*, 143–159.

Togarcheti, S. C., & Padamati, R. B. (2021). Comparative life cycle assessment of EPA and DHA production from microalgae and farmed fish. *Clean Technologies, 3*(4), 699–710. https://doi.org/10.3390/cleantechnol3040042, www.mdpi.com/journal/cleantechnol.

Yaakob, M. A., Mohamed, R. M. S. R., Al-Gheethi, A., Aswathnarayana Gokare, R., & Ambati, R. R. (2021). Influence of nitrogen and phosphorus on microalgal growth, biomass, lipid, and fatty acid production: An overview. *Cells, 10*(2), 393. https://doi.org/10.3390/cells10020393.

Zaimes, G. G., & Khanna, V. (2015). Life cycle sustainability aspects of microalgal biofuels. In *Assessing and measuring environmental impact and sustainability*. United States: Elsevier Inc, 255–276. http://doi.org/10.1016/B978-0-12-799968-5.00008-7, http://www.sciencedirect.com/science/book/9780127999685.

Zhang, Y., Wang, Y., Yang, J., Yang, W., Wang, X., Wu, C., & Song, Y. (2022). Improved γ-Linolenic acid production from cellulose in Mucor circinelloides via coexpression of cellobiohydrolase and delta-6 desaturase. *Journal of Agricultural and Food Chemistry, 70*(14), 4373–4381.

Ziegler, F., & Hilborn, R. (2023). Fished or farmed: Life cycle impacts of salmon consumer decisions and opportunities for reducing impacts. *Science of The Total Environment, 854*, 158591. https://doi.org/10.1016/j.scitotenv.2022.158591.

Zlaugotne, B., Sanchez, F. D., Pubule, J., & Blumberga, D. (2023). Life cycle assessment of fish feed for oil alternatives-environmental impact of microalgae, rapeseed and fish oil. *Agronomy Research, 21*(3), 1351–1360. https://doi.org/10.15159/AR.23.074, https://agronomy.emu.ee/index.php/category/volume-21-2023/number-3-volume-21-2023/?aid=9888&sa=0.

Chapter 26

Environmental sustainability in polyunsaturated fatty acid sourcing and production

Shreelekha Manthiri and Pavithra Palanisamy
ICAR-Central Institute of Brackishwater Aquaculture, Chennai, Tamil Nadu, India

26.1 Introduction

The environmental sustainability of polyunsaturated fatty acid (PUFA) sourcing and production is a critical area of research, due to the acknowledged increase in global demand for these essential nutrients with recognized ecological impacts of sources (Mukherjee et al., 2024; Zhou et al., 2023). When 12 carbon atoms or more are present, they are called long-chain fatty acids, and 22 or more carbon atoms are called as very long-chain fatty acids (Bazinet & Layé, 2014). Hydrocarbon chain and carboxylic group bounded with glycerol turn out to be unsaturated (mono and poly) or saturated (no double bonds) (Rubio-Rodríguez et al., 2010). The human body cannot synthesize most of the PUFA, so they must be obtained from their food, hence called essential fatty acids. Whereas, the human body can synthesize the nonessential fatty acids (saturated and monounsaturated fatty acids) (Bajpai et al., 1992). PUFAs are classified as omega-3 and omega-6, which are determined by the position of first double bond nearest to the methyl terminal end (Saini & Keum, 2018). Linoleic acid is the parent omega-6 fatty acid from which arachidonic acid is synthesized Fig. 26.1. Similarly, α-linolenic acid is the parent omega-3 fatty acid from which eicosapentaenoic acid (EPA), and docosahexaenoic acid (DHA) can be synthesized. However, conversion from alpha-linolenic acid (ALA) to EPA, docosapentaenoic acid, and DHA are low, so they can only be derived from diet, which is necessary for human health (WHO, 1994).

EPA and docosahexaenoic acid (DHA) play a vital role in vasoprotection, neurological function, inflammation modulation (Mukherjee et al., 2024), cardiac arrhythmia, myocardial infarction, and thrombosis (Lee et al., 2009). Many of the nutritionists advise that consumption of fish and green vegetables prevents humans from most of the ailments. It is very difficult to change the traditional food habits of the society, so nutritional supplements have been developed to reach a good n-6:3 ratio in blood without making changes in the diet. Life cycle assessment serves as a pivotal tool for systematically quantifying the environmental impacts (EI) across the life cycle of products and processes, enabling sustainable innovation and comparative analysis of different sourcing methods (Nitkiewicz & Cappelletti, 2022; Qin et al., 2023; Togarcheti & Padamati, 2021). This chapter analyzes the ecological crises inherent in PUFA sourcing and production, mapping the development from marine resource extraction towards economic systems that merge sustainability and biomass that might align nutritional needs with ecological integrity.

26.2 Recommended intake of polyunsaturated fatty acids

EFSA Panel on Nutrition, Novel Foods and Food Allergens states that total fat consumption should not exceed 20%–35% of energy (E%) (EFSA J., 2010). For ALA, the adequate intake is established at 0.5 E%. EFSA Panel recommends 100 mg/d of EPA with DHA for 6 to 24 months children and 250 mg/d for adults due to the health benefits of avoiding death from congenital heart disease (CHD) and sudden heart attacks (EFSA J., 2010). The panel also suggested adding 100–200 mg of DHA to ensure a sufficient supply of very long-chain polyunsaturated fatty acids (VLC-PUFAs) during pregnancy and breastfeeding. Additionally, National Institute of Medicine recommends that 10% of ALA intake come from EPA and DHA (Thompson et al., 2019). WHO suggested that adults should consume 200–500 mg of EPA and DHA

Omega-3 and Omega-6 Polyunsaturated Fatty Acids in Food Systems. DOI: https://doi.org/10.1016/B978-0-443-43810-3.00035-X

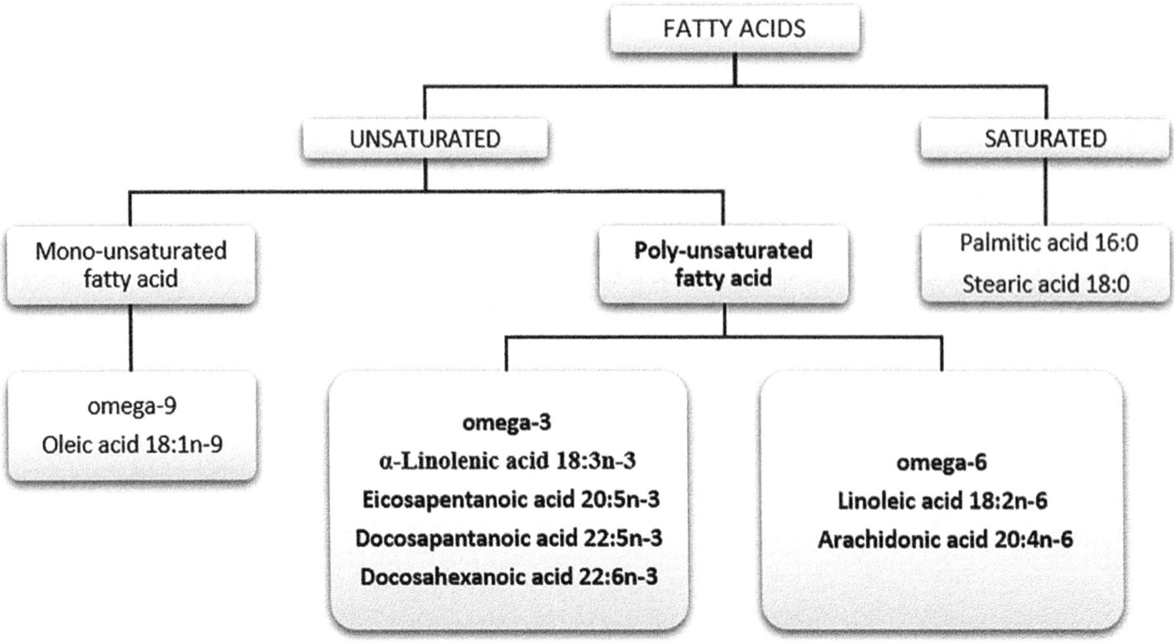

FIGURE 26.1 Classification of fatty acids.

(WHO study, 2003). Additionally, it advises vegetarians to consume enough plant-based ALA (WHO study, 2003). The body's n-3 FA status is determined by the n-3 index, which is the red blood cell (RBC), EPA, and DHA contents expressed as a percentage of total FAs (Harris & von Schacky, 2004).

According to Harris and von Schacky (2004), when the RBC n-3 index is greater than or equal to 8%, it is a realistic initial aim for lowering the risk of CHD. An increase in fish and fish oil supplement consumption is recommended to boost this index (Harris, 2009). Besides, this option is not feasible for vegetarians since they take supplements from plant or microbial sources. In accordance with the available data, the necessary amounts of PUFAs are not consumed by people all over the world, particularly vegans and vegetarians (Burns-Whitmore et al., 2019; Sarter et al., 2015; Lane et al., 2021; Thompson et al., 2019).

The report from National Health and Nutrition Examination Survey taken between 2003 and 2014 showed considerable differences in EPA and DHA intake by gender, age, and pregnancy status. Especially children and women who are advised to eat more are eating less than the recommended daily intake. As stated by IOM and WHO, children between the ages of 6 and 11 consume roughly 4.5%–27% of the recommended daily allowance of the EPA and DHA (Thompson et al., 2019). According to recent research, compared to people who consume fish and marine-derived fatty acids, vegans and vegetarians have significantly lower dietary n-3 intakes and total n-3 erythrocyte/plasma fatty acids (Lane et al., 2021). This has also been studied by Sarter et al. (2015), where they say that the vegan diet has 50%–60% less EPA and DHA than the nonvegetarian group. The biotransformation were VLC-PUFAs are converted from ALA is influenced by genetic variations in PUFA metabolism, particularly mutations in the FADS1–3 gene cluster that restrict the conversion to omega-3 fatty acids (Schulze et al., 2020). Therefore these aspects should be taken into consideration before recommending ALA, EPA, and DHA intake.

Circular bioeconomy methods: Strategies for circular production can enhance sustainability:

- Using waste from fish processing rather than the intended harvest
- Turning agricultural waste into substrates for fermentation
- Reusing CO_2 emissions for algae growth
- Combining systems for algae production with aquaculture
- Waste is decreased, resource efficiency is improved, and environmental impact is reduced with circular bioeconomy models (Geissdoerfer et al., 2017).

26.3 Natural sources of polyunsaturated fatty acid and production

26.3.1 Fish and fisheries derived oils

The conventional sources of marine PUFAs remain fish oil extracted from small pelagic species such as sardines, mackerel, herring, menhaden, and anchovy. These fishes accumulate EPA and DHA in their tissues by consuming PUFA-rich diets, resulting in variations in fatty acid profiles depending on the species, diet, habitat and environmental conditions. Besides whole fish, processed by products like heads, viscera, frames and skin are an important source of marine lipids which serve as a strategic resource for oil production (John et al., 2025; Zheng et al., 2025). Marine fishes are unique and rich dietary source of PUFAs for humans. Fishes don't synthesize fatty acids instead they obtain them through their diet which contains microalgae (Tocher, 2009). The fish oil source, which is the important conventional source of n-3 fatty acids, emphasizes high ecological impact, damage, or degradation.

26.3.2 Marine invertebrates

Crustaceans (krill, shrimp) and mollusks (mussels, oysters) are notable sources with a unique lipid profile. Krill oil in particular has gained attention because its PUFAs are bound to phospholipids rather than triglycerides, potentially offering enhanced absorption and bioavailability compared to fish oil. Studies on sponges, cnidarins, mollusks, crustaceans, and echinoderms have identified key enzymes and genes involved in PUFA metabolism, suggesting that some invertebrates can modify dietary PUFAs or synthesize them de novo to meet their physiological needs (John et al., 2025; Wang & Ding., 2021).

26.3.3 Marine microorganisms

The original producers of long-chain PUFAs are microalgae, bacteria, protists, fungi, and dinoflagellates. They synthesize EPA and DHA through dedicated biosynthetic pathways and are the most sustainable and scalable source of marine PUFAs. Thraustochytrids are suitable for industrial PUFA production because they can accumulate high concentrations of lipids particularly DHA. For commercial production, *Schizochytrium, Parietichytrium,* and *Thraustochytrium* synthesize PUFAs through polyketide synthase (PKS)-like enzymes employing fatty acid elongases and desaturases in a stepwise manner with a distinct pathway (Ishibashi et al., 2025; Literáková et al., 2024). Other important PUFA-producing microorganisms include marine bacteria such as *Shewanella, Moritella,* and *Photobacterium* (Tian et al., 2024).

26.4 Production technologies for marine polyunsaturated fatty acids

Conventional fish oil production primarily depends on wet rendering, that is, wet pressing process, a thermal separation process that has been optimized over the past few decades. This process involves five stages, starting from cooking to refinement. The raw material, which may be whole fish or by products, is initially heated at a temperature of 90°C–95°C for protein coagulation to extract oil and water from the tissues via indirect steam. The second step after cooking is pressing, where the material is pressed to divide the fluid phase (oil and water) from the solid portion (press cake). The next step is centrifugation, where crude oil is recovered from the aqueous phase, which also yields protein-rich stick water that can be concentrated into fishmeal. Then the oil is purified by removing the impurities (Pigott, 1967) (see Fig. 26.2.

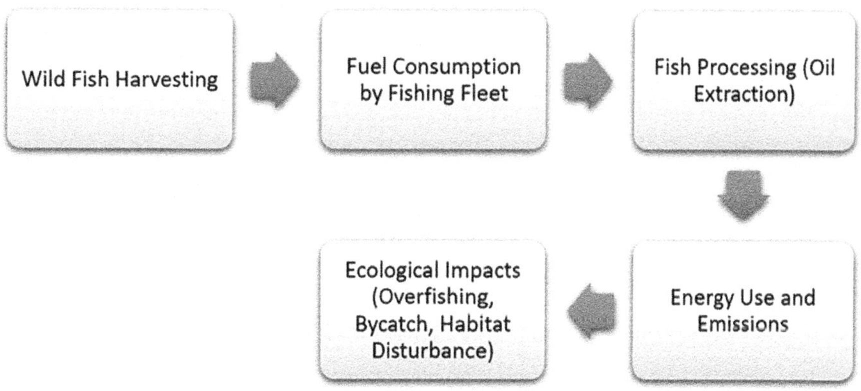

FIGURE 26.2 Environmental pathway of marine polyunsaturated fatty acid production.

Crude fish oil requires extensive refining to produce a palatable, stable, and safe product suitable for human consumption. The refining process typically includes:

- Degumming: Phosphoric or citric acid is used to remove phospholipids and mucilaginous materials.
- Neutralization: Alkali treatment (usually sodium hydroxide) to remove free fatty acids.
- Bleaching: Adsorption of pigments, oxidation products, and residual impurities using bleaching earth or activated carbon under vacuum.
- Winterization: By controlling the temperature to crystallize and remove high-melting-point saturated fats (stearine), it yields a liquid oil (olein) enriched in PUFAs that remains clear at refrigerator temperatures.
- Deodorization: Steam distillation in high vacuum and temperature to clear volatile compounds responsible for fishy odors and tastes.

While effective, traditional processing faces challenges including oxidative degradation of sensitive PUFAs, high energy consumption, and environmental concerns related to wastewater and by-product management (John et al., 2025; Zheng et al., 2025).

26.5 Environmental sustainability of marine sources

One of the most noteworthy ecological concerns is overfishing, including bycatch, habitat destruction, and the release of greenhouse gases (GHG) (Lucas et al., 2021). Fish oil production is mainly dependent on wild fish populations, which led to the depletion of numerous fisheries worldwide, threatening marine biodiversity by ripple effects on the marine food web and ecological balance (Rizzo et al., 2023; Tocher, 2009). The Intergovernmental Science-Policy Platform on Biodiversity and Ecosystem Services has highlighted that biodiversity loss in the marine environment is mainly because of the predominant overfishing habit (Tocher, 2009). The impact of fishery and aquaculture products in regions like France, for instance, highlights the potential for damage transfer from terrestrial to marine ecosystems (Lucas et al., 2021).

Indicating the fishing grounds' footprint, fisheries production is identified as an environmental degradation factor. Marine capture fisheries, which are the primary source of these valuable compounds, have led to overfishing, ecosystem degradation, and the environmental footprint of aquaculture. This has spurred the development of different and more sustainable production pathways (Lucas et al., 2021; Zhou et al., 2023). Aquaculture, while reducing pressure on wild stock, on the other hand, has its own ecological issues that include GHG emissions, particularly from marine shrimp monoculture, and the generation of significant wastewater that can lead to ecological problems if not managed effectively (Lucas et al., 2021). Removal of foundational species destroys the marine food web, so the predators prey on seabirds, and mammals. Fishing with nets like purse seines and bottom trawls heavily disrupts the trophic chain since most of the nontargeted species are captured in these types of fishing.

The supply chain for traditional fish oil is fundamentally unviable. According to scientific literature, global oceanic fish stocks either experience environmental contamination or reach the limits of sustainable management, prohibiting further extraction. This issue worsened by the extraordinary expansion of aquaculture in 2013, where fish farming, as opposed to wild capture, provided the majority (51%) of all fish consumed by humans. Aquaculture of marine species requires dietary supplementation with n-3 LC-PUFAs, creating a cycle of capture, extraction, and feed preparation that places continuous pressure on wild fish populations (Usher et al., 2015). Traditional fish oil faces contamination with environmental pollutants such as persistent organic pollutants and heavy metals, which accumulate in marine food chains. The search for alternative sources that are widely scalable and really sustainable by these criteria taken together (West et al., 2021).

Another crucial issue associated with marine-derived PUFAs is the possibility of contamination. Fish, especially those higher up in the food chain, can accumulate environmental toxins such as PCB like persistent organic pollutants and heavy metals from their diet (Oliver et al., 2020) (Table 26.1). These contaminants pose health risks to consumers and, moreover, reflect broader issues of marine pollution. There is a strong need to look into alternatives because of the inherent restrictions in sustainably increasing supply from marine sources and the fluctuation in quality (Chi et al., 2022).

26.6 Plant-based polyunsaturated fatty acid sources

Plants are excellent sources of ALA, a precursor to longer-chain omega-3 PUFAs, while most traditional oilseed crops do not produce EPA or DHA naturally (Yang et al., 2025). For instance, flaxseed oil, chia, canola, and soybean oils are rich in ALA, and sacha inchi oil is notable for its high omega-3 content, making it a promising novel vegetable source (Maurer et al., 2012). This metabolic bottleneck means that while plant-based ALA sources are beneficial, they cannot fully meet the physiological requirements for preformed EPA and DHA, especially in populations with higher needs or impaired

TABLE 26.1 Detailed polyunsaturated fatty acid (PUFA) levels in various marine-derived sources and their uses.

Source	Type	PUFA level	Total fat (g/100 g)	Total PUFA (g/100 g)	Key PUFAs present (mg/100 g)	Notes
Mackerel (Atlantic)	Fish (fatty)	32.1% of total fat	13.89	4.46	EPA: 504, DHA: 699	One of the highest sources of omega-3 FAs (Salma et al., 2016).
Anchovy (European)	Fish (fatty)	31.4% of total fat	4.84	1.52	EPA: 538, DHA: 647	Small fish are often consumed whole; very high EPA/DHA concentration relative to size (Karslı et al., 2025).
Salmon (Atlantic, wild)	Fish (fatty)	38.2% of total fat	6.34	2.42	EPA: 411, DHA: 1104	Wild salmon has a slightly different profile than farmed, often with a higher ratio of DHA (Fabian et al., 2015).
Salmon (Atlantic, farmed)	Fish (fatty)	36% of total fat	13.42	4.83	EPA: 862, DHA: 1447	Farmed salmon is often higher in total fat and total PUFAs due to the feed (Fabian et al., 2015).
Sardine (Pacific)	Fish (fatty)	37.9% of total fat	6.31	2.39	EPA: 473, DHA: 740	Highly sustainable source of marine PUFAs.
Tuna (bluefin)	Fish (fatty)	33.2% of total fat	4.9	1.63	EPA: 363, DHA: 890	Highly variable depending on the cut (e.g., toro vs lean) (Fabian et al., 2015).
Herring (Atlantic)	Fish (fatty)	20.2% of total fat	9.04	1.83	EPA: 523, DHA: 805	Often pickled or smoked; excellent source of EPA (Fabian et al., 2015).
Seabass (European, farmed)	Fish (lean/farmed)	29.9% of total fat	4.75	1.42	EPA: 278, DHA: 506	Farmed seabass has higher fat content than wild, boosting PUFA levels (Fabian et al., 2015; Tsopelakos et al., 2021).
Cod (Atlantic)	Fish (lean)	30.5% of total fat	0.67	0.2	EPA:38, DHA: 100	Low in total fat, so total PUFAs are low despite the high percentage in fat (Fabian et al., 2015).
Haddock	Fish (lean)	31% of total fat	0.6	0.19	EPA:35, DHA: 92	Similar to cod, lean white fish.
Shrimp	Crustacean	36.1% of total fat	0.51	0.18	EPA: 68, DHA: 70	Low in total fat, but the fat they have is highly polyunsaturated (Fabian et al., 2015; Traina et al., 2024).
Mussels (blue)	Mollusk	35.8% of total fat	1.79	0.64	EPA: 129, DHA: 202	Bivalves are good sources of marine PUFAs with a lower ecological footprint.
Oysters (Eastern, wild)	Mollusk	34.4% of total fat	1.26	0.43	EPA:122, DHA: 103	Highly variable by season; generally, a good source of EPA (Fabian et al., 2015).
Squid	Mollusk	28% of total fat	1.07	0.30	EPA: 56, DHA: 195	Often consumed fried, which alters the fat profile.

(Continued)

TABLE 26.1 (Continued)

Source	Type	PUFA level	Total fat (g/100 g)	Total PUFA (g/100 g)	Key PUFAs present (mg/100 g)	Notes
Krill oil	Crustacean	Variable	~100	~30	EPA, DHA	PUFAs are bound to phospholipids, which may enhance absorption.
Cod liver oil	Fish oil	22.5% of total fat	100	22.5	EPA:6897, DHA: 10768	A concentrated supplement source, also high in vitamin A and D.
Seaweed (kelp, raw)	Algae	45% of total fat	0.56	0.25	Trace amounts	Low in total fat, small amount of EPA.

conversion capabilities (Ouyang et al., 2016). The plant-based route (e.g., flax, soybean) contends with issues of land use change, water consumption, and pesticide use. Considering these factors, plant seeds containing PUFAs are being explored for commercial production of vegan n-3 PUFAs (Adarme-Vega et al., 2012) (see Fig. 26.3

Flaxseed (*Linum usitatissimum*) or linseed, is one of the rich plant sources of the omega-3 fatty acid ALA, with ALA comprising approximately 50%–60% of its total fatty acids. The oil content of flaxseed typically ranges from 40%–45%, making it a premier source of plant-based omega-3 for both human consumption and industrial applications.

Soybean (*Glycine max*) is the world's most extensively farmed oilseed crop, with an oil content of approximately 18%–22%. Soybean oil contains both LA (approximately 50%–55% of total fatty acids) and ALA (approximately 6%–10%), providing a balanced source of omega-6 and omega-3 PUFAs.

Rapeseed (*Brassica napus*) and its derivative canola are major oilseed crops with oil contents ranging from 40%–45%. Canola oil is valued for its favorable fatty acid profile, containing approximately 19% LA and 9% ALA, with low saturated fat content.

Sunflower (*Helianthus annuus*) and **safflower (*Carthamus tinctorius*)** are rich sources of LA, with traditional varieties containing 65%–70% LA in their oils. These oils are important dietary sources of omega-6 PUFAs.

Peanut (*Arachis hypogaea*) and **sesame (*Sesamum indicum*)** also contribute significant amounts of PUFAs to the human diet, primarily in the form of LA, with their oil contents ranging from 45%–50% (Yang et al., 2025).

Chia seeds (*Salvia hispanica*) have gained popularity as a rich plant source of ALA, with approximately 60% of their oil content being ALA. The seeds themselves contain 25%–35% oil, making them an excellent whole-food source of omega-3.

Perilla (*Perilla frutescens*), an herb cultivated primarily in Asia, produces seeds with oil containing up to 60% ALA, rivaling flaxseed as an omega-3 source.

Walnuts (*Juglans regia*) are notable among tree nuts for their high PUFA content, with approximately 70% of their fat being PUFAs, predominantly LA and ALA.

Hemp seeds (*Cannabis sativa*) contain approximately 25%–35% oil, with a favorable ratio of LA to ALA (approximately 3:1) and the presence of minor amounts of other PUFAs.

Garden cress (*Lepidium sativum*L.) seed oil has recently gained attention as a promising vegan source of PUFAs. Research by Dhara et al. (2023) demonstrated that garden cress seed oil extraction using hexane yields approximately 38% PUFA content. Optimized supercritical carbon dioxide (SC-CO_2) extraction with 350 bar pressure, a temperature of 60°C, and a flow rate of 30 g/min, the PUFA concentration can be increased to almost 50%. Under these approximate conditions, the tocopherol levels significantly increased from 486 to 1138 ppm, and the oil is enriched with unsaponifiable components (2.3%) like phytosterols. The advantages of the SC-CO_2 extraction method are that it eliminates the necessity for the use of toxic solvents like hexane, operates at a lower temperature than traditional methods, which minimizes oxidative degradation and enables selective extraction of desired compounds. Significantly, SC-CO_2 extraction targets oil extraction specifically, while discarding phospholipids, thereby removing a refining step and rendering the process cost-effective (Dhara et al., 2023).

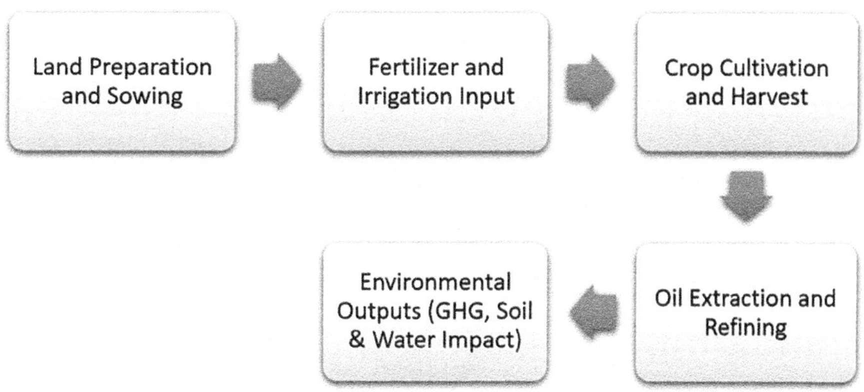

FIGURE 26.3 Environmental inputs in plant-based polyunsaturated fatty acid production.

26.6.1 Microalgae: primary producers of polyunsaturated fatty acids

As we all are aware that marine organisms like fish and shrimp are high in PUFAs, since they consume microalgae. The limitations of traditional marine and plant-based sources have propelled significant research and development into alternative, more sustainable methods for PUFA production. Microalgae have turned out to be a highly promising and sustainable "bio factory" for producing diverse high-value bioactive compounds, including n-3 and n-6 PUFAs (Santos-Sánchez et al., 2016; Ummalyma et al., 2019; Mukherjee et al., 2024; Ward & Singh, 2005).

Production of microalgae involves two pathways: desaturation and elongation pathways. Desaturation pathways involve desaturases, which introduce double bonds in the chain. Next, the elongases elongate the chain. Factors like temperature, nutrients (nitrogen and phosphorus), light intensity, salinity, and carbon dioxide supply affect the production of microalgae. The disadvantages are that the production cost of microalgae is higher due to extraction, and a controlled environment is needed for their culture (Zakaria et al., 2025). The most promising sustainable solution lies in advanced algal oil production, which bypasses many of these issues by producing key PUFAs like EPA and DHA directly from microalgae in controlled bioreactors. The major species cultured are *Phaeodactylum tricornutum, Chlorella vulgaris, Dunaliella sp, Nannochloropsis oceanica,* etc.

Membrane components and storage lipids are the major classes of lipids in algae, which vary depending on the algae. The overall fatty acid profile varies due to growth conditions, seasons, and developmental stages. Algae can be grown even in deserts, saltwater, and wastewater, and even orders of magnitude are far higher than traditional oilseed crops. Algal oil is absolutely pure, vegan, and also marine contaminants are not found Fig. 26.4

These unicellular organisms offer several advantages over traditional marine sources:

1. **Sustainability and scalability**: Microalgae cultivation can be carried out in controlled environments, reducing reliance on finite marine resources and minimizing ecosystem disruption. They are considered a scalable solution to address current and future shortages of food and nutrition (Mukherjee et al., 2024).
2. **Reduced environmental footprint**: Heterotrophic cultivation of microalgae for PUFA has substantially fewer EI than fish-based sources, as demonstrated by the life cycle assessment studies (Togarcheti & Padamati, 2021). To demonstrate this point, the primary energy demand and EI of heterotrophic PUFA production from microalgae are

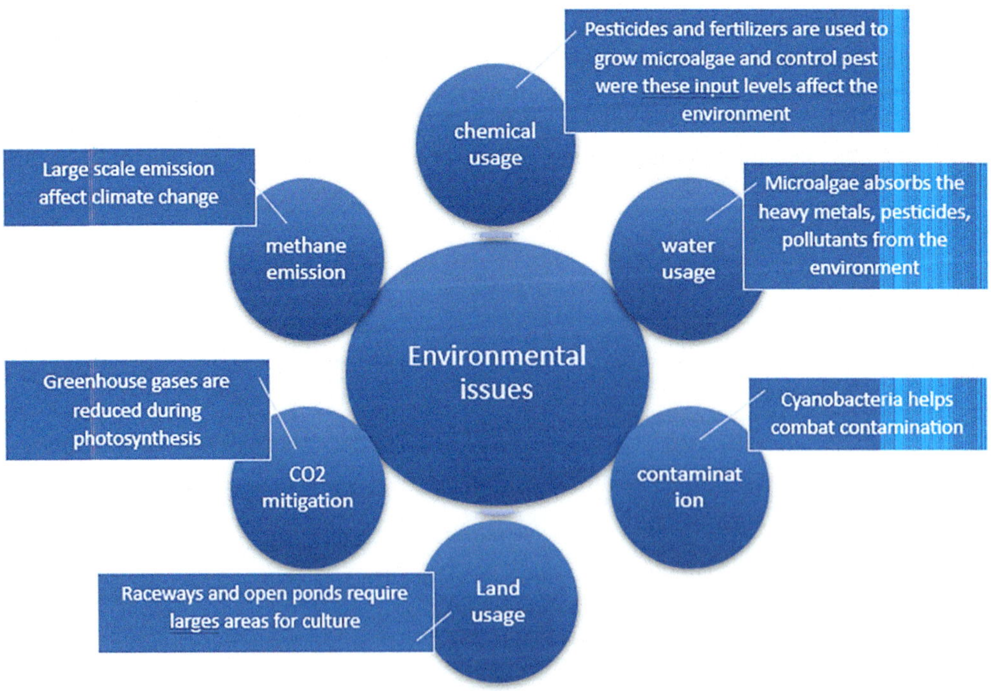

FIGURE 26.4 Environmental issues related to the use of microalgal sources of polyunsaturated fatty acid.

noticeably lower compared to photoautotrophy and fish oil production (Togarcheti & Padamati, 2021). This includes reduced carbon footprints, land use, and freshwater consumption (Qin et al., 2023).

3. **High purity and quality**: Microalgae-derived PUFAs offer higher purity and are less susceptible to contamination by persistent environmental pollutants compared to fish oils (Mukherjee et al., 2024). The ability to control cultivation conditions allows for tailoring the fatty acid profile and minimizing undesirable compounds (Santos-Sánchez et al., 2016).
4. **Vegan-friendly option**: Microbial PUFAs provide a vegan-friendly alternative for consumers who avoid animal products (Mukherjee et al., 2024).

26.7 Biosynthetic pathway for marine polyunsaturated fatty acids

26.7.1 Aerobic fatty acid synthase pathway

The aerobic pathway, found in microalgae, fungi, plants, and most aerobic microorganisms, requires molecular oxygen and involves a series of desaturase and elongase enzymes. This pathway begins with saturated fatty acids (typically C16:0 palmitic acid) synthesized by the fatty acid synthase complex, which contains multiple catalytic domains are acyl carrier protein (ACP), ketoacyl synthase (KS), ketoacyl reductase (KR), malonyl palmitoyl transferase, dehydratase (DH), enoyl reductase (ER) and thioesterase (Tian et al., 2024). The synthesis proceeds through iterative cycles of condensation, reduction, and dehydration. Desaturases add double bonds at designated locations, with Δ9, Δ12, and Δ15 desaturases progressively transforming stearic acid into oleic acid, linoleic acid, and α-linolenic acid. There are two primary pathways for synthesizing PUFAs: the Δ6 pathway, which employs Δ6 desaturase to convert substrates into γ-linolenic acid and stearidonic acid, followed by elongation and Δ5 desaturation to generate arachidonic acid and EPA; and the Δ8 pathway, mainly occurring in protists, that utilizes Δ9 elongase followed by Δ8 desaturase to reach the same intermediates (Tian et al., 2024).

26.7.2 Anaerobic polyunsaturated fatty acid synthase pathway

The anaerobic pathway, referred to as the PUFA synthase or PKS-like pathway, functions both in the presence and absence of oxygen, and is commonly found in marine bacteria as well as certain eukaryotic microalgae. This pathway is deemed more energy-efficient compared to the aerobic method, as it requires a lower amount of NADPH to synthesize long-chain PUFAs. PUFA synthases are large enzyme complexes made up of multiple subunits, usually comprising three or four subunits (identified as PfaA, PfaB, PfaC, etc.) that contain various catalytic domains. These domains include ACP, malonyl-CoA: ACP transacylase, DH, ER, acyltransferase, KS, KR, and chain length factor domains. The biosynthetic pathway begins with acetyl-ACP and involves successive cycles of condensation, ketoreduction, dehydration, and enoyl reductions, with the domain structures influencing the ultimate length of the fatty acid chain and the arrangement of double bonds. Research on the marine bacterium *Photobacterium profundum* has revealed that the PUFA synthase genes are clustered and coordinately regulated, with five genes (pfaA through pfaE) encoding the complete biosynthetic machinery. Interestingly, some studies have demonstrated a linkage between PUFA biosynthesis and polyunsaturated hydrocarbon production, mediated by enzymes like OleA that interact with ACP domains to divert intermediates toward alternative products (Tian et al., 2024) (see Table 26.2).

The growing of conventional oilseed crops also brings about various environmental issues, such as alterations in fertilizer use, pesticide use, land use, and water usage, which may lead to soil degradation, water contamination, and GHG emissions (Rizzo et al., 2023). While these impacts are different from those of marine sourcing, they still necessitate careful consideration in a comprehensive sustainability assessment.

26.7.3 Biosynthetic pathways for plant polyunsaturated fatty acids

The bacterial type II fatty acid synthase system in plants produces fatty acids in the plastids. Acetyl-CoA carboxylase starts the process by carboxylating acetyl-CoA to malonyl-CoA. The developing acyl chain is subsequently extended by two carbons in each of the repetitive cycles of condensation, reduction, dehydration, and more reduction that are catalyzed by the fatty acid synthase complex. Palmitic acid and stearic acid bound to ACP are the main products of this process. Stearoyl-ACP Δ9 desaturase can desaturate stearoyl-ACP before it is released, resulting in oleoyl-ACP (18:1Δ9). These acyl-ACP molecules are then hydrolyzed by fatty acyl-ACP Thioesterases, releasing free fatty acids that are exported from the plastid to the ER for further modification and incorporation into complex lipids (Yang et al., 2025).

TABLE 26.2 Detailed polyunsaturated fatty acid (PUFA) levels in various marine-derived sources and their uses.

Source	Type	Total PUFA (g/100 g)	Notes
Flaxseed oil (linseed)	Oil	67.8	One of the most loaded plant sources of omega-3 ALA. The n-6:n-3 ratio is low (0.2:1) (Rizzo et al., 2023).
Chia seeds (dried)	Seed	~23.7	Whole seeds are excellent sources of ALA (Rizzo et al., 2023).
Hemp seed (hulled)	Seed	~36	Provides a good balance of n-6 and n-3 with a ratio of 3:1.
Walnuts (dried/ grounded)	Nut	63.3 as oil	Walnut oil is rich in PUFA.
Soybean oil	Oil	57.7	A very common cooking oil high in omega-6 LA (Rizzo et al., 2023).
Sunflower oil	Oil	40.1–62	Values are significantly based on standards (Rizzo et al., 2023).
Corn oil	Oil	54.68	Omega-6 linoleic acid is predominantly present (Meyer et al., 2003).
Cottonseed oil	Oil	51.9	High in omega-6 LA but less in ALA.
Canola oil	Oil	28.1	Often considered a balanced oil with n-3 and n-6 (Rizzo et al., 2023).
Wheat germ oil	Oil	~60.4	55.1 g omega-6 LA/100 g but moderate ALA.
Olive oil	Oil	10.5	Celebrated for its monounsaturated fat (Meyer et al., 2003).
Coconut oil	Oil	1.7–3	Predominantly composed of saturated fats (Meyer et al., 2003).

26.7.4 Aerobic desaturation pathway

The conversion of oleic acid to PUFAs occurs while the fatty acids are esterified to glycerolipids, primarily phosphatidylcholine (PC) in the ER or monogalactosyldiacylglycerol (MGDG) in the plastids. Biosynthesis of linoleic acid: The introduction of the second double bond at the Δ12 position converts oleic acid to linoleic acid. This reaction is catalyzed by Δ12 desaturases (oleoyl desaturases), which are membrane-bound enzymes that use cytochrome b5 as an electron donor. In the ER pathway, the FAD2 gene encodes the microsomal Δ12 desaturase that acts on oleoyl groups esterified to PC. In the plastidial pathway, the FAD6 gene encodes a Δ12 desaturase that acts on oleoyl groups attached to MGDG and other chloroplast lipids. Biosynthesis of α-Linolenic Acid: The introduction of the third double bond at the Δ15 position, α-linolenic acid converted from linoleic acid. This reaction is catalyzed by omega-3 desaturases (linoleoyl desaturases), which introduce a double bond three carbons from the methyl end. Three genes encode omega-3 desaturases in plants: FAD3 (ER-localized), FAD7 (plastid-localized, constitutively expressed), and FAD8 (plastid-localized, cold-inducible). These enzymes act on linoleoyl groups esterified to lipids, producing ALA.

26.8 Sustainability of plant-based polyunsaturated fatty acids

Plant-derived omega-3s decrease the environmental footprint compared to fish-based diets. Genetically modified oil crops protect biodiversity by reducing the pressure on wild fish populations and the depletion of marine resources. Microalgae fermentation and seeds rich in PUFAs generate emits low GHG in comparison with fish oil production. They are found to be a safer and cleaner profile of nutrition since pollutant bioaccumulation is not found (Napier & Betancor, 2023). Waste materials like molasses hydrolysates, which are used as substrates for the growth of algae and microbes, by which valuable nutrients are produced from ecological liabilities. Bioengineered crops and algal production eliminate the risk of contamination by heavy metals, which is a very common problem in marine sources (Napier & Betancor, 2023).

Because of the existing agricultural infrastructure, transgenic oilseed crops have an added advantage of high scalability that can replace fish oil production faster than any other alternatives. The major disadvantage is the consumer acceptance of genetically modified crops, which requires communication, transport, and consumers in markets. The lowest carbon footprint can only be produced through microalgae cultivation. The contrast between autotrophic and heterotrophic production is that traditional pond cultivation, that is, autotrophic, involves less control, whereas the latter involves an organic carbon source in the dark, requiring less space.

Large-scale cultivation drives deforestation, leading to biodiversity loss and the release of carbon from forests. Intensive water supply is required for cultivation of a few oilseed crops; for instance, significant stress is created because of soy cultivation. Additionally, a large amount of pesticides and fertilizers are added, leading to degradation of soil, water eutrophication. Drastically, there is a reduction in huge varieties of species due to cultivation of a single crop in bulk quantities.

26.9 Comparative sustainability assessment

Several key themes emerge regarding the comparative sustainability of marine and plant-derived PUFA sources from the available evidence:

Climate impact: When integrated with waste valorization, microalgae-based PUFA synthesis emits less GHG than fish oil. The use of renewable energy in cultivation systems can further reduce climate impacts, though a comprehensive assessment must consider trade-offs across multiple impact categories.

Resource efficiency: Microalgae cultivated heterotrophically achieve excess productivity per unit land area by utilizing waste streams as feedstocks. Transgenic oilseed crops offer high resource efficiency across large land areas influenced by existing agricultural infrastructure and photosynthetic capacity, potentially.

Biodiversity: Microalgae and plant-based systems, at the same time, avoid direct pressure on marine ecosystems by reducing the biodiversity impacts associated with fish oil production. This is particularly crucial since fishmeal from small pelagic fish reduces their availability for artisanal fishing catches and marine wildlife feed, which support food security in low-income coastal nations.

Water use: LCA studies indicate that microalgae-based protein production can have lower water use impacts than fishmeal. Circular systems that repurpose water for irrigation or integrate algae cultivation with wastewater treatment promote responsible water management.

Land use: The one impact category where fishmeal outperforms microalgae is land use. Microalgae cultivation requires land area for ponds or photobioreactors, while fishmeal production utilizes ocean areas that are not typically accounted for in land use metrics. Transgenic oilseed crops similarly require agricultural land, creating potential competition with food production.

Pollution and toxicity: Plant-based systems avoid the accumulation of marine contaminants such as persistent organic pollutants and heavy metals. However, they may introduce other environmental trade-offs, such as fertilizer runoff and pesticide use in agricultural systems (McKuin et al., 2023; Thi et al., 2025; Togarcheti & Padamati, 2021).

26.10 Future directions and research needs

26.10.1 Technological optimization

Continued research improves the productivity and efficiency of both marine and plant-based PUFA production systems. For microalgae, priorities include strain improvement through adaptive evolution and genetic engineering, optimization of cultivation parameters (temperature, salinity, nutrient composition), and development of more energy-efficient harvesting and extraction technologies. The finding that lower temperatures enhance omega-3 production suggests opportunities for process optimization in temperate regions. For transgenic oilseeds, priorities include developing more efficient transformation methods, optimizing gene expression cassettes, and selecting elite germplasm with enhanced agronomic performance. Recent breakthroughs in n-3 LC-PUFA oilseed production provide a foundation for continued improvement (Lee Chang & Nichols, 2024).

26.10.2 Integration with circular bioeconomy

The most promising sustainability pathways involve integration with circular economy systems. This includes utilizing agricultural and food processing by products as fermentation feedstocks, coupling algae cultivation with renewable energy generation, and designing biorefinery approaches that coproduce multiple value-added products from microbial or plant biomass. The convergence of marine and plant-based approaches—using plant-derived waste streams to cultivate marine microalgae—exemplifies the integrated thinking needed for sustainable production. Similarly, the use of vegetative crop residues for insect production demonstrates how diverse biomass streams can be valorized (Patel et al., 2019).

26.10.3 Comprehensive sustainability assessment

Future research should employ comprehensive sustainability assessment frameworks that consider multiple environmental impact categories, economic viability, and social implications. Life cycle assessment should be expanded to include biodiversity impacts, water footprint, and social indicators such as food security implications for coastal communities. Standardized methodologies would facilitate comparison across production systems and guide policy decisions.

26.10.4 Regulatory and market development

Realizing the sustainability potential of alternative PUFA sources requires supportive regulatory frameworks and market development. This includes streamlined approval processes for safe and effective products, clear labeling standards, and policies that internalize the environmental costs of conventional fish oil production. Regulatory insights from recent oilseed production breakthroughs will be valuable as products move toward commercialization (Lee Chang & Nichols, 2024).

26.11 Conclusion

Marine-derived PUFA, particularly EPA and DHA, are essential nutrients with well-documented health benefits that position them as increasingly important components of functional foods and nutraceuticals. While traditional fish oil production from small species and processing by products has served as the primary source for decades, concerns over sustainability, environmental impact, and product quality are driving a fundamental transformation of the industry. The emergence of microbial production platforms, particularly using thraustochytrids and other marine microorganisms, represents a paradigm shift toward controlled, scalable, and environmentally sustainable PUFA production. Understanding the distinct biosynthetic aerobic FAS pathway and anaerobic PUFA synthase pathway has enabled metabolic engineering strategies that enhance yields and expand product profiles. Recent advances in bioprocess engineering, including chemical inhibitor strategies and abiotic stress manipulation, have demonstrated significant improvements in PUFA productivity. Furthermore, the development of transgene-free genome editing technologies opens new possibilities for tailored production of specific PUFAs, including rare fatty acids with potentially unique bioactivities.

References

Adarme-Vega, T. C., Lim, D. K., Timmins, M., Vernen, F., Li, Y., & Schenk, P. M. (2012). Microalgal biofactories: A promising approach towards sustainable omega-3 fatty acid production. *Microbial Cell Factories, 11*(1), 96.

Bajpai, P. K., Bajpai, P., & Ward, O. P. (1992). Optimisation of culture conditions for production of eicosapentaenoic acid by Mortierella elongate NRRL 5513. *Journal of Industrial Microbiology and Biotechnology, 9*(1), 11–17.

Bazinet, R. P., & Layé, S. (2014). Polyunsaturated fatty acids and their metabolites in brain function and disease. *Nature Reviews. Neuroscience, 15*(12), 771–785.

Burns-Whitmore, B., Froyen, E., Heskey, C., Parker, T., & San Pablo, G. (2019). Alpha-linolenic and linoleic fatty acids in the vegan diet: Do they require dietary reference intake/adequate intake special consideration? *Nutrients, 11*, 2365.

Chi, G., Xu, Y., Cao, X., Li, Z., Cao, M., Chisti, Y., & He, N. (2022). Production of polyunsaturated fatty acids by *Schizochytrium* (*Aurantiochytrium*) *spp. Biotechnology Advances, 55*, 107897.

Dhara, O., Azmeera, T., Eanti, A., & Chakrabarti, P. P. (2023). Garden cress oil as a vegan source of PUFA: Achieving through optimized supercritical carbon dioxide extraction. *Innovative Food Science & Emerging Technologies, 84*, 103283.

Fabian, C. J., Kimler, B. F., & Hursting, S. D. (2015). Omega-3 fatty acids for breast cancer prevention and survivorship. *Breast Cancer Research, 17*(1), 62.

FSA Panel on Dietetic Products, Nutrition, and Allergies (NDA). (2010). Scientific opinion on dietary reference values for fats, including saturated fatty acids, polyunsaturated fatty acids, monounsaturated fatty acids, trans fatty acids, and cholesterol. *EFSA Journal, 8*, 1461.

Geissdoerfer, M., Savaget, P., Bocken, N. M., & Hultink, E. J. (2017). The circular economy–A new sustainability paradigm? *Journal of Cleaner Production, 143*, 757–768.

Harris, W. S. (2009). The omega-3 index: From biomarker to risk marker to risk factor. *Current Atherosclerosis Reports, 11*, 411.

Harris, W. S., & von Schacky, C. (2004). The omega-3 index: A new risk factor for death from coronary heart disease? *Preventive Medicine, 39*, 212–220.

Ishibashi, Y., Tanimura, R., Ataka, Y., Kumagai, A., Honda, D., Ito, M., & Okino, N. (2025). Transgene-free protein-based genome editing in thraustochytrids enables customizable modulation of long-chain polyunsaturated fatty acid profiles. *Chemical Engineering Journal*, 171156.

John, R. M., Raj, A. L. T., Dinakarkumar, Y., Romauld, S. I., Selvaraj, A., Siddiqui, N., & Radhakrishnan, M. (2025). Marine lipids: A review of sources, extraction methods, characterization, and food applications. *Food and Humanity*, 100945.

Karslı, B., Öğretmen, Ö. Y., & Emanet, M. (2025). Proximate composition, fatty acid characteristics, and amino acid profile of European anchovy (Engraulis encrasicolus L. 1758): Monthly and seasonal influences. *Frontiers in Nutrition, 12*, 1684958.

Lane, K. E., Wilson, M., Hellon, T. G., & Davies, I. G. (2021). Bioavailability and conversion of plant-based sources of omega-3 fatty acids—A scoping review to update supplementation options for vegetarians and vegans. *Critical Reviews in Food Science and Nutrition*, 1–16.

Lee Chang, K. J., & Nichols, P. D. (2024). Marine biotechnology for sustainability of ecologically significant resources. *Sustainability, 16*(23), 10664.

Lee, J. H., O'keefe, J. H., Lavie, C. J., & Harris, W. S. (2009). Omega-3 fatty acids: Cardiovascular benefits, sources and sustainability. *Nature Reviews Cardiology, 6*(12), 753–758.

Literáková, P., Zavřel, T., Búzová, D., Kaštánek, P., & Červený, J. (2024). Marine microalgae Schizochytrium demonstrates strong production of essential fatty acids in various cultivation conditions, advancing dietary self-sufficiency. *Frontiers in Nutrition, 11*, 1290701.

Lucas, S., Soler, L. G., Irz, X., Gascuel, D., Aubin, J., & Cloâtre, T. (2021). The environmental impact of the consumption of fishery and aquaculture products in France. *Journal of Cleaner Production, 299*, 126718.

Maurer, N. E., Hatta-Sakoda, B., Pascual-Chagman, G., & Rodriguez-Saona, L. E. (2012). Characterization and authentication of a novel vegetable source of omega-3 fatty acids, sacha inchi (*Plukenetia volubilis* L.) oil. *Food Chemistry, 134*(2), 1173–1180.

McKuin, B., Kapuscinski, A. R., Sarker, P. K., Cheek, N., Lim, J., & Sabarsky, M. (2023). Comparative life cycle assessment of marine microalgae, *Nannochloropsis* sp. and fishmeal for sustainable protein ingredients in aquaculture feeds. *Elementa: Science of the Anthropocene, 11*(1), 00083.

Meyer, B. J., Mann, N. J., Lewis, J. L., Milligan, G. C., Sinclair, A. J., & Howe, P. R. (2003). Dietary intakes and food sources of omega-6 and omega-3 polyunsaturated fatty acids. *Lipids, 38*(4), 391–398.

Mukherjee, S., Mohanty, A. K., Rao, U., & Poddar, A. (2024). Microbial polyunsaturated fatty acids (PUFAs) for human health: A comprehensive review of evidence from in vivo preclinical models. *Discover Applied Sciences, 6*(10). https://doi.org/10.1007/s42452-024-06238-w.

Napier, J. A., & Betancor, M. B. (2023). Engineering plant-based feedstocks for sustainable aquaculture. *Current Opinion in Plant Biology, 71*, 102323.

Nitkiewicz, T., & Cappelletti, G. M. (2022). Verification of circular economy solutions and sustainability of products with life cycle assessment. In *Sustainable products in the circular economy*. Routledge, 36–52.

Oliver, L., Dietrich, T., Marañón, I., Villarán, M. C., & Barrio, R. J. (2020). Producing omega-3 polyunsaturated fatty acids: A review of sustainable sources and future trends for the EPA and DHA market. *Resources, 9*(12), 148.

Ouyang, X., Zhou, T., Li, S., Zhang, P., Gan, R., & Li, H. (2016). Resources and bioactivities of polyunsaturated fatty acids. *International Journal of Modern Biology and Medicine, 7*(1), 1–11.

Patel, A., Matsakas, L., Hrůzová, K., Rova, U., & Christakopoulos, P. (2019). Biosynthesis of nutraceutical fatty acids by the oleaginous marine microalgae Phaeodactylum tricornutum utilizing hydrolysates from organosolv-pretreated birch and spruce biomass. *Marine Drugs, 17*(2), 119.

Pigott, G. M. (1967). *Production of fish oil* (277). US Department of the Interior, Fish and Wildlife Service, Bureau of Commercial Fisheries.

Qin, Z. H., Hu, X., Mou, J. H., He, G. H., Ye, G. B., Li, H. Y., & Wang, X. (2023). Environmental profiling microalgae-based eicosapentaenoic acid production along the technical advancement via life cycle assessment. *Journal of Cleaner Production, 397*, 136477.

Rizzo, G., Baroni, L., & Lombardo, M. (2023). Promising sources of plant-derived polyunsaturated fatty acids: A narrative review. *International Journal of Environmental Research and Public Health, 20*(3), 1683.

Rubio-Rodríguez, N., Beltrán, S., Jaime, I., de Diego, S. M., Sanz, M. T., & Carballido, J. R. (2010). Production of omega-3 polyunsaturated fatty acid concentrates: A review. *Innovative Food Science & Emerging Technologies, 11*(1), 1–12.

Saini, R. K., & Keum, Y. S. (2018). Omega-3 and omega-6 polyunsaturated fatty acids: Dietary sources, metabolism, and significance—A review. *Life Sciences, 203*, 255–267.

Salma, E. O., Cyrine, D., & Nizar, M. (2016). Fatty acids and amino acids contents in Scomber scombrus fillets from the South East of Tunisia. *African Journal of Biotechnology, 15*(24), 1246–1252.

Santos-Sánchez, N. F., Valadez-Blanco, R., Hernández-Carlos, B., Torres-Ariño, A., Guadarrama-Mendoza, P. C., & Salas-Coronado, R. (2016). Lipids rich in ω-3 polyunsaturated fatty acids from microalgae. *Applied Microbiology and Biotechnology, 100*(20), 8667–8684.

Sarter, B., Kelsey, K. S., Schwartz, T. A., & Harris, W. S. (2015). Blood docosahexaenoic acid and eicosapentaenoic acid in vegans: Associations with age and gender and effects of an algal-derived omega-3 fatty acid supplement. *Clinical Nutrition (Edinburgh, Scotland), 34*, 212–218.

Schulze, M. B., Minihane, A. M., Saleh, R. N. M., & Risérus, U. (2020). Intake and metabolism of omega-3 and omega-6 polyunsaturated fatty acids: Nutritional implications for cardiometabolic diseases. *Lancet Diabetes Endocrinol, 8*, 915–930.

Thi, S. S., Cokro, A. A., Santillan, E., Selão, T. T., Vethathirri, R. S., Case, R. J., & Wuertz, S. (2025). Reusing bioreactor effluent as a circular bioresource strategy for cultivating marine microalgae and producing Omega-3 polyunsaturated fatty acids. *Bioresource Technology*, 133433.

Thompson, M., Hein, N., Hanson, C., Smith, L. M., Anderson-Berry, A., Richter, C. K., Stessy Bisselou, K., Kusi Appiah, A., Kris-Etherton, P., Skulas-Ray, A. C., et al. (2019). Omega-3 fatty acid intake by age, gender, and pregnancy status in the United States: National health and nutrition examination survey 2003–2014. *Nutrients, 11*, 177.

Tian, L., Chi, G., Lin, S., Ling, X., & He, N. (2024). Marine microorganisms: Natural factories for polyunsaturated fatty acid production. *Blue Biotechnology, 1*(1), 15.

Tocher, D. (2009). Issues surrounding fish as a source of omega-3 long-chain polyunsaturated fatty acids. *Lipid Technology, 21*(1), 13–16. https://doi.org/10.1002/lite.200800079.

Togarcheti, S. C., & Padamati, R. B. (2021). Comparative life cycle assessment of EPA and DHA production from microalgae and farmed fish. *Clean Technologies, 3*(4), 699–710. https://doi.org/10.3390/cleantechnol3040042.

Traina, A., Quinci, E. M., Sabatino, N., Del Core, M., Bellante, A., Bono, G., & D'Agostino, F. (2024). Protein, essential amino acid, and fatty acid composition of five target fishery species of Central Mediterranean Sea. *Animals, 14*(15), 2158.

Tsopelakos, A., Zogopoulou, E., Panagiotaki, P., & Miliou, H. (2021). Combined effects of dietary n-3 long-chain polyunsaturated fatty acid levels and saturated to monounsaturated fatty acid ratios on growth, fillet composition and blood parameters of European sea bass, *Dicentrarchus labrax* L. *Aquaculture Research, 52*(11), 5213–5228.

Ummalyma, S. B., Sindhu, R., Binod, P., Pandey, A., & Gnansounou, E. (2019). Production and applications of polyunsaturated fatty acids. *High Value Fermentation Products, 2*, 2109.

Usher, S., Haslam, R. P., Ruiz-Lopez, N., Sayanova, O., & Napier, J. A. (2015). Field trial evaluation of the accumulation of omega-3 long chain polyunsaturated fatty acids in transgenic *Camelina sativa*: Making fish oil substitutes in plants. *Metabolic Engineering Communications, 2*, 93–98.

Wang, H., & Ding, J. (2021). Mechanism of polyunsaturated fatty acids biosynthesis and metabolism in marine invertebrates; a review.

Ward, O. P., & Singh, A. (2005). Omega-3/6 fatty acids: Alternative sources of production. *Process Biochemistry, 40*(12), 3627–3652.

West, A. L., Miles, E. A., Lillycrop, K. A., Napier, J. A., Calder, P. C., & Burdge, G. C. (2021). Genetically modified plants are an alternative to oily fish for providing n-3 polyunsaturated fatty acids in the human diet: A summary of the findings of a Biotechnology and Biological Sciences Research Council funded project. *Nutrition Bulletin, 46*(1), 60–68.

WHO. (2003). *WHO technical report series 916*. The World Health Organisation.

World health organisation (WHO). 1994. Fats and oils in human nutrition.

Yang, Z., Chen, Y., Ma, S., Zhang, M., Tang, T., & Du, C. (2025). Bioengineering of long-chain polyunsaturated fatty acids in oilseed crops. *Progress in Lipid Research, 99*, 101333.

Zakaria, M. F., Zaidi, F. N. A. M., Kamal, A. H. A., Aleng, N. A., Abd Wahid, M. E., Katayama, T., & Jusoh, M. (2025). PUFA from microalgae: Challenges, factors affecting high production and industrial application. *Aquaculture and Fisheries, 10*(4), 545–555.

Zheng, B., Wen, H., Zheng, B., Tang, S., Su, W., & Xiang, X. (2025). Current research on the processing, safety evaluation and functional properties of aquatic-derived lipids considering the sustainable processing of omega-3 polyunsaturated fatty acids: A critical review. *Critical Reviews in Food Science and Nutrition*, 1–19.

Zhou, X. R., Yao, Z. J., Benedicto, K., Nichols, P. D., Green, A., & Singh, S. (2023). New sustainable oil seed sources of omega-3 long-chain polyunsaturated fatty acids: A journey from the ocean to the field. *Sustainability, 15*(14), 11327.

Further reading

Mariamenatu, A. H., & Abdu, E. M. (2021). Overconsumption of omega-6 polyunsaturated fatty acids (PUFAs) versus deficiency of omega-3 PUFAs in modern-day diets: the disturbing factor for their "balanced antagonistic metabolic functions" in the human body. *Journal of Lipids, 2021*(1), 8848161.

Spreafico, F., Sales, R. C., Gil-Zamorano, J., Medeiros, P. D. C., Latasa, M. J., Lima, M. R., & Dávalos, A. (2018). Dietary supplementation with hybrid palm oil alters liver function in the common Marmoset. *Scientific Reports, 8*(1), 2765.

Tyagi, R., Rastogi, R. P., Babich, O., Awasthi, M. K., & Tiwari, A. (2023). New perspectives of omega-3 fatty acids from diatoms. *Systems Microbiology and Biomanufacturing, 4*(2), 528–541. https://doi.org/10.1007/s43393-023-00202-2.

Section VI

Advances in technology

Chapter 27

Emerging technologies and trends in polyunsaturated fatty acid research and application

Rama Prabha M.[1]**, Srinivasan Krishnamoorthy**[2]**, James Elegbeleye**[3]**, and Venkatachalapathy Natarajan**[4]

[1]*Vellore Institute of Technology, Vellore, Tamil Nadu, India,* [2]*National Institute of Food Technology Entrepreneurship and Management - Thanjavur, Thanjavur, Tamil Nadu, India,* [3]*University of Pretoria, Pretoria, South Africa,* [4]*National Institute of Food Technology Entrepreneurship and Management-Thanjavur, Thanjavur, Tamil Nadu, India*

27.1 Introduction

Polyunsaturated fatty acids (PUFAs) are important lipids for various physiological functions in the human body that include the cardiovascular and nervous systems, and are reported to help in the symptomatic relief of various diseases such as depression, arthritis, and asthma. PUFAs constitute commercial fatty acids such as omega-3 (n-3) and omega-6 (n-6). It has been decades since the recommended daily allowance of nutrients, specifically scientists, have suggested an optimal intake of n-6 PUFAs by adjusting the diet in such a way that there is a higher intake of n-3 PUFAs. However, despite having adequate knowledge about the nutritional aspects and the required diet balance of n-6 PUFAs by incorporation of n-3 fatty acids, the South Asian population has not been able to achieve the dietary balance, due to the large consumption of n-6 rich vegetable oils, which may be one of the contributing factors for the high level of metabolic inflammation seen in the urban Indian population (Zongo et al., 2021). Long-chain omega-3 fatty acids such as eicosapentaenoic acid (EPA; C20:5n-3) and docosahexaenoic acid (DHA; C22:6n-3) are the essential PUFAs that cannot be synthesized by higher organisms (Krishnamoorthy et al., 2021). They are very important for several human health functions, ranging from maintenance of cardiovascular health to providing symptomatic relief in conditions like depression, arthritis, and asthma, etc.

PUFAs are highly vulnerable to oxidative degradation as those compounds have multiple double bonds (Joseph et al., 2021). A hydroxyl radical (-OH) can remove a bis-allylic hydrogen and some O_2 and may result in the formation of a lipid peroxyl radical that kicks off the chain. Those peroxyls can grab an electron to form peroxides, which then break apart on their compound structure and subsequently decompose. The human body preserves arachidonate (ARA, omega-6) and docosahexaenoate (DHA, omega-3), where dropping levels of one ought to free up more radicals to disturb the other. In worst cases, these fatty acids may turn into nasty by-products such as reactive carbonyl compounds that can transform into lipid peroxidation end-products (Sambra et al., 2021). Hence, numerous research works and novel strategies that can protect PUFA from oxidative cleavage and decomposition are underway.

Human overexploitation of marine resources causes huge stress on aquatic ecosystem and would lead to unsustainable utilization of biological resources, contradicting the UN Sustainable Development Goals (Rodrigues et al., 2024). Moreover, there is also a high risk of mercury and other harmful substances, such as dioxins and lead, in fish-based lipids (Qin et al., 2023). Using insect-derived fish oil can avoid the odor developed from aquatic sources, which is a big concern for vegetarians.

As krill and cold-water fish resources decline over time, researchers have turned their attention to alternative sources such as bacteria, fungi, plants, and microalgae (Rethinavelu et al., 2023). Fungi capable of producing EPA/DHA are a possible substitute, but they are limited to the use of organic feedstocks and have longer culturing times. Plants are not considered as a viable farmland source to produce long-chain omega-3 fatty acids as they require extensive genetic

Omega-3 and Omega-6 Polyunsaturated Fatty Acids in Food Systems. DOI: https://doi.org/10.1016/B978-0-443-43810-3.00031-2

modifications for high-stable PUFA production. Microalgae are another viable source to produce DHA/EPA. They are one of the key primary producers of EPA/DHA in the marine food chain and are known to accumulate a large amount of EPA/DHA under varied light and nutrient conditions. Furthermore, the autotrophic strains of microalgae have the potential to capture CO_2 as they can be cultivated on marginal farmland with a shorter harvesting time compared to other sources, thereby giving higher productivity rates (Theagarajan et al., 2021).

The heterotrophic production of DHA for infant formulas and health mix applications has already been on a commercial scale by several companies. DHA is also commonly manufactured for other applications, such as pigments, vitamins, and feed applications, cosmetics, and pharma (Krishnamoorthy & Buys, 2025). However, the heterotrophic production of omega-3 fatty acids, specifically EPA, has not yet fulfilled the global needs for sustainable and clean sources. Scalable processes for heterotrophic EPA and DHA production that can meet the increasing global demand remain to be developed.

Hence, this chapter covers the following topics: (1) PUFAs' nutritional value and health-promoting functions; (2) the main issues with PUFA production and use, such as sustainability, instability, cost, and safety considerations; (3) investigating alternative sources and substrates for PUFA production with an emphasis on sustainability; (4) reviewing recent developments in extraction, stabilization, and delivery techniques that maintain PUFA quality and increase bioavailability; (5) summarizing advancements in genetic and metabolic engineering approaches for enhanced PUFA synthesis; and (6) identifying important areas for future research aimed at enabling large-scale, economical, and ecologically friendly PUFA production.

27.2 Nutritional significance of polyunsaturated fatty acid and its beneficial health effects

PUFAs are popularly known for their medicinal benefits, in particular cardiovascular protection. Many cohort studies have decoded the physiological mechanisms of omega-3 fatty acids, such as their capacity to reduce circulating low-density lipoprotein, very low-density lipoprotein (VLDL), and triglycerides (TG) (Jiang et al., 2021). Subsequently, it will reduce blood pressure and lessen the risk of cardiac arrhythmias. Moreover, the PUFAs have been an integral part of the cellular membranes, which are crucial for cellular signaling, transport processes, and many other molecular communications between and within the cells (Priyanka Yashwant et al., 2021). Furthermore, PUFAs such as EPA and DHA promote brain growth, especially in early child growth and in developing the cognitive abilities of the neural system throughout the entire lifetime. These essential fatty acids also play key roles in pregnancy and cut down the possibilities of neurodevelopment issues during the childhood stages (Rajput et al., 2023). Meanwhile, for older adults, PUFA can prevent prognosis of developing Alzheimer's or dementia-like late-stage diseases (Kumaravel & Srinivasan, 2017). Other beneficial health effects include support for stronger muscles, blood clotting, and nerve signals.

Considering the health benefits and ongoing research progress in PUFA's role in alleviating obesity, type 2 diabetes, rheumatoid arthritis, and some cancer diseases, nutrition advisors keep advocating the intake of PUFA-rich foods for long-term well-being.

27.3 Challenges in polyunsaturated fatty acid production and applications

PUFAs, particularly members of the omega-3 and omega-6 families, play crucial roles in human nutrition, health maintenance, and a range of industrial uses. Despite the numerous benefits and advantages of these essential fatty acids, large-scale production from a sustainability point of view is far from straightforward. The process is hindered by a combination of technical limitations, financial considerations, and regulatory requirements that must be addressed simultaneously. To provide a structured perspective, this section discusses the key bottlenecks under five closely linked themes: production sustainability, oxidative instability, downstream recovery and purification, techno-economic limitations, and possible adverse effects (Table 27.1).

27.3.1 Sustainability of polyunsaturated fatty acid production

PUFAs are available from several sources, which include marine fish, microalgae, certain fungus species, and genetically modified oilseed crops. The prevailing source of global production of PUFAs has traditionally been from fish oil, which accounts for the highest abundance of EPA and DHA. However, current demands for PUFAs have been increased by the depletion of natural stocks, pollution, and the overremoval of fish, thus creating a need to find other sources in the near future (Qin et al., 2023).

TABLE 27.1 Major challenges in the production sustainability of polyunsaturated fatty acids (PUFAs).

Challenge area	Key factors	Recent insights	References
Sustainability of production	Marine fish, microalgae, fungi, and transgenic crops	Fish oil dominates (>1 million tonnes/year), but depleted stocks and contamination drive alternatives; microalgal production is ~20,000 tonnes/year currently.	Qin et al. (2023)
Biomass availability and demand	Supply constraints, market growth, and industrial scale-up	Global PUFA market valued > USD 6 billion; forecasted AA capacity ~410,000 tonnes (2025), omega-3 shortage >1 million tonnes yearly.	PUFA Market Size (2025)
Oxidative stability	PUFA structure with multiple double bonds	Life extension of PUFAs via encapsulation can reduce oxidation rate by up to 90%, improving shelf life considerably.	Karthik and Anandharamakrishnan (2016)
Downstream extraction & purification	Cell wall resistance, solvent use, complexity	Extraction accounts for 30%–50% of production cost; solvent removal > 99.9% purity demanded; up to 50%–80% energy savings possible using green methods.	Prasad et al. (2022)
Techno-economic constraints	Capital and operational expenditures	Capital expenditure and operating expenditure can comprise 60%–80% of overall cost; price ranges from €400–€1500/kg for EPA/DHA, up to €5000/kg for high-purity DHA.	Okeke et al. (2022)
Regulatory and safety issues	Pollutants, contaminants	Heavy metals like mercury in fish oils often exceed permissible limits by >10%; algal oils show undetectable levels.	Brodziak-Dopierała et al. (2023)
Consumer acceptance and market dynamics	GMO concerns, acceptance	Up to 45% of consumers express hesitancy toward GMO-derived ingredients; labeling transparency improves acceptance by 30%.	Srinivasan and Kumaravel (2016)
Strain productivity and genetic engineering	Metabolic improvements, clustered regularly interspaced short palindromic repeats	Editing efficiencies >90% reported in microbial PUFA biosynthesis; genetically modified strains can double PUFA yield.	Shi et al. (2022)
Environmental impact and lifecycle	Resource consumption, carbon footprint	Algal PUFA production can cut greenhouse gas emissions by 80%–90% versus fish oil; water use is reduced by 50%.	Sahena et al. (2009)
Product formulation and delivery	Bioavailability, stability, innovative carriers	Nanoencapsulation improves bioavailability by 2–3x; layered emulsions can extend PUFA shelf life from weeks to months.	Karthik and Anandharamakrishnan (2016)

27.3.2 Biomass availability and demand pressure

The value of the worldwide PUFAs market has already exceeded USD 6 billion, and it is still increasing fast, mainly due to the rising use of pills, breakfast cereals, infant foods, and medicines (PUFA Market Size, 2025). The production from marine oils is still predominant, but not enough to satisfy the increasing demand. It is estimated that the global production capacity for Arachidonic acid will be about 410,000 tons in 2025, lower than the predicted demand and the deficiency of omega-3 PUFAs, which shall be more than 1 million tons/year (Qin et al., 2023). Microbes and microalgae as alternative sources could give higher outputs or volume ratio and would avoid overexhaustion of marine stocks. Life cycle analysis shows that, driven by an optimized microalgae system, airborne or waterborne greenhouse gases and resource consumption could be reduced by 80%–90%, without the risk of contamination by heavy metals or persistent organic pollutants as in fish oils (Wolf et al., 2024).

27.3.3 Oxidative stability of polyunsaturated fatty acids

Although the extensive unsaturation and double bonds of PUFAs give enormous health benefits, it also makes them chemically unstable. Exposure to oxygen, heat, light, or trace metals can trigger oxidation, producing lipid peroxides and undesirable metabolic breakdown products that negatively affect flavor, quality, and safety (Sahena et al., 2009). Ensuring stability during the entirety of extraction, transportation, and food or supplement processing is still a major challenge, particularly for DHA and other highly unsaturated lipids.

27.3.4 Downstream extraction and purification

The extraction and formulation of PUFAs for commercial application is a resource-intensive process that ultimately influences the cost and final product quality. The challenging part is the rigid cell walls of PUFA-rich sources such as microalgae and fungi. Intensive chemical and mechanical disruption processes are required to get high yield at economic rates. More importantly, different species of these eukaryotic microorganisms require tailored treatments, which limit the universal common process design. Meanwhile, the usage of solvents such as chloroform, hexane, and other nonpolar solvents can cause severe environmental and food safety hazards (Navina et al., 2025).

27.3.5 Purification complexity

The purification of PUFAs from biological sources generally necessitates sequential refinement steps. Some of the major techniques include molecular distillation, urea complexation, low-temperature crystallization, silver-ion complexation, and supercritical extraction, where each technique varies in efficiency, cost, and environmental impact. For example, though the silver-ion method is efficient in the separation of PUFAs, the opportunity for heavy metal contamination is equally high (Nida et al., 2024).

27.3.6 Techno-economic constraints

The economic affordability of PUFA production and market availability is influenced by both capital expenditure and operational expenditure. Notwithstanding, the biomass generation cost alone is estimated at around 60%–80% of total expenses, which are closely tied to the system scaling-up approach, growth rate, nutrient supply, and equipment expenditures. Current pricing can range from INR 43,000/kg of EPA/DHA sourced from algal or fish oil, whereas a very high-purity algal DHA supplements exceeding INR 540,000/kg (Ferreira et al., 2025).

Overall, growing and extraction of PUFAs that meet the global demand without compromising the safety and quality, keeping sustainability in focus, remains a challenge as well as future research scope. The key solution will be to align novel bioprocess engineering technologies with market and regulatory requirements to deliver sustainable, affordable, and high-quality omega-3 and omega-6 products.

27.4 Trends in substrates and sources of polyunsaturated fatty acid

Animal-derived and byproduct sources form the major traditional sources of PUFAs. The majority of these are from marine life, mostly from oily fish and krill (Wei et al., 2025a, 2025b). Besides the fact that the production of fish oils is resource-intensive and environmentally unsustainable, fish also bioaccumulate toxins. This has led to a paradigm shift towards microbially-derived PUFAs. This approach is more environmentally sustainable, using a combination of novel biotechnology tools such as precision fermentation, leveraging on synthetic biology tools such as clustered regularly interspaced short palindromic repeats (CRISPR) Cas9, which allows for controlled, all-year-round production of PUFAs from waste-derived substrates. Some of the strategies used in the production of these oils include the overexpression of critical enzymes, inhibition of competing metabolic pathways, and reprogramming the metabolism for enhanced accumulation of DHA/EPA using chemical inhibitors or abiotic cold (Duan et al., 2025). Fig. 27.1 depicts the trends and innovations in PUFA sources and production systems.

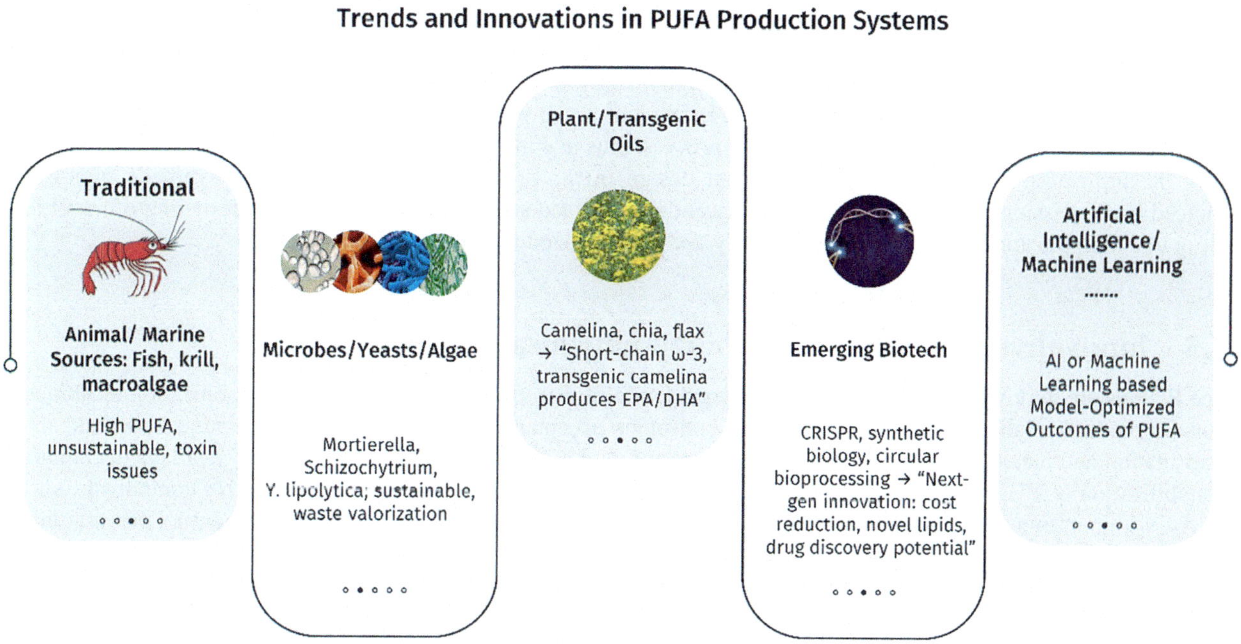

FIGURE 27.1 Trends and innovations in polyunsaturated fatty acid (PUFA) production systems.

An example of this shift is the production of omega-3 PUFAs, such as EPA and DHA, using alternative sources such as microalgae, fungi, and plant-based oils. Marine microbes such as *Shewanella* and *Vibrio* are important sustainable bioproducers of PUFAs. Other oleaginous microbes include some fungi and engineered yeasts such as *Yarrowia lipolytica* (Gemperlein et al., 2019). *Mortierella* fungi and *Aurantiochytrium* have been shown to accumulate approximately 30%–50% of their biomass as lipids, such as EPA-rich oil (Deeba et al., 2020; Kalidasan et al., 2021). These microorganisms can grow on inexpensive substrates, such as agro-industrial wastes, lignocellulosic hydrolysates, aquaculture by-products, and sometimes crude glycerol, making the option more attractive. Other sources include algal sources, such as microalgal strains, such as *Nannochloropsis*, *Phaeodactylum*, and *Schizochytrium*, which have been proven to bioaccumulate high concentrations of omega-3 lipids under optimized culture conditions (Duan et al., 2025).

A recent study confirmed that *Schizochytrium* fermentation yields a total of 50% approximately of EPA+DHA oil, comparable to fish-oil levels of long-chain PUFAs, hence its suitability and usage in the production of DHA-rich infant formula (Deeba et al., 2020). The advantage of the microalgal source for PUFAs is that it is perennial and can be easily cultivated in photobioreactors, producing PUFAs without the challenge of marine toxins. Macroalgae (such as seaweeds) are not often used in the biosynthesis of PUFAs because they produce only trace amounts of these compounds. Moreso, their fibrous nature and pigment-rich biomass also make the extraction process complicated. Nevertheless, innovative extraction techniques like microwave, supercritical, and ultrasound-assisted methods have been applied to improve the effectiveness and sustainability of extracting PUFAs from macroalgae (Carpena et al., 2023).

Unlike in microalgae, most terrestrial plant-derived PUFAs are short-chained (Määttänen et al., 2020). To address the issue of short-chain plant-derived PUFAs, transgenic oilseeds were developed that can accumulate approximately 11% EPA and 6% DHA in their seed oil. A good example of this transgenic plant is *Camelina sativa*. Human feeding trials showed that oil from such GM *Camelina* raises blood EPA+DHA levels as effectively as fish oil (West et al., 2020). Other examples of plant-derived PUFAs are from oilseeds like flax, chia, *Camelina*, *Perilla*, and *Sacha inchi*. These are rich in alpha-linolenic acid, an omega-3 that humans poorly metabolize into the more bioavailable EPA/DHA. Whereas *Echium* and *Buglossoides* accumulate stearidonic acid, which is a rare omega-3 that circumvents a metabolic step that is easily biotransformed into EPA (Saini et al., 2021).

Besides the innovations in the use of alternative sources such as microalgae in the biomanufacturing of PUFAs and the immense potential for scalability, there is a major challenge in the cost of the yeast-based fermentation media used in the process. This challenge is overcome using the valorization of waste streams into a low-cost feedstock in alignment with the principles of a circular bioeconomy. This approach was used in a recent study where cellular residues from

Aurantiochytrium and *Mortierella alpina* during the production of microbially-derived PUFAs were hydrolyzed enzymatically (Chauhan et al., 2023). The outcome was used as a nitrogen source during the fermentation of DHA and ARA instead of the expensive yeast medium, significantly reducing the cost by approximately 67% during DHA biomanufacturing. This innovative strategy utilizes a circular loop in which by-products from the growth process are later used as raw materials during the biomanufacturing process, thus making the process competitively economical. This trend shows the utilization of innovative and intelligent design in the production process, utilizing synthetic biology and advanced bioprocessing platforms. This trend transcends simple accumulation of PUFAs to the designing of novel lipids with potential applications in novel drug discovery and personalized nutrition (Yin et al., 2024).

27.5 Innovative techniques to stabilize polyunsaturated fatty acid

Since PUFAs are highly susceptible to oxidative degradation, it is imperative to develop some stabilization techniques to maintain product quality, nutritional value, and consumer acceptance. Such stabilization techniques include microencapsulation and nanoencapsulation. Though microencapsulation is a widely used, commercially available technique for the stabilization of PUFAs (Islam et al., 2023). Both techniques involve the enclosure of bioactive compounds, such as PUFAs, within carrier materials or matrices that form a protective barrier against environmental factors that may trigger the degradation (Khoshnoudi-Nia et al., 2022).

Fundamentally, the principle of microencapsulation involves the conversion of the unstable oil into a powder form, which makes it easier to incorporate into food products, thus protecting it from oxidation and loss of sensory properties. The process utilizes spray drying, which is a cost-effective method for producing microencapsulated products and is well-adapted for large-scale production (Srinivasan & Sivasubramanian, 2015). Other methods of microencapsulation are lyophilization/freeze drying and complex coacervation. Unlike spray drying, which involves the atomization of PUFA oil emulsion at high temperatures (100°C–300°C), freeze drying and complex coacervation do not involve high temperatures (Timilsena et al., 2017). Choosing between the methods of microencapsulation is a trade-off between spray drying, which presents the risks of thermal degradation. While spray drying presents an opportunity for industrial scalability and cost-efficiency, freeze drying, on the other hand, preserves the sensitive PUFAs but at a much higher cost and with a longer processing time. The optimal method, therefore, depends on the specific product requirements, the thermal sensitivity of the PUFA and other components, as well as economic considerations (Yang et al., 2024).

The effectiveness of the microencapsulation process outcome is not solely dependent on the method used, but also on the type of wall materials. The wall material must act as a robust barrier against oxygen, light, and moisture, while also contributing to the desired functional and sensory properties of the final product. Those wall materials are used as single or in combinations, and they include proteinaceous materials (e.g., sodium caseinate, whey protein, gelatin) and polysaccharide materials (e.g., maltodextrin, gum arabic, chitosan), with polysaccharide–protein–based wall materials proving to be more effective for fish oil (Khoshnoudi-Nia et al., 2022).

Conversely, nanoencapsulation represents the next level of PUFA delivery, tailor-made for enhanced delivery bioavailability and controlled release at the nanoscale level (typically below 100 nm), which normally alters the physicochemical properties of the encapsulated materials (Noore et al., 2024). The interactions between these lipophilic PUFAs and water matter in PUFA stability. Because the fatty acids have a higher surface area compared to their volume, their solubility in water improves a lot. This makes it easier to mix them into watery foods and drinks. But it's not just about solubility. These nanostructured carriers also protect the PUFAs from breaking down when exposed to heat or oxygen. That's a big deal because PUFAs are usually sensitive.

One of the main ways to deliver PUFAs like this is through nanoemulsions (Barradas & de Holanda e Silva, 2021). These are basically tiny droplets of oil spread out in water, held together by surfactants. Nanoemulsions help increase how well these compounds dissolve and get absorbed by the body. They make nanoemulsions using things like liposomes, solid lipid nanoparticles, and nanostructured lipid carriers. Notably, this method also allows combining omega-3s with other fat-loving compounds like vitamin D3 or alpha-tocopherol. This coencapsulation approach can create a kind of matrix effect, boosting the overall health benefits (Vieira et al., 2022). Hence, nanoemulsions not only improve solubility and absorption but also protect these sensitive compounds and help mix them with other useful nutrients. It's a neat way to get more out of PUFAs in food and supplements.

Besides the external encapsulation of PUFAs or PUFA-rich food products, other physical barrier methods have been developed and are usually based on proteins or polysaccharides. These include edible films and coatings. An external barrier technology that provides a direct surface-level defense, along with the internal stabilization of PUFAs, edible films can be incorporated with plant extracts that are rich in antioxidants to create an active packaging material. An edible film composed of whey protein was tested and proved to be very effective in reducing lipid oxidation in fish. It was also used to inhibit the growth of microorganisms in meat products and to reduce moisture loss (Shirai et al., 2025).

27.6 Novel delivery systems for polyunsaturated fatty acid

Generally, people need 0.25 to 2 g of EPA and DHA each day. The amount can go up or down with age, health, pregnancy, or if someone has a higher chance of heart problems (Van Dael, 2021). Many people do not get enough of this essential fatty acid from regular food. Even foods like fish oil only give about one-third of the lipid that people need in a normal diet (Lewis et al., 2025). This shortfall happens because many people do not eat fish. The amount of omega-3 in fish depends on the type and source of fish. These days, people across all generations prefer food with more PUFA. This change might directly affect the food environment as well as the economy. Hence, it becomes essential to find other options and supplements to get enough EPA and DHA. To bridge the gap in dietary intake, various chemical formulations of omega-3 fatty acids have been developed. These include fish oil TG, n-3 ethyl esters, and re-esterified fish oil TG synthesized chemically for achieving required dosages. While these formulations allow for concentrated doses, their handling poses serious challenges. Fig. 27.2 depicts the modern PUFA delivery systems.

Notably, the oxidative instability of PUFA requires theinclusion of antioxidants, controlled storage conditions, and innovative formulation technologies to protect PUFA integrity. Absorption and bioavailability of PUFAs are as critical as their quantity. Factors such as the size and surface area of lipid droplets, the presence of emulsifiers, and the physical state of the formulation impact enzymatic access and efficiency. Smaller droplets with increased surface area enhance lipase action and hence absorption (Navina et al., 2025). Additionally, the physicochemical properties of the delivery vehicle modulate solubility and mucosal penetration.

To address the dual challenges of oxidative deterioration and poor bioavailability, multiple delivery technologies have been invented and extensively researched. (1) Emulsions: the emulsion systems break down PUFAs into tiny droplets by mixing two liquids that are immiscible, such as oil and water. These smaller droplets boost the body's enzymes, "lipases," to break down the available fat faster and more efficiently for enhanced absorption. (2) Self-emulsifying drug delivery systems (SEDDS): SEDDS are mixtures of oils, surfactants, and other substances that form fine emulsions automatically when they contact digestive fluids. These molecules enhance the solubility and permeability of PUFAs through the intestinal tissues. Remarkably, the capacity to engineer droplet size meticulously in SEDDS is vital for bioavailability.

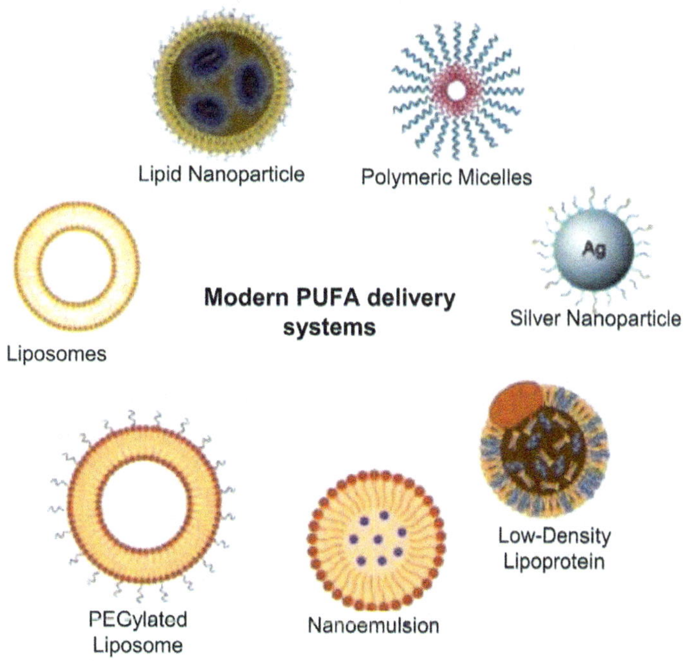

FIGURE 27.2 Emerging polyunsaturated fatty acid (PUFA) delivery systems.

(3) Gelled emulsions and liquid crystalline nanoparticles: gelled emulsions and liquid crystalline nanoparticles add extra stability and control how PUFAs get released in the gut. They also protect the fats from oxidizing, which is important because oxidation messes up the fatty acids. In addition, they help the PUFAs stay longer in the digestive tract, giving more time for absorption.

While these novel scientific breakthroughs make PUFA safe and stable until reaching the human digestive system, other PUFA protective techniques also include (4) salt formation, enteric-coated capsules, microencapsulation, and micellar matrices: these formulations protect PUFAs from the harsh stomach environment, so less gets destroyed before absorption. They also help target delivery to the right spots in the intestines and hide any bad taste. (5) High-energy processes (HEP) and low-energy processes (LEP): HEP uses machines such as homogenizers and ultrasonicators to smash droplets down to nano size, such as 10 to 100 nm. This huge surface area means digestion is superefficient. LEP uses strategic formulation of surfactants and oils to enable emulsification with improved stability and production scalability.

All these techniques focus on improving how PUFAs survive digestion and get absorbed, which is crucial for their health benefits. Literature survey revealed that phospholipid-based and amphiphilic emulsifiers were found to have better bioavailability and effectiveness compared with simple oils (Hu et al., 2021; Karthik & Anandharamakrishnan, 2016). EPA and DHA are the dietary fatty acids that are must for enhancing cardiovascular and neurological health. They are also essential for maintaining overall health. Although they are available in limited quantities in dietary sources, poor stability of these fatty acids towards oxidation is the major concern, which makes them unsuitable for oral administration (Krishnamoorthy et al., 2024). Therefore their stability, along with bioavailability and efficacy, can be enhanced using emulsions, SEDDS, and encapsulation. To enhance their bioavailability, the optimization of the droplet size, surface area, and their exact chemical form for better absorption in different segments of the gastrointestinal tract is required. Continuing research in these areas promises improved nutritional interventions in populations at risk of deficiency and chronic diseases.

27.7 Successful genetic engineering approaches for high production of polyunsaturated fatty acid

Owing to the limitations regarding yield, sustainability, and extraction cost. Genetic engineering approaches offer a promising alternative by enabling microbial or plant hosts to produce high levels of PUFAs through metabolic pathway modification.

1. Oleaginous microorganisms as PUFA producers
   Oleaginous yeasts and fungi are particularly suited for PUFA production due to their natural ability to accumulate lipids intracellularly. Among these, *Y. lipolytica* stands out because of its adaptive growth under industrial fermentation conditions and its intrinsic capacity to synthesize 4%–19% PUFA by dry cell weight depending on cultivation optimization, such as glucose supply and nitrogen availability. PUFA biosynthesis in *Y. lipolytica* and similar microbes occurs mainly via the aerobic desaturase/elongase pathway, though the polyketide synthase (PKS) pathway is also involved in some species (Liu et al., 2021).
2. CRISPR/Cas9 for precision metabolic engineering
   The CRISPR/Cas9 genome editing technique has revolutionized the genetic engineering of PUFA-producing microorganisms. It uses a Cas9 enzyme that's guided by a single-guide RNA (sgRNA), to cut DNA at specific spots. This lets you knock out, insert, or change genes exactly where the modification is required (Shi et al., 2022). Now, in *Y. lipolytica*, things are getting interesting because it repairs DNA breaks using nonhomologous end joining, not the usual homologous recombination. So, CRISPR/Cas9 works well here for gene editing.
   The sgRNA is made by combining two RNAs: the mature CRISPR RNA and the tracer RNA. They form one RNA scaffold that guides Cas9 to the exact target. This setup lets you disrupt or tweak genes involved in making PUFAs. That means you can boost production of EPA, DHA, or their precursors. Transformation efficiency is impressive. Single gene disruptions often hit over 92%, and some experiments even reach 100% editing success. That shows how solid and reliable CRISPR is for this kind of work (Schwartz et al., 2016).
3. Pathway engineering and production enhancement
   CRISPR/Cas9 genetic systems can be used to change the metabolic pathways, including knocking out unnecessary pathways or up and downregulating key enzymes such as desaturases and elongases. For example, if the fatty acid synthase (FAS) pathway is altered, the cell makes more EPA. If the PKS pathway is improved, the cell makes more DHA. Dual pathway engineering exploits both PKS and FAS routes for enhanced yields of PUFAs (Liu et al., 2024). CRISPR edits genes faster than the classical techniques. CRISPR also targets certain genes more accurately without

affecting other gene clusters. High accuracy means unwanted DNA changes may not happen. This property obviously lowers the chances of problems in the genome. Scientists use CRISPR in industrial fermentation to make strains with more PUFA.

Apart from yeasts such as *Y. lipolytica* and other species, CRISPR/Cas9 gene editing was also applied to various plants, such as *C. sativa*, soybean, and oil palm, to produce seed oils containing omega-3 fatty acids. By targeting specific genes, such as fatty acid desaturase 2 (FAD2) and fatty acid elongase 1, the oleic acid content of seed oils was increased and the PUFA profile was tailored for enhanced oxidative stability while retaining nutritional value (Jiang et al., 2017). Thus marine resources are less threatened. Metabolic engineering using CRISPR/Cas9 technologies is emerging as a key biotechnology tool to produce PUFAs (poly and unsaturated fatty acids) in microorganisms and plants. Currently, there are few sources of lipids that contain PUFAs that are of economic or nutritional value. It is expected that by applying CRISPR/Cas9 editing to lipid metabolism, it will be possible to engineer bacteria, yeast, algae, crop plants, and oilseed plants to accumulate various desired lipids, including the accumulation of EPA and DHA in quantities sufficient for the derivation of new sustainable nutritional, pharmaceutical, and bioproduct resources.

27.8 AI-enabled gains in polyunsaturated fatty acid yield and process efficiency

Recent studies demonstrate that artificial intelligence (AI) and machine learning (ML) techniques substantially accelerate the identification of cultivation and genetic strategies that increase lipid and PUFA productivity (Table 27.2).

1. ML-guided optimization of microalgal cultivation
   Recent advances demonstrate that ML can remarkably accelerate optimization of microalgal cultivation parameters such as light intensity, pH, nutrient profiles, and CO_2, which are crucial variables governing lipid and PUFA accumulation. By training ensemble models (e.g., random forests) on high-resolution photobioreactor datasets, researchers predict optimal regimes that maximize lipid productivity while reducing experimental trials. Although explicit PUFA yield data remain sparse, the methodological precedent is strongly transferable, promising streamlined tuning of stress phases that induce omega-3/omega-6 biosynthesis. Predictive control of microalgal biorefineries using ML models allows for faster scale-up and operation. The predictive controller indicates how to control the process in real time and decreases the need for empirical adjustments (Syed et al., 2024). Pilot-scale predictive control significantly reduced optimization time by more than 50% relative to empirical control and is particularly relevant to strains of interest, such as *Nannochloropsis* and *Thraustochytrium*, to produce PUFA. Cultures using ML models and sensor networks with feedback control will be able to monitor online and control the culture parameters in real time to maintain high lipid content and desired lipid profiles that will act as a basis for high-value PUFA process operations.
2. Reinforcement learning and time-series ML for spirulina scale-up
   Notably, in a recent multiscale study on *Arthrospira platensis* (commonly referred to as spirulina), time-series ML models such as long short-term memory (LSTM) networks and random forests are employed through reinforcement learning for optimizing the harvesting time, dynamic feeding, and light regime. This "smart control" upon scaling up from lab scale to large outdoor culture ponds (2019–24), it was observed that an increase in biomass productivity (around 40%) with tighter process control was achieved. Although PUFA enrichment was not assessed in spirulina, the approach can be very readily applied to microalgae strains that have enhanced PUFA content. In situations such as temporal stress induction, such as nitrogen deprivation or highlight pulses, the activity of FADs increases, which results in high-quality PUFA production. Applying the ML-based smart control to *Nannochloropsis* or *Schizochytrium* would give shorter optimization time, longer time to maintain lipid-rich culture, and therefore optimal stress timing (Syed et al., 2024).
3. Oleaginous yeast *Y. lipolytica*—metabolic engineering gains
   In another research work, Kamineni et al. built a *Y. lipolytica* strain with a heterologous Xpk/Pta pathway that leads the carbon from the pentose phosphate pathway to build up to acetyl-CoA. This strain showed up to 19% higher lipid yield and 78% higher cell-specific lipid productivity in a 1 L bioreactor culture compared with the control strains (Kamineni et al., 2021). Furthermore, the authors showed that the genome-scale model of *Y. lipolytica* suggested that the combination of expression of desaturases with the Xpk/Pta pathway and oxygen starvation in combination with nitrogen starvation led to an increase of lipid content by 67% (up to 39% dry weight biomass) and more than two-fold increase in TAG yield (up to 104 mg TAG/g glucose) (Kavšček et al., 2015). This confirms that constraint-based strain-design methodologies (such as OptDesign and GEM-based simulations) can be very useful for designing strains for PUFA production. Overexpressing desaturases in a strain engineered to produce EPA/DHA could further direct more carbon flux towards EPA/DHA. The increase in lipid yield and cell-specific lipid productivity in this study could serve

TABLE 27.2 Artificial intelligence or machine learning (ML)-based model-optimized outcomes of polyunsaturated fatty acid.

Case/system	Baseline metric	AI/model-optimized outcome	Improvement	References
Yarrowia *lipolytica* Xpk/Pta pathway (1 L bioreactor)	Lipid yield baseline (control)	↑ 19% in lipid yield	+19%	Kamineni et al. (2021)
Same system—cell-specific productivity	Productivity baseline (control)	↑ 78% cell-specific productivity	+78%	Kamineni et al. (2021)
GEM + aeration and N-starvation in *Y. lipolytica*	Lipid content (baseline)	39% DW (↑ 67%)	+67% lipid content	Kavščěk et al. (2015)
Same system—TAG yield	50 mg/g glucose	104 mg/g glucose	+108% (more than 2×)	Kavščěk et al. (2015)
Isochrysis galbana fucoxanthin prediction via ML	Model R^2 baseline (without hormone descriptors)	$R^2 = 0.839$ with descriptors	Improved prediction accuracy	Manochkumar et al. (2024)

as a reference point for developing high-titer strains for EPA/DHA production and for estimating the achievable titer in subsequent downstream processes.

4. Computational strain design and development of PUFA pathways
Genome-scale metabolic models and constraint-based modeling approaches have been used for strain design of yeast with improved lipid production. By combining metabolic model and process model and by optimizing the impact of aeration reduction and nitrogen starvation, lipid content increased by 67% in relation to dry weight (39% of dry weight) and TAG yield of 104 mg/g glucose (more than double that of the wild type) (Kavšček et al., 2015). Using these tools, one can expedite the design-build-test-learn cycle by prioritizing mutations and/or environmental perturbations in a design step before they are validated experimentally. For the PUFA production process, these tools can be used to forecast the most promising gene modifications, such as desaturases/elongases overexpression and inhibitors/competitive pathways inactivation, as well as the optimal culture conditions to direct the metabolism towards the desired EPA/DHA. By integrating ML-based expression predictors with computational strain design, the number of experimental validations can be strongly reduced to a limited set of high-promising designs, thus increasing the R&D productivity and the resource use efficiency.
5. Integrating omics with ML for regulatory insights
A growing number of studies integrate transcriptomic, proteomic, or metabolomic datasets with ML to identify regulatory nodes that control lipid or PUFA synthesis. These integrative ML frameworks reveal key enzymes or transcription factors (e.g., specific desaturases, elongases, stress-response regulators) that correlate with high PUFA content and suggest cultivation triggers (e.g., nutrient shifts, hormone supplementation) to activate them. Though few of these studies report concrete PUFA titers, their methodology has yielded testable hypotheses that reduce blind engineering. As a parallel, work predicting the effect of phytohormones on fucoxanthin in *Isochrysis galbana* reached high R^2 predictive accuracy (up to 0.839) when hormone descriptors were included in the random forest model, demonstrating how ML-omics synergy can accelerate identification of cultivation levers for high-value compounds. Applying this to PUFA-rich microalgae stands to expedite the discovery of lipid regulation networks and informed design of stress regimes (Manochkumar et al., 2024).
6. Reviews & synthesis highlighting AI's process-automation gains
Several review papers covering ML and AI for microalgae and oleaginous microbes have been published in the recent past. Some of them are focused on the control of bioreactor cultivation (Syed et al., 2024; Hu et al., 2024), on microalgae species selection, and on bioreactor real-time monitoring, harvesting strategies, and process parameter optimization. They all seem to suggest that the use of AI can dramatically reduce the time required for R&D activities, minimize the number of experimental runs, and therefore improve the predictability of the whole process from lab to full scale. None of them provides the specific PUFA composition of the strains that they are referring to, but all are aligned with the fact that the production of PUFAs in microalgae and oleaginous microbes can be improved using closed-loop ML control, hybrid (mechanistic data-driven) models,and omics-based design. Several journals have also published recently articles on the use of omics-based design, data-driven models, and ML/AI to produce PUFAs. All seem to agree that the integration of these tools can equip the PUFA biotechnology process with the right decision-making tools at every stage, from strain selection to process scale-up. In summary, AI seems to be a key catalyst for the PUFA biotechnology process improvement soon.

27.9 Future research directions

A multidisciplinary approach integrating synthetic biology, bioprocess engineering, advanced formulation, environmental sustainability, clinical science, and digital innovation is essential for overcoming current limitations and fully realizing the health and commercial potential of PUFAs in the decades ahead.

1. Exploitation of multiple sources of PUFA
The exploration of novel microbial sources, such as different species of microalgae (like *Schizochytrium* and *Aurantiochytrium*) and various species of filamentous fungi, is a very sustainable approach to produce LC-PUFAs like EPA and DHA in large quantities. These microorganisms have already evolved sophisticated lipid biosynthetic pathways and can produce large amounts of omega-3 fatty acids when cultivated under optimized conditions (Chauhan et al., 2023). Hence, efficient bioreactor technology for the economic production of omega-3 fatty acids using waste biomass (like agro-industrial residues or lignocellulosic hydrolysates) will be crucial in lowering production costs and thus contributing towards achieving the goals of a circular bioeconomy. In addition, investigations on extremophilic PUFA-producing microorganisms that can produce omega-3 fatty acids at high salinity and temperature will ensure that

PUFA production processes are operational at all times of the year under any conditions, thereby enhancing the robustness and resilience of the PUFA production processes.

2. Advanced genetic and metabolic engineering
The future demand for specific lipids can be met by developing lipid biosynthesis pathways in oilseed crops using CRISPR/Cas9 and other genome editing technologies. Future oilseed crops can be engineered to have improved PUFA profiles and oil content by overexpressing desaturases/elongases. Multiplex genome editing is also being explored to develop oilseed crops like *Camelina* and soybean to produce bespoke oils tailored to specific nutritional and functional requirements. Such development could include oils with improved stability and nutrition, as well as regulatory approval, thereby meeting the emerging bioeconomy challenges.
3. Stabilization and delivery innovations
Another area of research needed is future research opportunities in nano- and micro-encapsulation to enhance the stability of PUFAs. Nano- and micro-encapsulation formulations with enhanced bioavailability can be developed by selecting the most suitable core materials (Krishnamoorthy et al., 2024; Srinivasan & Sivasubramanian, 2015). Thus, multifunctional delivery systems would help in coencapsulating PUFAs with synergistic bioactive molecules such as antioxidants and vitamins, which would impart multiple therapeutic benefits. In addition, the use of edible films, active packaging, and surface coatings with natural antioxidants to prolong the stability of PUFAs by controlling oxidation in foods and increasing shelf life without deteriorating the sensory attributes of food products is a research area that needs to be explored. Similarly, optimization of self-emulsifying systems, nanoemulsions, and gelled emulsions with on-demand switch-on and switch-off actuation in response to different stimuli is required for the bioavailability enhancement of lipid-based drugs and for their site-specific targeting in the gastrointestinal tract.
4. Life cycle and economic assessments
A thorough life cycle assessment (LCA) of all traditional marine sources and microbial, algal, and engineered crop-derived PUFAs will need to be carried out to understand the environmental profile of the PUFA products. LCA will also aid in quantifying the carbon footprint and resource consumption associated with lipid production. Bioprocess optimization using integrated renewable energy, waste conversion, and coproduct application is a key step to meet future demands. The economic feasibility of novel energy-intensive technologies for large-scale production and compliance, consumer acceptance, and logistics will be a major focus.
5. Clinical and nutritional validation
Further large, well-designed studies are required on novel sources and products of fatty acids to be able to fully assess their impact on human health for a broad spectrum of human populations and life groups. The impact of PUFAs on emerging issues such as immunomodulation, neuroinflammation, metabolic syndrome, and personal nutrition needs to be elucidated. A better insight into PUFA metabolism and physiological functions can be gained by identifying relevant biomarkers and metabolomics tools for better assessing bioavailability and the large interindividual variability of the human response to varying dietary fatty acid consumption.
6. Regulatory and consumer acceptance strategies
Research works on genetically modified organisms should be done with reduced dependence on transgenic genome editing (such as DNA-free CRISPR/Cas9 or ribonucleoprotein complex delivery). New products are expected to come to the market quickly, potentially reducing controversy and GMO regulatory hurdles with consumers and government agencies. Better traceability, quality control measures for purity and safety, and product traceability from the farm to the consumer plate would also be needed for foods enriched in n-3 and n-6 PUFAs.
7. Integration of digital and AI technologies
The implementation of AI and ML strategies for strain optimization, fermentation management, and predictive modeling could speed up the production process and thus reduce costs for PUFA biomanufacturing (Manochkumar et al., 2024). The application of computational tools could assist in the development of optimized formulations for PUFA-based delivery systems that provide improved stability, solubility, and controlled release properties validated in vitro. In addition, the application of big data analytics employing omics-integrated approaches to identify new genes and regulatory elements that could be involved in PUFA biosynthesis, leading to the development of novel metabolic engineering tools.

27.10 Conclusion

PUFAs are important fatty acids that help the heart stay healthy, support brain growth, and help the body fight sickness. Marine lipids are the primary sources of PUFA; however, exhausting marine resources seriously affects the ecosystem. Meanwhile, microalgae, fungi, and oilseed crops are used as alternative sources for the extraction of PUFA. Recent work in metabolic engineering and CRISPR/Cas9 genome editing controls how microbes and plants make fat with more accuracy. These tools help make high-quality PUFA lipid profiles and less dependency on marine sources. Scientists employ encapsulation and targeted delivery systems to facilitate effective utilization of these omega fatty acids; otherwise it may be degraded due to oxidation. It becomes important to work out cost economics to introduce new techniques for the commercial production of essential fatty acids. Regulatory guidelines for the new methodology and scaling-up strategies need to be monitored before the industrial launch of these novel energy-efficient technologies. Integration of multiple field experts, especially from AI, microbial, and clinical sciences, will help to produce PUFA meeting the evolving global demands.

References

Barradas, T. N., & de Holanda e Silva, K. G. (2021). Nanoemulsions of essential oils to improve solubility, stability and permeability: A review. *Environmental Chemistry Letters, 19*(2), 1153–1171. https://doi.org/10.1007/s10311-020-01142-2, https://www.springer.com/journal/10311.

Brodziak-Dopierała, B., Fischer, A., Chrzanowska, M., & Ahnert, B. (2023). Mercury exposure from the consumption of dietary supplements containing vegetable, cod liver, and shark liver oils. *International Journal of Environmental Research and Public Health, 20*(3), 2129. https://doi.org/10.3390/ijerph20032129.

Carpena, M., Garcia-Perez, P., Garcia-Oliveira, P., Chamorro, F., Otero, P., Lourenço-Lopes, C., Cao, H., Simal-Gandara, J., & Prieto, M. A. (2023). Biological properties and potential of compounds extracted from red seaweeds. *Phytochemistry Reviews, 22*(6), 1509–1540. https://doi.org/10.1007/s11101-022-09826-z.

Chauhan, A. S., Patel, A. K., Chen, C. W., Chang, J. S., Michaud, P., Dong, C. D., & Singhania, R. R. (2023). Enhanced production of high-value polyunsaturated fatty acids (PUFAs) from potential thraustochytrid *Aurantiochytrium* sp. *Bioresource Technology, 370*, 128536. https://doi.org/10.1016/j.biortech.2022.128536.

Deeba, F., Kumar, K. K., & Gaur, N. A. (2020). Overview of microbial production of omega-3-polyunsaturated fatty acid. In *Nutraceutical fatty acids from oleaginous microalgae: A human health perspective*. India: wiley, 145–164. https://www.wiley.com/en-us/Nutraceutical+Fatty+Acids+from+Oleaginous+Microalgae%3A+A+Human+Health+Perspective-p-9781119631712.

Duan, Y., Chen, L., Ma, L., Zhai, Y., Hu, Y., Li, G., Chen, G., & Li, D. (2025). CRISPR/Cas9-mediated metabolic engineering for enhanced PUFA production in *Schizochytrium limacinum*. *Chemical Engineering Journal, 517*, 164320. https://doi.org/10.1016/j.cej.2025.164320.

Ferreira, F., Ortigueira, J., Reis, A., & Lopes, T. F. (2025). Benchmarking commercially available value-added fractions with potential for production via microalgae-based biorefineries: Is it worth it? *Biotechnology for Biofuels and Bioproducts, 18*(1). https://doi.org/10.1186/s13068-025-02633-6, https://biotechnologyforbiofuels.biomedcentral.com/.

Gemperlein, K., Dietrich, D., Kohlstedt, M., Zipf, G., Bernauer, H. S., Wittmann, C., Wenzel, S. C., & Müller, R. (2019). Polyunsaturated fatty acid production by *Yarrowia lipolytica* employing designed myxobacterial PUFA synthases. *Nature Communications, 10*(1). https://doi.org/10.1038/s41467-019-12025-8, https://www.nature.com/ncomms/.

Hu, X., Karthik, P., & Chen, J. (2021). Enhanced oral oil release and mouthfeel perception of starch emulsion gels. *Food Research International, 144*, 110356. https://doi.org/10.1016/j.foodres.2021.110356.

Hu, Z., Qian, J., Wang, Y., & Ye, C. (2024). Current status and applications of genome-scale metabolic models of oleaginous microorganisms. *Food Bioengineering, 3*(4), 492–511. https://doi.org/10.1002/fbe2.12113.

Islam, F., Imran, A., Nosheen, F., Fatima, M., Arshad, M. U., Afzaal, M., Ijaz, N., Noreen, R., Mehta, S., Biswas, S., Rasool, I. F. U., Aslam, M. A., Usman, I., Zahra, S. M., Segueni, N., & Amer Ali, Y. (2023). Functional roles and novel tools for improving-oxidative stability of polyunsaturated fatty acids: A comprehensive review. *Food Science and Nutrition, 11*(6), 2471–2482. https://doi.org/10.1002/fsn3.3272, onlinelibrary.wiley.com/journal/10.1002/%28ISSN%292048-7177.

Jiang, L., Wang, J., Xiong, K., Xu, L., Zhang, B., & Ma, A. (2021). Intake of fish and marine n-3 polyunsaturated fatty acids and risk of cardiovascular disease mortality: A meta-analysis of prospective cohort studies. *Nutrients, 13*(7). https://doi.org/10.3390/nu13072342.

Jiang, W. Z., Henry, I. M., Lynagh, P. G., Comai, L., Cahoon, E. B., & Weeks, D. P. (2017). Significant enhancement of fatty acid composition in seeds of the allohexaploid, *Camelina sativa*, using CRISPR/Cas9 gene editing. *Plant Biotechnology Journal, 15*(5), 648–657. https://doi.org/10.1111/pbi.12663, http://www.wiley.com/bw/journal.asp?ref=1467-7644.

Joseph, S. M., Krishnamoorthy, S., Paranthaman, R., Moses, J. A., & Anandharamakrishnan, C. (2021). A review on source-specific chemistry, functionality, and applications of chitin and chitosan. *Carbohydrate Polymer Technologies and Applications, 2*, 100036. https://doi.org/10.1016/j.carpta.2021.100036.

Kalidasan, K., Vinithkumar, N. V., Peter, D. M., Dharani, G., & Dufossé, L. (2021). Thraustochytrids of mangrove habitats from andaman islands: Species diversity, PUFA profiles and biotechnological potential. *Marine Drugs, 19*(10). https://doi.org/10.3390/md19100571, https://www.mdpi.com/1660-3397/19/10/571/pdf.

Kamineni, A., Consiglio, A. L., MacEwen, K., Chen, S., Chifamba, G., Shaw, A. J., & Tsakraklides, V. (2021). Increasing lipid yield in Yarrowia lipolytica through phosphoketolase and phosphotransacetylase expression in a phosphofructokinase deletion strain. *Biotechnology for Biofuels, 14*(1). https://doi.org/10.1186/s13068-021-01962-6, http://www.biotechnologyforbiofuels.com/.

Karthik, P., & Anandharamakrishnan, C. (2016). Enhancing omega-3 fatty acids nanoemulsion stability and in-vitro digestibility through emulsifiers. *Journal of Food Engineering, 187*, 92–105. https://doi.org/10.1016/j.jfoodeng.2016.05.003.

Kavščeк, M., Bhutada, G., Madl, T., & Natter, K. (2015). Optimization of lipid production with a genome-scale model of *Yarrowia lipolytica*. *BMC Systems Biology, 9*(1), 72. https://doi.org/10.1186/s12918-015-0217-4.

Khoshnoudi-Nia, S., Forghani, Z., & Jafari, S. M. (2022). A systematic review and meta-analysis of fish oil encapsulation within different micro/nanocarriers. *Critical Reviews in Food Science and Nutrition, 62*(8), 2061–2082. https://doi.org/10.1080/10408398.2020.1848793, https://www.tandfonline.com/loi/bfsn20.

Krishnamoorthy, S., & Buys, E. M. (2025). Identification and characterisation of β-carotene and retinol-producing commensal probiotic bacteria from liver, intestine and rumen tissues of grass-fed cattle. *Beneficial Microbes,* 1–12. https://doi.org/10.1163/18762891-bja00098.

Krishnamoorthy, S., Leena, M. M., Moses, J. A., & Anandharamakrishnan, C. (2024). Approaches for improved delivery of nutrients. In *Emerging technologies for the food industry*. Apple Academic Press, 157–187. https://doi.org/10.1201/9781003413660-6.

Krishnamoorthy, S., Moses, J. A., & Anandharamakrishnan, C. (2021). COVID-19, Food safety, and consumer preferences: Changing trends and the way forward. *Journal of Culinary Science & Technology,* 1–18. https://doi.org/10.1080/15428052.2021.2016526.

Kumaravel, S., & Srinivasan, K. (2017). Antioxidant and antimicrobial activity of silver nanoparticles synthesized using cinnamomum zeylanicum. *Indo American Journal of Pharmaceutical Sciences, 4*(1), 8–12.

Lewis, E., Steenson, S., Haslam, R. P., Mcdonald, E., Sharman, M., Traka, M., Stanton, A., Napier, J. A., Sweeting, A., Saleh, R. N. M., Hornberger, M., Givens, D. I., Calder, P. C., & Minihane, A. M. (2025). Sustainable and available sources of omega-3 fatty acids for health: Are the current dietary recommendations, food sources and legislation fit for purpose? *Nutrition Research Reviews*. https://doi.org/10.1017/S0954422425100127, http://journals.cambridge.org/NRR.

Liu, H., Song, Y., Fan, X., Wang, C., Lu, X., & Tian, Y. (2021). *Yarrowia lipolytica* as an oleaginous platform for the production of value-added fatty acid-based bioproducts. *Frontiers in Microbiology, 11*. https://doi.org/10.3389/fmicb.2020.608662, https://www.frontiersin.org/journals/microbiology#.

Liu, Y., Han, X., Chen, Z., Yan, Y., & Chen, Z. (2024). Selectively superior production of docosahexaenoic acid in *Schizochytrium* sp. through engineering the fatty acid biosynthetic pathways. *Biotechnology for Biofuels and Bioproducts, 17*(1), 75. https://doi.org/10.1186/s13068-024-02524-2.

Määttänen, P., Lurz, E., Botts, S. R., Wu, R. Y., Robinson, S. C., Yeung, C. W., Colas, R., Li, B., Johnson-Henry, K. C., Surette, M. E., Dalli, J., & Sherman, P. M. (2020). Plant- and fish-derived n-3 PUFAs suppress citrobacter rodentium–induced colonic inflammation. *Molecular Nutrition and Food Research, 64*(6). https://doi.org/10.1002/mnfr.201900873, http://onlinelibrary.wiley.com/journal/10.1002/(ISSN)1613-4133.

Manochkumar, J., Jonnalagadda, A., Cherukuri, A. K., Vannier, B., Janjaroen, D., Chandrasekaran, R., & Ramamoorthy, S. (2024). Machine learning-based prediction models unleash the enhanced production of fucoxanthin in *Isochrysis galbana*. *Frontiers in Plant Science, 15*. https://doi.org/10.3389/fpls.2024.1461610, https://www.frontiersin.org/journals/plant-science.

Navina, B., Velmurugan, N. K., Joseph, P. J., Krishnamoorthy, S., & Rajamani, M. (2025). Novel extraction technologies for nutrient recovery from edible insects: A review. *Food and Humanity*, 100896. https://doi.org/10.1016/j.foohum.2025.100896.

Nida, S., Krishnamoorthy, S., Moses, J. A., & Anandharamakrishnan, C. (2024). Applications of ozone in food processing. In *Emerging technologies for the food industry*. Apple Academic Press, 215–237. https://doi.org/10.1201/9781003413615-7.

Noore, S., Pathania, S., Fuciños, P., O'Donnell, C. P., & Tiwari, B. K. (2024). *Nanoencapsulation of bioactive compounds*. Cham: Springer, 49–61. https://doi.org/10.1007/978-3-031-57488-7_7.

Okeke, E. S., Ejeromedoghene, O., Okoye, C. O., Ezeorba, T. P. C., Nyaruaba, R., Ikechukwu, C. K., Oladipo, A., & Orege, J. I. (2022). Microalgae biorefinery: An integrated route for the sustainable production of high-value-added products. *Energy Conversion and Management: X, 16*, 100323. https://doi.org/10.1016/j.ecmx.2022.100323.

Prasad, W., Wani, A. D., Khamrui, K., Hussain, S. A., & Khetra, Y. (2022). Green solvents, potential alternatives for petroleum based products in food processing industries. *Cleaner Chemical Engineering, 3*, 100052. https://doi.org/10.1016/j.clce.2022.100052.

Priyanka Yashwant, C., Krishnmoorthy, S., Loganathan, M. A. R., Anandharaj, A., Baskaran, N., & Vignesh, S. (2021). Biotransformation of food waste to starter culture biomass: An investigation of antibiotic resistance-free lactic acid bacteria from dairy and household food waste. *The Pharma Innovation Journal, 10*(10S), 601–607. https://www.thepharmajournal.com/special-issue?year=2021&vol=10&issue=10S&ArticleId=8203.

PUFA Market Size. (2025, February 16). *Insights, Trends & SWOT & Forecast 2033*. Verified Market Reports.

Qin, J., Kurt, E., LBassi, T., Sa, L., & Xie, D. (2023). Biotechnological production of omega-3 fatty acids: current status and future perspectives. *Frontiers in Microbiology, 14*. https://doi.org/10.3389/fmicb.2023.1280296, https://www.frontiersin.org/journals/microbiology#.

Rajput, E., Rawson, A., Krishnamoorthy, S., & Rangarajan, J. (2023). Jackfruit byproducts: Functional properties and scope of utilization as unleavened flat bread. *Journal of Culinary Science & Technology, 21*(6), 1018–1040. https://doi.org/10.1080/15428052.2022.2027307.

Rethinavelu, G., Manoharan, L., Krishnamoorthy, S., Baskaran, N., & Sivanandham, V. (2023). Edible lichens and its unique bioactives: A review of its pharmacological and food applications. *Food and Humanity, 1*, 1598–1609. https://doi.org/10.1016/j.foohum.2023.11.007.

Rodrigues, M., Rosa, A., Almeida, A., Martins, R., Ribeiro, T., ânia, Pintado, M., Gonçalves, R. F. S., Pinheiro, A. C., Fonseca, A. J. M., Maia, M. R. G., Cabrita, A. R. J., Barros, L., & Caleja, C. (2024). Omega-3 fatty acids from fish by-products: Innovative extraction and application in food and feed. *Food and Bioproducts Processing, 145*, 32–41. https://doi.org/10.1016/j.fbp.2024.02.007.

Sahena, F., Zaidul, I. S. M., Jinap, S., Saari, N., Jahurul, H. A., Abbas, K. A., & Norulaini, N. A. (2009). PUFAs in fish: Extraction, fractionation, importance in health. *Comprehensive Reviews in Food Science and Food Safety, 8*(2), 59–74. https://doi.org/10.1111/j.1541-4337.2009.00069.x.

Saini, R. K., Prasad, P., Sreedhar, R. V., Akhilender Naidu, K., Shang, X., & Keum, Y.-S. (2021). Omega–3 polyunsaturated fatty acids (PUFAs): Emerging plant and microbial sources, oxidative stability, bioavailability, and health benefits—A review. *Antioxidants, 10*(10), 1627. https://doi.org/10.3390/antiox10101627.

Sambra, V., Echeverria, F., Valenzuela, A., Chouinard-Watkins, R., & Valenzuela, R. (2021). Docosahexaenoic and arachidonic acids as neuroprotective nutrients throughout the life cycle. *Nutrients, 13*(3), 986.

Schwartz, C. M., Hussain, M. S., Blenner, M., & Wheeldon, I. (2016). Synthetic RNA polymerase III promoters facilitate high-efficiency CRISPR-Cas9-mediated genome editing in *Yarrowia lipolytica. ACS Synthetic Biology, 5*(4), 356–359. https://doi.org/10.1021/acssynbio.5b00162, http://pubs.acs.org/journal/asbcd6.

Shi, J., Ni, X., Huang, J., Fu, Y., Wang, T., Yu, H., & Zhang, Y. (2022). CRISPR/Cas9-mediated gene editing of BnFAD2 and BnFAE1 modifies fatty acid profiles in *Brassica napus. Genes, 13*(10), 1681. https://doi.org/10.3390/genes13101681.

Shirai, M. A., Baú, T. R., Zanela, J., & Pimentel, T. C. (2025). Microalgae as an innovative active ingredient for edible films and coatings for food applications. *Algal Research, 86*, 103959. https://doi.org/10.1016/j.algal.2025.103959.

Srinivasan, K., & Kumaravel, S. (2016). Unraveling the potential phytochemical compounds of gymnema sylvestre through GC-MS STUDY. *International Journal of Pharmacy and Pharmaceutical Sciences, 8*(1), 450–453. http://innovareacademics.in/journals/index.php/ijpps/article/viewFile/6498/pdf.

Srinivasan, K., & Sivasubramanian, C. (2015). A study on the retention of pyrroloquinazoline alkaloid vasicine in nutraceutical formulations of adhatoda vasica. *World Journal of Pharmacy and Pharmaceutical Sciences, 4*(5).

Syed, T., Krujatz, F., Ihadjadene, Y., Mühlstädt, G., Hamedi, H., Mädler, J., & Urbas, L. (2024). A review on machine learning approaches for microalgae cultivation systems. *Computers in Biology and Medicine, 172*, 108248. https://doi.org/10.1016/j.compbiomed.2024.108248.

Theagarajan, R., Krishnamoorthy, S., Moses, J. A., & Anandharamakrishnan, C. (2021). 1 - Advanced applications of green materials in food applications. In S. Ahmed (Ed.). *Applications of advanced green materials* (pp. 1–31). Woodhead Publishing. https://doi.org/10.1016/B978-0-12-820484-9.00001-5.

Timilsena, Y. P., Wang, B., Adhikari, R., & Adhikari, B. (2017). Advances in microencapsulation of polyunsaturated fatty acids (PUFAs)-rich plant oils using complex coacervation: A review. *Food Hydrocolloids, 69*, 369–381. https://doi.org/10.1016/j.foodhyd.2017.03.007, https://www.journals.elsevier.com/food-hydrocolloids.

Van Dael, P. (2021). Role of n-3 long-chain polyunsaturated fatty acids in human nutrition and health: review of recent studies and recommendations. *Nutr Res Pract, 15*(2), 137–159. https://doi.org/10.4162/nrp.2021.15.2.137.

Vieira, M.da C., Vieira, S. A. G., Skupien, J. A., & Boeck, C. R. (2022). Nanoencapsulation of unsaturated omega-3 fatty acids as protection against oxidation: A systematic review and data-mining. In *Critical reviews in food science and nutrition, Vol. 62*, Taylor and Francis Ltd, 4356–4370. https://doi.org/10.1080/10408398.2021.1874870 Number 16.

Wei, W., Cheng, Z., Wang, X., Chang, M., Xie, D., Sun, C., Guo, X., & Li, B. (2025a). *The Potential of marine oils as functional foods: Nutritional composition, health benefits, applications, and future perspectives*. Taylor & Francis. https://doi.org/10.1080/87559129.2025.2528083.

Wei, W., Cheng, Z., Wang, X., Chang, M., Xie, D., Sun, C., Guo, X., & Li, B. (2025b). *The potential of marine oils as functional foods: Nutritional composition, health benefits, applications, and future perspectives*. Food Reviews International, 1–32. http://doi.org/10.1080/87559129.2025.2528083.

West, A. L., Miles, E. A., Lillycrop, K. A., Han, L., Napier, J. A., Calder, P. C., & Burdge, G. C. (2020). Dietary supplementation with seed oil from transgenic *Camelina sativa* induces similar increments in plasma and erythrocyte DHA and EPA to fish oil in healthy humans. *British Journal of Nutrition, 124*(9), 922–930. https://doi.org/10.1017/S0007114520002044.

Wolf, J., Chapman, R., D, C., P, M., B, S., & Ben, H. (2024). High-throughput screening to accelerate microalgae-based phycochemical production. In S. Abomohra Abdelfatah, & Ende (Eds.). *Value-added products from algae: Phycochemical production and applications* (pp. 273–319). Springer International Publishing. https://doi.org/10.1007/978-3-031-42026-9_10.

Yang, M., Li, L., Zhu, X., Liang, L., Chen, J., Cao, W., Liu, W., Duan, X., Ren, G., & Liu, Z. (2024). Microencapsulation of fish oil by spray drying, spray freeze-drying, freeze-drying, and microwave freeze-drying: Microcapsule characterization and storage stability. *Journal of Food Science, 89*(6), 3276–3289. https://doi.org/10.1111/1750-3841.17098.

Yin, F. W., Huang, J., Zhan, C. T., Sun, X. L., Zheng, W. L., Luo, X., Zhang, Y. Y., Yin, L. F., & Fu, Y. Q. (2024). Recycling fermentation strategy for waste cellular residues in the production of polyunsaturated fatty acids. *Fermentation, 10*(2). https://doi.org/10.3390/fermentation10020081, www.mdpi.com/journal/fermentation.

Zongo, K., Krishnamoorthy, S., Moses, J. A., Yazici, F., Çon, A. H., & Anandharamakrishnan, C. (2021). Total conjugated linoleic acid content of ruminant milk: The world status insights. *Food Chemistry, 334*. https://doi.org/10.1016/j.foodchem.2020.127555, www.elsevier.com/locate/foodchem.

Chapter 28

Techno-economic analysis of polyunsaturated fatty acid production and processing

K. Shobana[1], Asma Moideen[2], Sandhiya S.[3], and Balasasirekha R.[4]

[1]*Department of Food Technology, Faculty of Engineering, Karpagam Academy of Higher Education, Coimbatore, Tamil Nadu, India,* [2]*CMS College of Science and Commerce, Coimbatore, Tamil Nadu, India,* [3]*Vellore Institute of Technology, Vellore, Tamil Nadu, India,* [4]*Avinashilingam Institute for Home Science and Higher Education for Women, Coimbatore, Tamil Nadu, India*

28.1 Introduction

Polyunsaturated Fatty Acids (PUFAs), especially the long-chain fatty acids of omega-3, Docosahexaenoic Acid (DHA) and Eicosapentaenoic Acid (EPA) are considered the most important dietary substances for the heart, brain, eyes, and to a certain extent, cancer treatment by the above factors, leading to their diverse applications in dietary supplements, fortified foods, infant nutrition, and clinical nutrition (Banaszak et al., 2024). Over the past two decades, robust epidemiological evidence, clinical studies, and evolving dietary recommendations have driven a global rise in omega-3 PUFA consumption, which coincides with an aging population, lifestyle-related chronic illnesses, and increasing consumer interest in preventive healthcare, establishing these lipids as favored components in the food, nutraceutical, and medicinal industries (Noor et al., 2025). Research indicates that the worldwide market of omega-3 PUFA has nearly doubled cost-wise over the past decade and is expected to continue to grow at a period of time (Sivakumar et al., 2022).

28.1.1 Background on polyunsaturated fatty acid significance and market drivers

PUFAs have become a major component in the market for supplements, infant formula, functional foods, and clinical nutrition. Market reports hold the combined omega-3/omega-6 segment to be worth approximately 10.5 billion USD in 2024, then increasing to around 16 billion USD by 2030 with a Compound Annual Growth Rate (CAGR) of approximately 7.3, while the broader market for PUFAs is estimated to grow from 6.69 billion USD in 2025 to 11.42 billion USD by 2035 (CAGR ~5.5%) (Nandoskar et al., 2026). The main factors that play a vital role in the development of the PUFA market are the increasing scientific evidence for the benefits of EPA/DHA (Khalili et al., 2021), increasing lifestyle-related diseases (Tsao et al., 2023), preventive nutrition policies and consumer practices, and increasing demand for marine and alternative PUFA sources (Banaszak et al., 2024).

28.1.2 Historical context of polyunsaturated fatty acid production routes

The pathway of PUFA production has undergone significant changes, from maximizing the utilization of marine resources to creating supply chains of EPA and DHA that are scientifically targeted and increasingly engineered. The historical timeline starts back in the 8th century, when the Romans were producing garum; this fermented fish sauce accidentally turned out to be a source of concentrated omega-3s (Aquerreta et al., 2002). PUFA production history is illustrated in Table 28.1.

It runs to the 19th century when Peter Möller's advancements in the extraction, purification, and marketing of cod liver oil led to fish oil being recognized as a major industrial commodity (Burr & Burr, 1930). The biochemical era was marked by George and Mildred Burr's finding of Linoleic Acid (LA) followed by α-Linolenic Acid (ALA) as fatty acids that are

Omega-3 and Omega-6 Polyunsaturated Fatty Acids in Food Systems. DOI: https://doi.org/10.1016/B978-0-443-43810-3.00029-4

TABLE 28.1 History of polyunsaturated fatty acid (PUFA) production.

Ancient	**8th century**	**The Romans made garum, a fish sauce that was fermented, and it was an early concentrated source of omega-3 fats.**
Industrialization	1850	Peter Möller developed improved extraction, purification, and large-scale marketing methods for cod liver oil.
Essential fatty acids discovery	1929–30	Linoleic acid (and subsequently linolenic acid) was identified as an essential fatty acid by George and Mildred Burr.
The gap period	Post-1940s	Research attention concentrated on cholesterol and omega-6 metabolism, and previous omega-3s were largely neglected.
Discovery	1953	Docosahexaenoic Acid (DHA) was discovered (Abu-Nasr & Holman, 1954).
Omega-3 revolution	1978	Dyerberg and Bang linked high eicosapentaenoic acid and DHA intake in Greenland Inuit to very low coronary heart disease incidence.
Clinical validation	1980s	Clinical studies expanded, confirming omega-3 benefits for cardiovascular health, thrombosis, and inflammation.
Contemporary	Current	Marine oils represent about 75% of the omega-3 market, raising concerns about the sustainability of marine resources.
Future production	Current	Research focuses on heterotrophic fermentation and microalgae cultivation to provide sustainable PUFA sources.

essential, which occurred in 1929–30 (Mukhopadhyay, 2012). DHA itself was recognized as a separate long-chain omega-3 during the late 1950s, although the study carried out for decades largely moved towards omega-6 metabolism and cholesterol.

During the 1970s, government support diminished after the Bureau of Commercial Fisheries got its new name, the National Marine Fisheries Service, and importantly, the S.K. financing ceased. However, the clinical evidence continued to accumulate. The 19-year study by Dr. Averly Nelson in Seattle, published in 1972, found that patients with heart disease who ate fish at least three times a week suffered almost 4.5 times fewer recurrent heart attacks than those who ate fish rarely. These findings, despite being initially neglected, actually foreshadowed the enormous omega-3 research explosion that came after the Dyerberg–Bang Greenland Inuit studies. During the 1980s, clinical trials in Europe, North America, and Japan, conducted by major American researchers, including William E. M. Lands and groups at the Oregon University Health Sciences Center, were proving that fish oil PUFAs positively affect cardiovascular risk, thrombosis, and inflammatory responses.

28.1.3 Current market demand and sustainability imperatives

The dominant PUFA sector faces a major contradiction: marine fisheries sustainability is deteriorating, yet global demand is increasing. According to the 2021 report, only 62.3% of ocean fish stocks are still ecologically viable, indicating a significant decline in fish populations. Climate change predictions state that global DHA levels might drop by 10%–58% by the year 2100 because of the decline in microalgal production. During this time, the market share by volume of marine-derived oils has reached a whopping 75.11%, despite the sustainability concerns that keep rising. Thus the gap between demand and supply has prompted research into alternative production methods like heterotrophic fermentation (*Schizochytrium* species), phototrophic microalgae cultivation, and genetic engineering.

28.1.4 Rationale for techno-economic analysis

The process of strategic capital allocation entails the examination of the economic feasibility of new PUFA manufacturing methods. In the case of biotech systems, the production costs represent 62%–80% of the total costs of manufacturing, and a considerable amount is spent on bioreactors as well as equipment used for extraction and purification. In a comparative techno-economic assessment, all the factors, such as biomass productivity, purification efficiency, feedstock availability, energy consumption, and regional differences, need to be considered. Life-cycle costing techniques help to point out the most critical economic factors that influence the cost of items sold and the viability of a commercialization plan. The understanding of the economic situation of the competing production methods is necessary for the industries willing to take advantage of the ever-increasing PUFA market to make correct investment decisions and devise commercialization plans accordingly.

28.2 Significance of omega-6 and omega-3 polyunsaturated fatty acids in health and nutrition

ALA (n-3) and LA (n-6) are Essential Fatty Acids (EFAs), and can not be synthesized by the body in animals and humans and therefore must be obtained through the diet (Watts, 2016). In the human body, the above fatty acids pave the way for the production of EPA (n-3), DHA (n-3) and Arachidonic Acid (AA) (ARA) (n-6) that contribute major roles in homeostasis regulation (Watts, 2016). The above-mentioned FAs were segregated into locally mediating bioactive signaling lipids called eicosanoids and also regulate the various body homeostasis. Collectively, EPA and DHA help to develop ARA and antiinflammatory properties, whereas ARA assists in the development of proinflammatory eicosanoids (Watts, 2016). High intake of omega-3 PUFA may prevent inflammatory conditions, Cardiovascular Diseases (CVDs), chronic illness, and cancer (Saini & Keum, 2018).

28.2.1 Nutritional and health benefits

Saturated Fatty Acids (SAs) were altered with PUFAs, resulting in enhanced health benefits (Qi et al., 2004). Omega-6 PUFA has higher LA, which reduces the plasma Low-density Lipoprotein (LDL) cholesterol and total serum cholesterol by inducing the hepatic LDL receptor (LDLR) (Bishehkolaei & Pathak, 2024). LA modulates the binding elements which regulate the sterol and cholesterol homeostasis through LDLR. Reduction in LDL cholesterol in the body reduces the occurrence of CVD (Djuricic & Calder, 2021). ALA is an most EFAs present under the category of omega-3 PUFA and is abundantly present in flaxseed and walnut.

Studies by Gramlich et al., 2019, revealed that reduced intake of ALA will cause deficiency of EFAs. With adequate consumption, ALA will improve the cardiovascular health, thereby reducing the occurrence of CVD (Bishehkolaei & Pathak, 2024). The importance of ALA (EFA) for mental health and physical health is based on its role in elevating DHA, reducing LDL, and raising HDL (Sala-Vila et al., 2022). Omega-6 PUFA exhibits antiinflammatory properties in severe skin conditions such as atopic dermatitis (AD) that causes dryness, irritation, and skin rashes. Omega-6 PUFA ingestion improved the skin external barrier in the AD patients. Dyslipidemia was significantly improved while omega-6 PUFA was incorporated instead of SAs. The LDLR is induced by LA that regulates the total cholesterol by reducing the LDL (Djuricic & Calder, 2021).

28.2.2 Market drivers and global demand projections

New technologies, population changes, political developments, environmental changes, and global economic linkages cause disturbance in the markets. These factors together are fostering trends in health and food and also the relation among them. In relation to this, products of omega-3 procure more chances of elevating their market share, as much scientific evidence supports the efficiency of omega-3 in improving the wellness of humans (Oliver et al., 2020). In 2019, the worldwide revenue of omega-3 products was 2.49 billion USD, and during the period of 2020–27, the CAGR of these supplements was estimated to rise up to 7% (Schade, 2020). In recent times, nutraceuticals and functional foods sector became a functional area in the market and is expected to achieve sustained growth in future. Numerous chronic conditions were proven to be improved by the intake of omega-3, and that would be a key factor to enhance the sales of the omega-3 supplements in the medical industry as nutritional supplements (Size, 2020).

The constant support and encouragement from reliable sources facilitate the day-to-day consumption of omega-3 PUFAs, and it may improve the market share of omega-3 PUFAs in the nutraceuticals, pharma industry, and functional foods. The market of omega-3 is restricted at times as the recommended dosage is not disclosed officially. The recommended dosage differs from one scientific body to another. As an example, Food and Agriculture Organization and World Health Organization (WHO) proposed RDA of 250 mg of EPA and DHA, which should ensure a sufficient level of protection against infections, but International Society of the Study of Fatty Acids and Lipids (ISSFAL) and Global Organization of EPA and DHA omega-3s (GOED) indicated that a daily dose of 500 mg of EPA and DHA is needed to protect the cardiovascular system of normal adults (Oliver et al., 2020). The rapid growth of new technologies and the higher use of blue-light screens in everyday life are contributing to a rise in eye problems across all age groups (Ren et al.,

2022). Studies have proven that DHA helps in the healthy vision by supporting the retina cells and providing nourishment to them (Johnson et al., 2008).

Environmental and social trends should be kept in consideration while the omega-3 PUFA constituents are showcased as an emerging market among the group of functional ingredients. Finding alternative source of fish products is not solely because of the rise in omega-3 PUFA supplement demand. An emerging trend influencing the use of omega-3 PUFA ingredients in the food and beverage industry is the rising demand for animal-free products. As preference of consumers change continuously, there is an increasing need to develop alternative sources that do not rely on fish oil in order to meet demand and align with the altering dietary preferences (Oliver et al., 2020). Additionally, consumers are willing to pay for omega-3 supplements because of their proven health benefits, that have proven to provide long-term health and wellness benefits.

28.3 Polyunsaturated fatty acid production sources: Marine, plant, biotechnological, and novel routes

Producing genetically engineered omega-3 LC-PUFA in long-time viable oilseeds into fish oil-standard omega-3 LC-PUFA using multiple gene pathways has been difficult. The results of 20 years of joint effort have yielded oilseed crops with similar levels of fish oil omega-3 LC-PUFA, and, most importantly, a higher level of omega-3/omega-6 ratio (Zhou et al., 2023). Microalgae of different variants naturally developed LC-PUFA, and they are regarded as economically viable. Specifically in the marine culture and nutraceuticals sectors, the biosynthesis of active components from microalgae, specifically attention toward omega-3 fatty acids has been high lately. Studies also confirmed that microalgae can produce PUFAs (Dhanya et al., 2020).

28.3.1 Traditional marine sources

Conventionally, a variety of fish, including crustaceans, anchovies, shellfish, and sardines have been the main sources of DHA and EPA. Due to the limited access to marine sources and other dietary choices, it became difficult to meet the recommended daily intake (RDI) demand only from marine food sources. Accordingly, LC-PUFAs are commercially available worldwide as supplements originated from fish and krill oil (Tocher et al., 2019). Signature lipid compositions were revealed in all sources by the class-resolved mapping of DHA and EPA. While >90% of DHA was present in triacylglycerols in fish and *Schizochytrium*, 60%–80% of EPA occurred in glycolipids in microalgae.

About 70% of the high phospholipid profiles localized in krill oils were phosphatidylcholine-bound DHA. Notable differences were exhibited in nutritional characteristics. Algal oils derived from *Schizochytrium* have been exhibited to outperform fish and fish oils in terms of their PUFA to SA ratio (>0.45) and hypocholesterolemic to hypercholesterolemic ratio (>1) (Makay et al., 2025). Traditionally, the main dietary sources of LC-PUFA are fatty fish like salmon and small fishes like sardines, mackerel, anchovies, herring, and eel, all of which are of animal origin. They are also available in the flesh of land animals in a minimum amount (Givens & Gibbs, 2008).

28.3.2 Plant based sources

Plant seed oil bioengineering delivers an adequate supply of LC-PUFA and might be permissible to those who exclude fish from their diet. Besides, the algae aquaculture formulation may act as an innovative source for fish oils with high LC-PUFA content, but it is not cost-effective (Pandey et al., 2025). Echium oil supplements and increased dosage of flaxseeds did not increase the omega-3 index and some other research revealed that the values decreased. The sources of ALA which are of plant origin include flax, chia, canola, hemp, echium, walnut, and perilla seed oils and it has many health benefits (Nguyen, 2018). ALA is only abundant in particular items including chia seeds or oil, hemp seeds, flaxseed/linseed oil, and flaxseed. There are also other foods that contain sufficient ALA and also contain greater LA. It elicits a dilemma of taking adequate ALA without adding more LA to the diet because most ALA-rich foods are abundant in LA (Lane et al., 2022).

On the contrary, in the majority of studies, the enrichment of the diet with microalgal oil increased the index of omega-3. ALA is the most vital and ubiquitous vegetarian fatty acid, which is then transformed into more helpful DHA and EPA in the omega-3 metabolic process (Park et al., 2016). Seeds, nuts, and some kinds of vegetable oils such as soybean oil, corn oil, and safflower oil are the high sources of LA in vegan and vegetarian diets (Burns-Whitmore et al., 2019). Flaxseeds contain a specific high level of ALA, providing 39%–64% out of total fat and up to 50% w/w of lipid fraction. Also, 54% of LA is present by soybean oil (Zamani Ghaleshahi et al., 2020). When flaxseed oil was being assessed as a source of omega-3 fatty acids, researchers didn't look at it in isolation. They compared it with other oils such as maize oil, fish oil, sunflower oil, echium seed oil, maize oil, safflower oil, soybean oil, microalgal oil, and olive oil (Ryan & Symington, 2015).

28.3.3 Biotechnological polyunsaturated fatty acid production: microalgae and heterotrophic fermentation

Fish oil and porcine liver are the traditional sources of omega-3 and omega-6 fatty acids. On the other hand, oleaginous microorganisms comprise of bacteria, fungus, and algae, or single-cell oils, which showcase a potential source as well. These single-cell oils act as a perfect base for a bio-based economy as they can be converted into various chemical compounds that can contribute both to nutrition and as fuel sources (Ochsenreither et al., 2016). While comparing the usage of plant or animal sources, the microbial generation of SCO has a number of benefits. Microorganism cultures have minimal production times, are not affected by climate or location, and may be performed on a variety of substrates, including industrial waste. *Monodus* and *Phaeodactylum* are microalgae rich in EPA, but marine protists, and dinoflagellates are main sources of DHA-containing microbial groups such as *Thraustochytrium, Schizochytrium,* and *Crypthecodinum* (Ward & Singh, 2005).

Altered sources for the production of PUFA and the disadvantages of those methods are shown in Fig. 28.1 However, the production cost of both single-cell oils and seaweed oils is higher, while PUFA derived from stearidonic acid (SDA)-rich plants involves more steps, and the oils derived from genetically modified plants have lower acceptance among consumers.

Microalgal oils serve as an explicit plant-based alternative instead of fish oil consumption among vegetarians and vegans to meet omega-3 PUFAs (Craddock et al., 2017). Genetic modifications can be used to adjust the metabolic pathways involved in fatty acid breakdown and synthesis, enabling microalgae to produce higher levels of specific fatty acids. By directing these pathways toward the desired compounds, the overall production of targeted fatty acids can be enhanced (Sprague et al., 2017). Target suppression of genes participated in triacylglycerol catabolism is a genetic procedure that involves utilizing starchless mutants to disable the competitive carbon metabolic pathways (Li et al., 2010). An alternate approach is incorporating the new genes in the microorganism or microalgae to produce the fatty acid, and the regular approach involves a gene upregulation strategy (Ren et al., 2022).

Another approach is the transfer of novel genes into the microalgae or the microorganism to synthesize the fatty acid, where the most common one is the directed gene upregulation strategy. The Δ5-elongase of the *Ostreococcus tauri* and a glucose transporter (Ren et al., 2022) of the moss *Physcomitrella patens* make *Phaeodactylum tricornutum* encode the production of EPA and DHA of 23.6% and 36.5% of total fatty acids, respectively (Nichols et al., 2010).

With this, the technology of commercial-scale production of omega-3 EPA and DHA becomes more appealing (Sharma, Sharma et al., 2025). It is acknowledged that microbes have increased market production because of the higher concentration of PUFA along with a wide range of environmental tolerance. As a result, the most significant part of the

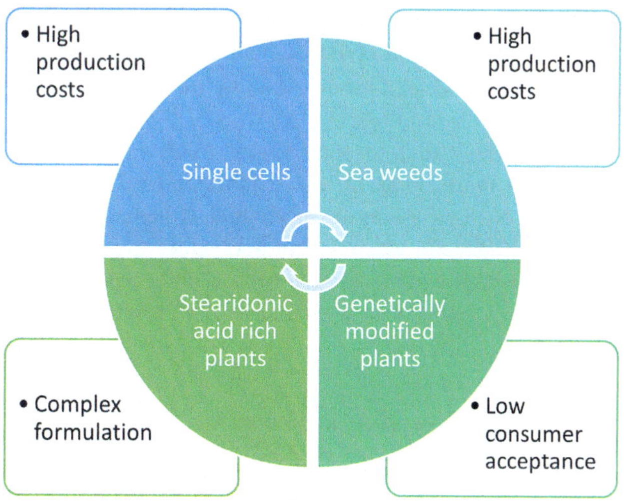

FIGURE 28.1 Alternate sources of polyunsaturated fatty acid production and its limitations.

research of metabolism of lipid in microbes is the interpretation of the mechanisms by which microalgae utilize and convert solar energy, that is of paramount value in the industrial synthesis of high-value n-3 EPA and DHA (Ren et al., 2022; Uma & Dineshbabu, 2020). In order to increase PUFA production in microalgae, they should be given adequate acetyl-CoA. Autotrophic, mixotrophic, and heterotrophic microalgae have either carbon dioxide (CO_2) or glucose as their source of carbon (Wu et al., 2019).

PUFA synthesis in microalgae occurs through two basically different processes: anaerobic and aerobic. The aerobic pathway includes a number of extensions and numerous desaturations, which are catalyzed by the alternating elongases and desaturases. The malonyl-CoA group is also carried to malonyl-ACP via acyl carrier protein transacylase. Chain elongation involves the use of acyl-ACP as a source of carbon. This is catalyzed by ketoacyl-ACP synthases (KASIII, KASI, and KASII) (Jovanovic, 2023). Each condensation undergoes a reduction, dehydration, and second reduction (Brown et al., 2009). The derived fatty acids are subjected to unsaturation and chain elongation in the presence of desaturases and elongases and are then carried into the cytoplasm of the cell, where the triacylglycerols are combined. For instance, in the production of PUFA, EPA, which is a long-chain omega-3 fatty acid is biosynthesized, and with the addition of two-carbon atoms, it is further elongated to stearic acid by a catalyzed reaction through an elongase enzyme in the main chain (Ren et al., 2022). When two double bonds have been incorporated, the first being in the third position in relation to the group of methyl, enzyme Stearoyl ACP desaturase catalyzes a reaction that changes stearic acid to ALA. The rearrangement of ALA to EPA is continued by Stearoyl ACP desaturase with the help of desaturase and elongase (Monroig et al., 2013).

Another way to biosynthesis fatty acids in microalgae is Polyketide Synthase (PKS) pathway (anaerobic pathway). It produces two specific fatty acids, including DHA and DPA. The PKS pathway involves 7 proteins that contain 3-ketoacyl synthase, 3-ketoacyl-ACP-reductase, dehydratase, enoyl reductase, dehydratase/*2-trans 3-cis* isomerase, dehydratase/2-*trans*, and 2-*cis* isomerase, and the addition of a double bond or two- carbon atoms. Because the formation of the double bonds is not accompanied by the participation of oxygen, there are malonyl-CoA and Acetyl-CoA as the major building blocks, which do not require the reduction of the intermediate in situ (Ren et al., 2022). The pathway takes place in *Schizochytrium* sp. and other *Thraustochytrid* organisms (Wu et al., 2019). The other microalgae culture growth technique that is more often applied in the commercial synthesis is the heterotrophic fermentation, where organic matter provides the energy (Ren et al., 2022). This ability of most species of microalgae to develop on reduced carbon sources enhances synthesis of lipids and PUFAs, including the use of glucose, which is easily absorbed and incorporated into acetyl-CoA significantly.

Currently, the major vegetarians worldwide take their n-3 PUFA from microalgae, which are developed through heterotrophic fermentation tanks. The frequently cultivated genera are *Dinophyceae, Schizochytrium sp.*, and *Thrustochytriaceae*, that contain 40%–60% lipid. When cultivated using glycerol or glucose as a carbon source, *Aurantiochytrium limacinum* SR21 may have lipid content of up to 84% (Li et al., 2015). Once the growth conditions are changed to optimum levels, a higher PUFA concentration may be obtained in microalgae, that may be utilized as a new form of EPA and DHA in nutritional supplements and food (Ren et al., 2022). The heterotrophic culture of microalgae could significantly increase cell mass and lipids (Najafabadi et al., 2015). In reference to photoautotrophy, it is possible to raise the biomass concentration to 18 g/L (Cheng et al., 2015) and 24 g/L (Nitsos et al., 2020; Chen & Walker, 2011). This represents 30%–50% of the total lipids (50 or 60 g/L) produced under the conventional commercial bioconversion by the yeast (Gayen et al., 2019).

Heterotrophic fermentation generates three to four times more lipids in comparison to autotrophic fermentation. Likewise, *Scenedesmus obliquus* formed more lipids in mixotrophic culture (11.6%–58.6%) than in photoautotrophic culture (7.14%) (Richa Katiyar et al., 2018). Studies revealed that (Bhatnagar et al., 2010), the microbial biomass produced by the mixotrophic growth of *Chlorella vulgaris* had 4.43 times more biomass compared to photoautotrophic growth. Besides dealing with the sterility environment, oxygen supply, and the source of organic carbon, the expenses are extremely high in developing this culture system. As an example, 1 ton of heterotrophic cultivation of microalgae needs 5 tons of sugar (Ren et al., 2022).

28.3.4 Genetic engineering and novel production routes

Through the modification and continuous expression of three genes encoding alternative Δ8-desaturation pathways components, high concentrations of very-long-chain polyunsaturated fatty acids (VLC-PUFAs), AA, and EPA were produced in a model higher plant A. thaliana. The specific C18-Δ9-fatty acyl elongating activity of the microalga I. galbana 28, Δ8 desaturase of E. gracilis29 and a Δ5-desaturase of the filamentous fungus M. alpina 26 are coded into the genes used (Qi et al., 2004). Production of AA in M. alpina would require the D6-desaturation pathway, although the first two of these genes developed in organisms in which the Δ8-evolved desaturation pathways can work. Nevertheless, conventional Δ6, as well as alternative Δ8-receptors differentiate at Δ5-desaturation. To facilitate the sequential transfer of the gene to A. thaliana, configurable resistance markers were utilized in Liberty herbicide, hygromycin, and kanamycin (Qi et al., 2004).

Ample amounts of EDA and ETrA were pooled in plants that expressed IgASE1 alone (Qi et al., 2004). In the past ten years, the majority of the primary genes of VLC-PUFA are found in various species, like aquatic animals, fungi, plants, and even animals. These genes can be classified into two different enzyme processes in which the basic synthesis is catalyzed (Venegas-Calerón et al., 2010). These encompass the first of them, called front-end PUFA desaturases, or microsomal fatty acid desaturases (Venegas-Calerón et al., 2010). In the past 15 years, a monumental scale of research has been conducted regarding the utilization of genetically modified plants that have been developed to produce huge amounts of VLC-PUFAs in their seed oil stores. To generate C20 PUFAs, including ARA and EPA, fatty acids of native plants are converted, which includes ALA and LA that need at least three consecutive nonnative enzyme reactions (Venegas-Calerón et al., 2010).

There is notable progress in the last few years amid the gene identification encoding the biosynthesis of VLC-PUFA in diverse sources of the activity, encompassing fungi, algae, plants, mammals, and mosses (Venegas-Calerón et al., 2010). It enables the first step of reverse engineering by introducing the target gene into a heterologous system such as a transgenic plant. The original results of low accumulation of EPA and ARA (Das et al., 2000) and resultant experiments (including extra genes) to formulate DHA (Meyer et al., 2004) provided supporting documents that the pathway of VLC-PUFA would be functional in transgenic host systems. Research has demonstrated that the transgenic expression of the LC-PUFA biosynthetic pathway in plants is feasible.

Initial assays of accumulating SDA and gamma-linolenic acid (GLA) in oilseed plants by expressing one gene, the D6-desaturase, also demonstrated how it could be possible to produce VLC-PUFAs in transgenic crops (Domergue et al., 2002). In the examples described above, VLC-PUFAs production in transgenic plants depended on the concurrent expression of elongases and desaturases in developing seeds (Venegas-Calerón et al., 2010). Promoters that drive seed-specific expression were usually obtained by storage protein biosynthesis and not the genes associated with oil production. Therefore higher levels of target VLC-PUFAs can be achieved by employing promoters that are active during the peak phase of oil synthesis and accumulation. In fact, the choice of promoter has been reported to play a major role in the wide range of VLC-PUFA levels detected in transgenic soybeans (Venegas-Calerón et al., 2010; Damude & Kinney, 2008).

28.4 Processing technologies for polyunsaturated fatty acid extraction, purification, and enrichment

Methods of chromatography such as counter-current and adsorption, low-temperature crystallization, solubility differences of the fatty acids, enzymatic splitting, supercritical fluid extraction, urea complexation, and fractional or molecular distillation are conducive to the production and marine oils omega-3 PUFA concentration. The current form of the omega-3 concentrates is Free Fatty Acids (FFAs), alkyl esters, and acylglycerols. While molecular distillation and urea complexation are often employed in producing omega-3 concentrates, the final products are typically in simple free acid or ester form. Enzymatic methods have obtained prominence recently because of the claimed benefits, and industrial production has increased (Wanasundara et al., 2002).

In order to develop various highly enhanced forms of n-3 PUFA concentrates, lipases are essential to catalyze esterification, transesterification, and hydrolysis reactions. The technique often followed to develop superior-quality n-3 PUFA structural acylglycerols is lipase-catalyzed alcoholysis or hydrolysis processes. Even though lipases have many significant benefits for enhancing n-3 PUFA, their high cost is not economically viable for industrial production. Other cutting-edge methods such as protein engineering and immobilization might be required to enrich the selectivity of lipases (Xie et al., 2023).

28.4.1 Biomass harvesting and dewatering

The harvesting strategy directly influences both the quantity and quality of microalgal biomass, as well as the overall feasibility of downstream product recovery. The potential of microalgae to produce high-value bioactive compounds is closely linked to the availability of cost-effective harvesting methods. Response surface methodology has been applied to optimize the use of cetytrimethylammonium bromide (CTAB) as an economic recovery agent by facilitating the dispersed air flotation process for *Schizochytrium* biomass. Under optimized conditions, CTAB concentration of 500 mg/L, air flow rate of 2 L/min, and a working volume of 600 mL, the process achieved approximately 91% biomass recovery with a 19-fold concentration factor (Watts, 2016; Alhattab & Puri, 2024).

However, an additional concentration stage is often required as a secondary step, which consumes nearly 70 times less energy compared with conventional centrifugation methods typically used for harvesting *Schizochytrium* species (Alhattab & Puri, 2024). This approach is particularly advantageous because it can be readily integrated into existing bioreactor systems that are already equipped with gas sprayers (Alhattab & Puri, 2024).

Similarly, effective harvesting outcomes have been reported using coagulation-flocculation strategies. Optimal harvesting efficiencies were observed for Bold's Basal medium at pH 11, with a coagulant concentration of 700 mg/L and a reaction time of 10 minutes, resulting in a recovery of 95.75%. In dairy wastewater medium, the best performance was achieved at pH 7 with the same coagulant concentration and a reaction time of 15 minutes, yielding 87.11% biomass recovery. The harvested microalgal biomass was subsequently utilized for lipid extraction (Pieber et al., 2012; Daneshvar et al., 2020).

28.4.2 Lipid extraction methods

EPA-enriched lipids were extracted from (Pieber et al., 2012), spray-dried biomass of *Nanochloropsis oceanica* using several solvent systems, including ethanol, dichloromethane methanol (DM), chloroform methanol (CM), and dichloromethane ethanol (Nichols et al., 2010). Among these methods, the conventional solvent mixtures DM and CM produced the highest lipid yields with similar extraction efficiencies, followed by DE (Hac İsa et al., 2022; Pieber et al., 2012).

Different solvent combinations such as CM, DM, DE, and ethanol were evaluated for their effectiveness in extracting EPA-rich lipids from *N. oceanica* biomass (Hac İsa et al., 2022). While the traditional CM and DM systems achieved the highest yields, ethanol extraction alone resulted in a total lipid recovery of 19.1% of the dry biomass. However, when ethanol extraction was combined with ultrasound treatment, the lipid yield increased significantly, with the ultrasound probe providing the most effective results (Pieber et al., 2012).

Furthermore, applying CM and DM solvent systems after ethanol extraction assisted by an ultrasound probe increased the EPA content by about 35% compared with extraction using ethanol alone, reaching levels comparable to those obtained with CM extraction (Pieber et al., 2012). These findings demonstrate that ethanol extraction aided by ultrasound is a promising approach for obtaining EPA-enriched lipid extracts from *N. oceanica*. This method offers advantages such as lower toxicity, the use of food-grade solvents and a more environmentally friendly extraction process (Pieber et al., 2012; Figueiredo et al., 2019).

28.4.3 Oil purification and polyunsaturated fatty acid enrichment

The fatty acids have been conventionally analyzed using gas chromatography (GC). The major difficulty in FFA separation in GC is the reduced volatility of the fatty acids, in particular those that are high in molecular weight and are highly polar, mainly hydroxy fatty acids. These considerations lead to peak tailing, and there was a need to use high temperatures, which causes thermal degradation of certain polyunsaturated FAs. There will be a financial necessity of cost-cutting techniques and skills to raise production of omega-3 fatty acids to cover the demands of large quantities of omega-products that have undergone extensive purging.

Supercritical fluid chromatography, high-performance liquid chromatography, and other chromatographic methods avoid the thermal degradation problems, but the key shortcomings include low sensitivity and inability to resolve complicated mixtures (Yves et al., 2016). The traditional method to procure crude fish oil at the industrial scale is the wet pressing method that is carried out on fresh fish (Rubio-Rodríguez et al., 2010). This process comprises several steps in the production of fish oil and fish meal, which is heating the raw material, pressing the cooked material, and finally, filtration or centrifugation to retrieve the oil in the miscella. A three-phase centrifuge can be used with a substantial number of stages that can be easily done after cooking (Rubio-Rodríguez et al., 2010).

28.5 Techno-economic analysis framework and methodologies

Techno-economic analysis (TEA) is a significant method that helps evaluate the technical feasibility of the production of PUFAs (Parsons et al., 2018). It combines mass and energy balance simulations with economic metrics to provide a standard for commercialization pathways. Modern TEA frameworks usually use computer-aided process design tools, like SuperPro Designer or Aspen Plus, to model each unit operation from feedstock intake to final product purification. The standard method divides the production facility into three main areas: upstream processing, which includes fermentation, inoculum preparation, and media sterilization; downstream processing (DSP), which includes harvesting, cell disruption, lipid extraction, and purification. Process utilities, which includes systems for steam generation, cooling water, compressed air, and wastewater treatment.

28.5.1 Capital expenditure analysis

Capital expenditure (CAPEX) refers to the essential fixed investments needed to design, build, and equip a production facility. In the case of microbial PUFA plants, CAPEX is heavily influenced by the production phase, which typically makes up about 76%–84% of the total equipment costs. To estimate fixed capital investment, the standard approach is to use the factorial method or Lang factor (f_L). This method connects the total delivered cost of major equipment items (C_e) to the overall plant cost (C_{TM}) through the equation: $C_{TM} = f_L \Sigma C_e$

For plants that primarily process fluids, which is common in large-scale fermentation, a f_L of 4.7 is usually applied. In contrast, mixed fluids–solids plants tend to use a factor of 3.6. Recent data from the industry regarding liquid processing plants indicates a more precise range of 3.00 to 5.33 for AACE Class 4 estimates. When it comes to equipment costs, these are adjusted for scale using scaling laws: $Cost_2 = Cost_1 \cdot \left(\frac{Size_2}{Size_1}\right)^n$

Here, the scaling exponent n generally falls between 0.6 and 0.7 for stainless steel bioreactors and DSP equipment. It's also crucial to factor in indirect costs like engineering design, construction fees, and contingency factors, which can push the basic equipment cost up by 35% or even more.

28.5.2 Operating expenditure analysis

Operating Expenditure (OPEX) refers to the costs that are incurred to operate the facility (Solutions, n.d.). Total production costs are divided into variable and fixed costs of operation. Variable costs comprises mainly raw materials and utilities. Feedstock, such as glucose or glycerol, is the biggest cost factor, often making up 70%–95% of the total production cost for biodiesel or bulk lipids. These costs can be minimized on average by 35% by using waste from the food industry. Utilities, especially the energy needed for agitation and aeration in high-density cultures, also play a significant role in driving costs.

Fixed costs include expenses like operating labor, maintenance, taxes, insurance, and plant overhead. Labor usually accounts for about 28%–36% of operational expenditures in large-scale algal systems. For a typical facility, it is common to assume a team of five operators for each main section, with wages adjusted based on local economic conditions (Castellini et al., 2021). Depreciation and taxes: facilities are generally depreciated over a period of 10 to 15 years using the straight-line method, with taxes estimated to be around 15% of the whole investment (Castellini et al., 2021). The minimum estimated selling price (MESP) is calculated at the point where the net present value (NPV) equals zero over the project's lifespan, which usually ranges from 10 to 20 years (Yu et al., 2022; Bhran, 2025).

28.6 Cost drivers and economic analysis of polyunsaturated fatty acid production

Economic viability of microbial PUFAs is very sensitive to the scale of production and valorization of feed.

28.6.1 Production cost components at different scales

Techno-economic analyzes reveal a strong economies of scale phenomenon. For example, the production of SCOs with oleaginous yeast *Metschnikowia pulcherrima* as a raw source exhibits a dramatic decrease in the MESP with scale (Parsons et al., 2018). A comparison of production scales and feedstocks is shown in Table 28.2.

Across all scales, the primary cost impact remain upstream (raw materials) and midstream processes (bioreactor utilities for agitation and aeration), while the intracellular nature of PUFA synthesis adds 20%–60% to total costs via downstream

TABLE 28.2 Comparison of production scales and feedstocks.

Production scale	Feedstock	MESP (€/ton)
100 tons/year	Sucrose	€14,000
10,000 tons/year	Sucrose	€4,000 – €8,000
10,000 tons/year	Wheat straw	€4,000 – €8,000

cell disruption and recovery. Larger-capacity plants (e.g., 100,000 tons/year) can bring biodiesel production costs down to $3.63/kg, making them competitive with traditional oils, provided lipid yields are high (e.g., 22%) (Castellini et al., 2021).

28.6.2 Break-even analysis and profitability projections

The break-even points for microbial PUFAs are more affected by the price of the feedstock than by the cost of auxiliary enzymes or nutrients. In the high-value segment, such as squalene production by Aurantiochytrium sp., the projects have shown strong financial viability with a NPV of $36.2 million over a 10-year time horizon. For profitable systems, the IRR values are expected to range between 9.5% and 22.1% for conventional commercial systems. In optimistic cases with circularity coefficients, the IRR values can reach 43%–48%. For advanced systems, the payback periods are estimated to vary between 1.41 and 1.57 years when using waste side-streams, as opposed to 3 years without integrating circularity concepts. The financial viability is very sensitive. The findings of the study indicate that a 20% reduction in net cash flow can decrease the NPV by almost 50% and the IRR from 42%–25%.

DSP contributes between 40% and 60% of the overall production cost of microbial oils. The high degree of unsaturation in PUFAs makes them highly sensitive to oxygen, light, and heat. Conventional lipid extraction typically involves hexane-based solvents. However, the current research cycle between 2021 and 2026 has witnessed a transition toward "green" and more efficient solvents. In 2025, a breakthrough showed that biphasic lipid extraction after pulsed electric field (PEF) processing was possible with lower energy requirements. The PEF processing breaks down the cell wall, enabling the gradual extraction of water-soluble proteins, followed by a smoother lipid extraction step. This method enables the energy consumption ratio to decrease to 1.6, compared with 9.9 in conventional monophasic extraction processes.

The use of CO_2 Table 28.3 at supercritical conditions enables extraction at low temperatures and in an oxygen-free atmosphere, thus retaining the oxidative stability of EPA and DHA (Ren et al., 2022). Although the process is energy-intensive and has high CAPEX costs, it is gaining popularity for high-purity pharmaceutical-grade PUFAs. Methods like urea inclusion, low-temperature crystallization, and molecular distillation are employed for the enrichment of particular fatty acids (Sharma, Das et al., 2025). Enzymatic approaches using lipases such as *Thermomyces lanuginosus* lipase provide a mild one-step process for concentrating PUFAs into glycerides, which are more bioavailable and amenable to human metabolism. For the microbial oils to be used in functional foods or dietary supplements, they need to be protected from auto-oxidation, which may cause the development of off-flavors (rancidity) and a reduction in nutritional quality. Microencapsulation is a process whereby the oil droplets are encapsulated in a polymeric matrix, represents the effect of various combinations of material utilized in oxidative stability and microencapsulation efficiency of PUFAs.

Studies have shown that a mixture of maltodextrin, modified starch, and gum arabic is the (Hussain et al., 2025) most effective combination in terms of strength, serving as a functional barrier against oxygen and moisture. Spray drying is more common large-scale tool of encapsulation because of its ability to operate on a continuous basis and its economic feasibility.

28.7 Heterotrophic *Schizochytrium* fermentation at pilot scale

Heterotrophic culture has been an extremely effective system for the industrial production of LC-PUFAs, mainly DHA. Although the economic viability of heterotrophic *Schizochytrium* fermentation is limited by the cost of substrate, with

TABLE 28.3 Effect of various combinations of material utilized in oxidative stability and microencapsulation efficiency of polyunsaturated fatty acid.

Wall material combination	Microencapsulation yield (%)	Microencapsulation efficiency (%)	Stability indicator (peroxide value)
Gum arabic (GA): maltodextrin (MD)	80.0%	85.0%	4.8 meq/kg (4 weeks)
GA: MD: modified starch (MS)	87.77%	90.11%	0.71–2.39 meq/kg (28 days @ 55°C)
Chitosan: whey protein	80.0%	87.73%	4.8 meq/kg (4 weeks)

glucose contributing about 70%–80% of overall cultivation costs (Oliver et al., 2020). This in turn causes changes in the cost of feedstock, to directly affect OPEX and minimum selling price (MSP) of DHA oil.

28.7.1 Process architecture and production performance

In contrast to photoautotrophic systems, heterotrophic fermentation excludes light as the main cause of growth restriction, enabling the growth in closed bioreactors under strictly regulated environmental conditions (Oliver et al., 2020). This shift from light-driven to substrate-driven metabolism allows much higher biomass concentrations and better volumetric productivity. In turn, the omega-3 productivities are said to be two to three orders higher than the autotrophic systems and surpass fungal or bacterial platforms, enhancing space-time yield and overall techno-economic efficiency (Oliver et al., 2020).

Schizochytrium species are one of the most commercially important heterotrophic DHA producers, accumulating 40%–60% lipids with high DHA content. Although other microalgae like *Crypthecodinium cohnii,* can also be utilized at an industrial scale, *Schizochytrium* is still favored because of its efficiency in metabolism, scalability, and food and feed regulatory acceptance (Ochsenreither et al., 2016). *Schizochytrium* is usually grown in fed-batch mode at pilot and precommercial scale to maximize biomass growth and lipids. With ideal conditions, biomass can be grown at 18–24 g/L with the high lipid content (Ren et al., 2022). In comparison to outdoor solar pond systems, fermentation-based production has a higher capability of sterility, reproducibility, and insensitivity to climatic variability, and facilitates geographically flexible implementation (Oliver et al., 2020).

28.7.2 Techno-economic cost structure, sensitivity, and scale-up considerations

Techno-economically, MSP relies upon annualized CAPEX, OPEX, and total DHA production. Thus growth in lipid productivity or substrate utilization lowers MSP, but a growth in substrate or energy expenditure disproportionately elevate production costs. The second significant cost driver is energy demand because lipid biosynthesis rate necessitates high oxygen transfer levels, which entail high aeration and agitation (Ren et al., 2022). The use of sterile operation also escalates CAPEX and OPEX by investing in bioreactor facilities and monitoring equipment. Further economic strains are provided by DSP, as the intracellular lipid recovery must use energy-demanding cell disruption and technologies like supercritical CO_2, expend more capital investment but better product quality (Ren et al., 2022; Ochsenreither et al., 2016).

Alternative feeds such as glycerol, molasses, and volatile fatty acids derived from waste streams have also been investigated to increase cost competitiveness (Oliver et al., 2020). Diversification of feedstock and optimization of the process can go a long way towards lowering the cost of production. Even though pilot-scale production determines technical feasibility, at the commercial scale, economies of scale and process integration help to build long-term competitiveness against marine-derived omega-3 sources.

28.7.3 Case study: Comparative cost analysis—Fish oil versus Microalgae production

Fish oil is now the commercial leader in the food and aquaculture markets in terms of LC-PUFAs. Nevertheless, the increase in the sustainability issues and pressure on supply has provoked the interest in considering microalgal production systems as alternative sources (McKuin et al., 2022; Togarcheti & Padamati, 2021).

28.7.3.1 Case background and cost benchmarking

Recent techno-economic studies have shown that the cost of microalgal biomass production varies between €3.4–5.96 per kg based on system arrangement and size (Ruiz et al., 2016; Norsker et al., 2011;). In conditions of underoptimal productivity, the cost can reduce to €0.68 per kg (Norsker et al., 2011), and within conditions of a 100-hectare plant, costs can be estimated to decrease to around €0.5 per kg in ten years because of the expansion of scale and intensification of the process (Ruiz et al., 2016). These forecasts show that although microalgal production in the present day is moving towards the competitiveness level, both technological development and scale have decisive roles in reducing the cost difference.

28.7.3.2 Economic trade-offs, integration potential, and strategic positioning

In addition to the cost of baseline production, there are system integration and environmental performance that affect the long-term techno-economic viability. A merit of microalgal systems is that the cost volatility is less compared to fish oil, which depends on capturing wild fish, and is subjected to fluctuations in marine yields (Davis et al., 2021; Cannon, 2009). On the other hand, fish oil has well-established supply chains, price stability, and control in production, which are frequently more powerful in the controlled microalgal cultivation systems.

There should also be the economic performance measured at the application level. Microalgae feed preparation costs around US$0.68/kg versus US$0.64/kg for reference feed under aquafeed formulation, but the economic ratio of conversion is favorable to microalgae, with costs of production of US$0.95/kg tilapia versus US$1.03/kg under traditional feeding regimes (Sarker et al., 2020). This implies that the cost saving from downstream efficiency can partially compensate for increased costs of biomass in the upstream. Integrated production models have been shown to have other economic benefits (Vázquez-Romero et al., 2023); a high-rate algal pond system of 6 m^3 used to treat aquaculture wastewater has been shown to recover up to 81% of costs by means of biomass valorization (Gupta & Bux, 2019). Effective production cost are also minimized by such integration, and resource efficiency is also promoted.

The systems are also differentiated in terms of environmental performance. Life-cycle analysis demonstrates that the production of microalgae can have the same or less harmful effects to the environment than fish fillet production (Schade et al., 2020), and it can decrease reliance on marine capture (Togarcheti & Padamati, 2021). Despite the cost benefits that fish oil maintains within developed systems of supply chains, microalgal systems provide superior stability to supply and scalability in the long term. On the whole, existing evidence indicates that production of microalgal PUFA is slightly more costly at present in most cases, but will reach cost-equivalence in the next 10 years as economies of scale, optimization of substrates, and combined production approaches are developed. This comparative techno-economic balance acts as an indicator of the short-term cost-effectiveness of fish oil systems and the long-term strategic advantage of microbial platforms.

28.7.4 Case study: Waste-based polyunsaturated fatty acid production via wastewater treatment integration

Wastewater-mediated PUFA formation through wastewater treatment implementation is another dual-purpose platform that produces PUFAs while also purifies nutrient-contaminated effluents. Multistage food waste fermentation and municipal wastewater treatment coupled with lipid-producing microorganisms have been shown to be feasible through integrated multistage systems. For example, combination processes involving oleaginous yeast (*Cryptococcus curvatus, Rhodotorula glutinis*) and microalgae (*Chlorella sorokiniana*) have resulted in final effluent nitrogen and phosphorus concentrations of 33–34 mg/L and 0.6–1.5 mg/L, respectively, with 1.1–1.5 g biomass of the yeast and 0.58–1.53 g biomass of algae, which contained 18.7%–28.6% lipids (Chi et al., 2011). These results ensure that nutrient remediation and lipid accumulation may take place simultaneously within a single operation.

The versatility of this approach is further supported by successful cultivation across diverse industrial and municipal waste streams. *Nannochloropsis oceanica* with a high EPA content has been cultivated in pesticide, pharmaceutical, municipal sewage, and petroleum wastewaters, with productivity of biomass of 21.78–27.78 mg/L/day (Mitra et al., 2016). Likewise, a culture system with fertilized *P. tricornutum* grown in the presence of food waste hydrolysate produced 0.87 g of EPA in a 2.8 L culture system (Wang et al., 2020; Wang et al., 2022). These works indicate that complex waste-based substrates can produce significant biomass and PUFAs without adversely affecting metabolic activity. Substrate-tailoring strategies have also been shown to enhance waste-derived lipid production. Growth of *Ochromonas danica* on wastewater-originated grease enhanced the PUFA content from 15%–67% with intracellular lipid accumulation of 48%–79% (Xiao & Ju, 2019), demonstrating the compositional upgrading potential of waste valorization.

Beyond production metrics, system-level integration strengthens environmental and economic positioning. The colocation of PUFA production plant and a wastewater treatment facility has been reported to lower net CO_2 emissions compared with standalone systems (Andersson et al., 2012). Concurrently, wastewater recycling methods minimize the volumes of discharge and costs of treatment (Song et al., 2017), while the valorization of waste fish oil can be added to the models of the circular economy in the seafood value chain (Monsiváis-Alonso et al., 2020). Collectively, these findings demonstrate that wastewater-integrated PUFA production is technically feasible across multiple waste streams and organism platforms. This integrated model could convert both the nutrient-rich effluents and organic residues into bioactive lipid resources.

28.8 Scale-up strategies and commercialization challenges

The production of PUFAs on a commercial scale using microbes is a major step from scientific investigation to practical application. Although microbial production is a more environmentally friendly alternative to traditional marine sources, technical challenges and economic inefficiencies still have to be overcome.

28.8.1 Technical scale-up barriers

The global scenario for PUFAs is currently undergoing a paradigm shift as biotechnology moves from lab-based innovation to commercial production. Large-scale fermentation requires a steady level of volumetric productivity and successful scale-up from the lab to fermenters. There are lots of technical challenges at present. Oxygen supply is the most critical limiting factor for high-density microalgal and fungal fermentation. In high-density fermentation, oxygen transfer is impeded by a physical "blocking effect" caused by the formation of thin layers of biosurfactants at the gas–iquid interface. This demands a constant volumetric mass transfer coefficient (KLa) and concentration of dissolved oxygen (DO).

The search for the optimal blend of the flow field and cell physiology is intricate. The simulation of *S. sp.* using the computational fluid dynamics (CFD) technique shows that a single arrowy blade in the middle and two straight blade disc turbines are better suited for biomass mixing and production (108.09 g/L). Conversely, two straight-blade disc turbines at the top and one six-arrowy blade disc turbine at the bottom, with a lower oxygen transfer rate, are better suited for the maximum DHA production (21.42 g/L) (Zakaria et al., 2025). Bioreactors produce large amounts of metabolic heat, especially in aerobic high-density bioreactors. It is necessary to maintain a thermostatic environment, as even small temperature variations (e.g., above 20°C) can be detrimental to the sensitive PUFAs. Advanced CFD simulations are currently employed to optimize fluid and thermal management in these reactors (Shaheen et al., 2025). Harvesting and extraction are still major energy-intensive steps. New technologies, such as surfactant-assisted dispersed air flotation for *Schizochytrium*, can use up to 70 times less energy than conventional centrifugation (Alhattab & Puri, 2024). Furthermore, biphasic lipid extraction after PEF processing has shown an energy ratio of 1.6, significantly lower than the traditional monophasic extraction's ratio of 9.9 (Zhang et al., 2024).

28.8.2 Regulatory and approval pathways

Regulatory and approval pathways for PUFA production are shown in Fig. 28.1. In particular, omega-3 EPA and DHA oils coming from fish, microalgae, and microorganisms work at multiple levels that ultimately influence commercialization, market positioning, and economic viability. At the ingredient level, new or nontraditional PUFA sources are generally evaluated via frameworks such as generally recognized as safe (GRAS) and New Dietary Ingredient notifications in the US, Novel Food procedures in the EU, and positive ingredient lists and product approval processes under FSSAI nutraceutical regulations in India, which all require in-depth data on composition, production, toxicity, and expected dietary exposure. Regulatory pathway for the introduction of a novel ingredient containing PUFAs is shown in Fig. 28.2.

After an ingredient is approved, product-level regulations control its application in dietary supplements, functional foods, infant formulas, and foods for special medical purposes, laying down purity standards, maximum allowed levels, and manufacturing conditions, while nutrition and health-claim regulations strictly control how the benefits of omega-3 PUFAs can be communicated to consumers. These combined requirements guarantee safety and honest communication, but also impose substantial lead times, dossier development costs, and scientific evidence demands that must be clearly considered in the discounted cash flow and scenario-based techno-economic models for PUFA production systems Fig. 28.2.

Recent advances in systems biology, synthetic biology, and bioprocess engineering have transformed the development strategy for PUFA production platforms, particularly microalgae, thraustochytrids, and engineered microbes. Rather than relying solely on strain screening and empirical process tuning, contemporary approaches combine rational metabolic engineering with model-based process optimization and biorefinery integration, with the explicit objective of improving techno-economic performance and environmental sustainability (Deepika et al., 2025).

28.9 Innovation and latest advantages in genetic engineering and bioprocess optimization

The main aim of metabolic engineering for PUFA production is to redirect the cellular carbon flux towards LC-PUFAs, increase total lipid content, and, finally, regulate the profiles of fatty acids, according to product specifications (Patel et al., 2021).

28.9.1 Metabolic engineering approaches

In the case of microalgae, major targets comprise desaturase and elongase enzymes, which transform C18 precursors into DHA and EPA through the conventional Δ6/Δ5 pathway or via alternative Δ8 routes and package those PUFAs into triglycerides with the help of acyltransferases. In Fig. 28.2, the desaturase/elongase pathway is depicted. The development of DHA through the biosynthesis pathway from precursor fatty acids also requires a combination of well-coordinated enzymatic modifications.

The pathway begins with the synthesis of intermediate fatty acids GLA (18:3 n-6), dihomo-gamma-linolenic acid (20:3 n-6), SDA (18:4 n-3), and eicosatetraenoic acid (20:4 n-3), from precursor fatty acids through the catalytic action of the Δ6- desaturase and the initial elongase enzyme (Wagner, 2015). These intermediate fatty acids are then used for the production of final omega-3 fatty acid through the action of the enzyme Δ5-desaturase. The aerobic desaturase or elongase route was given in Fig. 28.3. The enzyme attached a double bond at the fifth carbon in the fatty acid chain, resulting in the production of the omega-3 fatty acid EPA (20:5 n-3) (Watts, 2016) Fig. 28.3.

In the second phase of the pathway, the enzyme C20-specific elongase extends the omega-3 fatty acid chain by adding a two-carbon unit. The resulting omega-3 fatty acid is called DPA (22:5 n-3). Finally, the enzyme Δ4-desaturase is used in the final phase of the pathway to produce the end product DHA from the precursor omega-3 fatty acid DPA (Klińska-Bąchor et al., 2024). Overexpression of rate-limiting desaturases and elongases, knockdown of competing pathways (such as β-oxidation or storage of nonPUFA neutral lipids), and engineering of transcriptional regulators have all been shown to enhance PUFA content and alter the EPA/DHA ratio in several model strains.

Thraustochytrids and other associated heterotrophic protists are regarded as important research organisms because many of them are dependent on a PKS-like production pathway of DHA and other VLC-PUFAs. Among the different approaches in metabolic engineering, optimizing PKS gene clusters has been the most common, along with improving precursor and cofactor supplies (e.g., acetyl-CoA, malonyl-CoA, NADPH) and introducing heterologous PUFA biosynthetic pathways to enable a wider range of products. One prominent case was the incorporation of an EPA biosynthetic PKS module from *Shewanella japonica* into Aurantiochytrium, that resulted in approximately five-fold higher EPA production during fed-batch fermentation, showcasing the potential of rationally altering PUFA profiles for nutritional purposes. The use of synthetic biology tools is increasing in the development of strains that combine high PUFA productivity with characteristics desirable for industrial applications, such as resistance to shear, salinity, or fluctuating substrate quality, and these tools include modular gene assembly, CRISPR-based editing, and chassis engineering.

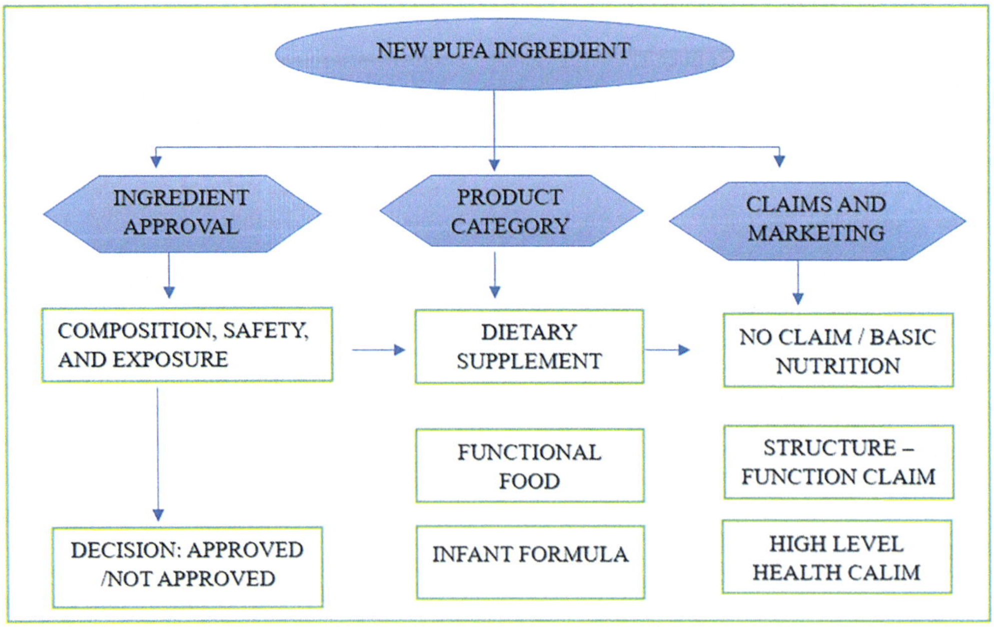

FIGURE 28.2 Regulatory pathway for the introduction of a novel ingredient containing polyunsaturated fatty acids (PUFAs).

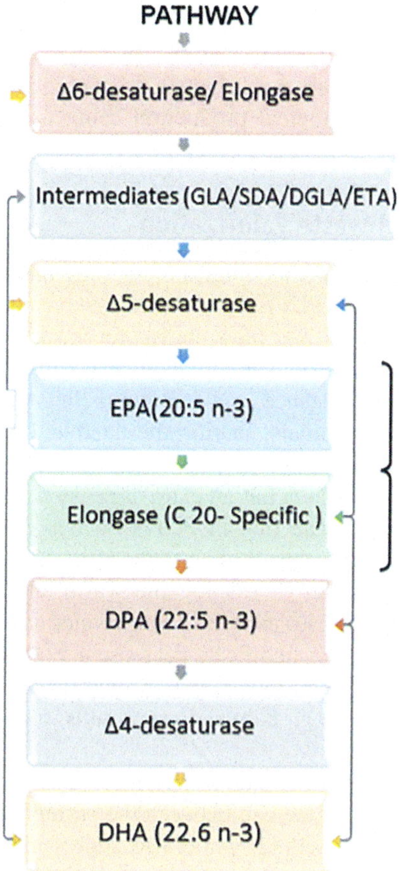

FIGURE 28.3 Aerobic desaturase/elongase route.

PUFA productivity, measured as g PUFA per liter per hour (g/L·h), quantifies production efficiency in microbial fermentations and is crucial for scaling processes. From a techno-economic point of view, advances made in metabolic engineering are very important because they enhance volumetric productivity (g PUFA/L·h), PUFA content (% of dry weight), and product selectivity, thereby decreasing the needed reactor volumes, downstream load per unit of PUFA, and the overall cost of goods. Nonetheless, the regulatory implications of using genetically modified production strains, especially in foods and nutraceuticals, must be taken into account, since they affect both market access and consumer acceptance.

28.9.2 Advanced fermentation strategies

Next to genetic modifications, sophisticated fermentation and growing methods have come out to be major factors in the uplifting of PUFA productivity and process economics. Heterotrophic methods (for instance, thraustochytrids) are increasingly favoring fed-batch and continuous rather than simple batch cultivation, which allows the separation of phases of growth and lipid accumulation, better control of carbon-to-nitrogen ratios, and prevention of substrate inhibition. Careful tailoring of the nutrients (kind and amount of carbon source, nitrogen source, micronutrients), in combination with management of DO, pH, salinity, and temperature, has brought about significant increases in DHA titers and yields of a few strains that are of industrial importance.

The use of process intensification strategies such as high-cell-density fermentation, oxygen-vector usage, and dynamic feeding algorithms, which are often supported by mechanistic or data-driven models, is likely to increase PUFA space-time yields and improve capital productivity. In addition, in phototrophic microalgae, there have been some advancements like better photobioreactor designs, optimized light distribution and mixing, and utilization of two-stage progress that involves isolation of biomass and lipid induction either in time or space to reduce productivity penalties. There is also a growing interest in hybrid systems using wastewater or effluent streams as nutrient sources combined with controlled heterotrophic or mixotrophic cultivation due to their medium reduction potential costs, and improve environmental behavior. Overall, these fermentation innovations mean higher productivities and lower unit costs in techno-economic assessments, resulting in the PUFA biotechnological production being nearer to the competitiveness of conventional fish oils.

28.9.3 Biorefinery integration and waste valorization

Biorefinery integration and waste valorization methodologies are getting more and more acknowledgment as vital to the economy and environmental sustainability of PUFA production systems. Modern concepts have moved away from treating biomass exclusively as a source of oil and have started to consider microalgae or thraustochytrid cultures as multiproduct platforms from which proteins, carbohydrates, pigments, carotenoids, terpenoids, and residual lipids along with EPA/DHA. Microalgal biorefineries, for instance, could combine PUFA extraction with the manufacturing of animal feed ingredients, biofertilizers, colorants, or biofuels, sharing the fixed and operating costs among the different product streams and thus enhancing the overall process economy.

The process of waste and side-stream valorization has an extra dimension: several recent investigations have proved the possibility of heterotrophic growth of microalgae rich in PUFA on hydrolysis from food waste, anaerobic digestate, molasses, and among others, low-cost substrates, thus leading to the removal of organic load and nutrients to a great extent while producing high-value lipids. This method of treating the waste and simultaneously getting the products is in accordance with the circular bioeconomy principles as it links wastewater purification or waste reduction with PUFA and byproduct production and consequently leads to a significant decrease in both substrate and treatment costs during techno-economic analyzes. Furthermore, the integration of microalgal or microbial PUFA biorefineries utilizing waste heat, CO_2, and effluents as inputs to these industrial sites (e.g., pulp and paper mills, food processing plants) has been suggested as a way of further improving the resource efficiency.

Together, metabolic engineering, advanced fermentation strategies, and biorefinery integration form a coherent path of innovation that is directed toward the closure of the gap between the current production costs of biotechnological PUFAs and the price structure needed for large-scale selling, while also addressing sustainability and the regulatory issues of modern lipid supply chains are being solved.

28.10 Regulatory frameworks and quality considerations

There are different laws governing the licensing and registration of omega-3 products across countries worldwide (Bhat et al., 2024). Moreover, depending on the laboratory methods required by a particular regulatory body, the safety and quality requirements for these mentioned products can change. In turn, these two elements have the power to change the regulatory regime of importing nations and they may prevent consumers to access such more quality products. Industries may develop new international voluntary standards and guidelines that are rigorous than local regulatory framework to enhance international trade. Making legal regulation on product compliance for a particular nation requires knowledge of the applicable rules and regulations. For example, based on the applicable tolerance or allowed limit, products may contain DHA + EPA quantities below a certain level stated on the label and still remain in compliance with local legislation (Bannenberg et al., 2020). Most marine oil omega-3 supplements sold in US market follow local laws.

28.10.1 International regulatory frameworks

Three key authorities considered leading regulators in this field are the Health Science Authority (HSA) Singapore, the Therapeutic Goods Administration (TGA) Australia, and (Health Canada, 2023; Bhat et al., 2024). There are two varieties in products of omega-3, such as natural health products, nutraceuticals, and complementary medicines respectively (Dighriri et al., 2022). Health Canada implies that licensing of health supplements must be performed as a legally licensable product in Canada. Conversely, the TGA indicates that the supplements are to be registered in the Australian Register of Therapeutic Goods (Therapeutic Goods Administration TGA, 2021). Therefore the HSA does not need licensing, and the dealers can report to the HSA that they are commercializing health supplements in Singapore (Health Science Authority HSA, 2018). Authorities impose rigorous requirements on manufacturers in terms of quality, safety/efficacy, claims requirements, and limitations. The HSA maintains quality of the product through regulations associated with storage, distribution conditions, manufacturing and packaging environments, labeling accuracy, stability and Good Manufacturing Practices.

Regulatory frameworks for complementary drugs and health supplements differ across countries, specifically regarding safety, claims, efficacy, and quality. Additionally, HAS restricts health supplements from making specific claims related to disease treatment properties and determines rigorous permissible limits, including specific criteria for microbiological and heavy metal contamination (Bhat et al., 2024). Likewise, Health Canada (2023) requires detailed documentation of the product and mandates all supplementary medications to follow GMP principles. Applicants should provide a thorough description of both medicinal and nonmedicinal compounds such as their dose, source, concentration, and their purpose of utilization. Reliable scientific data are obtained from clinical trials, pharmacopeial standards, peer-reviewed publications, or conventional references. The type and extent of evidence needed correlate with the risk level associated with the product and the proposed health claim (Bhat et al., 2024).

The Therapeutic Goods Administration TGA (n.d.) has a high-risk regulatory approach. When complementary drugs contain components that are not allowed in listed medications, have more extensive clinical properties or requires sterilization, it goes through full premarket evaluation. The type of claim and product risk classification are in accordance with the evidence criteria. Significantly, a "TGA assessed claim," may be demonstrated through licensed supplementary medicines, which indicates that the regulatory body has examined the application of the product (Bhat et al., 2024). Overall, all three authorities insist on evidence-based safety, efficacy assessment, and GMP compliance. HSA imposes stronger constraints on contaminant control and therapeutic claims, Health Canada (2023) emphasizes extensive scientific substantiation and documentation, and the TGA works within a defined risk-based framework with standard claim evaluation mechanisms (Bhat et al., 2024).

28.10.2 Quality standards and specifications

Evaluating the compliance for products sold in the US is challenging because of the inconsistent labeling requirements and absence of a government regulatory framework on the oxidation quality specific to functional foods. Even though it falls under the current permitted limits, 48% of the items had lower levels of EPA and DHA than then indicated on the label. Since there is no relationship between the chemical identifiers and expiration of product, adequate conditions for storage are suggested (Kim et al., 2015). Characteristics of the product quality, such as oxidative status and content label declarations must adhere to the relevant legislation or regulatory framework in the market where the product is sold (Bhat et al., 2024). Quality control is a compulsory process in the development of finished products, which comprises of n-3 FAs. This is normally done by conducting a quantitative chemical examination to ensure that pharmacopoeias and/or international standards are being adhered to.

Overall, a set of chemical analyses which falling under three main groups is crucial to identify the quality of products. At first, the analyses of active components like DHA and EPA and overall n-3 FAs are conducted. Moreover, the oxidation tests are established and calculated with the help of the anisidine value (AV) and peroxide value (PV). Finally, testing for environmental contaminants is carried out to ensure the safety and quality of omega-3 products. These tests generally include the analysis of harmful compounds such as polychlorinated biphenyls, dioxins, and heavy metals (Bhat et al., 2024). The measured levels of these substances can vary depending on the dosage form of active compounds such as ethyl esters, triglycerides, FFAs, or phospholipids, as well as the source of EPA, DHA, and total omega-3 fatty acids. Monitoring studies have shown clear differences among omega-3 sources. Fish and krill oils generally contain higher amounts of EPA, whereas algal oils are typically richer in DHA (Bhat et al., 2024).

To ensure that regulatory frameworks are adhered to, it is obligatory to see conformity to the reported EPA and DHA levels on product labels. For example, in New Zealand and Australia it is stipulated that a product needs to have at least 92% of the content it claims. On the other hand, n-FAs should possess minimum 80% of the label claim in US (Bhat et al., 2024), where they are categorized as natural products. Furthermore, a 20% tolerance for the nutrient is regarded as appropriate in the EU (Ritter et al., 2013; Kowalski et al., 2019). Subsequently, it became mandatory to enhance worldwide harmonization and/or consensus regarding the appropriate label claim for those supplements. Different pharmacopoeias state that to maintain the quality of the products containing omega-3 FAs oxidative stability should be tested. For instance, the maximum limit for acid value in the British Pharmacopoeia and the European Pharmacopoeia is NMT 2.0, however, the limit in the US Pharmacopoeia is NMT 3.0 (Bhat et al., 2024). Furthermore, different pharmacopoeias have separate maximum limits of oxidation tests for total oxidation value (TOTOX), AV, and PV.

28.11 Sustainability, circular bioeconomy, and environmental integration

In the long-term, seafood and fish oil are the major sources of omega-3 PUFA, in particular, DHA and EPA. As the world population is increasing continuously, there is growing interest in the omega-3 PUFA health benefits and improved socioeconomic conditions have led to increased demand, placing significant pressure on the supply chain and resulting in challenges related to insufficient production. In this regard, microalgae have been widely proposed as a promising alternative source of omega-3 PUFAs to help meet growing global demand. During the last 20 years, significant research has focused on exploiting microalgae as a starting resource for PUFA production, with encouraging progress in the commercial development of DHA-and EPA-rich oils from selected microalgal species (Liu et al., 2022). Many nations are stepping towards in restoring global fisheries and long-term viability; however, industrial fisheries need distinct strategies compared to small-scale fisheries (Howe et al., 2006).

The interesting note in the equation is that marine fisheries is have a much lesser environmental impact than animal protein produced by agriculture, whereby a clearance of forests is needed and, in most factors, a lesser effect than the vegetarian diets (Ray Hilborn, personal communication). The dietary sources rich in omega-3 PUFA content are prone to alterations in the global environment. Environmental factors such as pollutants, rising temperatures, eutrophication, and increased light intensity can significantly affect the production of algal omega-3 PUFAs. At the same time, these conditions tend to promote the growth of lower nutritional quality organisms, including green algae and cyanobacteria. Altogether, these variables may considerably reduce consumers' access to omega3 PUFAs and reduce their overall intake (Yan et al., 2024).

28.11.1 Life cycle assessment and environmental metrics

To evaluate the environmental impact of omega-3 production from heterotrophic algae, a comprehensive life cycle assessment (LCA) was conducted on two DHA omega-3 products derived from algae, available in both liquid and powder formulations. The assessment examined six environmental impact categories to provide a detailed evaluation of the overall sustainability of the production process. The industrial production of these products uses sugarcane as a feedstock for both production media. The results of the LCA for algae-derived DHA omega-3 indicate that sugarcane cultivation contributes significantly to most of the evaluated environmental impact categories. There were sensitive studies that disclosed that allocation methodology was not prominent in the outcomes, whether or not the sugar made significant contribution to the investment in DHA omega-3 yield and sugarcane yield. According to publicly available LCA databases, the two commercial algae-based DHA omega-3 supplements contribute only 30%–40% of the climate impact associated with fish oil (Davis et al., 2021).

Proper knowledge is deficient on the impacts of algal feed ingredients on the ecosystem (Cottrell et al., 2020). Even though the market demand for wild fish is reduced by algae-based ingredients, other environmental outcomes related to the industrial operations of these algae ingredients need to be assessed. The resilience of producing omega-3 PUFAs from algae requires a better understanding of the possible environmental trade-offs. LCA, a widely recognized methodology, provides a comprehensive approach to identifying trade-offs among environmental impacts and helps to prevent the transfer of environmental burdens across the value chain. Heterotrophic algae systems are evolving more and more popular due to their traits like rapid growth, high cell density, and higher lipid productivity (Parsons et al., 2018). However, according to studies, there are no LCAs of commercialized heterotrophic algae systems available in the public domain (Davis et al., 2021).

28.11.2 Fisheries sustainability and conservation benefits

Red meat, eggs, and some other foods also provide lesser levels of LC omega-3 oils per serving. There are minimum options to elevate seafood harvests due to the increasing worldwide population. Subsequently, innovative alternative sources are needed. Another challenge associated with long-chain omega-3 oils, despite their well-established health benefits, is the depletion of wild-caught fish stocks worldwide. Although this issue remains a subject of debate, it highlights the sustainability concerns of relying on marine sources for omega-3 production (Nichols et al., 2010). It was estimated in a widely known study (Myers & Worm, 2005) that still only 10% of the ocean's population of enormous fish persists compared to the preindustrial levels. In addition, it has been claimed that health of the fish stock and ocean is regarded to be under severe threat that the estimations predicted all seafood and commercial fish may collapse by 2048 (Mooney, 2002). There are various opinions on the status of the world's fisheries, but current developments have generated certain points of agreement between the frequently opposing viewpoints. Even though Australian marine resources are mostly well managed (Howe, 2002), the study carried out in Australia has also indicated that the stocks of as many as 60 species, including the eastern gemfish and snapper in New South Wales and Western Australia are overloaded by environmental degradation and overfishing (Hibbeln et al., 2007). Due to these decreases, the ongoing proliferation of the global aquaculture, growing global population, and growing seafood intake in Western diets, new sources of LC omega-3 oil will be required (Nichols et al., 2010).

Several recent studies have investigated global consumer demand for health-promoting long-chain omega-3 oils (Nichols et al., 2010; SACN/COT, 2004). Based on the widely RDI of 500 mg and considering an estimated global population of 8 billion by 2025 as per estimation by United Nations in 2007 and 2 to 5 mg per 100 g of fish oil, it has been projected that the current annual global fish harvest of 93 Mt would be insufficient to meet this demand (Nichols et al., 2010). Further calculations, assuming an average LC omega-3 content of 450 mg per 150 g serving of fish flesh, a total fish harvest of 70 Mt, and 50% a edible portion, also indicate that conventional fish resources alone would be unable to satisfy the projected global requirements for LC omega-3 fatty acids (Nichols et al., 2010). The inaccuracy of the processing is not considered in either of the estimations, which portrays a prediction of a declining fisheries catch that would meet the global demand of the exclusive and health-promoting LC omega-3 oils. The fish aquaculture has grown significantly in the past two decades. The marketed fish that is farmed will surpass wild fish in the near future. With the high pressure mentioned above on the stocks of wild fish, this looks like it would be quite eco-friendly.

Other than environmental issues, it is evident that the fish stocks available in the world may later be unable to sustain the nutritional requirements of human beings (Naylor et al., 2009). Therefore fish farming seems a better opportunity to improve worldwide production and helps to meet the global demand. In previous decades, as fish farming increased, most of the omnivorous and carnivorous fish were fed with fish-based products in tablet form that typically consist of fish oil and fish meal as major components or fed with other fish (tuna ranching). The farmed fish were provided as food for wild fish populations that were being harvested. With more providers starting to feed their fish on oils, plant-based and other sources of ingredients and oils because of environmental issues and the increased demand for fish oil globally (Glencross, 2009; Miller et al., 2008; Turchini et al., 2009). A major drawback of this process is that farmed fish cannot produce large quantities of LC omega-3 fatty acids, since wild fish obtain these compounds from aquatic plants and microalgae that form the base of the marine food chain (Nichols et al., 2010).

The LC omega-3 oils are then transferred through the food chain and eventually accumulate in fish tissues (Nichols et al., 2010). The primarily less beneficial short-chain (C18) omega-3 is generated by land plants. The fish that feed of land plants consist of short-chain ALA aggregate very less LC omega-3, and the customers may not benefit from similar health benefits (Nichols et al., 2010). In the meantime, it is possible to feed farmed fish with a diet rich in fish oil components to enhance the concentrations of LC omega-3, compared to wild fish. For example, compared with wild fish, major farmed species in Australia, such as Tasmanian Atlantic salmon from southern waters and barramundi from northern waters provide nearly 10times more LC omega-3 (Nichols et al., 2010).

28.11.3 Circular bioeconomy integration

Utilizing d-limonene as a green bio solvent, PUFA-rich fish oils are retrieved in maximum yield from anchovy filleting residue by a simplified solid–liquid extraction process that includes mechanical stirring, maceration, and limonene removal by evaporation under low pressure. This methodology creates a circular bioeconomy (CE) technique to generate valuable omega-3 extracts from biowaste that is accessible globally in several million t/year amount, since d-limonene is renewable and can be obtained from orange peel waste. By closing the material cycle, the technique enables the complete use of a significant biological resource that has previously been largely removed as waste (Ciriminna et al., 2019). Leading technological advancements in the CE comprise integrated multitrophic aquaculture, recirculating aquaculture systems, and fish waste valorization for bioenergy and fertilizer. To mainstream CE ideas in the industry, specific policy support, scalable technology investments, and the advancement of circular business models are essential (Osei et al., 2025).

28.12 Market outlook and future perspectives

The alterations in the population segment are another motivating factor in anticipation of increased share value of omega-3 in market as it possesses a positive health influence on individuals. According to the WHO, the ageing of the global population is largely attributed to a long-term reduction in birth rates along with increased life expectancy (Eurostat & Components, 2020). Numerous studies have demonstrated the significant role of omega-3 fatty acids in prevention and management of CVDs such as European Food Safety Authority, WHO or Institute of Medicine of USA, scientific associations like European Academy of Nutritional Sciences, American Heart Association or ISSFAL (Oliver et al., 2020) and industrial partners such as the GOED. Such bodies also imply the routine intake of omega-3 PUFA (EFSA Panel on Dietetic Products, Nutrition, and Allergies NDA, 2010).

28.12.1 Market growth projections

The emerging use of omega-3 fatty acid DHA in supplements of infants has highly increased its demand in the global market. Over the past decade, the omega-3 market has expanded considerably due to increasing awareness and consumption of these beneficial fatty acids. However, omega-3 PUFA production from traditional sources such as fish and vegetable oils encounters several challenges, including complex purification, unintentional contamination with marine contaminants, depletion or even disappearance of many fish stocks, and sustainability concerns. An alternative strategy for producing omega-3 PUFAs involves the use of microbial metabolism in organisms such as microalgae, yeast, and fungi (Finco et al., 2017).

28.12.2 Technology roadmap and development priorities

Omega-3 fatty acids are a main source of nutritional and therapeutic components, which underlines their immense commercial potential. The production of EFAs can be particularly enhanced by utilization of alternative microbial strains as cell factories. Strategies such as enhancing carbon flux, reducing by-product formation, and maintaining cofactor balance are critical for optimizing omega-3 fatty acid synthesis. These approaches not only increase the yield but also contribute to more cost-effective and efficient biomanufacturing processes. It can be carried out with the help of alternative sources of carbon, including cheap sugars, waste oils and fats, and CO_2-derived C1/C2 products (Qin et al., 2023). Continued progress in metabolic engineering, enabled by advanced molecular biology techniques, is expected to improve upstream production and efficiency of omega-3 fatty acid recovery. However, new technologies such as artificial intelligence-controlled fermentation and continuous fermentation are able to reduce operational and capital costs, high productivity, and improve downstream process engineering. These combined strategies can serve as the roadmap that will help to boost omega-3 PUFA production in a sustainable, cost-effective, and efficient way (Qin et al., 2023).

28.13 Limitations

The TEA of the challenges associated with PUFA production has varied sources, and consequently, the presence of such limitations is a reason for the cost estimates published in the past to be taken as indicative rather than predictable. In most existing TEA studies, laboratory or pilot-plant output (biomass productivity, lipid content, PUFA yield) is usually scaled up to industrial levels, but the losses related to light and mixing heterogeneity, contamination risk, long-term strain instability, and operational downtimes, which can considerably drive the actual capital and operating costs up as compared to the stated model ones, are not accounted for fully.

The processes for harvesting, cell disruption, extraction, and high-purity DHA/EPA concentration are simplified in TEA by the use of generic energy and efficiency factors and the coproduct credits in biorefinery scenarios (proteins, pigments, biofuels, fertilizers) are sometimes overstated due to the uncertainties over market volumes, logistics, and quality constraints, which have led to overestimation of the revenue potential from side streams. Also, the majority of TEA consider product prices, feedstock costs, and policy conditions as relatively stable, although omega-3 market prices, fish oil competition, sugar or waste-substrate costs, and carbon or sustainability policies are very dynamic and can thus very quickly change the competitiveness of algae or microbe-based PUFA processes.

Moreover, the costs related to regulatory and quality—which include the GRAS/Novel Food dossiers, toxicology and stability studies, health-claim substantiation, and very strict oxidation and contaminant specifications—are often not only partially accounted for but also ignored, even though their effect on time-to-market and NPV for high-purity PUFA ingredients is quite considerable. Disparities in methods between studies (various system boundaries, allocation rules, and functional units) impede the direct comparison of TEA results and make it unclear which processes are really more promising versus just being modeled under more favorable assumptions, thus highlighting the necessity for standardized, publicly disclosed TEA frameworks for PUFA production similar to those established for algal fuels and biorefineries.

28.14 Conclusion

The TEA of PUFA production highlights a critical transition from conventional marine-based supply toward diversified and innovation-driven production systems. While fish oil continues to dominate global EPA and DHA markets due to established infrastructure and cost familiarity, mounting sustainability concerns, fluctuating fish stocks, and increasing global demand expose long-term supply vulnerabilities. These pressures have accelerated the development of alternative production platforms, particularly heterotrophic microalgal fermentation and engineered biotechnological systems. Among emerging approaches, *Schizochytrium*-based heterotrophic fermentation demonstrates strong commercial feasibility, offering high lipid accumulation, controlled production environments and superior volumetric productivity compared to phototrophic systems. However, substrate costs especially glucose along with oxygen transfer energy requirements and downstream extraction processes remain key economic constraints.

Advancements in metabolic engineering, process optimization, and carbon source diversification are progressively reducing these cost barriers. Sustainability assessment further strengthens the case for microbial platforms. Life cycle analyzes suggest that algal DHA production can achieve lower climate impacts than conventional fish oil, particularly when integrated with waste valorization and circular bioeconomy models. Such integration enhances economic recovery while improving environmental performance. Overall future PUFA supply will likely rely on a hybrid model combining marine resources with scalable biotechnological production. Strategic investment, guided by rigorous techno-economic modeling and sustainability integration, will determine long-term competitiveness and ensure a resilient supply of essential nutritional lipids.

28.14.1 Key findings

The study identifies constant growth in omega-3 and omega-6 PUFA markets, driven by preventive healthcare trends, expanding nutraceutical applications, and aging populations. Currently, nearly 75% of omega-3 supply remains marine-derived, creating sustainability risks due to declining fish stocks and environmental pressures. Heterotrophic fermentation using *Schizochytrium* species achieves lipid contents of 40%–60% and high DHA productivity, outperforming phototrophic systems in process control and space-time yield. However, glucose accounts for approximately 70%–80% of cultivation costs, making feedstock price volatility the dominant economic sensitivity factor. Oxygen transfer requirements and energy-intensive DSP significantly influence operational expenditure and MSP. Comparative techno-economic models indicate that fish oil retains short-term advantages but with large-scale production, the use of alternative substrates, and advancements in process intensification, microbial oils have the potential to gradually lower production costs and move closer to price competitiveness with conventional oils within the next decade. Integration with wastewater treatment and circular bioeconomy frameworks improves environmental metrics and enhances economic recovery through biomass valorization. Metabolic engineering stratagies, targeting desaturase, elongase, and PKS pathways, substantially improve PUFA yield and volumetric productivity. Regulatory compliance, oxidative stability requirements and quality standards also impact commercialization timelines and investment decisions. Collectively, long-term competitiveness depends on integrated technological innovation, cost optimization, and sustainability alignment.

References

Abu-Nasr, A. M., & Holman, R. T. (1954). Highly unsaturated fatty acids. III. Isolation of methyl eicosapentaenoate, ethyl docosapentaenoate, and ethyl docosahexaenoate from cod liver oil esters by chromatography. *Journal of the American Oil Chemists' Society, 31*(2), 41–45.

Alhattab, M., & Puri, M. (2024). Harvesting optimization and Omega-3 recovery improvement from Schizochytrium DT3 using surfactant-aided dispersed air flotation: Response surface methodology. *Algal Research, 80*, 103512.

Andersson, V., Broberg, S., & Hackl, R. (2012). Integrated algae cultivation for municipal wastewater treatment and biofuels production in industrial clusters. In *Proceedings of WREF, Denver, USA*13–17.

Aquerreta, Y., Astiasarán, I., & Bello, J. (2002). Use of exogenous enzymes to elaborate the Roman fish sauce 'garum. *Journal of the Science of Food and Agriculture, 82*(1), 107–112. https://doi.org/10.1002/jsfa.1013.

Banaszak, M., Dobrzyńska, M., Kawka, A., Górna, I., Woźniak, D., Przysławski, J., & Drzymała-Czyż, S. (2024). Role of Omega-3 fatty acids eicosapentaenoic (EPA) and docosahexaenoic (DHA) as modulatory and anti-inflammatory agents in noncommunicable diet-related diseases – Reports from the last 10 years. *Clinical Nutrition ESPEN, 63*, 240–258. https://doi.org/10.1016/j.clnesp.2024.06.053.

Bannenberg, G., Rice, H. B., Bernasconi, A., Ferrari, A., Mallon, C., Navarrete, L., Hughes, R., Igarashi, J., Persons, K., Latynski, L., Phung, A., Wang, S., & Ismail, A. (2020). Ingredient label claim compliance and oxidative quality of EPA/DHA omega-3 retail products in the U.S. *Journal of Food Composition and Analysis, 88*, 103435. https://doi.org/10.1016/j.jfca.2020.103435.

Bhat, R. S., Alsuhaibani, A. S., Albugami, F. S., & Aldawsari, F. S. (2024). Omega 3 fatty acid as a health supplement: An overview of its manufacture and regulatory aspects. *Current Research in Nutrition and Food Science Journal, 12*(1), 70–90.

Bhatnagar, A., Bhatnagar, M., Chinnasamy, S., & Das, K. C. (2010). Chlorella minutissima—A promising fuel alga for cultivation in municipal wastewaters. *Applied Biochemistry and Biotechnology, 161*(1), 523–536.

Bhran, A. A. (2025). A comparative techno-economic analysis of waste cooking oils and chlorella microalgae for sustainable biodiesel production. *Processes, 13*(11), 3526.

Bishehkolaei, M., & Pathak, Y. (2024). Influence of omega n-6/n-3 ratio on cardiovascular disease and nutritional interventions. *Human Nutrition & Metabolism, 37*, 200275.

Brown, A. P., Slabas, A. R., & Rafferty, J. B. (2009). Fatty acid biosynthesis in plants—Metabolic pathways, structure and organization. In *Lipids in photosynthesis: Essential and regulatory functions*. Netherlands: Dordrecht: Springer, 11–34.

Burns-Whitmore, B., Froyen, E., Heskey, C., Parker, T., & San Pablo, G. (2019). Alpha-linolenic and linoleic fatty acids in the vegan diet: Do they require dietary reference intake/adequate intake special consideration? *Nutrients, 11*(10), 2365.

Burr, G. O., & Burr, M. M. (1930). On the nature and role of the fatty acids essential in nutrition. *Journal of Biological Chemistry, 86*(2), 587–621.

Cannon, D. (2009). From fish oil to microalgae oil… A win-win shift for humans and our habitat. *Explore: The Journal of Science and Healing, 5*(5), 299–303.

Castellini, M., Ubertini, S., Barletta, D., Baffo, I., Buzzini, P., & Barbanera, M. (2021). Techno-economic analysis of biodiesel production from microbial oil using cardoon stalks as carbon source. *Energies, 14*(5), 1473.

Chen, Y. H., & Walker, T. H. (2011). Biomass and lipid production of heterotrophic microalgae Chlorella protothecoides by using biodiesel-derived crude glycerol. *Biotechnology Letters, 33*(10), 1973–1983.

Cheng, Y. S., Labavitch, J., & VanderGheynst, J. S. (2015). Organic and inorganic nitrogen impact *Chlorella variabilis* productivity and host quality for viral production and cell lysis. *Applied Biochemistry and Biotechnology, 176*(2), 467–479.

Chi, Z., Zheng, Y., Jiang, A., & Chen, S. (2011). Lipid production by culturing oleaginous yeast and algae with food waste and municipal wastewater in an integrated process. *Applied Biochemistry and Biotechnology, 165*(2), 442–453.

Ciriminna, R., Scurria, A., Avellone, G., & Pagliaro, M. (2019). *A circular economy approach to omega-3 extraction.*

Cottrell, R. S., Blanchard, J. L., Halpern, B. S., Metian, M., & Froehlich, H. E. (2020). Global adoption of novel aquaculture feeds could substantially reduce forage fish demand by 2030. *Nature Food, 1*(5), 301–308.

Craddock, J. C., Neale, E. P., Probst, Y. C., & Peoples, G. E. (2017). Algal supplementation of vegetarian eating patterns improves plasma and serum docosahexaenoic acid concentrations and omega-3 indices: A systematic literature review. *Journal of Human Nutrition and Dietetics, 30*(6), 693–699.

Damude, H. G., & Kinney, A. J. (2008). Enhancing plant seed oils for human nutrition. *Plant Physiology, 147*, 962–968.

Daneshvar, E., Zarrinmehr, M. J., Kousha, M., & Bhatnagar, A. (2020). Performance evaluation of different harvesting methods and cultivation media on the harvesting efficiency of microalga and their fatty acids profile. *Fuel, 280*, 118592.

Das, T., Thurmond, J. M., Bobik, E., Leonard, A. E., Parker-Barnes, J. M., Huang, Y. S., & Mukerji, P. (2000). *Polyunsaturated Fatty Acid-specific Elongation Enzymes.*

Davis, D., Morão, A., Johnson, J. K., & Shen, L. (2021). Life cycle assessment of heterotrophic algae omega-3. *Algal Research, 60*, 102494. https://doi.org/10.1016/j.algal.2021.102494.

Deepika, C., Hankamer, B., & Ross, I. L. (2025). Can microalgal omega-3 PUFA production systems remain viable as GM plant sources emerge? *Bioresource Technology,* 133525.

Dhanya, B. S., Sowmiya, G., Jeslin, J., Chamundeeswari, M., & Verma, M. L. (2020). Algal biotechnology: A sustainable route for omega-3 fatty acid production. In *Microalgae biotechnology for food, health and high value products*. Singapore: Springer Singapore, 125–145.

Dighriri, I. M., Alsubaie, A. M., Hakami, F. M., Hamithi, D. M., Alshekh, M. M., Khobrani, F. A., & Tawhari, M. (2022). Effects of omega-3 polyunsaturated fatty acids on brain functions: A systematic review. *Cureus, 14*(10).

Djuricic, I., & Calder, P. C. (2021). Beneficial outcomes of omega-6 and omega-3 polyunsaturated fatty acids on human health: An update for 2021. *Nutrients, 13*(7), 2421.

Domergue, F., Lerchl, J., Zähringer, U., & Heinz, E. (2002). Cloning and functional characterization of *Phaeodactylum tricornutum* front-end desaturases involved in eicosapentaenoic acid biosynthesis. *European Journal of Biochemistry, 269*(16), 4105–4113.

Eurostat, G. D. P., & Components, M. Available online https://ec.europa.eu/eurostat/databrowser/view, *NAMQ_10_GDP/default/table*.

Figueiredo, A. R., da Costa, E., Silva, J., Domingues, M. R., & Domingues, P. (2019). The effects of different extraction methods of lipids from *Nannochloropsis oceanica*on the contents of omega-3 fatty acids. *Algal Research, 41*, 101556.

Finco, A. M., de, O., Mamani, L. D. G., Carvalho, J. C., de, de Melo Pereira, G. V., Thomaz-Soccol, V., & Soccol, C. R. (2017). Technological trends and market perspectives for production of microbial oils rich in omega-3. *Critical Reviews in Biotechnology, 37*, 656–671.

Gayen, K., Bhowmick, T. K., & Maity, S. K. (Eds.). (2019). *Sustainable downstream processing of microalgae for industrial application*CRC Press.

Givens, D. I., & Gibbs, R. A. (2008). Current intakes of EPA and DHA in European populations and the potential of animal-derived foods to increase them: Symposium on 'How can the n-3 content of the diet be improved?' *Proceedings of the Nutrition Society, 67*(3), 273–280.

Glencross, B. D. (2009). Exploring the nutritional demand for essential fatty acids by aquaculture species. *Reviews in Aquaculture, 1*(2), 71–124.

Gramlich, L., Ireton-Jones, C., Miles, J. M., Morrison, M., & Pontes-Arruda, A. (2019). Essential fatty acid requirements and intravenous lipid emulsions. *Journal of Parenteral and Enteral Nutrition, 43*(6), 697–707.

Gupta, S., & Bux, F. (2019). Application of microalgae in wastewater treatment. *1*.

Hac İsa, M., Metin, C., Ercan, E., & Alparslan, Y. (2022). Effect of different cell disruption methods on lipid yield of Schizochytrium sp. *Journal of the American Oil Chemists' Society, 99*(2), 129–139.

Hibbeln, J. R., Davis, J. M., Steer, C., Emmett, P., Rogers, I., Williams, C., & Golding, J. (2007). Maternal seafood consumption in pregnancy and neurodevelopmental outcomes in childhood (ALSPAC study): An observational cohort study. *The Lancet, 369*(9561), 578–585.

Howe, P. (2002). The omega workshop: Report and presentations. *Food Australia, 54*, 505–512.

EFSA Panel on Dietetic Products, Nutrition, and Allergies (NDA). (2010). Scientific opinion on dietary reference values for fats, including saturated fatty acids, polyunsaturated fatty acids, monounsaturated fatty acids, trans fatty acids, and cholesterol. *Efsa Journal, 8*(3), 1461.

Howe, P., Meyer, B., Record, S., & Baghurst, K. (2006). Dietary intake of long-chain ω-3 polyunsaturated fatty acids: Contribution of meat sources. *Nutrition, 22*(1), 47–53.

Hussain, M., Bisht, A., Khan, I., Chaudhary, M. N., Kanwal, N., Khalid, M. U., & Zou, X. (2025). Enhanced stability of n-3 PUFAs rich structured lipids via spray-dried microencapsulation with tailored wall materials. *Sustainable Food Technology, 3*(5), 1492–1504.

Johnson, E. J., Chung, H. Y., Caldarella, S. M., & Snodderly, D. M. (2008). The influence of supplemental lutein and docosahexaenoic acid on serum, lipoproteins, and macular pigmentation. *The American Journal of Clinical Nutrition, 87*(5), 1521–1529.

Jovanovic, G., S. (2023). Metabolic and regulatory network analysis of DHA-producing recombinant *Yarrowia lipolytica*.

Khalili, L., Valdes-Ramos, R., & Harbige, L. S. (2021). Effect of n-3 (Omega-3) polyunsaturated fatty acid supplementation on metabolic and inflammatory biomarkers and body weight in patients with type 2 diabetes mellitus: A systematic review and meta-analysis of RCTs. *Metabolites, 11*(11), 742.

Kim, S. K., Richmond, A., & Hu, Q. (2015). Handbook of microalgal culture. *Applied Phycology and Biotechnology, 2e*.

Klińska-Bąchor, S., Demski, K., Gong, Y., & Banaś, A. (2024). Metabolic engineering of omega-3 long chain polyunsaturated fatty acids in plants using differentΔ 6-andΔ 5-desaturases co-expressed with LPCAT from the marine diatom Phaeodactylum tricornutum. *Scientific Reports, 14*(1), 9512.

Health Canada. (2023, March 15). Fish Oil. retrieved from July 30, 2023.

Health Science Authority (HSA). (2018). *Regulatory overview of health supplements*. Published December 31 https://www.hsa.gov.sg/health-supplements/overview.

Katiyar, R., Bharti, R. K., Gurjar, B. R., Kumar, A., Biswas, S., & Pruthi, V. (2018). Utilization of de-oiled algal biomass for enhancing vehicular quality biodiesel production from *Chlorella* sp. in mixotrophic cultivation systems.

Kowalski, R., Kałwa, K., Wilczyński, K., & Kobus, Z. (2019). The fatty acids composition of selected fish oils used as dietary supplements. *Polish Journal of Natural Sciences, 34*(1), 115–126.

Lane, K. E., Wilson, M., Hellon, T. G., & Davies, I. G. (2022). Bioavailability and conversion of plant based sources of omega-3 fatty acids–a scoping review to update supplementation options for vegetarians and vegans. *Critical Reviews in Food Science and Nutrition, 62*(18), 4982–4997.

Li, J., Liu, R., Chang, G., Li, X., Chang, M., Liu, Y., & Wang, X. (2015). A strategy for the highly efficient production of docosahexaenoic acid by *Aurantiochytrium limacinum* SR21 using glucose and glycerol as the mixed carbon sources. *Bioresource Technology, 177*, 51–57.

Li, Y., Han, D., Hu, G., Sommerfeld, M., & Hu, Q. (2010). Inhibition of starch synthesis results in overproduction of lipids in *Chlamydomonas reinhardtii*. *Biotechnology and Bioengineering, 107*(2), 258–268.

Liu, Y., Ren, X., Fan, C., Wu, W., Zhang, W., & Wang, Y. (2022). Health benefits, food applications, and sustainability of microalgae-derived N-3 PUFA. *Foods, 11*(13), 1883.

Makay, K., Griehl, C., Schilling, S., & Grewe, C. (2025). Omega-3 source matters: Comparative lipid signatures and quantitative distribution of EPA/DHA across marine resources. *Marine Drugs, 24*(1), 4.

McKuin, B. L., Kapuscinski, A. R., Sarker, P. K., Cheek, N., Colwell, A., Schoffstall, B., & Greenwood, C. (2022). Comparative life cycle assessment of heterotrophic microalgae Schizochytrium and fish oil in sustainable aquaculture feeds. *Elementa: Science of the Anthropocene, 10*(1), 00098.

Meyer, A., Kirsch, H., Domergue, F., Abbadi, A., Sperling, P., Bauer, J., & Heinz, E. (2004). Novel fatty acid elongases and their use for the reconstitution of docosahexaenoic acid biosynthesis. *Journal of Lipid Research, 45*(10), 1899–1909.

Miller, M. R., Nichols, P. D., & Carter, C. G. (2008). n-3 Oil sources for use in aquaculture–alternatives to the unsustainable harvest of wild fish. *Nutrition Research Reviews, 21*(2), 85–96.

Mitra, M., Shah, F., Bharadwaj, S. V., Patidar, S. K., & Mishra, S. (2016). Cultivation of *Nannochloropsis oceanica* biomass rich in eicosapentaenoic acid utilizing wastewater as nutrient resource. *Bioresource Technology, 218*, 1178–1186.

Monroig, Ó., Tocher, D., & Navarro, J. (2013). Biosynthesis of polyunsaturated fatty acids in marine invertebrates: Recent advances in molecular mechanisms. *Marine Drugs, 11*, 3998–4018.

Monsiváis-Alonso, R., Mansouri, S. S., & Román-Martínez, A. (2020). Life cycle assessment of intensified processes towards circular economy: Omega-3 production from waste fish oil. *Chemical Engineering and Processing-Process Intensification, 158*, 108171.

Mooney, B. D. (2002). *Seafood the good food II: Oil profiles for further Australian seafoods, and influencing factors*. CSIRO Marine Research Vol. 2.

Mukhopadhyay, R. (2012). Essential fatty acids: The work of George and Mildred Burr. *Journal of Biological Chemistry, 287*(42), 35439–35441.

Myers, R. A., & Worm, B. (2005). Extinction, survival or recovery of large predatory fishes. *Philosophical Transactions of the Royal Society B: Biological Sciences, 360*(1453), 13–20. https://doi.org/10.1098/rstb.2004.1573.

Najafabadi, H. A., Malekzadeh, M., Jalilian, F., Vossoughi, M., & Pazuki, G. (2015). Effect of various carbon sources on biomass and lipid production of *Chlorella vulgaris* during nutrient sufficient and nitrogen starvation conditions. *Bioresource Technology, 180*, 311–317.

Nandoskar, S. D., Rana, S., & Singh, S. K. (2026). Polyunsaturated fatty acids in biotechnology and health: Sources, synthesis, applications, and market trends. *Archives of Microbiology, 208*(3), 142.

Naylor, R. L., Hardy, R. W., Bureau, D. P., Chiu, A., Elliott, M., Farrell, A. P., & Nichols, P. D. (2009). Feeding aquaculture in an era of finite resources. *Proceedings of the National Academy of Sciences, 106*(36), 15103–15110.

Nguyen, D. V. (2018). Nutritional supplementation with dietary omega-3 PUFA-rich flaxseed and canola oils enhances prime lamb performance and meat quality (Doctoral dissertation, James Cook University)..

Nichols, P. D., Petrie, J., & Singh, S. (2010). Long-chain omega-3 oils–an update on sustainable sources. *Nutrients, 2*(6), 572–585.

Nitsos, C., Filali, R., Taidi, B., & Lemaire, J. (2020). Current and novel approaches to downstream processing of microalgae: A review. *Biotechnology Advances, 45*, 107650.

Noor, N. M., Azmi, N. A. N., Hanifah, N. A., & Zamarudin, Z. (2025). Advances in lipid processing and utilization: Mechanisms, applications, and halalan toyyiban concept. *AIJR Books*, 89–106.

Norsker, N. H., Barbosa, M. J., Vermuë, M. H., & Wijffels, R. H. (2011). Microalgal production—A close look at the economics. *Biotechnology Advances, 29*(1), 24–27.

Ochsenreither, K., Glück, C., Stressler, T., Fischer, L., & Syldatk, C. (2016). Production strategies and applications of microbial single cell oils. *Frontiers in Microbiology, 7*, 1539.

Oliver, L., Dietrich, T., Marañón, I., Villarán, M. C., & Barrio, R. J. (2020). Producing omega-3 polyunsaturated fatty acids: A review of sustainable sources and future trends for the EPA and DHA market. *Resources, 9*(12), 148.

Osei, S. A., Ayisi, C. L., Boamah, G. A., & Mensah, G. D. (2025). The circular economy in aquaculture and fisheries: Enhancing sustainability and food security. *Circular Economy and Sustainability,* 1–50.

Pandey, A., Kamran, F., Choudhury, M., Li, L., Rahman, M. S., & Hussain, M. A. (2025). Omega-3 fatty acid fortification of plant-based beverages to enhance their nutritional profile. *Foods, 14*(9), 1602.

Park, H. G., Lawrence, P., Engel, M. G., Kothapalli, K., & Brenna, J. T. (2016). Metabolic fate of docosahexaenoic acid (DHA; 22: 6n-3) in human cells: direct retroconversion of DHA to eicosapentaenoic acid (20: 5n-3) dominates over elongation to tetracosahexaenoic acid (24: 6n-3). *FEBS Letters, 590*(18), 3188–3194.

Parsons, S., Chuck, C. J., & McManus, M. C. (2018). Microbial lipids: Progress in life cycle assessment (LCA) and future outlook of heterotrophic algae and yeast-derived oils. *Journal of Cleaner Production, 172,* 661–672.

Patel, A., Karageorgou, D., Katapodis, P., Sharma, A., Rova, U., Christakopoulos, P., & Matsakas, L. (2021). Bioprospecting of thraustochytrids for omega-3 fatty acids: A sustainable approach to reduce dependency on animal sources. *Trends in Food Science & Technology, 115,* 433–444.

Pieber, S., Schober, S., & Mittelbach, M. (2012). Pressurized fluid extraction of polyunsaturated fatty acids from the microalga *Nannochloropsis oculata*. *Biomass and Bioenergy, 47,* 474–482.

Qi, B., Fraser, T., Mugford, S., Dobson, G., Sayanova, O., Butler, J., & Lazarus, C. M. (2004). Production of very long chain polyunsaturated omega-3 and omega-6 fatty acids in plants. *Nature Biotechnology, 22*(6), 739–745.

Qin, J., Kurt, E., LBassi, T., Sa, L., & Xie, D. (2023). Biotechnological production of omega-3 fatty acids: Current status and future perspectives. *Frontiers in Microbiology, 14,* 1280296.

Ren, X., Liu, Y., Fan, C., Hong, H., Wu, W., Zhang, W., & Wang, Y. (2022). Production, processing, and protection of microalgal n-3 PUFA-rich oil. *Foods, 11*(9), 1215.

Ritter, J. C. S., Budge, S. M., & Jovica, F. (2013). Quality analysis of commercial fish oil preparations. *Journal of the Science of Food and Agriculture, 93*(8), 1935–1939.

Rubio-Rodríguez, N., Beltrán, S., Jaime, I., de Diego, S. M., Sanz, M. T., & Carballido, J. R. (2010). Production of omega-3 polyunsaturated fatty acid concentrates: A review. *Innovative Food Science & Emerging Technologies, 11*(1), 1–12.

Ruiz, J., Olivieri, G., De Vree, J., Bosma, R., Willems, P., Reith, J. H., & Barbosa, M. J. (2016). Towards industrial products from microalgae. *Energy & Environmental Science, 9*(10), 3036–3043.

Ryan, L., & Symington, A. M. (2015). Algal-oil supplements are a viable alternative to fish-oil supplements in terms of docosahexaenoic acid (22: 6n-3; DHA). *Journal of Functional Foods, 19,* 852–858.

Saini, R. K., & Keum, Y. S. (2018). Omega-3 and omega-6 polyunsaturated fatty acids: Dietary sources, metabolism, and significance—A review. *Life Sciences, 203,* 255–267.

Sala-Vila, J., Fleming, P., & Kris-Etherton, E. R. (2022). Impact of α-linolenic acid, the vegetable ω-3 fatty acid, on cardiovascular disease and cognition. *Advances in Nutrition Bethesda, Md, 13*(5), 1584–1602.

Sarker, P. K., Kapuscinski, A. R., McKuin, B., Fitzgerald, D. S., Nash, H. M., & Greenwood, C. (2020). Microalgae-blend tilapia feed eliminates fishmeal and fish oil, improves growth, and is cost viable. *Scientific Reports, 10*(1), 19328.

SACN/COT. (2004). Scientific Advisory Committee on Nutrition (SACN) and Committee on Toxicity (COT), Advice on Fish Consumption: Benefits and Risks; TSO: Norwich, UK,p. 204.

Schade, S. (2020). Distinct microalgae for human nutrition: comparative life cycle assessments and techno-economic analysis of microalgae cultivation; [kumulative Dissertation] (Doctoral dissertation)..

Schade, S., Stangl, G. I., & Meier, T. (2020). Distinct microalgae species for food—part 2: comparative life cycle assessment of microalgae and fish for eicosapentaenoic acid (EPA), docosahexaenoic acid (DHA), and protein. *Journal of Applied Phycology, 32*(5), 2997–3013.

Shaheen, S., Mahmood, T., Raja, M. A. Z., Al-Yarimi, F. A., Arain, M. B., & Hu, J. (2025). Machine learning-based investigation of activation energy for bio-convective boundary layer flow inspired by challenges in aerospace heat transfer systems. *Engineering Applications of Artificial Intelligence, 160,* 111917.

Sharma, N., Sharma, S. G., Kocher, G. S., & Dhir, A. (2025). Microalgae: A treasure house for polyunsaturated fatty acid (PUFA) production. *National Academy Science Letters,* 1–17.

Sharma, T., Das, N., Mehta Kakkar, P., Mohapatra, R. K., Pamidimarri, S., Singh, R. K., Kumar, M., Guldhe, A., & Nayak, M. (2025). Microalgae as an emerging alternative raw material of docosahexaenoic acid and eicosapentaenoic acid – A review. *Critical Reviews in Food Science and Nutrition, 65*(31), 7883–7902. https://doi.org/10.1080/10408398.2025.2486267.

Sivakumar, R., Sachin, S., Priyadarshini, R., & Ghosh, S. (2022). Sustainable production of eicosapentaenoic acid-rich oil from microalgae: Towards an algal biorefinery. *Journal of Applied Microbiology, 132*(6), 4170–4185.

Size, M. V. M. (2020). *Share & trends analysis report. URL* https://www.grandviewresearch.com/industry-analysis/automated-guided-vehicle-agv-market.

Song, X., Ma, Z., Tan, Y., Zhang, H., & Cui, Q. (2017). Wastewater recycling technology for fermentation in polyunsaturated fatty acid production. *Bioresource Technology, 235,* 79–86.

Sprague, M., Betancor, M. B., & Tocher, D. R. (2017). Microbial and genetically engineered oils as replacements for fish oil in aquaculture feeds. *Biotechnology Letters, 39*(11), 1599–1609.

Tocher, D. R., Betancor, M. B., Sprague, M., Olsen, R. E., & Napier, J. A. (2019). Omega-3 long-chain polyunsaturated fatty acids, EPA and DHA: Bridging the gap between supply and demand. *Nutrients, 11*(1), 89.

Togarcheti, S. C., & Padamati, R. B. (2021). Comparative life cycle assessment of EPA and DHA production from microalgae and farmed fish. *Clean Technologies, 3*(4), 699–710.

Therapeutic Goods Administration (TGA). (2021). *Overview of the regulation of listed medicines and registered complementary medicines*. Published July https://www.tga.gov.au/sites/default/files/overview-regulation-listed-medicines-and-registered-complementary-medicines.pdf.

Therapeutic Goods Administration (TGA). (n.d.). Registered complementary medicines. https://www.tga.gov.au/products/medicines/non-prescription-medicines/registered-complementary-medicines

Tsao, C. W., Aday, A. W., Almarzooq, Z. I., Anderson, C. A., Arora, P., Avery, C. L., & Martin, S. S. (2023). Heart disease and stroke statistics—2023 update: A report from the American Heart Association. *Circulation, 147*(8), e93.

Turchini, G. M., Torstensen, B. E., & Ng, W. K. (2009). Fish oil replacement in finfish nutrition. *Reviews in Aquaculture, 1*(1), 10–57.

Uma, V. S., & Dineshbabu, G. (2020). Biobased fats and oils from microalgae. In *Recent developments in bioenergy research*. Elsevier, 273–298.

Venegas-Calerón, M., Sayanova, O., & Napier, J. A. (2010). An alternative to fish oils: metabolic engineering of oil-seed crops to produce omega-3 long chain polyunsaturated fatty acids. *Progress in Lipid Research, 49*(2), 108–119.

Vázquez-Romero, B., Villar-Navarro, E., Perales, J. A., & Ruiz, J. (2023). *Profitability of using microalgae to treat effluents from fish RAS farming and replace fish meal: A case study*. SSRN. *Available at SSRN 4366476*.

Wagner, L. (2015). NMR metabolomics and lipid analyses in salmonid tissue. *Acta Universitatis Agriculturae Sueciae, 2015*(62).

Wanasundara, U. N., Wanasundara, J., & Shahidi, F. (2002). Omega-3 fatty acid concentrates: A review of production technologies. *Seafoods—Quality, Technology and Nutraceutical Applications,* 157–174.

Wang, X., Balamurugan, S., Liu, S. F., Zhang, M. M., Yang, W. D., Liu, J. S., & Lin, C. S. K. (2020). Enhanced polyunsaturated fatty acid production using food wastes and biofuels byproducts by an evolved strain of Phaeodactylum tricornutum. *Bioresource Technology, 296*, 122351.

Wang, X., Liu, S. F., Wang, Z. Y., Hao, T. B., Balamurugan, S., Li, D. W., & Lin, C. S. K. (2022). A waste upcycling loop: Two-factor adaptive evolution of microalgae to increase polyunsaturated fatty acid production using food waste. *Journal of Cleaner Production, 331*, 130018.

Ward, O. P., & Singh, A. (2005). Omega-3/6 fatty acids: Alternative sources of production. *Process Biochemistry, 40*(12), 3627–3652.

Watts, J. L. (2016). Using Caenorhabditis elegans to uncover conserved functions of omega-3 and omega-6 fatty acids. *Journal of Clinical Medicine, 5*(2), 19.

Wu, S., Gu, W., Huang, A., Li, Y., Kumar, M., Lim, P. E., & Wang, G. (2019). Elevated CO_2 improves both lipid accumulation and growth rate in the glucose-6-phosphate dehydrogenase engineered *Phaeodactylum tricornutum. Microbial Cell Factories, 18*(1), 161.

Xiao, S., & Ju, L. K. (2019). Conversion of wastewater-originated waste grease to polyunsaturated fatty acid-rich algae with phagotrophic capability. *Applied Microbiology and Biotechnology, 103*(2), 695–705.

Xie, D., Chen, Y., Yu, J., Yang, Z., Wang, X., & Wang, X. (2023). Progress in enrichment of n-3 polyunsaturated fatty acid: A review. *Critical Reviews in Food Science and Nutrition, 63*(32), 11310–11326.

Yan, K., Guo, F., Kainz, M. J., Li, F., Gao, W., Bunn, S. E., & Zhang, Y. (2024). The importance of omega-3 polyunsaturated fatty acids as high-quality food in freshwater ecosystems with implications of global change. *Biological Reviews, 99*(1), 200–218.

Yu, J., Xu, Z., Chen, S., Yu, Y., Zhang, C., Chen, X., & Jin, M. (2022). DLCA (ch) pretreatment brings economic benefits to both biomass logistics and biomass conversion for low cost cellulosic ethanol production. *Fuel, 311*, 122603.

Yves, H., Korma, S. A., Ali, A. H., Tuyishime, M. A., Habinshuti, I., & Abed, S. M. (2016). Extraction, refining and purification of ω-3 PUFA through different techniques—A review. *Am. J. Food Sci. Nutr. Res, 4*, 18–26.

Zakaria, M. F., Mat Zaidi, F. N. A., Ahmad Kamal, A. H., Aleng, N. A., Abd Wahid, M. E., Katayama, T., & Jusoh, M. (2025). PUFA from microalgae: Challenges, factors affecting high production and industrial application. *Aquaculture and Fisheries, 10*(4), 545–555. https://doi.org/10.1016/j.aaf.2025.01.004.

Zamani Ghaleshahi, A., Ezzatpanah, H., Rajabzadeh, G., & Ghavami, M. (2020). Comparison and analysis characteristics of flax, perilla and basil seed oils cultivated in Iran. *Journal of Food Science and Technology, 57*(4), 1258–1268.

Zhang, Z. X., Xu, Y. S., Li, Z. J., Xu, L. W., Ma, W., Li, Y. F., & Huang, H. (2024). Turning waste into treasure: A new direction for low-cost production of lipid chemicals from Thraustochytrids. *Biotechnology Advances, 73*, 108354.

Zhou, X. R., Yao, Z. J., Benedicto, K., Nichols, P. D., Green, A., & Singh, S. (2023). New sustainable oil seed sources of omega-3 long-chain polyunsaturated fatty acids: A journey from the ocean to the field. *Sustainability, 15*(14), 11327.

Chapter 29

Challenges and solutions in scaling up polyunsaturated fatty acid production for industrial use

Harish Sharma[1], Pankaj Sharma[1], Vinay Jain[2], Apoorwa Pathak[1], and Anjaneyulu Vinukonda[3]
[1]*Department of Pharmaceutics, Shriram College of Pharmacy, Morena, Madhya Pradesh, India,* [2]*Department of Pharmacognosy, ShriRam College of Pharmacy, Morena, Madhya Pradesh, India,* [3]*Formulation and Process Development, Strides Pharma Inc, New York, NY, United States*

29.1 Introduction

Polyunsaturated fatty acids (PUFAs) are a crucial group of lipids that are essential to human health, physiological normal functioning, and the prevention of diseases. The omega-3 and omega-6 fatty acids are among them and have received a remarkable scientific, clinical, and industrial interest because of their essentiality and extensive biological functions. The enzymatic ability of humans to add the additional double bonds after position D9 of the fatty acid chain is absent, which is why omega-3 and omega-6 fatty acids are nutritionally required and can only be supplied through the diet (Calder, 2017). Epidemiological, clinical, and mechanistic evidence has grown in the last 10 years supporting the health benefits of proper consumption of omega-3 and omega-6 PUFAs. The omega-3 fatty acids were associated with lower cardiovascular risk, better lipid metabolism, neuroprotective effects, cognitive development, and suppression of chronic inflammatory disorders. Omega-6 fatty acids play a central role in normal growth, skin barrier protection, immune responses, and reproductive health (Calder, 2020a, 2020b). Their presence in pharmaceutical preparations and nutraceutical supplements, functional foods, infant formulas, and cosmetics has largely been propelled by this robust scientific basis and has greatly enhanced their industrial applications and commercial importance (Bimbo et al., 2020; Shahidi, 2021). The increased usage of omega-3 and omega-6 PUFAs has consequently led to a significant growth in the worldwide demand for these products in the past decade. The market of products based on PUFA has been active due to the increasing number of aged individuals, the rising consumer awareness of preventive care, and the continuously increasing number of chronic diseases related to lifestyle (Sprague et al., 2017). Also, industrial demand has increased by regulatory authorization of docosahexaenoic acid (DHA) and arachidonic acid (ARA) fortification in infant food and medical food, creating a lot of pressure on current production systems. As such, the stability, scalability, and sustainability of the supply of high-quality PUFAs have become an important industrial issue. Despite its effectiveness, this reliance on marine resources is increasingly considered unsustainable under the conditions of overfishing, draining wild stocks of fish, disrupting the ecosystem, and being susceptible to climate change (Ganesan et al., 2018). Moreover, fish oils are also subject to heavy metal, dioxin, and polychlorinated biphenyl contamination, which require more refining and purifying processes, making production more expensive and even more harmful to the environment (Ruiz, 2021; Shahidi & Zhong, 2021). There are limitations to plant-based sources of omega-6, such as land-use, changes in oil composition, agricultural inputs, and competing food and feed production systems (Patel, 2021).

All these sustainability, safety, and supply-chain issues have prompted research across the globe to find alternative production platforms of PUFA. Microbial and algal systems have also become especially promising alternatives because of their high growth rates, their ability not to be reliant on arable land and marine ecosystems, and their susceptibility to controlled cultivation conditions (Adarme-Vega et al., 2020; Ratledge, 2019). Microalgae, filamentous fungi, yeasts, and genetically engineered bacteria can accumulate large intracellular lipid levels with custom fatty acid composition, so they can be promising sources of the PUFA industry (Lee et al., 2019; Zhou et al., 2022). Although this is a promising venture,

Omega-3 and Omega-6 Polyunsaturated Fatty Acids in Food Systems. DOI: https://doi.org/10.1016/B978-0-443-43810-3.00026-9

the transfer of microbial and algal PUFA production at laboratory scale or pilot scale into industrial production is a complicated and expensive task. Low volumetric productivity is one of the most critical obstacles that directly influences the economics of the processes and their commercial viability (López, 2020; Morales, 2023). Mass-produced bioreactor processes also pose other issues, such as oxygen transfer rate, ineffective mixing, heat loss, and shear stress sensitivity of PUFA-producing organisms, and they may affect the yield and product consistency (Ganesan et al., 2018; Ruiz, 2021). Downstream processing is also another significant bottleneck of PUFA industrialization. A significant percentage of the total production costs may be due to cell harvesting, lipid extraction, purification, and concentration (Bimbo et al., 2020; Patel, 2021). Traditional solvent-based extraction techniques have issues that are associated with the toxicity of the solvents, efficiency, and low environmental sustainability, but on the other hand, the alternative green extraction techniques often consume large amounts of capital. What is more, it is the number of multiple oxidative bonds that makes PUFAs particularly vulnerable to oxidative degradation, requiring strict control of the conditions of processing, storage, and formulation to maintain the quality of the products and their bioactivity (Shahidi, 2021; Shahidi & Zhong, 2021). Regulation is also an added complexity in industrial PUFA manufacturing. Pharmaceutical, infant nutrition, and medical food products should have high-purity, safety, traceability, and stability indices in accordance with the international standards). To become approved by the regulation at an industrial level, approved production processes, developed quality management systems, and elaborate risk assessment instruments must be considered, which significantly become more complex and cost-intensive to run (Morales, 2023).

The economic feasibility is still a conclusive factor that determines the use of alternative PUFA production technologies. Despite the current improvement of the production system through the use of strain engineering and optimization of bioprocess, microbial and algal production systems of PUFA tend to be more costly than the traditional fish oil extraction (Ruiz, 2021; Zhou et al., 2022). The cost of feedstock, energy needs, capital expenditure on bioreactor systems, and postprocessing costs are all factors that influence the structure of the costs of industrial activity. There is thus a need to address these economic limitations in order to allow large-scale commercialization. The latest technological changes provide promising solutions to these problems. PUFA biosynthetic pathways have also been redesigned using metabolic engineering and synthetic biology tools to increase carbon flux towards target fatty acids and the capacity of strains to survive and work under industrial conditions (Lee et al., 2019; López, 2020). Sustainability concerns have been gaining a lot of focus on PUFA industrialization. The research of life-cycle assessment suggests that the use of conventional marine-derived PUFA production is related to a high carbon footprint, and next-generation microbial and algal platforms, especially when combined with renewable feedstocks and principles of a circular bioeconomy, have lower carbon footprints (Morales, 2023). It is also a scientific and industrial necessity to align the production of PUFA with the global goals of sustainability.

Nevertheless, despite all the advances, the literature on the topic is typically more fragmented, covering separate biological, engineering, or regulatory factors related to the issues of production of PUFA. What is missing is the combination of what can be termed as integrated analysis that addresses biological systems, process engineering, downstream processing, regulatory compliance, economic feasibility, and environmental sustainability in an integrated manner. This loophole highlights the importance of a thorough assessment of the issues of scale-up and the plans for a solution.

In this regard, the purpose of this chapter is to conduct a systematic and integrative evaluation of the issues and remedies in scaling up the production of omega-3 and omega-6 PUFA to be utilized in industries. The priority is paid to processes of the last 10 years with specific references to microbial and algal production systems, bioprocess engineering practices, stabilization, and sustainability-oriented innovations. Through the integration of recent scientific and industrial developments, this chapter aims to provide a consistent perspective of the future of scalable, economical, and environmentally friendly production of PUFA.

29.2 Present-day situation and literature review

In the last 10 years, the industrial synthesis of omega-3 fatty acids and omega-6 fatty acids (PUFAs) has tremendously changed in line with the increased demand for these fatty acids by pharmaceutical, nutraceutical, food, and cosmetic products. Traditional marine-based production methods and plant-derived PUFA in the initial production phases had a lot of reliance on the traditional sources, but growing concerns about sustainability, quality, and scalability have transformed the world of PUFA production (Sprague et al., 2017). Modern studies and industrial activities are placing more emphasis on alternative biological sources, superior bioprocess technologies, as well as integrated production systems in a bid to maintain a steady and sustainable supply of PUFA.

29.2.1 Traditional sources of polyunsaturated fatty acids: the present state of affairs and the limitations

Industrial extraction of PUFA still relies on oily fish (anchovy, sardine, mackerel, etc.) as a raw material because these fish naturally contain a large amount of omega-3 (Ganesan et al., 2018; Shahidi & Zhong, 2021). Although technology has led to higher extraction and purification efficiency, the overexploitation of fish stocks, the ecological disequilibrium, and exposure to fluctuations in the marine ecosystem based on climate conditions are also posing an increasing challenge to the use of marine resources (Ruiz, 2021).

Fish-derived PUFAs have quality and safety issues besides environmental sustainability issues. Oils of marine origin are prone to oxidative deterioration and heavy metal contamination, dioxin, and persistent organic pollutant contamination, and thus require intense refining, deodorization, and stabilization (Bimbo et al., 2020; Shahidi, 2021). The extra processing involved raises the cost of production and may have adverse effects on the nutritional value of PUFAs. More so, the preferences of consumers are slowly moving to the vegetarian and vegan options, which further hinder the sustainability of fish oil-derived PUFA supply chains in the long term (Patel, 2021).

The primary sources of omega-6 fatty acids and short-chain omega-3 fatty acids like α-linolenic acid (ALA) are plant-based sources, especially the oil-bearing crops (e.g., soybean, sunflower, flax, etc.). Although these sources are renewable and abundant, their use in the production of long-chain PUFAs is minimal because of low levels of the effectiveness of the conversion of ALA to eicosapentaenoic acid (EPA) and DHA in the human body. Additionally, land, climatic unpredictability, pesticides, and food and feed competition also limit agricultural production of oilseed crops, which casts doubt on scalability and sustainability (Morales, 2023; Patel, 2021).

29.2.2 Growth of microbial and algal polyunsaturated fatty acid production systems

Microbial and algal systems have become a significant and promising alternative to the traditional sources of PUFA as a result of their restriction. Microalgae are the most important sources of long-chain omega-3 PUFAs in marine food webs, and thus offer a biologically reasonable and sustainable food source alternative to fish (Adarme-Vega et al., 2020). By growing microalgae industrially, it is possible to produce EPA and DHA in a controlled environment without depending on wild fish stocks, which is an important solution to significant sustainability issues (López, 2020; Ratledge, 2019). In addition to microalgae, oleaginous microorganisms have been shown to have a high ability to produce and accumulate PUFA, including fungi (e.g., *Mortierella* species), yeasts, and genetically engineered bacteria (Lee et al., 2019; Ratledge, 2019). The advantages of these systems are high lipid productivity, rapid growth rates, nondependence on climatic conditions, and the ability to use these systems on a large-scale fermentation (Morales, 2023; Zhou et al., 2022). Improvements in metabolic engineering have further improved the capacity of microbial systems to synthesize a given profile of PUFA to meet industrial demand. Nevertheless, microbial and algal production of PUFA on a commercial scale has not been achieved despite promising laboratory-scale production. The problems with the current industrial processes are connected with the robustness of the strain, the stability of the productivity, and the competitive performance in the economy in comparison with the existing fish oil extraction methods (Patel, 2021; Ruiz, 2021).

29.2.3 Polyunsaturated fatty acids biosynthesis and strain engineering (2015–25) advances

In the last 10 years, there has been a great deal of success in designing PUFA biosynthetic pathways and manipulating them. The desaturase and elongase enzymes are key to the transformation of the precursory fatty acids into the long-chain PUFAs, and the targeted regulation of these pathways has been a top priority in recent research (Lee et al., 2019). The precision of routing metabolic systems has been made possible through synthetic biology and genome-editing tools, which have led to higher yields of PUFA and a higher efficacy of carbon flux (López, 2020; Zhou et al., 2022). These innovations have led to the accumulation of lipid, less production of by-products, and tolerance to stresses associated with processes (oxygen demand and shear forces). However, the issues of genetic stability and acceptance regulation of genetically modified microorganisms are major obstacles to wide industry implementation.

29.2.4 Bioprocess and scale-up innovations in the present-day industrial environment

Bio process engineering has become a key factor in determining the success of PUFA production in industries. The recent works focus on the need to maximize fermentation regimes, such as batch, fed-batch, and continuous ones, to increase productivity and scalability (Ganesan et al., 2018; Zhou et al., 2022). In the case of microorganisms involved in the PUFA production, in particular, oxygen transfer efficiency, nutrient feeding, and temperature regulation play a particularly important role in the lipid buildup and fatty acid structure (Morales, 2023; Ruiz, 2021). In spite of technological advances, the laboratory to industrial bioreactor scaling-up processes tend to lead to a decrease in yields and erratic product quality. The issues of hydrodynamic stress, oxygen shortage, and heat loss are even more severe at a large scale, and advanced reactor design and process control systems are required (López, 2020; Patel, 2021). These problems suggest the enduring disconnect between the innovation and implementation of laboratories and industry.

29.2.5 Downstream processing and stability problems

Downstream processing is also among the most expensive processes in manufacturing PUFA. More than half of total production costs can be attributed to cell harvesting, lipid extraction, purification, and stabilization, especially microbial and algal systems (Bimbo et al., 2020; Ruiz, 2021). Traditional solvent-based extraction methods are not only good but also evoke concerns about solvent recovery, safety, and environmental consequences, which have led to the increasing popularity of other green extraction technologies (Patel, 2021; Shahidi & Zhong, 2021). Another significant issue is oxidative instability because PUFAs are very prone to oxidation during processing and storage. The recent research points to the increasing role of antioxidant addition, encapsulation, and sophisticated formulation approaches to maintain the quality of PUFA and additionally increase their shelf life (Morales, 2023; Shahidi, 2021). The developments are vital in guaranteeing the incorporation of industrial quality standards and consumer expectations.

29.2.6 Market and regulatory trends that are defining the present situation

The regulatory standards on PUFA manufacturing and commercialization have grown tighter within the past 10 years, especially with regard to the use of the product in the pharmaceutical and infant food sectors. The safety assessment, traceability records, and constant product quality pose challenges to the emergent production platforms and are obligatory by the regulatory agencies. Meeting these needs is frequently an indicator of the viability of the scaling of new technologies of PUFA production. In market terms, the demand for sustainably produced and vegetarian PUFAs is steadily growing, as consumers are more aware of these products, and companies have a corporate responsibility towards sustainability). The trend is likely to continue enhancing the pace of innovation in the microbial and algal PUFA-based production systems despite the prevailing technical and economic challenges.

29.2.7 Overview of the prevailing situation

In short, the modern-day picture of PUFA production demonstrates a shift in the traditional sources of production, which are based on the ocean and agriculture, towards the new microbial and algal sources that are able to be supported by biotechnology and process engineering. Although this has improved a lot during the last 10 years, industrial-scale production still experiences the issue of productivity, cost, stability, regulatory compliance, and sustainability. To solve these interrelated problems, it is necessary to approach these issues with combined measures that combine biological innovation, engineering optimization, and regulatory alignment.

29.3 Principles and methodology of polyunsaturated fatty acid production scale-up to an industrial level

The process of expanding the production of omega-3 and omega-6 PUFAs from laboratory or pilot levels to industrial levels would require thorough knowledge of the biological systems, process engineering principles, and economic limitations. The scale-up of industrial processes does not correlate with laboratory processes; instead, it entails multidimensional interactions in terms of microbial physiology, hydrodynamics of bioreactors, mass and heat transfers, and efficiency in downstream processing (Ganesan et al., 2018; López, 2020). The extensive commercialization of PUFA production technologies to industry scale is thus pegged on a well-knit approach that takes into account upstream and downstream issues.

29.3.1 Biological support of polyunsaturated fatty acid biosynthesis

A cascade of enzyme reactions that are highly regulated controls the synthesis of PUFA in microorganisms and algae, via fatty acid desaturases and elongases. These enzymes add the number of double bonds and long carbon chains, making it possible to convert precursor fatty acids into long-chain PUFAs, including EPA, DHA, and ARA (Lee et al., 2019). Nobody can be sure of backing up intracellular lipid accumulation or ultimate PUFA production without the efficiency of these biosynthetic pathways, and thus metabolic control is an important factor to be considered during scale-up. At the industrial level, cellular metabolism is highly dependent on environmental factors, including nutrient level, oxygen level, temperature, and pH. The change of such parameters can modify the activity of enzymes, the distribution of metabolic fluxes, and the composition of lipids, which can cause inconsistencies in the production of PUFA (Morales, 2023; Ratledge, 2019). As a result, the preservation of metabolic stability across large-volume bioreactors is a principle of the industrial production of PUFA.

29.3.2 Strain improvement and selection strategies

The adoption of strong and productive strains is a foundation of the scalable production of PUFA. High lipid accumulation capabilities are found in naturally oleaginous microorganisms, including microalgae, filamentous fungi, and some yeasts; nevertheless, their inherent productivity of PUFA is frequently below that needed to be competitive in the industry (Adarme-Vega et al., 2020; Ruiz, 2021). Consequently, the improvement of strain has come to be the center of interest in industrial PUFA scale-up approaches.

The metabolic engineering strategies are designed to reintroduce the carbon flow into PUFA production through overexpression of the major desaturase and elongase enzymes, inhibition of alternative pathways, and improvement of the precursors (Lee et al., 2019; López, 2020).

29.3.3 Process and mode fermentation design

The mode of production of the type of PUFA is usually rooted in the principles of submerged fermentation used in the batch, fed-batch, or continuous modes of cultivation, each having distinct benefits and drawbacks (Ganesan et al., 2018; Patel, 2021). Simple batch processes are simple in terms of operations, but in most cases are limited by nutrient depletion and low productivity. The quantity of nutrients fed to the organism is controlled with fed-batch systems, which promote biomass and lipid growth. Sustained fermentation is also the topic of investigation that will allow achieving volumetric productivity and overall process efficiency, but the longevity of the culture and the ability to maintain the composition of PUFA are also the primary concern (Ruiz, 2021; Zhou et al., 2022). Various technical and operational limits play a major role in determining the yield and quality of PUFA during scale-up. In Table 29.1, the key scale-up problems in the upstream, the reasons behind them, the consequences in the production of PUFA, and mitigation measures are summarized. The choice of a suitable mode of fermentation should thus be a trade-off between productivity, operational stability and economic viability, especially at the industrial level.

29.3.4 Constricted oxygen transfer and mixing

The availability of oxygen is one of the most crucial parameters that affect the production of PUFA because the desaturase enzyme that includes double bonds to the fatty acid chains is an oxygen-dependent enzyme. Although oxygen constraint is not often a big issue with laboratory scale because of the smaller working volumes and effective agitation, it is a major constraint in industrial-scale operations (Ganesan et al., 2018; López, 2020). Oxygen gradient, inadequate mass transfer, low mixing efficiency, and localized hypoxia can occur in large bioreactors and adversely influence the growth of microbes and lipid accumulation. In order to overcome these limitations, agitation rate, aeration rate, and reactor geometry should be optimized to promote higher oxygen transfer rates (OTR). Nevertheless, such adaptations have to be well-balanced to ensure that shear stress is minimized to avoid harming delicate PUFA-bearing microorganisms and lowering the overall productivity (Morales, 2023; Patel, 2021). To overcome the scale-up issues, especially those inherent in the traditional stirred-tank reactors, alternative reactors design that include air-lift reactors and bubble column reactors have been suggested. These systems enhance the mass transfer between gases and liquids and decrease the shear caused by the mechanisms, thus being appropriate in large-scale PUFA fermentation processes (Ruiz, 2021; Zhou et al., 2022). The industrial PUFA production workflow, as shown in Fig. 29.1, combines several steps, such as strain engineering towards greater lipid productivity, large-scale fermentation under regulated oxygen availability, downstream processing to obtain lipid products that need extraction and purification, and the ultimate step of formulating it into either a pharmaceutical, nutraceutical, or food-grade product (Ganesan et al., 2018; López, 2020; Morales, 2023).

29.3.5 Optimization of nutrient feeding and carbon source

Lipid accumulation and PUFA composition depend on the strength of the carbon and nitrogen availability. To achieve an optimal scale-up of nutrient feeding strategies in industrial settings is essential to achieve the highest PUFA production with the minimal amount of substrates wasted and production cost (Bimbo et al., 2020; Ratledge, 2019). The carbon-rich environments and nitrogen-limited environments are usually used to promote lipid build-up, but the over-nutrient-limited

TABLE 29.1 Critical upstream scale-up threats and mitigation strategies in polyunsaturated fatty acid (PUFA) manufacturing.

Scale-up challenge	Underlying cause affecting PUFA production	Impact on PUFA yield/quality	Mitigation/reduction strategies	Citations
Poor volumetric productivity	Metabolic bottlenecks; nutrient imbalance	Reduced PUFA yield; increased production cost	Metabolic engineering; fed-batch fermentation strategies	López (2020), Ratledge (2019)
Limitations in oxygen transfer	High cell density; large bioreactor volumes	Incomplete fatty acid desaturation; reduced LC-PUFA synthesis	Optimized aeration rates; improved bioreactor design	Ganesan et al. (2018), Ruiz (2021)
Sensitivity to shear stress	High agitation and aeration rates	Cell damage, lipid leakage, and loss	Use of air-lift reactors; development of shear-tolerant strains	Patel (2021), Zhou et al. (2022)
Nutrient variability	Use of low-cost or complex feedstocks	Batch-to-batch variability; inconsistent PUFA profiles	Adaptive and controlled feeding strategies	Morales (2023), Ratledge (2019)

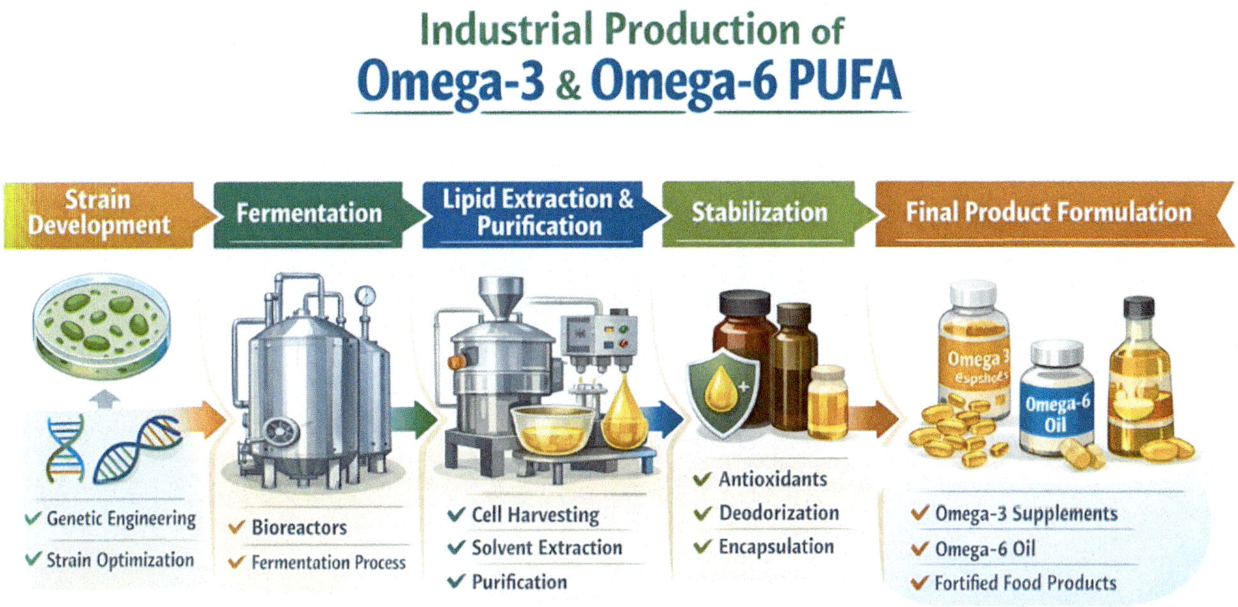

FIGURE 29.1 Shows the overall workflow that is usually used in industrial polyunsaturated fatty acid (PUFA) creation, which includes strain engineering, mass fermentation, downstream processing, and formulation.
Source: From Ganesan, B., Brothersen, C., & McMahon, D. J. (2018). Fortification of foods with omega-3 polyunsaturated fatty acids. Critical Reviews in Food Science and Nutrition, 58(1), 1–13. https://doi.org/10.1080/10408398.2016.1164126 López, S., et al. (2020). Industrial fermentation strategies for omega-3 production. Biotechnology Advances, 43, 107552. https://doi.org/10.1016/j.biotechadv.2020.107552 Morales, D., et al. (2023). Sustainable microbial lipid production for food and nutraceutical applications. Trends in Food Science & Technology, 134, 25–38. https://doi.org/10.1016/j.tifs.2023.02.006.

environments may decrease the cell viability and productivity when used on a large scale. Although promising, the utilization of alternative feedstocks implies that the composition and possible inhibitory compounds vary and require solid process control approaches in the industrial deployment (Patel, 2021; Ruiz, 2021).

29.3.6 Scale-up requirements and process control

The identification and preservation of major scale-up criteria, e.g., constant power input per unit volume, oxygen transfer coefficient (kLa), or mixing time, are essential to scale-up PUFA production processes successfully (Ganesan et al., 2018; Zhou et al., 2022). Nevertheless, there is no universal criterion chosen to implement all PUFA production systems, and it is critical to optimize the case. The level of process monitoring and control systems is of high significance in the industrial production of PUFA. Such technologies will be especially useful when it comes to ensuring PUFA quality and consistency between production batches.

29.3.7 Downstream processing methodologies

A significant portion of the overall production costs is incurred by the cell harvesting, lipid extraction, purification, and concentration (Bimbo et al., 2020; Ruiz, 2021). According to the data in Table 29.2, the downstream processing procedures, including centrifugation, solvent extraction, molecular distillation, and oxidation control, play an important role in determining the overall cost framework and commercial viability of the PUFA production process. Mass production of PUFA, therefore needs effective downstream strategies to be economically viable. As an example, traditional centrifugation as a form of cell harvesting is an energy-consuming process that significantly increases the cost of operation, whereas the implementation of membrane filtration methodologies is gaining popularity as scalable alternatives that are more energy-efficient (Ruiz, 2021; Morales, 2023). On the same note, the conventional direct organic solvent extraction techniques, although commonly used, owing to their superior extraction rate, evoke issues regarding the toxicity of solvents, environmental issues, and legal requirements. Table 29.2 shows that the extraction of supercritical CO_2 is being considered a safer and greener way to extract with better selectivity and lower solvent residue (Shahidi & Zhong, 2021). Molecular distillation is also a conventional method in the purification step, but it is expensive and capital-intensive and characterized by a high cost of operation. The development of membrane-based purification systems as

TABLE 29.2 Downstream processing and polyunsaturated fatty acid stabilization methodologies.

Processing stage	Traditional solution	Limitations	Scalable/advanced alternatives	References
Cell harvesting	Centrifugation	High energy consumption; operational cost	Membrane filtration techniques	Ruiz (2021), Morales (2023)
Solvent extraction	Direct organic solvent extraction	Solvent toxicity; environmental and safety concerns	Supercritical CO_2 extraction	Shahidi and Zhong (2021)
Purification	Molecular distillation	Capital-intensive; high operational cost	Membrane-based purification systems	Patel (2021)
Oxidation control	Synthetic antioxidants	Regulatory restrictions; consumer safety concerns	Encapsulation technologies; natural antioxidants	Shahidi (2021), Bimbo et al. (2020)

cost-effective and scalable systems is also becoming popular in the industrial sphere (Patel, 2021). In addition, one of the most important aspects when it comes to the preservation of PUFA is the oxidation control. Although the use of synthetic antioxidants has long been a traditional method, the desire to mitigate this tendency by regulatory requirements and the need to ensure the safety of the products have promoted the development of interest in encapsulation technologies and natural antioxidants as less dangerous forms of stabilization (Bimbo et al., 2020; Shahidi, 2021). Downstream Processing and PUFA stabilization methodologies, the adoption of alternative methods of PUFA production, where traditional methods are replaced by scalable and sustainable methods, is a necessity to enhance the economic feasibility and industrial scalability of PUFA production processes.

29.3.8 Polyunsaturated fatty acid stability and oxidation control during processing

The chemical composition of PUFAs makes them very vulnerable to oxidative degradation when it comes to processing and storage. Not only does oxidation decrease the nutritional value, but it also forms off-flavors and potentially toxic oxidation products, which are serious quality and safety issues (Shahidi, 2021; Shahidi & Zhong, 2021). PUFA stability is also improved by encapsulation and advanced delivery systems; therefore they are combined with the scale-up approaches in the industrial use of PUFA (Patel, 2021; Shahidi, 2021).

29.3.9 Scale-up economic and sustainability issues

Microbial and algal systems have sustainability benefits, but their production is commonly more expensive than the traditional fish oil extraction systems, which limits their competitiveness on the market. Life-cycle analysis and other forms of sustainability assessment have become important in the process of making scale-up decisions in industry. The research continues to show that optimized systems of microbial and algal production of PUFA can result in a smaller environmental footprint in the case of renewable energy sources and the principles of a circular bioeconomy (Morales, 2023). Sustainability indicators in scale-up methodologies are hence necessary in the long-term industrial achievement.

The algal-derived DHA has attained very high momentum within the nutraceutical sector because of its vegetarian-derived source, lack of marine pollutants, and the uniformity of fatty acid profile (Adarme-Vega et al., 2020; Zhou et al., 2022). Even though omega-6 fatty acids are highly abundant in plant oils, they are gradually being integrated into balanced omega-3/omega-6 supplements to restore the ideal ratios of the fats in the diet (Calder, 2017; Simopoulos, 2020). The industrial encapsulation technologies are instrumental in the case of enhancing shelf stability, hiding odor, and bioavailability of the nutraceutical PUFA products (Patel, 2021; Shahidi & Zhong, 2021).

29.3.10 Economic sustainability in scale-up

The economic feasibility of the PUFA production technologies is a solution to determine whether the proposed technologies have a good chance to be scaled up successfully. Microbial and algal systems have many advantages in terms of sustainability, but the cost of production is usually higher than conventional fish oil extraction, which also restricts their competitiveness in the market. Sustainability evaluations, such as analysis of life-cycle, have assumed more significance in the process of making decisions on industrial scale-up. The literature shows that microbial and algal PUFA production systems, which are optimized, would be able to produce lower environmental footprints when incorporated with renewable energy sources and circular bioeconomy principles (Morales, 2023). The integration of sustainability metrics in the scale-up practices is hence necessary in order to be successful in the industries in the long-term perspective.

29.3.11 Systemic approach to scale-up in industrial-scale

Strain engineering, bioprocess optimization, downstream innovation, and sustainability assessment are all parts and parcels of an integrated approach needed to overcome the multifaceted challenges of PUFA industrialization. Individual process components can be optimized in a fragmented manner, but when the processes are implemented in an integrated manner, they can produce synergies in their productivity, quality, and cost efficiency (López, 2020; Morales, 2023). The recent literature gives increased focus to the interplay between biotechnology, process engineering, and digitalization in the production of PUFA used in industries. The future of scale-up strategies has a strong role in advanced modeling, real-time monitoring, and data-based optimization tools, which will allow making industrial processes more predictable and controllable (Morales, 2023; Zhou et al., 2022).

29.4 Omega-3 and omega-6 polyunsaturated fatty acids as industrial applications

29.4.1 Introduction to industrial polyunsaturated fatty acids applications

The scientifically proven health benefits and versatile application as functional ingredients in a variety of industries have made omega-3 and omega-6 PUFAs no longer niche nutritional constituents (Calder, 2020a, 2020b; Shahidi & Ambigaipalan, 2018). They have uses in pharmaceuticals, nutraceuticals, functional foods, infant nutrition, cosmetics, animal feed, and novel medical nutrition treatments; thus large-scale production of PUFA is a strategic priority of the world industries (Ganesan et al., 2018; Swanson et al., 2019). Regarding industries, high-value health markets are dominated by omega-3 fatty acids, namely, EPA and DHA, and omega-6 fatty acids, including ARA, are of significant importance in infant nutrition and clinical preparations (Calder, 2017; Ratledge, 2019). The variety of alternative sources of PUFA that have been achieved by means of microbial and algal systems rather than the traditional fish oil has greatly increased the use options as they guarantee sustainability, purity, and stability of the supply chain (Adarme-Vega et al., 2020; Zhou et al., 2022).

29.4.2 Pharmaceutical and clinical nutrition applications

In cardiovascular, inflammatory, neurological, and metabolic diseases, the pharmaceutical industry is one of the most controlled and at the same time profitable applications of omega-3 and omega-6 PUFA (Calder, 2020a, 2020b; Shahidi & Zhong, 2021). The production of PUFA in large amounts thus needs to fulfill the necessary purity of pharmaceutical grade, oxidation, and batch-to-batch consistency (López, 2020; Patel, 2021). The use of omega-6 fatty acids and, specifically, ARA as clinically important nutrients in neonatal and parenteral nutrition is supported by promoting immune development, cell membrane integrity, and the production of eicosanoids (Calder, 2017; Koletzko, 2020). Fermentation platforms based on microorganisms have become the technology of choice to produce pharmaceutical-grade ARA because it is capable of producing lipids that are free of contaminants with specific fatty acid profiles (Morales, 2023; Ratledge, 2019). The growing significance of PUFA-based lipid emulsions in intravenous nutrition only enhances the fact that scalable, sterile, regulatory-compliant production systems are significantly needed (Ruiz, 2021; Shahidi & Ambigaipalan, 2018).

29.4.3 Nutraceutical and dietary supplement industry

The biggest commercial consumer of omega-3 fatty acids is the nutraceutical market, as more consumers are becoming aware of the benefits of preventive healthcare and the management of lifestyle-related illnesses (Calder, 2020a, 2020b; Swanson et al., 2019). Omega-3 products for cardiovascular health, cognitive support, joint health, and immune modulation in the form of capsules, soft gels, emulsions, and powders are commonly sold in the market (Nichols, 2019; Shahidi, 2021). On an industrial scale, the issues of scalability directly impact the affordability and accessibility of the products, so PUFA production based on cost-optimization is a necessary factor in the market sustainability (López, 2020; Morales, 2023).

29.4.4 Functional foods and beverage uses

The addition of omega-3 and omega-6 PUFAs to functional foods can be discussed as one of the most rapidly developing areas of application due to the growing popularity of everyday health-promoting food among consumers (Ganesan et al., 2018; Swanson et al., 2019). Nutritional fortification of dairy products, bakery products, beverages, edible oils, spreads, and meat analogs mainly involves the use of DHA and linoleic acid (LA) by functional foodstuffs. Such fortification approaches boost the nutritional content without making any major change in the sensory attributes when well-designed (Shahidi, 2021; Shahidi & Ambigaipalan, 2018). Nevertheless, massive inclusion of PUFAs into food systems poses serious technological issues, especially thermal unstable nature of products and oxidative degradation during processing and storage, as shown in Table 29.3 (Ganesan et al., 2018; Morales, 2023). To overcome these limitations, more and more protective technologies are used within industries in order to combat them including microencapsulation, nano-emulation systems, and spray-drying methods. These methods stabilize PUFAs by reducing the exposure to oxygen, light, and heat, and retain the bioactivity of the active compounds, allowing the release of these compounds to be controlled in complex food systems (Patel, 2021; Zhou et al., 2022). Omega-6 fats also add functionality other than nutrition. They modify texture, mouthfeel, and caloric density and promote neurodevelopment as well as immune modulation in combination with DHA and ARA in infant foods and specialized nutrition products, as demonstrated under the infant formula industry in Table 29.3 (Calder, 2017; Koletzko, 2020; Ratledge, 2019). However, compliance with the regulation and high purity

TABLE 29.3 Key industrial application areas of omega-3 and omega-6 polyunsaturated fatty acids, formulation strategies, and scale-up challenges.

Application sector	Key PUFA type	Functional role	Industrial form	Major scale-up challenges	References
Pharmaceuticals	DHA, EPA	Antiinflammatory activity; triglyceride reduction	Capsules, emulsions, injectables	Requirement for high purity; oxidation control	Calder (2020a, 2020b), Skulas-Ray (2021)
Nutraceuticals	EPA, DHA	Cardiovascular protection; cognitive health support	Soft gels, powders	Cost of production; shelf-life stability	Nichols (2019), Shahidi (2021)
Functional foodstuffs	DHA, LA	Nutritional fortification	Dairy products, bakery items, beverages	Thermal instability; oxidative degradation	Ganesan et al. (2018), Morales (2023)
Infant formula	DHA, ARA	Neurodevelopment; immune modulation	Oil blends, microencapsulated forms	Regulatory compliance; stringent purity standards	Koletzko (2020), Ratledge (2019)
Cosmetics	LA, ALA	Skin barrier enhancement; antiaging effects	Creams, lotions, serums	Odor masking; oxidation prevention	Shahidi and Zhong (2021)
Animal nutrition	DHA, EPA	Growth promotion; immune enhancement	Feed oils, pellets	Cost-effective large-scale production	Tacon and Metian (2020)

remain key scale-up factors in this segment. In addition to the functional foods, Table 29.3 also captures the other important industrial sectors such as pharmaceuticals, nutraceuticals, and cosmetics. Formulations to be used as pharmaceuticals, including capsules, emulsions, and injectables, need a high degree of purity and control over oxidation of DHA and EPA (Calder, 2020a, 2020b; Skulas-Ray et al., 2021; Skulas-Ray, 2021). Nutraceuticals are subjected to issues regarding the cost of production and the shelf-life stability (Nichols, 2019; Shahidi, 2021), whereas cosmetic formulations have to deal with the problem of odor masking and oxidative stability (Shahidi & Zhong, 2021). Key industrial application areas of omega-3 and omega-6 PUFAs, formulation strategies, and scale-up challenges. Scalable stabilization technologies and highly regulatory-approved food-grade antioxidants should be obligatory to make sure that the product will be stable, safe, and successful (Morales, 2023; Shahidi & Zhong, 2021).

29.4.5 Infant formula and early-life nutrition

Infant formula is one of the most strictly controlled and scientifically important spheres of application of omega-3 and omega-6 PUFAs (Calder, 2017; Koletzko, 2020). The main PUFAs were introduced into infant nutrition products because of their essential functions in brain development, vision, immune system development, and cellular growth (Calder, 2020a, 2020b; Ratledge, 2019). The synthesis of PUFAs that are to be used in infant formula must meet very high standards of purity, a set of ratios of fatty acids, and global regulatory standards, including those developed by the European Food Safety Authority and the Codex Alimentarius Commission (López, 2020; Morales, 2023). These standards control the maximum contaminants, oxidative stability, and composition requirements in order to maintain the safety of infants. DHA and ARA produced through fermentation by microorganisms are now the choice in industrial sources of infant formula. The production of oils through fermentation avoids the risks of heavy metals and environmental contaminants and guarantees the consistency of supplies and controlled fatty acid compositions in comparison with marine-derived oils (Adarme-Vega et al., 2020; Zhou et al., 2022). The PUFA value chain has shifted to large-scale fermentation, downstream purification, stabilization, and formulation strategies to satisfy the global market. Microbial production systems are scalable, which is especially significant when it comes to the uninterrupted supply of these products in developing economies, where the demand for fortified infant nutrition products is ever-growing (Ruiz, 2021; Swanson et al., 2019). Nevertheless, processing and storage that occurs through oxidative degradation is a significant technical issue. Thus the downstream purification methods and stabilization technologies are highly developed, such as microencapsulation and the use of antioxidants, to preserve the integrity of the products, as can be seen in Fig. 29.2. Flow chart of PUFA value chain demonstrating the transition to the large-scale production and integrated downstream processing (Patel, 2021; Shahidi & Ambigaipalan, 2018). In this way, infant formula is a highly controlled but fast-growing industry in which technology, regulatory adherence, and production on a large scale have to closely interact with each other in order to provide safety and effectiveness in nutritional value.

29.4.6 Cosmetic and personal care applications

The use of omega-3 and omega-6 fatty acids is slowly becoming a trend in cosmetic and personal care formulations because of their skin barrier repair, antiinflammatory, and moisturizing effects (Calder, 2020a, 2020b; Shahidi, 2021). LA is an omega-6 fatty acid that is essential in epidermal maintenance and in the prevention of transepidermal water loss, whereas omega-3 fatty acids play a role in antiaging and photoprotective (Morales, 2023; Simopoulos, 2020). A stable and odor-neutral PUFA ingredient with nonoxidizing properties is needed in the cosmetic industry, and it all directly affects the industrial processing strategies (Patel, 2021; Ruiz, 2021).

PUFAs produced by biotechnology are especially appealing to cosmetic use because they can be traced, which is more sustainable, and because they can be used in clean labeling (Adarme-Vega et al., 2020; Zhou et al., 2022). The industrial encapsulation systems allow the use of PUFAs in creams, serums, and lotions without affecting their shelf life, sensory characteristics, or other properties (Morales, 2023; Shahidi & Zhong, 2021). The commercial feasibility of such technologies depends on their scalability when used in mass-market cosmetic products (Ganesan et al., 2018; López, 2020).

29.4.7 Feeding of livestock and aquaculture

Examples of significant consumers of omega-3 PUFA and, in particular, DHA and EPA are aquaculture and the animal feed industry, which require them to develop, maintain immunity, and improve fillet quality (Nichols, 2019; Tacon & Metian, 2020). Reduction in the supply of fish oil has increased the use of microbial and algal sources of PUFA as sustainable feeds (Adarme-Vega et al., 2020; Zhou et al., 2022). The production of PUFA on an industrial scale allows the

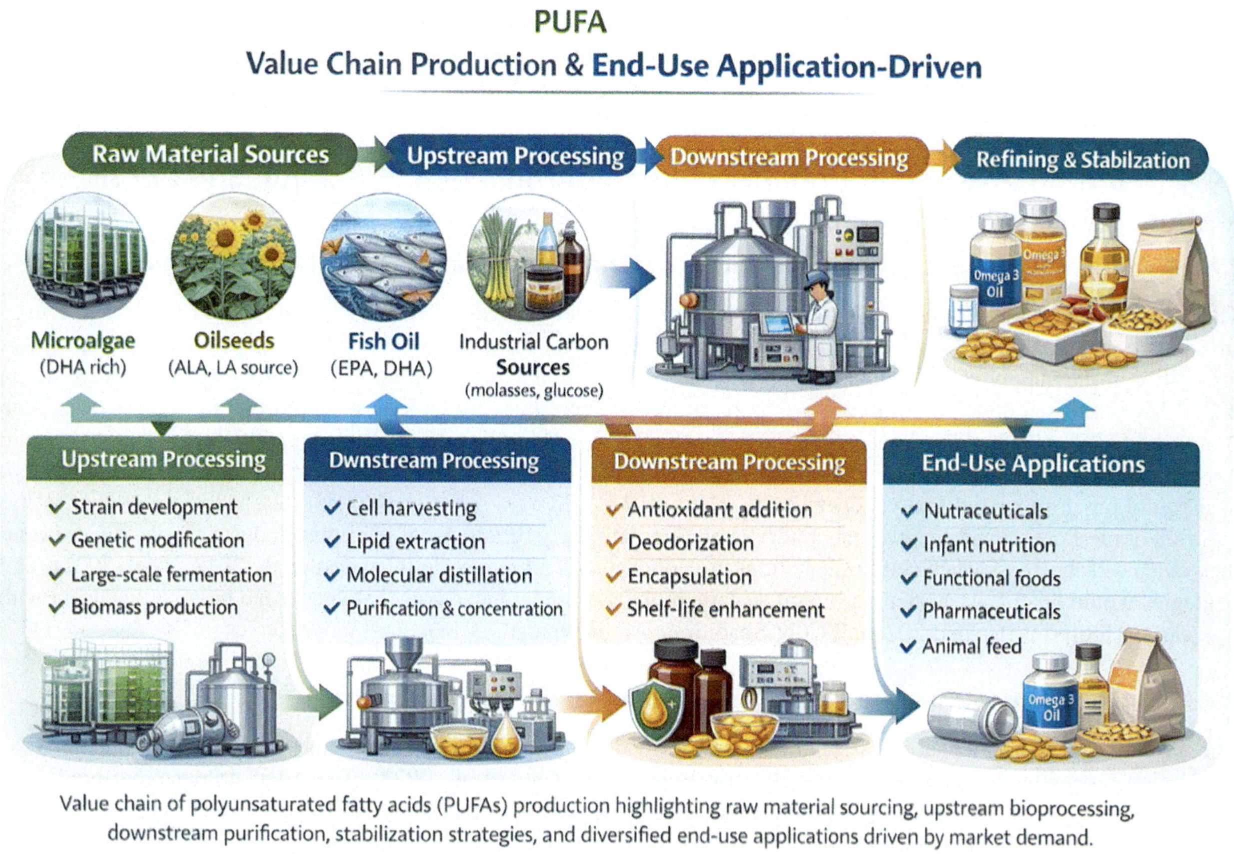

FIGURE 29.2 Flow chart of polyunsaturated fatty acid (PUFA) value chain showing the shift of the large-scale microbial/algal production to downstream processing, stabilization, formulation, and sector-specific uses such as pharmaceuticals, functional foods, infant nutrition, cosmetics, and animal feed.

Source: From López, S. et al. (2020). Industrial fermentation strategies for omega-3 production. Biotechnology Advances, 43, 107552. https://doi.org/10.1016/j.biotechadv.2020.107552 Shahidi, F., & Ambigaipalan, P. (2018). Omega-3 polyunsaturated fatty acids and their health benefits. Annual Review of Food Science and Technology, 9, 345–381. https://doi.org/10.1146/annurev-food-111317-095850 Zhou, Y., et al. (2022). Synthetic biology approaches for omega-3 production. Metabolic Engineering, 69, 1–14. https://doi.org/10.1016/j.ymben.2021.10.003.

active supply of high-quality lipids in the composition of aquafeed and decreases the pressure on marine ecosystems (López, 2020; Morales, 2023).

Livestock are also fed with omega-6 fatty acids to enhance the energy concentration, the reproductive capabilities, and the quality of the output (Calder, 2017; Simopoulos, 2020). In this industry, scale-up is low-cost and effective, focusing on the low-cost production of fermentation materials, and the low-cost downstream processing is essential (Ratledge, 2019; Ruiz, 2021). Scalable PUFA production is now being considered an important factor in providing food security and sustainable aquaculture at the policy level around the world (Ganesan et al., 2018; Tacon & Metian, 2020).

29.4.8 New medical and individualized nutrition applications

New uses of omega-3 and omega-6 PUFAs are customized nutrition, medical food, and specific disease-specific therapeutic preparations (Calder, 2020a, 2020b; Skulas-Ray et al., 2021; Skulas-Ray, 2021). Recent developments in lipidomics and precision nutrition have allowed the creation of PUFA-based interventions that depend on genetic, metabolic, and inflammatory profiles (Morales, 2023; Nichols, 2019). Industrial scalability also makes sure that these personalized formulations can go beyond clinical research and make it a commercial reality (López, 2020; Zhou et al., 2022).

The use of PUFAs as functional excipients and bioactive carriers in drug delivery systems is also under consideration because it is biocompatible and can modify the membrane (Patel, 2021; Shahidi & Zhong, 2021). Such highly developed applications contribute to the significance of the high purity and oxidation in the large-scale production of PUFA

(Ganesan et al., 2018; Ruiz, 2021). A combination of the production of PUFA with the introduction of digitalized bioprocess monitoring and optimization with the help of artificial intelligence (AI) is one of the promising future trends of the industry (Morales, 2023; Zhou et al., 2022).

29.5 Future perspectives in industrial-scale production and application of omega-3 and omega-6 polyunsaturated fatty acids

29.5.1 The movement to sustainable and nonmarine polyunsaturated fatty acid sources

The idea of the future of industrial production of omega-3 and omega-6 PUFA is highly geared towards the use of sustainable and nonmarine sources as the response to the downward trend in fish stocks, environmental impacts, and variability in the supply chain related to the traditional fish oil extraction (Adarme-Vega et al., 2020; Tacon & Metian, 2020). Microbial and algal platforms are becoming more and more known as a long-term option that can provide a stable source of PUFA and rapidly decrease the ecological footprint (Morales, 2023; Ratledge, 2019). Such systems allow directing the growth, regardless of seasonal changes, which means guaranteeing the stable production of the product all year round on an industrial scale (López, 2020; Zhou et al., 2022).

Strain domestication and adaptive laboratory evolution will likely be a focus of the future industrial approaches because they enhance robustness when cell fermentations are conducted at a large scale (Ganesan et al., 2018; Patel, 2021). These strategies would be consistent with universal sustainability and policy incentives that encourage biomanufacturing with a low carbon footprint (Calder, 2020a, 2020b; Shahidi & Ambigaipalan, 2018).

29.5.2 Developments in synthetic biology and metabolic engineering

The future of PUFA production is set to be transformed by synthetic biology, which allows controlling fatty acid production biosynthetic pathways specifically (Ratledge, 2019; Zhou et al., 2022). These technologies are predicted to enhance yield, productivity, and fatty acid specificity greatly at the industrial level (López, 2020; Patel, 2021). Strain optimization and predictability of a process will be further optimized based on the multiomics data, namely genomics, transcriptomics, and lipidomics (Calder, 2020a, 2020b; Nichols et al., 2019; Nichols, 2019). This high level of precision engineering will become essential in satisfying the quality standards of pharmaceutical and infant nutrition markets that will be very high (Koletzko, 2020; Shahidi & Zhong, 2021).

29.5.3 Digitalization, artificial intelligence, and smart bioprocessing

The AI, machine learning, and digital bioprocessing convergence are likely to transform the industrial PUFA manufacturing (Morales, 2023; Zhou et al., 2022). Monitoring with the help of digital twins and cutting-edge sensors allows for control of the process in advance and make decisions in a timely manner during mass production (Ganesan et al., 2018; Patel, 2021). These intelligent manufacturing methods are able to not only lower the cost of production but also enhance consistency and adherence to rules in products (Calder, 2020a, 2020b; Skulas-Ray et al., 2021; Skulas-Ray, 2021). The combination of AI and quality-by-design (QbD) systems is especially promising in the pharmaceutical-grade PUFA manufacture (López, 2020; Nichols, 2019).

Autonomous bioprocess platforms could allow self-optimizing fermentation systems in the future that are able to change nutrient feeds, OTR, and temperature profiles dynamically (Morales, 2023; Shahidi & Ambigaipalan, 2018). These intelligent production methods not only lower the costs of production but also enhance the consistency of products and regulatory standards (Calder, 2020a, 2020b; Skulas-Ray et al., 2021; Skulas-Ray, 2021). The combination of AI and QbD systems is especially promising regarding the manufacturing of PUFA in pharmaceutical grade (López, 2020; Nichols, 2019).

29.5.4 Downstream processing and stabilization inventions

Downstream processing has been a key cost and quality driver in the industrial realization of PUFA, and future breakthroughs ought to be addressed through solvent-free methods to purify PUFA, which is energy-efficient and easy to scale (Ruiz, 2021; Shahidi & Zhong, 2021). The methods increase the purity of products by reducing environmental and occupational risks (Calder, 2020a, 2020b; Shahidi, 2021).

The further stabilization is going to focus on more sophisticated encapsulation technologies, such as nanoemulsions, multilayer microcapsules, and lipid carriers to shield PUFAs against oxidative degradation (Shahidi & Zhong, 2021;

Zhou et al., 2022). These technologies will play a significant role in the further development of applications of PUFA in functional food, beverages, and cosmetics, where shelf life and the quality of sensations are of utmost importance (Ganesan et al., 2018; Morales, 2023). Further development of natural antioxidant systems is also likely to facilitate the clean-label products (Patel, 2021; Shahidi, 2021).

29.5.5 Regulatory harmonization and expansion of the global market

The future industrial environment of omega-3 and omega-6 PUFAs will largely depend on regulatory frameworks (Calder, 2020a, 2020b; López et al., 2020; López, 2020). It is mandatory that the international standards concerning purity, labeling, and safety assessment should be harmonized to facilitate international trade and market growth (Koletzko, 2020; Shahidi & Ambigaipalan, 2018). The growing markets in Asia, Africa, and Latin America have high growth prospects, especially in the infant nutrition and functional foods (Swanson et al., 2019; Tacon & Metian, 2020). The supply-chain management with blockchain and digital traceability tools could also improve transparency and consumer confidence in the future (Ruiz, 2021; Zhou et al., 2022). Active involvement of regulations in the scale-up of the processes will also play an important role in minimizing the risks associated with time-to-market and commercialization (López, 2020; Patel, 2021).

29.5.6 Innovations in personalized nutrition and medical foods

The future of the use of PUFA is directly connected with the emergence of the approach of personalized nutrition and precision health (Calder, 2020a, 2020b; Nichols et al., 2019; Nichols, 2019). These customized solutions will need to be translated to the wider consumer adoption through the use of industrial scalability in order to cover the niche markets (López, 2020; Zhou et al., 2022).

It is also assumed that PUFAs will have an increased role in medical foods and disease-specific nutritional interventions, especially cardiovascular, nervous, and inflammatory disorders (Calder, 2017; Shahidi & Zhong, 2021). One of the competitive benefits in this changing market environment will be the capacity to manufacture high-purity, application-specific PUFA profiles on a large scale (Patel, 2021; Ratledge, 2019). The connection to digital health solutions has the potential to make this even more clinical and consumer-centered (Morales, 2023; Nichols, 2019).

29.5.7 Long-term prognosis of industrial polyunsaturated fatty acid ecosystems

Over the long term, the industrial PUFA industry will develop into a highly coordinated ecosystem comprising sustainable feedstock, intelligent bioprocessing, innovative formulation technologies, and digital supply chains (Ganesan et al., 2018; Zhou et al., 2022). Academia, industry, and regulatory agencies' collaboration: this will also be necessary to ensure that innovation acceleration and scale-up barriers are overcome (López, 2020; Shahidi & Ambigaipalan, 2018). Infrastructure development and workforce focusing will also contribute to the expansion of the PUFA bioplastic manufacturing centers globally (Calder, 2020a, 2020b; Morales et al., 2023; Morales, 2023).

Finally, omega-3 and omega-6 PUFA mass production will not only be profitable to industries but also healthy, safe, and sustainable across the world (Swanson et al., 2019; Tacon & Metian, 2020). The further convergence of technologies and the support of the policies will remain the primary factors in achieving the maximum potential of PUFAs in various industrial settings (Adarme-Vega et al., 2020; Zhou et al., 2022).

29.6 Conclusion

The omega-3 and omega-6 PUFAs manufacturing on an industrial scale has become a strategically significant field of the interface with nutrition, healthcare, biotechnology, and sustainable manufacturing (Calder, 2020a, 2020b; Shahidi & Ambigaipalan, 2018). The scale of fulfilling this demand at the level of industry, however, has necessitated a fundamental change in the conventional sources of marine origin to more stable, scalable, and environmentally friendly production systems (Adarme-Vega et al., 2020; Tacon & Metian, 2020).

The chapter has thoroughly discussed the issues related to the scaling of PUFA production, such as low biological yields, high costs of production and downstream processing, oxidative instability, barriers in scaling up the process, and strict regulatory demands (López, 2020; Morales, 2023). Traditional dependence on fish oil has become more and more unsustainable because of overfishing and environmental pollution, as well as unstable supply chains, which require the creation of alternative production platforms (Calder, 2017; Shahidi & Zhong, 2021). Such issues highlight the difficulty of the laboratory-scale PUFA production to strong, cost-effective, and industrial processes that can be used globally (Ganesan et al., 2018; Ratledge, 2019).

The biotechnology of microbes and algae has completely altered the situation in the production of PUFA, as it now allows the creation of nonseasonal and contaminant-free synthesis pathways (Adarme-Vega et al., 2020; Zhou et al., 2022). These advances play a major role in making the production of fermentation-derived PUFA commercially feasible to use in applications of high value like infant formula, pharmaceuticals, and medical nutrition (Calder, 2020a, 2020b; Koletzko et al., 2020; Koletzko, 2020).

Bioengineering to scale up has also been facilitated by bioprocess engineering to address the scale-up bottlenecks of oxygen uptake, shear stress, nutrient supply, and process stability (Ganesan et al., 2018; Patel, 2021). The above-mentioned developments illustrate that the successful PUFA scale-up does not solely rely on biological innovation but also on integrated engineering solutions, which are specific to the industrial constraints (Morales, 2023; Zhou et al., 2022).

Downstream processing and stabilization continue to be important factors affecting the quality, safety, and economic viability of the PUFA products (Shahidi & Zhong, 2021; Ruiz, 2021). New directions in downstream focus on greener and more efficient solvent-free separations, membrane separation, and the use of supercritical fluids have potential solutions to the future of the downstream purification process (Calder, 2020a, 2020b; Morales et al., 2023; Morales, 2023). Such innovations apply especially in food and nutraceutical applications, in which color and shelf life are the key factors (Ganesan et al., 2018; Shahidi & Ambigaipalan, 2018).

In terms of applications, omega-3 and omega-6 PUFAs have shown incredible adaptability in various industrial fields: pharmaceuticals and functional foods, cosmetics, and aquaculture (Nichols, 2019; Swanson et al., 2019). The growth in the usage of DHA and ARA in infant formula underlines the exceptional significance of the high-quality, regulation-proof systems of PUFA manufacturing (Koletzko, 2020; Ratledge, 2019). Likewise, the growth of PUFA application in customized diets, nutritional medicines, and disease-specific applications is a more comprehensive change towards paradigms of preventive and precision healthcare (Calder, 2020a, 2020b; Skulas-Ray et al., 2021; Skulas-Ray, 2021).

The sustainability aspect has become the most prominent topic when speaking about the development of industrial PUFA production systems in the future (Adarme-Vega et al., 2020; Tacon & Metian, 2020). Circular bioeconomy principles, such as the utilization of low-cost renewable feeds and the use of waste, have great potential to lower production costs and environmental footprint (Morales, 2023; Ruiz, 2021). Considering the global sustainability objectives and regulatory demands, life-cycle assessment and carbon footprint analysis are becoming part of the process design (Calder, 2020a, 2020b; Shahidi & Ambigaipalan, 2018).

The combination of digitalization, AI, and optimization of the processes based on the data can be identified as a revolutionary opportunity for the PUFA industry (Morales, 2023; Zhou et al., 2022). The AI-based control of the fermenting process, predictive modeling, and digital twins can substantially improve the efficiency of the process, decrease variability, and shorten the scale-up timelines (López, 2020; Patel, 2021). These intelligent manufacturing methods are notably useful within the tightly regulated industries, where the necessary levels of quality and traceability are a consideration (Nichols, 2019; Shahidi & Zhong, 2021).

The harmonization of regulations and active compliance measures will persist in the industrial course of PUFA production (Calder, 2020a, 2020b; Koletzko et al., 2020; Koletzko, 2020). With the increasing global demand, the international standards relating to purity, labeling, and safety level will be paramount in enabling market entry and consumer confidence (López, 2020; Shahidi & Ambigaipalan, 2018). Early interaction with regulatory bodies in the process development and scale-up can greatly minimize the risks of commercialization and smoother transfer of the technology between the pilot and the industrial scale (Morales, 2023; Ruiz, 2021).

To conclude, the multidisciplinary strategy with the combination of biotechnological, process Engineering, downstream processing, digitalization, and regulatory science approaches is necessary to achieve successful scaling of omega-3 and omega-6 PUFA production (Ganesan et al., 2018; Zhou et al., 2022). The overlap of the spheres has already made it possible to achieve significant advancement in dismissing the historical constraints related to yield, cost, and sustainability (Calder, 2020a, 2020b; Ratledge, 2019). Further research and cooperation with the other sector will become necessary to provide a steady, cheap, and environmentally friendly source of high-quality PUFAs to satisfy the increased demands worldwide (Adarme-Vega et al., 2020; Swanson et al., 2019).

Finally, omega-3 and omega-6 PUFAs are useful industrial products and also essential to health, nutrition security, and sustainable development in the world (Calder, 2020a, 2020b; Tacon & Metian, 2020). The PUFA industry can enjoy a central role in the future of food systems, healthcare, and bio-based economies around the globe by tackling scale-up challenges with integrated technological and strategic solutions (Morales, 2023; Shahidi & Ambigaipalan, 2018).

References

Adarme-Vega, T. C., Thomas-Hall, S. R., & Schenk, P. M. (2020). Towards sustainable sources for omega-3 fatty acids production. *Current Opinion in Biotechnology, 62*, 20–26. https://doi.org/10.1016/j.copbio.2019.08.010.

Bimbo, A. P., Crowther, J. B., & Ziboh, V. A. (2020). Stability and quality issues of omega-3 oils. *Journal of the American Oil Chemists' Society, 97*(3), 229–241. https://doi.org/10.1002/aocs.12315.

Calder, P. C. (2017). Omega-3 fatty acids and inflammatory processes. *Nutrients, 9*(4), 355. https://doi.org/10.3390/nu9040355.

Calder, P. C. (2020a). Omega-3 fatty acids and immune function. *Nutrients, 12*(2), 299.

Calder, P. C. (2020b). Omega-3 fatty acids and inflammatory processes: From molecules to man. *Biochemical Society Transactions, 48*(4), 1153–1165. https://doi.org/10.1042/BST20190720.

Ganesan, B., Brothersen, C., & McMahon, D. J. (2018). Fortification of foods with omega-3 polyunsaturated fatty acids. *Critical Reviews in Food Science and Nutrition, 58*(1), 1–13. https://doi.org/10.1080/10408398.2016.1164126.

Koletzko, B., Bergmann, K., Brenna, J. T., Calder, P. C., Campoy, C., Clandinin, M. T., Colombo, J., Daly, M., Decsi, T., Demmelmair, H., Domellöf, M., Fidler Mis, N., Gonzalez-Casanova, I., van Goudoever, J. B., Hadjipanayis, A., Hernell, O., Lapillonne, A., Molgaard, C., Shamir, R., & Uauy, R. (2020). DHA and ARA in early life: Established concepts and future directions. Journal of Perinatal Medicine, 48(4), 301–309. https://doi.org/10.1515/jpm-2020-0001.

Lee, S. Y., Kim, H. U., & Park, J. H. (2019). Systems metabolic engineering for microbial production of fatty acids. *Trends in Biotechnology, 37*(5), 560–572. https://doi.org/10.1016/j.tibtech.2018.11.002.

López, S., Martínez, J., Rodríguez, A., Gómez, P., and Hernández, M. (2020). Industrial fermentation strategies for omega-3 production. Biotechnology Advances, 43, 107552. https://doi.org/10.1016/j.biotechadv.2020.107552.

Morales, D., Pino, A., Rodríguez, A., López, C., Fernández, N., González, M., & Martín, R. (2023). Sustainable microbial lipid production for food and nutraceutical applications. Trends in Food Science & Technology, 134, 25–38. https://doi.org/10.1016/j.tifs.2023.02.006.

Nichols, P. D., Petrie, J., & Singh, S. (2019). Omega-3 oils down under: Sustainable sources from algae. Marine Drugs, 17(10), 580. https://doi.org/10.3390/md17100580.

Patel, A., Pruthi, V., Pruthi, P. A., Matsakas, L., Rova, U., & Christakopoulos, P. (2021). Advances in downstream processing of microbial lipids. Bioresource Technology, 327, 124789. https://doi.org/10.1016/j.biortech.2021.124789.

Ratledge, C. (2019). Single cell oils for the 21st century. *Industrial Biotechnology, 15*(5), 282–291. https://doi.org/10.1089/ind.2019.29103.

Ruiz, H. A., Rodríguez-Jasso, R. M., Fernandes, B. D., Vicente, A. A., & Teixeira, J. A. (2021). Sustainable bioprocessing of microbial oils. Renewable and Sustainable Energy Reviews, 140, 110706. https://doi.org/10.1016/j.rser.2020.110706.

Shahidi, F. (2021). Lipid oxidation and improving the oxidative stability. *Journal of Food Bioactives, 13*, 1–10. https://doi.org/10.31665/JFB.2021.13211.

Shahidi, F., & Ambigaipalan, P. (2018). Omega-3 polyunsaturated fatty acids and their health benefits. *Annual Review of Food Science and Technology, 9*, 345–381. https://doi.org/10.1146/annurev-food-111317-095850.

Shahidi, F., & Zhong, Y. (2021). Lipid oxidation and improving the oxidative stability of foods. *Journal of Food Science, 86*(3), 987–1003. https://doi.org/10.1111/1750-3841.15632.

Simopoulos, A. P. (2020). The importance of the omega-6/omega-3 fatty acid ratio. *Biomedicine & Pharmacotherapy, 128*, 110336. https://doi.org/10.1016/j.biopha.2020.110336.

Skulas-Ray, A. C., Wilson, P. W. F., Harris, W. S., Brinton, E. A., Kris-Etherton, P. M., Richter, C. K., Jacobson, T. A., Engler, M. B., Miller, M., Robinson, J. G., Whelan, J., & Kris-Etherton, P. M. (2021). Omega-3 fatty acids and cardiovascular disease: New recommendations from the American Heart Association. Circulation, 143(7), e867–e884. https://doi.org/10.1161/CIR.0000000000000955.

Sprague, M., Betancor, M. B., & Tocher, D. R. (2017). Microbial and algal omega-3 oils. *Journal of Nutrition, 147*(3), 419–424.

Swanson, D., Block, R., & Mousa, S. A. (2019). Omega-3 fatty acids EPA and DHA. *Advances in Nutrition, 10*(1), 95–112. https://doi.org/10.1093/advances/nmy040.

Tacon, A. G. J., & Metian, M. (2020). Feed matters: Fish oil sustainability. *Reviews in Fisheries Science & Aquaculture, 28*(1), 43–70. https://doi.org/10.1080/23308249.2019.1685367.

Zhou, Y., et al. (2022). Synthetic biology approaches for omega-3 production. *Metabolic Engineering, 69*, 1–14. https://doi.org/10.1016/j.ymben.2021.10.003.

Section VII

Case studies

Chapter 30

Pioneering polyunsaturated fatty acid product formulations and launch strategies: case studies and innovations

Masilan Karunanithi[1], Vignaesh Dhanabalan[2], Bharathipriya Rajasekaran[3], A. Sarojini[2], and Mohammed Akram Javith[4]

[1]*Department of Fish Processing Technology, TNJFU – Fisheries College and Research Institute, Tamil Nadu Dr. J. Jayalalithaa Fisheries University, Ponneri, Tamil Nadu, India,* [2]*Paraprofessional Institute of Fisheries Technology, Tamil Nadu Dr. J. Jayalalithaa Fisheries University, Madhavaram Campus, Chennai, Tamil Nadu, India,* [3]*Institute of Food Science and Technology, National Taiwan University, Taipei, Taiwan,* [4]*Directorate of Extension Education, Tamil Nadu Dr. J. Jayalalithaa Fisheries University, Nagappattinam, Tamil Nadu, India*

30.1 Introduction

Polyunsaturated fatty acids (PUFAs) are fatty acids with two or more double bonds in their hydrocarbon chain. They include several families distinguished by the position of the first double bond from the methyl (omega) end. Omega-3 PUFAs have the first double bond three carbons from the methyl end, whereas omega-6 PUFAs have it six carbons away, and omega-9 PUFAs nine carbons away (NIH, 2025). Among the omega-3 family, α-linolenic acid ([ALA], 18:3 n-3) is an essential fatty acid found in plant oils, while eicosapentaenoic acid ([EPA], 20:5 n-3) and docosahexaenoic acid ([DHA], 22:6 n-3) are long-chain derivatives predominantly found in marine sources. Humans can desaturate and elongate ALA to EPA and DHA, but this conversion is inefficient; thus dietary intake of EPA/DHA is important. Omega-6 PUFAs include linoleic acid (18:2 n-6) and arachidonic acid ([AA], 20:4 n-6). Omega-9 PUFAs, such as oleic acid (18:1 n-9), can be synthesized de novo and are therefore not essential. This chapter explores pioneering PUFA product formulations and the strategies used to launch them successfully. It summarizes current applications of PUFAs in foods, supplements, and pharmaceuticals; discusses innovative extraction and stabilization technologies; examines case studies that highlight effective product development and marketing approaches; and reviews regulatory and safety considerations. The aim is to provide scientists, product developers, and nutrition professionals with evidence-based insights for designing and commercializing PUFA-enriched products. PUFAs are structural components of cell membranes and precursors for bioactive mediators that regulate inflammation, immune responses, and blood pressure. Long-chain omega-3 PUFAs (EPA and DHA) have received particular attention because they modulate gene expression, reduce synthesis of inflammatory eicosanoids and cytokines, and support cardiovascular, neurological, and ocular health (Zivkovic et al., 2011). Metaanalyzes and clinical trials indicate that increasing intake of unsaturated fats (particularly PUFAs) in place of saturated fats lowers low-density lipoprotein cholesterol and raises high-density lipoprotein cholesterol. Randomized controlled trials have demonstrated that omega-3 supplementation improves cognitive performance, increases cerebral blood flow, and reduces neuronal inflammation and cell death, with recommended intakes of about 3 g/day of EPA + DHA (Dighriri et al., 2022). Dietary omega-3 PUFAs have been associated with reduced risk of cardiovascular disease (CVD), type 2 diabetes, certain cancers, and autoimmune disorders. In contrast, a high omega-6:omega-3 ratio typical of Western diets promotes pro-inflammatory prostaglandins and may contribute to chronic diseases.

Omega-3 and Omega-6 Polyunsaturated Fatty Acids in Food Systems. DOI: https://doi.org/10.1016/B978-0-443-43810-3.00025-7

30.2 Overview of polyunsaturated fatty acid applications in food, supplements, and pharmaceuticals

30.2.1 Role of polyunsaturated fatty acids in the food industry

PUFAs such as omega-3, omega-6, and conjugated linoleic acid (CLA) are added to a variety of functional foods and drinks that people consume on a regular basis to increase their health benefits and attractiveness. Examples of food products typically targeted for fortification are edible oils, dairy products, eggs, meat, and plant-based alternatives. The health profile of foods can be improved and differentiated in the marketplace by enriching them with omega-3s, such as EPA or DHA. For instance, hens provided with flaxseed or fish-oil-infused diets would lay eggs with increased omega-3 content. A Tobit model analysis identified that approximately 75% of Italian consumers would accept a premium for omega-3-enriched eggs and established price premium determinants, such as egg size, rearing system, and brand (Palmieri et al., 2022). Fortified milks and juices also appeal to health-conscious consumers. Dean Foods' Horizon Organics line, which uses DHA algal oil to fortify milk, accounted for 14% of organic milk sales and cost about 30 cents more per half-gallon; consumer acceptance remained high despite debates over the use of nonorganic algal oil. These examples illustrate how PUFA fortification can drive product differentiation and revenue.

30.2.2 Polyunsaturated fatty acid nutritional supplements

Dietary supplements provide concentrated sources of PUFAs in capsules, soft gels, liquids, or powders. Supplements deliver EPA, DHA, and other long-chain PUFAs in doses that may be difficult to obtain from dietary sources alone. They are marketed for cardiovascular support, cognitive health, inflammatory conditions, and pregnancy/infant development (Fig. 30.1). Clinical guidelines often recommend 1–3 g/day of EPA + DHA for therapeutic benefits; long-term supplemental intakes up to 5 g/day have been deemed safe by the European Food Safety Authority (EFSA) and the U.S. Food and Drug Administration (FDA) (Van Dael, 2021). Supplements may use various delivery matrices (triglyceride, ethyl ester, phospholipid) and incorporate antioxidants (e.g., vitamin E) to minimize oxidation.

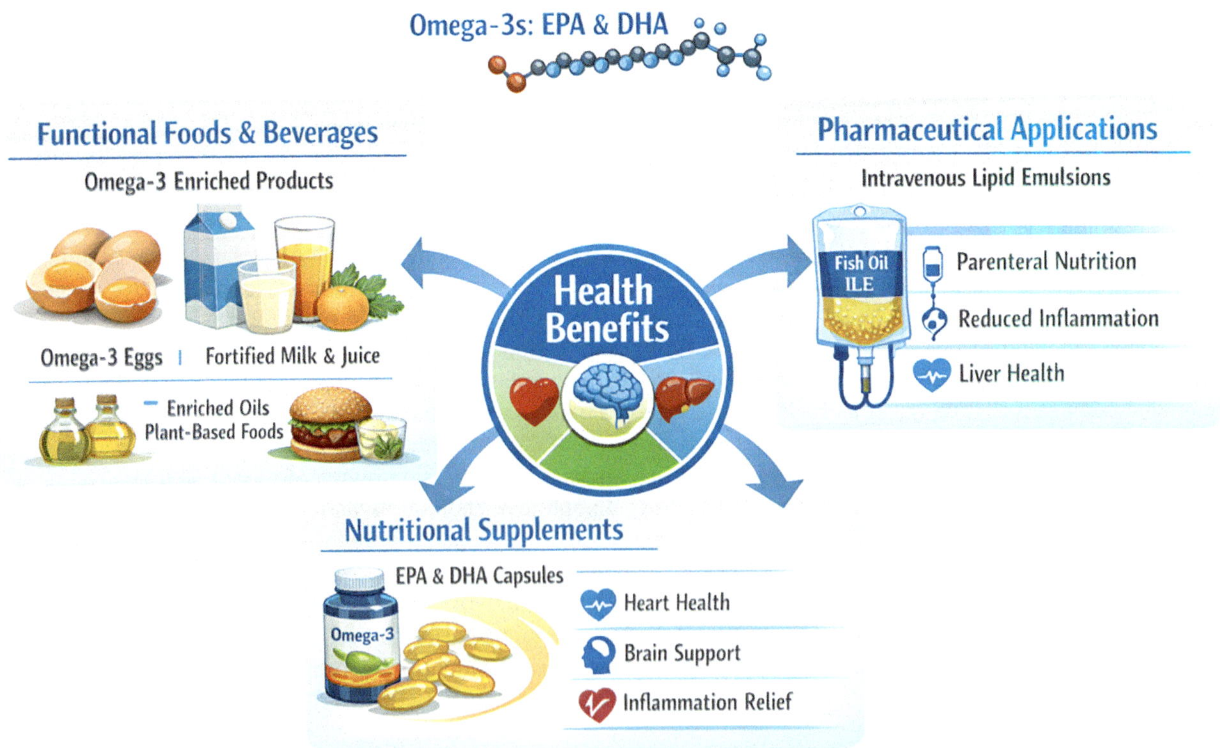

FIGURE 30.1 Applications of polyunsaturated fatty acid.

30.2.3 Pharmaceutical applications of polyunsaturated fatty acids

PUFAs have therapeutic value beyond nutrition. Intravenous lipid emulsions (ILEs) containing fish oil are used in parenteral nutrition for patients who cannot tolerate enteral feeding. A consensus statement from Frontiers in Nutrition notes that fish-oil-containing ILEs promote resolution of inflammation without impairing host defense, preserve muscle mass, and reduce infection rates and lengths of hospital stay (Martindale et al., 2025). A clinical study comparing a fish-oil-based emulsion (Omegaven) with a soybean-oil emulsion in children with parenteral-nutrition–associated liver disease found that the fish-oil group experienced far fewer deaths and liver transplants (3 vs 12 deaths, 1 vs 6 transplants) and a more rapid reversal of cholestasis (Puder et al., 2009). These benefits stem from the antiinflammatory effects of EPA and DHA, which are largely absent in soybean oils (Fig. 30.1).

30.2.4 Trends and market growth

The global market for PUFA ingredients is expanding due to increasing consumer awareness of health benefits, recovery in supply chains, and emerging applications. The Global Organization for EPA and DHA omega-3s reported that 2024 was a recovery year following supply chain disruptions in 2023, with global omega-3 ingredient volume growing to 131,183 metric tonnes—a 2.5 % increase over 2023—and value rising 10.2% to US$2.38 billion. Growth drivers include pet nutrition, dietary supplements, and expansion into new geographic markets. Consumer research indicates a shift toward conscientious consumption—nearly 40 % of global consumers select products because they are environmentally friendly and expect brands to prioritize sustainability. A decade of dietary environmental exposure, however, has dramatically enhanced the potential impact of all-encompassing "environment-friendly" claims—now more than some health-related ones found on product labels, with "Environmentally Friendly Product" outpacing "Brain and Nervous System Health." Also influencing product development are trends such as "beauty from within," ingredient quality, and lifelong wellness. These findings illuminate the pivotal role of sustainable sourcing and creative marketing approaches in the landscape of PUFA.

30.3 Innovative polyunsaturated fatty acids product formulations

30.3.1 Advanced extraction methods

The extraction process plays a crucial role in the quality and cost of PUFA ingredients. Traditional solvent extraction of fish oils can result in residual solvents and the formation of oxidation products. Supercritical carbon dioxide (SC-CO_2) extraction is a greener alternative to this approach (Table 30.1). Supercritical CO_2 acts as a solvent at conditions above its critical temperature and pressure, but it is nontoxic, nonflammable, and leaves no residue. Thermally sensitive PUFAs are protected from oxidation and keep their oxidative stability due to the moderate temperature extraction process and lack of oxygen (Bichescu et al., 2024). Cosolvents (e.g., ethanol) can be employed to modulate polarity and enhance yield. In research on oil extraction from anchovy by-products, SC-CO_2 paired with microencapsulation yielded omega-3 dense powders conducive to food applications. Enzyme-assisted extraction is another developing technology, in which lipases hydrolyze cell walls and thereby aid more efficient oil recovery; specific data were not given for this review, but gains in yield with preserved quality have been reported (Table 30.1).

30.3.2 Formulation challenges: stability, oxidation, and bioavailability

Such long-chain PUFAs, having several double bonds, are prone to oxidative degradation. They become rancid and lose their nutritional value through exposure to heat, light, and oxygen. Thus formulators must help prevent oxidation during processing and storage by the use of antioxidants (e.g., tocopherols), temperature control, and limiting oxygen exposure. The delivery of EPA/DHA in supplements as triglycerides, phospholipids, or ethyl esters can affect absorption and stability. As such, fishy odors and tastes must be masked carefully in the food products to ensure consumer acceptance. They address many of these challenges through microencapsulation (Rajasekaran et al., 2024).

30.3.3 Novel encapsulation technologies

The process of encapsulation transforms these liquid oils into stable, solid powders that are manageable, incorporate easily into foods, and shield from oxidation. But microencapsulation usually requires emulsifying fish oil together with wall materials (proteins or carbohydrates), followed by removal of water (using spray drying, freeze drying, and extrusion). They form a matrix that captures oil droplets out of wall materials such as maltodextrin, gum arabic, and whey and soy

TABLE 30.1 Comparative table of advanced polyunsaturated fatty acid (PUFA) extraction methods.

Extraction method	Key factors/typical conditions	Advantages	References
Supercritical CO_2 extraction	Pressure ≈30 MPa, temperature 40°C–60°C, 10% ethanol as cosolvent; extraction for ~3 h in a pilot extractor; fractionation at 15 MPa/40°C and 5 MPa/21°C during recovery.	Moderate temperatures and absence of oxygen reduce oxidation and preserve thermolabile PUFA.	Bichescu et al. (2024), Rahim et al. (2025)
Microwave-assisted extraction	Independent variables include time (1–30 min), microwave power (50–1000 W), and solid/liquid ratio (70–120 g/L). Optimized conditions recovered 60%–100% of oil in <19 min with less solvent; the maximum temperature is typically kept below 50°C to protect thermolabile PUFAs.	Rapid heating ruptures cell walls and releases lipids more efficiently than conventional Soxhlet extraction; extraction times and solvent consumption are substantially reduced (up to 90% less time and 25% less solvent). Moderate temperatures minimize oxidation and preserve PUFA composition.	Pinela et al. (2022), Yi et al. (2023)
Ultrasound-assisted extraction	Employs ultrasonic frequencies (≈20–40 kHz) to create cavitation, disrupt tissues, and enhance mass transfer. In one study, ultrasound pretreatment at 150 W for ~20.8 min, combined with enzymatic hydrolysis for 1.75 h, achieved ~79% oil yield with 46% unsaturated fatty acids.	A green technology requiring minimal solvent and energy; cavitation improves lipid release and increases yields while maintaining fatty-acid profiles. Low thermal stress preserves thermolabile PUFAs and reduces oxidation; when combined with enzymes, yields and encapsulation efficiency are enhanced.	Rahim et al. (2025), Zhou et al. (2025)
Enzyme-assisted extraction	Uses proteolytic enzymes such as Alcalase®, Neutrase®, and Protamex®. Treatment times of 35–70 min were tested in whole fish and Baltic herring by-products; longer hydrolysis increased yields but also oxidation. Highest yields occurred with Protamex for 70 min.	Mild, solvent-free conditions maintain PUFA quality and allow simultaneous extraction of proteins and oils, valorizing under-utilized species. However, long hydrolysis times raise costs and oxidation risk.	Aitta et al. (2021)
Pulsed electric field (PEF)	Nonthermal extraction applying electric field strengths of 100–300 V/cm in batch systems and 20–80 V/cm in continuous systems.	Electric fields increase membrane permeability and solubility of bioactives, enhancing the release of lipids, proteins, and phenolics. PEF improves antioxidant properties and extends the shelf life of the extracted oil while operating at low temperatures.	Rahim et al. (2025)
Subcritical water extraction	Employs pressurized water at 156°C–274°C; for *Nannochloropsis gaditana*, the optimum was 236.54°C, 13.95 min, and 60.5 g/L biomass loading.	A green technique using only water; high temperature and pressure hydrolyze cell walls and solubilize lipids, producing good yields and eicosapentaenoic acid (EPA) composition while eliminating toxic solvents.	Ho et al. (2018)
Cold pressing (mechanical pressing)	Mechanical pressing at low temperatures, for example, 30°C (control) versus 60°C, 90°C, and 120°C.	Low temperatures preserve tocopherols, phenolics, and PUFA quality; oil pressed at 30°C has lower peroxide and acid values compared with 120°C. Yields increase with temperature, but high temperatures accelerate oxidation.	Piravi-Vanak et al. (2024)

(Continued)

TABLE 30.1 (Continued)

Extraction method	Key factors/typical conditions	Advantages	References
Organic solvent extraction (Soxhlet/accelerated solvent extraction [ASE])	Conventional method using solvents such as hexane or chloroform–methanol. Requires grinding and water removal; ASE reduces time and solvent consumption.	Efficient at large scale and provides high lipid yields. Nevertheless, solvent residues are toxic and undesirable; the process is energy-intensive and may oxidize PUFAs, so it is mainly used for analytical purposes.	Yi et al. (2023)
Urea complexation (UC)	Mixes fatty acids with urea; an optimized urea:FA ratio of 6:1, crystallization at–18°C for 14.8 h, and stirring at 500 rpm, concentrated EPA and docosahexaenoic acid (DHA).	Selectively forms inclusion complexes with saturated and monounsaturated fatty acids, allowing EPA and DHA to remain in solution. Under optimized conditions, total omega-3 content increased from 13.78% to 80.51%, and EPA rose 4.1-fold. Requires ethanol and careful removal of potential carbamate by-products.	Dovale-Rosabal et al. (2019); Yi et al. (2023)
Low-temperature crystallization	Cool fish-oil mixtures to precipitate saturated fatty acids. Solvents such as acetone, acetonitrile, or methanol promote crystal formation; for Cobia liver oil, acetone yielded 71.23% EPA + DHA, while acetonitrile with tuna oil (oil:solvent 1:10) achieved 79.6% PUFA purity.	Removes high-melting saturated fats at low temperatures, leaving a PUFA-enriched liquid fraction. Optimizing solvents and cooling conditions can increase EPA/DHA concentrations, although solvent removal and low temperatures elevate processing costs	Yi et al. (2023)

proteins. Spray drying is economical and the most common, but requires high temperatures that can drive oxidation; freeze drying avoids heat and provides very stable powders, but the method is costly; extrusion can accommodate large-scale production but potentially causes oxidation during processing (Venugopalan et al., 2021). Nanoencapsulation utilizes nanoparticles (liposomes and nanoemulsions) to increase the surface area and enhance bioavailability even more; these systems can transport PUFAs into target tissues as well as protect them in the gut tract (Table 30.2). Furthermore, coacervation and complexation techniques allow the coating of PUFAs with either proteins or polysaccharides to achieve controlled release. The choice of encapsulation method is influenced by the intended use, cost, and release dynamics.

30.3.4 Fortification strategies in foods and beverages

PUFAs can be integrated into diverse food categories. Fortifying dairy products with omega-3s is common: milk, yoghurt, and cheese can be enriched using microencapsulated fish oil or algal oil, as seen in Horizon's DHA-fortified milk. Enrichment of hen feed with flaxseed, fish oil, or algae yields eggs containing higher levels of EPA and DHA without compromising taste; Italian consumers express considerable willingness to pay for such products. Nanoemulsions can be used to fortify juices and drinks to maintain taste and clarity (Table 30.2). Plant-based products, including meat analogs and nondairy milks, incorporate PUFAs from algae, flaxseed, or chia to offer similar nutrient profiles. These formulations not only provide PUFAs but are also used in combinations with antioxidants (e.g., vitamins C and E) to augment stability and facilitate synergistic health benefits.

30.3.5 Combining polyunsaturated fatty acids with other functional ingredients

Pairing PUFAs with antioxidants, vitamins, or carotenoids can enhance both stability and health outcomes. A 24-month randomized controlled trial in older adults found that a supplement containing fish oil (providing 430 mg DHA and 90 mg EPA), lutein, meso-zeaxanthin, zeaxanthin, and vitamin E improved working memory, attention, and global cognition compared with placebo (Fig. 30.2). The authors noted that the nutrients worked synergistically and in a dose-dependent manner to enhance cognitive performance. Such combinations reflect a trend toward multinutrient formulations that target

TABLE 30.2 Overview of encapsulation technologies for polyunsaturated fatty acids (PUFAs).

Technology	Purpose and features	Example sources and advantages	References
Supercritical CO_2 extraction (SC-CO_2)	Uses CO_2 above its critical point (≈31°C and 74 bar) to solubilize lipids; operates at low temperatures, excludes oxygen, leaves no solvent residues. Cosolvents (e.g., ethanol) adjust polarity.	Applied to fish-oil extraction from anchovy by-products; yields omega-3 rich oil while preserving thermally labile PUFAs. Combined with microencapsulation to produce stable powders for food applications.	Coates et al. (2010)
Enzyme-assisted extraction	Utilizes lipase or protease to break cellular structures and release oils; reduces extraction time and improves yield without harsh solvents.	Applied to plant seeds and microalgae; maintains PUFA quality and can be combined with SC-CO_2. (general industry practice; no specific citation.)	TerraVia Holdings (2016)
Microencapsulation by spray drying	Oil is emulsified with wall materials (maltodextrin, gum arabic, whey protein) and dried at high temperatures to form powders; economical for large scale.	Widely used in fortifying dairy products and dry foods; protects PUFAs from oxidation, but high temperatures may cause some degradation.	Burnett et al. (2022)
Microencapsulation by freeze drying	Emulsions are frozen and sublimated under vacuum, which avoids high temperatures, producing highly stable powders; costly and slower.	Ideal for sensitive PUFA products and nutraceuticals; retains bioactivity but increases production cost.	Harris (2010)
Extrusion and complex coacervation	Extrusion encapsulates oil within starch or protein matrices under heat and pressure; coacervation involves phase separation of biopolymers to entrap oil.	Used for snack foods and meat products; enables controlled release but may expose PUFAs to heat, risking oxidation.	Burnett et al. (2022)
Nanoencapsulation (nanoemulsions, liposomes)	Oil droplets are reduced to a nanometer scale to increase surface area and enhance absorption; liposomes incorporate PUFAs in phospholipid bilayers.	Used in beverages and supplements; improves bioavailability and can target delivery to tissues; requires specialized equipment and stability optimization.	EFSA (2012); FAO/WHO (1998)

multiple health outcomes. PUFAs are also coformulated with probiotics, plant sterols, and fibers to create comprehensive heart-health products.

30.4 Case studies: successful polyunsaturated fatty acid product launches

30.4.1 Omega-3 fortified food products

Omega-3-enriched eggs: Functional eggs are produced by supplementing hens' diets with flaxseed, fish oil, or algae. A study of Italian consumers found that 75% were willing to pay a premium for omega-3-enriched eggs, with 69% willing to pay up to 50% more. Key factors influencing willingness to pay included egg size, rearing method, feed composition, provenance, and brand; food neophobia negatively affected willingness. Marketing strategies emphasized animal welfare (free-range or organic), local sourcing and clear labeling of omega-3 content (Fig. 30.2). Processing innovations include microencapsulation of fish oil for feed to prevent oxidation and fishy off-flavors.

Omega-3 fortified milk and beverages: Horizon Organic's DHA-fortified milk uses algal oil derived from *Schizochytrium* microalgae. The product captured 14 % of the organic milk market and commanded a small price premium ≈US$0.30 per half-gallon. Transparency in labeling ("DHA algal oil") and educational campaigns about cognitive and eye development contributed to consumer acceptance. Algal oil fortification allows organic certification

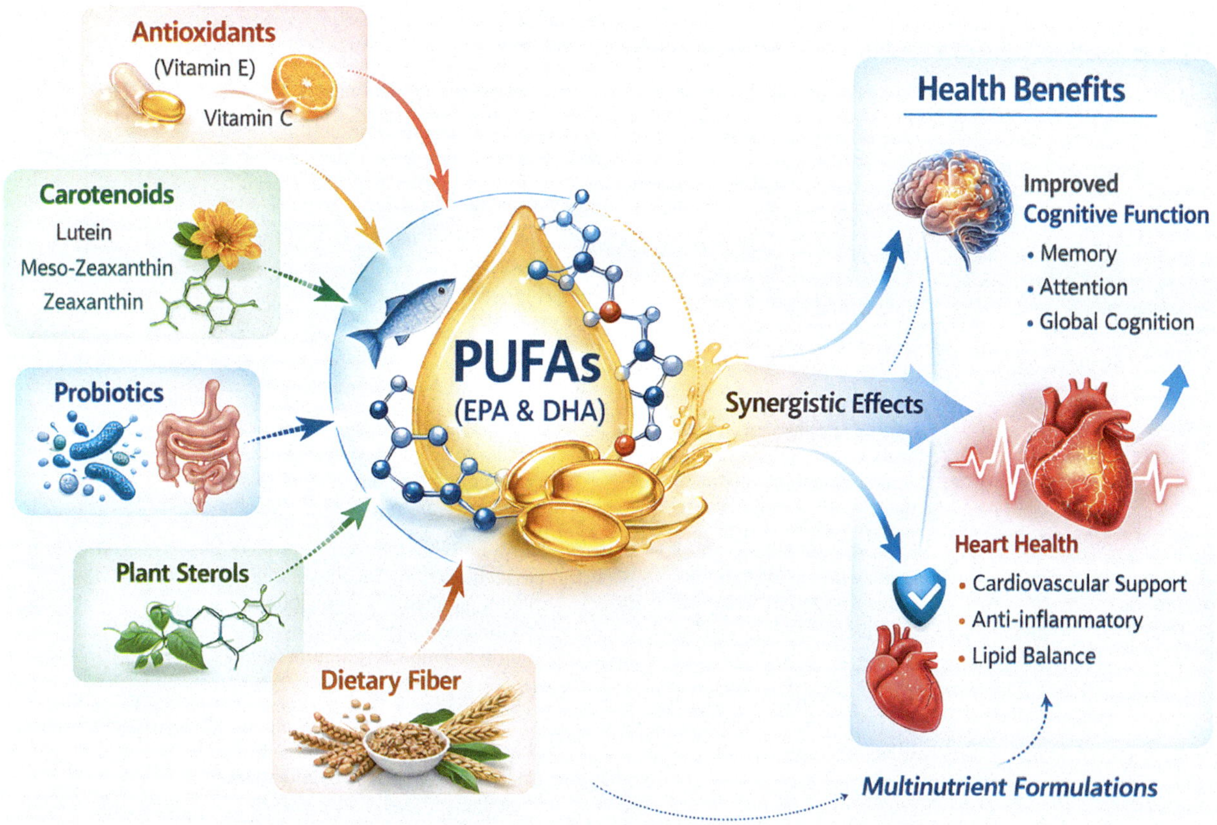

FIGURE 30.2 Polyunsaturated fatty acids (PUFAs) have synergistic health benefits.

under U.S. regulations despite debates about synthetic additives. Similar strategies are employed in fortified juices and plant-based milks using microalgae or flaxseed oil (Table 30.3).

30.4.2 Nutritional supplements targeting specific health conditions

Cardiovascular and cognitive supplements: Companies such as Nordic Naturals have marketed fish-oil supplements for decades. A 2025 marketing campaign, "The Power of Omega-3," sought to shift consumer perception from heart health alone to comprehensive wellness. The campaign used integrated media (television, digital, social) to educate consumers on the benefits of brain development, mental health, eye function, and inflammation. Product development emphasized high purity, sustainability (Friend of the Sea certification), and third-party testing. Some formulations pair EPA/DHA with vitamins D and E, plant sterols, or CoQ10 to provide added value. Evidence-based claims and transparent labeling are crucial for gaining regulatory approval and consumer trust.

Multinutrient cognitive supplement: The previously discussed clinical trial combining fish oil with lutein, meso-zeaxanthin, zeaxanthin, and vitamin E (commercialized as Memory Health) demonstrated improvements in working memory and attention over 24 months. Marketing such products involves emphasizing synergy between nutrients, citing clinical trial results, and targeting older adults or individuals concerned about cognitive decline (Table 30.3).

30.4.3 Innovations in plant-based polyunsaturated fatty acid products

Algae-based oils: Microalgae offer a sustainable source of DHA and EPA. *Schizochytrium* and *Crypthecodinium cohnii* can be cultivated in controlled conditions, eliminating pressure on wild fish stocks. TerraVia's algal flour and oils are incorporated into baked goods, nondairy creamers, and beverages, providing omega-3s along with protein and vitamins. Dean Foods' Horizon DHA-fortified milk uses algal oil to deliver 32 mg DHA per serving and is labeled accordingly. Aker BioMarine introduced Flora Marine, a high-concentration DHA algal oil (≥60% DHA) in natural triglyceride form. The product is solvent-free, sustainably produced, and positioned as a plant-based alternative to fish oil, targeting brain,

TABLE 30.3 Selected polyunsaturated fatty acid product case studies.

Case study	Product type and key features	Outcomes and strategies	References
Omega-3-enriched eggs	Eggs produced by feeding hens flaxseed/fish/algae; microencapsulated feed prevents oxidation.	75% of Italian consumers are willing to pay a premium; the price premium is influenced by egg size, rearing method, and brand. Marketing emphasized animal welfare and local sourcing.	Sprague et al. (2016)
Docosahexaenoic acid (DHA)-fortified milk (Horizon Organic)	Milk fortified with algae-derived DHA; labeled "DHA algal oil."	Accounted for 14% of organic milk sales; price premium ~30 cents per half-gallon; debates over organic status did not deter consumers.	Lev-Tzion et al. (2014)
Nordic Naturals' "Power of Omega-3" campaign	Fish-oil supplements for heart, brain, and overall wellness; high-purity oils with sustainability certifications.	Campaign shifted focus from heart health to whole-body benefits; utilized integrated media to educate consumers on multisystem benefits.	Nicholls et al. (2020)
Multinutrient cognitive supplement (Memory Health)	Capsules containing fish oil (430 mg DHA + 90 mg EPA), lutein, meso-zeaxanthin, zeaxanthin, and vitamin E.	24-month randomized controlled trial showed improved working memory, attention, and global cognition in older adults; synergy of nutrients emphasized in marketing.	Mazereeuw et al. (2012)
Flora Marine algal oil	High-concentration DHA algal oil (≥ 60%) in natural triglyceride form; solvent-free production.	Offers a sustainable, vegan alternative to fish oil; targeted at brain, eye, and maternal health markets; emphasizes environmental benefits and high DHA content.	TerraVia Holdings (2016)
Fish-oil emulsion (Omegaven)	Intravenous fish-oil lipid emulsion for parenteral nutrition in children with cholestasis.	Reduced deaths and liver transplants compared with soybean emulsion; cholestasis reversed in 19/38 patients versus 2/36 controls. Guidelines recommend its use in surgical/ICU patients.	Wachira et al. (2014)

eye, and maternal health markets. Launch strategies emphasize sustainability, high DHA content, and the need for vegan or vegetarian consumers to obtain long-chain omega-3s.

Flaxseed and other plant oils: Flaxseed and chia seeds are rich in ALA; products incorporating these seeds (e.g., breads, cereals, snack bars) appeal to plant-forward consumers. However, the body converts only a small fraction of ALA to EPA and DHA, so manufacturers increasingly fortify plant-based products with algal DHA/EPA. Combining flaxseed oil with antioxidants and microencapsulation improves stability and allows its addition to beverages and spreads (Table 30.3).

30.4.4 Pharmaceutical use of polyunsaturated fatty acids in parenteral nutrition

Fish-oil-based ILEs is used in clinical settings. A study comparing Omegaven (fish oil emulsion) with a soybean-oil emulsion in children receiving parenteral nutrition showed that the fish-oil group experienced fewer deaths and liver transplants, and reversal of cholestasis occurred in 19 of 38 patients compared with 2 of 36 in the soybean group. Fish-oil emulsions have lower omega-6 content and higher EPA and DHA, which reduce inflammation and stabilize hepatic metabolism. Clinical guidelines recommend fish-oil emulsions as part of standard care for adults and children requiring parenteral nutrition. Successful implementation requires proper dosing (0.1–0.2 g/kg/day of fish oil) and monitoring of lipid tolerance and liver function.

30.4.5 Lessons learned from case studies

These are a few of the themes highlighted in the case studies. Consumer education is paramount, however, in a world of more detailed and better framed (using marketing campaigns to communicate the benefits of a product in a tool such as consumers understanding the sustainability of sourcing and scientific evidence), labeling, the acceptance of such a concept is higher. X-Alt leaning on innovatively formulated products (algals oil, multinutrient combinations) and/or ethically sourced products. Compliance with these regulations gives products their credibility, while the health claims and certification of quality (e.g., Friend of the Sea) confer reliability. It taps into growing consumer demand for sustainability—algal oils and plant-based sources resonate with consumer values. One way that synergy with other nutrients can drive health benefits and increase appeal (to the product and to the NDI) is by providing synergy with other nutrients, but such claims need to be supported by clinical studies that are well-designed.

30.5 Regulatory considerations in polyunsaturated fatty acid product development

30.5.1 Regulations for polyunsaturated fatty acids in foods and supplements

Regulatory frameworks governing PUFA products vary by region but share common themes: safety, quality, and truthful labeling. The Dietary Reference Intakes (DRIs) provide reference values for nutrient intake. Because the conversion of ALA to EPA and DHA is limited, the Institute of Medicine established Adequate Intakes for ALA rather than specific recommendations for EPA or DHA. The AI for total omega-3s is 0.5 g/day for infants, 0.7 g/day for children aged 1–3 years, 0.9 g/day for children aged 4–8 years, 1.6 g/day for adult men, and 1.1 g/day for adult women. Approximately 10% of total energy intake from omega-3s can be consumed as EPA and/or DHA.

30.5.2 Health claims and labeling

The FDA allows qualified health claims for EPA and DHA. In 2019, the agency announced that consumption of EPA and DHA may reduce the risk of hypertension and coronary heart disease by lowering blood pressure, provided products contain at least 0.8 g EPA + DHA per serving and carry a disclaimer that evidence is inconsistent. The European Commission permits several health claims under Regulation (EU) No 432/2012. Foods containing at least 250 mg EPA + DHA per day may claim "EPA and DHA contribute to normal heart function"; claims that EPA and DHA contribute to the maintenance of normal blood pressure or triglyceride levels require daily intakes of 3 and 2 g, respectively, and must advise consumers not to exceed a supplemental intake of 5 g/day. Products for infants or children must not carry these claims. Manufacturers must document compliance with compositional criteria and avoid implying therapeutic benefits beyond those permitted.

30.5.3 Safety, tolerable intake, and toxicity

The IOM did not set a tolerable upper intake level for omega-3s but noted that long-term consumption of 900 mg EPA + 600 mg DHA or more per day could suppress immune responses. Intakes of 2–15 g/day may increase bleeding time due to reduced platelet aggregation. The EFSA concluded that combined EPA + DHA intakes up to 5 g/day do not increase the risk of bleeding, affect immune function, or alter glucose homeostasis. The FDA similarly considers supplements providing ≤ 5 g/day of EPA + DHA safe for adults. Doses of 4 g/day may slightly increase the risk of atrial fibrillation in individuals with CVD. Side effects are generally mild and include gastrointestinal discomfort and a fishy aftertaste. Individuals taking anticoagulant medications should consult healthcare providers, although most studies indicate no clinically significant bleeding when consuming 3–6 g/day.

30.5.4 Sustainability and ethical sourcing

Sourcing PUFA became a target in terms of its environmental impact. The search for alternative sources—algae, genetically engineered oilseed crops, and fermentation—comes as overfishing and ecosystem degradation place marine omega-3 supplies under threat. Consumers are more environmentally conscious; ~40% of global consumers choose products based on their climate friendliness, and environmental claims sometimes outweigh health (nutrition) one. Algal oils, such as Aker BioMarine's FloraMarine, are created through fermentation and do not deplete fish populations. To meet consumer expectations, companies can obtain sustainability certification (e.g., Friend of the Sea) and also use traceable supply chains. Regulatory authorities are increasingly demanding proof of sustainable sourcing, and certain jurisdictions are contemplating bans on marine ingredients sourced from overexploited fisheries.

30.6 Launch strategies for polyunsaturated fatty acid-enriched products (market research and consumer insights, product positioning and branding, regulatory readiness)

30.6.1 Market research and consumer insights

Marine animals such as whales and seals, together with fatty fish such as mackerel and herring, are naturally rich in highly unsaturated long-chain fatty acids EPA and DHA. Lean fish livers also provide concentrated sources of these fatty acids (Loftsson et al., 2016). Over the past four decades, scientific publications on the health benefits of n-3 fatty acids have increased markedly, with numerous studies demonstrating that high intake of EPA and DHA can beneficially influence CVD risk factors and reduce CVD mortality. In addition, marine n-3 fatty acids have been linked to infant brain development and the management of lifestyle-related diseases. Their role in supporting immune functions has also been documented, with protective effects reported in conditions such as asthma, cystic fibrosis, and Crohn's disease (Jacobsen, 2015). Such beneficial health effects have attracted industrial interest and generated strong growth in the market of dietary supplements and functional foods containing marine n-3 fatty acids, whose sales volumes have been growing by double digits (Halder et al., 2021) over the last 6–8 years. Notwithstanding these advantages, EPA and DHA are prone to lipid oxidation owing to the polyunsaturated structure, which generates unpleasant fishy or rancid off-flavors that can cause consumer rejection of enriched products. Additionally, in the US and some European countries, the intake of PUFAs from food, is still below recommendations, with average daily ingestion between 88 and 226 mg, far behind the consumption needed to trigger beneficial effects (Lopes et al., 2023). Supplementation is therefore considered essential. There are multiple barriers that limit adequate intake from food sources, including dietary habits (low overall fish consumption), concerns with the presence of methyl mercury in certain fish species, and the high cost and instability of fish oils in food matrices. The sustainability challenges make things more complicated, as stocks of wild and farmed fish are finite, raising ecological questions. Thus alternative sources for PUFA are being sought through the cultivation of microalgae, as this methodology has shown potential for auto-sustainable and ecological benefits (Kumar et al., 2019). Consequently, dietary supplements provide a reasonable pathway to enhance health outcomes, especially for senior citizens, as these products guarantee safe, stable, and consistent access to EPA and DHA.

30.6.2 Product positioning and branding

The EFSA has extensively evaluated the scientific evidence on the effects of EPA and DHA in relation to CVD risk markers, concluding that DHA contributes to the maintenance of normal blood triglyceride levels and blood pressure. EFSA has also confirmed a cause-and-effect relationship between DHA and brain function, thereby permitting health claims on foods that provide at least 250 mg DHA per serving. A similar recognition has been granted for DHA in maintaining normal vision, with the same requirement of 250 mg DHA per serving for products to bear the claim (Jacobsen, 2015). The formation of structured lipids for obtaining new PUFA-rich formulations with health-promoting effects is a promising way. The structured lipids can be applied as functional oils for the metabolism of triacylglycerol, which may prevent fatty liver, obesity, atherosclerosis, and age-related chronic diseases. Medium-long-medium structured lipids with medium-chain fatty acids on the sn-1 and sn-3 positions, and long-chain omega-3 PUFAs on the sn-2 position, compared to conventional long-chain triacylglycerols, have special physiological properties; they provide rapid as well as sustained release of energy (Kim & Akoh, 2015). In particular, it was emphasized that such structured lipids may be useful in analogs of human milk fat used in infant formulas (especially when supplemented with performed DHA to increase the nutritional value). In addition, oleogelation has also been proposed as a beneficial delivery system for the delivery of fatty acids. Oleogelation is an encountered food structuring technology, and the type of vegetable oil incorporated into oleogels greatly affects physicochemical properties and functional characteristics of a formulation inside a food matrix, hence it provides versatility in developing functional foods with enhanced stability and bioavailability (Manzoor et al., 2022). EFSA recognition of DHA health benefits and development of structured lipid technologies together outline the textile process of regulatory validation and technological nourishments for PPPTex to humans.

30.6.3 Regulatory readiness and launch strategies

Based on this science, the EFSA has issued a scientific opinion supporting approved structure-function claims for DHA, including that it contributes to the maintenance of normal blood triglyceride levels and to normal blood pressure. Low DHA intake can impair brain function and vision. Nonetheless, although there is a higher ingredient loading from the supplementation with lipids compared to currently established ingredients for hepatic care (155), oxidation products of lipid components could risk one's health; namely, because they are easily prone to oxidative processes, such as peroxidation, and so require stabilization strategies in order to achieve regulatory approval and also consumer safety. Multiple approaches are used to combat oxidation. Optimizing processing conditions by controlling temperature, exposure to oxygen, and handling steps minimizes lipid oxidation initiation (Jacobsen, 2015). Physical protection of EPA and DHA is also provided by various delivery systems (e.g., encapsulation, emulsions, oleogels, and structured lipid matrices) that further improve oxidative and sensory stability. Furthermore, the inclusion of antioxidants adds an extra layer of protection: primary antioxidants (e.g., tocopherols, ascorbic acid, caffeic acid, chlorogenic acid, BHT, BHA, propyl gallate) donate hydrogen atoms to stabilize the radicals; secondary antioxidants (e.g., EDTA, polyphosphate s phytate caseinate and lactoferrin) inhibit hydroperoxide decomposition act as oxygen scavengers; multifunctionantioxidants such as polyphenols link together radical scravenging and chelation metals. Certain secondary antioxidants can also regenerate primary antioxidants, thereby improving overall stability (Rajasekaran et al., 2024). In addition, the right choice is also needed because some compounds, such as α-tocopherol, β-carotene, and soy isoflavones, may show pro-oxidant properties under certain conditions. Antioxidants can enhance the stability of structured triacylglycerols, and are essential because consumption of oxidized lipids has been demonstrated to impair lipid metabolism, increase oxidative stress, and negatively impact vascular function. The stability of structured fat molecules (triacylglycerols) supplemented with antioxidants has not been reported so far. One particularly sensitive product category is infant formulations for whom AA and DHA are commonly supplemented to aid growth and development, specifically for preterm newborns (Halder et al., 2021). But commercial formulations have positional distribution differing from that of human milk fat. Structured lipids, for example, human milk fat analogs, were developed to deliver AA, DHA, and other long-chain PUFAs in a physiologically relevant form. Oxidation of EPA and DHA results in the formation of volatile aldehydes, ketones, and alcohols with very low sensory thresholds, which has been a problematic factor to be overcome for a long time. These compounds develop fishy, rancid, or metallic off-flavors at ng/g levels and can lead to decreased consumer acceptance and market opportunity (Loftsson et al., 2016).

30.7 Future trends and innovations (personalized nutrition and AI, sustainable production, integration into new product categories, smart packaging, and sensors)

Nutritional lipids have transitioned from being solely dietary fats to multifunctional ingredients important in food, medicine, and nutraceuticals—with pivotal roles in modulating inflammatory, cognitive, metabolic, and cardiovascular health. Essential fatty acids, phospholipids, and fat-soluble vitamins are primarily derived from daily foods. Fatty fish, nuts, seeds, dairy products, and plant oils have been the common sources (Jala et al., 2025). To combat deficiencies, fortification strategies have been the focus of research, including omega-3-enriched eggs (high in ALA), phytosterol-fortified margarines, and DHA-enhanced dairy products. Concentrated lipid supplements (e.g., fish oil capsules and vitamin D3 tablets) offer a bioavailable alternative for people with restrictive diets, malabsorption, or certain health conditions (Guo et al., 2026). While emerging technologies (e.g., the use of nanoencapsulation and structured lipid formulations) are improving stability and absorption, soft capsules are still widely used as a vehicle for delivering functional lipids such as omega-3 fatty acids, CLA, and tocotrienols (Fig. 30.3). Empowered by reincarnations such as enteric coatings, multilayer lipid systems, and smart capsules, they harness targeted release and enhanced bioavailability (Zhang & Xu, 2025). Omega-3 fatty acids, phytosterols, structured triglycerides, and lipid-based delivery of vitamins and antioxidants via nanoemulsion and microencapsulation continue to find their way into functional foods and beverages. What does every infant need in terms of nutrition: structured lipids such as sn-2 palmitate that correspond to human milk fat, with DHA and AA supplementation. For medical nutrition support of recovery, immune function, and gut health, tailored lipids mainly including medium-chain triglycerides as well as structured lipids with immunomodulatory properties were employed, while parenteral emulsions also containing fish oil-derived PUFAs exerted antiinflammatory and hepatic-protective effects (Yuan et al., 2022). And it is even possible that information about brain energy can be used to target cryptic pathways throughout the body, as seen in some novel sports nutrition supplementation products that provide medium-long chain triglycerides and emulsified lipids for endurance (and fat oxidation) supported by research, based upon emergence of novel products with cognitive and antifatigue properties including CLA, phosphatidylserine (PS), neuropeptides, nitric oxide donors and choline. Custom lipid formulations (e.g., algal DHA for eye and brain health, CLAs for body composition, diacylglycerols for weight control) enhance personalized and preventive nutrition but also deliver bioactive polyphenols and fat-soluble vitamins in lipid-based carriers that may also reduce long-term disease risk (Ma et al., 2023). All of these advancements collectively reflect the diverse chemical nature and, therefore metabolic flexibility of lipids, positioning lipids for pivotal innovation in traditional, clinical, and personalized nutrition. New delivery systems are enabling PUFA to be included in novel product categories (Fig. 30.3). Microencapsulation uses

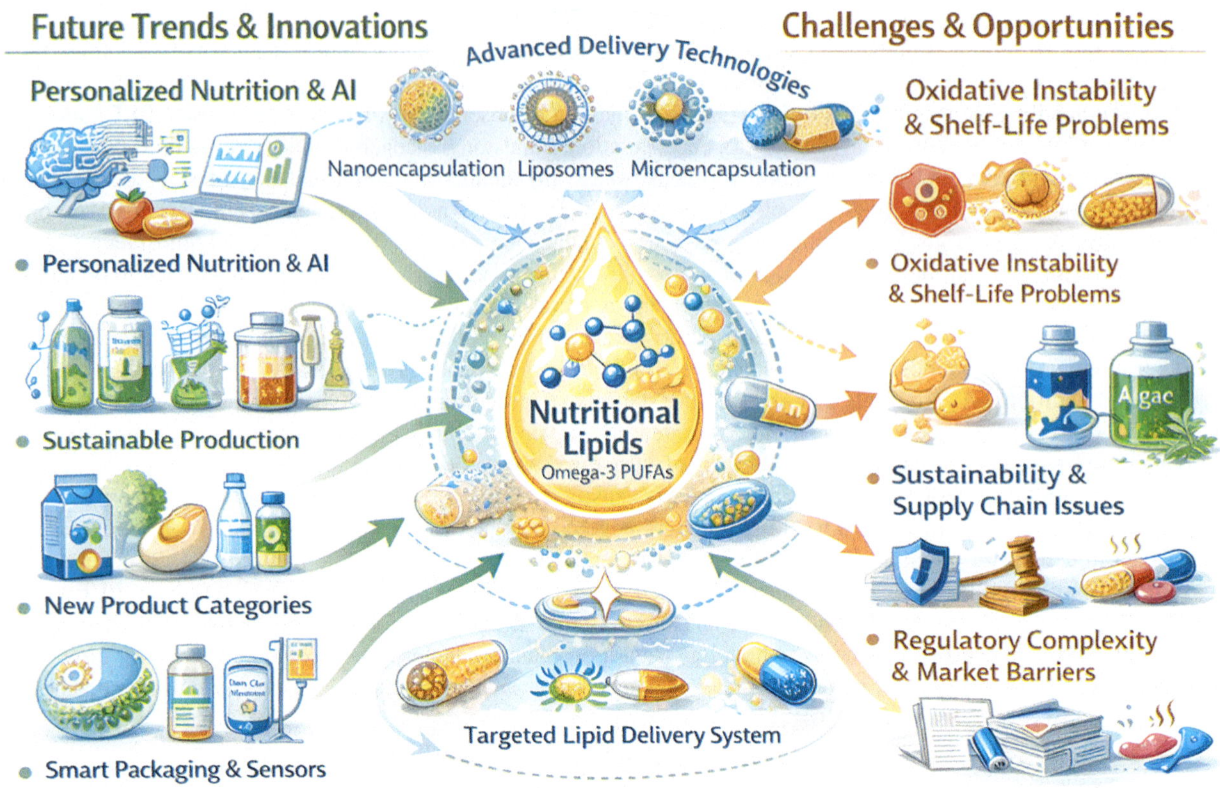

FIGURE 30.3 Future trends and opportunities of polyunsaturated fatty acids (PUFAs).

natural wall materials, which provide protective barriers around the bioactive compounds, promote stability properties, and controlled release during processing activities, storage, and digestion (Zhang & Xu, 2025). Liposomes, biomimetic systems composed of phospholipid bilayers, allow simultaneous encapsulation of both hydrophilic and hydrophobic compounds that provide excellent biocompatibility and high cellular uptake efficiency. Plant sterol-based liposomal formulations of algal-derived DHA have reached a significantly greater conversion than nonencapsulated oils. Characterized by the synergy between liposomes' biomimetic features and microcapsules capable of controlled release, nano delivery systems grew into intelligent carriers that function through the unique nanoscale size complemented with surface functionalization to revolutionize poorly soluble and nontargeted lipophilic bioactives. Cell, tissue, and organ niche responsive nanoparticles, in particular pH- and reactive oxygen species-sensitive systems, allow for precise release kinetics (Filipczak et al., 2020), site-specific delivery and targeting, including localized sites such as mitochondria, which is achievable via astaxanthin nanoparticles that can afford reduced levels of oxidative stress and inflammation both in vitro and in vivo (Filipczak et al., 2020). Altogether, these smart delivery technologies are extending the use of sensitive compounds to functional foods, nutraceuticals, and therapeutic formulations spanning a wide array of applications in health promotion, prevention, and treatment. Specifically, the intelligent response systems represent an innovative leap that integrates lipid science into personalized nutrition, preventative medicine, and targeted therapies. Precision nutrition also constitutes a significant frontier in food sciences, which has the goal of customizing meal interventions greatly based on individual genomic background, metabolic properties, lifestyle, and environmental influences, being primarily aimed at blocking disease or optimizing health and precision treatment. Genomics, metabolomics, and microbiomics are targeted to generate an accurate molecular basis for assessing individual nutritional requirements (Kupikowska-Stobba et al., 2025), while phenotyping allows integration of omics data with clinical outcomes and body measurements to optimize intervention strategies. Examples of this in precision nutrition include the fermented spirulina probiotic compositions and analysis via untargeted metabolomics for fatty liver disease prevention, as well as cerebrospinal fluid biomarkers used in patients with prodromal dementia. The utilization of artificial intelligence and machine learning in this field is expected to attract attention by incorporating multiomics data, phenotypic factors, food intake patterns, as well as lifestyle and exercise habits to develop dynamic personalized plate plans, recipes, and dietary supplements in the form (e.g., tailored revising omega-6:omega-3 ratio in lipid formulations (Hu et al., 2024)). These strategies can be implemented into feasible products with the help of compound nutrients and formulation technologies, further empowered by 3D printing to achieve customizable morphologies, dosages, and nutrient combinations according to consumer preference (e.g., multicolor oral dissolvable film containing anthocyanins, phycocyanin, chitosan starch/carrageen). Complementary to these advances are microfluidic technologies, which offer miniaturized and high-throughput testing platforms for nutritional formulas in simulated human environments, enabling low-cost portable point-of-care devices for biomarker monitoring and therapeutic applications (e.g., hydrogel microbeads that can be rapidly screened for the diagnosis of colitis or probiotic-loaded beads used in photothermal nano system treatments) (Guo et al., 2026). Altogether, precision nutrition, multiomics, AI, advanced formulation technologies, and microfluidics will redefine personalized nutrition with increasingly specific dietary solutions that adapt to individual health needs and future changes in the fields of functional foods and nutraceuticals.

30.8 Challenges and opportunities (technological and stability challenges, sustainability and supply chain, market penetration and consumer trust, packaging and shelf-life solutions)

However, with increasingly globalized supply chains for nutritional lipids, the sustainability of supply chains is a looming critical concern. Hurdles imposed by regulations, such as stringent labeling requirements and approval processes of novel lipid sources, slow down product development. While health concerns have led to an increased emphasis on dietary guidelines to focus on healthy fats, consumer hesitancy remains alongside technological barriers that lead to instability of unsaturated lipids and, more specifically, EPA and DHA in terms of shelf life (Lopes et al., 2023). Encapsulation, incorporation of antioxidants, and packaging under an inert atmosphere are strategies utilized to overcome these issues; however, stability is still challenging. Sensory characteristics provide challenges as fish oil, phytosterols, and structured lipids often confer off-tastes, odors, or mouthfeel, leading to lowered consumer acceptance. Formulation technologies such as microencapsulation, emulsification, and masking agents are implemented to provide harmony between health gimmickry and palatability. Further, this can generate another layer of complexity related to production and scalability, given that processes such as enzymatic interesterification, high-pressure homogenization and microfluidization may be cost increasing or quality complicating (higher capital investment and increased monitoring needed for the process), limiting their uptake in price-sensitive markets (Fig. 30.3). The complexity of regulatory processes further confines innovation, while well-characterized compounds such as DHA, AA and phytosterols have global approval whereas newer lipids with potential health benefits such as odd-chain fatty acids and structured fats share uncertain regulatory pathways, compounded by regional discrepancies in frameworks (Guo et al., 2026). Alleviation of such inter-individual variation with respect to genetic polymorphisms and their influence on lipid metabolism, as well as age, health status, and gut microbiota composition, greatly complicates product design and efficacy, thereby emphasizing the need for truly personalized approaches to address these challenges whilst extending our knowledge into lipid-gene interplay as well as lipid-microbiome interactions. But the environment and sustainability are equally important, because the growing demand for fish oil raises questions about biodiversity loss and carbon footprints, requiring sustainable sourcing, alternative feedstocks including algae and microbial oils, as well as circular production models to align innovations with global sustainability objectives. Meanwhile, opportunities for innovation in demand advances of encapsulation, changes in precision fermentation, and AI-assisted formulation become the main driving force behind industry growth, while strategic collaborations between food companies and biotech startups can scale sustainable production (Zhang & Xu, 2025). The development of future clean products will be driven by consumer demand for clean-label, plant-based and functional foods with precision lipid nutrition matched to genotype and metabolism, while bioactive functional synergies and digital health technology integration for personalized delivery and monitoring are on the horizon (Fig. 30.3). Together, these challenges and opportunities highlight the need for interdisciplinary coordination across food technology, regulatory science, sensory science, and sustainability to assure efficacy, safety, and consumer confidence in harnessing the full extent of nutritional lipids.

30.9 Conclusions

PUFAs itself is an evolving and complex area. Consumers have learned more about the beneficial effects of long-chain omega-3s on health and are willing to pay premiums for omega-3 fortified foods and higher quality supplements. New extraction and encapsulation technologies - especially supercritical CO_2 extraction and microencapsulation—allow producers to provide stable, bioavailable PUFA inputs with a fraction of the ecological footprint. Case studies show that success lies in blending scientific evidence, transparent communication, sustainability, and innovative marketing. Regulatory frameworks ensure safe and truthful labeling, and new guidelines are emerging that underscore sustainable sourcing. Future innovations are expected to interlace PUFAs with other bioactives, harness plant-based fermentation and gene-edited oilseed crops, and optimize products for personalized nutrition. By exploring the science, technology, and market dynamics described in this chapter, researchers and product developers can lay the groundwork for the next generation of PUFA-enriched foods, supplements, and pharmaceutical formulations.

References

Aitta, E., Marsol-Vall, A., Damerau, A., & Yang, B. (2021). Enzyme-assisted extraction of fish oil from whole fish and by-products of Baltic herring (*Clupea harengus membras*). *Foods, 10*(8), 1811.

Bichescu, C. I., Mihalcea, L., Raimondo, R., Cotârleț, M., Păcularu-Burada, B., Barbu, V., Râpeanu, G., Bahrim, G. E., & Stănciuc, N. (2024). Supercritical CO_2 fluid extraction and microencapsulation of oil from anchovy (*Engraulis mordax*) by-products. *Food Technology and Biotechnology, 62*(3), 302–313.

Burnett, A., Ahmmed, M. K., Carne, A., Tian, H. S., Ahmed, I. A. M., Al-Juhaimi, F. Y., & Bekhit, A. E. A. (2022). Effect of pulsed electric fields on the lipidomic profile of lipid extracted from hoki fish male gonad. *Foods, 11*(4), 610 21.

Coates, P. M., Betz, J. M., Blackman, M. R., et al. (2010). Omega-3 fatty acidsIn *Encyclopedia of dietary supplements* (2nd ed.). Informa Healthcare, 577–586.

Dighriri, I. M., Alsubaie, A. M., Hakami, F. M., Hamithi, D. M., Alshekh, M. M., Khobrani, F. A., Dalak, F. E., Hakami, A. A., Alsueaadi, E. H., Alsaawi, L. S., Alshammari, S. F., Alqahtani, A. S., Alawi, I. A., Aljuaid, A. A., & Tawhari, M. Q. (2022). Effects of omega-3 polyunsaturated fatty acids on brain functions: A systematic review. *Cureus, 9*(10), e30091 14.

Dovale-Rosabal, G., Rodríguez, A., Contreras, E., Ortiz-Viedma, J., Muñoz, M., Trigo, M., ... Espinosa, A. (2019). Concentration of EPA and DHA from refined salmon oil by optimizing the urea–fatty acid adduction reaction conditions using response surface methodology. *Molecules, 24*(9), 1642.

EFSA Panel on Dietetic Products, Nutrition and Allergies. (2012). Scientific opinion on the tolerable upper intake level of eicosapentaenoic acid (EPA), docosahexaenoic acid (DHA) and docosapentaenoic acid (DPA). *EFSA Journal, 10*(7), 2815.

Filipczak, N., Pan, J., Yalamarty, S. S. K., & Torchilin, V. P. (2020). Recent advancements in liposome technology. *Advanced Drug Delivery Reviews, 156*, 4–22.

Food and Agriculture Organization/World Health Organization (FAO/WHO). (1998). Fish oil specifications. In *Joint FAO/WHO Expert Committee on Food Additives*: Compendium of Food Additive Specifications (FAO Food and Nutrition Paper 52). (Provides peroxide and anisidine value limits for fish oils.)

Guo, W., Wang, H., Bai, Y., & Tan, M. (2026). Global patent landscape of marine functional foods: Technological trends, hotspots, and future challenges. *Trends in Food Science & Technology*, 105555.

Halder, T., Mehta, P., & Acharya, N. (2021). Trends in the functional food market and nutraceutical product development. In *Nutraceuticals for aging and anti-aging*. CRC Press, 1–26.

Harris, W. S. (2010). Omega-3 fatty acidsIn *Encyclopedia of dietary supplements* (2nd ed.). Informa Healthcare, 577–586.

Ho, B. C. H., Kamal, S. M. M., Danquah, M. K., & Harun, R. (2018). Optimization of subcritical water extraction (SWE) of lipid and eicosapentaenoic acid (EPA) from Nannochloropsis gaditana. *BioMed Research International, 2018*(1), 8273581.

Hu, Y., Li, W., Cheng, X., Yang, H., She, Z. G., Cai, J., ... Zhang, X. J. (2024). Emerging roles and therapeutic applications of arachidonic acid pathways in cardiometabolic diseases. *Circulation Research, 135*(1), 222–260.

Jacobsen, C. (2015). Some strategies for the stabilization of long chain n-3 PUFA-enriched foods: A review. *European Journal of Lipid Science and Technology, 117*(11), 1853–1866.

Jala, R. C. R., Zhang, H., Yang, M., Guo, R., Li, S., Xu, X., ... Xu, X. (2025). Encapsulation of DHA oils for better bioavailability: A review from the practical aspect. *Journal of the American Oil Chemists' Society, 102*(7), 1089–1112.

Kim, B. H., & &Akoh, C. C. (2015). Recent research trends on the enzymatic synthesis of structured lipids. *Journal of Food Science, 80*(8), C1713–C1724.

Kumar, B. R., Deviram, G., Mathimani, T., Duc, P. A., & &Pugazhendhi, A. (2019). Microalgae as rich source of polyunsaturated fatty acids. *Biocatalysis and Agricultural Biotechnology, 17*, 583–588.

Kupikowska-Stobba, B., Niu, H., Klojdová, I., Agregán, R., Lorenzo, J. M., & Kasprzak, M. (2025). Controlled lipid digestion in the development of functional and personalized foods for a tailored delivery of dietary fats. *Food Chemistry, 466*, 142151.

Lev-Tzion, R., Griffiths, A. M., Leder, O., & Turner, D. (2014). Omega 3 fatty acids (fish oil) for maintenance of remission in Crohn's disease. *Cochrane Database of Systematic Reviews, 2*, CD006320.

Loftsson, T., Ilievska, B., Asgrimsdottir, G. M., Ormarsson, O. T., & Stefansson, E. (2016). Fatty acids from marine lipids: Biological activity, formulation and stability. *Journal of Drug Delivery Science and Technology, 34*, 71–75.

Lopes, P. A., Alfaia, C. M., Pestana, J. M., & Prates, J. A. (2023). Structured lipids engineering for health: Novel formulations enriched in n-3 long-chain polyunsaturated fatty acids with potential nutritional benefits. *Metabolites, 13*(10), 1060.

Ma, Q., Zhang, X., Li, X., Liu, L., Liu, S., Hao, D., ... Li, J. (2023). Novel trends and challenges in fat modification of next-generation infant formula: Considering the structure of milk fat globules to improve lipid digestion and metabolism of infants. *Food Research International, 174*, 113574.

Manzoor, S., Masoodi, F. A., Naqash, F., & Rashid, R. (2022). Oleogels: Promising alternatives to solid fats for food applications. *Food Hydrocolloids for Health, 2*, 100058.

Martindale, R. G., Evans, D. C., Waitzberg, D., Warren, M., Mundi, M. S., Klek, S., Wischmeyer, P. E., & Rosenthal, M. D. (2025). Parenteral nutritional support in surgical patients: Expert consensus statements regarding intravenous lipid emulsions containing omega-3 fatty acids. *Frontiers in Nutrition, 12*, 1546089.

Mazereeuw, G., Lanctot, K. L., Chau, S. A., Swardfager, W., & Herrmann, N. (2012). Effects of omega-3 fatty acids on cognitive performance: A meta-analysis. *Neurobiology of Aging, 33*(7), 1482 e17–1482.e29.

Nicholls, S. J., Lincoff, M., Garcia, M., et al. (2020). Effect of high-dose omega-3 fatty acids vs corn oil on major adverse cardiovascular events in patients at high cardiovascular risk: The STRENGTH randomized clinical trial. *Journal of the American Medical Association, 324*(22), 2268–2280.

NIH. (2025). Omega-3 fatty acids - health professional fact sheet. https://ods.od.nih.gov/factsheets/Omega3FattyAcids-HealthProfessional/

Palmieri, N., Stefanoni, W., Latterini, F., & Pari, L. (2022). Factors influencing Italian consumers' willingness to pay for eggs enriched with omega-3-fatty acids. *Foods, 11*(4), 545.

Pinela, J., Fuente, B. D. L., Rodrigues, M., Pires, T. C., Mandim, F., Almeida, A., ... Barros, L. (2022). Upcycling fish by-products into bioactive fish oil: The suitability of microwave-assisted extraction. *Biomolecules, 13*(1), 1.

Piravi-Vanak, Z., Dadazadeh, A., Azadmard-Damirchi, S., Torbati, M., & Martinez, F. (2024). The effect of extraction by pressing at different temperatures on sesame oil quality characteristics. *Foods, 13*(10), 1472.

Puder, M., Valim, C., Meisel, J. A., Le, H. D., de Meijer, V. E., Robinson, E. M., Zhou, J., Duggan, C., & Gura, K. M. (2009). Parenteral fish oil improves outcomes in patients with parenteral nutrition-associated liver injury. *Annals of Surgery, 250*(3), 395–402.

Rahim, M. A., Uzma, M., Al-Asmari, F., Koraqi, H., Ramadan, M. F., Castro-Muñoz, R., & Zongo, E. (2025). A comprehensive review on nutritional traits, extraction methods, oxidative stability, encapsulation technologies, food applications and health benefits of omega fatty acids. *Food Science and Nutrition, 28*(10), e71008 13.

Rajasekaran, B., Gulzar, S., Gopalrajan, S., Karunanithi, M., & Benjakul, S. (2024). Omega-3 enriched fish and shellfish oils: Extraction, preservation, and health benefits. In *Fish waste to valuable products*. Singapore: Springer Nature Singapore, 195–229.

Sprague, M., Dick, J. R., & Tocher, D. R. (2016). Impact of sustainable feeds on omega-3 long-chain fatty acid levels in farmed Atlantic salmon, 2006–2015. *Scientific Reports, 6*, 21892.

TerraVia Holdings. (2016). *Microalgae: A new source of nutrition*. (Press release summarising uses of microalgae in foods and beverages.)

Van Dael, P. (2021). Role of n-3 long-chain polyunsaturated fatty acids in human nutrition and health: Review of recent studies and recommendations. *Nutrition Research and Practice, 15*(2), 137–159.

Venugopalan, V. K., Gopakumar, L. R., Kumaran, A. K., Chatterjee, N. S., Soman, V., Peeralil, S., Mathew, S., McClements, D. J., & Nagarajarao, R. C. (2021). Encapsulation and protection of omega-3-rich fish oils using food-grade delivery systems. *Foods, 10*(7), 1566.

Wachira, J. K., Larson, M. K., & Harris, W. S. (2014). n-3 fatty acids affect haemostasis but do not increase the risk of bleeding: Clinical observations and mechanistic insights. *British Journal of Nutrition, 111*(9), 1652–1662.

Yi, M., You, Y., Zhang, Y., Wu, G., Karrar, E., Zhang, L., ... Wang, X. (2023). Highly valuable fish oil: Formation process, enrichment, subsequent utilization, and storage of eicosapentaenoic acid ethyl esters. *Molecules, 28*(2), 672.

Yuan, T., Wang, L., Jin, J., Mi, L., Pang, J., Liu, Z., ... Wang, X. (2022). Role medium-chain fatty acids in the lipid metabolism of infants. *Frontiers in Nutrition, 9*, 804880.

Zhang, H., & Xu, X. (2025). Nutritional lipids: An overview of nutritional progress and market trends. *Journal of Food Bioactives, 31*, 8–30.

Zhou, Y., Guo, Z., Chang, S. K., Zhang, Y., Hong, H., Luo, Y., & Tan, Y. (2025). Ultrasound-assisted, machine learning-optimized extraction of silver carp viscera fish oil and microencapsulation via complex coacervation. *Ultrasonics Sonochemistry, 120*, 107452.

Zivkovic, A. M., Telis, N., German, J. B., & Hammock, B. D. (2011). Dietary omega-3 fatty acids aid in the modulation of inflammation and metabolic health. *California Agriculture (Berkeley), 65*(3), 106–111.

Chapter 31

Commercialization strategies for polyunsaturated fatty acid products with case study analysis: From concept to market

Sunayan Sharma and Soumi Chakraborty
Amity Institute of Food Technology, Amity University, Noida, Uttar Pradesh, India

31.1 Introduction

Polyunsaturated fatty acids (PUFAs) are one of the fatty acids that play a plethora of significant roles in human physiology, specifically in managing cardiovascular health, neural development, immune modulation, and inflammatory regulation (Calder, 2015). PUFAs are structural components of cell membranes, which influence the fluidity, receptor activity, gene expression, and intracellular signaling pathways (Swanson et al., 2012). Among several PUFAs, omega-3 (n-3) and omega-6 (n-6) fatty acids have been highly commercialized because they cannot be synthesized de novo in adequate quantities by humans and must therefore be obtained through diet or supplementation (Calder, 2015). Recent clinical studies have suggested that adequate intake of eicosapentaenoic acid (EPA) and docosahexaenoic acid (DHA) is correlated with reducing the risk of cardiovascular diseases, improving neurodevelopmental outcomes in infants, and potential protective effects against chronic inflammatory and metabolic disorders (Calder, 2017; Mozaffarian & Wu, 2011). It has been found that populations consuming fish-rich diets show lower rates of coronary heart disease (Mozaffarian & Wu, 2011), later it is postulated that the correlation is only with fatty fish consumption, and the beneficial effects are not evident from lean fish consumption. Subsequently, clinical and mechanistic studies analyzed the roles of PUFAs in lipid metabolism, endothelial function, inflammation resolution, and neural development, further supporting their incorporation into functional foods, dietary supplements, and pharmaceutical formulations (Calder, 2017). Studies on nearly all bodily functions and a broad range of illnesses have been illustrated in Fig. 31.1.

PUFAs are chemically unstable because of their multiple double bonds, which make them susceptible to oxidation during processing, storage, and distribution (Granato et al., 2020). Such oxidative changes compromise the nutritional quality, sensory attributes, and consumer safety. With growing demand, the commercialization of PUFA products presents different technical and strategic challenges (Jacobsen, 2015). However, sustainability concerns, fluctuating marine resources, potential contamination with environmental pollutants, and sensory issues (odor and taste) are the challenges for consumer acceptance (Nicholas et al., 2014). In this aspect, the use of different technologies such as microencapsulation, bio-fortification, and controlled packaging can offer higher shelf stability and consumer acceptability (Granato et al., 2020). Algal oils, plant-derived precursors such as alpha-linolenic acid (ALA), and biotechnologically produced fatty acids have been introduced in the market. The aforesaid PUFA-alternatives are ethical, shelf-stable, and offered dietary preferences, particularly among vegetarian and vegan consumers, while also improving product consistency and supply chain stability (Nicholas et al., 2014).

It has been found from market surveys that commercialization achievement depends on the scientific evidence, consumer perception, pricing strategies, branding, and sustainability. With increasing awareness of environmental issues has been an increased demand for responsibly sourced omega-3 products, principally those derived from algae or sustainably managed fisheries (Tocher, Betancor, Sprague, Olsen, Napier, 2019). Consequently, PUFAs have emerged as

Omega-3 and Omega-6 Polyunsaturated Fatty Acids in Food Systems. DOI: https://doi.org/10.1016/B978-0-443-43810-3.00034-8

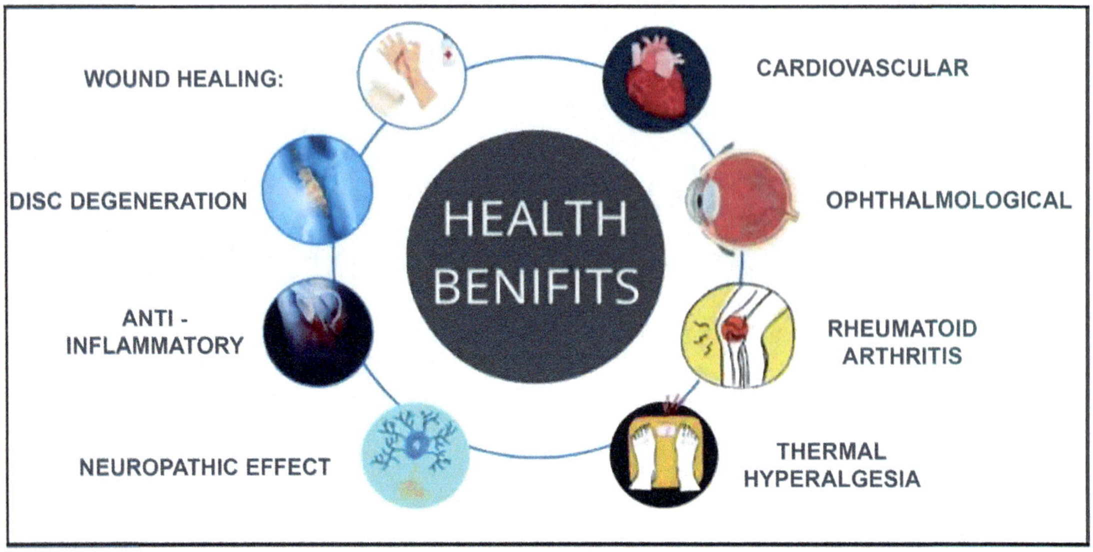

FIGURE 31.1 Benefits of polyunsaturated fatty acid-enriched food in various diseases.
Source: From Patted, et. al., 2024.

central components in the rapidly expanding functional lipid market, linking nutritional science with food innovation, biotechnology, and global health promotion.

31.2 Biochemical characteristics, sources, health functions, and commercial relevance of omega-3 and omega-6 fatty acids

Omega-3 PUFAs (n-3 PUFAs) represent a critical class of essential fatty acids widely recognized for their physiological, clinical, and commercial importance. Structurally, omega-3 fatty acids are characterized by the first double bond occurring at the third carbon atom from the methyl (omega) end of the fatty acid chain. As human lack Δ12 and Δ15 desaturases enzymes, because of which omega-3 does not get synthesized endogenously and is obtained from dietary intake (Calder, 2017). ALA, EPA, and DHA play a vital role in cardiovascular health and neurological homeostasis. Thereby, driving substantial commercial interest in food, pharmaceutical, and nutraceutical industries (Shahidi & Ambigaipalan, 2018a, 2018b; Swanson et al., 2012). Table 31.1 illustrates the biochemical classification of omega-3 fatty acids.

Omega-6 PUFAs (n-6 PUFAs) constitute a major class of essential fatty acids widely distributed in plant oils, animal products, and processed food systems. They are characterized by the presence of the first double bond at the sixth carbon from the methyl end of the fatty acid chain. The principal omega-6 fatty acids of nutritional and commercial importance include linoleic acid (LA; 18:2 n-6), gamma-linolenic acid (18:3 n-6), dihomo-gamma-linolenic acid (20:3 n-6), and arachidonic acid (AA; 20:4 n-6) (Simopoulos, 2016). LA acts as the primary dietary precursor for AA, involved in the synthesis of prostaglandins, leukotrienes, and thromboxane-bioactive lipid mediators essential for immune response and inflammatory signaling (Calder, 2017). AA is specifically important in infant nutrition due to its involvement in brain growth, visual acuity, and immune system maturation. It has been found that AA is frequently incorporated along with DHA in infant formula products (Koletzko et al., 2020). Table 31.2 illustrates the biochemical classification of omega-6 fatty acids.

31.3 From concept to commercial product: strategic framework

31.3.1 Market analysis and consumer positioning

The successful commercialization of PUFA products requires a multidisciplinary marketing strategy that integrates scientific validation, branding innovation, and effective distribution networks. The functional health positioning of PUFA products requires marketing approaches that emphasize credibility, transparency, and sustainability while addressing consumer perceptions, competitive differentiation, and evolving nutritional trends. There has been growing awareness of the role of PUFA products in the global market (Calder, 2015; Nicholas et al., 2014). Fig. 31.2 illustrates the market

TABLE 31.1 Classification, sources, functions, and commercial applications.

Type of n-3 polyunsaturated fatty acid	Details	Food sources	Commercial/health significance	References
Alpha-linolenic acid	Short-chain plant-derived omega-3 fatty acid; precursor to EPA and DHA with limited conversion efficiency.	Flaxseed, chia seeds, walnuts, soybean oil, canola oil	Widely used in vegetarian supplements and functional edible oils; important in plant-based nutrition markets.	Burdge and Calder (2015)
Eicosapentaenoic acid (EPA)	Long-chain omega-3 fatty acid primarily from marine organisms; regulates inflammation and cardiovascular function.	Fish oils, krill oil, microalgae	Used in cardiovascular supplements, antiinflammatory nutraceuticals, and pharmaceutical formulations.	Calder (2017)
Docosahexaenoic acid (DHA)	Structural fatty acid in brain and retina; critical for neurodevelopment and vision.	Fatty fish, algal oil, fortified infant formula	Essential ingredient in infant nutrition, prenatal supplements, and cognitive health products. Algal and biotechnological sources are sustainable alternative sources produced via fermentation or biotechnology. The sources are microalgae DHA oil, engineered oilseed crops, etc., which have been in high demand because these are vegan sources (Adarme-Vega et al., 2012).	Koletzko et al. (2020)

TABLE 31.2 Classification, sources, and commercial health significance of omega-6 fatty acids.

Category of omega-6 fatty acids	Description	Food sources	Commercial health significance	References
Linoleic acid (LA)	Major essential omega-6 fatty acid serves as a precursor to longer-chain omega-6 fatty acids. Widely consumed through vegetable oils.	Soybean oil, sunflower oil, safflower oil, corn oil, sesame oil	Dominant dietary polyunsaturated fatty acid globally; extensively used in the edible oil industry and processed foods.	Shahidi and Ambigaipalan (2018)
Gamma-linolenic acid (GLA)	Metabolite of LA with antiinflammatory potential; often used therapeutically.	Evening primrose oil, borage oil, blackcurrant seed oil	Used in nutraceutical supplements targeting inflammatory conditions, skin health, and hormonal balance.	
Dihomo-gamma-linolenic acid	Intermediate omega-6 metabolite with potential antiinflammatory properties.	Formed metabolically from GLA	Interest in pharmaceutical and clinical nutrition applications.	Calder. (2017)
Arachidonic acid	Long-chain omega-6 fatty acid involved in eicosanoid production and immune responses.	Meat, poultry, eggs, dairy products; infant formula fortification	Essential for infant brain development, immune function, and inflammatory response regulation.	Koletzko et al. (2020)

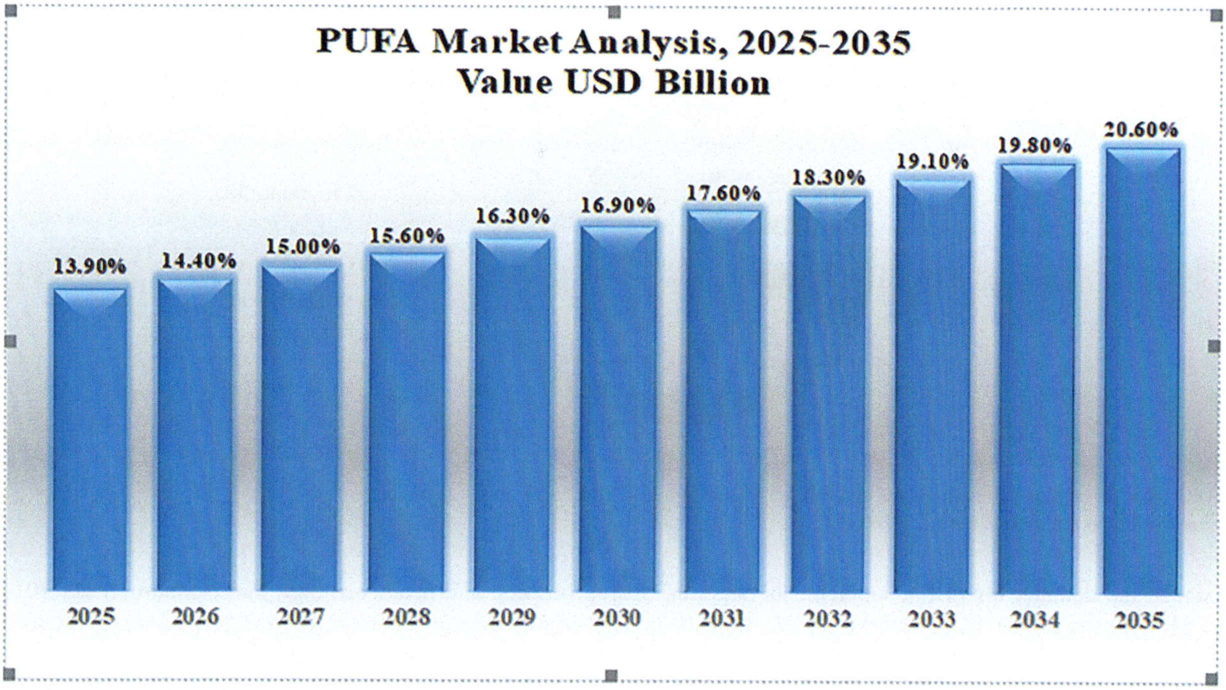

FIGURE 31.2 Growth of polyunsaturated fatty acid (PUFA) market from 2025–35.
Source: From Market Research Future, 2026.

research future analysis, the PUFAs market size increased from USD 48.2 billion in 2024 to USD 50.38 billion in 2025 to USD 78.38 billion by 2035, which exhibits a compound annual growth rate (CAGR) of 4.52% during the forecast period 2025–35.

31.3.1.1 Consumer health awareness and preventive nutrition

Effective segmentation allows manufacturers to tailor product formulations, packaging, pricing, and distribution channels to specific consumer needs, thereby enhancing market penetration (Kotler & Keller, 2016; Verbeke et al., 2007). PUFAs are primarily marketed within functional food, nutraceutical, and pharmaceutical domains; consumer purchasing decision get affected by multiple factors, such as health awareness, lifestyle factors, and demographic characteristics.

31.3.1.2 Maternal and infant nutrition

DHA, a long-chain omega-3 fatty acid, plays a critical role in immune response, fetal brain development, and retinal development. Subsequently, pregnant and lactating women represent a key target market for PUFA supplementation. DHA-enriched infant formulas are widely commercialized because of evidence linking adequate intake with improved cognitive and visual outcomes among infants (Koletzko et al., 2020). DHA intakes have a significant impact on visual and cognitive development in breastfed infants. Recommended for term infants for DHA from 0.2% to 0.4% of fatty acid (Mitmesser & Jensen, 2007).

31.3.1.3 Adults and performance and fitness consumers

Physically active adults are increasingly seeking preventive nutrition solutions for cardiovascular health, metabolic wellness, and stress management. Omega-3 fatty acids have been associated with reduced cardiovascular disease risk, making the group a primary market segment for supplements and fortified foods (Mozaffarian & Wu, 2011). Evidence has broadly supported the beneficial effects of EPA/DHA supplementation for athletes, the efficacy of EPA/DHA supplementation for improved endurance capacity, and delayed onset of muscle soreness, as well as on markers related to enhanced recovery and immune modulation (Thielecke & Blannin, 2020). Athletes and physically active enthusiasts often consume omega-3 fatty acids for their antiinflammatory effects, potential recovery benefits, and support for muscle function and endurance performance (Philpott et al., 2019). Older adults often use PUFA products for maintenance of cognitive health, joint health, inflammation control, and chronic disease prevention. Aging populations globally have

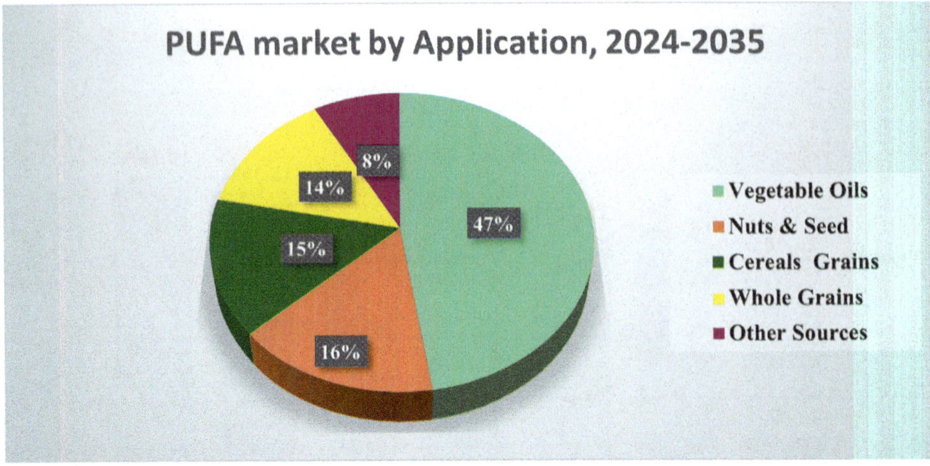

FIGURE 31.3 The polyunsaturated fatty acids (PUFAs) market by application, 2024–35 (USD billion).
Source: From Market Research Future, 2026.

expanded the demand for PUFA supplements targeting neuroprotection and healthy aging (Yurko-Mauro et al., 2010). Fig. 31.3 illustrates the PUFA market application in dietary supplements in contrast to food and beverages. Dietary supplements have the largest share among health-conscious consumers to enhance their nutritional intake.

31.3.1.4 Environmentally conscious consumers

Recent concerns have raised the demand for plant-based or algae-derived omega-3 products. Purchasing behavior has been influenced by ethical sourcing, carbon footprint considerations, and marine ecosystem protection (Hamilton et al., 2020). With advances in synthetic biology, biotechnological production of omega-3 fatty acids via engineered microbial cell factories still offers the best solution to provide a more stable, sustainable, and affordable source of omega-3 fatty acids by overcoming the major issues associated with conventional sources (Qin et al., 2023).

31.3.2 Market growth projections and economic trends

The growth of PUFA-enriched food product market in USD 6686.9 million in 2025 and it will growth to USD 11,422.3 million by 2035 which is expanding at a CAGR of 5.5% over the forecasted period due to worldwide focus on cardiovascular health, cognitive development, and immune support resulting in the consumption of PUFA across diets, pharmaceuticals, and functional food. Fig. 31.4 illustrates the country growth CAGR from 2025 to 2035.

The regional dietary patterns, economic development, and cultural attitudes toward supplements influence PUFA product demands. Moreover, income and education are certain factors significantly affecting the purchasing behavior for PUFA-enriched products. Latin America and the Asia-Pacific regions have reported high-growth markets due to the rise in disposable income, urbanization, and increasing health awareness. In 2025, North America holds a dominant 30.78% share of the market, bolstered by its advanced regulatory frameworks. Meanwhile, the Asia-Pacific region is on rapid ascent, which is projected to grow at a 6.85% CAGR through 2032, which us fueled by an uptick in health consciousness. Japan and South Korea are continuing to take the lead with the highest global omega-3 index scores, which reflect the strong consumer awareness and consumption patterns. On the contrary, Chinese consumers are showing interest in fish oils, which signals the growing market potential. Europe has robust growth in the PUFAs market, holding approximately 30% of the global share. This increased have been showcased with an increase in consumer awareness regarding health benefits, specifically in cardiovascular health, and stringent regulations promoting the use of omega-3 fatty acids in food products. Fig. 31.5 illustrates the market size in USD billion in Middle East, Asia-Pacific, Europe, and North America.

31.4 Commercialization pathway: from concept to market

The commercialization of PUFA products involves a multidisciplinary process that integrates the scientific research, product development, regulatory compliance, marketing strategy, and supply chain management. With the sensitivity of

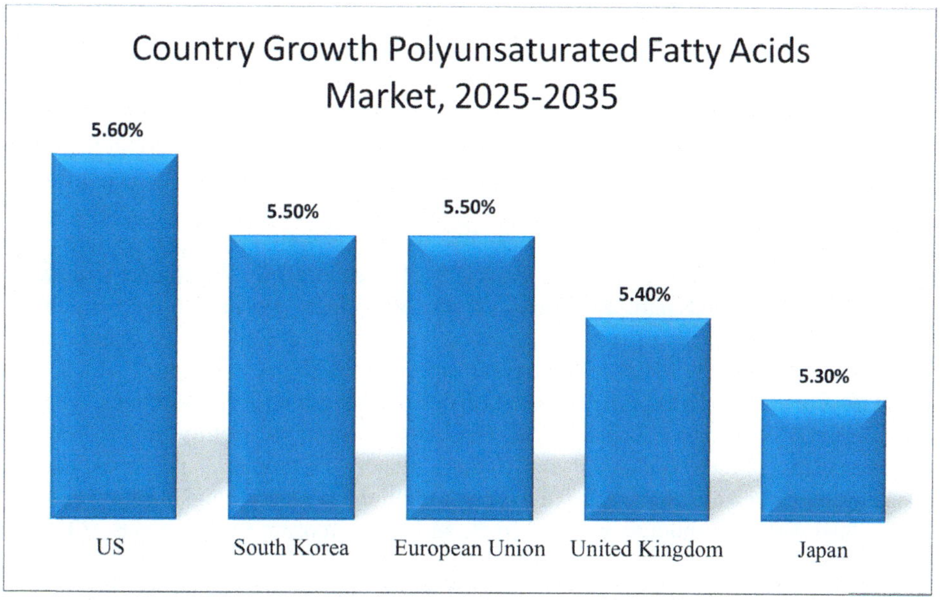

FIGURE 31.4 Polyunsaturated fatty acid-enriched product compound annual growth rate growth from 2025 to 2035.
Source: From Future Market Insights, 2025.

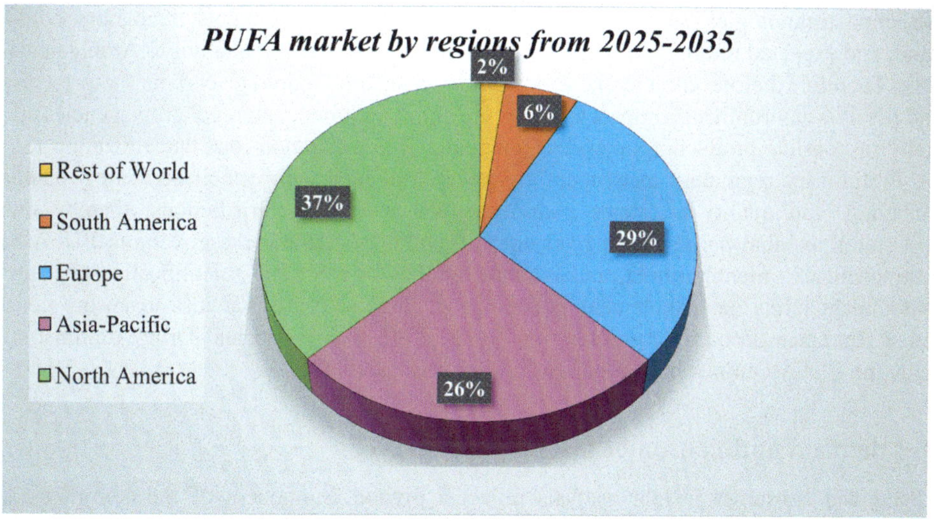

FIGURE 31.5 Polyunsaturated fatty acid (PUFA) market by regions from 2025–35, in USD billion.
Source: From Market Research Future, 2026.

PUFAs to oxidation, regulatory scrutiny over health claims, and increasing consumer demand for functional foods, a systematized pathway is crucial for assessment, product development, regulatory approval, branding and marketing, and distribution scale-up.

31.4.1 Research and feasibility assessment

A critical preliminary stage in the commercialization of PUFA products, as it explains the scientific validity, technological practicality, economic sustainability, regulatory readiness, and market acceptance of a product before large-scale commercialization investments are made. This process typically begins with the identification and evaluation of appropriate PUFA sources, such as marine fish oils in EPA and DHA, microalgae-derived oils regarded as sustainable vegetarian alternatives, plant-based oils including flax seed, chia seeds, and canola oil which are rich in ALA and emerging microbial or genetically engineered oilseed sources produced via biotechnology. The above concern has raised the demand for microalgae biotechnology as a renewable and controlled source of high-quality omega-3 fatty acids, although production cost and scale-up challenges remain significant considerations (Kunj et al., 2025; Schneider, et al., 2025). While selecting the raw material, it also requires a detailed evaluation of the composition of fatty acid, contaminant risks such as heavy metals, supply consistency, and environmental sustainability (Calder, 2020; Shahidi & Ambigaipalan, 2018a, 2018b). Recent clinical and cohort studies demonstrated that omega-3 fatty acids also contribute to cardiovascular health by reducing fatal coronary heart disease risk, improving lipid metabolism, modulating inflammation, and supporting metabolic regulation, while emerging evidence also suggests potential roles in cognitive function maintenance and healthy aging (Banaszak et al., 2024; Djuricic & Calder, 2025; Lee et al., 2026). Recent systematic reviews further highlighted that PUFA-enriched food may encompass protective effects against chronic inflammatory conditions, neurological conditions, and in reinforcing the significance of preventive nutrition and development of functional foods (Patted et al., 2024). There has been a crucial technological aspect of feasibility assessment which includes the stability evaluation because PUFAs are highly susceptible to oxidation due to their multiple double bonds, which leads to rancidity, nutrient loss, and decreased consumer acceptability. Consequently, some feasibility studies analyzed and included peroxide value measurements, accelerated shelf-life testing, sensory evaluation, and investigation of stabilization strategies such as encapsulation technologies, antioxidant incorporation, advanced emulsification systems, and innovative packaging solutions, which help to minimize oxygen, light, and heat exposure (McClements, 2015; Shahidi & Zhong, 2010; Waraho et al., 2011).

The market feasibility also examines consumer awareness, demographic trends, dietary patterns, purchasing power, and competitive product landscapes. With an increase in global interest in preventive healthcare, functional foods, personalized nutrition, and sustainable dietary patterns have been significantly integrated PUFA products into nutraceuticals, pharmaceuticals, infant nutrition, and functional food sectors (Bleakley & Hayes, 2017; Calder, 2020; Shahidi & Ambigaipalan, 2018a, 2018b). Economic feasibility analysis evaluates the cost of production, which includes raw material procurement, extraction technologies, stabilization methods, packaging requirements, regulatory compliance expenses, scalability potential, and expected return on investment, etc. (McClements, 2015; Shahidi & Ambigaipalan, 2018a, 2018b; Venugopal, 2008). Therefore before commercialization, the sustainable sourcing, carbon footprint assessment, ethical supply chains, and lifestyle environmental impact analyzes are highly required, and regulatory agencies are also focusing on the environmentally responsible production practices (International Organization for Standardization ISO, 2006; Poore & Nemecek, 2018). Preliminary regulatory assessment ensures compliance with established safety standards, permissible health claims, labeling, and quality assurance parameters across various jurisdictions, thereby minimizing delays, reformulation costs, and potential barriers to market entry. Regulatory frameworks governing PUFA-based products—specifically in nutraceuticals, infant formula, and functional foods—necessitate scientifically substantial health claims, adherence to contaminant limits, and implementation of good manufacturing practices to ensure consumer safety and product consistency (European Food Safety Authority EFSA, 2012; U.S. Food and Drug Administration FDA, 2022). Fig. 31.6 illustrates the PUFA commercialization feasibility assessment.

31.4.2 Market demand and consumer insight analysis

The market demand and consumer insight analysis reflect a pivotal component of the commercialization of PUFA products, as successful market entry depends not only on scientific validity but also on consumer awareness, acceptance, purchasing behavior, and evolving nutritional trends. In recent years, PUFA-enriched functional foods, dietary supplements, pharmaceuticals, and infant nutrition products. PUFA-enriched foods are widely recognized for their potential roles in the management of human health, making them highly attractive to health-conscious consumers seeking evidence-based entry interventions (Calder, 2015; Swanson et al., 2012). This demand is further strengthened by increasing public access to nutrition awareness campaigns, which have enhanced consumer knowledge of functional ingredients and encouraged proactive dietary choices (Calder, 2020; Ventola, 2014). Demographic factors also significantly shape PUFA market demand; aging populations in many countries have heightened interest in products that support the physical and physiological health, while younger consumers increasingly adopt functional foods as part of fitness, mental wellness, and preventive health lifestyles (Calder, 2015; Swanson et al., 2012). With growing awareness of nutrition science, consumption of PUFA-enriched food has encouraged proactive dietary habits for stress management, cognitive performance, and physical recovery (Shahidi & Ambigaipalan, 2018a, 2018b). Moreover, increasing urbanization, higher disposable income among working-age populations, and lifestyle changes favor convenient functional foods such as fortified beverages and dietary supplements. Thereby, expanding the PUFA consumer base across varied demographic groups. Hence, demographic profiling and consumer segmentations must be widely recognized as critical

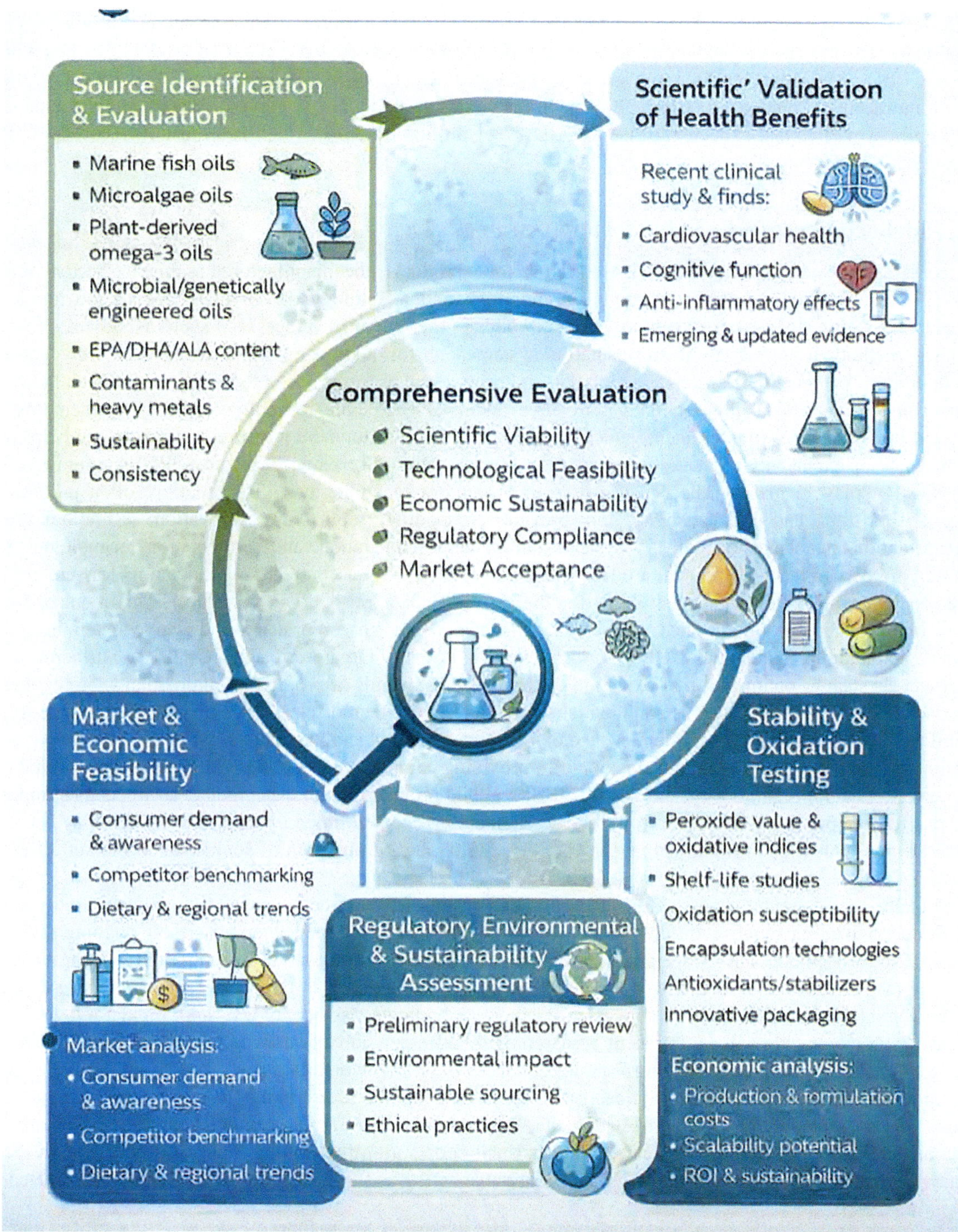
Source Identification & Evaluation
Marine fish oils
Microalgae oils
Plant-derived omega-3 oils
Microbial/genetically engineered oils
EPA/DHA/ALA content
Contaminants & heavy metals
Sustainability
Consistency
Scientific' Validation of Health Benefits
Recent clinical study & finds:
Cardiovascular health
Cognitive function
Anti-inflammatory effects
Emerging & updated evidence
Comprehensive Evaluation
Scientific Viability
Technological Feasibility
Economic Sustainability
Regulatory Compliance
Market Acceptance
Market & Economic Feasibility
Consumer demand & awareness
Competitor benchmarking
Dietary & regional trends
Market analysis:
Consumer demand & awareness
Competitor benchmarking
Dietary & regional trends
Regulatory, Environmental & Sustainability Assessment
Preliminary regulatory review
Environmental impact
Sustainable sourcing
Ethical practices
Stability & Oxidation Testing
Peroxide value & oxidative indices
Shelf-life studies
Oxidation susceptibility
Encapsulation technologies
Antioxidants/stabilizers
Innovative packaging
Economic analysis:
Production & formulation costs
Scalability potential
ROI & sustainability

FIGURE 31.6 Polyunsaturated fatty acid commercialization feasibility assessment (Schneider, et al., 2025; Lee et al., 2026).

determinants of success in the PUFA-enriched products (Bleakley & Hayes, 2017; Shahidi & Ambigaipalan, 2018a, 2018b; Kotle & Keller, 2016).

The global demographic projections indicate the proportion of people aged 65 years and older is expected to rise from about 9% in 2019 to nearly 12% by 2030 and approximately 16% by 2050, which creates substantial demand for functional foods and nutraceuticals targeting age-related health conditions (News Medical, 2050). Subsequently, the market reach of omega-3 supplements was valued at USD 7.68 billion in the year 2024. Further, it may grow up to USD

12.89 billion by the end of 2030 and almost USD 13.3 billion by 2035 because of buyers' interest in omega-3-enriched functional food products (Future Market Insights, 2025). As per the recent estimate, the food product fortified with PUFA may exceed USD 388 billion by 2025 and gradually may progress to USD 901 billion by 2035, reflecting the global demand for nutraceutical innovations (Fact., 2025). On the contrary, the Indian market of omega-3 supplements is around USD 425 million in 2023 and expected to rise to USD 879.1 million by 2030, which is almost 10.9% of CAGR (Grand View Research, 2024).

31.4.3 Intellectual property and innovation strategy

For a successful commercialization of PUFA-enriched food products, the manufacturer requires effective intellectual property (IP) and innovation strategies that are competitive and technology driven that concern the nutraceuticals, pharmaceutical, and food sectors. Such novelties implicate the complex processes, such as advanced extraction technologies, methods for stabilization, encapsulation systems, and formulative optimization (Teece, 1986. To safeguard these technologies, patents, trade secrets, trademarks, and proprietary processes need to be required, which helps the firm secure its competitive advantages, facilitate more investment, and expedite technology transfer partnerships. Having strong IP aids the companies to internment values from research and development to prevent imitation and helps to ensure the maintenance of exclusivity in market segmentation (Teece, 1986). For patent protection, PUFA commercialization, patent protection plays a pivotal role because it is important for technological differentiation, often product quality, stability of shelf-life, and bioavailability. To prevent competitive replication, innovation technologies such as microencapsulation, nanoemulsion delivery systems, antioxidant stabilization, and fermentation technologies for algal fermentation are certain technologies that are frequently patented to prevent competitive replication (Kassem et al., 2025. Trade secrets are another key component of IP for the commercialization of PUFA products. This requires full public disclosure in exchange for time-limited exclusivity, this help to protect proprietary knowledge indefinitely with the provision of maintaining confidential needs (World Intellectual Property Organization WIPO, 2020). Furthermore, several crucial processes such as optimization of oxidation control systems, blends of proprietary antioxidants, protocol related to quality control are to be safeguarded as confidential savoir-faire rather than disclosed while filing patent. Due to the high susceptibility of PUFAs products that often leads to oxidative degradation and rancidity, companies should develop unique stabilization and different processing methods to aid in providing competitive advantages in shelf-life, bioavailability, and sensory quality (Shahidi & Ambigaipalan, 2018a, 2018b). While protecting with these methods, it becomes important for trade secrets to help prevent competitors from reverse-engineering detailed process parameters so that they become more accessible through patent publication, helping in stability, purity, and formulation of sophisticated market differentiation (Grandstand, 2000).

To maintain the competitiveness of changing pharmaceutical, nutraceutical, and functional food industries, PUFA commercialization requires different innovative strategies that lay special emphasis on ongoing technological and research advancement and cooperative partnerships. In order to optimize bioavailability, improve oxidative stability, improvised extraction technology to validate health benefits. Various nutraceutical industries have interdisciplinary knowledge that enhances nutrition science, food technology, biotechnology, and regulatory affairs, which are crucial to integrate internal environment research with different collaborators (Chesbrough, 2003). To improve innovation efficiency, science-driven sectors should collaborate with networks that can promote knowledge sharing and low technical uncertainty. With joint clinical trials, to re-develop the stabilization technologies, sustainable source programs, for example, algal or microbial omega-3 production, and IP agreements become necessary for the commercialization of PUFAs. There is a need for consistent cooperation for ongoing innovation that boosts the market legitimacy so as to create a unique PUFA product that satisfies the health needs and legal requirements of consumers (Powell et al., 1996).

The integrated IP strategy helps to align the market trends, regulatory constraints, and sustainability priorities. With increased regulatory scrutiny of environmental effect, product safety, and verified health claims, businesses need to integrate the sustainable-driven innovation with IP planning. The synthesis of omega-3 algal production has drawn a lot of attention towards sustainable substitutes for conventional fish oil sources, because they provide scalable and controlled production systems while reducing the negative impact on marine ecosystems. Technological originality and process complexity are developing technologies that frequently offer better patent positioning (Ryckebosch et al., 2014). The majority of the time business are well equipped with strong IP protection measures that can satisfy the changing regulatory requirements, enhance brand credibility, and guarantee long-term commercial viability. Therefore with strategic IP management, a vital business tool promotes innovation leadership, market differentiation, and long-term growth to the PUFA industry (World Intellectual Property Organization WIPO, 2020).

31.5 Branding approaches in polyunsaturated fatty acid commercialization

With different branding approaches, various translating scientific value of PUFAs integrated consumer trust, perceived efficacy, and buying behavior. PUFA products often fall within the functional food or nutraceutical category- where health benefits are intangible and preventive rather than immediate-brand strategy must reduce uncertainty, communicate scientific credibility, and create emotional resonance (Kotler & Keller, 2016). In the context of PUFAs, particularly omega-3 and omega-6 fatty acids, certain brands incorporate evidence-based messages, clinical endorsement, transparent sourcing, for example, marine versus plant-based origin, and plant certification (e.g., third-party testing) can strengthen perceived efficacy with regulatory frameworks further to enhance credibility.

31.5.1 Evidence-centric branding

This represents as the critical differentiation strategies in commercialization of PUFA products, as they are more preventive rather than immediate perceptible. Consumer majorly reply on scientific credibility to evaluate the product efficacy (Grunert, 2010). Such type of branding highlights clinical trial outcomes, research summaries, transparent labeling of EPA/DHA content, and obtaining third-party certification such as pharmaceutical-grade purity testing (Annunziata & Vecchio, 2013). In the nutraceutical sector, associations with clinical validation enhance perceived reliability and reduce consumer uncertainty. Henceforward, corporations recurrently cooperate with healthcare professionals, research institutions, and regulatory bodies to authenticate declarations, thereby there is an accumulative buyer trust and brand loyalty.

31.5.2 Sustainability-focused branding

Sustainability-focused branding has emerged as a decisive dimension for PUFA commercialization, particularly because of concerns related to ecological surroundings as in the case of marine oil extraction. Environmentally responsible positioning needs to be adopted for consumer scrutiny of fish oil sourcing otherwise it can lead to overfishing, biodiversity loss, and climate impacts. For this reason, certain brands lay emphasis on environmental centric practices such as certified sustainable fisheries, traceable supply chain, alternative sources which includes algal-derived omega-3 fish oils, as are considered ecological sustainable (Nicholas et al, 2014). Such of mentioned branding majorly enhance consumer trust, ethical appeal, and perceived product quality, influencing the purchasing criteria of functional food and nutraceutical markets. Evidence have indicated that adopting environmentally friendly branding may also improves the purchasing intentions and consumer trust, specifically for younger demographics (Hartmann & Apaolaza, 2006).

31.5.3 Clean label and transparency branding

Product label or clean-label branding depicts the growing consumer demand, as it encourages transparency of ingredients, authenticity, specifically for functional and nutraceuticals where buyers' trust can be validated for perceived health benefits. Furthermore, such strategies highlight the processing technologies, no use of any artificial additives, limiting the genetically modified ingredients, and sourcing disclosure and purity testing (Asioli et al., 2017). This helps to address the consumers' concerns related to any risks of contamination such as heavy. Metals or oxidation specifically in marine oils and highlighting the enhanced perceived product safety and quality standards (Nicholas et al, 2014). Explicit reporting of EPA/DHA content, raw materials, and third-party testing certifications can reduce the skepticism, which is majorly related to dietary labeling, brand credibility, and purchase intentions.

31.5.4 Life-stage and targeted segment branding

Market segmenting branding upholds the relevance and effectiveness of PUFA commercialized products since the requirement of nutritional and perceived health support can vary in different stages of life. With targeted branding communication, brands can align the product aiding to the physiological needs and perception of risks for certain demographic groups, which can enhance the perceived personal relevance and purchase intention (Kotler & Keller, 2016). For instance, during prenatal development, consumption of DHA supplementation is encouraged because of impacts leads to cognitive and visual concerns. The maternal DHA consumption has been correlated with improved cognitive functioning and visual acuity among infants (Innis, 2007; Koletzko et al., 2008). PUFA-enriched food in pediatrics frequently focuses on cognitive development, whereas elderly-targeted formulations emphasize antiinflammatory and neuroprotective properties (Kotler & Keller, 2016). Targeted branding reduces the cognitive overload by providing clear usage contexts, thereby increasing purchase confidence (Annunziata & Vecchio, 2013). Brands can improve perceived efficacy and personal relevance by customizing message, such as "active ageing," "prenatal brain development," or "heart health support." This increases consumer trust, engagement, and buying intention. In the markets for functional foods and nutraceuticals, where the benefits are preventive and demand greater levels of customer confidence, targeted health communication is especially crucial (Grunert, 2010). Therefore segment-specific branding combines demographic targeting techniques with scientific data to enhance market uniqueness and emotional resonance while bolstering brand credibility in the cutthroat PUFA industry (Kotler & Keller, 2016).

31.5.5 Premium and pharmaceutical-grade branding

Nutraceutical industries often employ premium positioning branding to commercialize PUFA-enriched products as to communicate superior quality, which can support higher prices of the product. Omega-3-enriched products often require credibility evidence, such as bioavailability of the product, ingredient purity, and premium branding, which serves to lower perceived risk and enhance the perception value. Apart from these, certain diseases such as cardiovascular or cognitive functioning, require higher concentrations of EPA and DHA, highlighted as markers of potency and efficacy. Enteric-coated capsules are intended to increase the bioavailability and improve gastrointestinal tolerance capacity. Thus third-party certifications, heavy metal screening, molecular distillation, and purification procedures emphasize safety and pharmaceutical-grade quality (Nicholas et al., 2014). Such aspects serve as extrinsic signals that support perceived brand equity and provide justification for higher price in product categories enhancing health condition (Kotler & Keller, 2016).

31.5.6 Digital and direct-to-consumer branding

PUFA-commercialized products have substantial transition due to digital transformation, allowing more direct, personalized, and having more interactive customer contact. With more individualized advice, subscription-based supplement services, and ongoing consumer education via blogs, webinars, and digital health content, direct-to-consumer platforms that enables firm to increase customer retention services and perceived value (Chaffey & Ellis-Chadwick, 2019). Social media marketing or campaigns have emerged as crucial branding strategies for PUFA products. In recent times, buyers' demand relies on expert recommendation,evaluation by peers and online forums assessing the legitimacy of functional foods or nutraceuticals, majorly focusing on long-term health benefits (Hajli, 2014). That's why, digital transformation is a key element of recent PUFA commercialization because digital engagement maneuverers not only increase market reach but to inculcate trust, transparency, and brand loyalty.

31.6 Postmarket surveillance and product improvement

Postmarket surveillance (PMS) reflects a crucial stage in the commercialization lifecycle of PUFA products, that ensures the ongoing product safety, efficacy, regulatory compliance, and brand credibility after the market launch. Unlike pharmaceutical products that undergo extensive pre-market clinical evaluation, several PUFA-based products, specifically functional foods, nutraceuticals, and dietary supplements. Consequently, systematic monitoring followed by commercialization becomes essential to identify adverse effects, evaluate real-world performance, ensure product stability and generate insights for continuous innovation (Gliklich et al., 2014). Fig. 31.7 illustrates the PMS and product improvement for PUFA products.

One of the primary components of PMS involves safety monitoring and adverse event reporting. Although PUFA-enriched products are generally recognized as safe, excessive intake with medication such as anticoagulants may lead to mild gastrointestinal disturbances, bleeding risks, or allergic responses in sensitive populations. With constant monitoring, such physiological factors may help manufacturers to detect emerging safety signals early. Regulatory authorities such as the FDA, European Food Safety Authority, and FSSAI constantly emphasize postmarket reporting to strengthen the consumer framework. Such proactive safety surveillance improves transparency and reduces legal and reputational risks (Gliklich et al., 2014). Quality stability monitoring is the inherent susceptibility of PUFAs to oxidative degradation. Oxidation leads to deterioration of nutritional efficacy, leads to unpleasant sensory characteristics, and sometimes leads to potentially injurious oxidative compounds. Henceforth, manufacturer is required to assess peroxide value and total oxidation (TOTOX) indices the shelf life of the product. The Global Organization for EPA and DHA Omega-3 ensures the regular quality verification, ensuring compliance with industry standards. The perceived product quality majorly gets influenced by brand equity and purchasing behavior of the consumers which can impact the quality assurance (Aaker, 1991). The consumer feedback analysis can enable digital transformation with real-time monitoring of consumer

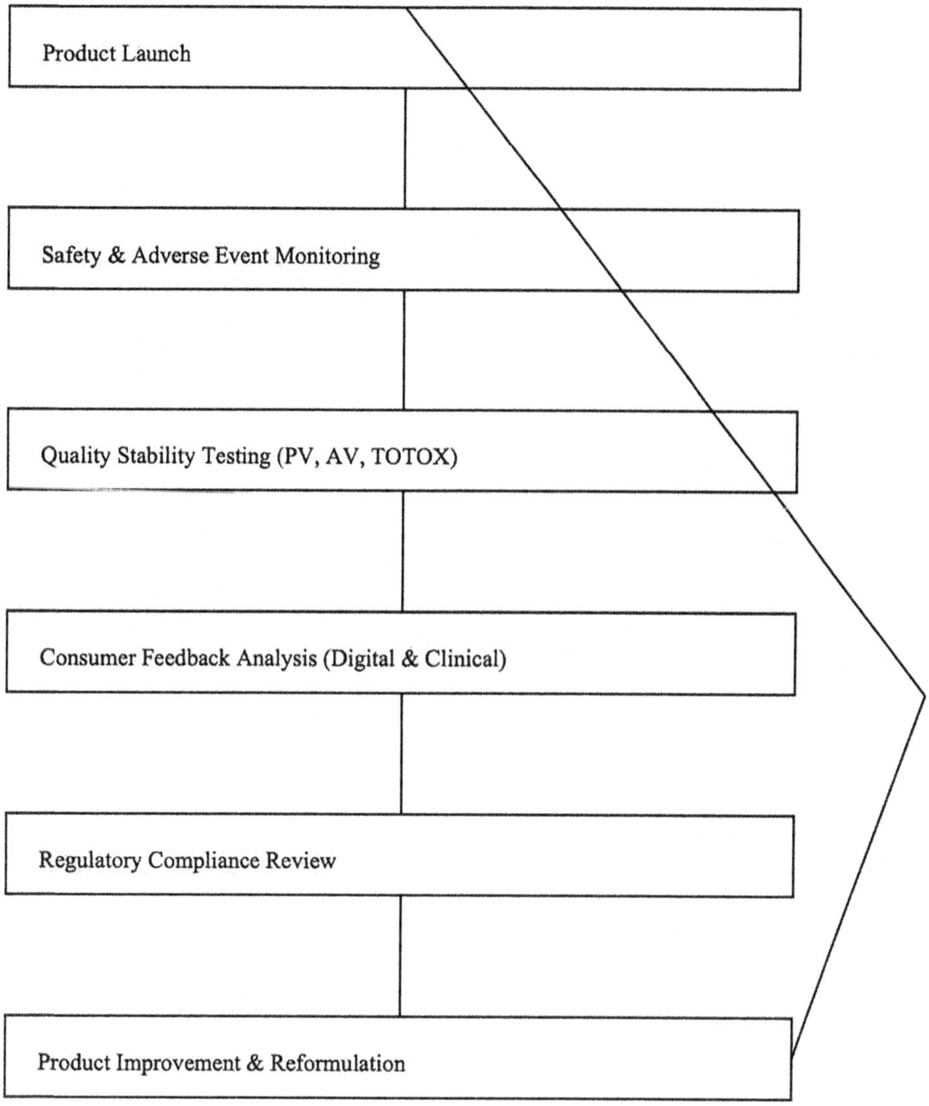

FIGURE 31.7 Postmarket surveillance (PMS) and product improvement framework for polyunsaturated fatty acid Products.

perception with the help of online reviews or ratings, social media discussion, and postpurchase surveys. Such feedback helps to provide valuable insights into sensory acceptability, packaging functionality, and dosage clarity (Chevalier & Mayzlin, 2006). Feedback helps to curb certain issues related to fishy aftertaste, discomfort that can be caused by the size of the capsule and other sustainability sourcing.

Product reformulation and innovation are supported by postmarket surveillance, which is essential to maintain the competition in rapidly growing nutraceutical markets. The insights from stability testing, feedback from consumers, and growing clinical evidence help product improvement. The reformulation strategies may incorporate antioxidant systems that can improve the oxidative stability, can adopt microencapsulation technology that can reduce sensory issues, and can use optimization strategies for EPA/DHA ratios based on updated clinical research. To address sustainability concerns, a transition to algal-derived omega-3 sources can be adopted (Napoli et al., 2014). For effective postmarket systems, crisis management and recall preparedness can be incorporated. Regardless of rigorous quality control, misleading information that can lead to errors, contamination incidents, or adverse reactions may require product recalls. With such structured recalls, the protocol should include traceability mechanisms, risk communication strategies, and corrective action plans that are crucial for reducing health risks and reputational damage. Transparent crisis communication depicted the mitigation of negative brand perception at the time of adverse events (Coombs, 2007). Another increasingly critical element is supply-chain evaluation and sustainable monitoring. Sourcing of PUFA-enriched products, particularly marine-derived omega-3 oil, faces environmental sustainability, geopolitical instability, and contamination risks. To ensure consistent product quality and ethical sourcing practices, there should be periodic supplier autism traceability systems, particularly for marine-derived omega-3 oils (Hartmann & Apaolaza, 2006).

Last of all, companies should incorporate a framework for continuous improvement, such as methodical collection of data analysis, remedial measures, and strategic decision-making, which should be adopted to guide postmarket surveillance. Initially developed by (Deming, 1986).

A continuous improvement framework that incorporates methodical data collection and analysis as a quality management method, the plan-do-check-act (PDCA) cycle, and philosophy has been widely accepted to guarantee a systematic and iterative improvement process in various businesses, which includes the nutraceuticals sector as well. Corporate organizations can transition from reactive compliance to proactive quality enhancement by incorporating the PDCA model for the purpose of postmarketing monitoring systems. Various crucial inputs for risk assessment and evaluation of performance may come from market analysis for the maintenance of consumer feedback, safety measures, and regulatory compliance. The information regarding the corrective and preventive actions (CAPA) to maintain the quality management remedial measures, and strategic decision-making should guide postmarket surveillance. Originally developed by Deming as a quality management method, the Plan–Do–Check–Act (PDCA) cycle is widely used to guarantee systematic and iterative improvement processes in a variety of businesses, including the food and nutraceutical sectors (Deming, 1986). Organizations can transition from reactive compliance to proactive quality enhancement by integrating PDCA principles into postmarket monitoring systems. Critical inputs for risk assessment and performance evaluation come from market analytics, adverse event reporting, consumer feedback, safety monitoring systems, and regulatory inspections. To inform CAPA within quality management systems, these insights can be methodically examined to find trends, underlying causes, and areas for improvement (International Organization for Standardization ISO, 2015). PMS and product improvement are indispensable components of PUFA commercialization. It ensures ongoing safety, regulatory compliance, quality stability, consumer satisfaction, and sustainable sourcing practices. More importantly, they provide actionable insights for continuous innovation and brand differentiation.

31.7 Case study analysis

31.7.1 Case study 1: algal docosahexaenoic acid Infant formula commercialization

31.7.1.1 Background and market context

Algal-derived DHA in the development of infant formula feeding is one of the major innovative strategies in the PUFA nutraceutical sector. During early life stages, requirement of DHA is crucial for infants' neurodevelopment, visual acuity and immune function. Traditionally, DHA sources are marine fish oils. However, there have been growing concerns about contamination risks, sustainability concerns, and vegetarian dietary preferences have created obstructions in the acceptance of the microalgae-derived DHA. Due to these reasons, the product has faced commendation from international health organizations that emphasize the importance of long-chain omega-3 fatty acids for recommended nutritional requirements during infancy (Koletzko et al., 2020). The market analyzes depicted that omega-3 fatty acids used in infant nutrition are growing gradually with rising awareness of early-life situations.

31.7.1.2 Sustainability and ethical branding

Algal DHA has benefits, including:

- Controlled cultivation environments
- Reduces risk of heavy metal contamination
- Compatibility with vegetarian/vegan preferences
- Lower ecological impact compared with marine harvesting

Such attributes can be leveraged in branding strategies that emphasize sustainability and purity.

31.7.1.3 Product differentiation

Companies are introducing premium infant formula feeding products that are enriched with algal DHA, with organic and clean-label variants, and are specialized in producing formulas that can target preterm infants or allergy-sensitive populations. Although the premium orientation has enabled a higher price while reinforcing perceived quality.

31.7.1.4 Market impact and performance

There has been growing demand for functional infant nutrition among consumers because of parental awareness of infant development. Research has indicated that with growing parents' awareness of health literacy and preventive healthcare, there is an increase in DHA-inclusive ingredients in formula feeding for infants. Henceforth, algal DHA has expanded the market with more plant-based food, particularly in regions such as India, Europe, and parts of North America. So, manufacturer have gained attention about infant formula that is enriched with DHA, but it also commands premium pricing, which is relative to standard formulation ,leading to higher margins of profits, majorly because of health benefits such as cognitive functioning. Companies that are adopting algal DHA technology have gained the competitive advantages through the product differentiation and regulatory compliance. The conceptual trends have reflected the incorporation of DHA into infant formula products because of scientific evidence that is linked to DHA consumption and its benefits of neurodevelopment, visual acuity, and immune functioning during infancy (Koletzko et al., 2020).

31.7.1.5 Challenges

Irrespective of commercial success, several barriers remain, which are:

- Higher production costs compared with fish oil DHA
- Regulatory scrutiny of health claims
- Consumer education requirements
- Supply chain scalability for microalgae cultivation

Scientific validation, sustainable positioning, and targeted branding have proved successful for the commercialization of PUFA-enriched products, which is enhancing technological advances while reducing the cost barriers. Continued growth of plant-based nutritional trends and expanded health awareness globally have highlighted the alignment of regulatory compliance, consumer education, and technological innovation in the functional food market.

31.7.2 Case study 2: omega-3 fortified edible oil in emerging markets

31.7.2.1 Background and market rationale

Public health concerns related to omega-3 fatty acid deficiency have been a major concern in many developing countries, particularly areas away from the coastline, due to low seafood consumption and also because of dietary imbalances that favor omega-6 fatty acids. Recent public health strategies have focused on the fortification of commonly consumed edible oils with omega-3 fatty acids, which is also cost-effective. The fortified staple food needs to reach a wide population without changes in behavioral aspects (Ganesan et al., 2014). Due to urbanization, lifestyle patterns, metabolic disorders, and consumer literacy on cardiovascular health conditions have increased the demand for PUFA-fortified food in the emerging markets of Asia, Latin America, and Africa. These manufacturing industries have indicated the steady growth in the functional edible oils that are enriched with omega-3 fatty acids, which is expanding globally.

31.7.2.2 Commercialization strategy

31.7.2.2.1 Mass fortification approach

The targeted markets have widely consumed soybean, sunflower, mustard oil, and other vegetable or seed oils in cooking. This has led to ensuring:

- High population reach
- Regular consumption patterns
- Public health alignment

The fortified edible oils often contain microencapsulated omega-3 fatty acids to maintain stability during storage and cooking.

31.7.2.2.2 Pricing and accessibility

Some of the fortified oils are being positioned as within the affordable functional products as compared to premium expensive supplements. The competitive pricing strategies are facilitating and making easier for middle-income household to adopt while maintaining the acceptable profit margins with high sales volume.

31.7.2.2.3 Health education campaigns

Certain manufacturing companies frequently collaborated with:

- Public health organizations
- Nutrition awareness campaigns
- Retail promotion initiatives.

31.7.2.2.4 Market performance and consumer acceptance

Emerging research has indicated that the health benefits have been made evident; while maintaining the sensory qualities, consumers are more inclined towards the adoption of fortified staple foods. A major factor that influences the acceptability is fortified neutrality, that is lack of fishy taste or smell. Urban consumers have adopted more, particularly those who are conscious of maintaining their physical health. Institutional purchasers, including government-imposed nutritional programs, hospitals, and schools, have been largely expanded.

31.7.2.2.5 Challenges

Technological obstacles and commercialization of fortified edible oils have adversely impacted the following:

- Oxidative instability when cooking at high temperatures
- Low consumer awareness of the advantages of omega-3
- Encapsulation technology costs
- Differences in regulations between nations

Even though omega-3 retention has been constantly used for cooking, there is still a requirement for research to be conducted for technological advancement. Public health interventions and business opportunities have adopted the edible oils enriched with omega-3 fatty acids as functional food fortification. This has shown a potential approach for addressing the nutritional inadequacies at the population level, even though its low implementation continues the ongoing success of such fortified food technological advancements.

31.8 Future perspective

With rapid development in biotechnology, sustainability concerns and consumer behavior, and digital transformation, progress has been made in consumer health awareness with respect to the commercialization of PUFA-enriched products. To expand awareness and understanding of PUFA products related to health benefits such as cognitive ageing, metabolic disorders, immune modulation, and personalized nutrition, more clinical evidence should emerge that focuses on preventive healthcare that can further strengthen the demand for PUFA-enriched functional foods. An ageing population and an increase in lifestyle disorder have led a demographic shift in long-term market growth, especially in Asia-Pacific and other developing countries where health awareness and disposable income are rising. Technological innovation has been integral to the commercialization of PUFA products. Other than this, recent emulsification technologies, smart packaging, nanoencapsulation, biotechnologically driven technologies, microalgae cultivation, microbial fermentation, and genetically engineered oilseed crops focus on sustainability challenges and have been associated with marine sources that can ensure a consistent supply and quality. These alternative innovative production technologies have not only reduced costs and time but also enabled broader access to consumer reach to food systems and clinical nutrition sectors.

Continued technology advancement serving successful commercialization in the formulation of product stability, innovative strategy systems, and enhanced bioavailability has served as a foundation for PUFA-enriched products. Since PUFAs are highly susceptible to oxidative breakdown, it has an adverse impact on their nutritive value, sensory properties, and shelf life. Future research made in the direction of next-generation encapsulation methods, nanoemulsion-based delivery, usage of synergistic antioxidants, and smart packaging should be designed to protect the product from oxygen and light. These advancements have enabled an effective integration of PUFAs in a wide variety of food products, from beverages and dairy to baked goods and also medically advised nutraceuticals. That can broaden the conventional supplement formats. Furthermore, advances in nutrigenomics, wearable health monitoring, and digital health integration have enabled PUFA supplementation which is based on genetic information, nutritional status, and lifestyle factors. PUFA product brand engagement should adhere to more practices towards e-commerce platforms, more digital engagement, and direct-to-consumer marketing. The commercialization of PUFA should intersect public health initiatives that can adopt fortification methods of staple foods with PUFA, specifically omega-3 fatty acids that improve the health outcomes.

Such strategies should combine together towards cost-effective production and consumer education. Some of these efforts can enhance both market expansion and societal health benefits. For evolved global health needs, integration of technological innovation, sustainability, rigorous regulatory compliance, and strategic marketing should be adopted for PUFA commercialization.

PUFA commercialization reflects a conventional shift from nutritional supplementation, integrating an ecosystem that encompasses digital engagement, advanced food technology, and sustainable production. For such integration, companies require transparency in public alignment, maintaining scientific credibility, consumer trust, and environmental responsibility, helping sustained growth and leadership in the evolving global functional PUFA-enriched food market. Furthermore, there should be collaborations among academic institutions, biotechnology firms, food manufacturers, and regulatory agencies, helping to accelerate innovation that will reduce the development costs and technical uncertainties. Public-private partnerships, research platforms, and innovation models enhance the production development of PUFA-enriched food products.

31.9 Conclusion

The commercialization of PUFA-enriched products is a potent progressive market in food technology, biotechnology, nutrition and also strategic marketing. Both omega-3 and omega-6 fatty acids indicated significant physiological changes in cardiovascular health, cognitive development, certain inflammation modulation, and regulation in bodily metabolism. In the wake of such progressive changes, they have been incorporated into pharmaceuticals, functional foods, nutraceuticals, and formula feeding. The demographic changes, such as an ageing population and growing health concerns, and growing buyers awareness about preventive healthcare have increased the global demand for PUFA-enriched products in the market. The comprehensive strategies integrate research and development, regulatory compliance, stability, and branding, as well as market intelligence that goes beyond scientific validation for effective commercialization. Significant technological factors, such as significant formulation and shelf-life issues, have been brought by the oxidative instability for PUFAs, which is necessary for the use of futuristic strategies for stabilization such as microencapsulation, antioxidant inclusion, packaging, and optimization of supply chain management. Earlier, the procurement of marine oil having sustainable concerns spurred the innovative technologies that alternate to PUFA sources such as microalgae, plant-based precursors, and different biotechnological production systems. With such emerging advances can accelerate the long-term supply of oxidation stability that can address ethical and environmental concerns at the same time. Certain crucial constituents' branding tactics, such as consumer segmentation and branding strategies of PUFA commercialization from a market point of view. Evidence-centric branding such as clean-label transparency, life-stage marketing, and sustainable positioning can uphold the consumer confidence and product effectiveness within the market. Furthermore, digital transformation and direct-to-consumer platforms, personal communication, and brand engagement have facilitated customer input, quality monitoring, and research findings in product cycle improvement. Apart from these, quality monitoring, incorporating customers' inputs, and PMS have pivotal roles in maintaining the product safety and regulatory compliance. The case study of algal DHA infant formula demonstrated how scientific validation can lead to sustainable, driven innovations that can generate premium market prospects, specifically in the field of maternal and newborn nutrition. The process of fortification, for example, omega-3-enriched edible oils, caters to nutritional inadequacies.

References

Aaker, D. A. (1991). *Managing brand equity: Capitalising on the value of a brand name.* New York: The Free Press, 411–423.

Adarme-Vega, T. C., Lim, D. K., Timmins, M., Vernen, F., Li, Y., & Schenk, P. M. (2012). Microalgal bio-factories: A promising approach toward sustainable omega-3 fatty acid production. *Microbial Cell Factories, 11*, 96.

Annunziata, A., & Vecchio, R. (2013). Consumer perception of functional foods: A conjoint analysis with probiotics. *Food Quality and Preference, 28*(1), 348–355. https://doi.org/10.1016/j.foodqual.2012.10.009.

Asioli, D., Aschemann-Witzel, J., Caputo, V., Vecchio, R., Annunziata, A., Næs, T., & Varela, P. (2017). Making sense of the "clean label" trends: A review of consumer food choice behavior and discussion of industry implications. *Food Research International, 99*, 58–71. https://doi.org/10.1016/j.foodres.2017.07.022, www.elsevier.com/inca/publications/store/4/2/2/9/7/0.

Banaszak, M., Dobrzyńska, M., Kawka, A., Górna, I., Woźniak, D., Przysławski, J., & Drzymała-Czyż, S. (2024). Role of Omega-3 fatty acids eicosapentaenoic (EPA) and docosahexaenoic (DHA) as modulatory and anti-inflammatory agents in noncommunicable diet-related diseases – Reports from the last 10 years. *Clinical Nutrition ESPEN, 63*, 240–258. https://doi.org/10.1016/j.clnesp.2024.06.053, https://www.sciencedirect.com/science/journal/24054577.

Bleakley, S., & Hayes, M. (2017). Functional foods, nutraceuticals, and PUFA enrichments: Trends and prospects. *Foods, 6*(11), 95.

Burdge, G. C., & Calder, P. C. (2015). Conversion of alpha-linolenic acid to longer-chain omega-3 fatty acids. *Reproduction, Nutrition, Development, 45*, 581–597.

Calder, P. C. (2015). Functional roles of fatty acids and their effects on human health. *Journal of Parenteral and Enteral Nutrition, 39*, 18–32. https://doi.org/10.1177/0148607115595980, http://onlinelibrary.wiley.com/journal/10.1002/(ISSN)1941-2444.

Calder, P. C. (2017). Omega-3 fatty acids and inflammatory processes: From molecules to man. *Biochemical Society Transactions, 45*(5), 1105–1115. https://doi.org/10.1042/BST20160474, http://www.biochemsoctrans.org/content/45/5/1105.full-text.pdf.

Calder, P. C. (2020). Omega-3 fatty acid and inflammatory processes: From molecules to man. *Biochemical Society Transaction, 48*(1), 1–17.

Chaffey, D., & Ellis-Chadwick, F. (2019). *Digital marketing* (7th ed.). Pearson.

Chesbrough, H. W. (2003). *Open innovation: The new imperative for creating and profiting from technology*. Harvard Business School Press.

Chevalier, J. A., & Mayzlin, D. (2006). The effect of word of mouth on sales: Online book reviews. *Journal of Marketing Research, 43*(3), 345–354. https://doi.org/10.1509/jmkr.43.3.345, https://journals.sagepub.com/home/mrj.

Coombs, W. T. (2007). Protecting organization reputations during a crisis: The development and application of situational crisis communication theory. *Corporate Reputation Review, 10*(3), 163–176. https://doi.org/10.1057/palgrave.crr.1550049, http://www.palgrave-journals.com/crr/index.html.

Deming, W. E. (1986). *Out of the crisis*. MIT Press.

Djuricic, I., & Calder, P. C. (2025). N-3 fatty acids (EPA and DHA) and cardiovascular health-updated review of mechanisms and clinical outcomes. *Current Atherosclerosis Reports, 27*(1), 116.

European Food Safety Authority (EFSA) (2012). Scientific opinion on the substantiation of health claims related to omega-3 fatty acids. *EFSA Journal, 10*(7), 2815.

Fact. M. R. (2025). Functional foods market size and share forecast outlook 2025 to 2035.

Ganesan, B., Brothersen, C., & McMahon, D. J. (2014). Fortification of foods with omega-3 polyunsaturated fatty acids. *Critical Reviews in Food Science and Nutrition, 54*(1), 98–114. https://doi.org/10.1080/10408398.2011.578221.

Gliklich, R. E., Dreyer, N. A., & Leavy, M. B. (2014). Registries for evaluating patient outcomes: A user's guide. *Effective Health Care Program*, 233–315 (3rd ed.).

Granato, D., Barba, F. J., Bursać Kovačević, D., Lorenzo, J. M., Cruz, A. G., & Putnik, P. (2020). Functional foods: Product development, technological trends, efficacy testing, and safety. *Annual Review of Food Science and Technology, 11*, 93–118. https://doi.org/10.1146/annurev-food-032519-051708, http://www.annualreviews.org/journal/food.

Grandstand, O. (2000). *The economics and management of intellectual property: Towards intellectual capitalism*. Edward Elgar Publishing.

Grunert, K. G. (2010). European consumers' acceptance of functional foods. *Annals of the New York Academy of Sciences, 1190*(1), 166–173. https://doi.org/10.1111/j.1749-6632.2009.05260.x.

Grand View Research. (2024). Omega-3 markets size and supplements market analysis reports. https://www.grandviewresearch.com/industry-analysis/omega-3-supplement-market.

Hajli, N. (2014). A study of the impact of social Media on consumers. *International Journal of Market Research, 56*(3), 387–404.

Hamilton, H. A., Newton, R., Auchterlonie, N. A., & Muller, D. B. (2020). Sustainable omega-3 production. *Nature Food, 1*, 230–237.

Hartmann, P., & Apaolaza, V. (2006). Green value added. *Marketing Intelligence, 24*(7), 673–680. https://www.factmr.com/report/functional-foods-market.

International Organization for Standardization (ISO) (2006). ISO 14040:2006 Environmental Management-Life cycle assessment: Principles and framework. (2nd Edi.). https://www.cscses.com/uploads/2016328/20160328110518251825.pdf.

International Organization for Standardization (ISO). (2015). ISO 9001:2015. Quality Management Systems-Requirements. International Organization for Standardization (ISO). (2015). *ISO 9001:2015 quality management systems—Requirements*. ISO.

Innis, S. M. (2007). Dietary (n-3) fatty acids and brain development. *Journal of Nutrition, 137*(4), 855–859. https://doi.org/10.1093/jn/137.4.855, http://jn.nutrition.org/cgi/reprint/137/4/855.

Jacobsen, C. (2015). Some strategies for the stabilization of long chain n-3 PUFA enriched foods: A review. *European Journal of Lipid Science and Technology, 117*(1), 1853–1866.

Koletzko, B., Lien, E., Agostoni, C., Bohles, H., Compoy, C., Cetin, I., Decsi, T., Dudebhausen, J. W., Dupont, C., Forsyth, S., Hoesli, I., Holzgreve, W., Lapillonne, A., Putet, G., Secher, N. J., Symonds, M., Szajewska, H., Willatts, P., & Uauy, R. (2008). The roles of long-chain polyunsaturated fatty acids in pregnancy, lactation and infancy: Review of current knowledge and consensus recommendations. *Journal of Perinatal Medicine, 36*(1), 5–14.

Kassem, J. M., Abdulqahar, E. W., Zaky, A. A., Boulkrane, M. S., Darwish, A., Farouk, A., Ozcelik, B., Magouz, O., Liu, X., & El-Messery, T. M. (2025). Micro and nano capsulation of omega-3 fatty acids: Functional applications and future perspective in food systems. *Food Safety and Health, 00*, 1–19.

Koletzko, B., Carlson, S. E., & van Goudoever, J. B. (2020). DHA and arachidonic acid in infant nutrition. *Annals of Nutrition and Metabolism, 76*(3), 137–147.

Kotler, P., & Keller, K. L. (2016). *Marketing management* (15th ed.). Pearson.

Kunj, P., Sahu, S., Singh, G., & Arya, S. K. (2025). A review on algal oils as a sustainable source of essential omega-3 fatty acids. *Bioresource Technology Reports, 30*, 102154. https://doi.org/10.1016/j.biteb.2025.102154.

Lee, W. M., Ryu, S. I., Lim, M. N., Han, J. W., Bae, J. B., Kim, T. H., Kwak, K. P., Kim, B. J., Kim, S. G., Kim, J. L., Moon, S. W., Park, J. H., Ryu, S. H., Lee, D. W., Lee, S. B., Lee, J. J., Lee, D. Y., Kim, K. W., & Jhoo, J. H. (2026). Association between omega-3 supplement use and cognitive function in korean older adults: An 8-year longitudinal cohort study. *Journal of Nutrition, Health and Aging, 30*(1). https://doi.org/10.1016/j.jnha.2025.100739, https://www.sciencedirect.com/journal/the-journal-of-nutrition-health-and-aging.

Mitmesser, S. H., & Jensen, C. (2007). Roles of long-chain polyunsaturated fatty acids in the term infant: Developmental benefits. *Neonatal Network, 26*(4), 229–234.

McClements, D. J. (2015). Encapsulation, protection and delivery of omega-3 fatty acids using emulsion-based delivery systems. *Annual reviews of Food Science and Technology, 6*, 299–327.

Mozaffarian, D., & Wu, J. H. Y. (2011). Omega-3 fatty acids and cardiovascular disease: Effects on risk factors, molecular pathways, and clinical events. *Journal of the American College of Cardiology, 58*(20), 2047–2067. https://doi.org/10.1016/j.jacc.2011.06.063, www.elsevier.com/locate/jacc.

Napoli, J., Dickinson, S. J., Beverland, M. B., & Farrelly, F. (2014). Measuring consumer-based brand authenticity. *Journal of Business Research, 67*(6), 1090–1098. https://doi.org/10.1016/j.jbusres.2013.06.001.

Nicholas, P. D., Petrie, J., & Singh, S. (2014). Long-chain omega-3 oils: An update on sustainable sources. *Nutrients, 6*(9) 3727-2733.

Patted, P. G., Masareddy, R. S., Patil, A. S., Kanabargi, R. R., & Bhat, C. T. (2024). Omega-3 fatty acids: A comprehensive scientific review of their sources, functions and health benefits. *Future Journal of Pharmaceutical Sciences, 10*(1). https://doi.org/10.1186/s43094-024-00667-5.

Philpott, J. D., Witard, O. C., & Galloway, S. D. R. (2019). Applications of omega-3 polyunsaturated fatty acid supplementation for sport performance. *Research in Sports Medicine, 27*(2), 219–237. https://doi.org/10.1080/15438627.2018.1550401, http://www.tandf.co.uk/journals/titles/15438627.html.

Poore, J., & Nemecek, T. (2018). Reducing food's environmental impacts through producers and consumers. *Science (New York, N.Y.), 360*(6392), 987–992. https://doi.org/10.1126/science.aaq0216.

Powell, W. W., Koput, K. W., & Smith-Doerr, L. (1996). Interorganizational collaboration and the locus of innovation: Networks of learning in biotechnology. *Administrative Science Quarterly, 41*(1), 116–145. https://doi.org/10.2307/2393988, http://asq.sagepub.com/content/current.

Qin, J., Kurt, E., LBassi, T., Sa, L., & Xie, D. (2023). Biotechnological production of omega-3 fatty acids: Current status and future perspectives. *Frontiers in Microbiology, 14*. https://doi.org/10.3389/fmicb.2023.1280296, https://www.frontiersin.org/journals/microbiology#.

Ryckebosch, E., Bruneel, C., Termote-Verhalle, R., Goiris, K., Muylaert, K., & Foubert, I. (2014). Nutritional evaluation of microalgae oils rich in omega-3 long chain polyunsaturated fatty acids as an alternative for fish oil. *Food Chemistry, 160*, 393–400. https://doi.org/10.1016/j.foodchem.2014.03.087, www.elsevier.com/locate/foodchem.

Schneider, A. T., Machado, R. L. S., Dutra, D. A., Machado, E. F., Dias, R. R., Depra, M. C., Zepka, L. Q., & Lopes, E. J. (2025). Microalgae biotechnology and its role in sustainable and health food design. *Frontiers Bioengineering Biotechnology, 13*, 1716473.

Shahidi, F., & Ambigaipalan, P. (2018a). Omega-3 polyunsaturated fatty acids and health benefits. *Annual Review of Food Science and technology, 3*, 1–7.

Shahidi, F., & Ambigaipalan, P. (2018b). Omega-3 polyunsaturated fatty acids and their health benefits. *Annual Review of Food Science and Technology, 9*(1), 345–381. https://doi.org/10.1146/annurev-food-111317-095850.

Shahidi, F., & Zhong, Y. (2010). Lipid oxidation and improving the oxidative stability. *Chemical Society Reviews, 39*(11), 4067. https://doi.org/10.1039/b922183m.

Simopoulos, A. P. (2016). An increase in the omega-6/omega-3 fatty acid ration increases chronic disease risk. *Nutrients, 8*(3), 128.

Swanson, D., Block, R., & Mousa, S. A. (2012). Omega-3 fatty acids EPA and DHA: Health benefits throughout life. *Advances in Nutrition, 3*(1), 1–7. https://doi.org/10.3945/an.111.000893, http://advances.nutrition.org/content/3/1/1.full.pdf.

Tocher, D. R., Betancor, M. B., Sprague, M., Olsen, R. E., & Napier, J. A. (2019). Omega-3 long chain polyunsaturated fatty acids, EPA and DHA: Bridging the gap between supply and demand. *Nutrients, 11*(1), 89.

Teece, D. J. (1986). Profiting from technological innovation: Implications for integration, collaboration, licensing and public policy. *Research Policy, 15*(6), 285–305. https://doi.org/10.1016/0048-7333(86)90027-2.

Thielecke, F., & Blannin, A. (2020). Omega-3 fatty acids for sport performance—Are they equally beneficial for athletes and amateurs? A narrative review. *Nutrients, 12*(12), 3712. https://doi.org/10.3390/nu12123712.

U.S. Food and Drug Administration (FDA) (2022). Guidance for industry: Nutrition and supplement labelling regulations. U.S. Department of Health and Human Services.

Ventola, C. L. (2014). Social media and health care professionals: Benefits, risks and best practices. *Pharmacy and Therapeutics, 39*(7), 491–520.

Venugopal, V. (2008). *Marine products for healthcare: Functional and bioactive nutraceutical compounds from the ocean marine products for healthcare: Functional and bioactive nutraceutical compounds from the ocean*. India: CRC Press, 1–527. https://www.taylorfrancis.com/books/e/9781420052640.

Verbeke, W., Sioen, I., Pieniak, Z., Van Camp, J., & De Henauw, S. (2007). Consumer perception of omega-3 health benefits. *Public Health Nutrition, 8*(4), 422–429.

World Intellectual Property Organization (WIPO). (2020). WIPO intellectual property handbook: Policy, law and use. WIPO publishing.

Waraho, T., McClements, D. J., & Decker, E. A. (2011). Mechanisms of lipid oxidation in food dispersions. *Critical Reviews in Food Science and Nutrition, 51*(10), 915–930.

Yurko-Mauro, K., McCarthy, D., Rom, D., Nelson, E. B., Ryan, A. B., Salem, N., Stedman, M., & Investigators., M. I. D. A. S. (2010). Beneficial effects of docosahexaenoic acid on cognition in age-related cognitive decline. *Alzheimer's Dementia, 6*(6), 456–464.

Chapter 32

Polyunsaturated fatty acids-based nutraceuticals and supplements: case studies and application in modern healthcare

Laureana de Quevedo Barcelos, Sergio Roberto Mortari, Elisângela Colpo, and Carina Rodrigues Boeck
Universidade Franciscana, Programa de Pós-graduação em Nanociências, Mestrado em Ciências da Saúde e da Vida, Santa Maria, Rio Grande do Sul, Brazil

32.1 Introduction

Characterized as concentrated sources of nutrients, supplements are designed to augment daily intake with minerals, vitamins, and fatty acids to perform nutritional or physiological roles safely (Brasil, 2018; FDA, 2024). They are offered in capsules, tablets, gummies, powders, liquids, or food-like formats, as long as they do not replace meals or are classified as conventional foods (Fernandes et al., 2025).

The formulations aim to meet the specific needs of populations with nutritional deficiencies, higher metabolic demand, or clinical conditions that compromise nutrient intake or absorption (Cederholm et al., 2017; EFSA, 2024). When indicated, supplementation can help maintain health, prevent illness, and provide therapeutic support, and should be individualized and supervised to ensure safety and effectiveness (FDA, 2024; WHO, 2023).

Nutraceuticals are bioactive compounds naturally present in foods that exert specific physiological effects when isolated and administered in therapeutic doses (Puri et al., 2022). Eicosapentaenoic acid (EPA) and docosahexaenoic acid (DHA), omega-3 (n-3) polyunsaturated fatty acids (PUFAs), are obtained from fish, microalgae, or seeds, and act as targeted recommended nutraceuticals by international guidelines (Lichtenstein et al., 2021; Skulas-Ray et al., 2019; WHO, 2020, 2023; United States, 2020), and different supplementation forms (Swanson et al., 2012; Venugopalan et al., 2021) (Fig. 32.1). While dietary supplements replace isolated nutrients in cases of deficiency, nutraceuticals maintain their dietary origin and act on specific mechanisms associated with health and/or disease (Jain et al., 2022; Puri et al., 2022).

Marine organisms (fatty fish and microalgae), plant-based derivatives (seeds and vegetable oils), and processed options (fortified foods and emulsions) constitute the main dietary and technological pathways to increase the availability of these PUFAs.

In clinical contexts, essential fatty acids act as antiinflammatory, cardioprotective, neuroprotective, and immunomodulatory (Aglago et al., 2020; Patted et al., 2024). Humans cannot endogenously synthesize fatty acids with unsaturation preceding the ninth carbon. The low hepatic conversion of α-linolenic acid (ALA) to n-3 EPA, and subsequently to DHA, occurs at rates of less than 15%. Thus ALA and n-6 linoleic acid (LA) require consumption through diet or supplementation (Patted et al., 2024; Shahidi & Ambigaipalan, 2018; Soares et al., 2023). This strategy constitutes an effective strategy to ensure bioavailability, especially in populations with higher metabolic demand or nutritional risk (Krupa et al., 2024; Patted et al., 2024; Punia et al., 2019; Shahidi & Ambigaipalan, 2018; WHO, 2020).

32.1.1 Safety of dietary supplements

Food safety is ensured by regulatory agencies through standards to guarantee the safety, efficacy, and labeling of supplements, covering authorized ingredients, usage limits, permitted health claims, and presentation forms to the

Omega-3 and Omega-6 Polyunsaturated Fatty Acids in Food Systems. DOI: https://doi.org/10.1016/B978-0-443-43810-3.00033-6

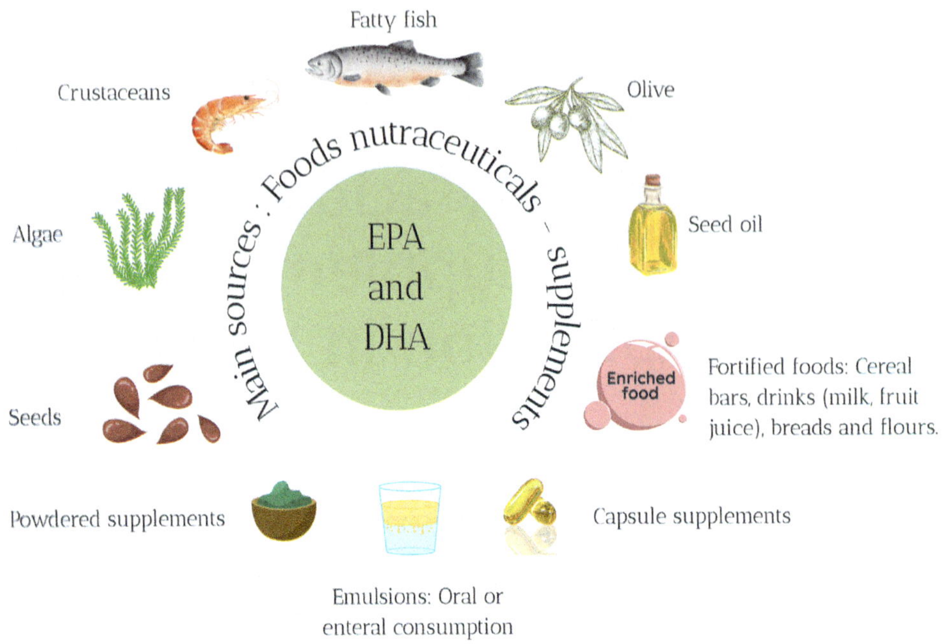

FIGURE 32.1 Natural sources of n-3 and their initial forms as supplements and nutraceuticals.

consumer. The Dietary Supplement Health and Education Act (1994) (United States [EUA], 1994) from the United States establishes that the manufacturers are responsible for ensuring the safety and label accuracy of the supplements. The Food and Drug Administration (FDA) monitors the market and intervenes when it identifies health risks, applying sanctions when necessary (FDA, 2023; WHO, 2023, United States, 2020). Directive 2002/46/EC harmonizes standards among member countries in the European Union. In addition, the Codex Alimentarius, developed by the Food and Agriculture Organization (FAO) and the World Health Organization (WHO, 2023), guides countries in legislation development (European Union EU, 2002; FAO/WHO Codex Alimentarius Commission, 2005). In Brazil, the National Health Surveillance Agency (Agência Nacional de Vigilância Sanitária [ANVISA], 2024) operates under a preventive regulatory framework that mandates the notification of all supplements, enhancing transparency for the consumer (Agência Nacional de Vigilância Sanitária [ANVISA], 2024). The health benefits of EPA and DHA are well-established. However, the doses recommended by regulatory agencies differ according to the target audience profile. Tables 32.1 and 32.2 present the main international guidelines, highlighting convergences and differences between them.

32.2 Applications: polyunsaturated fatty acids in modern healthcare

Fig. 32.2 presents the main approaches of this study based on the application areas of PUFAs, as determined by international recommendations and scientific evidence. Potential applications of PUFAs (n-3 and n-6) in different clinical contexts, main raw materials, and presentation forms.

32.2.1 Polyunsaturated fatty acids in inflammation and immune modulation

The Western transition of dietary patterns has reduced the diversity of whole foods, microbial exposure, and n-3 intake, while increasing the n-6/n-3 ratio (Mariamenatu & Abdu, 2021). This scenario compromises immune maturation and favors dysfunctional immune responses and chronic low-grade inflammation, which are typical of metabolic, immunological, and aging disorders (Tingö et al., 2022). The interaction between inflammation and oxidative stress generates a feedback loop that amplifies tissue damage. This occurs because inflammatory signals stimulate reactive oxygen species (ROS) production, which in turn promotes inflammation through the activation of the nuclear factor kappa B pathway and the NLRP3 inflammasome (Biswas, 2016; Stiefvatter et al., 2022). The result is the sustained secretion of pro-inflammatory cytokines, specifically tumor necrosis factor alpha (TNF-α), which amplifies ROS production and perpetuates the mechanisms of pain, inflammation, and oxidative damage (Zhang & An, 2007).

TABLE 32.1 Overview of international recommendations for adults and older adults of eicosapentaenoic acid (EPA): docosahexaenoic acid (DHA).

Organization/year	Adults	Older adults
FAO, 2010	Polyunsaturated fatty acids (PUFA) total: 6–11% E. Minimum of 2.5% E linoleic acid (LA) and 0.5% E alpha-linolenic acid (ALA). EPA + DHA: ≥ 250 mg/day.	250 mg/day of EPA + DHA
[1]EFSA (2010)	EPA + DHA: 250 mg/day. **ALA:** 0.5–1.2 g/day. **LA:** 4.5–10 g/day.	
[2]DGE Günther et al. (2015)	PUFA total: 7–10% E	
[3]NNR Blomhoff et al. (2023)	PUFA total: 5–10 E%; n-3: ≥1 E%; ALA: ≥0.5 E%; PUFA + MUFA (cis): ≥⅔ of the total fatty acids	Same recommendations as for adults. Emphasis is placed on the quality of fat and maintaining PUFA and MUFA intake with aging.
[4]ESC/EAS, 2011–2021 Reiner et al. (2011); Visseren et al. (2021)	2011: n-6 PUFAs <10 E%.	
	2021: to reduce triglycerides in hypertriglyceridemia >135 mg/dL = 4 g/day of EPA + DHA	
[5]AFSSA (2010)	To prevent the cardiovascular risk: 500 mg/day of EPA + DHA	
[6]FSA (2007)	Average intake of 6.5 E%.	
[7]Scientific Advisory Committee on Nutrition SACN, sory Committee on Nutrition SACN (2008)		
[8]DGAC, 2020–2025 United States (2020)	≥8 oz (227 g) of seafood/week, equivalent to approximately 325–500 mg/day of EPA + DHA	
Academy of Nutrition and Dietetics, Vannice and Rasmussen (2014)	Rising intake of n-3 PUFA	
[9]Institute of Medicine – atualmente National Academy of Medicine OIM, 2005 (2005)	5–10 E% and 0.6–1.2 E%	

[1] European Food Safety Authority.
[2] Deutsche Gesellschaft für Ernährung.
[3] Nordic Nutrition Recommendations.
[4] European Society of Cardiology/European Atherosclerosis Society.
[5] Agence Française de Sécurité Sanitaire des Aliments.
[6] Food Standards Agency.
[7] Scientific Advisory Committee on Nutrition.
[8] Dietary Guidelines Advisory Committee.
[9] Institute of Medicine. % E: total energy percentage. MUFA: monounsaturated fatty acids; AI: Adequate Intake, E%: percentage of dietary energy. Parte superior do formulário.

The inflammatory modulation promoted by n-3 has been extensively studied in the cardiovascular health of older adults, including when combined with antioxidant micronutrients such as vitamin D and probiotics (Table 32.3). Although combined supplementation did not reduce interleukin-6 (IL-6), intake of n-3 increases in IL-10 and valeric acid were observed, as well as reductions in arachidonic acid (AA), homocysteine, and high-sensitivity C-reactive protein, and improvement in the n-6/n-3 ratio (Birudaraju et al., 2020; Costenbader et al., 2019; Martucci et al., 2020; Tingö et al., 2022). *Phaeodactylum tricornutum* microalga, a source of EPA, fucoxanthin, and β-glucans, showed promising effects in healthy older adult individuals, decreasing IL-6 and the n-6/n-3 ratio even with a reduced EPA intake (63mg/day). The antiinflammatory effect suggests a synergistic action between its bioactive compounds, indicating potential as a functional supplement in controlling inflammation associated with aging (Stiefvatter et al., 2022).

TABLE 32.2 Overview of international recommendations for children and pregnant women regarding eicosapentaenoic acid (EPA): docosahexaenoic acid (DHA).

Organization/year	Children	Pregnant women
FAO (2010)	≥2.5 E% linoleic acid (LA) and 0.5 E% alpha-linolenic acid (ALA); total polyunsaturated fatty acid (PUFA) 2.5–3.5 E%.	≥ 300 mg/day of EPA + DHA, ≥200 mg/day of DHA.
EFSA (2010)	7–24 months of age: 100 mg/day of DHA. 2–18 years: 250 mg/day of EPA + DHA.	≥250 mg/day of EPA + DHA, + 100–200 mg/day of DHA during pregnancy and lactation.
NNR, Blomhoff et al. (2023)	>6 months: total PUFA: 5–10 E% n-3: ≥1 E% ALA: ≥0.5 E% PUFA + monounsaturated fatty acid (cis): ≥⅔ of total fatty acids	Total PUFA: 5–10 E% n-3: ≥1 E% DHA: 200 mg/day (within the E% of n-3) Essential fatty acids (n-6 + n-3): ≥5 E% (including ≥0.5 E % de ALA)
ESC/EAS, 2011–21, Reiner et al. (2011); Visseren et al. (2021)	It is recommended to adjust the proportional EPA + DHA requirements according to age and body weight.	
AFSSA (2010)	0 to 6 months: LA 2.7% of E%. ALA: 0.45% of E%. DHA: 0.32% fatty acids for milk, contributing with 70 kcal and 3.4 g of total lipids per 100 mL reconstituted. 6 months–3 years: 70 mg DHA. 3–9 years: 250 mg EPA + DHA. 10–18 years: 500 mg/day EPA + DHA.	500 mg/day of n-3
DAGC, 2020–2025 United States (2020)	1–2 servings/week of seafood (28–85 g); approximately 50–150 mg/day of EPA + DHA	8–12 oz (227–340 g) / week of seafood; approx. 250 mg/day of EPA + DHA, with emphasis on ≥200 mg/day of DHA.
National Academy of Medicine OIM, 2005 (2005)	≥1 year old, and adults: 5–10 E% (n-6) and 0.6–1.2 E% (ALA)	

Parenteral lipid emulsions are efficient strategies in premature infants for providing energy not derived from carbohydrates and reducing osmotic overload. Formulations previously only based on soybean oil have evolved to incorporate olive and fish oil blends along with medium-chain fatty acids, which are capable of modulating inflammation and rebalancing the lipid profile (Stiefvatter et al., 2022). These effects include reducing pro-inflammatory cytokines, such as IL-6 and IL-8, as well as improving the n-6/n-3 ratio (Skouroliakou et al., 2016). Enteral supplementation with EPA, DHA, and α-tocopherol intensified antiinflammatory responses even in the face of the clinical conditions of prematurity, increasing oleic acid and reducing the n-6/n-3 ratio and IL-6, suggesting synergy between lipids and antioxidants (Papandreou et al., 2020).

32.2.2 Cardiometabolic diseases

Body composition, lipid metabolism, and cardiometabolic parameters are significantly impacted by the levels of n-3 and n-6, with effects that vary according to the ingestion timing and the isomer administered, determined by bioavailability (Konishi et al., 2021; Mądry et al., 2016; Shahidi & Ambigaipalan, 2018). EPA and DHA supplementation showed incorporation into phospholipids of subcutaneous adipose tissue, increased highly unsaturated triglycerides, and contributed to remodeling the body lipid profile (Stanley et al., 2017). Although the most consistent effects are observed with marine n-3, n-6 compounds such as conjugated LA have also been associated with improved anthropometric markers (Mądry et al., 2016).

Microalgae-based DHA formulations may influence cardiometabolic prevention with responses modulated by genetic factors. Although maternal supplementation does not directly modify the offspring's metabolic syndrome score, variants in desaturase genes significantly influence the cardiometabolic trajectory (Wimalasena et al., 2024). Furthermore, genetic polymorphisms modulate the clinical response to n-3, as demonstrated in individuals with the GG genotype with lower endogenous conversion of PUFAs, who showed greater benefit in ventricular remodeling and inflammatory markers after

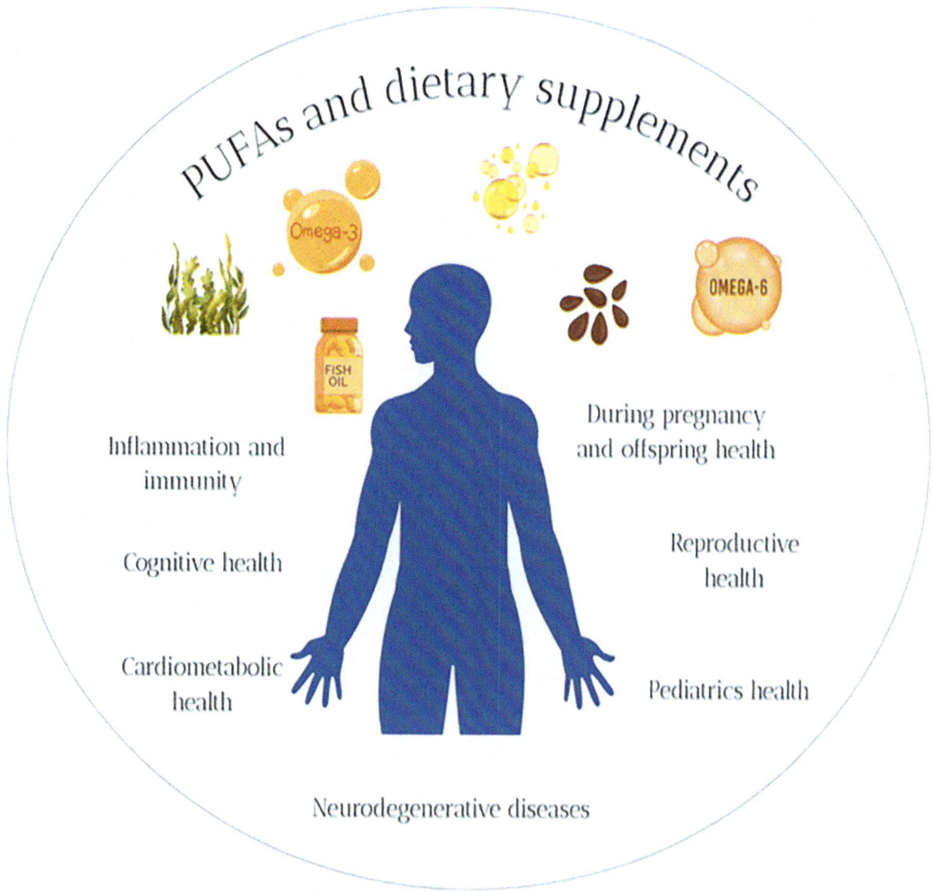

FIGURE 32.2 Polyunsaturated fatty acids (PUFAs) and applications in human health.

acute myocardial infarction (Kwong et al., 2019). These findings reinforce the potential of genotyping to guide personalized therapeutic strategies with n-3 (Table 32.4).

In nonalcoholic fatty liver disease (NAFLD), PUFAs reduce lipid accumulation and liver inflammation through suppressing lipogenesis and stimulating fatty acid oxidation via modulation of transcription factors (Nogueira et al., 2016; Walker, West, et al., 2015). Formulations with concentrated EPA and DHA, including microalgae oils, promote an improved lipid profile, greater systemic antioxidant capacity, and reductions in triglycerides, total cholesterol, glycemia, blood pressure, and inflammatory markers (García-Maldonado et al., 2023; Peña-de-la-Sancha et al., 2023; Zeng et al., 2017). Supplements rich in PUFAs, specifically shark liver lipids, also elevate plasma n-3 and increase high-density lipoprotein, while lowering CRP in healthy individuals. Ethyl ester forms of EPA and DHA boost erythrocyte n-3, reduce the n-6/n-3 ratio, and mitigate liver fat in adults with NAFLD, while in children and adolescents, there is an improvement of AST, GGT, and adiponectin. Taken together, the evidence indicates that PUFAs robustly modulate hepatic and lipid parameters associated with NAFLD in different age groups (Janczyk et al., 2015; Nogueira et al., 2016; Tobin et al., 2018; Walker, Decker, et al., 2015; Zakrzewska et al., 2021).

Ethyl ester formulations of EPA (including icosapent ethyl) and EPA + DHA (approved by the FDA) are indicated to reduce serum triglycerides by ≥30%, with doses of 2–4 g/day. The hypolipidemic action results from decreased hepatic triglyceride synthesis, increased mitochondrial and peroxisomal β-oxidation, and improved clearance of triglyceride-rich lipoproteins (Krupa et al., 2024; Skulas-Ray et al., 2019). EPA supplementation in the reduction of cardiovascular events with EPA intervention trial study reduced major cardiovascular events by 25%, being attributed to lipid reduction and the antiinflammatory and pro-resolution action mediated by EPA-derived oxylipins (Bhatt et al., 2019).

Long-term n-3 formulations (3.36 g/day for 30 months) have consistently reduced serum triglycerides among individuals diagnosed with coronary artery disease (Amangurbanova et al., 2024). Ethyl esters of EPA + DHA in young

TABLE 32.3 Characteristics of studies that evaluated inflammation and immune modulation.

Author and year	Target	Formulation
Tingö et al. (2022)	Both sexes; n = 76; average age: 71 years	2 capsules/day: 1100 mg of fish oil (300 mg eicosapentaenoic acid (EPA) + 220 mg docosahexaenoic acid (DHA) + 200 IU vitamin D) + 2 capsules of multistrain probiotic; 8 weeks
Stiefvatter et al. (2022)	Both sexes; n = 19; mean age: 67.7 ± 6.5 years	*Phaeodactylum tricornutum* lyophilized + β-1,3-glucan supernatant; EPA: 288 mg, DHA: 5 mg; total n-3: 295 mg; 2 weeks
Birudaraju et al. (2020)	Both sexes; n = 70; mean age: 48.8 ± 16 years	2 softgel capsules, twice a day: 500 mg of curcumin + 450 mg of EPA + 100 mg of DHA + 125 mg of other n-3, 3 mg of astaxanthin, 9.5 mg of GLA, 12.5 mg of mixed tocotrienols, 6.25 mg of hydroxytyrosol, 1000 IU of vitamin D, and 12.75 mg of K; 4 weeks
Costenbader et al. (2019)	Both sexes; n = 1561; mean age: 55 years	Vitamin D capsules 2000 IU/day and 460 mg EPA + 380 mg DHA; 1 year
Martucci et al. (2020)	Both sexes; n = 48; mean age: 70 ± 4.5 years	Fortified milk: EPA + DHA 350 mg; vitamin D 7.5 μg, E 12.5 mg, C 47.5 mg, B6 1.6 μg, B12 2.5 μg, B9 200 μg; if 55 μg; Zn 10 mg; 12 weeks
Skouroliakou et al. (2016)	Premature neonates: n = 51; gestational age 29 weeks; intervention initiated on the 1st–2nd day of life	IVFE, 1–3 g/kg/day, until oral intake reaches ≥80% of total energy: 30% MCT, 30% soy, 25% olive, 15% fish (≈ 0.6 g EPA + 0.4 g DHA/100 mL; α-tocoferol 200 mg/L)
Papandreou et al. (2020)	Premature neonates: n = 92; gestational age <32 weeks	IVFE, 1–3 g/kg/day for 15 days: ≈ 50 mg of EPA + DHA per g of lipid (≈ 0.6 g EPA + 0.4 g DHA/100 mL)

GLA: gamma-linolenic acid; MCT: medium-chain triglycerides; Se: selenium; Zn: zinc; IQR: interquartile range.

men exposed to acute inflammatory stimuli increased the biosynthesis of antiinflammatory oxylipins and incorporation of these PUFAs into triglyceride-rich lipoproteins, promoting vascular protection (Walker et al., 2023).

32.2.3 Polyunsaturated fatty acids and brain health

32.2.3.1 Children and adolescents

Perinatal supplementation with fish oil has shown promising effects on infant neurodevelopment, especially in domains such as attention and communication (Table 32.5). Benefits were observed in pregnant women supplemented in the second half of pregnancy, particularly with DHA, regarding specific aspects of neurocognitive development, including communicative skills and sustained attention in the first months of life, reinforcing the potential of PUFAs in early neurological programming (Ostadrahimi et al., 2018).

EPA and DHA supplementation, alone or combined with GLA (n-6), has been investigated as a complementary intervention in managing attention deficit hyperactivity disorder (ADHD) (Barragán et al., 2017; Carucci et al., 2022; Checa-Ros et al., 2019; Johnson et al., 2017; Roach et al., 2021; Tammam et al., 2016). The concurrent administration of EPA and DHA as an adjunct to methylphenidate resulted in improved behavioral symptoms, attention, and core symptoms of ADHD, and greater tolerability and safety compared to the exclusive use of the drug, suggesting an additional effect of fatty acids (Barragán et al., 2017; Checa-Ros et al., 2019).

These benefits extend to children with subclinical symptoms of inattention, demonstrating progress in reading and learning skills (Johnson et al., 2017). Correcting nutritional deficits through synergistically combining bioactive compounds with antioxidant and neuromodulatory action can reduce behavioral symptoms and promote sociability in adolescents with low baseline levels of these nutrients, as well as improve scores for atypical behavior (Tammam et al., 2016). Furthermore, new technologies, such as microencapsulation, have been adopted to increase the stability and absorption of PUFAs, especially in preschoolers, aiming to improve behavioral self-regulation, which is fundamental to neurocognitive development (Roach et al., 2021).

TABLE 32.4 Polyunsaturated fatty acids formulations applied to cardiometabolic health.

Author and year	Target	Formulation
Wimalasena et al. (2024)	Both sexes; n = 203, average age: babies up to 11 years; mothers supplemented during pregnancy	Prenatal supplementation with 400 mg/day of docosahexaenoic acid (DHA) from algae until delivery
Kwong et al. (2019)	Both sexes, n = 312; average age 59 ± 10 years	4 g/day eicosapentaenoic acid (EPA) + DHA; 6 months
Konishi et al. (2021)	Both sexes, n = 20; average age: 20 to 60 years.	Enriched sausages; fish oil (DHA 1010 mg + EPA 240 mg/day); 8 weeks
Stanley et al. (2017)	n-3 group: n = 20; both sexes; average age: 52 ± 13 years	Fish oil capsules equivalent to 4 servings of fish/week (13.08 g n-3; 6 g EPA + 7.08 g DHA); 6 or 12 months
Nogueira et al. (2016)	Both sexes, total n = 50; average age: 52.5 ± 7.2 years	3 capsules/day (0.945 g/day; 64% ALA, 16% EPA, 21% DHA from flaxseed and fish oils); 6 months
Walker, West, et al. (2015)	Both sexes; n = 163; average age: 20 to 80 years	6 fish oil capsules equivalent to 1 serving of fish/day (1.5 g EPA + 1.77 g DHA); 12 months
Zeng et al. (2017)	Both sexes; n-3: n = 211; average age: 43.0 ± 9.7 years	2 capsules/day (182 mg EPA + 129 mg DHA/capsule) = 0.62 g/day + 1000 ppm tocopherol; 3 months
Peña-de-la-Sancha et al. (2023)	Both sexes; n = 18, mean age: 42.5 ± 6.2 years	Capsules: 1.68 g n-3; 920 mg EPA + 760 mg DHA/ day; for 5 weeks
García-Maldonado et al. (2023)	Both sexes; n = 116, mean age: 42 years	Capsules with DHA 250 mg/day; 5 weeks
Zakrzewska et al. (2021)	Female; n = 27; mean age: 23.9 ± 2.0 years	Shark liver oil; 1500 mg/day; 6 weeks and 12 weeks
Tobin et al. (2018)	Both sexes; n = 176; mean age: ~55 years	Capsules; 1.38 g EPA + 1.14 g DHA/day; 24 weeks
Janczyk et al. (2015)	Both sexes; n = 64; mean age: 13 years	450 mg DHA + 1300 mg EPA/day; 6 months
Bhatt et al. (2019)	Both sexes; n = 8179; mean age: 64 ± 9 years	Icosapent ethyl (EPA-ethyl esters) 4 g/day: 2 g twice daily; 4.9 years
Amangurbanova et al. (2024)	Both sexes; n = 139; mean age: 62 ± 8 years	EPA + DHA capsules 3.36 g/day; 30 months
Walker et al. (2023)	Men; n = 17, mean age: 23 years	Ethyl esters; 4 capsules/day; 460 mg EPA + 380 mg DHA; 8 to 12 weeks

ppm: parts per million.

32.2.3.2 Older adults

PUFAs, especially EPA and DHA, reduce inflammatory processes and promote neuroplasticity, stimulating synapses and modulating cell signaling (Fotuhi et al., 2009; Kermack et al., 2020; Peña-de-la-Sancha et al., 2023; Simonetto et al., 2019; Stavrinou et al., 2020). The combination with vitamins can enhance these effects, especially in individuals with cognitive impairment (Stavrinou et al., 2020; Sueyasu et al., 2023). Antioxidants help neutralize reactive oxygen and nitrogen species, whose excessive production increases with aging and impairs neurological and muscular functions (Pasini et al., 2022; Stavrinou et al., 2020).

The concurrent intake of n-3 with antioxidants in older adults followed for a long period was linked to better cognitive performance (Assmann et al., 2018). In addition, the inclusion of carotenoids, such as lutein and zeaxanthin, in a formulation with PUFAs in older adults with complaints of amnesia did not benefit the overall sample, but improved the performance of participants with cognitive decline, suggesting the influence of baseline status (Sueyasu et al., 2023). Moreover, high doses of n-3/n-6 with antioxidant vitamins improved cognition, functionality, and quality of life among older adults with mild cognitive impairment (Stavrinou et al., 2020). In turn, the combination of ALA-rich oil with citrus fruit antioxidants in healthy older adults resulted in greater cognitive gains and increased DHA than the use of the oil alone, possibly due to its greater antioxidant potential (Hashimoto et al., 2022).

TABLE 32.5 Polyunsaturated fatty acids (PUFA) formulations are applied for cognitive health in children and older adults.

Author and year	Sample	Formulation
Ostadrahimi et al. (2018)	Pregnant women: n = 150; average age: 18–35 years; 20th week to 30 days postpartum; babies evaluated at 4–6 months	Fish oil: 1 capsule/day: eicosapentaenoic acid (EPA) 180 mg and docosahexaenoic acid (DHA) 120 mg; up to 1 month postpartum
Barragán et al. (2017)	Both sexes; n = 90; average age 6–12 years	6 capsules/day: EPA 558 mg + DHA 174 mg + gamma-linolenic acid (GLA) 60 mg; 12 months
Checa-Ros et al. (2019)	Both sexes; n = 40; average age: 7–15 years	Methylphenidate 1 mg/kg/day + EPA 70 mg/day and DHA 250 mg/day; 1 month
Johnson et al. (2017)	Both sexes; n = 154; average age: 9–10 years	3 capsules 2x/day; EPA 558 mg + DHA 174 mg + GLA 60 mg; 3 months
Tammam et al. (2016)	Both sexes; n = 196; average age 13 to 16 years	EPA 165 mg and DHA 116 mg/day + multivitamin supplement; 12 weeks
Stavrinou et al. (2020)	Both sexes; n = 36; average age 78.8 ± 7.3 years	20 mL/day (EPA 810 mg + DHA 4140 mg; GLA 1800 mg + linolenic acid 3150 mg; vitamin A 0.6 mg; vitamin E 22 mg; γ-tocopherol 760 mg); 6 months
Sueyasu et al. (2023)	Both sexes; n = 71; average age: 65.0 ± 0.8 years	LCPUFA + LZ: 6 capsules/day (ARA 120 mg + DHA 300 mg + EPA 100 mg + lutein 10 mg + zeaxanthin 2 mg); 24 weeks
Assmann et al. (2018)	Both sexes; n = 3362; average age 65.5 ± 4.6 years	Dietary intake of monounsaturated fatty acid and n-3/n-6 PUFA (24-h recalls) + antioxidant supplement (vitamin C, vitamin E, β-carotene, selenium, and zinc); 7 years
Hashimoto et al. (2022)	Both sexes; n = 44; Average age: 68.7 ± 1.2 years.	Capsules: PO 1.47 mL/day (ALA 0.88 g) or PO + ponkan powder 1.12 g (nobiletin 2.91 mg); 12 months

LCPUFA: Long-chain polyunsaturated fatty acids; ARA: Arachidonic acid; LZ: Lutein + zeaxanthin; PO: Ponkan oil.

32.2.4 Pregnancy, lactation, and neonatal development

Maternal supplementation with PUFAs, especially DHA, has shown relevant benefits in reducing early preterm births (Table 32.6). An amount of 600 mg/day of DHA reduced preterm births in the KUDOS study, while DHA supplementation in the DOMInO trial generated an average savings of AUS$92 per pregnancy and a potential annual savings of AUS$ 15 to 51 million, attributed to the lower incidence of prematurity and neonatal complications (Ahmed et al., 2015; Shireman et al., 2016). Prenatal supplementation with high DHA doses increases maternal and fetal serum levels, promotes maintenance of pregnancy, and reduces prematurity risk, especially in black women with low baseline DHA levels or in conditions such as type 1 diabetes, which also require EPA (Defranco et al., 2024; Ivanisevic et al., 2021).

At the inflammatory level, maternal n-3 supplementation modulates eicosanoid pathways and pro-resolution mediators, increasing precursors such as 18-HEPE and 17-HDHA in cord blood and indicating activation of resolvin pathways at birth (Valentine et al., 2021). In addition, n-3 use in overweight or obese pregnant women reduced inflammatory activation in adipose tissue and placenta, with lower expression of Toll-4 (TLR4) and cytokines such as IL-6, IL-8, and TNF-α (Haghiac et al., 2015; See et al., 2016). Gestational DHA was associated with immunological profiles consistent with a higher probability of term pregnancy, including a smaller drop in advanced glycation end products (sRAGE) at delivery and greater increases in IL-6 throughout pregnancy (Haghiac et al., 2015). Furthermore, PUFA supplementation combined with vitamin D and olive oil increased embryonic quality markers in couples undergoing in vitro fertilization when performed in the preconception period, suggesting an influence on fetal development programming (Kermack et al., 2020).

The inclusion of fish oil in parenteral emulsions in premature infants increased EPA and reduced serum AA; although DHA increased slightly, there was beneficial modulation of the long-chain polyunsaturated fatty acids profile (Nilsson et al., 2019). These effects may vary according to polymorphisms in desaturase genes, such as FADS2, which modulate

TABLE 32.6 Polyunsaturated fatty acids formulations applied to perinatal and neonatal development.

Author and year	Sample	Formulation
Shireman et al. (2016)	Pregnant women and their babies, n = 197; mean maternal age 25.4 years	3 capsules/day of DHA (600 mg/day); 26 weeks
Ahmed et al. (2015)	Pregnant women <20 weeks; n = 2342	Fish oil capsules; 800 mg docosahexaenoic acid (DHA)/day until delivery
Defranco et al. (2024)	Pregnant women: n = 1032	Prenatal DHA 200 mg/day or 1000 mg/day; prenatal follow-up until delivery
Ivanisevic et al. (2021)	Pregnant women: n = 84; mean age: 30.5 ± 5.2; NB, n = 84	Fish oil capsules 2x/day; eicosapentaenoic acid (EPA) 120 mg + DHA 616 mg; 11th–12th week until delivery
Valentine et al. (2021)	Female: n = 1100; 12 to 20 weeks of gestation	1000 mg/day of DHA: capsules of (800 mg DHA) + 200 mg from prenatal; 12th week until delivery
Kermack et al. (2020)	Couples: n = 111; female, mean age: 33.4 ± 4.2 years; male: 36.0 ± 5.5 years	Daily enriched drink (EPA 800 mg + DHA 1200 mg + vitamin D 10 μg) + olive oil; Preconception intervention (6 weeks)
See et al. (2017)	Pregnant women: n = 83; mean age: 31 years; and children followed up at birth and at 12 years of age	4 capsules/day (1 g each; total 3.7 g n-3; DHA 2.07 g; EPA 1.03 g); from the 20th week until delivery
Haghiac et al. (2015)	Pregnant women, n = 25; mean age: 27 ± 5 years	4 capsules/day, 2x/day: 2 g EPA + DHA; 10th–16th week until term
Nilsson et al. (2019)	Postpartum women: n = 78; NB premature infants, both sexes: n = 90; GA<28 weeks	Parenteral nutrition: mixed emulsion (30% soy, 30% medium-chain triglycerides, 25% olive, 15% fish; EPA 5.64 mg/mL; DHA 5.65 mg/mL; arachidonic acid 0.54 mg/mL)
Gonzalez-Casanova et al. (2021)	Pregnant women: n = 1094; 26 ± 5 years; children: n = 622 at 5 years (female 46% and male 54%)	Algae oil capsules: 400 mg/day of DHA; from the 18th–22nd week until delivery
Gonzalez-Casanova et al. (2015)	Pregnant women: n = 654; infants: n = 654	Algae oil capsules: 400 mg/day of DHA; from the 18th–22nd week until delivery
Angoa et al. (2022)	Lactating mothers: n = 461; very premature infants: n = 528 (<29 weeks GA; female n = 253; male n = 275; mean GA 26.5 ± 1.6 weeks; birth weight 895 ± 240 g; 16 NICUs)	DHA 1.2 g/day (start <72 h postpartum until 36 weeks postmenstrual)
Sheppard et al. (2017)	Premature infants; N = 27; both sexes; mean age: 30 months corrected	Oral supplementation: EPA 338 mg, DHA 225 mg, gamma-linolenic acid (GLA) 83 mg, linoleic acid 280 mg, algae oil: 306 mg; 3 months
Boone et al. (2020)	Premature infants (<35 weeks without GA), both sexes; mean age 10–16 months (corrected)	DHA 200 mg + arachidonic acid 200 mg/day; 180 days
Keim et al. (2022)	Both sexes; N = 70; mean age: 2 to 6 years	n-3/n-6 liquid (25/50/100 mg/kg/day; EPA 112 mg/mL; DHA 67 mg/mL; GLA 32 mg/mL); 90 days

NB: newborn; GA: gestational age.

the impacts of DHA on fetal growth and neurodevelopment (Gonzalez Casanova et al., 2021; Gonzalez-Casanova et al., 2015). DHA in breast milk during lactation influenced the development of premature infants, with distinct responses according to the baby's sex, reinforcing the importance of individualized strategies (Angoa et al., 2022).

Neuroimaging and biomarker evidence indicate that adequate DHA levels are associated with healthier brain development and better organization of more structured early cognitive functions (McNamara et al., 2010; Weiser et al., 2016). Deficiency of n-3, especially DHA, can compromise neuronal formation, impairing synaptogenesis, plasticity, and signaling between neurons (Ostadrahimi et al., 2018). Thus, an adequate supply of EPA and DHA during

TABLE 32.7 Polyunsaturated fatty acids (PUFA) formulations applied to gastrointestinal health and carcinogenesis.

Author and year	Target	Formulation
Djuric et al. (2017)	N = 38; both sexes; mean age 47 ± 14 years	1 g/capsule (eicosapentaenoic acid [EPA] 530 mg + docosahexaenoic acid [DHA] 150 mg + 101 mg other n-3); dose adjusted for EPA:AA ratio ≈ 1:2; (2 test + 10 intervention); mean 5.5 ± 2.0 g/day (2–10 g/day); 12 weeks
Wilson et al. (2018)	Both sexes; n = 47; mean age: 47 ± 12 years	Dose adjusted by serum EPA:AA ratio; mean dose 5.5 ± 2.0 g/day of EPA + DHA; 12 weeks
Murff et al. (2022)	Both sexes, n = 141	n-3 capsules: 2.5 g/day; 6 months
Watson et al. (2018)	Both sexes, n = 22; mean age: 50 ± 9 years	4 g/day EPA + DHA in soft capsules or drink; 8 weeks
Dolatkhah et al. (2017)	Both sexes, n = 34; mean age: 56 ± 11 years	PUFAs: 3600 mg/day, orally with chemotherapy (cisplatin, 3 cycles)
Schmidt et al. (2020)	Both sexes; n = 41; mean age: 63 ± 8 years	Fish oil: 10 capsules/day (4.8 g) or 400 mL/day nutritional drink (4.0 g); 4 weeks

critical developmental windows supports brain maturation and reduces the risk of deficits in vulnerable populations (Clandinin et al., 1980; Johnson et al., 2017; McNamara et al., 2010).

Clinical trials show positive effects of PUFA supplementation in premature infants at risk of autism spectrum disorder (ASD), including improvements in behavioral symptoms, language (use of gestures), internalizing behaviors, and adaptive skills (Boone et al., 2020; Briggs-Gowan, 2004; Keim et al., 2018; Sheppard et al., 2017). As ASD involves neuroinflammatory processes, modulation by PUFAs appears relevant: elevated erythrocyte levels of EPA and DHA, and a decline in IL-2 suggest an immunoinflammatory effect associated with behavioral improvement. This mechanism may involve competition of EPA and DHA with AA in eicosanoid membranes and pathways, reducing AA-derived pro-inflammatory mediators and favoring the synthesis of resolvins and neuroprotective protectins (Keim et al., 2022).

32.2.5 Effect of polyunsaturated fatty acids on gastrointestinal health and carcinogenesis

Next, n-3 PUFAs supplemented in gastrointestinal cancer influence inflammatory markers, proliferation, apoptosis, and gut microbiota composition (Table 32.7). Clinical trials have demonstrated that n-3s reduce prostaglandin E2 (PGE2) production involved in colonic inflammation and carcinogenesis, with reductions of up to 50% when supplementation is personalized by the EPA: AA ratio (Djuric et al., 2017; White et al., 2019). Interpersonal variability is significant: factors such as BMI, genomic expression, and modifications in the fatty acid profile in the colon explain about 48% of the difference in PGE2 reduction (Wilson et al., 2018). The effects of n-3 mainly result from modulating the inflammatory microenvironment and eicosanoids, accompanied by an increase in *Bifidobacterium*, *Roseburia*, and *Lactobacillus* genera, which are producers of short-chain fatty acids (Murff et al., 2022; Watson et al., 2018).

PUFAs increase the expression of caspases-3 and 9 in patients with gastrointestinal cancer, indicating an adjuvant effect to chemotherapy (Dolatkhah et al., 2017). The supplement presentation form also influences adherence: fish oil capsules tend to be better accepted than nutritional drinks, although flavor, texture, and the number of capsules impact acceptability without significantly altering the lipid profile or nutritional status (Schmidt et al., 2020). Moreover, n-3 generally exerts a multifaceted influence on gastrointestinal wellness and oncology prevention. They function by modulating eicosanoids (PGE2, PGE-M), cell proliferation and apoptosis, as well as promoting beneficial changes in the intestinal microbiome and lipid metabolism (Djuric et al., 2017; Dolatkhah et al., 2017; Watson et al., 2018; White et al., 2019).

32.3 Future perspectives: technological advances in polyunsaturated fatty acid delivery in micro and nanostructures

The evolution of formulations stems from limitations of conventional supplements marked by oxidative instability, which compromises chemical integrity, bioavailability, and the correspondence between labeled and actual EPA and DHA levels

(Albert et al., 2015; Bannenberg et al., 2017; Jackowski et al., 2015; Pasini et al., 2022). Market assessments reveal variability between brands and the occasional presence of contaminants, reinforcing the need for analytical standardization and good manufacturing practices (Jairoun et al., 2020; Opperman et al., 2011). External factors such as light, heat, oxygen, and metals accelerate oxidation and generate off-flavors, even with antioxidants and stability monitoring (Khoshnoudi-Nia et al., 2022).

Industrial processes such as refining and re-esterification alter molecular profiles, and although measures such as barrier packaging, antioxidants, and monitoring PV, p-AV, and TOTOX are employed, they often do not prevent advanced degradation (Pasini et al., 2022; Yenipazar & Şahin-Yeşilçubuk, 2023). In addition, physiological conditions such as aging, intestinal inflammation, and dysbiosis also reduce efficiency (Dmytriv et al., 2024; Sanders et al., 2023). In this context, supplementation with PUFAs not only requires attention to the dose but also to the stability and delivery method, opening space for micro and nanometric systems capable of protecting bioactive compounds and improving their absorption (Altemimi et al., 2024; Heller et al., 2019; Lane et al., 2014; McClements & Öztürk, 2021).

Microencapsulation transforms oil into powder through microparticles of 1–200 μm encapsulated by proteins or polysaccharides (such as gum arabic, chitosan, maltodextrin, gum arabic, or soy and whey protein isolates). The technique increases oxidative stability, reduces off-flavors, and facilitates incorporation into foods and supplements (Charles et al., 2021; Ozkan et al., 2019). Molecular inclusion with β-cyclodextrin in enriched yogurt preserved sensory acceptance and reduced peroxides (Ghorbanzade et al., 2022). Hollow solid lipid systems increased the stability and bioaccessibility of enriched milk (40.4% vs 27.4% of free oil) (Yang et al., 2024). Microencapsulation of flaxseed oil in baked goods reduced oxidizing volatiles and thermal contaminants such as acrylamide (Gökmen et al., 2011).

Self-emulsifying systems act as preconcentrates for capsules and targeted oral use, which form micro or nanodroplets in situ upon contact with the aqueous gastrointestinal environment, and reduce dependence on food intake (Maki et al., 2018). Crossover trials in healthy adults demonstrated increases in the area under the curve and with the maximum concentration (C_{max}) of EPA/DHA versus nonemulsified ethyl ester, including in the fasting state (Hayashida et al., 2022; Maki et al., 2018). Independent studies confirmed greater blood incorporation after a single dose and with repeated use, with an increase in n-3 for up to 12 weeks (Maki et al., 2018; Qin et al., 2017).

Nanoscale platforms optimize lipid digestion and intestinal micellization. Lyotropic liquid-crystalline phase nanoparticles have increased the systemic exposure of EPA and DHA compared to conventional capsules, with good tolerability (Kang et al., 2023). In the nutritional field, PEGylation of DHA reorganizes nanoparticle structure, favoring the transition to the lamellar phase, generating more stable vesicles with prolonged circulation (Bor et al., 2022). Nano systems such as nanoemulsions, lipid nanoparticles, nanoliposomes, nanocapsules, and Pickering emulsions operate between 20–200 nm, accelerating digestion and micellization (Venugopalan et al., 2021; Vieira et al., 2020). Nanoemulsions stand out for increasing the interfacial area for lipases and enabling coencapsulation of antioxidants, delaying autoxidation (McClements & Öztürk, 2021; Shehzad et al., 2021). Liposomes and protein–polysaccharide complexes show good stability in juices and yogurts, while Pickering emulsions offer interfaces that are more resistant to pro-oxidants, reducing the need for surfactants (Altemimi et al., 2024; Ghorbanzade et al., 2022; Ilyasoglu & El, 2014).

32.4 Discussion

PUFAs play a cross-cutting role in human health throughout life, acting on fertility, pregnancy, neurocognitive development, memory, cardiometabolic health, and inflammation (Amangurbanova et al., 2024; Ivanisevic et al., 2021; Papandreou et al., 2020; Stavrinou et al., 2020; Zeng et al., 2017). However, conventional products face limitations such as oxidation, quality variability, and irregular bioavailability, which shift the emphasis from "how much to supplement" to "how to preserve and deliver" the active ingredient, integrating dose, formulation, and analytical control (Khoshnoudi-Nia et al., 2022). International recommendations indicate approximately 250 mg/day of EPA + DHA for adults, plus 100–200 mg/day of DHA in pregnant and lactating women; targets in pediatrics range from 100 mg/day of DHA in infants to 250 mg/day of EPA + DHA in childhood (AFSSA, 2010; EFSA, 2010; FAO, 2010). In turn, 2–4 g/day are used in therapeutic applications, especially for triglyceride reduction, while interventions aimed at cognitive and gestational support range from 0.5 to 2 g/day (Amangurbanova et al., 2024; Carucci et al., 2022; Gonzalez-Casanova et al., 2015; Kwong et al., 2019; Reiner et al., 2011; Tobin et al., 2018). Efficacy depends on the bioavailability of the formulations and on genetic and metabolic factors, reinforcing personalized approaches, especially in the perinatal period, where immunometabolic modulation influences future health. PUFAs consistently reduce inflammatory and lipid markers and support in managing cardiovascular, metabolic, and ADHD diseases, with safety and a low incidence of adverse effects (Barragán et al., 2017; Checa-Ros et al., 2019; Johnson et al., 2017).

Microencapsulation aims to improve stability and acceptability, while nanostructured systems improve digestion and systemic exposure (Charles et al., 2021; Ozkan et al., 2019). The choice between micro and nanostructures should consider clinical objectives, matrix, tolerability, and regulatory requirements. The sustainable adoption of these technologies requires integrating biopharmaceutical performance, nutritional safety, and regulatory compliance, prioritizing appropriate excipients, minimal emulsifiers, and efficient processing routes to ensure consistent benefits (Altemimi et al., 2024; Ghorbanzade et al., 2022; Kang et al., 2023).

32.5 Conclusion

The evolution of nutritional and technological approaches applied to PUFAs reveals a rapidly expanding field where materials science, biopharmaceuticals, and nutrition converge to enhance efficacy and safety. Incorporating micro and nanotechnology tools enables overcoming traditional limitations and unlocking the potential of n-3 through highly targeted and individualized strategies. In this context, the future of EPA and DHA-based nutraceuticals will depend on the ability to integrate innovation, sustainability, and regulatory rigor, creating formulations that broaden clinical impact and strengthen the role of PUFAs as pillars of modern human health.

References

AFSSA. (2010). *OPINION of the French Food Safety Agency on the update of French population reference intakes (ANCs) for fatty acids 1. Review of the request.*

Aglago, E. K., Huybrechts, I., Murphy, N., Casagrande, C., Nicolas, G., Pischon, T., Fedirko, V., Severi, G., Boutron-Ruault, M.-C., Fournier, A., Katzke, V., Kühn, T., Olsen, A., Tjønneland, A., Dahm, C. C., Overvad, K., Lasheras, C., Agudo, A., Sánchez, M.-J., ... Gunter, M. J. (2020). Consumption of fish and long-chain n-3 polyunsaturated fatty acids is associated with reduced risk of colorectal cancer in a large European cohort. *Clinical Gastroenterology and Hepatology, 18*(3), 654–666.e6. https://doi.org/10.1016/j.cgh.2019.06.031.

Agência Nacional de Vigilância Sanitária (ANVISA). (2024). *Constituintes autorizados para uso em suplementos alimentares.* https://www.Gov.Br/Anvisa/Pt-Br/Assuntos/Alimentos/Paineis-de-Consulta-de-Alimentos/Constituintes-Autorizados-Para-Uso-Em-Suplementos-Alimentares.

Ahmed, S., Makrides, M., Sim, N., McPhee, A., Quinlivan, J., Gibson, R., & Umberger, W. (2015). Analysis of hospital cost outcome of DHA-rich fish-oil supplementation in pregnancy: Evidence from a randomized controlled trial. *Prostaglandins, Leukotrienes, and Essential Fatty Acids, 102–103*, 5–11. https://doi.org/10.1016/j.plefa.2015.08.002.

Albert, B. B., Derraik, J. G. B., Cameron-Smith, D., Hofman, P. L., Tumanov, S., Villas-Boas, S. G., Garg, M. L., & Cutfield, W. S. (2015). Fish oil supplements in New Zealand are highly oxidised and do not meet label content of n-3 PUFA. *Scientific Reports, 5*(1), 7928. https://doi.org/10.1038/srep07928.

Altemimi, A. B., Farag, H. A. M., Salih, T. H., Awlqadr, F. H., Al-Manhel, A. J. A., Vieira, I. R. S., & Conte-Junior, C. A. (2024). Application of nanoparticles in human nutrition: A review. *Nutrients, 16*(5), 636. https://doi.org/10.3390/nu16050636.

Amangurbanova, M., Daher, R., Asbeutah, A. A., Vemuri, B., Mirza, H., Waseem, S., Malik, A., & Welty, F. K. (2024). Higher epicardial adipose tissue volume is associated with higher coronary fatty plaque volume and is regulated by waist circumference but not EPA+DHA supplementation. *Journal of Clinical Lipidology, 18*(5), e773–e786. https://doi.org/10.1016/j.jacl.2024.06.006.

Angoa, G., Pronovost, E., Ndiaye, A. B. K. T., Lavoie, P. M., Lemyre, B., Mohamed, I., Simonyan, D., Qureshi, M., Afifi, J., Yusuf, K., Sériès, T., Guillot, M., Piedboeuf, B., Fraser, W. D., Nuyt, A.-M., Mâsse, B., Lacaze-Masmonteil, T., & Marc, I. (2022). Effect of maternal docosahexaenoic acid supplementation on very preterm infant growth: Secondary outcome of a randomized clinical trial. *Neonatology, 119*(3), 377–385. https://doi.org/10.1159/000524147.

Assmann, K. E., Adjibade, M., Hercberg, S., Galan, P., & Kesse-Guyot, E. (2018). Unsaturated fatty acid intakes during midlife are positively associated with later cognitive function in older adults with modulating effects of antioxidant supplementation. *The Journal of Nutrition, 148*(12), 1938–1945. https://doi.org/10.1093/jn/nxy206.

Bannenberg, G., Mallon, C., Edwards, H., Yeadon, D., Yan, K., Johnson, H., & Ismail, A. (2017). Omega-3 long-chain polyunsaturated fatty acid content and oxidation state of fish oil supplements in New Zealand. *Scientific Reports, 7*(1), 1488. https://doi.org/10.1038/s41598-017-01470-4.

Barragán, E., Breuer, D., & Döpfner, M. (2017). Efficacy and safety of omega-3/6 fatty acids, methylphenidate, and a combined treatment in children with ADHD. *Journal of Attention Disorders, 21*(5), 433–441. https://doi.org/10.1177/1087054713518239.

Bhatt, D. L., Steg, P. G., Miller, M., Brinton, E. A., Jacobson, T. A., Ketchum, S. B., Doyle, R. T., Juliano, R. A., Jiao, L., Granowitz, C., Tardif, J.-C., & Ballantyne, C. M. (2019). Cardiovascular risk reduction with icosapent ethyl for hypertriglyceridemia. *New England Journal of Medicine, 380*(1), 11–22. https://doi.org/10.1056/NEJMoa1812792.

Birudaraju, D., Cherukuri, L., Kinninger, A., Chaganti, B. T., Shaikh, K., Hamal, S., Flores, F., Roy, S. K., & Budoff, M. J. (2020). A combined effect of cavacurcumin, eicosapentaenoic acid (omega-3s), astaxanthin and gamma –linoleic acid (omega-6) (CEAG) in healthy volunteers- a randomized, double-blind, placebo-controlled study. *Clinical Nutrition ESPEN, 35*, 174–179. https://doi.org/10.1016/j.clnesp.2019.09.011.

Biswas, S. K. (2016). Does the Interdependence between oxidative stress and inflammation explain the antioxidant paradox? *Oxidative Medicine and Cellular Longevity, 2016*(1). https://doi.org/10.1155/2016/5698931.

Blomhoff, R., Andersen, R., Arnesen, E. K., Christensen, J. J., Eneroth, H., Erkkola, M., Gudanaviciene, I., Halldórsson, Þl., Høyer-Lund, A., Lemming, E. W., Meltzer, H. M., Pitsi, T., Siksna, I., Þórsdóttir, I., & Trolle, E. (2023). *Nordic nutrition recommendations 2023*. Nordic Council of Ministers. https://doi.org/10.6027/nord2023-003.

Boone, K. M., Parrott, A., Rausch, J., Yeates, K. O., Klebanoff, M. A., Norris Turner, A., & Keim, S. A. (2020). Fatty acid supplementation and socioemotional outcomes: Secondary analysis of a randomized trial. *Pediatrics, 146*(4). https://doi.org/10.1542/peds.2020-0284.

Bor, G., Lin, J.-H., Lin, K.-Y., Chen, H.-C., Prajnamitra, R. P., Salentinig, S., Hsieh, P. C. H., Moghimi, S. M., & Yaghmur, A. (2022). PEGylation of phosphatidylglycerol/docosahexaenoic acid hexosomes with <scp>d</scp> -α-tocopheryl succinate poly(ethylene glycol) 2000 induces morphological transformation into vesicles with prolonged circulation times. *ACS Applied Materials & Interfaces, 14*(43), 48449–48463. https://doi.org/10.1021/acsami.2c14375.

Brasil. (2018). *Resolução da Diretoria Colegiada – RDC no 243, de 26 de julho de 2018.*

Briggs-Gowan, M. J. (2004). The brief infant-toddler social and emotional assessment: Screening for social-emotional problems and delays in competence. *Journal of Pediatric Psychology, 29*(2), 143–155. https://doi.org/10.1093/jpepsy/jsh017.

Carucci, S., Romaniello, R., Demuru, G., Curatolo, P., Grelloni, C., Masi, G., Liboni, F., Mereu, A., Contu, P., Lamberti, M., Gagliano, A., & Zuddas, A. (2022). Omega-3/6 supplementation for mild to moderate inattentive ADHD: A randomised, double-blind, placebo-controlled efficacy study in Italian children. *European Archives of Psychiatry and Clinical Neuroscience, 272*(8), 1453–1467. https://doi.org/10.1007/s00406-022-01428-2.

Cederholm, T., Barazzoni, R., Austin, P., Ballmer, P., Biolo, G., Bischoff, S. C., Compher, C., Correia, I., Higashiguchi, T., Holst, M., Jensen, G. L., Malone, A., Muscaritoli, M., Nyulasi, I., Pirlich, M., Rothenberg, E., Schindler, K., Schneider, S. M., de van der Schueren, M. A. E., ... Singer, P. (2017). ESPEN guidelines on definitions and terminology of clinical nutrition. *Clinical Nutrition, 36*(1), 49–64. https://doi.org/10.1016/j.clnu.2016.09.004.

Charles, A. L., Abdillah, A. A., Saraswati, Y. R., Sridhar, K., Balderamos, C., Masithah, E. D., & Alamsjah, M. A. (2021). Characterization of freeze-dried microencapsulation tuna fish oil with arrowroot starch and maltodextrin. *Food Hydrocolloids, 112*, 106281. https://doi.org/10.1016/j.foodhyd.2020.106281.

Checa-Ros, A., Haro-García, A., Seiquer, I., Molina-Carballo, A., Uberos-Fernández, J., & Muñoz-Hoyos, A. (2019). Early monitoring of fatty acid profile in children with attention deficit and/or hyperactivity disorder under treatment with omega-3 polyunsaturated fatty acids. *Minerva Pediatrica, 71*(4). https://doi.org/10.23736/S0026-4946.18.04975-7.

Clandinin, M. T., Chappell, J. E., Leong, S., Heim, T., Swyer, P. R., & Chance, G. W. (1980). Intrauterine fatty acid accretion rates in human brain: Implications for fatty acid requirements. *Early Human Development, 4*(2), 121–129. https://doi.org/10.1016/0378-3782(80)90015-8.

Costenbader, K. H., MacFarlane, L. A., Lee, I.-M., Buring, J. E., Mora, S., Bubes, V., Kotler, G., Camargo, C. A., Manson, J. E., & Cook, N. R. (2019). Effects of one year of vitamin D and marine omega-3 fatty acid supplementation on biomarkers of systemic inflammation in older US adults. *Clinical Chemistry, 65*(12), 1508–1521. https://doi.org/10.1373/clinchem.2019.306902.

Defranco, E. A., Valentine, C. J., Carlson, S. E., Sands, S. A., & Gajewski, B. J. (2024). Racial disparity in efficacy of docosahexaenoic acid supplementation for prevention of preterm birth: Secondary analysis from a randomized, double-blind trial. *American Journal of Obstetrics & Gynecology MFM, 6*(5), 101358. https://doi.org/10.1016/j.ajogmf.2024.101358.

Djuric, Z., Turgeon, D. K., Sen, A., Ren, J., Herman, K., Ramaswamy, D., Zhao, L., Ruffin, M. T., Normolle, D. P., Smith, W. L., & Brenner, D. E. (2017). The anti-inflammatory effect of personalized omega-3 fatty acid dosing for reducing prostaglandin E2 in the colonic mucosa is attenuated in obesity. *Cancer Prevention Research, 10*(12), 729–737. https://doi.org/10.1158/1940-6207.CAPR-17-0091.

Dmytriv, T. R., Storey, K. B., & Lushchak, V. I. (2024). Intestinal barrier permeability: The influence of gut microbiota, nutrition, and exercise. *Frontiers in Physiology, 15*. https://doi.org/10.3389/fphys.2024.1380713.

Dolatkhah, H., Movahedian, A., Somi, M.-H., Aghaei, M., Samadi, N., Mirza-Aghazade, A., & Esfahani, A. (2017). Effect of PUFAs oral administration on the amount of apoptotic caspases enzymes in gastric cancer patients undergoing chemotherapy. *Anti-cancer Agents in Medicinal Chemistry, 17*(1), 93–101. https://doi.org/10.2174/1871520616666160520113503.

EFSA. (2024). *Dietary reference values*. https://www.Efsa.Europa.Eu/En/Topics/Topic/Dietary-Reference-Values?Utm_source=chatgpt.Com.

EFSA. (2010). Scientific opinion on dietary reference values for fats, including saturated fatty acids, polyunsaturated fatty acids, monounsaturated fatty acids, trans fatty acids, and cholesterol. *EFSA Journal, 8*(3). https://doi.org/10.2903/j.efsa.2010.1461.

European Union (EU). (2002). Directive 2002/46/EC of the European Parliament and of the Council of 10 June 2002 on food supplements. https://Eur-Lex.Europa.Eu/Eli/Dir/2002/46/Oj/Eng.

FAO. (2010). *Food and Agriculture Organization of the United Nations Fats and fatty acids in human nutrition.*

FAO/WHO Codex Alimentarius Commission. (2005). *Guidelines for vitamin and mineral food supplements (CXG 55-2005)*. https://www.Fao.Org/Fao-Who-Codexalimentarius/Codex-Texts/Guidelines/En/. https://www.fao.org/fao-who-codexalimentarius/codex-texts/guidelines/en/.

FDA. (2023). Notifications for structure/function and related claims in dietary supplement labeling. https://www.fda.gov/food/information-industry-dietary-supplements/notifications-structurefunction-and-related-claims-dietary-supplement-labeling.

FDA. (2024). Dietary Supplements. https://www.fda.gov/food/dietary-supplements.

Fernandes, P., Castilho, D. N., Castro, A. K. F. D., Schreiner, L. L., Almeida, R., Ana, S., Marquim, C., Araújo, F. D., Araújo, C., V., Cary, R., Reis, D., Homero, M., Machado, F., Gomes, L. B., Oliveira, C., Menezes, E., … Tozetto, B. (2025). *Elaboração Gerência-Geral de Alimentos (GGALI).*

Fotuhi, M., Mohassel, P., & Yaffe, K. (2009). Fish consumption, long-chain omega-3 fatty acids and risk of cognitive decline or Alzheimer disease: A complex association. *Nature Reviews Neurology, 5*(3), 140–152. https://doi.org/10.1038/ncpneuro1044.

FSA (2007). FSA nutrient and food based guidelines for UK institutions. www.food.gov.uk.

García-Maldonado, E., Alcorta, A., Zapatera, B., & Vaquero, M. P. (2023). Changes in fatty acid levels after consumption of a novel docosahexaenoic supplement from algae: A crossover randomized controlled trial in omnivorous, lacto-ovo vegetarians and vegans. *European Journal of Nutrition, 62*(4), 1691–1705. https://doi.org/10.1007/s00394-022-03050-3.

Ghorbanzade, T., Akhavan-Mahdavi, S., Kharazmi, M. S., Ibrahim, S. A., & Jafari, S. M. (2022). Loading of fish oil into β-cyclodextrin nanocomplexes for the production of a functional yogurt. *Food Chemistry: X, 15*, 100406. https://doi.org/10.1016/j.fochx.2022.100406.

Gonzalez Casanova, I., Schoen, M., Tandon, S., Stein, A. D., Barraza Villarreal, A., DiGirolamo, A. M., Demmelmair, H., Ramirez Silva, I., Feregrino, R. G., Rzehak, P., Stevenson, I., Standl, M., Schnaas, L., Romieu, I., Koletzko, B., & Ramakrishnan, U. (2021). Maternal FADS2 single nucleotide polymorphism modified the impact of prenatal docosahexaenoic acid (DHA) supplementation on child neurodevelopment at 5 years: Follow-up of a randomized clinical trial. *Clinical Nutrition, 40*(10), 5339–5345. https://doi.org/10.1016/j.clnu.2021.08.026.

Gonzalez-Casanova, I., Stein, A. D., Hao, W., Garcia-Feregrino, R., Barraza-Villarreal, A., Romieu, I., Rivera, J. A., Martorell, R., & Ramakrishnan, U. (2015). Prenatal supplementation with docosahexaenoic acid has no effect on growth through 60 months of age. *The Journal of Nutrition, 145*(6), 1330–1334. https://doi.org/10.3945/jn.114.203570.

Gökmen, V., Mogol, B. A., Lumaga, R. B., Fogliano, V., Kaplun, Z., & Shimoni, E. (2011). Development of functional bread containing nanoencapsulated omega-3 fatty acids. *Journal of Food Engineering, 105*(4), 585–591. https://doi.org/10.1016/j.jfoodeng.2011.03.021.

Günther, W., Bechthold, A., Boeing, H., Dinter, J., Ellinger, S., Hauner, H., Kroke, A., Leschik-Bonnet, E., Linseisen, J., Lorkowksi, S., Schulze, M., & Stehle, P. (2015). Evidenzbasierte Leitlinie Fettzufuhr und Prävention ausgewählter ernährungsmitbedingter Krankheiten Autoren bzw. *Mitglieder der Leitlinienkommission der DGE*.

Haghiac, M., Yang, X., Presley, L., Smith, S., Dettelback, S., Minium, J., Belury, M. A., Catalano, P. M., & Hauguel-de Mouzon, S. (2015). Dietary omega-3 fatty acid supplementation reduces inflammation in obese pregnant women: A randomized double-blind controlled clinical trial. *PLoS ONE, 10*(9), e0137309. https://doi.org/10.1371/journal.pone.0137309.

Hashimoto, M., Matsuzaki, K., Maruyama, K., Hossain, S., Sumiyoshi, E., Wakatsuki, H., Kato, S., Ohno, M., Tanabe, Y., Kuroda, Y., Yamaguchi, S., Kajima, K., Ohizumi, Y., & Shido, O. (2022). *Perilla* seed oil in combination with nobiletin-rich ponkan powder enhances cognitive function in healthy elderly Japanese individuals: A possible supplement for brain health in the elderly. *Food & Function, 13*(5), 2768–2781. https://doi.org/10.1039/D1FO03508H.

Hayashida, M., Ishii, Y., Adachi, T., Imai, R., Uotsu, N., & Yui, K. (2022). Pharmacokinetics of a single intake of a self-emulsifying drug delivery system containing the triglyceride form of DHA: A randomized, double-blinded, crossover study. *Current Developments in Nutrition, 6*(9), nzac122. https://doi.org/10.1093/cdn/nzac122.

Heller, M., Gemming, L., Tung, C., & Grant, R. (2019). Oxidation of fish oil supplements in Australia. *International Journal of Food Sciences and Nutrition, 70*(5), 540–550. https://doi.org/10.1080/09637486.2018.1542666.

Ilyasoglu, H., & El, S. N. (2014). Nanoencapsulation of EPA/DHA with sodium caseinate–gum arabic complex and its usage in the enrichment of fruit juice. *LWT - Food Science and Technology, 56*(2), 461–468. https://doi.org/10.1016/j.lwt.2013.12.002.

Institute of Medicine – atualmente National Academy of Medicine (OIM, 2005). (2005). *Dietary reference intakes for energy, carbohydrate, fiber, fat, fatty acids, cholesterol, protein, and amino acids*. National Academies Press. https://doi.org/10.17226/10490.

Ivanisevic, M., Horvaticek, M., Delmis, K., & Delmis, J. (2021). Supplementation of EPA and DHA in pregnant women with type 1 diabetes mellitus. *Annals of Medicine, 53*(1), 848–859. https://doi.org/10.1080/07853890.2021.1936151.

Jackowski, S. A., Alvi, A. Z., Mirajkar, A., Imani, Z., Gamalevych, Y., Shaikh, N. A., & Jackowski, G. (2015). Oxidation levels of North American over-the-counter *n* -3 (omega-3) supplements and the influence of supplement formulation and delivery form on evaluating oxidative safety. *Journal of Nutritional Science, 4*, e30. https://doi.org/10.1017/jns.2015.21.

Jain, N., Radhakrishnan, A., & Kuppusamy, G. (2022). Review on nutraceuticals: Phase transition from preventive to protective care. *Journal of Complementary and Integrative Medicine, 19*(3), 553–570. https://doi.org/10.1515/jcim-2022-0026.

Jairoun, A. A., Shahwan, M., & Zyoud, S. H. (2020). Fish oil supplements, oxidative status, and compliance behaviour: Regulatory challenges and opportunities. *PLoS ONE, 15*(12), e0244688. https://doi.org/10.1371/journal.pone.0244688.

Janczyk, W., Lebensztejn, D., Wierzbicka-Rucińska, A., Mazur, A., Neuhoff-Murawska, J., Matusik, P., & Socha, P. (2015). Omega-3 fatty acids therapy in children with nonalcoholic fatty liver disease: A randomized controlled trial. *The Journal of Pediatrics, 166*(6), 1358–1363.e3. https://doi.org/10.1016/j.jpeds.2015.01.056.

Johnson, M., Fransson, G., Östlund, S., Areskoug, B., & Gillberg, C. (2017). Omega 3/6 fatty acids for reading in children: A randomized, double-blind, placebo-controlled trial in 9-year-old mainstream schoolchildren in Sweden. *Journal of Child Psychology and Psychiatry, 58*(1), 83–93. https://doi.org/10.1111/jcpp.12614.

Kang, K.-M., Jeon, S.-W., De, A., Hong, T.-S., & Park, Y.-J. (2023). A randomized, open-label, single-dose, crossover study of the comparative bioavailability of EPA and DHA in a novel liquid crystalline nanoparticle-based formulation of ω-3 acid ethyl ester versus omacor® soft capsule among healthy adults. *International Journal of Molecular Sciences, 24*(24), 17201. https://doi.org/10.3390/ijms242417201.

Keim, S. A., Boone, K. M., Klebanoff, M. A., Turner, A. N., Rausch, J., Nelin, M. A., Rogers, L. K., Yeates, K. O., Nelin, L., & Sheppard, K. W. (2018). Effect of docosahexaenoic acid supplementation vs placebo on developmental outcomes of toddlers born preterm. *JAMA Pediatrics, 172*(12), 1126. https://doi.org/10.1001/jamapediatrics.2018.3082.

Keim, S. A., Jude, A., Smith, K., Khan, A. Q., Coury, D. L., Rausch, J., Udaipuria, S., Norris, M., Bartram, L. R., Narayanan, A. R., & Rogers, L. K. (2022). Randomized controlled trial of omega-3 and -6 fatty acid supplementation to reduce inflammatory markers in children with autism spectrum disorder. *Journal of Autism and Developmental Disorders, 52*(12), 5342–5355. https://doi.org/10.1007/s10803-021-05396-9.

Kermack, A. J., Lowen, P., Wellstead, S. J., Fisk, H. L., Montag, M., Cheong, Y., Osmond, C., Houghton, F. D., Calder, P. C., & Macklon, N. S. (2020). Effect of a 6-week "Mediterranean" dietary intervention on in vitro human embryo development: The Preconception Dietary Supplements in Assisted Reproduction double-blinded randomized controlled trial. *Fertility and Sterility, 113*(2), 260–269. https://doi.org/10.1016/j.fertnstert.2019.09.041.

Khoshnoudi-Nia, S., Forghani, Z., & Jafari, S. M. (2022). A systematic review and meta-analysis of fish oil encapsulation within different micro/nanocarriers. *Critical Reviews in Food Science and Nutrition, 62*(8), 2061–2082. https://doi.org/10.1080/10408398.2020.1848793.

Konishi, T., Takahashi, Y., Shiina, Y., Oike, H., & Oishi, K. (2021). Time-of-day effects of consumption of fish oil–enriched sausages on serum lipid parameters and fatty acid composition in normolipidemic adults: A randomized, double-blind, placebo-controlled, and parallel-group pilot study. *Nutrition, 90*, 111247. https://doi.org/10.1016/j.nut.2021.111247.

Krupa, C. N., Fritz, C., & Parmar, M. (2024). Ácidos graxos ômega-3. StatPearls Publishing.

Kwong, R. Y., Heydari, B., Ge, Y., Abdullah, S., Fujikura, K., Kaneko, K., Harris, W. S., Jerosch-Herold, M., Antman, E. M., Seidman, J. G., & Pfeffer, M. A. (2019). Genetic profiling of fatty acid desaturase polymorphisms identifies patients who may benefit from high-dose omega-3 fatty acids in cardiac remodeling after acute myocardial infarction—Post-hoc analysis from the OMEGA-REMODEL randomized controlled trial. *PLoS ONE, 14*(9), e0222061. https://doi.org/10.1371/journal.pone.0222061.

Lane, K. E., Li, W., Smith, C., & Derbyshire, E. (2014). The bioavailability of an omega-3-rich algal oil is improved by nanoemulsion technology using yogurt as a food vehicle. *International Journal of Food Science & Technology, 49*(5), 1264–1271. https://doi.org/10.1111/ijfs.12455.

Lichtenstein, A. H., Appel, L. J., Vadiveloo, M., Hu, F. B., Kris-Etherton, P. M., Rebholz, C. M., Sacks, F. M., Thorndike, A. N., Van Horn, L., & Wylie-Rosett, J. (2021). 2021 Dietary guidance to improve cardiovascular health: A scientific statement from the American Heart Association. *Circulation, 144*(23). https://doi.org/10.1161/CIR.0000000000001031.

Maki, K. C., Palacios, O. M., Buggia, M. A., Trivedi, R., Dicklin, M. R., & Maki, C. E. (2018). Effects of a self–micro-emulsifying delivery system formulation versus a standard ω-3 acid ethyl ester product on the bioavailability of eicosapentaenoic acid and docosahexaenoic acid: A study in healthy men and women in a fasted state. *Clinical Therapeutics, 40*(12), 2065–2076. https://doi.org/10.1016/j.clinthera.2018.10.014.

Mariamenatu, A. H., & Abdu, E. M. (2021). Overconsumption of omega-6 polyunsaturated fatty acids (PUFAs) versus deficiency of omega-3 PUFAs in modern-day diets: The disturbing factor for their "balanced antagonistic metabolic functions" in the human body. *Journal of Lipids, 2021*, 1–15. https://doi.org/10.1155/2021/8848161.

Martucci, M., Conte, M., Bucci, L., Giampieri, E., Fabbri, C., Palmas, M., Izzi, M., Salvioli, S., Zambrini, A., Orsi, C., Brigidi, P., Santoro, A., Capri, M., Monti, D., & Franceschi, C. (2020). Twelve-week daily consumption of ad hoc fortified milk with ω-3, D, and group B vitamins has a positive impact on inflammaging parameters: A randomized cross-over trial. *Nutrients, 12*(11), 3580. https://doi.org/10.3390/nu12113580.

McClements, D., & Öztürk, B. (2021). Utilization of nanotechnology to improve the handling, storage and biocompatibility of bioactive lipids in food applications. *Foods, 10*(2), 365. https://doi.org/10.3390/foods10020365.

McNamara, R. K., Able, J., Jandacek, R., Rider, T., Tso, P., Eliassen, J. C., Alfieri, D., Weber, W., Jarvis, K., DelBello, M. P., Strakowski, S. M., & Adler, C. M. (2010). Docosahexaenoic acid supplementation increases prefrontal cortex activation during sustained attention in healthy boys: A placebo-controlled, dose-ranging, functional magnetic resonance imaging study. *The American Journal of Clinical Nutrition, 91*(4), 1060–1067. https://doi.org/10.3945/ajcn.2009.28549.

Murff, H. J., Shrubsole, M. J., Cai, Q., Su, T., Dooley, J. H., Cai, S. S., Zheng, W., & Dai, Q. (2022). N-3 long chain fatty acids supplementation, fatty acids desaturase activity, and colorectal cancer risk: A randomized controlled trial. *Nutrition and Cancer, 74*(4), 1388–1398. https://doi.org/10.1080/01635581.2021.1955286.

Mądry, E., Chudzicka-Strugała, I., Grabańska-Martyńska, K., Malikowska, K., Grebowiec, P., Lisowska, A., Bogdański, P., & Walkowiak, J. (2016). Twelve weeks CLA supplementation decreases the hip circumference in overweight and obese women. A double-blind, randomized, placebo-controlled trial. *Acta Scientiarum Polonorum Technologia Alimentaria, 15*(1), 107–113. https://doi.org/10.17306/J.AFS.2016.1.11.

Nilsson, A. K., Löfqvist, C., Najm, S., Hellgren, G., Sävman, K., Andersson, M. X., Smith, L. E. H., & Hellström, A. (2019). Influence of human milk and parenteral lipid emulsions on serum fatty acid profiles in extremely preterm infants. *Journal of Parenteral and Enteral Nutrition, 43*(1), 152–161. https://doi.org/10.1002/jpen.1172.

Nogueira, M. A., Oliveira, C. P., Ferreira Alves, V. A., Stefano, J. T., Rodrigues, L. S.dos R., Torrinhas, R. S., Cogliati, B., Barbeiro, H., Carrilho, F. J., & Waitzberg, D. L. (2016). Omega-3 polyunsaturated fatty acids in treating non-alcoholic steatohepatitis: A randomized, double-blind, placebo-controlled trial. *Clinical Nutrition, 35*(3), 578–586. https://doi.org/10.1016/j.clnu.2015.05.001.

Opperman, M., Marais, D. W., & Benade, A. J. S. (2011). Analysis of omega-3 fatty acid content of South African fish oil supplements. *Cardiovascular Journal of Africa, 22*(6), 324–329. https://doi.org/10.5830/CVJA-2010-080.

Ostadrahimi, A., Salehi-pourmehr, H., Mohammad-Alizadeh-Charandabi, S., Heidarabady, S., & Farshbaf-Khalili, A. (2018). The effect of perinatal fish oil supplementation on neurodevelopment and growth of infants: A randomized controlled trial. *European Journal of Nutrition, 57*(7), 2387–2397. https://doi.org/10.1007/s00394-017-1512-1.

Ozkan, G., Franco, P., De Marco, I., Xiao, J., & Capanoglu, E. (2019). A review of microencapsulation methods for food antioxidants: Principles, advantages, drawbacks and applications. *Food Chemistry, 272*, 494–506. https://doi.org/10.1016/j.foodchem.2018.07.205.

Papandreou, P., Gioxarı, A., Ntountaniotis, D., Korda, O.-N., Skouroliakou, M., & Siahanidou, T. (2020). Administration of an intravenous fat emulsion enriched with medium-chain triglyceride/ω-3 fatty acids is beneficial towards anti-inflammatory related fatty acid profile in preterm neonates: A randomized, double-blind clinical trial. *Nutrients, 12*(11), 3526. https://doi.org/10.3390/nu12113526.

Pasini, F., Gómez-Caravaca, A. M., Blasco, T., Cvejić, J., Caboni, M. F., & Verardo, V. (2022). Assessment of lipid quality in commercial omega-3 supplements sold in the french market. *Biomolecules, 12*(10), 1361. https://doi.org/10.3390/biom12101361.

Patted, P. G., Masareddy, R. S., Patil, A. S., Kanabargi, R. R., & Bhat, C. T. (2024). Omega-3 fatty acids: A comprehensive scientific review of their sources, functions and health benefits. *Future Journal of Pharmaceutical Sciences, 10*(1). https://doi.org/10.1186/s43094-024-00667-5.

Peña-de-la-Sancha, P., Muñoz-García, A., Espínola-Zavaleta, N., Bautista-Pérez, R., Mejía, A. M., Luna-Luna, M., López-Olmos, V., Rodríguez-Pérez, J.-M., Fragoso, J.-M., Carreón-Torres, E., & Pérez-Méndez, Ó. (2023). Eicosapentaenoic and docosahexaenoic acid supplementation increases HDL content in n-3 fatty acids and improves endothelial function in hypertriglyceridemic patients. *International Journal of Molecular Sciences, 24*(6), 5390. https://doi.org/10.3390/ijms24065390.

Punia, S., Sandhu, K. S., Siroha, A. K., & Dhull, S. B. (2019). Omega 3-metabolism, absorption, bioavailability and health benefits–A review. *PharmaNutrition, 10*, 100162. https://doi.org/10.1016/j.phanu.2019.100162.

Puri, V., Nagpal, M., Singh, I., Singh, M., Dhingra, G. A., Huanbutta, K., Dheer, D., Sharma, A., & Sangnim, T. (2022). A comprehensive review on nutraceuticals: Therapy support and formulation challenges. *Nutrients, 14*(21), 4637. https://doi.org/10.3390/nu14214637.

Qin, Y., Nyheim, H., Haram, E. M., Moritz, J. M., & Hustvedt, S. O. (2017). A novel self-micro-emulsifying delivery system (SMEDS) formulation significantly improves the fasting absorption of EPA and DHA from a single dose of an omega-3 ethyl ester concentrate. *Lipids in Health and Disease, 16*(1), 204. https://doi.org/10.1186/s12944-017-0589-0.

Reiner, Z., Catapano, A. L., De Backer, G., Graham, I., Taskinen, M.-R., Wiklund, O., Agewall, S., Alegria, E., Chapman, M. J., Durrington, P., Erdine, S., Halcox, J., Hobbs, R., Kjekshus, J., Filardi, P. P., Riccardi, G., Storey, R. F., Wood, D., Bax, J., ... Zamorano, J. L. (2011). ESC/EAS guidelines for the management of dyslipidaemias: The task force for the management of dyslipidaemias of the European Society of Cardiology (ESC) and the European Atherosclerosis Society (EAS). *European Heart Journal, 32*(14), 1769–1818. https://doi.org/10.1093/eurheartj/ehr158.

Roach, L. A., Byrne, M. K., Howard, S. J., Johnstone, S. J., Batterham, M., Wright, I. M. R., Okely, A. D., de Groot, R. H. M., van der Wurff, I. S. M., Jones, A., & Meyer, B. J. (2021). The feasibility of the "omega kid" study protocol: A double-blind, randomised, placebo-controlled trial investigating the effect of omega-3 supplementation on self-regulation in preschool-aged children. *Nutrients, 13*(1), 213. https://doi.org/10.3390/nu13010213.

Sanders, L. M., Goltz, S., & Maki, K. C. (2023). Resiliency of the digestive system during aging and the impact of diet. *Nutrition Today, 58*(4), 165–174. https://doi.org/10.1097/NT.0000000000000616.

Schmidt, N., Møller, G., Bæksgaard, L., Østerlind, K., Stark, K. D., Lauritzen, L., & Andersen, J. R. (2020). Fish oil supplementation in cancer patients. Capsules or nutritional drink supplements? A controlled study of compliance. *Clinical Nutrition ESPEN, 35*, 63–68. https://doi.org/10.1016/j.clnesp.2019.12.004.

See, V. H. L., Mas, E., Burrows, S., O'Callaghan, N. J., Fenech, M., Prescott, S. L., Beilin, L. J., Huang, R. C., & Mori, T. A. (2016). Prenatal omega-3 fatty acid supplementation does not affect offspring telomere length and F2-isoprostanes at 12 years: A double blind, randomized controlled trial. *Prostaglandins, Leukotrienes, and Essential Fatty Acids, 112*, 50–55. https://doi.org/10.1016/j.plefa.2016.08.006.

Scientific Advisory Committee on Nutrition (SACN). (2008). *The nutritional wellbeing of the British population : Scientific Advisory Committee on Nutrition 2008*. TSO.

See, V. H. L., Mas, E., Prescott, S. L., Beilin, L. J., Burrows, S., Barden, A. E., Huang, R.-C., & Mori, T. A. (2017). Effects of prenatal *n* -3 fatty acid supplementation on offspring resolvins at birth and 12 years of age: A double-blind, randomised controlled clinical trial. *British Journal of Nutrition, 118*(11), 971–980. https://doi.org/10.1017/S0007114517002914.

Shahidi, F., & Ambigaipalan, P. (2018). Omega-3 polyunsaturated fatty acids and their health benefits. *Annual Review of Food Science and Technology, 9*(1), 345–381. https://doi.org/10.1146/annurev-food-111317-095850.

Shehzad, Q., Rehman, A., Jafari, S. M., Zuo, M., Khan, M. A., Ali, A., Khan, S., Karim, A., Usman, M., Hussain, A., & Xia, W. (2021). Improving the oxidative stability of fish oil nanoemulsions by co-encapsulation with curcumin and resveratrol. *Colloids and Surfaces B: Biointerfaces, 199*, 111481. https://doi.org/10.1016/j.colsurfb.2020.111481.

Sheppard, K. W., Boone, K. M., Gracious, B., Klebanoff, M. A., Rogers, L. K., Rausch, J., Bartlett, C., Coury, D. L., & Keim, S. A. (2017). Effect of omega-3 and -6 supplementation on language in preterm toddlers exhibiting autism spectrum disorder symptoms. *Journal of Autism and Developmental Disorders, 47*(11), 3358–3369. https://doi.org/10.1007/s10803-017-3249-3.

Shireman, T. I., Kerling, E. H., Gajewski, B. J., Colombo, J., & Carlson, S. E. (2016). Docosahexaenoic acid supplementation (DHA) and the return on investment for pregnancy outcomes. *Prostaglandins, Leukotrienes, and Essential Fatty Acids, 111*, 8–10. https://doi.org/10.1016/j.plefa.2016.05.008.

Simonetto, M., Infante, M., Sacco, R. L., Rundek, T., & Della-Morte, D. (2019). A novel anti-inflammatory role of omega-3 PUFAs in prevention and treatment of atherosclerosis and vascular cognitive impairment and dementia. *Nutrients, 11*(10), 2279. https://doi.org/10.3390/nu11102279.

Skouroliakou, M., Konstantinou, D., Agakidis, C., Kaliora, A., Kalogeropoulos, N., Massara, P., Antoniadi, M., Panagiotakos, D., & Karagiozoglou-Lampoudi, T. (2016). Parenteral MCT/ω-3 polyunsaturated fatty acid–enriched intravenous fat emulsion is associated with cytokine and fatty acid profiles consistent with attenuated inflammatory response in preterm neonates. *Nutrition in Clinical Practice, 31*(2), 235–244. https://doi.org/10.1177/0884533615602011.

Skulas-Ray, A. C., Wilson, P. W. F., Harris, W. S., Brinton, E. A., Kris-Etherton, P. M., Richter, C. K., Jacobson, T. A., Engler, M. B., Miller, M., Robinson, J. G., Blum, C. B., Rodriguez-Leyva, D., de Ferranti, S. D., & Welty, F. K. (2019). Omega-3 fatty acids for the management of hypertriglyceridemia: A science advisory from the american heart association. *Circulation, 140*(12). https://doi.org/10.1161/CIR.0000000000000709.

Soares, V. M., Silva, T. C.da, & Santos, P. P.dos (2023). Papel do Ômega-3 e do Ômega-6 sobre Fatores de Risco Cardiovasculares: Importância da Fonte da Dieta e da Estrutura do Lipídio. *Arquivos Brasileiros de Cardiologia, 120*(11). https://doi.org/10.36660/abc.20230753.

Stanley, E. G., Jenkins, B. J., Walker, C. G., Koulman, A., Browning, L., West, A. L., Calder, P. C., Jebb, S. A., & Griffin, J. L. (2017). Lipidomics profiling of human adipose tissue identifies a pattern of lipids associated with fish oil supplementation. *Journal of Proteome Research, 16*(9), 3168–3179. https://doi.org/10.1021/acs.jproteome.7b00161.

Stavrinou, P. S., Andreou, E., Aphamis, G., Pantzaris, M., Ioannou, M., S. Patrikios, I., & D. Giannaki, C. (2020). The effects of a 6-month high dose omega-3 and omega-6 polyunsaturated fatty acids and antioxidant vitamins supplementation on cognitive function and functional capacity in older adults with mild cognitive impairment. *Nutrients, 12*(2), 325. https://doi.org/10.3390/nu12020325.

Stiefvatter, L., Frick, K., Lehnert, K., Vetter, W., Montoya-Arroyo, A., Frank, J., Schmid-Staiger, U., & Bischoff, S. C. (2022). Potentially beneficial effects on healthy aging by supplementation of the EPA-rich microalgae phaeodactylum tricornutum or its supernatant—A randomized controlled pilot trial in elderly individuals. *Marine Drugs, 20*(11), 716. https://doi.org/10.3390/md20110716.

Sueyasu, T., Yasumoto, K., Tokuda, H., Kaneda, Y., Obata, H., Rogi, T., Izumo, T., Kondo, S., Saito, J., Tsukiura, T., & Nakai, M. (2023). Effects of long-chain polyunsaturated fatty acids in combination with lutein and zeaxanthin on episodic memory in healthy older adults. *Nutrients, 15*(13), 2825. https://doi.org/10.3390/nu15132825.

Swanson, D., Block, R., & Mousa, S. A. (2012). Omega-3 fatty acids EPA and DHA: Health benefits throughout life. *Advances in Nutrition, 3*(1), 1–7. https://doi.org/10.3945/an.111.000893.

Tammam, J. D., Steinsaltz, D., Bester, D. W., Semb-Andenaes, T., & Stein, J. F. (2016). A randomised double-blind placebo-controlled trial investigating the behavioural effects of vitamin, mineral and *n* -3 fatty acid supplementation in typically developing adolescent schoolchildren. *British Journal of Nutrition, 115*(2), 361–373. https://doi.org/10.1017/S0007114515004390.

Tingö, L., Hutchinson, A. N., Bergh, C., Stiefvatter, L., Schweinlin, A., Jensen, M. G., Krüger, K., Bischoff, S. C., & Brummer, R. J. (2022). Potential modulation of inflammation by probiotic and omega-3 supplementation in elderly with chronic low-grade inflammation—A randomized, placebo-controlled trial. *Nutrients, 14*(19), 3998. https://doi.org/10.3390/nu14193998.

Tobin, D., Brevik-Andersen, M., Qin, Y., Innes, J. K., & Calder, P. C. (2018). Evaluation of a high concentrate omega-3 for correcting the omega-3 fatty acid nutritional deficiency in non-alcoholic fatty liver disease (CONDIN). *Nutrients, 10*(8), 1126. https://doi.org/10.3390/nu10081126.

United States. (2020). *Dietary guidelines for Americans*. https://www.dietaryguidelines.gov/sites/default/files/2020-12/Dietary_Guidelines_for_Americans_2020-2025.pdf?utm_source.

United States (EUA). (1994). *Dietary supplement health and education act of 1994 (DSHEA), Pub. L*103–417. https://Ods.Od.Nih.Gov/About/DSHEA_Wording.Aspx.

Valentine, C. J., Khan, A. Q., Brown, A. R., Sands, S. A., Defranco, E. A., Gajewski, B. J., Carlson, S. E., Reber, K. M., & Rogers, L. K. (2021). Higher-Dose DHA supplementation modulates immune responses in pregnancy and is associated with decreased preterm birth. *Nutrients, 13*(12), 4248. https://doi.org/10.3390/nu13124248.

Vannice, G., & Rasmussen, H. (2014). Position of the academy of nutrition and dietetics: Dietary fatty acids for healthy adults. *Journal of the Academy of Nutrition and Dietetics, 114*(1), 136–153. https://doi.org/10.1016/j.jand.2013.11.001.

Venugopalan, V. K., Gopakumar, L. R., Kumaran, A. K., Chatterjee, N. S., Soman, V., Peeralil, S., Mathew, S., McClements, D. J., & Nagarajarao, R. C. (2021). Encapsulation and protection of omega-3-rich fish oils using food-grade delivery systems. *Foods, 10*(7), 1566. https://doi.org/10.3390/foods10071566.

Vieira, M. C., Bakof, K. K., Schuch, N. J., Skupien, J. A., & Boeck, C. R. (2020). The benefits of omega-3 fatty acid nanocapsulation for the enrichment of food products: A review. *Revista de Nutrição, 33*. https://doi.org/10.1590/1678-9865202033e190165.

Visseren, F. L. J., Mach, F., Smulders, Y. M., Carballo, D., Koskinas, K. C., Bäck, M., Benetos, A., Biffi, A., Boavida, J.-M., Capodanno, D., Cosyns, B., Crawford, C., Davos, C. H., Desormais, I., Di Angelantonio, E., Franco, O. H., Halvorsen, S., Hobbs, F. D. R., Hollander, M., ... Williams, B. (2021). 2021 ESC guidelines on cardiovascular disease prevention in clinical practice. *European Heart Journal, 42*(34), 3227–3337. https://doi.org/10.1093/eurheartj/ehab484.

Walker, C., West, A., Browning, L., Madden, J., Gambell, J., Jebb, S., & Calder, P. (2015). The pattern of fatty acids displaced by EPA and DHA following 12 months supplementation varies between blood cell and plasma fractions. *Nutrients, 7*(8), 6281–6293. https://doi.org/10.3390/nu7085285.

Walker, R., Decker, E. A., & McClements, D. J. (2015). Development of food-grade nanoemulsions and emulsions for delivery of omega-3 fatty acids: Opportunities and obstacles in the food industry. *Food & Function, 6*(1), 41–54. https://doi.org/10.1039/C4FO00723A.

Walker, R. E., Richter, C. K., Skulas-Ray, A. C., Flock, M. R., Harsch, B. A., Annevelink, C. E., Kris-Etherton, P. M., Jensen, G. L., & Shearer, G. C. (2023). Effect of omega-3 ethyl esters on the triglyceride-rich lipoprotein response to endotoxin challenge in healthy young men. *Journal of Lipid Research, 64*(5), 100353. https://doi.org/10.1016/j.jlr.2023.100353.

Watson, H., Mitra, S., Croden, F. C., Taylor, M., Wood, H. M., Perry, S. L., Spencer, J. A., Quirke, P., Toogood, G. J., Lawton, C. L., Dye, L., Loadman, P. M., & Hull, M. A. (2018). A randomised trial of the effect of omega-3 polyunsaturated fatty acid supplements on the human intestinal microbiota. *Gut, 67*(11), 1974–1983. https://doi.org/10.1136/gutjnl-2017-314968.

Weiser, M., Butt, C., & Mohajeri, M. (2016). Docosahexaenoic acid and cognition throughout the lifespan. *Nutrients, 8*(2), 99. https://doi.org/10.3390/nu8020099.

White, M. N., Shrubsole, M. J., Cai, Q., Su, T., Hardee, J., Coppola, J.-A., Cai, S. S., Martin, S. M., Motley, S., Swift, L. L., Milne, G. L., Zheng, W., Dai, Q., & Murff, H. J. (2019). Effects of fish oil supplementation on eicosanoid production in patients at higher risk for colorectal cancer. *European Journal of Cancer Prevention, 28*(3), 188–195. https://doi.org/10.1097/CEJ.0000000000000455.

WHO. (2020). *Word Health Organization: Healthy diet*. https://wTableww.Who.Int/News-Room/Fact-Sheets/Detail/Healthy-Diet?Utm_source, https://www.who.int/news-room/fact-sheets/detail/healthy-diet?utm_source.

WHO. (2023). *Saturated fatty acid and trans-fatty acid intake for adults and children: WHO guideline*. https://iris.who.int/bitstream/handle/10665/370419/9789240073630-eng.pdf?sequence=1.

Wilson, M. J., Sen, A., Bridges, D., Turgeon, D. K., Brenner, D. E., Smith, W. L., Ruffin, M. T., & Djuric, Z. (2018). Higher baseline expression of the PTGS2 gene and greater decreases in total colonic fatty acid content predict greater decreases in colonic prostaglandin-E2 concentrations after dietary supplementation with ω-3 fatty acids. *Prostaglandins, Leukotrienes, and Essential Fatty Acids, 139*, 14–19. https://doi.org/10.1016/j.plefa.2018.11.001.

Wimalasena, S. T., Ramírez Silva, C. I., Gonzalez Casanova, I., Rivera, J. A., Sun, Y. V., Stein, A. D., Ferranti, E. P., Alvarez, J. A., Demmelmair, H., Koletzko, B., & Ramakrishnan, U. (2024). Maternal and offspring fatty acid desaturase variants, prenatal DHA supplementation, and dietary n–6:n–3 fatty acid ratio in relation to cardiometabolic health in Mexican children. *The Journal of Nutrition, 154*(5), 1540–1548. https://doi.org/10.1016/j.tjnut.2024.03.004.

Yang, J., Ciftci, D., & Ciftci, O. N. (2024). Fortification of milk with omega-3 fatty acids using novel bioactive-carrier hollow solid lipid micro- and nanoparticles for improved omega-3 stability and bioaccessibility. *ACS Food Science & Technology, 4*(4), 813–820. https://doi.org/10.1021/acsfoodscitech.3c00141.

Yenipazar, H., & Şahin-Yeşilçubuk, N. (2023). Effect of packaging and encapsulation on the oxidative and sensory stability of omega-3 supplements. *Food Science & Nutrition, 11*(3), 1426–1440. https://doi.org/10.1002/fsn3.3182.

Zakrzewska, K., Oszajca, K., Zep, W., Piekarska, A., & Sidorkiewicz, M. (2021). The impact of short-term shark liver oil supplementation on the fatty acid composition of erythrocyte membranes. *Nutrients, 13*(10), 3329. https://doi.org/10.3390/nu13103329.

Zeng, Q., Dong, S.-Y., Liu, Y.-P., Fu, J., Shuai, P., Zhao, Z.-M., & Li, T.-X. (2017). Effects of fish oil-derived fatty acids on suboptimal cardiovascular health: A multicenter, randomized, double-blind, placebo-controlled trial. *Nutrition, Metabolism, and Cardiovascular Diseases, 27*(11), 964–970. https://doi.org/10.1016/j.numecd.2017.09.004.

Zhang, J.-M., & An, J. (2007). Cytokines, inflammation, and pain. *International Anesthesiology Clinics, 45*(2), 27–37. https://doi.org/10.1097/AIA.0b013e318034194e.

Chapter 33

Polyunsaturated fatty acid utilization in emerging food sectors: case studies on technological advancement

Sureshkumar Sujithra[1], Ravi Sanjana[1], Kalaiselvi Krishnamoorthy[2], Safreena Kabeer[1], Kumar P. Kiran[3], Karthikeyan Velayutham[1,4], and Pothiyappan Karthik[1]

[1]*Department of Food Technology, Faculty of Engineering, Karpagam Academy of Higher Education, Coimbatore, Tamil Nadu, India,* [2]*Centre for Herbal Pharmacology and Environmental Sustainability, Chettinad Hospital and Research Institute, Chettinad Academy of Research and Education, Chennai, Tamil Nadu, India,* [3]*Department of Chemistry, Seshadripuram Institute of Technology, Mysuru, Karnataka, India,* [4]*Centre for Nanotechnology, Karpagam Academy of Higher Education, Coimbatore, Tamil Nadu, India*

33.1 Introduction

Fatty acids (FAs) are classified into three groups based on the number of double bonds present in their side chains: saturated fatty acids (SFAs), monounsaturated fatty acids, and polyunsaturated fatty acids (PUFAs). Among them, PUFAs contain two or more double bonds; they are long-chain FAs that are residues from lipids and are categorized into two types, omega-3 and omega-6. Both are essential nutrients and are naturally obtained from the regular diet. The global dietary guidelines recommend regular consumption of sea-based food products, which provide an enriched level of omega-3, and consumption of nuts and seeds, that provides the omega-6 sources (Xu, Molenaar, et al., 2025; Bhashira & Gopalakrishnan, 2025). Alpha-linolenic acid (ALA), eicosapentaenoic acid (EPA), and docosahexaenoic acid (DHA) are the types of omega-3 PUFAs, while linoleic acid (LA), arachidonic acid , and dihomo-gamma-linolenic acid are representatives of omega-6 PUFAs (Le et al., 2009; Cholewski et al., 2018) (Fig. 33.1). Both FAs play an important role in human health, such as regulation of metabolism, antiinflammatory activities, gene expression, heart function, brain development and function, and cardiac function (Kaur et al., 2014). Omega-3, particularly EPA and DHA, relates to maintaining the cardiovascular system by monitoring plasma triglyceride ratios, reducing the risk of atherosclerosis, and improving vascular elasticity (Sherratt et al., 2022; Zanetti et al., 2015). DHA is vital for neurological growth and cognition, particularly for infants and kids, whose brain development and retinal health greatly depend on regular consumption (Lauritzen et al., 2016). Both EPA and DHA have antiinflammatory activities that are essential to controlling cytokine production and lowering the risk of chronic illnesses, including diabetes, inflammatory bowel disease, and arthritis. Although they can be found in excess in modern diets, omega-6 FAs are also necessary for skin health, development, and immunological function (Mallick et al., 2023; Geetha et al., 2025; Silva et al., 2018).

Nutrition-based research in recent years has focused on PUFA integration into food products, which leads to various food fortification methods and novel product developments (Finco et al., 2016; Mannucci et al., 2023; Rizzo et al., 2023). The increasing consumption of processed, high-energy, and low-nutrient foods, as well as changing lifestyles and industrialized food systems, has made it more significant than ever to include PUFA in modern diets (Fig. 33.2). Though fish and seafood are still significant sources of long-chain omega-3 FAs, their accessibility varies globally and is sometimes limited by factors such as expense, traditions, and concerns regarding sustainability (Kitessa et al., 2014). Furthermore, there is a greater need for nonmarine sources of PUFAs due to the growing popularity of vegetarian and vegan diet culture (Saini et al., 2021). To fill nutritional gaps, researchers are currently looking into oils made from sunflower, flaxseed, canola, soybeans, and chia, as well as oils made from algae and products of microbial fermentation.

Omega-3 and Omega-6 Polyunsaturated Fatty Acids in Food Systems. DOI: https://doi.org/10.1016/B978-0-443-43810-3.00023-3

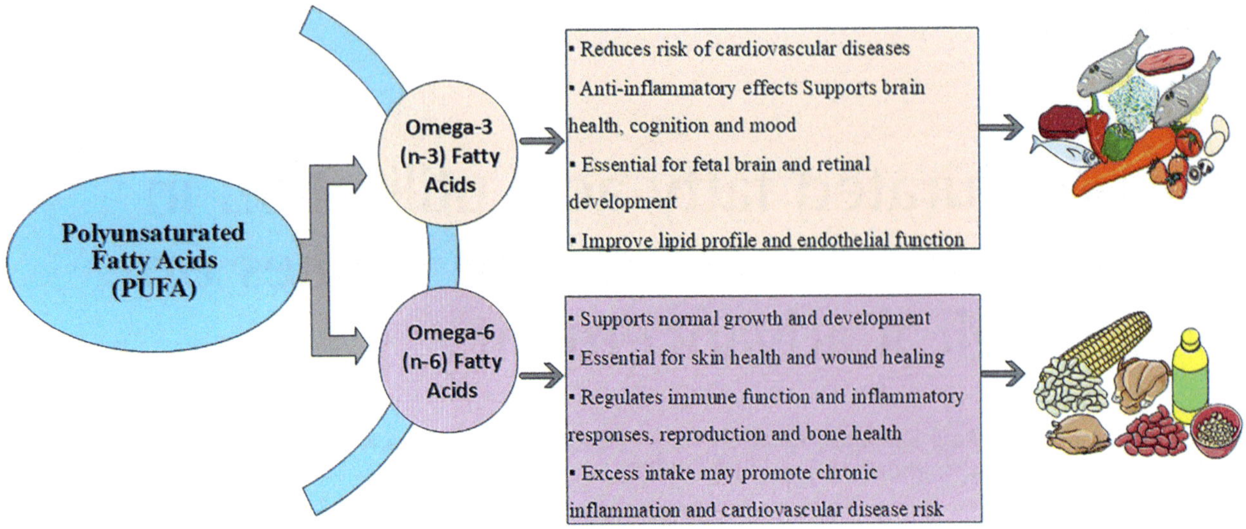

FIGURE 33.1 Polyunsaturated fatty acid (PUFA) classifications and their major sources.

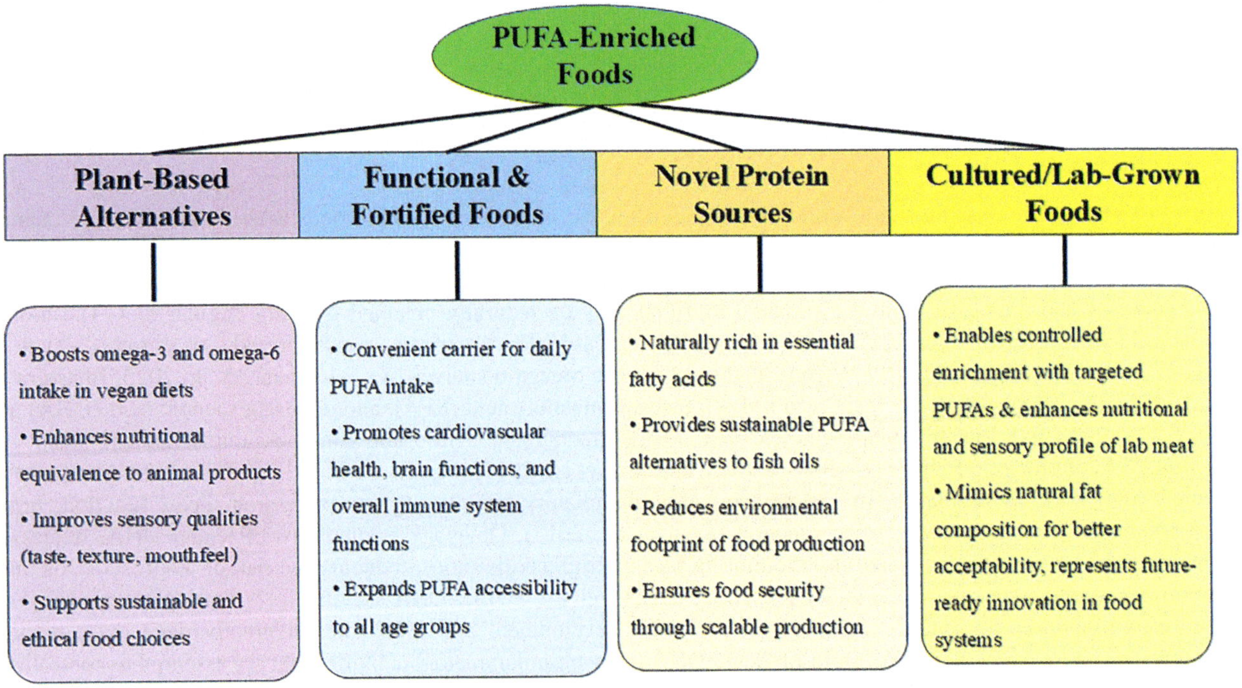

FIGURE 33.2 Illustration of polyunsaturated fatty acid (PUFA)-enriched foods and their benefits.

Numerous opportunities for the incorporation of PUFA in food production are presented by the developing food industry. Plant-based alternatives to meat, dairy, and egg-based products are becoming increasingly common because of consumer desire for sustainable and ethical food choices (Alcorta et al., 2021; Liu et al., 2022a). Generally, these products are usually improved by PUFA-rich oils to get nutritional benefits, as well as animal-based products in parallel. PUFA incorporation into the food products can enhance the health benefits as well as sensory qualities such as flavor and good mouthfeel. In functional food preparations, PUFA play an important role, such as in yogurts, drinks, baked goods, and snack bars, where PUFA act as a nutritional and taste-improving carrier (Zhang et al., 2024).

Novel protein sources such as algae and edible insects are getting more attention due to their highest PUFA content and protein levels (Quintieri et al., 2023; Moura et al., 2023; Azizi et al., 2025). The increased awareness of the health importance linked with PUFA has been getting more attention in functional foods enriched with omega-3 and 6.

Concurrently, the development in biotechnology, algal production, genetic engineering-based oil crop production, and aquaculture techniques is creating new and sustainable avenues for large-scale PUFA availability (Zhao, Wang, et al., 2025). If in the future, the integration of consumer preferences, new technologies, and scientific projections indicates that PUFA-based novel foods will remain the new transformation in the forthcoming food system. Overall, the current chapter provides the nutritional benefits and drawbacks of incorporating PUFAs into food production, also describing the benefits brought forth by developments in fermentation, biotechnology, and sustainable agriculture.

33.2 Polyunsaturated fatty acid sources and extraction technologies

FAs function as fundamental components that create lipids, which serve as vital elements for all living organisms according to the metabolism of FA (Shyam et al., 2025). They function as essential components that provide energy, support signaling mechanisms, and form the foundation of cellular structures. The health effects of fats show distinct patterns according to their unsaturation levels and carbon chain length, while trans fats display different characteristics that create particular health effects according to Hegazy et al. (2025). There are different sources of FAs. The essential FAs present in fatty fish and dairy products constitute animal sources that include omega-3s. Plant sources, including nuts and seeds, offer beneficial monounsaturated and polyunsaturated FAs. Omega-3s, which serve as vital nutrients for cardiovascular health, exist in high concentrations in marine sources that include fish and algae, according to Yeung et al. (2025). PUFAs, particularly omega-3 and omega-6 FAs, are essential bioactive lipids with significant physiological and industrial importance according to Usturoi et al. (2025).

Long-chain omega-3 PUFAs, EPA, and DHA from marine sources have been historically obtained from fatty fish and krill, which serve as the main sources. The search for alternative sources has become urgent because overfishing, environmental contaminants, and sustainability issues raise concerns. The primary producers of aquatic food webs produce EPA and DHA, which marine microalgae offer as a sustainable solution for their production. In parallel, plant-based oils such as flaxseed, chia, and canola provide ALA, while sunflower and soybean oils are rich in LA (Ahmed et al., 2026). Although plant sources are widely available and economically viable, their limited capacity to provide long-chain omega-3 PUFAs due to low conversion efficiency in humans remains a challenge. The comparative evaluation of major PUFA sources with respect to dominant FAs, sustainability, cost, and scalability is presented in Table 33.1

33.2.1 Natural sources

Natural sources of PUFAs are predominantly obtained from marine organisms and terrestrial plants. They serve as the primary reservoirs of essential omega-3 and omega-6 FAs in the human diet. Marine sources such as fatty fish and microalgae are rich in long-chain omega-3 PUFAs such as EPA and DHA (Mititelu et al., 2024). These compounds are directly bioavailable and associated with cardiovascular, neurological, and antiinflammatory health benefits. Fish accumulate FAs through the consumption of PUFA-producing microalgae (Xu, Molenaar, et al., 2025). This makes marine ecosystems the original biological source of long-chain omega-3s. In contrast, plant-based sources include flaxseed, chia seeds, walnuts, soybean, and sunflower oils. They primarily provide short-chain PUFAs such as ALA and LA. When compared to fish oil, plant oils are widely accessible, cost-effective, and sustainable (Özyurt et al., 2026). The conversion of ALA to EPA and DHA in humans is metabolically limited. Therefore, natural PUFA sources collectively contribute to nutritional security. Thus, marine organisms help to provide long-chain omega-3s, whereas plant-based products provide essential FAs required for maintaining physiological functions (García-Cervantes et al., 2026).

33.2.2 Marine sources

Marine sources are considered the most important natural reservoir of long-chain omega-3 PUFAs, predominantly EPA and DHA (Glencross et al., 2025). Fatty fish such as salmon, mackerel, sardines, and tuna are rich in these bioactive lipids (Tufail et al., 2025). They constitute the primary dietary source of preformed EPA and DHA for humans. These FAs originate from marine microalgae at the base of the aquatic food chain. Microalgae are subsequently accumulated in fish tissues through trophic transfer (Zhao, Wang, et al., 2025). In addition, fish, krill, and other marine invertebrates also provide significant amounts of omega-3 PUFAs (Glencross et al., 2025). Marine microalgae themselves are increasingly recognized as a sustainable and direct source of EPA and DHA (Panchal et al., 2025). They have several advantages, such as controlled cultivation and reduced risk of environmental contaminants. These products are suitable for vegetarian and vegan applications. Marine-derived PUFAs are still widely used in the nutraceutical, pharmaceutical, and functional food industries due to their high bioavailability and recognized health benefits (Wei et al., 2025).

TABLE 33.1 Comparative evaluation of major polyunsaturated fatty acid (PUFA) sources based on predominant fatty acids, sustainability, production cost, and scalability.

Types of sources	Major PUFA	Sustainability	Cost	Scalability	References
Fish oil	Eicosapentaenoic acid (EPA), docosahexaenoic acid (DHA)	Moderate	Medium	High	Mititelu et al. (2024)
Krill oil	EPA, DHA (PL form)	Moderate	High	Medium	Glencross et al. (2025)
Microalgae	DHA, EPA	High	Medium-high	High	Mititelu et al. (2024)
Plant oils	Alpha-linolenic acid, linoleic acid	High	Low	Very high	Özyurt et al. (2026)
Engineered crops	EPA, DHA	High	Medium	High	Jia et al. (2021)
Microbial fermentation	DHA, arachidonic acid	Very high	Medium	High	Moi et al. (2018)

33.2.3 Plant-based sources

Plant-based sources are an important and sustainable supply of PUFAs, particularly short-chain omega-3 and omega-6 FAs. Oilseeds and vegetable oils such as flaxseed, chia seed, canola, soybean, sunflower, walnut, evening primrose, and borage are rich in ALA and LA (Xu, Zhang, et al., 2025). γ-Linolenic acid (GLA) can be seen in certain specialty oils. These essential FAs cannot be synthesized by the human body and must be obtained through the diet (Latifi et al., 2025). They serve as precursors for longer-chain PUFAs involved in inflammatory regulation, cell membrane structure, and metabolic signaling. Although the bioconversion of ALA to EPA and DHA in humans is limited. Plant-derived oils remain highly valuable due to their wide availability, affordability and environmental sustainability (Rajendran et al., 2025). They are suitable for vegetarian and vegan populations. Consequently, plant-based PUFA sources play a vital role in meeting global nutritional demands and supporting overall physiological functions (Vergara Nieto et al., 2025).

33.2.4 Novel microbial/lab-based sources

Novel microbial and lab-based sources have emerged as viable alternatives for the long-term and controlled production of PUFAs, mainly long-chain omega-3 and omega-6 FAs (Ayub et al., 2025). Under optimized fermentation conditions, oleaginous microorganisms, including marine microalgae, fungi, and yeast, are capable of accumulating substantial amounts of lipids rich in specific PUFAs (Mohamed et al., 2026). Species such as *Schizochytrium* and *Crypthecodinium cohnii* are widely used for DHA production (Umar et al., 2025). *Mortierella alpina* is recognized for the synthesis of amino acids (Zhao, Ding, et al., 2025). In addition, genetically engineered microorganisms and oilseed crops have been developed through metabolic engineering approaches to enable the biosynthesis of EPA and DHA (Assefa et al., 2025). These technologies provide benefits such as year-round production, less reliance on the marine environments, regulated quality, and scalability, making microbial and lab-based systems increasingly important for nutraceutical, pharmaceutical, and infant nutrition applications.

33.2.5 Sustainable and eco-friendly extraction methods

The extraction of PUFAs from marine, plant, and microbial sources is a crucial step to obtain high-quality oils with preserved bioactivity (Rahim et al., 2025). The standard extraction methods for this process use two techniques, which are mechanical pressing and solvent extraction. The processing of plant oils uses mechanical methods, which include both cold pressing and expeller pressing (Babu et al., 2025). The process produces moderate quantities of active compounds, which remain in the environment friendly system. The process of solvent extraction with organic solvents such as hexane results in better lipid extraction. The process needs to remove all remaining solvents in a careful manner. The process needs to maintain control because any failure will result in PUFA oxidation (Lima-Pereira et al., 2025).

The improvement of yield, selectivity, and sustainability requires advanced extraction techniques, which have been created (Ayele et al., 2025). Supercritical CO_2 extraction operates as an environmentally friendly method that does not need solvents to extract marine oils, microalgae, and krill. The products provide high purity, which results in minimal thermal degradation and safe environmental impact (Mirzaee Kalaei., et al., 2025). Enzyme-assisted extraction uses cellulases, pectinases, or proteases to destroy cell walls in plants and microbial biomass. The process enables oil extraction through better oil release while maintaining PUFA protection (Priyadarshini & Kataria, 2025). Advanced methods combine with each other to achieve better results in both recovery and quality of products.

The production of stable high-purity PUFA oils requires downstream purification to follow extraction (Yin et al., 2025). The process uses degumming, neutralization, molecular distillation, winterization, and microencapsulation to remove contaminants from the material. The methods enable researchers to extract desired FAs from their sources while safeguarding them from oxidative deterioration (Alao, 2025). The process of microbial PUFA production uses fermentation to extract lipids from cells, which undergo destruction before their contents undergo solvent or supercritical extraction and purification (Pabba et al., 2026). The system enables continuous production while it allows users to generate specific FA profiles and expand operations to meet industrial demands. The combination of extraction and purification techniques enables the effective utilization of PUFAs from different sources in nutraceutical and pharmaceutical products as well as functional food applications (Rahim et al., 2025).

33.3 Technological advancements in polyunsaturated fatty acid stabilization

Technical progression in the stabilization of PUFAs has been principally focused on overcoming the effect of oxidation, which degrades their nutritional quality and stability. One of the most promising technologies developed is the encapsulation technology, which offers a shield to PUFAs-rich oils against ecological factors, enhances their solubility, removes off-flavors, and improves their stability in emulsions. Encapsulation techniques include the use of nanoparticles, hydrogels, oleogels, nanocrystals, and nanofibers, which effectively protect PUFAs from oxidative degradation during processing, storage, and digestion (Jurić et al., 2020; Karthik, 2016). Additionally, microencapsulation techniques utilizing polymeric matrices, mostly polysaccharides, permit controlled release of omega-3 FAs and increase oxidative stability. The encapsulation approaches, as shown in Fig. 33.3, ease the integration of PUFAs into various food systems with maximum stability while protecting the FA composition (Ruiz Ruiz et al., 2017). In addition, to encapsulation technologies, biological advancements also contribute to PUFA stabilization. In certain studies, PUFA production has been improved by employing optimization of biosynthetic pathways, metabolic regulation, and genome editing techniques with the usage of microorganisms such as *Yarrowia lipolytica,* employing methods such as optimization of biosynthetic pathways, metabolic regulation, and (Jia et al., 2021). Another technological frontier, spotted on sustainable production with least contamination compared to traditional fish oil sources, is the utilization of marine bacteria (Moi et al., 2018).

33.3.1 Challenges in polyunsaturated fatty acid degradation: oxidation and shelf-life issues

PUFAs possess major challenges in degradation, potentially due to oxidation, which may reduce the stability and functionality when fortified or integrated in foods and supplements. Due to the presence of multiple double bonds, a tedious process targeting PUFAs is oxidative degradation or lipid peroxidation, which leads to primary products such as hydroperoxides and subsequent secondary reactive products, including lipid free radicals, as shown in Fig. 33.4. These reactive species will accelerate further oxidation of lipids and damage proteins and nucleic acids, causing health concerns (Prisacaru, 2016). During processing, transportation, and storage, due to the presence of multiple unsaturated bonds, they are highly susceptible to oxidation, which in turn results in decreased consumer acceptance, nutritional value, and stability with the presence of harmful oxidation products (Prisacaru, 2016; Ruiz Ruiz et al., 2017). For instance, without protective measures, omega-3 PUFAs in vegetable oils rapidly degrade and cause the oil to be unsuitable for incorporation into longer shelf-life foods (Ruiz Ruiz et al., 2017).

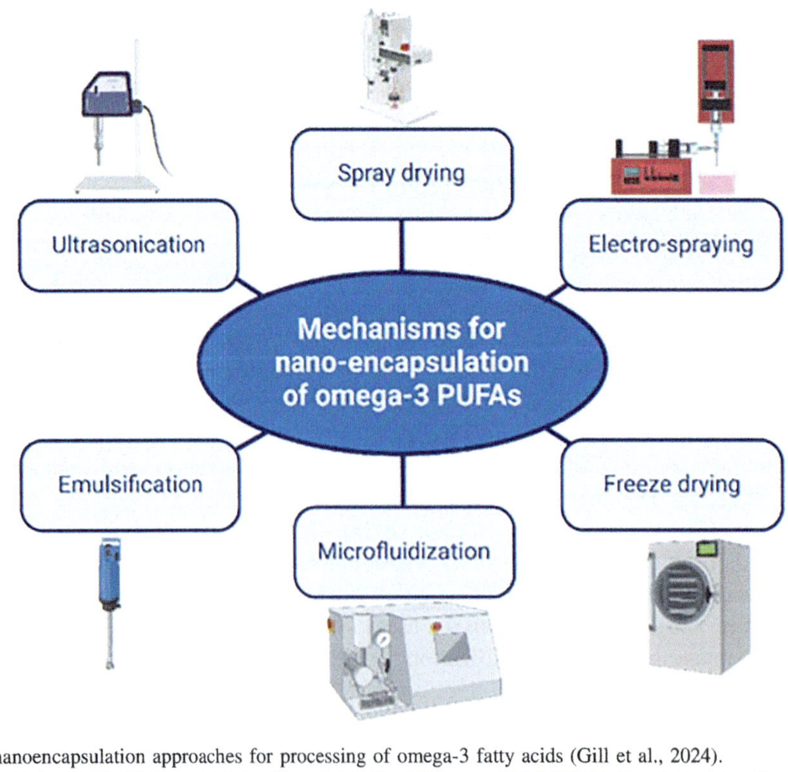

FIGURE 33.3 Different nanoencapsulation approaches for processing of omega-3 fatty acids (Gill et al., 2024).
From Gill, R., Al-Badr, M., Alghouti, M., Mohamed, N.A., Abou-Saleh, H. & Rahman, M.M. (2024). Revolutionizing Cardiovascular Health with Nano Encapsulated Omega-3 Fatty Acids: A Nano-Solution Approach. Marine Drugs, 22(6). https://doi.org/10.3390/md22060256.

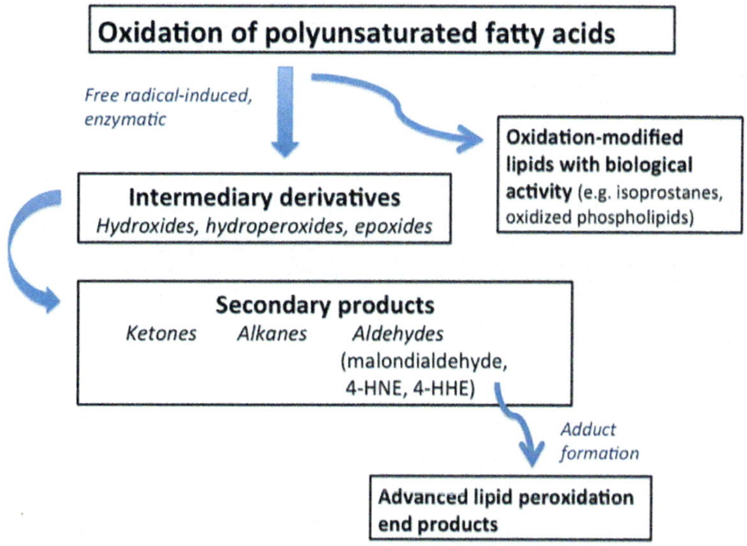

FIGURE 33.4 Formation of lipid oxidative product during lipid peroxidation (Ahotupa, 2024).
From Ahotupa, M. (2024). Lipid oxidation products and the risk of cardiovascular diseases: Role of lipoprotein transport. Antioxidants, 13(5), 512. https://doi.org/10.3390/antiox13050512.

Diverse strategies have been developed to increase the oxidative stability and enhance the shelf life of PUFA-incorporated and rich products. One such strategy is the integration of antioxidants, which minimize oxidative damage by scavenging free radicals and inhibiting the propagation of lipid peroxidation. Phenolic compounds, a type of natural antioxidant present in extra virgin olive oil, have been shown to recover PUFA stability by decreasing the degradation rate when mixed with oils rich in PUFAs. The presence of extra virgin olive oil offers slower PUFA degradation and minimizes the formation of secondary oxidation compounds during transportation and storage (González-Hedström et al., 2020)

Another key technique to enhance oxidative stability is the design of emulsion-based delivery systems and encapsulation techniques. Emulsions such as multilayer, gelled, and Pickering emulsions can be customized in terms of interfacial and structural properties to defend PUFAs during storage and transportation. Crucial factors influencing the interfacial barrier against oxidation are the selection and modification of emulsifiers (Wang et al., 2020). Moreover, PUFAs located at the sn-2 position are more prone to oxidation, and the positional distribution of FAs in triacylglycerides influences oxidative stability. With higher PUFA contents, they tend to have lower oxidative stability and shorter shelf-life, which is indicated through thermal decomposition studies, but natural antioxidants present in some kinds of oils can retard this effect (Gao & Birch, 2016). In recent times, chemically reinforced PUFAs such as deuterated polyunsaturated fatty acids have been researched, and found that modified PUFAs slow oxidation via the kinetic isotope effect, inhibiting lipid peroxidation and reactive oxygen species accumulation, thus potentially enhancing stability and decreasing oxidation (Beaudoin-Chabot et al., 2019).

33.3.2 Encapsulation technologies

Stabilization of PUFAs through technological advancements has largely influenced encapsulation techniques, namely, nanoemulsion, microencapsulation, liposomes, and nanogels. These techniques address the major challenges, such as oxidation, instability, and poor water solubility. Nanoemulsions are a promising technology for stabilization of PUFA, as their ability to encapsulate fat-soluble bioactives below 200 nm is very effective. This strategy enhances the chemical and physical stability of PUFAs by minimizing the oxidative condition and can enhance bioavailability (Ezhilarasi et al., 2013; Karthik & Anandharamakrishnan, 2016). Protein-based nanoemulsion with the use of an emulsifier such as lactoferrin has enhanced protection of omega-3 PUFAs against stability and oxidation and releases PUFAs in a controlled manner depending on pH, showing stability at lower temperatures (Nunes et al., 2020). Nanoemulsions made with pinenut oil formulated with phospholipid stabilizers have been used for drug delivery as well as to protect and target the bioactive delivery (Tiwari et al., 2006). Nanoemulsion technologies such as high-pressure homogenization and ultrasonication have enabled the formation of nanoemulsions with improved stability and efficiency in encapsulating sensitive PUFAs

(Banasaz et al., 2020). Fusion of nanomaterials combining liposomes and nanogels has been fabricated to create structures that offer controlled release and enhance biostability with potential application in nutrient preservation and delivery of drugs (Sugawara et al., 2006).

Cross-linked polymer networks in the nanoscale range are nanogels, which are emerging vehicles for bioactive encapsulation, such as PUFAs, due to their high swelling capacity, surface functional capabilities to enhance encapsulation efficiency, and tunable size. Certain research and studies indicate that nanogels can increase the bioavailability and stability of encapsulated substances and also develop stimuli-responsive and targeted delivery abilities (Neamtu et al., 2017; Vinogradov, 2006). Furthermore, nanogels are beneficial in preventing microbial spoilage with the integration of natural compounds (Abdollahi et al., 2024). Incorporation of structural elements such as phytosterols in nanoemulsion has decreased off-flavor and oxidation in PUFA-rich oils such as algae oil, which improves organoleptic and storage properties (Chen et al., 2016).

33.3.3 Smart packaging technologies to enhance polyunsaturated fatty acid shelf-life

Nowadays, the shelf-life of PUFA is significantly enhanced by smart packaging technologies through incorporating intelligent and active systems to increase food quality and safety. Critical factors such as PUFA oxidation and stability are delayed with the help of active packaging integrated with additives such as antimicrobial agents, moisture absorbers, antioxidants, and oxygen scavengers (Nasution et al., 2023; Kadirvel et al., 2024). Delaying lipoxidation for PUFA-rich sources can be enhanced by embedding antioxidants derived from natural extracts in matrices made of polylactic acid, which creates an active packaging material. This kind of strategy physically protects oxidation and chemically stabilizes the shelf-life and protects nutritional value (Nasution et al., 2023). In intelligent packaging, sensors and smart labels are used in PUFA integrated product packaging that helps in monitoring quality, freshness, gas composition, and provides real-time information about the product packed. Due to real-time monitoring, intelligent packaging aids in the detection of oxidation and spoilage and helps in managing proper storage and reducing contamination (Biji et al., 2015; Mkhari et al., 2025). Combined usage of modified atmospheric package and smart packaging, which contains antimicrobial and antioxidant compounds, will protect products such as fish and seafood rich in PUFA from oxidation, improve stability, and reduce microbial growth (Tsironi & Taoukis, 2018).

33.4 Polyunsaturated fatty acid integration into emerging food sectors

PUFA has become an emerging constituent for food fortification to overcome nutritional deficiencies and to improve the nutritional value in multiple food sectors. Modern and fast foods in many countries use saturated fats that cause multiple metabolic diseases, including cardiovascular disorders, diabetes, and obesity, etc. To overcome these detrimental effects, many foods are being incorporated with PUFA to improve the health benefits (Shahidi and Ambigaipalan, 2018; Vijaykrishnaraj et al., 2024). PUFAs extracted from seeds such as flax, chia, etc., are used in plant-based alternatives. In functional food systems such as beverages and bars, emulsion and encapsulation in nano and micro ranges provide an enhanced delivery mechanism. PUFA integration is also widely seen in insect and algae-based foods and cultured meat with optimized texture and flavor. Fermented microalgal oils can be used as an excellent PUFA source for fortification. Supplements in capsule form are widely present, but their bioavailability is questionable due to various biological factors. Alternatively, nanoemulsions of 50–500 nm sizes and encapsulated forms have better viability of PUFA in the food systems (Sun et al., 2015).

33.4.1 Plant-based and vegan alternatives

Omega-3 oils used in different Chinese recipes, including flaxseed oil (for ALA) in a citrus-based salad, perilla seed oil (for ALA) in steamed tofu, and seaweed (for EPA) based nori buns, thisplant-based foods improved heart health, brain health, cognitive and memory power, etc. Emulsified and encapsulated PUFA are incorporated in beverages to overcome the lipophilicity of the PUFA in aqueous systems. Inapurapu et al. (2020) and Gulotta et al. (2014) reported that the "colloidal delivery system" was effective in beverages to improve the clarity of the product. Algal-DHA oil in emulsified form has been granted generally recognized as safe (GRAS) status and is used as a vegan alternative to PUFA in food fortification. "OceansOmega," a USA-based company, has stabilized a DHA-based PUFA source for juices, water, and other carbonated fizzy drinks (Saini et al., 2021). Plant-based beverages are used as a substitute for dairy for vegans. Although they lack multiple nutrients, including protein, PUFA, vitamins, and minerals, etc. Some research has documented that the use of fish oil in vegetable or fruit juice negatively affected palatability (Pandey et al., 2025).

33.4.2 Functional foods and beverages

Eggs are nutrient-dense and are considered "effective nutrient carriers of dietary bioactives" due to their structure, of containing both hydrophilic and hydrophobic ends. Hence, they can be used to produce PUFA fortified functional eggs (Ma et al., 2026). Introducing fish oil, algal oil, or other omega-3 PUFA-rich seed oils, such as flax or chia, into the yolk increases the EPA and DHA content of the food component. Other than this, eggs are rich in choline, protein, selenium, and other major trace minerals. These benefits enable such functional eggs as fortifiers in the maternal diet and carriers in beverages, supplements, etc. (Lemahieu et al., 2015). Kralik et al. (2021) reported that the incorporation of 1.5% of fish oil enhanced the PUFA content to 327 mg/100 g of egg from 205 mg/100 g of egg. Microalgal oil provides high-purity DHA. Similarly, plant seed oils such as flaxseed and linseed oil provide high-quality ALA. When compared with multiple PUFA sources for egg fortification, fish oil provides the highest DHA/EPA, but it may negatively impact the flavor and sensory quality and oxidative stability (Bailey et al., 2024).

Similarly, Lipilina and Ganji (2009) reported improved PUFA (linolenic and LA) and fiber in bread. Apart from nutritional enrichment, flaxseed gum enhanced the viscosity and other crucial parameters of bread, such as loaf volume and palatability, and decreased the staling of bread (Wang et al., 2010). Matumoto-Pintro et al. (2011) utilized flax lignin to improve the oxidative stability of dairy beverages. With similar benefits, chia seed oil can be used as an emulsifier and stabilizer in dairy and baked goods. Dawczynski et al. (2010) studied the health effects of PUFA supplementation in dairy products. Approximately 50 participants in a double-blind controlled trial, split into two groups, were fed with PUFA-supplemented and control dairy beverages. The lipid levels were tested to understand that the total cholesterol and low-density lipoprotein/high-density lipoprotein ratio were lowered significantly. These results showed the potential of PUFA-supplemented products to improve cardio health.

Saini et al. (2021) reported that future research should focus on producing PUFA-rich vegan-based mayonnaise, smoothies, ice creams, salads, etc. Various microalgae used in dairy products were documented by Andrade-Bustamante et al. (2025). *Chlorella vulgaris* and *Sargassum wightii* improved the antioxidant capacity and other micro-minerals such as zinc, potassium, iron, etc. *Pavlova lutheri* was used as a source of PUFA in yogurt and also enhanced antiinflammatory activity. *Schizochytrium sp.* was used to extract DHA oil to be incorporated in candy, jam, and jellies. Similarly, DHA oil from the powder of *Dunaliella salina* was incorporated into bread, cookies, crackers, and fermented products, such as tofu. While DHA oil from *Auxenochlorella protothecoides*was used in beverages such as soups, juices, sauces, and oil (Sidari & Tofalo, 2019).

Incorporation of PUFA in foods enhances the nutritional aspect of the functional foods and beverages. During fortification, techniques such as emulsion and encapsulation improve the stability and bioavailability of the food. Many PUFA sources, such as fish oil and algal oil, leave off-flavors that impact the sensory result. This aspect during product development is to be checked and improved. Multiple case studies and randomized control trials on the PUFA-enriched and fortified functional foods and beverages should be done to demonstrate the efficacy of the health benefits.

33.5 Case studies on polyunsaturated fatty acid-enriched product development

PUFAs, particularly omega-3 FAs such as EPA and DHA, are increasingly incorporated into novel food products to address dietary deficiencies linked to cardiovascular health and cognitive function. This chapter elaborates case studies on PUFA-enriched product development, drawing from academic research to illustrate technological innovations in emerging sectors.

33.5.1 Microalgae polyunsaturated fatty acid in chicken patties

PUFAs derived from microalgae sources are progressively used as effective components to fortify the meat products, including chicken patties, to increase their omega-3 FAs profile and complete nutritional value. A current case study validated that PUFAs extracted from microalgae can be integrated into chicken patty interpretations at varying levels (e.g., 1%-3%), leading to a measurable increase in fat content and omega-3 FAs fortification while maintaining acceptable physicochemical properties during frozen storage. These outcomes and the feasibility of using microalgae PUFAs as an ecological substitute to traditional animal-based or fish oil sources for increasing the health-promoting potential of treated meat products (Santin et al., 2022; Zaman et al., 2023). From a quality stability perspective, the case study showed that PUFA-enhanced patties experienced a minor rise in lipid oxidation markers (such as thiobarbituric acid reactive substances) throughout storage, replicating the natural susceptibility of unsaturated fats to oxidation. Humidity content also changed over time, with the control (nonsupplemented) patties holding more humidity initially, while the higher-PUFA treatments demonstrated slightly lower humidity at the end of storage. Although these changes, the microbiological safety and basic textural aspects remained within tolerable limits, indicating that the microalgae PUFAs can be incorporated into chicken patties without major compromise to product shelf life under normal glacial conditions (Remize et al., 2021).

Sensory assessment exposed that increasing PUFA levels from microalgae led to a steady decline in overall tolerability scores, likely due to refined off-flavors or texture modifications associated with higher lipid oxidation. However, the sensory scores for all PUFA-supplemented treatments still fell within a standard range compared with the control, suggesting moderate consumer tolerability if used at optimized levels. The case study therefore recommends that microalgae-PUFA-supplemented chicken patties be combined with suitable antioxidants or enhanced processing protocols to reduce oxidation and maintain palatability, thereby positioning them as feasible functional meat products for health-oriented consumers (Liu and Ren, 2022b).

33.5.2 Fish oil dairy fortification

Dairy products highlight efforts to enhance nutritional profile, achieved through the incorporation of omega-3 FAs, such as EPA and DHA, into items such as milk, yogurt, cheese, and butter. Researchers experienced purified fish oil in several dairy matrices, finding that solid, high-fat products, such as processed cheese and spreadable fresh cheese tolerated higher fortification levels (up to levels providing 180 mg of long-chain omega-3 per 30 g serving) without major sensory issues, particularly when additives masked off-notes. Yogurt-like semiliquid products were limited to 1–5 g/kg fish oil to maintain tolerability over 4 weeks of storage (Soto-Méndez et al., 2019).

In recent years, there have been improvements in milk fortification with new methods, such as using quite solid lipid micro and nanoparticles made with supercritical CO_2; this makes the milk more stable and easier to absorb. With these methods, the body absorbed 92.8% of the fish oil and kept EPA/DHA levels up for about three weeks, compared to regular fish oil, which only lasted about a week. This lab test also displayed that encapsulated omega-3 had 40% bioavailability, compared to 27% for normal forms. These techniques can help allow for a clean, easy mix into drinks while also reducing oxidation and fishy taste (Yang et al., 2024).

33.5.3 Microalgae single-cell oil (docosahexaenoic acid) infant formula

Algae-based single-cell oil, which contains a lot of DHA, is increasingly being used as a good alternative to fish oil DHA in infant formula. The oils with 40% to 43% DHA are obtained by reliable and secure strains such as *Schizochytrium limacinum* and *Crypthecodinium cohnii* under optimized conditions. These can be mixed with other oils and put into baby formula at about the same amount as what is in human milk, usually 20 to 50 mg of DHA per 100 kcal. Groups such as the European Food Safety Authority (EFSA) and FSANZ have checked out these algae oils and said they aren't bad for you, work just like other DHA sources, and are okay to put in baby formula without messing with growth (Turck et al., 2023).

Microalgae-based DHA is great for product development and the market because it skips the marine gunk and allergens you get with fish oil. If you're a vegetarian or have allergies, this is for you. Plus, it's easier on our fish populations. A study of healthy babies showed that formulas with algal DHA are just as good for growth and digestion as regular formulas, a nutritious ingredient. Microalgae single-cell oil is a cool thing in baby food. It's safe, works well, and is good for the environment. It fits right into what people want now in baby formula (Ochsenreither et al., 2016).

33.5.4 Algal polyunsaturated fatty acid aquaculture feed

This study looks at ways to replace fish oil in margarine-type stuff with sustainable options. Certain microbes, such as *Mortierella alpina* and *Yarrowia lipolytica*, can make cool PUFAs, such as arachidonic acid , GLA, and EPA. They do this by fermentation when things are tweaked just right, such as limiting nitrogen, and can end up with up to 40% fat. Plants, such as flaxseed or chia seed, give us α-linolenic acid (ALA), and modified crops are getting better at turning stearidonic acid into stuff we can use (Ferreira et al., 2021). These alternatives allow us to create heart-healthy spreads with lower inflammation, avoiding that fishy taste and the concern about catching innumerable fish. It can also add probiotics to these vegetable oil spreads, and they'll stay good for a few weeks. Increasing the size of the fermentation tanks along with the modification of the microbes increases the yield, which makes it useful for food technology.

33.6 Regulatory and safety considerations

The quick development of the PUFA into functional foods, nutraceuticals, plant-based products, fortified food and beverage usage makes it stronger to link with the regulatory safety considerations. Due to their sensitivity to contamination issues and the oxidation process. Safety testing is mandatory for purity identifications, shelf life, and labeling identifications. Overall, to maintain the consumers' quality food consumption and technological innovations, the food industry and regulatory bodies need to maintain these risk evaluation methods for each manufacturer's product (Khan et al., 2023).

The Food and Drug Administration (FDA) in the US uses the GRAS framework to regulate PUFA compounds. For some dietary uses, long-chain omega-3 FAs such as EPA and DHA, which are frequently obtained from fish oil or microalgae, have been granted GRAS certification. Comprehensive scientific evidence, such as toxicological tests, compositional analysis, intake evaluation, and historical consumption data, proving safety under the intended circumstances of use, is necessary for GRAS determination. Manufacturers can alert the FDA for evaluation of GRAS status (Mititelu et al., 2024). Specific labeling is mandatory for the consumer, transparent, and regulatory management. At least the sources of the omega and their manufacturing details, expiry date, and instructions for consuming are necessary to be mentioned on the label of the product. Overall, the safety of the PUFA-based food products needs to fulfill the consumers' needs as well as organizations such as the FDA, EFSA, and FSSAI regulations. On the other hand, packaging and transportation are another important part of product development in food industries. Commonly, nitrogen flushing, cold-chain storage, light-protective containers, and oxygen-impermeable material technologies are used in industries (Hoppenbrouwers et al., 2019; Chang et al., 2023; Finco et al., 2016). Here, shelf life needs to be monitored due to the oxidation stability of the PUFAs presented in plant-based meat alternatives, dairy alternatives, and infant formula. Alternatively, technologies such as microencapsulation methods provide hope for the product sensitive FAs from the oxidation process while enhancing the sensory stability.

33.7 Consumer perception and market trends

Consumer demand for PUFAs, especially long-chain PUFAs such as EPA and DHA, is driven by increasing public awareness of their putative health benefits (such as cardiovascular, neurodevelopmental, and antiinflammatory effects), simultaneous growth in the development of functional food, and expanding the uses of nutraceutical and fortified foods (Li et al., 2022). Recent market analyses also indicate a very stable and steady growth in PUFA markets, with forecasts projecting compound annual growth rates in a mid-single-digit percentage range through the 2025–2035 horizon (Future Market Insights, 2025; Coherent Market Insights, 2025). These macro trends interact with consumer perceptions, regulatory contexts, and innovations in sustainable PUFA sourcing in products such as microalgae, microbial fermentation, and upcycled seafood by-products.

Considering the consumer knowledge, attitudes, and drivers, many surveys and observational studies show that most of the consumers perceive omega-3 PUFAs as "natural," safe, and beneficial, and these beliefs correlate strongly with supplement and fortified-food intakes (Hitl et al., 2024). Motivations for purchase vary by demographic: older adults tend to cardiovascular and cognitive health claims, while parents and those planning for pregnancy focus on developmental benefits for children and infants (Hitl et al., 2024; Li et al., 2022). However, there are still knowledge gaps that exist. Research reveals differences in knowledge on recommended doses, the research base for different purposes, and EPA versus DHA (Hitl et al., 2024). Prominently, high-profile observational and trial data indicate both benefits and potential risks (e.g., recent large observational reports linking certain fish-oil supplement patterns with a small increase in atrial fibrillation or stroke risk in some populations) have begun to nuance public perceptions, and clinical advice for increasing demand for clearer and more physician guidance (Albert, 2021). Thus trust and provenance are the two key parameters for purchase determinants. Consumers are increasingly valuing sustainability labels (certified sourcing, and traceability), and they evaluate food products not only on perceived health benefits, but also on sustainability-related labeling and transparency mechanisms, which significantly influence perceived product value and credibility (Grunert, 2011). In addition, "plant-based" positioning and third-party quality verification contribute to building consumer confidence, particularly among ethically and environmentally conscious segments (Hartmann & Siegrist, 2017).

33.7.1 Market segmentation and commercial trends

The PUFA market encompasses dietary supplements, infant and medical nutrition, functional foods (including fortified foods, dairy substitutes, and bread items), as well as feed and animal nutrition sectors. Market studies report a worldwide PUFA market size in the multibillion USD range, with significant expansion anticipated between 2025 and 2035, driven by increasing demand for functional foods, regulatory endorsement for fortification, and heightened interest in sustainable alternatives to fish oil. Thus the global market forecasts suggest the PUFA market projection to experience a steady growth, as given in Table 33.2 (Future Market Insights, 2025; Coherent Market Insights, 2025).

TABLE 33.2 Summarizes recently published projection estimates.

Sources	Reported 2025 estimate	Forecast horizon CAGR
Future Market Insights, (2025)	~USD 6.69 billion	CAGR ~5.5% to (2025–35)
Coherent Market Insights, (2025)	~USD 7.4 billion	Forecast to 2032 with ~8% CAGR
Market Research Future (2025)	~USD billion 50.38	CAGR ~4.52% (2025–35)

When it comes to supply-side innovations and changing market dynamics, the architecture of consumer choice is mainly evolving due to two supply-side trends. First, nonmarine sources of EPA/DHA that cater to the vegan and vegetarian markets are provided by microalgae and engineered microorganisms; their commercial introductions and increased production efficiency have led to increased retail availability (Omokaro et al., 2025; Swetha & Mathanghi, 2024). Second, advances in precision fermentation and metabolic engineering allow companies to produce tailored PUFA profiles (e.g., higher EPA or DHA ratios) and coproduce value-added coproducts in biorefinery models, potentially lowering the cost as the scale improves (Qin et al., 2023). Diverse regulatory environments exist; fortification regulations and acceptable claims impact product positioning; health claims for omega-3s are permitted in certain countries but prohibited in others. Additionally, new safety warnings and inconsistent train results have prompted regulators and doctors to communicate more cautiously (source, EPA/DHA content, third-party verification). Transparent labeling (source, EPA/DHA content, third-party verification) and unambiguous instructions on targeted demographics and dosages are now essential for consumer acceptability. Overall, the consumer perception of PUFA products is increasingly molded by three main themes: one, health efficacy as per the evolving clinical evidence; two, sustainability, provenance concerns, and trustworthiness that are signaled by quality testing with clear labeling. The second and third most significant impediments are the downstream processing. PUFAs are highly prone to oxidative degradation, which reduces nutritional value acceptability.

33.8 Future perspectives and challenges

Prospects and difficulties for the future, the combined demands of precision nutrition and sustainability are rapidly driving the research and commercialization of PUFA requirements. Although the long-term sustainability of PUFA supply will rely on technological and technical improvements, cost-effectiveness scaling, environmental accountability, and translational innovation, notwithstanding the notable advancements made in various sources of production systems. Coordinated integration is required, such as digital system usage, circular bioeconomy frameworks, and the integration of research in the above, which is necessary for future innovative developments.

33.8.1 Technological gaps and R&D directions, potential for AI and biotechnology in polyunsaturated fatty acid optimization

One of the primary technological challenges remains improving biosynthetic efficiency in alternative PUFA production platforms. Historically, marine fisheries, which are dominant in the omega-3 supply chain, have faced ecological limitations and variability in raw material quality. Consequently, the substitute to the above is the microalgae and oleaginous microorganisms that are gaining attention for scalable industries capable of producing EPA and DHA products under controlled conditions. As a result, microalgae and oleaginous microorganisms are also becoming more popular recently, since they are scalable enterprises that can produce DHA and EPA under regulated conditions (Karageorgou et al., 2023; Chang et al., 2023). However, the lipid accumulation is often caused by stress conditions under hindered growth rates, resulting in a trade-off between biomass productivity and PUFA production. The production of omega-3 LC-PUFAs from nonmarine hosts is now possible thanks to developments in metabolic engineering, specifically the targeted modulation of desaturase and elongase enzymes, which have increased the carbon flux towards long-chain FA synthesis in both microbial and heterogenous plant systems (Qin et al., 2023; Ruiz-López et al., 2012). Despite these gains, the industrial translation required improved genetic stability, resistance to contamination, and clarity in regulatory standards for the industrial translation.

The extreme sensitivity of long-chain PUFAs to oxidation, which can adversely affect the sensory qualities and nutritional values of oils, makes the downstream processing of PUFAs a considerable technological problem. With this context, recent research studies showed that the use of supercritical carbon dioxide extraction has been widely studied as a part of a greener alternative to solvent extraction, offering lower oxidation risk and improved selectivity and stability compared to traditional methods (Rubio-Rodríguez et al., 2012). Similar to that, another methodology that has been a very innovative approach, such as ultrasound and subcritical technologies, is also showing promise in improving yield and reducing oxidative degradation during the stage of processing (Marsol-Vall et al., 2022). With the growing need for food items that are both technologically sophisticated and nutritionally enriched, PUFAs, especially omega-3 FAs, have gained significant interest in the new generation of food industries. To maximize PUFA synthesis, stability, and functional usage, cutting-edge technologies such as artificial intelligence tools are being investigated. Recent advancements also indicate that artificial intelligence (AI) is beginning to support omega-3 FA research and food applications.

Omega-3 FAs, including ALA, EPA, and DHA, are essential nutrients obtained primarily through dietary sources such as fish and algae. The integration of AI with multiomics techniques can help to design for increased production efficiency, as well as generate system-level insights into organisms that produce omega-3 FAs (Puranik, 2025). In food processing contexts, artificial neural network (ANN) models have demonstrated strong capability to predict the optimization of nutritional quality parameters.

This demonstrates that the potential of AI-guided modeling can be used to maintain thermal processing on the quality of lipids. Beyond production and processing, machine learning approaches have also been used to assess correlations between dietary omega-3 consumption and biological ageing indicators, in addition, to synthesis and processing, highlighting the relevance of computational tools in nutritional evaluation (Yan et al., 2025). Collectively, these studies demonstrate and provide a positive approach that AI functions not just as a computational tool, but also enables a framework supporting PUFA optimization, quality preservation, and nutritional assessment within emerging food sectors. Table 33.3 shows technological advances in PUFA utilization.

33.8.2 Economic barriers and scale-up concerns, sustainability, and circular economy approaches

Economic scalability is another key consideration. Significant capital expenditure is required for microalgal cultivation systems, particularly for sterile-fermentation infrastructure and closed photobioreactors. Production costs are strongly influenced by energy input, source of nutrients, and downstream purification requirements. By facilitating the covalorization of proteins, pigments, and carbohydrates, and residual biomass in addition to PUFA extraction, the biorefinery idea presents a possible solution (Torres-Tiji et al., 2020). At the same time, price sensitivity remains an important moderating factor in retail decision-making. While a few segments of health-oriented and higher-income consumers demonstrate willingness to pay for premium products that have been significantly aligned with sustainability and health claims, in fact, the broader market has been constrained by price perceptions (Aschemann-Witzel & Zielke, 2017). Also, the large-scale production of microalgal omega-3 FAs has remained constrained by high cultivation and downstream processing costs, particularly in comparison with the conventional fish oil supply (Adarme-Vega et al., 2012). Hence, this evidence also suggests that although consumers express positive attitudes towards sustainable and high-quality food products, actual buying behavior frequently reflects a balance between ethical preference and economic affordability.

TABLE 33.3 Technological advances in polyunsaturated fatty acid (PUFA) utilization.

Technology	Application	Advantage	Key reference
Mircoalgal fermentation	Eicosapentaenoic acid/docosahexaenoic acid production	Nonmarine source	Chen et al. (2023)
Metabolic engineering	LC-PUFA synthesis	Host flexibility	Ruiz-Lopez et al. (2012)
Artificial neural network optimization	Thermal processing	Improved PUFA/saturated fatty acids	Sadhu et al. (2021)
Supercritical carbon dioxide extraction	Downstream purification	Reduced oxidation	Rubio-Rodríguez et al. (2012)

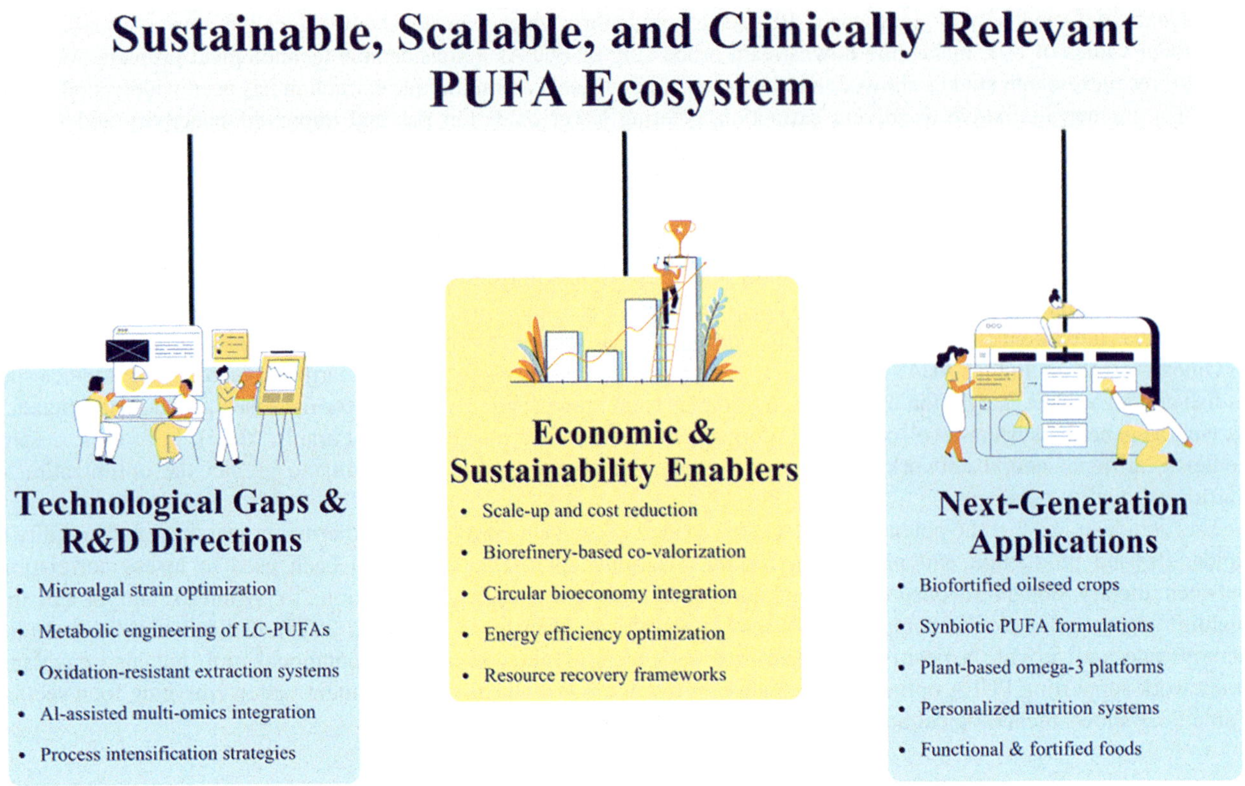

FIGURE 33.5 Future technological road map for integration of sustainable, economic, and next-generation applications.

33.8.3 Next-generation polyunsaturated fatty acid applications (biofortified crops and synbiotic polyunsaturated fatty acid products)

Beyond production challenges, biofortification of oilseed crops such as *Camelina sativa* with microalgal biosynthesis genes has enabled terrestrial production of long-chain omega-3 FAs, including EPA and DHA, reducing reliance on marine sources (Petrie et al., 2014). Engineered Camelina oils containing these PUFAs have shown compositional stability, efficacy, and acceptable applications compared to traditional fish oils. In addition to crop biofortification strategies, evolving innovations are also exploring and gaining increasing attention for enhancing stability, bioavailability, and metabolic outcomes of symbiotic PUFA formulations that combine omega-3 FAs with probiotic or prebiotic components, which increases the interaction between dietary omega-3 FAs and the gut microbiota. Thus, these compositions may influence inflammatory regulation and lipid metabolism (Costantini et al., 2017). Integrating the PUFA delivery system with probiotic carriers has therefore been proposed as one of the promising functional strategies, particularly for the personalized and preventive nutrition contexts. Such approaches may improve both intestinal absorption and simultaneously support gut health. Hence, expanding the therapeutic and commercial applications for next-generation PUFA-enriched foods (Gibson et al., 2017). Fig. 33.5 shows the future possible road map of integrating technological, economical, and next-generation applications for obtaining a sustainable, scalable, and clinically relevant PUFA ecosystem. Such advances will support the feasibility of plant-based omega-3 platforms for sustainable nutritional supply. However, unified regulatory guidelines, validated reports, and technologies are needed to translate these methods into consumer goods and clinical practice.

33.9 Conclusion

Due to their predominant health benefits, the development of innovative food products, and sustainability, PUFA gets more attention. At the same time, the increasing demand for the PUFAs highlights the need for sufficient, cost-effective, and environmentally sustainable sources. Moreover, an innovative opportunity to improve PUFA production will be possible in the future, which is a combination of genetic engineering, fermentation technologies, and modern biotechnology. When combined, these strategies not only increase the variety of PUFA sources but also provide economical and environmentally friendly ways for satisfying the growing demand worldwide. These developments will be crucial to meeting the demands of consumers for healthier foods, resolving global nutritional security, and preserving ecological balance. The future of PUFA use therefore depends on embracing multidisciplinary concepts that link health benefits, technological developments, and sustainability goals.

References

Abdollahi, A., Fereydouni, N., Moradi, H., Karimivaselabadi, A., Zarenezhad, E., & Osanloo, M. (2024). Nanoformulated herbal compounds: Enhanced antibacterial efficacy of camphor and thymol-loaded nanogels. *BMC Complementary Medicine and Therapies, 24*(1). https://doi.org/10.1186/s12906-024-04435-z.

Adarme-Vega, T. C., Lim, D. K. Y., Timmins, M., Vernen, F., Li, Y., & Schenk, P. M. (2012). Microalgal biofactories: A promising approach towards sustainable omega-3 fatty acid production. *Microbial Cell Factories, 11*. https://doi.org/10.1186/1475-2859-11-96Australia, http://www.microbialcellfactories.com/content/11/1/96.

Ahmed, Z. H. T., Singh, P., Shankar, R., Kumar, S., Sarkar, D., Noor Shah, U., & Hassan, S. (2026). *Unleashing the nutritional power of sunflower seeds, pumpkin seeds, chia seeds, flaxseeds, and hemp seeds*. Elsevier BV, 99–128. https://doi.org/10.1016/b978-0-443-33488-7.00003-5.

Ahotupa, M. (2024). Lipid oxidation products and the risk of cardiovascular diseases: Role of lipoprotein transport. *Antioxidants, 13*(5), 512.

Albert, C.M. (2021). Effect of long-term marine omega-3 fatty acids supplementation on the risk of atrial fibrillation in randomized controlled trials of cardiovascular outcomes: A systematic review and meta-analysis.

Alao, A. I. (2025). A critical review on vegetable oils refining: a case for local reagents application. *International Journal of Research and Scientific Innovation, 12*(10), 2865–2879. https://doi.org/10.51244/ijrsi.2025.1210000247.

Alcorta, A., Porta, A., Tárrega, A., Alvarez, M. D., & Vaquero, M. P. (2021). Foods for plant-based diets: challenges and innovations. *Foods, 10*(2), 293. 10.3390/foods10020293.

Andrade-Bustamante, G., Martínez-Ruiz, F. E., Ortega-García, J., Renganathan, P., Gaysina, L. A., Mahendhiran, M., & Puente, E. O. R. (2025). Microalgae-based functional foods: a blue-green revolution in sustainable nutrition and health. *Applied Microbiology, 5*(2), 39. 10.3390/applmicrobiol5020039.

Aschemann-Witzel, J., & Zielke, S. (2017). Can't buy me green? A review of consumer perceptions of and behavior toward the price of organic food. *Journal of Consumer Affairs, 51*(1), 211–251. https://doi.org/10.1111/joca.12092.

Assefa, M., Zhao, Y., Zhou, C., Song, Y., & Zhao, X. (2025). Advancements in crop PUFAs biosynthesis and genetic engineering: A systematic and mixed review system. *International Journal of Molecular Sciences, 26*(8), 3462. https://doi.org/10.3390/ijms26083462.

Ayub, A., Rahayu, F., Khamidah, A., Antarlina, S. S., Iswari, K., Supriyadi, K., Mufidah, E., Singh, A., Chopra, C., & Wani, A. K. (2025). Harnessing microalgae as a bioresource for nutraceuticals: Advancing bioactive compound exploration and shaping the future of health and functional food innovation. *Discover Applied Sciences, 7*(5). https://doi.org/10.1007/s42452-025-06916-3, https://link.springer.com/journal/42452.

Ayele, T. M., Abera, M. K., Yohannes, T. G., Amera, G. M., Sahlu, A. B., et al. (2025). *Green energy and technology,sustainable development research in manufacturing, process engineering, green infrastructure, and water resources*. Springer Nature Switzerland, 279–295. https://doi.org/10.1007/978-3-031-77339-6_17.

Azizi, R., Baggio, A., Capuano, E., & Pellegrini, N. (2024). Protein transition: focus on protein quality in sustainable alternative sources. *Critical Reviews in Food Science and Nutrition, 65*(18), 3401–3421. https://doi.org/10.1080/10408398.2024.2365339.

Babu, V. V. P., Gupta, M. S., & Khan, M. A. (2025). A review on development and performance evaluation of a cold pressed oil extraction machine. In *AIP conference proceedings, Vol. 3342*AIP Publishing020020 No. 1.

Bailey, E., Wojcik, J., Rahn, M., Roos, F., Spooren, A., & Koshibu, K. (2024). *Microalgal oil as an alternative source of essential nutrients omega-3 DHA and EPA*. Research Square. https://www.researchsquare.com/browse, https://doi.org/10.21203/rs.3.rs-5111519/v1.

Bhashira, R., & Gopalakrishnan, S. (2025). The association between seafood consumption and non-seafood consumption with serum levels of non-HDL cholesterol. *Romanian Journal of Diabetes Nutrition and Metabolic Diseases, 32*(2), 180–186.

Banasaz, S., Morozova, K., Ferrentino, G., & Scampicchio, M. (2020). Encapsulation of lipid-soluble bioactives by nanoemulsions. *Molecules (Basel, Switzerland), 25*(17), 3966. https://doi.org/10.3390/molecules25173966.

Biji, K. B., Ravishankar, C. N., Mohan, C. O., Srinivasa Gopal, T. K., et al. (2015). Smart packaging systems for food applications: a review. *Journal of Food Science and Technology, 52*(10), 6125–6135. https://doi.org/10.1007/s13197-015-1766-7.

Beaudoin-Chabot, C., Wang, L., Smarun, A. V., Vidović, D., Shchepinov, M. S., & Thibault, G. (2019). Deuterated polyunsaturated fatty acids reduce oxidative stress and extend the lifespan of C. Elegans. *Frontiers in Physiology, 10*(MAY). https://doi.org/10.3389/fphys.2019.00641, http://www.frontiersin.org/Physiology/archive/.

Chen, X. W., Chen, Y. J., Wang, J. M., Guo, J., Yin, S. W., & Yang, X. Q. (2016). Phytosterol structured algae oil nanoemulsions and powders: Improving antioxidant and flavor properties. *Food and Function, 7*(9), 3694–3702. https://doi.org/10.1039/c6fo00449k, http://www.rsc.org/Publishing/Journals/FO/about.asp.

Chen, W., Li, T., Du, S., Chen, H., Wang, Q., et al. (2023). Microalgal polyunsaturated fatty acids: Hotspots and production techniques. *Frontiers in Bioengineering and Biotechnology, 11*. https://doi.org/10.3389/fbioe.2023.1146881.

Chang, J. P.-C., Tseng, P.-T., Zeng, B.-S., Chang, C.-H., Su, H., Chou, P.-H., Su, K.-P., et al. (2023). Safety of supplementation of omega-3 polyunsaturated fatty acids: a systematic review and meta-analysis of randomized controlled trials. *Advances in Nutrition, 14*(6), 1326–1336. https://doi.org/10.1016/j.advnut.2023.08.003.

Cholewski, M., Tomczykowa, M., & Tomczyk, M. (2018). A comprehensive review of chemistry, sources and bioavailability of omega-3 fatty acids. *Nutrients, 10*(11), 1662.

Coherent Market Insights (2025). Polyunsaturated Fatty Acids Market Size, Trends, Analysis and Forecast 2025–2032..

Costantini, L., Molinari, R., Farinon, B., & Merendino, N. (2017). Impact of omega-3 fatty acids on the gut microbiota. *International Journal of Molecular Sciences, 18*(12), 2645. https://doi.org/10.3390/ijms18122645.

Dawczynski, C., Martin, L., Wagner, A., & Jahreis, G. (2010). n–3 LC-PUFA-enriched dairy products are able to reduce cardiovascular risk factors: A double-blind, cross-over study. *Clinical Nutrition, 29*(5), 592–599. https://doi.org/10.1016/j.clnu.2010.02.008.

Ezhilarasi, P. N., Karthik, P., Chhanwal, N., & Anandharamakrishnan, C. (2013). Nanoencapsulation techniques for food bioactive components: A review. *Food and Bioprocess Technology, 6*(3), 628–647. https://doi.org/10.1007/s11947-012-0944-0.

Ferreira, M., Fernandes, H., Peres, H., Oliva-Teles, A., Belo, I., & Salgado, J. M. (2021). Polyunsaturated fatty acids production by solid-state fermentation on polyurethane foam by *Mortierella alpina*. *Biotechnology Progress, 37*(3). https://doi.org/10.1002/btpr.3113, http://onlinelibrary.wiley.com/journal/10.1021/(ISSN)1520-6033.

Finco, A. M. de O., Mamani, L. D. G., Carvalho, J. C. de, de Melo Pereira, G. V., Thomaz-Soccol, V., & Soccol, C. R. (2016). Technological trends and market perspectives for production of microbial oils rich in omega-3. *Critical Reviews in Biotechnology, 37*(5), 656–671. https://doi.org/10.1080/07388551.2016.1213221.

Gao, F., & Birch, J. (2016). Oxidative stability, thermal decomposition, and oxidation onset prediction of carrot, flax, hemp, and canola seed oils in relation to oil composition and positional distribution of fatty acids. *European Journal of Lipid Science and Technology, 118*(7), 1042–1052. https://doi.org/10.1002/ejlt.201500208, http://onlinelibrary.wiley.com/journal/10.1002/(ISSN)1438-9312.

García-Cervantes, A. M., Ezzaitouni, M., Chileh-Chelh, T., Haddou, S., Ferjani, F. A., & Guil-Guerrero, J. L. (2026). Wild seeds as sustainable sources of C18-series bioactive fatty acids: Metabolic diversity, nutritional value, and functional applications. *Seeds (New York, N.Y.), 5*(1). https://doi.org/10.3390/seeds5010006, https://www.mdpi.com/journal/seeds.

Geetha, P., Bharathi, D., Deepa, N., Gopi, G., Begum, S., & Devi, T. (2025). Effectiveness of alpha lipoic acid in type 2 diabetes mellitus patients with cardiac autonomic neuropathy. *Asian Journal of Pharmacy and Technology, 15*(3), 286–288.

Glencross, B. D., Bachis, E., Betancor, M. B., Calder, P., Liland, N., Newton, R., & Ruyter, B. (2025). Omega-3 futures in aquaculture: Exploring the supply and demands for long-chain omega-3 essential fatty acids by aquaculture species. *Reviews in Fisheries Science and Aquaculture, 33*(2), 167–216. https://doi.org/10.1080/23308249.2024.2388563, http://www.tandfonline.com/loi/brfs20.

Gibson, G. R., Hutkins, R., Sanders, M. E., Prescott, S. L., Reimer, R. A., Salminen, S. J., Scott, K., Stanton, C., Swanson, K. S., Cani, P. D., Verbeke, K., Reid, G., et al. (2017). Expert consensus document: The International Scientific Association for Probiotics and Prebiotics (ISAPP) consensus statement on the definition and scope of prebiotics. *Nature Reviews Gastroenterology & Hepatology, 14*(8), 491–502. https://doi.org/10.1038/nrgastro.2017.75.

Gill, R., Al-Badr, M., Alghouti, M., Mohamed, N.A., Abou-Saleh, H. & Rahman, M.M. (2024). Revolutionizing Cardiovascular Health with Nano Encapsulated Omega-3 Fatty Acids: A Nano-Solution Approach. Marine Drugs, 22(6). https://doi.org/10.3390/md22060256..

González-Hedström, D., Granado, M., & Inarejos-García, A. M. (2020). Protective effects of extra virgin olive oil against storage-induced omega-3 fatty acid oxidation of algae oil. *NFS Journal, 21*, 9–15.

Grunert, K. G. (2011). Sustainability in the food sector: A consumer behaviour perspective. *International Journal on Food System Dynamics, 2*(3), 207–218. https://doi.org/10.18461/ijfsd.v2i3.232, www.centmapress.org.

Gulotta, A., Saberi, A. H., Nicoli, M. C., McClements, D. J., et al. (2014). Nanoemulsion-based delivery systems for polyunsaturated (ω-3) oils: formation using a spontaneous emulsification method. *Journal of Agricultural and Food Chemistry, 62*(7), 1720–1725. https://doi.org/10.1021/jf4054808.

Hartmann, C., & Siegrist, M. (2017). Consumer perception and behaviour regarding sustainable protein consumption: A systematic review. *Trends in Food Science & Technology, 61*, 11–25.

Hegazy, M. A, Vidovic, B., Abobakr, S., Zeljkovic, A., Stefanovic, A., Vekic, J., et al. (2025). Hidden industrial trans-fatty acids: mechanistic insights into dyslipidemia, cardiovascular disease, and metabolic dysfunction-associated steatotic liver disease. *International Journal of Molecular Sciences, 26*(23), 11715. https://doi.org/10.3390/ijms262311715.

Hitl, M., Kladar, N., Banović Fuentes, J., Bijelić, K., Đermanović, M., & Torović, L. (2024). Knowledge and consumption patterns of omega-3 fatty acids among the central Balkan population: A prospective cross-sectional study. *Nutrients, 17*(1), 122.

Hoppenbrouwers, T., Cvejić Hogervorst, J. H., Garssen, J., Wichers, H. J., Willemsen, L. E. M., et al. (2019). Long chain polyunsaturated fatty acids (LCPUFAs) in the prevention of food allergy. *Frontiers in Immunology, 10*. https://doi.org/10.3389/fimmu.2019.01118.

Inapurapu, S. P., Ibrahim, A., Kona, S. R., Pawar, S. C., Bodiga, S., Bodiga, V. L., et al. (2020). Development and characterization of ω-3 fatty acid nanoemulsions with improved physicochemical stability and bioaccessibility. *Colloids and Surfaces A: Physicochemical and Engineering Aspects, 606*, 125515. https://doi.org/10.1016/j.colsurfa.2020.125515.

Jia, Y.-L., Wang, L.-R., Zhang, Z.-X., Gu, Y., & Sun, X.-M. (2021). Recent advances in biotechnological production of polyunsaturated fatty acids by *Yarrowia lipolytica*. *Critical Reviews in Food Science and Nutrition, 61*(Suppl. 1), 8920–8934.

Jurić, S., Jurić, M., Siddique, M. A. B., & Fathi, M. (2020). Vegetable oils rich in polyunsaturated fatty acids: Nanoencapsulation methods and stability enhancement. *Food Reviews International, 38*(1), 32–69.

Kadirvel, V., Palanisamy, Y., & Ganesan, N. D. (2024). Active packaging system—An overview of recent advances for enhanced food quality and safety. *Packaging Technology and Science, 38*(2), 145–162.

Karageorgou, D., Rova, U., Christakopoulos, P., Katapodis, P., Matsakas, L., & Patel, A. (2023). Benefits of supplementation with microbial omega-3 fatty acids on human health and the current market scenario for fish-free omega-3 fatty acid. *Trends in Food Science & Technology*, 136, 169–180..

Karthik, P. (2016). *Micro and nanoencapsulation of omega-3 fatty acids by emulsion and spray-freeze-drying techniques* (Doctoral dissertation, PhD thesis, Academy of Scientific and Innovative Research, India).

Karthik, P., & Anandharamakrishnan, C. (2016). Enhancing omega-3 fatty acids nanoemulsion stability and in-vitro digestibility through emulsifiers. *Journal of Food Engineering, 187*, 92–105. https://doi.org/10.1016/j.jfoodeng.2016.05.003.

Kaur, N., Chugh, V., & Gupta, A. K. (2014). Essential fatty acids as functional components of foods: A review. *Journal of Food Science and Technology, 51*(10), 2289–2303.

Karageorgou, D., Rova, U., Christakopoulos, P., Katapodis, P., Matsakas, L., Patel, A., et al. (2023). Benefits of supplementation with microbial omega-3 fatty acids on human health and the current market scenario for fish-free omega-3 fatty acid. *Trends in Food Science & Technology, 136*, 169–180. https://doi.org/10.1016/j.tifs.2023.04.018.

Khan, I., Hussain, M., Jiang, B., Zheng, L., Pan, Y., Hu, J., Khan, A., Ashraf, A., & Zou, X. (2023). Omega-3 long-chain polyunsaturated fatty acids: Metabolism and health implications. *Progress in Lipid Research, 92*, 101255. https://doi.org/10.1016/j.plipres.2023.101255.

Kitessa, S. M., Abeywardena, M., Wijesundera, C., & Nichols, P. D. (2014). DHA-containing oilseed: A timely solution for the sustainability issues surrounding fish oil sources of the health-benefitting long-chain omega-3 oils. *Nutrients, 6*(5), 2035–2058. https://doi.org/10.3390/nu6052035, http://www.mdpi.com/2072-6643/6/5/2035/pdf.

Kralik, G., Kralik, Z., Grčević, M., Galović, O., Hanžek, D., & Biazik, E. (2021). Fatty acid profile of eggs produced by laying hens fed diets containing different shares of fish oil. *Poultry Science, 100*(10), 101379. 10.1016/j.psj.2021.101379.

Latifi, M., Jalali Bidgoli, F., Hajihassani, H., Hassani, D., Ingvarsson, P. K., & Farrokhi, N. (2025). Recent advances and future directions on GLA-producing organisms. *Frontiers in Bioengineering and Biotechnology, 13*. https://doi.org/10.3389/fbioe.2025.1567840, http://journal.frontiersin.org/journal/bioengineering-and-biotechnology#archive.

Lauritzen, L., Brambilla, P., Mazzocchi, A., Harsløf, L. B. S., Ciappolino, V., & Agostoni, C. (2016). DHA effects in brain development and function. *Nutrients, 8*(1). https://doi.org/10.3390/nu8010006, http://www.mdpi.com/2072-6643/8/1/6/pdf.

Le, H. D., Meisel, J. A., de Meijer, V. E., Gura, K. M., & Puder, M. (2009). The essentiality of arachidonic acid and docosahexaenoic acid. Prostaglandins, *Leukotrienes and Essential Fatty Acids*, 81(2–3), 165–170..

Lemahieu, C., Bruneel, C., Ryckebosch, E., Muylaert, K., Buyse, J., & Foubert, I. (2015). Impact of different omega-3 polyunsaturated fatty acid (n-3 PUFA) sources (flaxseed, Isochrysis galbana, fish oil and DHA Gold) on n-3 LC-PUFA enrichment (efficiency) in the egg yolk. *Journal of Functional Foods, 19*, 821–827. https://doi.org/10.1016/j.jff.2015.04.021.

Li, J. J., Dou, K. F., Zhou, Z. G., Zhao, D., Ye, P., Zhao, J. J., & Guo, L. X. (2022). Role of omega-3 fatty acids in the prevention and treatment of cardiovascular Diseases: A consensus statement from the Experts' Committee of National Society of Cardiometabolic Medicine. *Frontiers in Pharmacology, 13*. https://doi.org/10.3389/fphar.2022.1069992, http://www.frontiersin.org/Pharmacology.

Lima-Pereira, Y., de Souza, E. M. O., dos Reis, D. S., Barcellos-Silva, I. G. C., Miki, K. S. L., Veiga-Júnior, V. F., & Teixeira-Costa, B. E. (2025). Current perspectives on the extraction, isolation, and identification of fats and fatty acids using conventional and green methods. *Separations, 12*(6). https://doi.org/10.3390/separations12060160, www.mdpi.com/journal/separations.

Lipilina, E., & Ganji, V. (2009). Incorporation of ground flaxseed into bakery products and its effect on sensory and nutritional characteristics – a pilot study. *Journal of Foodservice, 20*(1), 52–59. https://doi.org/10.1111/j.1748-0159.2008.00124.x.

Liu, F., Li, M., Wang, Q., Yan, J., Han, S., Ma, C., Ma, P., Liu, X., & McClements, D. J. (2022a). Future foods: Alternative proteins, food architecture, sustainable packaging, and precision nutrition. *Critical Reviews in Food Science and Nutrition, 63*(23), 6423–6444. https://doi.org/10.1080/10408398.2022.2033683.

Liu, Y., Ren, X., Fan, C., Wu, W., Zhang, W., & Wang, Y. (2022b). Health benefits, food applications, and sustainability of microalgae-derived n-3 PUFA. *Foods, 11*, 1883.

Market Research Future. (2025). *Polyunsaturated fatty acids (PUFAs) market*. Market Research Future.

Mallick, R., Basak, S., Das, R. K., Banerjee, A., Paul, S., Pathak, S., & Duttaroy, A. K. (2023). Fatty acids and their proteins in adipose tissue inflammation. *Cell Biochemistry and Biophysics, 82*(1), 35–51. https://doi.org/10.1007/s12013-023-01185-6.

Ma, C., Azad, M. A. K., Yu, X., Sun, J., Zhang, H., Pi, J., & Wu, Y. (2026). Egg-based nutrient delivery system: Advances in omega-3, antioxidant, and micronutrient enrichment. *Frontiers in Nutrition, 13*. https://doi.org/10.3389/fnut.2026.1770381.

Marsol-Vall, A., Aitta, E., Guo, Z., & Yang, B. (2022). Green technologies for production of oils rich in n-3 polyunsaturated fatty acids from aquatic sources. *Critical Reviews in Food Science and Nutrition, 62*(11), 2942–2962. https://doi.org/10.1080/10408398.2020.1861426.

Matumoto-Pintro, P. T., Petit, H. V., Giroux, H. J., Côrtes, C., Gagnon, N., & Britten, M. (2011). Effect of flaxseed lignans added to milk or fed to cows on oxidative degradation of dairy beverages enriched with polyunsaturated fatty acids. *Journal of Dairy Research, 78*(1), 111–117.

Mititelu, M., Lupuliasa, D., Neacşu, S. M., Olteanu, G., Busnatu, Ş. S., Mihai, A., Popovici, V., Măru, N., Boroghină, S. C., Mihai, S., Ioniţă-Mîndrican, C. B., & Scafa-Udrişte, A. (2024). Polyunsaturated fatty acids and human health: A key to modern nutritional balance in association with polyphenolic compounds from food sources. *Foods, 14*(1), 46.

Mannucci, P. M., Jolliet, O., Meijaard, E., Slavin, J., Rasetti, M., Aleta, A., Moreno, Y., & Agostoni, C. (2023). Sustainable nutrition and the case of vegetable oils to match present and future dietary needs. *Frontiers in Public Health, 11*. https://doi.org/10.3389/fpubh.2023.1106083.

Mirzaee Kalaei, F., Hosseini, S. F., Rezaei, M., Yamini, Y., et al. (2025). Extraction of astaxanthin-rich lipid extracts from green tiger (*Penaeus semisulcatus*) shrimp by-products using supercritical CO_2 extraction. *Separation Science and Technology, 61*(6), 851–860. https://doi.org/10.1080/01496395.2025.2593386.

Mkhari, T., Adeyemi, J. O., & Fawole, O. A. (2025). Recent advances in the fabrication of intelligent packaging for food preservation: A review. *Processes, 13*(2), 539.

Mohamed, H., Zan, X., Naz, T., Eltoukhy, A., Ramadan, A. S., Abo-Kadoum, M. A., Hassane, A., Liu, Q., Feng, S., & Song, Y. (2026). Manipulation of oleaginous fungi to enhance biomass and sustainable lipid production: High cell density fermentation strategies, accumulation mechanism, and genetic engineering aspect. *Biomass Conversion and Biorefinery, 16*(4). https://doi.org/10.1007/s13399-025-07055-w, https://www.springer.com/journal/13399.

Moi, I. M., Leow, A. T. C., Ali, M. S. M., Rahman, R. N. Z. R. A., Salleh, A. B., & Sabri, S. (2018). Polyunsaturated fatty acids in marine bacteria and strategies to enhance their production. *Applied Microbiology and Biotechnology, 102*(14), 5811–5826. https://doi.org/10.1007/s00253-018-9063-9, https://link.springer.de/link/service/journals/00253/index.htm.

Moura, M. A. F. E., Martins, B. D. A., Oliveira, G. P. D., & Takahashi, J. A. (2023). Alternative protein sources of plant, algal, fungal and insect origins for dietary diversification in search of nutrition and health. *Critical Reviews in Food Science and Nutrition, 63*(31), 10691–10708.

Nasution, H., Harahap, H., Julianti, E., Safitri, A., & Jaafar, M. (2023). Smart packaging based on polylactic acid: The effects of antibacterial and antioxidant agents from natural extracts on physical–mechanical properties, colony reduction, perishable food shelf life, and future prospective. *Polymers, 15*(20), 4103. https://doi.org/10.3390/polym15204103.

Neamtu, I., Rusu, A. G., Diaconu, A., Nita, L. E., Chiriac, A. P., et al. (2017). Basic concepts and recent advances in nanogels as carriers for medical applications. *Drug Delivery, 24*(1), 539–557. https://doi.org/10.1080/10717544.2016.1276232.

Nunes, R., Pereira, B. D. A., Cerqueira, M. A., Silva, P., Pastrana, L. M., Vicente, A. A., Martins, J. T., & Bourbon, A. I. (2020). Lactoferrin-based nanoemulsions to improve the physical and chemical stability of omega-3 fatty acids. *Food and Function, 11*(3), 1966–1981. https://doi.org/10.1039/c9fo02307k, http://pubs.rsc.org/en/journals/journal/fo.

Ochsenreither, K., Glück, C., Stressler, T., Fischer, L., & Syldatk, C. (2016). Production strategies and applications of microbial single cell oils. *Frontiers in Microbiology, 7*. https://doi.org/10.3389/fmicb.2016.01539.

Omokaro, G. O., Nafula, Z. S., Iloabuchi, N. E., Chikukula, A. A., Osayogie, O. G., & Nnoli, E. C. (2025). Microalgae as biofactories for sustainable applications: Advancing carbon sequestration, bioenergy, and environmental remediation. *Sustainable Chemistry for Climate Action*100098.

Özyurt, G., Daday, M. T., Sakarya, Y., & Kuley, E. (2026). Wheat germ oil for enhanced stability of microencapsulated fish oil during spray drying and optimization of coating component ratios. *Food and Bioprocess Technology, 19*(1). https://doi.org/10.1007/s11947-025-04142-8, https://www.springer.com/journal/11947.

Pabba, M., Shah, A. M., Salim, M. H., Mettu, S., Talukder, M. M. R., & Puniredd, S. R. (2026). Engineering lignocellulosic biomass to single-cell oils: Microbial design, process intensification, and techno-economic constraints. *Industrial and Engineering Chemistry Research, 65*(6), 3027–3048. https://doi.org/10.1021/acs.iecr.5c04697, http://pubs.acs.org/journal/iecred.

Panchal, S. K., Heimann, K., & Brown, L. (2025). *Microalgae as sustainable and economic sources of omega-3 fatty acids. In* Omega-3 fatty acids: Keys to nutritional health and disease. Switzerland: Springer Nature, 43–52.

Pandey, A., Kamran, F., Choudhury, M., Li, L., Rahman, M. S., & Hussain, M. A. (2025). Omega-3 fatty acid fortification of plant-based beverages to enhance their nutritional profile. *Foods, 14*(9). https://doi.org/10.3390/foods14091602, www.mdpi.com/journal/foods.

Petrie, J. R., Shrestha, P., Belide, S., Kennedy, Y., Lester, G., Liu, Q., Divi, U. K., Mulder, R. J., Mansour, M. P., Nichols, P. D., & Singh, S. P. (2014). Metabolic engineering *Camelina sativa* with fish oil-like levels of DHA. *PLoS One, 9*(1). https://doi.org/10.1371/journal.pone.0085061, http://www.plosone.org/article/fetchObject.action?uri=info%3Adoi%2F10.1371%2Fjournal.pone.0085061&representation=PDF.

Prisacaru, A. E. (2016). Effect of antioxidants on polyunsaturated fatty acids - Review. *Acta Scientiarum Polonorum, Technologia Alimentaria, 15*(2), 121–129. https://doi.org/10.17306/J.AFS.2016.2.12, http://www.food.actapol.net/pub/1_2_2016.pdf.

Priyadarshini, L. A. S., & Kataria, R. (2025). Microbial synthesis and extraction of value-added metabolites by *Rhodotorula toruloides* from waste stream: A sustainable approach. *Microbial Cell Factories, 24*(1). https://doi.org/10.1186/s12934-025-02752-7.

Puranik, S. S. (2025). Artificial intelligence (AI) in omega-3 fatty acids. In *Omega-3 fatty acids: Keys to nutritional health and disease*. India: Springer Science+Business Media, 13–19. https://doi.org/10.1007/978-3-031-84200-9_2.

Qin, J., Kurt, E., LBassi, T., Sa, L., & Xie, D. (2023). Biotechnological production of omega-3 fatty acids: Current status and future perspectives. *Frontiers in Microbiology, 14*. https://doi.org/10.3389/fmicb.2023.1280296, https://www.frontiersin.org/journals/microbiology#.

Quintieri, L., Nitride, C., De Angelis, E., Lamonaca, A., Pilolli, R., Russo, F., & Monaci, L. (2023). Alternative protein sources and novel foods: benefits, food applications and safety issues. *Nutrients, 15*(6), 1509. https://doi.org/10.3390/nu15061509.

Rahim, M. A., Uzma, M., Al-Asmari, F., Koraqi, H., Ramadan, M. F., Castro-Muñoz, R., & Zongo, E. (2025). A comprehensive review on nutritional traits, extraction methods, oxidative stability, encapsulation technologies, food applications and health benefits of omega fatty acids. *Food Science & Nutrition, 13*(10). https://doi.org/10.1002/fsn3.71008.

Rajendran, S., Al-Samydai, A., Palani, G., Trilaksana, H., Sathish, T., Giri, J., Saravanan, R., Lalvani, J. I. J. R., & Nasri, F. (2025). Replacement of petroleum based products with plant-based materials, green and sustainable energy—A review. *Engineering Reports, 7*(4). https://doi.org/10.1002/eng2.70108.

Remize, M., Brunel, Y., Silva, J. L., Berthon, J. Y., & Filaire, E. (2021). Microalgae n-3 PUFAs production and use in food and feed industries. *Marine Drugs, 19*(2). https://doi.org/10.3390/MD19020113, https://www.mdpi.com/1660-3397/19/2/113/pdf.

Rizzo, G., Baroni, L., & Lombardo, M. (2023). Promising sources of plant-derived polyunsaturated fatty acids: A narrative review. *International Journal of Environmental Research and Public Health, 20*(3), 1683.

Rubio-Rodríguez, N., De Diego, S. M., Beltrán, S., Jaime, I., Sanz, M. T., & Rovira, J. (2012). Supercritical fluid extraction of fish oil from fish by-products: A comparison with other extraction methods. *Journal of Food Engineering, 109*(2), 238–248.

Ruiz Ruiz, J. C., Ortiz Vázquez, E. D. L. L., & Segura Campos, M. R. (2017). Encapsulation of vegetable oils as source of omega-3 fatty acids for enriched functional foods. *Critical Reviews in Food Science and Nutrition, 57*(7), 1423–1434.

Ruiz-López, N., Sayanova, O., Napier, J. A., & Haslam, R. P. (2012). Metabolic engineering of the omega-3 long chain polyunsaturated fatty acid biosynthetic pathway into transgenic plants. *Journal of Experimental Botany, 63*(7), 2397–2410.

Saini, Prasad, Sreedhar, Shang, & Keum (2021). Omega-3 polyunsaturated fatty acids (PUFAs): Emerging plant and microbial sources, oxidative stability, bioavailability, and health benefits—A review. *Antioxidants (Basel, Switzerland), 10*(10).

Sadhu, T., Banerjee, I., Lahiri, S. K., Chakrabarty, J., et al. (2021). Enhancement of nutritional value of fried fish using an artificial intelligence approach. *Environmental Science and Pollution Research, 29*(14), 20048–20063. https://doi.org/10.1007/s11356-021-13548-8.

Sidari, R., & Tofalo, R. (2019). A comprehensive overview on microalgal-fortified/based food and beverages. *Food Reviews International, 35*(8), 778–805.

Shahidi, F., & Ambigaipalan, P. (2018). Omega-3 polyunsaturated fatty acids and their health benefits. *Annual Review of Food Science and Technology, 9*(1), 345–381. https://doi.org/10.1146/annurev-food-111317-095850.

Santin, A., Balzano, S., Russo, M. T., Palma Esposito, F., Ferrante, M. I., Blasio, M., Cavalletti, E., Sardo, A., et al. (2022). Microalgae-based PUFAs for food and feed: current applications, future possibilities, and constraints. *Journal of Marine Science and Engineering, 10*(7), 844. https://doi.org/10.3390/jmse10070844.

Silva, J. R., Burger, B., Kühl, C. M., Candreva, T., Dos Anjos, M. B., & Rodrigues, H. G. (2018). Wound healing and omega-6 fatty acids: From inflammation to repair. *Mediators of Inflammation, 2018*, 2503950.

Sherratt, S. C. R., Libby, P., Budoff, M. J., Bhatt, D. L., & Mason, R. P. (2022). Role of omega-3 fatty acids in cardiovascular disease: the debate continues. *Current Atherosclerosis Reports, 25*(1), 1–17. https://doi.org/10.1007/s11883-022-01075-x.

Soto-Méndez, M. J., Rangel-Huerta, O. D., Ruiz-López, M. D., Martínez De Victoria, E., Anguita-Ruiz, A., & Gil, A. (2019). Role of functional fortified dairy products in cardiometabolic health: A systematic review and meta-analyses of randomized clinical trials. *Advances in Nutrition, 10*, S251. https://doi.org/10.1093/advances/nmz001, http://advances.nutrition.org/.

Shyam, H., Sahu, D. K., Mishra, A., Singh, S., Singh, N., et al. (2025). Metabolism of fatty acid. *In Metabolomics of Bladder Cancer*, 53. https://doi.org/10.1016/B978- 0-443-23881-9.00004-9.

Sugawara, A., Yamane, S., & Akiyoshi, K. (2006). Nanogel-templated mineralization: Polymer–calcium phosphate hybrid nanomaterials. *Macromolecular Rapid Communications, 27*(6), 441–446.

Sun, Y., Xia, Z., Zheng, J., Qiu, P., Zhang, L., McClements, D. J., & Xiao, H. (2015). Nanoemulsion-based delivery systems for nutraceuticals: Influence of carrier oil type on bioavailability of pterostilbene. *Journal of Functional Foods, 13*, 61–70. https://doi.org/10.1016/j.jff.2014.12.030, http://www.elsevier.com/wps/find/journaldescription.cws_home/717426/description#description.

Swetha, N., & Mathanghi, S. K. (2024). Towards sustainable omega-3 fatty acids production: A comprehensive review on extraction methods, oxidative stability and bio-availability enhancement. *Food Chemistry Advances, 4*, 100603.

Tiwari, S., Tan, Y.-M., & Amiji, M. (2006). Preparation and in vitro characterization of multifunctional nanoemulsions for simultaneous MR imaging and targeted drug delivery. *Journal of Biomedical Nanotechnology, 2*(3), 217–224.

Torres-Tiji, Y., Fields, F. J., & Mayfield, S. P. (2020). Microalgae as a future food source. *Biotechnology Advances, 41*, 107536.

Tsironi, T. N., & Taoukis, P. S. (2018). Current practice and innovations in fish packaging. *Journal of Aquatic Food Product Technology, 27*(10), 1024–1047. https://doi.org/10.1080/10498850.2018.1532479, http://www.tandfonline.com/toc/wafp20/current.

Tufail, T., Bader Ul Ain, H., Ashraf, J., Mahmood, S., Noreen, S., Ijaz, A., ikram, A., Arshad, M. T., & Abdullahi, M. A. (2025). Bioactive compounds in seafood: Implications for health and nutrition. *Food Science & Nutrition, 13*(4). https://doi.org/10.1002/fsn3.70181.

Turck, D., Bohn, T., Castenmiller, J., De Henauw, S., Hirsch-Ernst, K. I., Maciuk, A., Mangelsdorf, I., McArdle, H. J., Naska, A., Pelaez, C., Pentieva, K., Siani, A., Thies, F., Tsabouri, S., Vinceti, M., Aguilera-Gómez, M., Cubadda, F., Frenzel, T., Heinonen, M., ... Knutsen, H. K. (2023). Safety of oil from *Schizochytrium* sp. (strain CABIO-A-2) for use in infant and follow-on formula as a novel food pursuant to Regulation (EU) 2015/2283. *EFSA Journal, 21*(12). https://doi.org/10.2903/j.efsa.2023.8415 Available from: efsa.onlinelibrary.wiley.com/journal/18314732/.

Umar, A. W., Ahmad, N., & Xu, M. (2025). Hormonal cross-talk in DHA biosynthesis: Regulatory roles of auxin and jasmonic acid in *Schizochytrium* spp. and *Crypthecodinium cohnii*. *Algal Research*104316.

Usturoi, M. G., Rațu, R. N., Crivei, I. C., Veleşcu, I. D., Usturoi, A., Stoica, F., & Radu Rusu, R.-M. (2025). Unlocking the power of eggs: nutritional insights, bioactive compounds, and the advantages of omega-3 and omega-6 enriched varieties. *Agriculture, 15*(3), 242. https://doi.org/10.3390/agriculture15030242.

Vergara Nieto, Á. A., Díaz, A. H., Hernández Millán, M., & Sagredo, D. (2025). Molecular features, effective sources, and physiological effects of omega-3 unsaturated fatty acids on cardiovascular, neurological, and muscular health, and clinical relevance for several conditions: A Narrative Review. *Nutrition Reviews*. https://doi.org/10.1093/nutrit/nuaf201.

Vinogradov, S. V. (2006). Polymeric nanogel formulations of nucleoside analogs. *Expert Opinion on Drug Delivery, 4*(1), 5–17. https://doi.org/10.1517/17425247.4.1.5.

Vijaykrishnaraj, M., Kumar, P. K., & Karthik, P. (2024). Polyunsaturated fatty acid fortification. In *Food fortification*. CRC Press, 329–354.

Wang, C., Sun, C., Lu, W., Gul, K., Mata, A., & Fang, Y. (2020). Emulsion structure design for improving the oxidative stability of polyunsaturated fatty acids. *Comprehensive Reviews in Food Science and Food Safety, 19*(6), 2955–2971. https://doi.org/10.1111/1541-4337.12621.

Wang, Y., Li, D., Wang, L., & Adhikari, B. (2010). The effect of addition of flaxseed gum on the emulsion properties of soybean protein isolate (SPI). *Journal of Food Engineering, 104*(1), 56–62.

Wei, W., Cheng, Z., Wang, X., Chang, M., Xie, D., Sun, C., Guo, X., & Li, B. (2025). *The potential of marine oils as functional foods: Nutritional composition, health benefits, applications, and future perspectives*. Food Reviews International, 1–32. https://doi.org/10.1080/87559129.2025.2528083.

Xu, R., Molenaar, A. J., Chen, Z., & Yuan, Y. (2025). Mode and mechanism of action of omega-3 and omega-6 unsaturated fatty acids in chronic diseases. *Nutrients, 17*(9). https://doi.org/10.3390/nu17091540, http://www.mdpi.com/journal/nutrients/.

Xu, Y., Zhang, Z., Bian, Y., Wang, Y., Deng, Z., Luo, R., & Sun, D. (2025). Regulatory mechanisms of EPA and DHA proportions in a PUFA-producing microalga, *Schizochytrium* sp. ATCC 20888: From the biosynthesis and storage distribution aspects. *Journal of Agricultural and Food Chemistry, 73*(7), 4137–4151.

Yan, Z., Xu, Y., Peng, T., & Du, X. (2025). A clinical prediction model integrated with machine learning algorithms uncovers the associations between dietary omega-3, its components, and aging biomarkers. *Journal of Food Science, 90*(7). https://doi.org/10.1111/1750-3841.70334.

Yang, J., Ciftci, D., & Ciftci, O. N. (2024). Fortification of milk with omega-3 fatty acids using novel bioactive-carrier hollow solid lipid micro- and nanoparticles for improved omega-3 stability and bioaccessibility. *ACS Food Science & Technology, 4*(4), 813–820.

Yin, F., Sun, X., Luo, X., Zheng, W., Yin, L., Zhang, Y., & Fu, Y. (2025). A review on marine microbial docosahexaenoic acid production through circular economy, fermentation engineering, and antioxidant technology. *Marine Drugs, 23*(6), 256. https://doi.org/10.3390/md23060256.

Yeung, A. W. K., Solka, M., Jóźwik, A., Ksepka, N., Matin, M., Wysocki, K., Abdallah, E. M., Sundaram, A. S. M., Iantovics, L. B., Echeverría, J., Tewari, D., Horbańczuk, J. O., Lucarini, M., Durazzo, A., Stolarczyk, A., Adamska, O., Chandragiri, S. S., Tzvetkov, N. T., Matin, F. B., Łysek-Gładysinska, M., & Atanasov, A. G. (2025). Omega-3 fatty acids: dietary components for the promotion of human and animal health. *Animal Science Papers and Reports, 43*(3), 235–260. https://doi.org/10.2478/aspr-2025-0017.

Zaman, M. M., Farooq, Z., Hafeez, A., Sajid, M. W., Tariq, M. R., Ali, S. W., Ali, S., Shafiq, M., Iftikhar, M., Safdar, W., Ali, U., Kanwal, M., Umer, Z., & Basharat, Z. (2023). Supplementation of PUFA extracted from microalgae for the development of chicken patties. *PeerJ, 11*, e15355.

Zanetti, M., Grillo, A., Losurdo, P., Panizon, E., Mearelli, F., Cattin, L., & Carretta, R. (2015). Omega-3 polyunsaturated fatty acids: Structural and functional effects on the vascular wall. *BioMed Research International, 2015*, 791978.

Zhang, T., Zhang, X., Zhou, X., Tian, R., Tang, X., Zhang, Y., Jiang, L., & Sui, X. (2024). Plant-based fat substitutes with promising functional properties and health benefits. *Journal of the American Oil Chemists' Society, 101*(11), 1183–1196. https://doi.org/10.1002/aocs.12797.

Zhao, Q., Wang, F., Xiong, A., Li, S., Wang, Y., Lei, X., Deyholos, M. K., Wang, Y., Zhuang, J., Yu, H., & Zhang, J. (2025). Regulation of fatty acid synthesis in oilseed crops: Multidimensional insights and strategies for enhancing oil quality. *Critical Reviews in Biotechnology, 45*(8), 1737–1753. https://doi.org/10.1080/07388551.2025.2529591, http://www.tandfonline.com/loi/ibty20.

Zhao, R., Ding, J., Yang, Y., Huang, H., & Di, Y. (2025). Trophic-transferred hierarchical fragmentation of microplastics inducing distinct bio-adaptations via a microalgae–mussel–crab food chain. *Journal of Hazardous Materials, 489*, 137620.

Chapter 34

Polyunsaturated fatty acid-enriched foods in the market: case studies and strategies

Kalaivanan Rajalakshmi[1], Amit Ranjan[2], Govindharaj Sathishkumar[3], and Munusamy Ajithkumar[4]

[1]*Erode Bhavanisagar centre for Sustainable Aquaculture (EBCeSA), Tamil Nadu Dr. J. Jayalalithaa Fisheries University (TNJFU), Erode, Tamil Nadu, India,* [2]*Department of Fish Nutrition and Feed Technology, Tamil Nadu Dr. J. Jayalalithaa FIsheries University, Chennai, Tamil Nadu, India,* [3]*GKSM, Department of Fish Nutrition and Feed Technology, Research & Development Department, The Waterbase Limited, Nellore, Andhra Pradesh, India,* [4]*Department of Genetics, Benchmark Genetics, Bergen, Norway*

34.1 Introduction

The mind and body of people can be healthy through the intake of proper, balanced consumption of micro and macro nutrients. So, among these nutrients, lipids from food are essential. It is not only the source of energy but also important as structural and regulatory molecules in biological systems (Wiktorowska-Owczarek et al., 2015). At present, more attention has been given to n-3 polyunsaturated fatty acids (PUFA) because of its heart supporting function, inflammation modulation, and supporting eye and nervous system (Nowak, 2009). So, these functions elucidate the importance and value of PUFA from baby to adult.

Lipids have many classes of compounds that are made of carbon and hydrogen. Fatty acids, the basic units of many lipids, mainly have a hydrocarbon chain with 12–24C. It may be saturated, monounsaturated, or polyunsaturated, which is determined by double bonds within the presence of carbon chain (Das, 2006). PUFAs have omega-3 (n-3) and omega-6 (n-6) by their way of first double bond occurs if it counts from the methyl end (Nettleton, 1995). Docosahexaenoic acid (DHA) (C22:6ω-3) means 22C with six double bonds, and the first double bond is present 3C away from methyl terminus (Das, 2006). Main PUFA categories are DHA (C22:6n-3), eicosapentaenoic acid (EPA; C20:5n-3), and arachidonic acid (AA; C20:4n-6).

Humans can't synthesize Δ12- and Δ15-desaturase enzymes, and so endogenous products of linoleic acid (LA), α-linolenic acid (ALA), were prevented. And thereby it is classified as an essential amino acid (Tvrzicka et al., 2011). Even though elongation and desaturation of these precursors can produce EPA, DHA, and AA, this process of conversion is constrained to a certain extent, which is why it made long-chain derivatives conditionally essential under certain conditions (Kapoor et al., 2021). The PUFAs biological activity depends on their cis double bond configuration, which develops metabolic processes and immune system regulation (Li et al., 2020). Though mammals can't produce some essential fatty acids on their own, it has to be supplemented through diet, and that tells about its importance as a constraining factor in the nutrition of people (Brenna & Carlson, 2014).

The important EPA, DHA, and ALA are very crucial for human health because mammals don't have the ability to produce them on their own, hence they should be obtained through food consumption (Mane et al., 2024). The roles of PUFA range from less onset of heart problems, inflammation regulation, production of hormones, neural transmission, and prevention of severe disease stages before it occurs (Li et al., 2020). So, with all the above as a backdrop about PUFA, its enrichment of food products will be a fine idea to solve gaps and drawbacks that will lead to the development of people's health. This chapter explains and conveys the foundations of PUFAs, how they can be incorporated into food products, the challenges encountered, and the enrichment strategies, so that it will be a topic that gives an emerging good view of PUFA-enriched foods in the global market.

Omega-3 and Omega-6 Polyunsaturated Fatty Acids in Food Systems. DOI: https://doi.org/10.1016/B978-0-443-43810-3.00028-2

34.2 Categorization of polyunsaturated fatty acid

PUFAs are splatted as per its molecular configuration, extent of double-bond presence, carbon chain length, and the location of unsaturated linkages along the hydrocarbon framework. Fatty acids are organic acids consisting of a carbon chain attached to a terminal carboxyl functional group, which is identified as the first carbon atom in the structure. In the omega (ω or n) system, carbon numbering starts at the terminal methyl group, and the omega value denotes the position of the first double bond from that end. For instance, DHA (22:6n-3) has a 22-carbon chain with six double bonds, the first situated at the third carbon from the methyl terminus (Riediger et al., 2009). Chemically, fatty acids are divided into saturated and unsaturated forms based on the presence of carbon–carbon double bonds (Savatinova & Ivanova, 2024). Saturated fatty acids (SFAs) lack double bonds and are grouped by chain length as short-chain (C2–C4), medium-chain (C6–C10), long-chain (C12–C18), and very-long-chain (≥C20). Unsaturated fatty acids contain one or more double bonds and are classified as monounsaturated fatty acids (MUFA) or PUFA. MUFAs possess a single double bond, usually in the cis configuration, whereas PUFAs have two or more double bonds. PUFAs are further categorized into omega-3 (n-3) and omega-6 (n-6) families according to the location of the first double bond from the methyl end (Savatinova & Ivanova, 2024). Fig. 34.1 shows the categorization of fatty acids.

Fatty acids that cannot be synthesized in humans and must be obtained from the diet are termed essential (Burdge, 2010). In the n-3 series, ALA (18:3n-3) serves as the precursor. Human conversion of ALA to longer-chain derivatives is limited; therefore dietary intake is important (Riediger et al., 2009). Its principal metabolites are EPA (20:5n-3), DHA (22:6n-3), and docosapentaenoic acid (DPA; 22:5n-3), collectively known as long-chain n-3 PUFAs (Tvrzicka et al., 2011). In the n-6 pathway, LA (18:2n-6) is the parent compound and is converted to γ-linolenic acid (GLA), dihomo-γ-linolenic acid, arachidonic acid (AA), and other minor products (Tvrzicka et al., 2011). ALA and LA are considered essential because humans lack Δ12- and Δ15-desaturase enzymes required for their synthesis; moreover, conversion to long-chain products such as EPA, DHA, and AA is relatively inefficient (Burdge, 2010). Fig. 34.2 shows the types of PUFAs and their major biological functions.

Thus the categorization of PUFAs is grounded in structural chemistry but carries profound nutritional implications. The differentiation between saturated, monounsaturated, and PUFAs, and more specifically between n-3 and n-6 families, forms the biochemical basis for dietary recommendations, functional food development, and PUFA enrichment strategies. In the context of PUFA-enriched foods in the market, this classification underpins product formulation, labeling standards, health claims, and strategic fortification approaches that aim to address dietary insufficiencies and optimize the wellness of people.

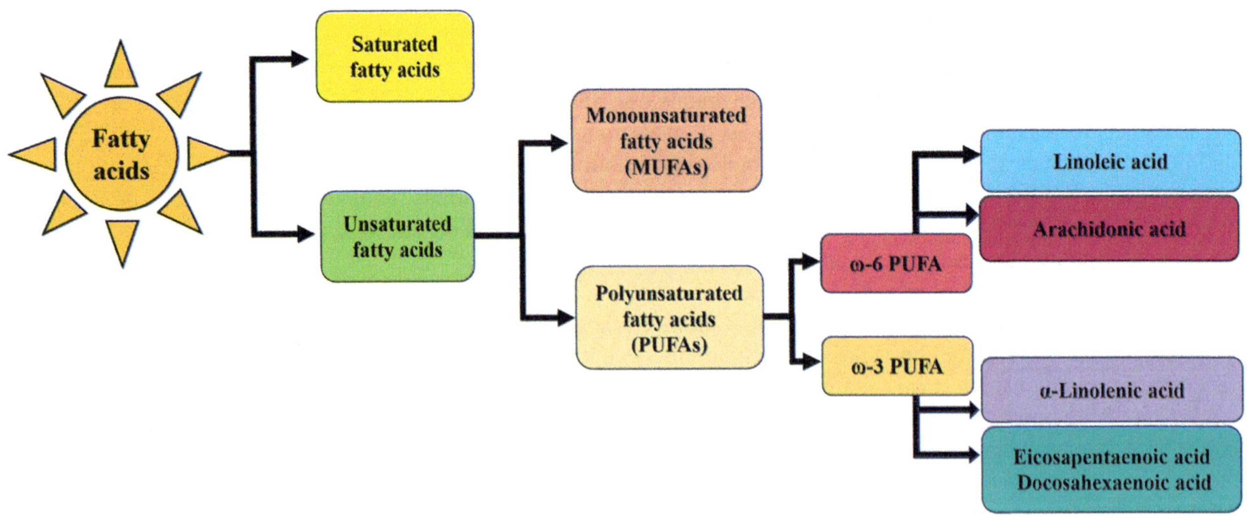

FIGURE 34.1 Categorization of fatty acids.

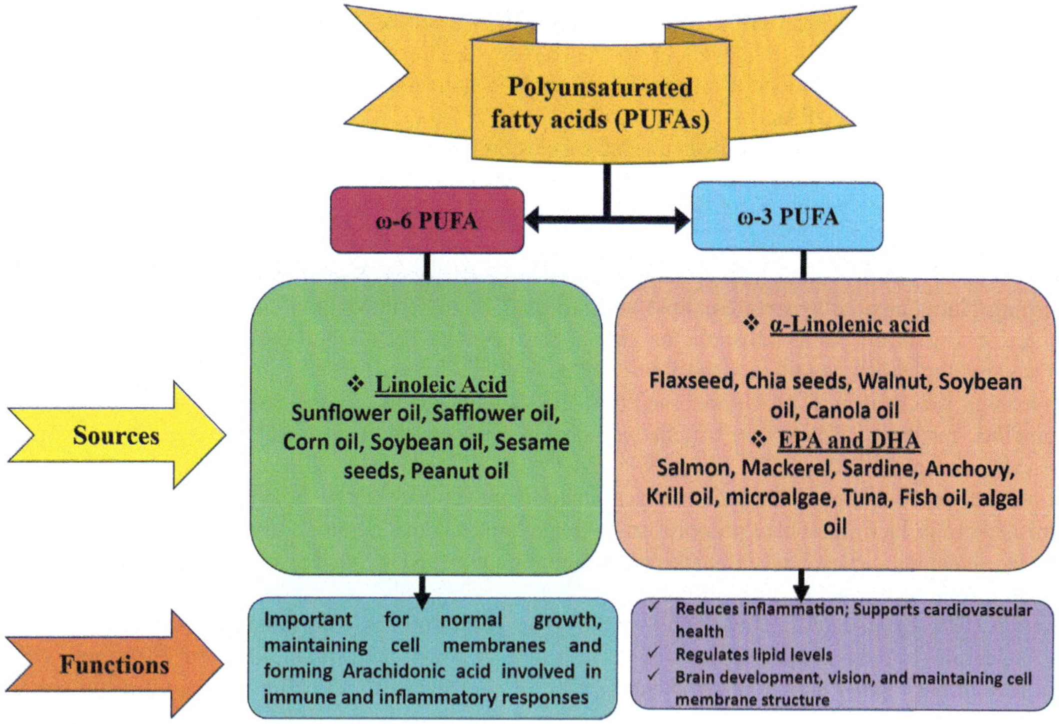

FIGURE 34.2 Types of polyunsaturated fatty acids (PUFAs) and their major biological functions.

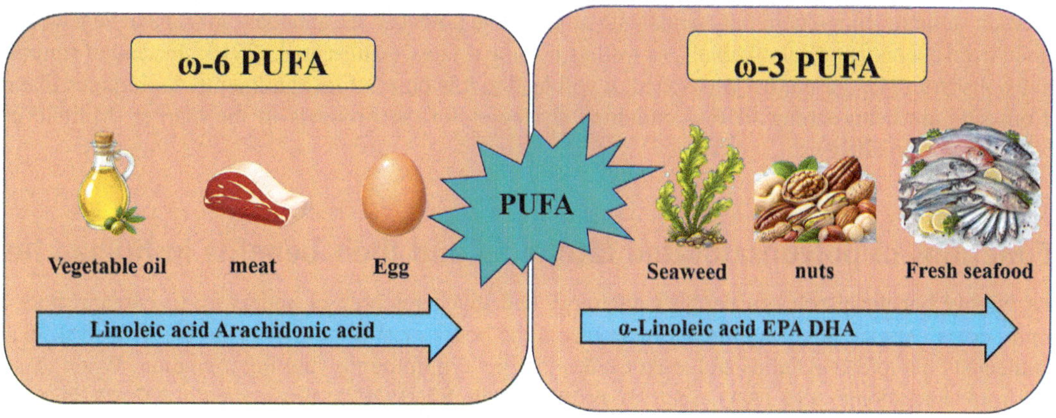

FIGURE 34.3 Some sources of n-3 and n-6 polyunsaturated fatty acids (PUFAs).

34.3 Availability of polyunsaturated fatty acids

PUFA supplemented in market foods are mainly from marine and plant sources, in which each was capable of giving a good number of fatty acids along with its benefits. Marine fish remain the principal dietary source of EPA and DHA. The fatty acid composition of fish, which determines their nutritional quality, varies according to species, habitat, feeding pattern, and environmental conditions. Comparative analyzes of freshwater species have shown variability in lipid classes, where barbel fillets contained higher MUFA (18.51%), whereas river mullet exhibited comparatively higher PUFA content (1.87%) and the greatest omega-3 proportion among the species studied (Gaffari & Khoshnood, 2021). Similarly, salmon demonstrated EPA (0.8%), DHA (1.6%), and total PUFA levels of 12.4%, while Russian sturgeon showed EPA (11.3%), DHA (0.7%), and total PUFA levels of 46.8% (Kyosev & Dragoev, 2009). These observations confirm the role of freshwater fish as notable providers of omega-3 fatty acids in humans (Gaffari & Khoshnood, 2021). Fig. 34.3 shows some sources of n-3 and n-6 PUFAs.

Most commercial fish oils are obtained from marine species, as marine ecosystems are rich reservoirs of EPA and DHA. They are highlighted for their numerous benefits in the aspects of health, such as heart, immune maintenance, and enhancement (Göksen et al., 2020). DHA in particular contributes to the brain and vision development of children and supports pregnant women (Calder, 2016).

Fishes obtain PUFAs from sources like microalgae and marine microbes (Napier et al., 2015). Variations in seasons and different fishing places also influence gross lipid and omega-3 PUFA composition (Jensen et al., 2007).

Oils that are obtained from plants tell about the important ALA. Like the marine source oils, oils from vegetable sources don't produce any unpleasant condition when it was added to food. Oilseeds from walnut, soy, flaxseed, canola, camelina are termed as high rich source of ALA (Ganesan et al., 2014). Fortification trials have demonstrated the effectiveness of linseed, camelina, raspberry, *Echium plantagineum*, and blackcurrant oils in enhancing omega-3 levels in yogurt, with respective ALA contents of 71%, 36%, 29%, 33%, and 14% (Dal Bello et al., 2015). LA (n-6) and ALA (n-3) serve as biosynthetic precursors for longer-chain derivatives, including EPA and DHA (Jakobsson and Westerberg, 2006). But, higher plants generally lack significant proportions of long-chain polyunsaturated fatty acids (HUFAs) which are mainly synthesized by algae and subsequently transferred through aquatic food webs (Hixson et al., 2015). Terrestrial vascular plants typically contain greater proportions of omega-6 fatty acids, whereas aquatic primary producers are richer in omega-3 forms (Gladyshev et al., 2013). While ALA from plant sources contributes to overall n-3 intake, evidence consistently indicates stronger associations between health benefits and marine-derived EPA and DHA. Clinical evaluations reveal that regular eating habit of fish or fish oil contributes to a decline in overall death risk and cardiac-related deaths, whereas similar benefits have not been conclusively demonstrated for ALA intake alone (Wang et al., 2006). Moreover, bioavailability and physiological efficacy of n-3 PUFAs are impacted by fatty acid type, food matrix, processing conditions, and storage stability, factors of considerable importance in the formulation and marketing of PUFA-enriched foods (Wang et al., 2006). Consequently, fish oil and the edible portions of heavy fish are still the plentiful providers of n-3 PUFAs in the food (Tvrzicka et al., 2011).

Also, to marine and plant oils, overall dietary fat composition must be considered when formulating PUFA-enriched products. Certain saturated long-chain fatty acids with atherogenic potential are abundant in tropical vegetable oils such as those obtained from coconut and palm kernels, as well as in animal fats (Akihisa et al., 2010). Instead of saturated lipids, if PUFA surplus oils from plant or marine was added, it will lead to low onset of heart ailments. So, sources like marine fish, algae, and oilseeds are being strong PUFA- enriching strategies for the products in the market (Mititelu et al., 2024; Shahidi & Ambigaipalan, 2018).

34.4 Functions of polyunsaturated fatty acid and their benefits in human health

PUFAs play highly beneficial roles in people's anatomy, and much research is underway to explain more about their functional properties. Among many significant functions in the body, most important is the PUFA's work in synthesis of signaling molecules like prostaglandins and leukotrienes that govern immunity and inflammation. When these mediators are derived from arachidonic acid (AA), such as prostaglandin E2 (PGE2), prostaglandin D2 (PGD2), and 4-series leukotrienes, they exert predominantly pro-inflammatory effects, mechanisms that are well described in scientific inquiries into the mode of naturally occurring therapeutic drug activity. In contrast, EPA and DHA generate fewer inflammatory derivatives and contribute to multiple protective biological processes. Investigational results demonstrate that EPA and DHA help maintain membrane fluidity, suppress inflammatory cascades, reduce monocytic wave of inflammatory cytokine factors and cells with immunity, decrease vulnerability to ventricular arrhythmias, enhance endothelial performance, inhibit platelet aggregation, and lower hepatic triglyceride synthesis (Nowak, 2009).

Omega-3 fatty acids exert pronounced benefits on lipid homeostasis. Supplementation with EPA and DHA has been documented to diminish plasma triglyceride levels by approximately 30%, and in severe hypertriglyceridemia by up to 80%, while simultaneously cutting down circulating cholesterol and LDL levels and elevating high-density lipoprotein concentrations (Strauss et al., 2005). Their antithrombotic properties are mediated through prolonged bleeding time, reduced platelet adhesion and aggregation, inhibition of thromboxane A2 and platelet-activating factor synthesis, decreased fibrinogen levels, and enhanced prostacyclin and tissue plasminogen activator activity (McEwen et al., 2013). Additionally, omega-3 PUFAs enhance responsiveness to antiplatelet therapies and suppress thrombin activity in individuals with coronary artery disease who are administered combination therapy with omega-3 PUFAs, aspirin, and clopidogrel; fibrin clots exhibited a looser structure and were more susceptible to breakdown (Gajos et al., 2011).

The proportion of n-6 to n-3 fatty acids is equally critical for optimal health. An intake ratio near 4:1 or lower is considered beneficial in minimizing chronic inflammatory processes (Mititelu et al., 2024). Excessive omega-6 consumption typical adherence to Western diets has been related to has been associated with persistent inflammation and related chronic diseases (Djuricic & Calder, 2021). LA and ALA are necessary, and they can be obtained from food. These are serving as precursors for the eicosanoids, which are bioactive and safeguard the onset of diseases of atherosclerosis (Simonetto et al., 2019). And even though ALA taken from plants can be converted to n-3 through metabolism, its virulence is reduced to a certain extent. So, the consumption of n-3 straight through marine oils suggests that it has a powerful connection with health benefits (Garg et al., 2006).

Collectively gathered saturated lipids reduce membrane fluidity and hinder insulin receptor performance, thereby fostering Insulin desensitization and raising type 2 diabetes risk (Mititelu et al., 2024). Moreover, saturated fat metabolism generates pro-inflammatory mediators, reinforcing the importance of omega-3-rich foods with antiinflammatory properties in chronic disease prevention (D'Angelo et al., 2020). The integrated biochemical actions of PUFAs include attenuation of inflammation, strengthening of antioxidant defenses, and support of cardiovascular, neurological, and metabolic health (Mititelu et al., 2024).

EPA and DHA have demonstrated benefits extending beyond cardiovascular protection. Evidence supports their role in preventing hypertension, diabetes, arthritis, autoimmune disorders, allergies, and certain cancers (Mnari et al., 2007). Positive outcomes have also been observed in platelet regulation, hyperlipidemia management, depression, dementia, including Alzheimer's disease, and systemic inflammation (Ruxton & Derbyshire, 2009). Population-wide increases in tissue levels of n-3 could therefore substantially lessen the global burden of chronic degenerative diseases (Hibbeln et al., 2006). n-3 PUFAs lead to a lower occurrence of brain problems (Lie, 2004). DHA is particularly helpful for good vision and brain functioning, especially in developing babies inside the mother's womb (Agostoni, 2008; Connor, 2000). From Scientific Advisory Committee on Nutrition (SACN) (2004) and European Food Safety Authority (EFSA) (2010), it is recommended at the level of 250–450 mg of EPA and DHA for pregnant women.

Therefore with consideration of all the multifunctional benefits, pointing out the idea of PUFA-enriched foods, which will take a step to mitigate nutrient deficiencies and promote the health of people.

34.5 Polyunsaturated fatty acid enriched foods: products in the market

The world's PUFA market is expected to grow wider because of demand and the importance of PUFA-enriched foods prevailing among people. The status will be recorded to be around USD 12.5 billion in 2023 and is expected to increase at a compound annual growth rate (CAGR) of almost 6% to reach nearly USD 21.3 billion by 2032 (PUFA (Polyunsaturated Fatty Acids) Market: Global Forecast 2025–2033 (Datalntelo)). Likewise, from various parts of the world, companies and sectors estimate that the market will be worth USD 5.53 billion in 2024 and it may move at a compound annual growth rate of 4.7% to attain USD 8.39 billion by 2033 (Business Research Insights, 2025-2033). Reports from markets specify that sources from marine and plant sides have huge production, whereas other applications are focused on food and beverages, dietary supplements, pharmaceuticals, and animal nutrition (Datalntelo, 2025–33). In the food industry, the addition of PUFA into different food products like dairy, bakery, edible oils, children's diet, beverages, and snack products. Because of its numerous health benefits for the heart, brain, and antiinflammation, it accelerated the interest of people towards the necessity of foods with the presence of PUFAs. So, from a business point of view, many shops like supermarkets and online retail areas move steps to get access to consumers to distribute their products (Datalntelo, 2025–33). Recently, a good finding from industry was implemented, which is the introduction of more concentrated n-3 oil Omevital by BASF SE derived from marine sources, and it is used for addition in dietary and functional foods 2033 (Business Research Insights, 2025-2033). So, these kind of advancements and ideas talks about how we have moved to very pure, stable PUFA ingredients that can be used for a high amount of food fortification. Many upcoming ideas, even more take high adoption of other sources of PUFA like algae and krill to address environmental sustainability issues, and for people with veg eating habits (Business Research Insights, 2025-2033). So, all these improvements lead to pathways for strategies to produce PUFA-enriched food products.

n-3 PUFAs have gained more attention to make foods with more health benefits. Foods such as breads, cereals, cookies, which give less activity of water and are found to be powerful carriers for n-3 addition. These also increase oxidative stability. Bread, because of its worldwide preference for eating, with less moisture and stable shortening systems, provides a favorable matrix for PUFA incorporation (Hernandez, 2013). Also, to mention here that from earlier times, bread was a commercially available source of n-3 fish oil.

n-3 PUFA are basic nutrients to tell a meal which perfectly has complete balanced nutrients that are needed for good growth, development, and other physiological conditions. But obtaining n-3 PUFA from the ocean remains not sufficient to fulfill the nutritional needs worldwide. Consequently, scientific focus has shifted toward developing foods intrinsically supplemented with omega-3 PUFAs and identifying alternative EPA and DHA sources (Tocher et al., 2019). Food fortification reports a long-lasting idea to enhance omega-3 consumption without necessitating substantial food modifications (Fraeye et al., 2012).

Now an assortment of omega-3-added items is available globally. Edible oils surplus in ALA, including canola, flaxseed, perilla, and soybean oils, are widely marketed, and reducing high-LA vegetable oils while favoring monounsaturated-rich oils improves the LA/ALA ratio (Simopoulos et al., 1999). Egg enrichment through dietary modification of hens using fish meal, fish oil, flaxseed, rapeseed oil, soybean oil, palm oil, or algal DHA results in the laying down of ALA, EPA, and DHA into egg yolk, reflecting the monogastric metabolism of poultry (Réhault-Godbert et al., 2019). Designer eggs can provide over 600 mg omega-3 PUFA and approximately 6 mg tocopherol, while achieving balanced omega-6/omega-3 and PUFA/SFA ratios near 1:1 (Miranda et al., 2015). Addition of flaxseed in hen diets has been shown to elevate ALA to around 200 mg and DHA to 90 mg per egg (Lemahieu et al., 2015), and achieving the correct quantity omega-6/omega-3 balance is important for meeting modern nutritional recommendations (Attia et al., 2024). The growing business with plentiful availability of eggs tells how much people have become aware of their heart and brain benefits (Shakoor et al., 2020).

The nutrition of newborn children has been focused on more now. The human milk in nature itself contains AA, DHA, and EPA, which is not the same as traditional cow milk. In dairy, native bovine milk fat has a minor amount of ALA and n-3 PUFA due to ruminal biohydrogenation (Frutos et al., 2018). Making changes in the diets of hoofed mammals with linseed, hemp seed, rapeseed, rubber seed, fish meal, fish oil, algal oil, or microalgae biomass importantly elevates the fatty acid composition of milk (Kliem et al., 2019). But, straight addition of dairy products leads to more accurate dosage and high n-3 levels in the final product outcome (Savatinova & Ivanova, 2024). Curd highly added with linseed or blackcurrant oil has depicted high n-3s, with flaxseed having more sensory analysis (Dal Bello et al., 2015). When fish oil was added at a rate of 1–5 g/kg in curd and cream, 20–60 g/kg in butter, processed cheese, and this has sensory qualities to cope with when 180–360 mg n-3 per 30 g of food (Savatinova & Ivanova, 2024).

Emerging sources of omega-3 PUFAs include microalgae, krill oil, calamari oil, fungi, and genetically modified crops (Mane et al., 2024). Microalgae are cultivated for PUFAs, pigments, antioxidants, polyphenols, and other bioactive compounds, and their biomass is utilized in feed, food, and nutraceutical applications (Mane et al., 2024). Cereal-based PUFA-enriched bioproducts have been developed through solid-state fermentation using fungi such as *T. elegans* and *M. alpina*, producing significant levels of GLA, AA, DGLA, and EPA and enabling optimization of x-6/x-3 PUFA ratios (Certik & Adamechova, 2009).

Salmonids, including trout and salmon, are recognized as natural functional foods due to their higher quantity of n-3 PUFAs (Usydus & Szlinder-Richert, 2012). Their fatty acid profile is obtained by diet, season, and aspects of their surroundings, and aquaculture feeding strategies enriched with omega-3 PUFAs can further enhance tissue concentrations (Roy et al., 2020).

According to Codex Alimentarius, food enrichment means adding important nutritive compounds to the food to mitigate deficiencies in people. So, in that sense, enriching food with PUFA was being seen as the best welcoming idea to fasten eating such foods and reduce the diseases mainly concerned with heart in people (Kolanowski, 2005). The effects on the body after eating enriched foods with PUFA depend on which chemical form the n-3 are included, in which particularly EPA and DHA taken from the ocean, has high benefits than ALA. The quality of fish oil, food, and its ingredients mainly tells about how the products and the food are functionally efficient (Kolanowski, 2005). So, as a whole, the expanding portfolio of PUFA-enriched products demonstrates a dynamic integration of nutritional science, technological innovation, and market-driven health strategies.

34.6 Case studies

34.6.1 Development of upcoming findings in plants and microbes

Many case studies are being done to explain the wide uses of n-3 PUFAs, especially EPA and DHA, mainly concerned with health and food products. Also, it has the tendency to give protection against noncontagious diseases. Nowadays, in the world, because of lifestyle changes, people are affected by many disorders. So, in those circumstances, the necessity for natural and eco-friendly ways for n-3 PUFAs increased. Oils obtained from plant sources like chia (*Salvia hispanica*), flax (*Linum usitatissimum*), and garden cress (*Lepidium sativum*) are mainly used to improve absorption of ALA through diet. In addition to all these, oils from *Echium plantagineum*, *Buglossoides arvensis*, and Ribes species are being chosen as high availability of stearidonic acid, and it is highly strong than ALA in elevating EPA and DHA in people. At present, for commercial production of veg n-3 oils, microalgae and thraustochytrids are being the food sources has high EPA and DHA. Therefore in the case study done by Saini et al. (2021), it has been shown that plant, micro, and macroalgae, thraustochytrids with respect to oxidative stability, bioavailability, and other aspects in the upcoming years are clearly depicted with nutrition and industry point of view.

34.6.2 Regulation of gut microbiota through foods enriched with omega-3

Prevailing evidence links gut microbes to the improvement of metabolic and inflammation disorders, and at this stage, diet acts as an important modulator for the microorganisms. The case study in which 45-year man who has taken 600 mg n-3 daily for nearly 14 days, with microbes found in fecal resulted in the finding of less occurrence of overall species, but on the other side with some more amount of butyrate- generating bacteria present. A decrease in the presence of *Faecalibacterium prausnitzii* and *Akkermansia* species was noted; the presence of microbes went to very low levels after the experimental 14-days duration. Noriega et al. (2016) showed that the benefits of n-3 might be affected by the production of butyrate-generating bacteria, so this study talks about a mechanism for its protection from deadly disorders and elucidated protocols for good nutrition strategies.

34.6.3 Bio accessibility analysis and carriage of n-3 through cells in incorporated meat products

The important aspect to focus on while producing foods enriched with PUFA is bioavailability. In the case study done by Solomando et al. (2024), it dealt with bioaccessibility in the intestine and the internal transport of fatty acids in the body from meat added with n-3 microcapsules, with joint static breakdown in a lab environment, with Caco-2 cell lineage evaluation. Parameters like presence of lipid level in extract of intestine, how long it is incubating, and the complete mixing nature are being examined. And when shaking the medium level SFAs consumption, it was found that a level of 30 mg fat and 8 hours intact time were interrogated as factors concerning fatty acid movement from one place to another and its absorption. Mainly, EPA and DHA were highly absorbed and without leaving Caco-2 monolayer integrity, which justifies and tells that digestion cell model as a whole will be an easy and fine method to check fatty acid bioavailability in enriched meat food items.

34.6.4 Restoring n-3 polyunsaturated fatty acids through marine foods

Forghani et al. (2023) analyzed the combined flocculation–dissolved air flotation to restore high protein and lipid presence from presalting and spice brine of herring (*Clupea harengus*). Hence, flocculation methods that are done with the help of carrageenan usage typically elevated protein and lipid restoration when compared to only the process of acidification. The final output reveals that the presence of some extent of amino acids and 16% n-3 PUFAs is observed. The source of brine decides the sensory characteristics, and presalting brine, which gives like gel forming nature. This idea talks about how by-products with nutritive value that were thrown away can be converted to useful functional food components.

34.6.5 Omega-3 and omega-6 fatty acids in brain cancer progression

The importance and benefit of PUFAs in cancer treatment have undergone many evaluations. Due to the changes in the PUFA dissemination and composition, oxylipin signaling, the onset of brain cancer with more deaths is encountered. Proofs are there to tell that diets surplus with n-6 may support tumor formation, but n-3 acts against it. Montecillo-Aguado et al. (2020) conducted research in the lab and in living animals and interpreted that n-3 and its metabolites affect tumor cell multiplication, apoptosis, angiogenesis, invasion, and immune modulation. With the controllable factors of chemotherapeutic drug penetration across the blood–brain barrier, modulation of the omega-3/omega-6 ratio presents a promising adjunct strategy in brain cancer management.

34.6.6 Natural antioxidant strategies to improve polyunsaturated fatty acid stability

The major difficulty to resolve is the oxidative instability of PUFAs. To point out this particular thing, Araújo Rodrigues et al. (2024) interrogated the stabilization in the oil, which is enriched with PUFA, and this was obtained from sardine fish cooking wastewater with the help of phenolic extract taken from the shells of acorns. The extract obtained has been shown to have more phenolic composition and high antioxidant activity, with some main constituents found are ellagic acid, epicatechin, procyanidin B2, and azelaic acid. Less occurrence of peroxide generation and resistance to oxidation of LA,

EPA, and DHA was due to application of the isolate. The concept of converting waste with a sustainable point of view encourages the implementation of strong, natural, antioxidant techniques for functional ingredients surplus with PUFA.

34.6.7 Dietary polyunsaturated fatty acid balance and breast cancer modulation

The balance of fatty acids has received more importance in the research of breast cancer. Many studies in animals and cell culture resulted in findings that n-3 PUFAs slow and reduce tumor than n-6 does. So, in the case study by Zanoaga et al. (2018), it was listed with the processes that act against cancer as membrane remodeling, modulation of signaling cascades, gene expression regulation, antiangiogenic and antimetastatic activities, and microRNA modulation. So, in context, De Lorgeril & Salen (2012) showed that a food chart similar to food from mediterranean have a less saturated and n-6 consumption. Also, plant and marine n-3 consumption in moderate amounts reduces the risk of heart problems and breast cancer, especially by way of developing a ratio of n-3 and n-6.

34.6.8 Resistance of inflammation in kidney transplant patients through n-3 foods

The inflammation-resisting quality of n-3-stuffed diets was supported by many proofs in medical science. Sabbatini et al. (2013) showed that patients experiencing reduced omega-6/omega-3 ratios, decreased plasma cholesterol, triglycerides, C-reactive protein, and interleukin-6 levels, and a 50% lower in proteinuria and microalbuminuria without changes in glomerular filtration rate when they have taken omega-3 surplus foods naturally. The therapeutic potential of dietary n-3 strategies in transplant care was underscored by nonsignificant performance in the control group.

34.6.9 Reproductive behavior in fish through intake of polyunsaturated fatty acid-enriched foods

In a case study undertaken by Asturiano et al. (2001), it was shown that fish had qualities like more weight gain, higher volume of milt and sperm density, and improved survival of embryo and larva. Therefore this kind of results leads to the understanding of the fact that through PUFA-enriched foods, reproduction can be enhanced in the broodstock of fish.

34.6.10 Omega-3 intake and oxidative stress in mild cognitive impairment

PUFAs resolved the problem of mild cognitive impairment (MCI) in people, especially older people, in terms of giving neuroprotection benefits. Lee et al. (2013) interpreted that the lipid peroxidation was occurring at very low levels in MCI patients' plasma, and this example suggests the world that how protective PUFA can act against the process of nerve degeneration.

34.6.11 Supplementation of n-3 polyunsaturated fatty acid into beverages

García-Alonso et al. (2012) explained that if a women eat tomato beverage that is supplemented with PUFA regularly for nearly two weeks, it has been found with positive outcomes like uplifted antioxidant capacity, less lipid peroxidation and homocysteine levels, decreases in cell-binding molecules such as vascular cell adhesion molecule (VCAM)-1 and intercellular adhesion molecule (ICAM)-1, which leads to good protection of the heart, and all these benefits are due to n-3 PUFAs and antioxidants in tomato. Here, Table 34.1 shows some case studies and outcomes related to PUFAs.

34.7 Challenges in polyunsaturated fatty acids incorporation

Even though PUFA foods have a good place in the market, PUFA supplementation in foods has some challenges, such as oxidative instability, degradation risk, and marine oils contamination. So, steps to resolve all these have now become a major task (Business Research Insights, 2025-2033).

34.7.1 Unequal proportion of n-3 and n-6 in current nutrition foods

Many proofs talk about cytokine-stimulating eicosanoid production with respect to n-6. On the other side, inflammation-reducing pathways supported by n-3, and that leads to the execution of balance for health regulation (Simopoulos, 2010). Now, because of the imbalance of n-6 and n-3, people are facing heart problems, cancer, and other severe impacts (Simopoulos, 2010). Through medical science, it has been shown that a 4:1 ratio reduces heart attack and stroke deaths; a 2:1 to 3:1 ratio suppresses inflammatory problems like rheumatoid arthritis, and a 5:1 ratio has benefits with asthma patients. For prolonged health benefits, ratios near 10:1 (Simopoulos, 2010).

TABLE 34.1 Case studies and outcomes related to polyunsaturated fatty acids (PUFAs).

Case study	Findings	References
Sustainable sources	Plant oils (chia, flax) and microalgae are emerging eco-friendly sources of omega-3 (EPA and DHA) for functional foods.	Saini et al. (2021)
Gut health	Omega-3 intake can modify gut bacteria and support metabolic and antiinflammatory benefits.	Noriega et al. (2016)
Bioavailability	Fortified foods can effectively deliver EPA and DHA when absorption and stability are optimized.	Solomando et al. (2024)
Waste recovery	Marine processing by-products can be reused to extract valuable long-chain omega-3 fatty acids.	Forghani et al. (2023)
Cancer research	Higher omega-3 and balanced omega-6/omega-3 ratios may help reduce tumor progression.	Montecillo-Aguado et al. (2020), Zanoaga et al. (2018)
Oxidative stability	Natural antioxidants improve the stability of PUFA-rich oils and prevent oxidation.	Araújo-Rodrigues et al. (2024)
Clinical benefits	Omega-3-rich diets reduce inflammation and improve health markers in patients.	Sabbatini et al. (2013)
Aquaculture	PUFA-enriched diets enhance reproductive performance in fish broodstock.	Asturiano et al. (2001)
Cognitive health	Increased omega-3 intake may lower oxidative stress and protect brain function.	Lee et al. (2013)
Functional beverages	Omega-3 fortification in drinks improves antioxidant status and heart-health markers.	García-Alonso et al. (2012)

34.7.2 Technological constraints in bakery fortification

Providing n-3 fatty acids through food has become a challenge nowadays because of lipids, which is high effectively taken to temperature breakdown and oxidative damage during preparation and storage. But, now many building techniques of n-3 activity are taken to the combination aspect of marine and microalgal oil into baked items, and that projects to the encapsulation and antioxidant quality developed to preserve stability in food (Savatinova & Ivanova, 2024).

34.7.3 Sensory and oxidative stability challenges of marine oils

Oils obtained from marine sources with n-3 have distinctive taste, smell, and qualities that affect preference by consumers when it is supplemented to functional food products. The level of taste and smell is mainly determined by how much level is added and which fish species is chosen. Especially fish oil has a high risk of oxidative changes. In addition to this, high temperature and moisture also disturb the quality of food. So, strong measures need to be taken during the manufacture and preservation of marine oils and food items to maintain their quality (Savatinova & Ivanova, 2024).

34.7.4 Contaminant concerns in marine-derived omega-3 sources

n-3 taken from the ocean has many impurities that will affect the environment and get collected inside the fish body, and cause problems if not removed. So, at this stage, we can go for bleaching-like processes to encounter this issue. If it has been exposed to those impurities for so long, then it will lead to neurodevelopmental deficits, endocrine disruption, immune suppression, reproductive impairment, and increased carcinogenic risk. So, people, especially children, pregnant women, and women after delivery, have to be very careful in choosing marine foods for consumption (Simopoulos, 2010).

34.7.5 Dietary transitions and sustainability implications

The high importance given to processed foods having low levels of fatty acids was a drawback in nutrition. Therefore measures have to be adopted to maintain and regulate good metabolism by the utilization of traditional ingredients that will elevate sustainable nutrition with prolonged stable health and environment (Simopoulos, 2010).

34.7.6 Multifaceted challenges in polyunsaturated fatty acid-fortified food development

The criteria followed during processing, packing, and preservation techniques decide the shelf life of products and their bioavailability. So, the idea of adding fish oil during initial mixing of dough has led to high resistance to oxidation in enriched products, which highlights the maximizing efficiency of PUFA- enriched foods (Savatinova & Ivanova, 2024).

34.7.7 Production and scalability constraints in omega-enriched eggs

To produce eggs with high PUFAs mainly depends on what kind of nutritionally compiled feed is being fed to egg-producing hens. So, feed has to be prepared and fed to hens to give them good health and production of eggs. Complexes such as feed profile, environment concerns, and hen management are present to encounter. So, nutrition has to be focused beyond all these complexes, and so that the quality egg production with a good nutritional profile and availability over time can be ensured (Burdge, 2010; Simopoulos, 2010).

34.8 Strategies for effective polyunsaturated fatty acid enrichment

34.8.1 Eggs as a major supplier of n-3 polyunsaturated fatty acid

Egg is being the most preferred food product to accelerate n-3 consumption among people. Because lipids are more in egg (>4/egg) and also their metabolism within laying hens, which allows rapid modification of yolk fatty acid composition through dietary intervention (Alagawany et al., 2019).

34.8.2 Importance of egg supplementation with polyunsaturated fatty acid

The essential fatty acids are very important for regulating health. So, providing eggs supplemented with PUFA plays a major role in the development of nutritive food products (Mens et al., 2022). Fortified eggs provide a simple way to boost omega-3 intake in fish-averse diets. The integration of bioactive components and advancements in enrichment strategies has positioned eggs as bioactive foods able to address significant public health challenges (Herranz et al., 2024).

34.8.3 Technological approaches to overcome oxidation and sensory limitations

From a technological standpoint, one of the primary solutions to issues such as lipid oxidation, undesirable aroma, and off-flavors associated with fish oil incorporation is encapsulation technology. The inclusion of naturally derived antioxidant agents such as rosemary (Siejak et al., 2021), chamomile (Avula et al., 2014), beetroot, and ginger extracts (Srivastava et al., 2015) has also been explored to enhance oxidative stability.

34.8.4 Incorporation in familiar food products of people with fish oil

The best idea to encourage people to take n-3 in their diet is through the addition of pure fish oil in the foods. So, in that aspect for PUFA incorporation, food products like bread, dairy, pasta, ice cream, milkshake can be preferred because of their short shelf life, and also the problems like odor and taste will be maintained when fish oil can be straight away incorporated in these foods. Apart from this, another way is through microencapsulation, in which what happens is that the fine grind of liquid fish oil enhances oxidative stability and facilitates incorporation into products such as bakery items and infant nutritional formula.

34.8.5 Application technologies and antioxidant systems

Many synthetic antioxidants are being used, but to a certain level, due to food safety concerns. Nowadays, antioxidants from natural origin like from plants such as rosemary and oregano, are used along with tocopherol, and this is more effective than synthetic antioxidants in safeguarding PUFAs in food from oxidative adverse effects (Shahidi & Zhong, 2010).

34.8.6 Microencapsulation and processing considerations

Microcapsulation is adopted to the maximum to protect the n-3 from oxidative processes and ensure the complete availability of PUFAs in food (Kolanowski et al., 2007). Therefore before stabilizing this, the oils to be added to foods have to be thoroughly processed to get rid of impurities (Hernandez, 2019). Also, n-3 oils can be administered along with olive oil, palm oil, canola oil, and high-oleic sunflower oil to improve the resistance capacity to prevent oxidative breakdown and damage (Sundram et al., 1999).

34.8.7 Sustainable aquaculture and fatty acid optimization

In aquaculture, fatty acids can be greatly mediated through feed. So, choosing lipid sources to incorporate in feed mainly influences fatty acids with nutrition and health benefits (Alasalvar et al., 2002). Also, fish obtained from aquaculture are eco-friendly and have better nutrients incorporated than the wild capture ones. Therefore these should be in equilibrium in the maintenance of the environment and nutrition requirements (Pauly et al., 2005).

34.8.8 Dietary strategies to enhance omega-3/omega-6 proportion

People who prefer veg can go for ALA-rich plant-sourced foods (Swanson and Block, 2012). If food consumed didn't fulfill the dietary requirement, oils like fish oil, krill oil, and algal oil can be preferred for proper PUFA supplementation. In case of n-6, olive, avocado, and coconut can be preferred at a medium level (Yamashima et al., 2020). Therefore foods like greens, nuts, seeds, walnuts, and flaxseeds uplift PUFA intake (Cena & Calder, 2020).

34.8.9 Synergistic interaction of polyunsaturated fatty acids and polyphenols

Polyphenols, along with fruits and greens, maximize n-3 intake in the body. Because it prevents peroxidation that occurs through lipids. For example, chia with berries has given the best health results with important bioactive components present in them (Mititelu et al., 2024).

34.8.10 Micro- and nano-encapsulation approaches

Micro- and nano-encapsulation uses both plant and animal wall items to safeguard PUFAs from environmental factors to give good shelf life of foods (Jurić et al., 2022). The effectiveness of this process is mainly influenced by the external layer and the shell (Mane et al., 2024).

34.8.11 Encapsulation techniques and industrial feasibility

Most frequently used processes include atomization drying, phase separation encapsulation, atomized cooling solidification, solvent removal technique, fluidized bed coating method, emulsion formation process, supercritical fluid processing, electrospinning, and extrusion (Bakry et al., 2016).

34.8.12 Bioavailability of microalgal omega-3

Gastrointestinal availability of n-3 LC-PUFA from *Nannochloropsis* sp. was reported at 13%, increasing to 27%–29% following breaking of cells (Bernaerts et al., 2020), highlighting the importance of processing for enhancing nutrient availability.

34.8.13 Use of n-3 in microencapsulated nutrition goods

Growing awareness of PUFA benefits has driven widespread incorporation of microencapsulated n-3 PUFAs into dairy products, beverages, bakery items, infant foods, and animal feeds. Fish oil remains the predominant source, followed by flaxseed and other vegetable oils. However, vegan considerations have encouraged the use of plant-based omega-rich oils. Microencapsulated oils in gel or granular form have proven effective in producing oxidatively stable fortified foods (Mane et al., 2024).

34.8.14 Oleo-gels and powdered Oil systems in fortification

Oleo-gels have been explored as alternatives to products containing trans and saturated lipid spreads, chocolates, dairy, meat items, and desserts. Oleo-gels manufactured with sunflower oil and 2% shellac demonstrated four-month stability due to wax crystallization (Patel et al., 2014), while spreads formulated with virgin olive oil and 7% monoglycerides exhibited three-month stability and textural properties comparable to commercial margarine (Ögütcü & Yilmaz, 2014). Complex coacervation has been used to encapsulate fish oil for omega-3-enriched yogurt, maintaining physicochemical and sensory quality over 21 days (Tamjidi et al., 2012). Fortification of milk with flaxseed oil powder maintained acceptable sensory properties for up to five days (Goyal et al., 2015), and microencapsulated garden cress oil has been included incookies as an n-3 product (Umesha et al., 2015).

34.8.15 Augmentation of n-3 and n-6 in eggs: market and regulation

Modifying the breeding chicken's nutrition to produce eggs augmented with n-3 and n-6 has attracted strong consumer interest in functional foods (Djuricic & Calder, 2021). EPA and DHA support heart function, cognitive performance, and antiinflammatory responses, whereas n-6 plays key roles in cellular signaling and membrane integrity (Kpomasse et al., 2023; Zamani et al., 2024). Enriched eggs can contain markedly higher omega-3 concentrations reported up to 12 times greater than conventional eggs, making them attractive to individuals who do not consume fish, despite higher cost and ongoing discussion about the ideal n-3/n-6 ratio under regulatory guidance (Zamani et al., 2024). Fig. 34.4 shows some strategies to increase PUFA in food.

34.9 Future recommendation

Forecast data from 2025–33 indicates sustained expansion driven by health awareness, plant-based dietary shifts, sustainable sourcing innovations, and technological advancements in extraction and microencapsulation (DataIntelo,

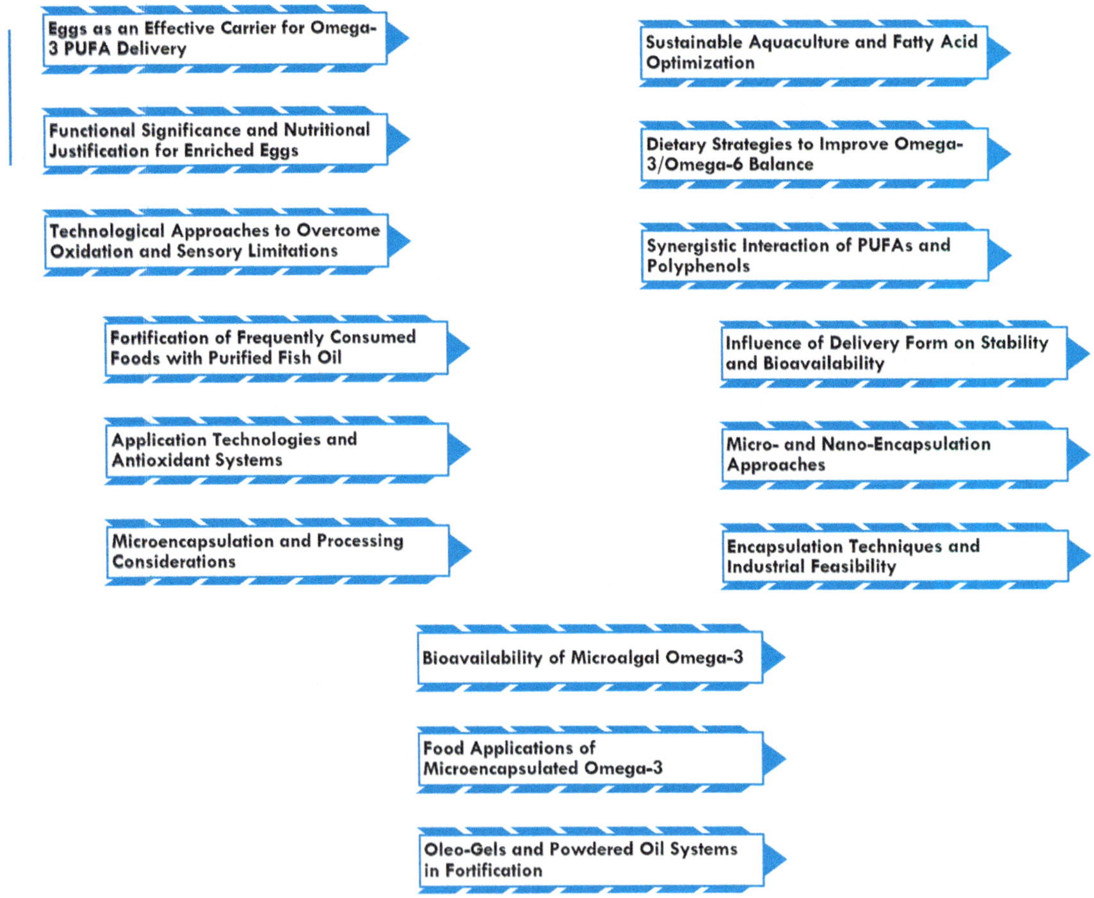
Eggs as an Effective Carrier for Omega-3 PUFA Delivery
Functional Significance and Nutritional Justification for Enriched Eggs
Technological Approaches to Overcome Oxidation and Sensory Limitations
Fortification of Frequently Consumed Foods with Purified Fish Oil
Application Technologies and Antioxidant Systems
Microencapsulation and Processing Considerations
Sustainable Aquaculture and Fatty Acid Optimization
Dietary Strategies to Improve Omega-3/Omega-6 Balance
Synergistic Interaction of PUFAs and Polyphenols
Influence of Delivery Form on Stability and Bioavailability
Micro- and Nano-Encapsulation Approaches
Encapsulation Techniques and Industrial Feasibility
Bioavailability of Microalgal Omega-3
Food Applications of Microencapsulated Omega-3
Oleo-Gels and Powdered Oil Systems in Fortification

FIGURE 34.4 Strategies to increase polyunsaturated fatty acid (PUFA) in food.

2025–33). The convergence of functional food demand and sustainability-driven product development is expected to further diversify PUFA-enriched food portfolios globally. Awareness has to be given to people about PUFA and its health benefits in the body. With techniques like encapsulation, microorganisms and their nutritional benefits, further steps can lead to technologies that will accelerate yield improvement and broaden commercial applications, ultimately strengthening the input of PUFA-enriched diets to people's nutrition, overall health, and sustainable food system development.

34.10 Conclusion

From analyzing the value and importance of PUFAs in human health, formulation of food products, their dietary efficiency, enrichment methods, it has become clear and pivotal to focus more on the preparation of PUFA-enriched foods in the market by considering all these aspects. This will automatically lead it as the natural medicine for various outbreaks of disease and also being a sustainable utilization of resources around us to make and give this for people like children, pregnant women, sports people, and adults in a good way that has highly beneficial activity.

References

Agostoni, C. (2008). Role of long-chain polyunsaturated fatty acids in the first year of life. *Journal of Pediatric Gastroenterology and Nutrition, 47*, 41–44.

Akihisa, T., Kojima, N., Katoh, N., Ichimura, Y., Suzuki, H., Fukatsu, M., Maranz, S., & Masters, E. T. (2010). Triterpene alcohol and fatty acid composition of shea nuts from seven African countries. *Journal of Oleo Science, 59*(7), 351–360.

Alagawany, M., Elnesr, S. S., Farag, M. R., Abd El-Hack, M. E., Khafaga, A. F., Taha, A. E., Tiwari, R., Yatoo, M. I., Bhatt, P., Khurana, S. K., & Dhama, K. (2019). Omega-3 and omega-6 fatty acids in poultry nutrition: Effect on production performance and health. *Animals, 9*(8), 573.

Alasalvar, C., Taylor, K. D. A., Zubcov, E., Shahidi, F., & Alexis, M. (2002). Differentiation of cultured and wild sea bass (*Dicentrarchus labrax*): Total lipid content, fatty acid and trace mineral composition. *Food Chemistry, 79*(2), 145–150.

Araújo-Rodrigues, H., Ribeiro, T. B., Machado, M., Pereira, C. D., & Pintado, M. E. (2024). The potential of acorn extract treatment on PUFAs oxidative stability: A case study on fish cooking wastewater. *Foods, 13*(6), 935.

Asturiano, J. F., Sorbera, L. A., Carrillo, M., Zanuy, S., Ramos, J., Navarro, J. C., & Bromage, N. (2001). Reproductive performance in male European sea bass (*Dicentrarchus labrax, L.*) fed two PUFA-enriched experimental diets: A comparison with males fed a wet diet. *Aquaculture, 194*(1-2), 173–190.

Attia, Y., Al Sagan, A. A., Hussein, E. S. O., Olal, M. J., Ebeid, T. A., Alabdullatif, A. A., Alhotan, R. A., Qaid, M. M., Tufarelli, V., Pugliese, G., & Asiry, K. A. (2024). Enhancing the nutritional values of egg yolks of laying hens by different dietary sources of omega-3 fatty acids, vitamin e and trace elements. *Livestock Science, 289*, 105573.

Avula, B., Wang, Y. H., Wang, M., Avonto, C., Zhao, J., Smillie, T. J., Rua, D., & Khan, I. A. (2014). Quantitative determination of phenolic compounds by UHPLC-UV–MS and use of partial least-square discriminant analysis to differentiate chemo-types of Chamomile/Chrysanthemum flower heads. *Journal of Pharmaceutical and Biomedical Analysis, 88*, 278–288.

Bakry, A. M., Abbas, S., Ali, B., Majeed, H., Abouelwafa, M. Y., Mousa, A., & Liang, L. (2016). Microencapsulation of oils: A comprehensive review of benefits, techniques, and applications. *Comprehensive Reviews in Food Science and Food Safety, 15*(1), 143–182.

Bernaerts, T. M., Verstreken, H., Dejonghe, C., Gheysen, L., Foubert, I., Grauwet, T., & Van Loey, A. M. (2020). Cell disruption of *Nannochloropsis* sp. improves in vitro bioaccessibility of carotenoids and ω3-LC-PUFA. *Journal of Functional Foods, 65*, 103770.

Brenna, J. T., & Carlson, S. E. (2014). Docosahexaenoic acid and human brain development: evidence that a dietary supply is needed for optimal development. *Journal of Human Evolution, 77*, 99–106.

Burdge, G. C. (2010). Polyunsaturated fatty acid intakes and α-linolenic acid metabolism. *The American Journal of Clinical Nutrition, 93*(3), 665–666.

Business Research Insights (2025-2033). https://www.businessresearchinsights.com/market-reports/pufa-market-112261.

Calder, P. C. (2016). Docosahexaenoic acid. *Annals of Nutrition and Metabolism, 69*(Suppl. 1), 8–21.

Cena, H., & Calder, P. C. (2020). Defining a healthy diet: evidence for the role of contemporary dietary patterns in health and disease. *Nutrients, 12*(2), 334.

Certik, M., & Adamechova, Z. (2009). Cereal-based bioproducts containing polyunsaturated fatty acids. *Lipid Technology, 21*(11-12), 250–253.

Connor, W. E. (2000). Importance of n– 3 fatty acids in health and disease. *The American Journal of Clinical Nutrition, 71*(1), 171–175.

Dal Bello, B., Torri, L., Piochi, M., & Zeppa, G. (2015). Healthy yogurt fortified with n-3 fatty acids from vegetable sources. *Journal of Dairy Science, 98*(12), 8375–8385.

D'Angelo, S., Motti, M. L., & Meccariello, R. (2020). ω-3 and ω-6 polyunsaturated fatty acids, obesity and cancer. *Nutrients, 12*(9), 2751.

Das, U. N. (2006). Essential fatty acids-A review. *Current Pharmaceutical Biotechnology, 7*(6), 467–482.

De Lorgeril, M., & Salen, P. (2012). New insights into the health effects of dietary saturated and omega-6 and omega-3 polyunsaturated fatty acids. *BMC Medicine, 10*(1), 50.

Djuricic, I., & Calder, P. C. (2021). Beneficial outcomes of omega-6 and omega-3 polyunsaturated fatty acids on human health: An update for 2021. *Nutrients, 13*(7), 2421.

EFSA Panel on Dietetic Products, Nutrition, and Allergies (NDA), (2010). Scientific Opinion on Dietary Reference Values for fats, including saturated fatty acids, polyunsaturated fatty acids, monounsaturated fatty acids, trans fatty acids, and cholesterol. Efsa Journal, 8(3), 1461.

Forghani, B., Mihnea, M., Svendsen, T. C., & Undeland, I. (2023). Protein and long-chain n-3 polyunsaturated fatty acids recovered from herring brines upon flocculation and flotation— A case study. *ACS Sustainable Chemistry & Engineering, 11*(17), 6523–6534.

Fraeye, I., Bruneel, C., Lemahieu, C., Buyse, J., Muylaert, K., & Foubert, I. (2012). Dietary enrichment of eggs with omega-3 fatty acids: A review. *Food Research International, 48*(2), 961–969.

Frutos, P., Toral, P. G., Belenguer, A., & Hervás, G. (2018). Milk fat depression in dairy ewes fed fish oil: Might differences in rumen biohydrogenation, fermentation, or bacterial community explain the individual variation? *Journal of Dairy Science, 101*(7), 6122–6132.

Gaffari, S. M., & Khoshnood, Z. (2021). Comparative study of the fatty acid composition of light/dark mixture musculature of five freshwater fish from the region of Dezful, Iran. *Food Science and Applied Biotechnology, 4*(1), 57–62.

Gajos, G., Zalewski, J., Rostoff, P., Nessler, J., Piwowarska, W., & Undas, A. (2011). Reduced thrombin formation and altered fibrin clot properties induced by polyunsaturated omega-3 fatty acids on top of dual antiplatelet therapy in patients undergoing percutaneous coronary intervention (OMEGA-PCI clot). *Arteriosclerosis, Thrombosis, and Vascular Biology, 31*(7), 1696–1702.

Ganesan, B., Brothersen, C., & McMahon, D. J. (2014). Fortification of foods with omega-3 polyunsaturated fatty acids. *Critical Reviews in Food Science and Nutrition, 54*(1), 98–114.

García-Alonso, F. J., Jorge-Vidal, V., Ros, G., & Periago, M. J. (2012). Effect of consumption of tomato juice enriched with n-3 polyunsaturated fatty acids on the lipid profile, antioxidant biomarker status, and cardiovascular disease risk in healthy women. *European Journal of Nutrition, 51*(4), 415–424.

Garg, M. L., Wood, L. G., Singh, H., & Moughan, P. J. (2006). Means of delivering recommended levels of long chain n-3 polyunsaturated fatty acids in human diets. *Journal of Food Science, 71*(5), 66–71.

Gladyshev, M. I., Sushchik, N. N., & Makhutova, O. N. (2013). Production of EPA and DHA in aquatic ecosystems and their transfer to the land. *Prostaglandins & Other Lipid Mediators, 107*, 117–126.

Göksen, G., Fabra, M. J., Ekiz, H. I., & López-Rubio, A. (2020). Phytochemical-loaded electrospun nanofibers as novel active edible films: Characterization and antibacterial efficiency in cheese slices. *Food Control, 112*, 107133.

Goyal, A., Sharma, V., Sihag, M. K., Tomar, S. K., Arora, S., Sabikhi, L., & Singh, A. K. (2015). Development and physico-chemical characterization of microencapsulated flaxseed oil powder: A functional ingredient for omega-3 fortification. *Powder Technology, 286*, 27–537.

Hernandez, E. (2019). Production, processing, and refining of oils. In *Healthful lipids*. AOCS Publishing (48-64).

Hernandez, E. M. (2013). Enrichment of baked goods with omega-3 fatty acids. In *Food enrichment with omega-3 fatty acids*. Woodhead Publishing (319-335).

Herranz, B., Romero, C., Sánchez-Román, I., López-Torres, M., Viveros, A., Arija, I., Álvarez, M. D., de Pascual-Teresa, S., & Chamorro, S. (2024). Enriching eggs with bioactive compounds through the inclusion of grape pomace in laying hens diet: Effect on internal and external egg quality parameters. *Foods, 13*(10), 1553.

Hibbeln, J. R., Nieminen, L. R., Blasbalg, T. L., Riggs, J. A., & Lands, W. E. (2006). Healthy intakes of n– 3 and n–6 fatty acids: Estimations considering worldwide diversity. *The American Journal of Clinical Nutrition, 83*(6), 1483S–1493S.

Hixson, S. M., Sharma, B., Kainz, M. J., Wacker, A., & Arts, M. T. (2015). Production, distribution, and abundance of long-chain omega-3 polyunsaturated fatty acids: A fundamental dichotomy between freshwater and terrestrial ecosystems. *Environmental Reviews, 23*(4), 414–424.

Jakobsson, A., Westerberg, R., & Jacobsson, A. (2006). Fatty acid elongases in mammals: Their regulation and roles in metabolism. *Progress in Lipid Research, 45*(3), 237–249.

Jensen, K. N., Jacobsen, C., & Nielsen, H. H. (2007). Fatty acid composition of herring (*Clupea harengus* L.): Influence of time and place of catch on n-3 PUFA content. *Journal of the Science of Food and Agriculture, 87*(4), 710–718.

Jurić, S., Jurić, M., Siddique, M. A. B., & Fathi, M. (2022). Vegetable oils rich in polyunsaturated fatty acids: Nanoencapsulation methods and stability enhancement. *Food Reviews International, 38*(1), 32–69.

Kapoor, B., Kapoor, D., Gautam, S., Singh, R., & Bhardwaj, S. (2021). Dietary polyunsaturated fatty acids (PUFAs): Uses and potential health benefits. *Current nutrition reports, 10*(3), 232–242.

Kliem, K. E., Humphries, D. J., Kirton, P., Givens, D. I., & Reynolds, C. K. (2019). Differential effects of oilseed supplements on methane production and milk fatty acid concentrations in dairy cows. *Animal, 13*(2), 309–317.

Kolanowski, W. (2005). Bioavailability of omega-3 PUFA from foods enriched with fish oil. *Polish Journal of Food and Nutrition Sciences, 55*(4), 335–340.

Kolanowski, W., Jaworska, D., Weißbrodt, J., & Kunz, B. (2007). Sensory assessment of microencapsulated fish oil powder. *Journal of the American Oil Chemists' Society, 84*(1), 37–45.

Kpomasse, C. C., Kouame, Y. A. E., N'nanle, O., Houndonougbo, F. M., Tona, K., & Oke, O. E. (2023). The productivity and resilience of the indigenous chickens in the tropical environments: Improvement and future perspectives. *Journal of Applied Animal Research, 51*(1), 456–469.

Kyosev, D., & Dragoev, S. (2009). *Technology of the fish and the fish products* (1st ed.). HVP. [In Bulgarian], 334 p. Print ISBN: 978-954-90533-6-4.

Lee, L. K., Shahar, S., Rajab, N., Yusoff, N. A. M., Jamal, R. A., & Then, S. M. (2013). The role of long chain omega-3 polyunsaturated fatty acids in reducing lipid peroxidation among elderly patients with mild cognitive impairment: A case-control study. *The Journal of Nutritional Biochemistry, 24*(5), 803–808.

Lemahieu, C., Bruneel, C., Ryckebosch, E., Muylaert, K., Buyse, J., & Foubert, I. (2015). Impact of different omega-3 polyunsaturated fatty acid (n-3 PUFA) sources (flaxseed, *Isochrysis galbana*, fish oil and DHA Gold) on n-3 LC-PUFA enrichment (efficiency) in the egg yolk. *Journal of Functional Foods, 19*, 821–827.

Li, M., Liu, Y., Li, Q., Yang, M., Pi, Y., Yang, N., Zheng, Y., & Yue, X. (2020). Comparative exploration of free fatty acids in donkey colostrum and mature milk based on a metabolomics approach. *Journal of Dairy Science, 103*(7), 6022–6031.

Lie, D. (2004). Dietary fatty acids may reduce risk of cognitive decline. *Neurology, 62*, 275–280.

Mane, S., Kumari, P., Singh, A., Taneja, N. K., & Chopra, R. (2024). Amelioration for oxidative stability and bioavailability of N-3 PUFA enriched microalgae oil: An overview. *Critical Reviews in Food Science and Nutrition, 64*(9), 2579–2600.

McEwen, B. J., Morel-Kopp, M. C., Chen, W., Tofler, G. H., & Ward, C. M. (2013). February. Effects of omega-3 polyunsaturated fatty acids on platelet function in healthy subjects and subjects with cardiovascular disease. In *Seminars in thrombosis and hemostasis, Vol. 39*Thieme Medical Publishers No. 01, 025-032.

Mens, A. J. W., Van Krimpen, M. M., Kar, S. K., Guiscafre, F. J., & Sijtsma, L. (2022). Enriching table eggs with n-3 polyunsaturated fatty acids through dietary supplementation with the phototrophically grown green algae Nannochloropsis limnetica: Effects of microalgae on nutrient retention, performance, egg characteristics and health parameters. *Poultry Science, 101*(6), 101869.

Miranda, J. M., Anton, X., Redondo-Valbuena, C., Roca-Saavedra, P., Rodriguez, J. A., Lamas, A., Franco, C. M., & Cepeda, A. (2015). Egg and egg-derived foods: Effects on human health and use as functional foods. *Nutrients, 7*(1), 706–729.

Mititelu, M., Lupuliasa, D., Neacşu, S. M., Olteanu, G., Busnatu, S., Mihai, A., Popovici, V., Măru, N., Boroghină, S. C., Mihai, S., & Ioniță-Mîndrican, C. B. (2024). Polyunsaturated fatty acids and human health: A key to modern nutritional balance in association with polyphenolic compounds from food sources. *Foods, 14*(1), 46.

Mnari, A., Bouhlel, I., Chraief, I., Hammami, M., Romdhane, M. S., El Cafsi, M., & Chaouch, A. (2007). Fatty acids in muscles and liver of Tunisian wild and farmed gilthead sea bream, *Sparus aurata. Food Chemistry, 100*(4), 1393–1397.

Montecillo-Aguado, M., Tirado-Rodriguez, B., Tong, Z., Vega, O. M., Morales-Martínez, M., Abkenari, S., Pedraza-Chaverri, J., & Huerta-Yepez, S. (2020). Importance of the role of ω-3 and ω-6 polyunsaturated fatty acids in the progression of brain cancer. *Brain Sciences, 10*(6), 381.

Napier, J. A., Usher, S., Haslam, R. P., Ruiz-Lopez, N., & Sayanova, O. (2015). Transgenic plants as a sustainable, terrestrial source of fish oils. *European Journal of Lipid Science and Technology, 117*(9), 1317–1324.

Nettleton, J. A. (1995). Omega-3 fatty acids and health. In *Omega-3 fatty acids and health.* Boston, MA: Springer US (64-76).

Noriega, B. S., Sanchez-Gonzalez, M. A., Salyakina, D., & Coffman, J. (2016). Understanding the impact of omega-3 rich diet on the gut microbiota. *Case Reports in Medicine*(1), 3089303 2016.

Nowak, J. Z. (2009). Wielonienasycone kwasy tłuszczowe omega-3 w siatkówce i praktyce medycznej–blaski i cienie. *Magazyn Lekarza Okulisty, 3*, 208–220.

Ögütcü, M., & Yilmaz, E. (2014). Oleogels of virgin olive oil with carnauba wax and monoglyceride as spreadable products. *Grasas y Aceites, 65*(3), 12.

Patel, A. R., Rajarethinem, P. S., Grędowska, A., Turhan, O., Lesaffer, A., De Vos, W. H., Van de Walle, D., & Dewettinck, K. (2014). Edible applications of shellac oleogels: Spreads, chocolate paste and cakes. *Food & Function, 5*(4), 645–652.

PUFA (Polyunsaturated Fatty Acids) Market (Global forecast from 2025 to 2033) [dataintelo.com]. https://r.search.yahoo.com/_ylt=AwrKDyYoOp1pKQIAjz67HAx.;_ylu=Y29sbwNzZzMEcG9zAzEEdnRpZAMEc2VjA3Ny/RV=2/RE=1773121320/RO=10/RU=https%3a%2f%2fdataintelo.com%2freport%2fpufamarket/RK=2/RS=e2m4EcXbC5ErHuu16PoFmce00wQ-.

Pauly, D., Watson, R., & Alder, J. (2005). Global trends in world fisheries: Impacts on marine ecosystems and food security. *Philosophical Transactions of the Royal Society B: Biological Sciences, 360*(1453), 5–12.

Réhault-Godbert, S., Guyot, N., & Nys, Y. (2019). The golden egg: Nutritional value, bioactivities, and emerging benefits for human health. *Nutrients, 11*(3), 684.

Riediger, N. D., Othman, R. A., Suh, M., & Moghadasian, M. H. (2009). A systemic review of the roles of n-3 fatty acids in health and disease. *Journal of the American Dietetic Association, 109*(4), 668–679.

Roy, J., Mercier, Y., Tonnet, L., Burel, C., Lanuque, A., Surget, A., Larroquet, L., Corraze, G., Terrier, F., Panserat, S., & Skiba, S. (2020). Rainbow trout prefer diets rich in omega-3 long chain polyunsaturated fatty acids DHA and EPA. *Physiology & Behavior, 213*, 112692.

Ruxton, C. H. S., & Derbyshire, E. (2009). Latest evidence on omega-3 fatty acids and health. *Nutrition & Food Science, 39*(4), 423–438.

Sabbatini, M., Apicella, L., Cataldi, M., Maresca, I., Nastasi, A., Vitale, S., Memoli, B., Postiglione, L., Riccio, E., Gallo, R., & Federico, S. (2013). Effects of a diet rich in N-3 polyunsaturated fatty acids on systemic inflammation in renal transplant recipients. *Journal of the American College of Nutrition, 32*(6), 375–383.

Saini, R. K., Prasad, P., Sreedhar, R. V., Akhilender Naidu, K., Shang, X., & Keum, Y. S. (2021). Omega– 3 polyunsaturated fatty acids (PUFAs): Emerging plant and microbial sources, oxidative stability, bioavailability, and health benefits—A review. *Antioxidants, 10*(10), 1627.

Savatinova, M., & Ivanova, M. (2024). Functional dairy products enriched with omega-3 fatty acids. *Food Science and Applied Biotechnology, 7*(1), 1–13.

Shahidi, F., & Ambigaipalan, P. (2018). Omega-3 polyunsaturated fatty acids and their health benefits. *Annual Review of Food Science and Technology, 9*, 345–381.

Shahidi, F., & Zhong, Y. (2010). Novel antioxidants in food quality preservation and health promotion. *European Journal of Lipid Science and Technology, 112*(9), 930–940.

Shakoor, H., Khan, M. I., Sahar, A., Khan, M. K. I., Faiz, F., & Basheer Ahmad, H. (2020). Development of omega-3 rich eggs through dietary flaxseed and bio-evaluation in metabolic syndrome. *Food Science & Nutrition, 8*(6), 2619–2626.

SACN, U. (2004). Advice on fish consumption: benefits & risks. Istituto Superiore di Sanit.

Siejak, P., Smułek, W., Fathordobady, F., Grygier, A., Baranowska, H. M., Rudzińska, M., Masewicz, Ł., Jarzębska, M., Nowakowski, P. T., Makiej, A., & Kazemian, P. (2021). Multidisciplinary studies of folk medicine "five thieves' oil"(*Olejek pięciu* złodziei) components. *Molecules, 26*(10), 2931.

Simonetto, M., Infante, M., Sacco, R. L., Rundek, T., & Della-Morte, D. (2019). A novel anti-inflammatory role of omega-3 PUFAs in prevention and treatment of atherosclerosis and vascular cognitive impairment and dementia. *Nutrients, 11*(10), 2279.

Simopoulos, A. P. (2010). The omega-6/omega-3 fatty acid ratio: Health implications. *Oléagineux, Corps Gras, Lipides, 17*(5), 267–275.

Simopoulos, A.P., Leaf, A., & Salem, N., Jr. (1999). Workshop on the essentiality of and recommended dietary intakes for omega-6 and omega-3 fatty acids. ISSFAL Newsletters, 6(2), 14–16.

Solomando, J. C., Antequera, T., Estaras, M., González, A., & Perez-Palacios, T. (2024). In vitro digestion and culture in Caco-2 cells to assess the bioavailability of fatty acids: A case study in meat matrix enriched with ω-3 microcapsules. *Food Science & Nutrition, 12*(9), 6338–6352.

Srivastava, P., Prasad, S. G. M., Ali, M. N., & Prasad, M. (2015). Analysis of antioxidant activity of herbal yoghurt prepared from different milk. *The Pharma Innovation, 4*(3, Part A), 18.

Strauss, M. H., Dorian, P., & Verma, S. (2005). Fish oil supplementation and arrhythmias. *JAMA, 294*(17), 2165–2166.

Sundram, K., Perlman, D., Hayes, K. C., & Brandeis University. (1999). *Blends of palm fat and corn oil provide oxidation-resistant shortenings for baking and frying* (U.S. Patent no. 5,874,117).

Swanson, D., Block, R., & Mousa, S. A. (2012). Omega-3 fatty acids EPA and DHA: Health benefits throughout life. *Advances in Nutrition, 3*(1), 1–7.

Tamjidi, F., Nasirpour, A., & Shahedi, M. (2012). Physicochemical and sensory properties of yogurt enriched with microencapsulated fish oil. *Food Science and Technology International, 18*(4), 381–390.

Tocher, D. R., Betancor, M. B., Sprague, M., Olsen, R. E., & Napier, J. A. (2019). Omega-3 long-chain polyunsaturated fatty acids, EPA and DHA: Bridging the gap between supply and demand. *Nutrients, 11*(1), 89.

Tvrzicka, E., Kremmyda, L. S., Stankova, B., & Zak, A. (2011). Fatty acids as biocompounds: Their role in human metabolism, health and disease–A review. Part 1: classification, dietary sources and biological functions. *Biomedical Papers of the Medical Faculty of the University Palacký, Olomouc, Czech Republic, 155*(2), 117–130.

Umesha, S. S., Manohar, R. S., Indiramma, A. R., Akshitha, S., & Naidu, K. A. (2015). Enrichment of biscuits with microencapsulated omega-3 fatty acid (Alpha-linolenic acid) rich Garden cress (*Lepidium sativum*) seed oil: Physical, sensory and storage quality characteristics of biscuits. *LWT-Food Science and Technology, 62*(1), 654–661.

Usydus, Z., & Szlinder-Richert, J. (2012). Functional properties of fish and fish products: A review. *International Journal of Food Properties, 15*(4), 823–846.

Wang, C., Harris, W. S., Chung, M., Lichtenstein, A. H., Balk, E. M., Kupelnick, B., Jordan, H. S., & Lau, J. (2006). n– 3 Fatty acids from fish or fish-oil supplements, but not α-linolenic acid, benefit cardiovascular disease outcomes in primary-and secondary-prevention studies: A systematic review. *The American Journal of Clinical Nutrition, 84*(1), 5–17.

Wiktorowska-Owczarek, A., Berezinska, M., & Nowak, J. Z. (2015). PUFAs: Structures, metabolism and functions. *Advances in Clinical and Experimental Medicine, 24*(6), 931–941.

Yamashima, T., Ota, T., Mizukoshi, E., Nakamura, H., Yamamoto, Y., Kikuchi, M., Yamashita, T., & Kaneko, S. (2020). Intake of ω-6 polyunsaturated fatty acid-rich vegetable oils and risk of lifestyle diseases. *Advances in Nutrition, 11*(6), 1489–1509.

Zamani, O., Bittmann, T., & Ortega, D. L. (2024). The effect of avian influenza outbreaks on retail price premiums in the United States poultry market. *Poultry Science, 103*(10), 104102.

Zanoaga, O., Jurj, A., Raduly, L., Cojocneanu-Petric, R., Fuentes-Mattei, E., Wu, O., Braicu, C., Gherman, C. D., & Berindan-Neagoe, I. (2018). Implications of dietary ω-3 and ω-6 polyunsaturated fatty acids in breast cancer. *Experimental and Therapeutic Medicine, 15*(2), 1167–1176.

Section VIII

Future opportunities

Chapter 35

Future directions in polyunsaturated fatty acid technology and product development

Saeid Jafari[1,2], Mahdi Ebrahimi[3], Dharmendra Mishra[1], and Kitipong Assatarakul[2]
[1]*Department of Food Science, Purdue University, West Lafayette, IN, United States,* [2]*Department of Food Technology, Faculty of Science, Chulalongkorn University, Bangkok, Thailand,* [3]*Department of Vet erinary Preclinical Sciences, Faculty of Veterinary Medicine, University Putra Malaysia, Serdang, Selangor, Malaysia*

35.1 Introduction

35.1.1 Overview of current polyunsaturated fatty acids applications

The omega-3 and omega-6 families of polyunsaturated fatty acids (PUFAs) are vital for maintaining cardiovascular health, brain function, and regulating inflammation. Given these benefits, compounds such as eicosapentaenoic acid (EPA) and docosahexaenoic acid (DHA) are key ingredients in functional foods and supplements, and are extensively used across food, pharmaceutical, and cosmetic applications (Jafari et al., 2022).

In the food industry, PUFAs are incorporated into fortified products, including infant formulas, dairy alternatives, and functional beverages, to enhance their nutritional value. Their role in maintaining heart health has also led to the widespread inclusion of omega-3-rich oils in processed foods and dietary supplements. In the pharmaceutical sector, PUFAs are utilized for their therapeutic potential, particularly in managing conditions such as cardiovascular diseases, arthritis, and cognitive decline. Prescription omega-3 formulations are available for patients with hypertriglyceridemia and other metabolic disorders (Kaka et al., 2023).

In addition, their nutritional and therapeutic uses, PUFAs are now prominent ingredients in cosmetic products, valued for their ability to nourish skin and combat signs of aging. Incorporated into skincare formulations, these bioactive lipids enhance hydration, diminish inflammation, and strengthen the skin's protective barrier. Continuous advancements in research and processing technologies are broadening PUFA applications, resulting in more effective delivery mechanisms, environmentally sustainable production, and innovative formulations that boost both their stability and performance.

35.1.2 Importance of innovation in polyunsaturated fatty acids technology

PUFAs are essential bioactive lipids with significant health benefits, widely utilized in food, pharmaceuticals, and cosmetics. However, their application is often challenged by issues such as oxidative instability, limited bioavailability, and sustainable sourcing. Innovations in PUFA technology are crucial to overcoming these limitations and enhancing their functionality, efficacy, and accessibility. Advancements in extraction, purification, and encapsulation techniques have improved the stability and delivery of PUFAs in various formulations (Jafari et al., 2023). Emerging technologies, such as nanotechnology-based delivery systems and structural modifications, are further optimizing PUFA absorption and bioactivity. Additionally, sustainable production methods, including algal and microbial fermentation, are addressing environmental concerns and reducing reliance on traditional marine sources.

Artificial intelligence and biotechnological approaches, such as genetic modification of microorganisms and plants, are revolutionizing PUFA production by enabling precision fermentation and bioengineering for enhanced yield and purity (Zhao et al., 2024). These innovations not only support a circular bioeconomy but also contribute to the development of high-value PUFA-enriched products with improved health benefits. As consumer demand for functional foods and

Omega-3 and Omega-6 Polyunsaturated Fatty Acids in Food Systems. DOI: https://doi.org/10.1016/B978-0-443-43810-3.00024-5

nutraceuticals grows, continuous advancements in PUFA technology will be essential in shaping the future of the industry. By leveraging cutting-edge research and technological breakthroughs, the next generation of PUFA-based products will offer superior stability, bioavailability, and sustainability, meeting both health and environmental goals (Ebrahimi et al., 2018).

This chapter explores advancements in PUFA technology and product development, focusing on improving extraction, purification, and stabilization methods. It examines sustainable sources like algal and microbial fermentation and the role of AI and bioengineering in optimizing PUFA production. Additionally, it reviews market trends, regulatory considerations, and emerging challenges and opportunities in the field. By addressing these areas, the chapter provides insights into the future of PUFA-enriched food, pharmaceutical, and cosmetic applications.

35.1.3 Emerging trends in polyunsaturated fatty acid research: advances in biosynthesis and biotechnology

The key advances in PUFA biosynthesis and biotechnology are as follows (Jia et al., 2022): (1) genetic engineering of microorganisms for PUFA production: genetic modification of microorganisms, including bacteria, yeast, and fungi, has emerged as a powerful strategy for producing PUFAs at scale. To achieve more efficient and sustainable production, microbial metabolic pathways are being genetically reprogrammed to overproduce specific PUFAs such as omega-3 and omega-6 fatty acids. By overexpressing rate-limiting enzymes, including desaturases and elongases, researchers can develop strains that deliver higher yields while lowering production costs and environmental impact compared to traditional methods. Genetic modification has enabled microorganisms like the lipid-rich yeast *Yarrowia lipolytica* to produce long-chain PUFAs (EPA, DHA). Similarly, engineered *Escherichia coli* and *Saccharomyces cerevisiae* strains achieve high omega-3 yields, offering a sustainable alternative to marine extraction. (2) Algal biotechnology for sustainable PUFA production: microalgae are considered one of the most sustainable and efficient sources of PUFAs, particularly for omega-3 fatty acids like EPA and DHA. Algal strains naturally produce these PUFAs, but advances in algal biotechnology have enabled significant improvements in their yield and productivity. Through selective breeding and genetic modification, algae strains are being developed with enhanced PUFA biosynthesis capabilities, allowing for large-scale, sustainable production in controlled environments such as photobioreactors (Harwood, 2019). Metabolic engineering is also being applied to algae to optimize the biosynthetic pathways for PUFAs. By introducing or enhancing the expression of specific genes responsible for PUFA synthesis, researchers have been able to increase the yield of desirable PUFAs in algal strains. The ability to produce high concentrations of EPA and DHA from algae offers a renewable and environmentally friendly alternative to fish oil, which is subject to overfishing concerns:

35.1.3.1 Plant-based polyunsaturated fatty acid production through genetic modification

Plants, particularly oilseed crops such as soybeans, canola, and flaxseed, have long been utilized for the production of omega-3 PUFAs, but their natural yields of these fatty acids are limited. Advances in plant biotechnology are addressing this limitation by genetically modifying crops to produce higher concentrations of PUFAs (Ruiz-Lopez et al., 2015). For instance, transgenic canola plants have been engineered to produce increased levels of α-linolenic acid (ALA), a precursor to omega-3 fatty acids, by introducing genes from algae and microorganisms that enhance omega-3 biosynthesis (Xue et al., 2023). In addition, the genetic modification of oilseeds to produce more desirable PUFAs, such as EPA and DHA, is also being explored. By introducing key desaturases and elongases from algae or microorganisms into plant genomes, researchers are developing oilseed crops capable of synthesizing PUFAs in higher quantities, providing an alternative source for human and animal nutrition.

35.1.3.2 Bioreactor and fermentation technologies for polyunsaturated fatty acid production

Bioreactors and fermentation systems are integral to scaling up PUFA production from genetically modified microorganisms, algae, and plants (Guo et al., 2018). Recent innovations in bioreactor design and fermentation techniques have led to more efficient, cost-effective, and sustainable PUFA production processes (Venkatraman et al., 2024). High-density fermentation systems, which allow for large-scale microbial growth in controlled environments, are being optimized to produce high concentrations of PUFAs. Furthermore, bioreactor systems are being tailored to specific production needs, such as the optimization of light conditions, nutrient availability, and temperature, to enhance the yield of PUFAs from microalgae. Fed-batch and continuous fermentation processes have also shown promise in improving the yield and productivity of PUFAs, while minimizing the environmental impact of traditional production methods.

35.1.3.3 Synthetic biology approaches to polyunsaturated fatty acid production

Synthetic biology is playing a transformative role in the production of PUFAs by enabling the construction of novel metabolic pathways that can produce PUFAs in microorganisms and plants (Jagadevan et al., 2018). This field combines principles from genetic engineering, metabolic engineering, and systems biology to design and construct new biological systems capable of synthesizing PUFAs more efficiently and at scale. One notable application of synthetic biology is the creation of engineered biosynthetic pathways in microorganisms that enable the production of uncommon or high-value PUFA derivatives (Xu et al., 2013). For example, researchers are using synthetic biology to produce high-value omega-3 fatty acids, such as EPA and DHA, in microbial platforms, reducing the reliance on marine sources and providing a more sustainable alternative (Qin et al., 2023).

35.1.3.4 Optimization of polyunsaturated fatty acid yield through metabolic engineering

Metabolic engineering is a key strategy for optimizing PUFA production in microbial and plant systems (Gong et al., 2014). To enhance the biosynthesis of target PUFAs and minimize by-product formation, scientists strategically redirect cellular metabolic pathways. This strategy involves pinpointing bottlenecks in the biosynthetic process and implementing genetic alterations to channel more precursor substrates toward PUFA synthesis. Contemporary tools like CRISPR-Cas9 genome editing facilitate the precise modification of genes governing PUFA metabolism, enabling targeted enhancements in production yield (Subedi et al., 2020). Through metabolic engineering, scientists are also developing new microbial strains and plant varieties with enhanced capacity to produce PUFAs, offering new sources of these essential lipids for food, pharmaceutical, and industrial applications.

Advances in biosynthesis and biotechnology are driving the future of PUFA production, making it more sustainable, efficient, and scalable. Genetic engineering of microorganisms, algae, and plants, along with innovations in bioreactor design, synthetic biology, and metabolic engineering, are revolutionizing PUFA production processes (Qin et al., 2023). These developments contribute to the goal of sustainability by reducing reliance on marine-derived sources and promoting environmentally friendly production methods. As these technologies continue to evolve, they hold the potential to reshape the PUFA industry, providing high-quality bioactive lipids for a wide range of applications.

35.1.4 Novel sources of omega-3 and omega-6 fatty acids

As mentioned earlier, omega-3 and omega-6 fatty acids play vital roles in human health, particularly in cardiovascular function, brain health, and the regulation of inflammation (Ebrahimi et al., 2018). Traditionally, these fatty acids have been sourced from fish oils, flaxseeds, and other plant-based oils. The escalating global demand for omega-3 and omega-6 products, coupled with mounting ecological pressures on conventional marine supplies, is driving significant research into viable alternative sources for these essential fatty acids. Some of the most promising avenues currently under exploration include:

35.1.4.1 Microalgae as a sustainable source of omega-3 and omega-6

Acknowledged for their sustainability and productivity, microalgae have emerged as a leading source for long-chain omega-3 fatty acids, notably EPA and DHA (Barta et al., 2021). Their cultivation in managed systems like photobioreactors offers a production route with a reduced ecological impact relative to traditional fisheries.

Furthermore, specific strains of microalgae, such as *Schizochytrium* and *Nannochloropsis*, have been identified for their high DHA and EPA yields (Lopes et al., 2017). Advances in algal biotechnology, including selective breeding and genetic modification, have led to increased production rates of omega-3s, making algae a viable, renewable, and eco-friendly alternative to fish oils. Microalgae also offer an opportunity to produce omega-6 fatty acids, such as arachidonic acid (AA), which is important for inflammatory response and cellular function.

35.1.4.2 Genetically modified plants for omega-3 and omega-6

Another promising approach to developing novel sources of omega-3 and omega-6 fatty acids involves the genetic modification of plants. Conventional plant sources such as flaxseed, chia, and hemp provide omega-3 in the form of ALA, but their conversion into longer-chain omega-3s like EPA and DHA is inefficient in humans (Abozid & Ayimba, 2014). To overcome this limitation, genetic engineering of oilseed crops like canola, soybean, and camelina is underway to increase the content of omega-3 fatty acids directly. For instance, transgenic canola plants have been developed that produce higher levels of ALA and even longer-chain omega-3s, such as EPA and DHA, by incorporating genes from algae or other organisms that biosynthesize these fatty acids (Deckelbaum & Torrejon, 2012). This approach not only improves the omega-3 content of plants but also provides a more cost-effective, land-based alternative to marine-sourced omega-3s. Concurrently, scientific efforts are directed toward biofortifying crops to elevate their omega-6 fatty acid levels, including γ-linolenic acid (GLA) and dihomo-gamma-Linolenic acid, through genetic modification (Saini & Keum, 2018). Such advancements hold potential for enriching the nutritional value of widespread plant-based oils, including those from soybean, sunflower, and safflower.

35.1.4.3 Insects as an emerging source of omega-3 and omega-6 fatty acids

Edible insects—including crickets, mealworms, and black soldier fly larvae—are emerging as a novel source of omega-3 and omega-6 fatty acids. These species contain appreciable levels of PUFAs and represent a promising, sustainable nutritional resource (Lumanlan, et al., 2022). Insects naturally accumulate omega-3 and omega-6 fatty acids in their tissues, particularly in their fat bodies, which makes them an appealing option for inclusion in food products and animal feeds. The nutritional composition of insect fats can vary depending on their diet, with some species, like crickets, naturally containing significant amounts of omega-3s, especially ALA, as well as omega-6s (Riekkinen et al., 2022). The efficient rearing of insects on organic waste streams underscores their role in a circular economy, positioning them as a resource-efficient and ecological option for omega fatty acid production compared to traditional animal agriculture.

35.1.4.4 Marine microorganisms for omega-3 fatty acids

Marine microorganisms, including bacteria and fungi, are emerging as novel sources of omega-3 fatty acids. Certain strains of marine bacteria, such as *Marinobacter* and *Phaeobacter*, are known to produce omega-3 fatty acids, including EPA and DHA (Giordano et al., 2015). These microorganisms can be cultured in bioreactors, offering a sustainable, controlled environment for large-scale production. Fungi, particularly marine-derived species like *Mortierella* and *Thraustochytrium*, are also capable of producing significant amounts of omega-3s, particularly DHA (Soni et al., 2023). These organisms can be cultivated on low-cost substrates, such as agricultural by-products, and offer an alternative to fish oils for omega-3 production. The development of marine-based microorganisms as commercial sources of omega-3s offers a promising avenue for sustainable fatty acid production without the environmental concerns associated with overfishing.

35.1.4.5 Fermentation-based production of omega-3 and omega-6 fatty acids

Fermentation processes, particularly those involving engineered yeasts and bacteria, have also emerged as a novel method for producing omega-3 and omega-6 fatty acids. Through the application of synthetic biology and metabolic engineering, microorganisms can be designed to biosynthesize high concentrations of omega-3s and omega-6s. For example, engineered strains of *S. cerevisiae* (baker's yeast) and *E. coli* have been developed to produce high amounts of EPA and DHA (Gong et al., 2014). In these systems, fermentation conditions are optimized to maximize the yield of these fatty acids, offering a cost-effective and scalable solution to PUFA production. This approach also allows for the production of novel omega-6 derivatives like GLA, which has important health benefits, especially for skin health and inflammation management.

35.1.4.6 Seaweeds and other marine plants

While microalgae are well-known for their high omega-3 content, other marine plants, such as seaweeds, have also emerged as valuable sources of omega-3s and omega-6s. Certain species of brown and red seaweeds, such as *Undaria pinnatifida* and *Porphyra*spp., are rich in omega-3 fatty acids, particularly ALA, and provide an additional sustainable source of PUFAs (Martinsson, 2016). Seaweeds also contain significant amounts of omega-6 fatty acids, such as linoleic acid, contributing to their potential as a source of both omega-3 and omega-6 fatty acids. As research into seaweed-based nutritional products advances, seaweeds could become a valuable raw material for PUFA-rich functional foods, dietary supplements, and bioactive compounds.

As the demand for omega-3 and omega-6 fatty acids grows, novel sources of these essential lipids are playing an increasingly important role in ensuring sustainable, efficient production. From microalgae and genetically modified plants to insects, marine microorganisms, and fermentation technologies, these alternative sources offer promising solutions to meet global demand while minimizing the environmental impact of traditional omega-rich products. Continued research and innovation in these areas will be key to developing new, sustainable, and bioavailable omega fatty acid sources for human and animal nutrition.

35.2 Precision fermentation and microbial production of polyunsaturated fatty acids

Precision fermentation and microbial production of PUFAs represent cutting-edge approaches that promise to revolutionize the production of essential fatty acids (Augustin et al., 2024). This innovative technology involves using genetically engineered microorganisms, such as bacteria, yeast, and fungi, to produce high-value PUFAs, including omega-3 and omega-6 fatty acids, with greater efficiency, sustainability, and scalability than traditional methods. Here, we discuss the principles, advancements, and potential of precision fermentation in microbial production of PUFAs.

35.2.1 Principles of precision fermentation

Precision fermentation is a highly controlled process in which microorganisms are engineered to produce specific compounds of interest. Unlike traditional fermentation, which relies on the natural fermentation pathways of microorganisms, precision fermentation involves the use of synthetic biology and metabolic engineering to design microorganisms with enhanced capabilities for producing target metabolites—in this case, PUFAs. By manipulating microbial metabolic pathways through genetic modifications, the efficiency and yield of PUFA production can be significantly increased. In the context of PUFA production, microorganisms such as *E. coli*, *S. cerevisiae* (baker's yeast), and various fungi and bacteria are used as microbial cell factories (Patel et al., 2020). These microorganisms are engineered to produce omega-3 (such as EPA and DHA) and omega-6 (such as AA) fatty acids. Precision fermentation ensures that the growth conditions—such as temperature, pH, nutrient supply, and oxygen levels—are optimized for maximum PUFA yield, thereby enhancing the overall efficiency of production.

35.2.2 Microbial strains engineered for polyunsaturated fatty acid production

Synthetic biology has facilitated the engineering of microorganisms with enhanced productivity for omega-3 and omega-6 fatty acids. Employing genetic strategies such as targeted gene insertion, controlled overexpression, and metabolic pathway fine-tuning optimizes the cellular machinery for more efficient PUFA biosynthesis.

1 Bacterial strains: Engineered strains of *E. coli* and other bacteria have been utilized to produce omega-3 fatty acids. By introducing genes for key enzymes involved in the omega-3 biosynthesis pathway—such as desaturases and elongases—scientists have successfully created bacterial strains capable of producing EPA and DHA (Xie et al., 2015). These fatty acids are usually obtained from marine sources, but microbial production offers a more sustainable and scalable alternative.
2 Yeast strains: Yeasts like *S. cerevisiae* and *Y. lipolytica* have been engineered to produce both omega-3 and omega-6 fatty acids, as these microorganisms naturally possess the ability to accumulate lipids (Zhu & Jackson, 2015). Researchers have genetically modified yeasts to produce high amounts of EPA, DHA, and ALA, allowing for efficient fermentation-based production. Yeasts have the advantage of being easy to culture in large fermenters and are more versatile compared to other microorganisms, such as algae or bacteria.
3 Fungal strains: Fungi, particularly those from the *Mortierella* and *Thraustochytrium* genera, have been engineered to produce omega-3 fatty acids, especially DHA (dos Reis et al., 2024). These fungi naturally accumulate lipids, making them well-suited for PUFA production. Genetic engineering has further enhanced their production capacity by optimizing the enzymes involved in the PUFA biosynthesis pathway.

35.2.3 Advancements in polyunsaturated fatty acid production using precision fermentation

Recent advancements in microbial production of PUFAs have focused on increasing the yield and quality of omega-3 and omega-6 fatty acids through various strategies:

1 Metabolic pathway engineering: One of the key advancements in precision fermentation is the optimization of the metabolic pathways responsible for PUFA biosynthesis. By enhancing the expression of desaturase and elongase genes, researchers can increase the flow of fatty acids into the PUFA pathway, resulting in higher yields of target fatty acids. Additionally, the use of biosynthetic pathway shunting can prevent the formation of unwanted by-products, further improving the efficiency of PUFA production.
2 Cofermentation and mixed cultures: Some advancements in fermentation technology involve the use of cofermentation or mixed microbial cultures to produce multiple PUFAs simultaneously. For example, different strains of bacteria or yeasts can be used in tandem to produce both omega-3 and omega-6 fatty acids, thereby reducing the need for separating fermentation processes. This approach can improve efficiency and reduce production costs.

3 Optimized fermentation conditions: Precision fermentation systems are designed to closely control the environmental conditions that affect microbial growth and PUFA production. For instance, researchers are optimizing nutrient feeding strategies, fermentation duration, and aeration to maximize the production of omega-3 and omega-6 fatty acids. Additionally, process intensification techniques, such as fed-batch or continuous fermentation, are being explored to increase overall productivity.
4 High-throughput screening: High-throughput screening methods are being applied to identify and isolate microbial strains with superior PUFA production capabilities. By screening large numbers of microbial strains and genetic variants, researchers can rapidly identify those that produce the highest yields of PUFAs, allowing for faster optimization and scaling of the fermentation process.

35.2.4 Advantages of precision fermentation for PUFA production

There are some advantages of precision fermentation for PUFA production, which will be discussed as follows: (1) Sustainability: Microbial production of PUFAs through precision fermentation offers a highly sustainable solution to the growing demand for omega-3 and omega-6 fatty acids. Unlike traditional sources, such as fish and flaxseeds, which can be limited by environmental factors and resource depletion, microbial production systems are more flexible, can be operated in controlled environments, and do not require large land areas or significant water resources. (2) Scalability: Precision fermentation enables the large-scale production of PUFAs in fermenters, providing a cost-effective and efficient alternative to traditional production methods. The scalability of microbial fermentation processes makes it possible to meet the global demand for omega-rich products used in food, pharmaceuticals, and nutraceuticals. (3) Reduced environmental impact: As microbial systems can be grown on renewable, nonfood substrates, the environmental impact of PUFA production is significantly reduced compared to traditional methods that rely on marine sources. Furthermore, precision fermentation does not contribute to overfishing or habitat destruction, making it an environmentally friendly alternative to fish-derived omega-3s. (4) Customization and precision: Precision fermentation allows for the production of specific, high-quality PUFAs with tailored profiles. Through genetic modifications and metabolic engineering, it is possible to optimize the composition of omega-3 and omega-6 fatty acids to meet the specific needs of different applications, from food enrichment to pharmaceutical use.

Despite the promising advances in precision fermentation and microbial production of PUFAs, several challenges remain. These include the need for continued optimization of microbial strains and fermentation conditions to maximize PUFA yields, reduce production costs, and improve scalability. Moreover, regulatory approval and consumer acceptance of genetically engineered microorganisms for PUFA production may pose hurdles. Looking ahead, the integration of synthetic biology, artificial intelligence, and data-driven optimization techniques could further accelerate the development of precision fermentation processes for PUFA production. The continuous innovation in this field holds the potential to transform the PUFA industry, providing a sustainable, cost-effective solution to meet the global demand for these essential fatty acids.

Through genetic engineering, metabolic pathway optimization, and controlled fermentation processes, researchers are advancing the ability to produce these essential nutrients in a sustainable, efficient, and scalable manner. The continued advancement of these biotechnologies positions them as crucial solutions for satisfying global PUFA requirements, providing an environmentally responsible substitute for conventional marine sourcing.

35.3 Nanoencapsulation and microencapsulation technologies of polyunsaturated fatty acids

35.3.1 Nanoencapsulation of polyunsaturated fatty acids

Nanoencapsulation involves the use of nanometer-sized carriers (less than 1000 nm) to encapsulate bioactive compounds like PUFAs. These nanocarriers offer several advantages, including enhanced stability against oxidation, protection from environmental factors (e.g., temperature and UV light), and the ability to target specific delivery sites in the body. The small size of the nanoparticles allows for better absorption and higher bioavailability compared to conventional delivery methods.

35.3.1.1 Types of nanoencapsulation systems

Types of nanoencapsulation systems for PUFAs are as follows:

1 Lipid-based nanoencapsulation (Mozafari et al., 2006): a. Nanostructured lipid carriers (NLCs): NLCs are composed of a blend of solid and liquid lipids, offering superior stability and flexibility. These carriers help to encapsulate PUFAs in a stable matrix, protecting them from oxidative degradation and improving their release profiles in food or pharmaceutical applications. b. Solid lipid nanoparticles (SLNs): SLNs consist of solid lipids and offer controlled release and enhanced

stability of PUFAs, which are otherwise prone to oxidation. They can be used to encapsulate oils containing high concentrations of omega-3 fatty acids.

2 Polymeric nanoencapsulation (Jurić et al., 2022): a. Polymeric nanoparticles: Nanoparticles made from natural and synthetic polymers (such as chitosan, alginate, and PLGA) provide a stable matrix for the encapsulation of PUFAs. These polymers offer controlled release, biocompatibility, and low toxicity, making them ideal for pharmaceutical and nutraceutical formulations. b. Lipid-polymer hybrid nanoparticles: These nanoparticles combine both lipid and polymer components to improve the stability and controlled release of PUFAs, making them useful for improving the therapeutic effects of omega-3 fatty acids.

3 Self-assembled nanocarriers (Visentini et al., 2019): Liposomes and micelles: Liposomes (lipid bilayer vesicles) and micelles (self-assembled amphiphilic molecules) are widely used for encapsulating hydrophobic compounds like PUFAs. Liposomes provide an ideal system for the delivery of PUFAs due to their ability to form bilayers, which can protect and solubilize hydrophobic molecules. Micelles are another promising nanocarrier that facilitates the solubilization and absorption of PUFAs.

35.3.1.2 Nanoencapsulation techniques

There are three main nanoencapsulation techniques: (1) High-pressure homogenization: This method involves subjecting a lipid or polymeric solution containing PUFAs to high pressure to break the system into nanosized particles. The technique is commonly used to produce SLNs and NLCs. (2) Solvent evaporation: This technique uses an organic solvent to dissolve the lipids or polymers and the PUFAs, followed by the evaporation of the solvent under reduced pressure to form the nanoparticles, and (3) Microemulsion: A microemulsion-based method uses a surfactant to create nanoscale droplets, in which the PUFAs are encapsulated. This method ensures the formation of stable and uniform nanocarriers.

35.3.2 Microencapsulation of polyunsaturated fatty acids

Microencapsulation refers to the process of encapsulating bioactive compounds in microsized carriers (typically in the range of 1–1000 μm). Unlike nanoencapsulation, microencapsulation involves larger carrier systems that offer stability, controlled release, and protection of the encapsulated material (Table 35.1). Microencapsulation of PUFAs is commonly used in the food and nutraceutical industries to improve shelf life, enhance sensory properties, and ensure that PUFAs are delivered effectively in functional products.

35.3.2.1 Types of microencapsulation systems

Types of microencapsulation systems for PUFAs are: (1) Spray drying: One of the most widely used techniques for the microencapsulation of PUFAs, spray drying involves converting a liquid feed (containing PUFAs and encapsulating agents like maltodextrin or gum arabic) into a powder by spraying it into a hot air stream. This process produces microcapsules that protect PUFAs from oxidation while allowing for easy incorporation into food products, and (2) Coacervation: Coacervation is a phase separation process where the encapsulating material (typically a polymer) forms a coating around the PUFAs. This method produces microcapsules with good stability and controlled release properties, often used in nutraceutical applications.

TABLE 35.1 Key differences between nanoencapsulation and microencapsulation for the delivery of polyunsaturated fatty acid (Khoshnoudi-Nia et al., 2022).

Aspect	Nanoencapsulation	Microencapsulation
Particle size and delivery mechanism	Particles range from 10 to 1000 nm, offering faster absorption and more efficient delivery.	Particles range from 1–1000 μm, with slower release profiles.
Stability	Superior oxidative protection and stability due to the smaller size and higher surface-to-volume ratio of nanocarriers.	Less oxidative protection compared to nanoencapsulation, but still offers good stability.
Bioavailability and release	More effective in enhancing bioavailability due to smaller size and potential for targeted delivery.	Provides more controlled release, ideal for sustained delivery over time.

Source: From Khoshnoudi-Nia, S., Forghani, Z., & Jafari, S.M. (2022). A systematic review and meta-analysis of fish oil encapsulation within different micro/nanocarriers. Critical Reviews in Food Science and Nutrition, 62(8), 2061–2082.

Nanoencapsulation and microencapsulation technologies have revolutionized the delivery of PUFAs by enhancing their stability, bioavailability, and controlled release. These technologies hold immense potential for improving the therapeutic and nutritional benefits of PUFAs, particularly in the food, pharmaceutical, and nutraceutical industries. As encapsulation techniques continue to evolve, it is expected that more efficient and sustainable methods will emerge, further expanding the application of PUFAs in various health-related products. While both nanoencapsulation and microencapsulation offer benefits in the protection and delivery of PUFAs, they differ significantly in terms of particle size, stability, release mechanisms, and applications.

In terms of applications of nano and microencapsulation in food, pharmaceutical, and nutraceutical industriesboth nano and microencapsulation technologies have vast applications in various sectors such as (1) Food industry: Encapsulated PUFAs can be added to functional foods and beverages to enhance nutritional value and prevent oxidation, ensuring a longer shelf life without compromising the sensory properties, (2) Pharmaceutical industry: In drug formulations, nanoencapsulation allows for targeted delivery of omega-3 and other PUFAs, improving their therapeutic effects and minimizing side effects and (3) Nutraceutical industry: Encapsulated PUFAs are commonly used in dietary supplements, where they improve the bioavailability of omega-3s and protect them from degradation during storage and digestion.

35.3.3 Liposomes and emulsions for enhanced bioavailability of polyunsaturated fatty acids

PUFAs are prone to oxidation, degradation, and poor solubility, which limits their bioavailability when administered in conventional forms. To address these challenges, liposomes and emulsions have emerged as effective delivery systems to enhance the bioavailability of PUFAs (Table 35.2).

35.3.3.1 Liposomes

Liposomes are nanoscale structures characterized by their spherical shape, formed from single or multiple concentric phospholipid bilayers that encapsulate a central water-filled compartment. These structures are highly versatile and have been widely used as drug delivery systems, particularly for encapsulating hydrophobic substances such as PUFAs. Liposomes mimic biological membranes, offering numerous benefits in improving the bioavailability and stability of encapsulated compounds. Liposomes function by encapsulating PUFAs within their lipid bilayers or aqueous core, depending on the nature of the liposome (Zelikina et al., 2022). The lipid bilayers protect the encapsulated PUFAs from oxidative degradation, while also improving the solubility of hydrophobic compounds. Liposomes enhance the absorption of PUFAs by facilitating their transport across cellular membranes, thereby increasing their bioavailability. Furthermore, liposomes offer controlled release of PUFAs, ensuring that they are delivered efficiently to the target site in the body. There are some benefits of liposomes in PUFA delivery: (1) Oxidative stability: Liposomes provide a protective barrier for PUFAs, reducing the risk of oxidation that can lead to a loss of nutritional value, (2) Improved solubility: Liposomes enhance the solubility of PUFAs, making them more bioavailable when consumed, (3) Targeted delivery: Liposomes can be engineered to target specific tissues or organs, enhancing the therapeutic potential of PUFAs, particularly in

TABLE 35.2 Comparative analysis of liposomes and emulsions for polyunsaturated fatty acid (PUFA) delivery.

Aspect	Liposomes	Emulsions
Encapsulation Mechanism	PUFAs are encapsulated within lipid bilayers or an aqueous core.	PUFAs are dispersed as oil droplets in an aqueous phase.
Stability	Offers high stability by protecting PUFAs from oxidation.	Protects PUFAs from oxidation, but is less stable than liposomes.
Bioavailability	Increases bioavailability through enhanced solubility and absorption.	Improves solubility and absorption by reducing droplet size.
Controlled release	Provides sustained release of PUFAs.	Can be designed for controlled release, but typically has a faster release.
Targeted delivery	Can be engineered for targeted delivery to specific tissues.	Limited targeted delivery capability.
Applications	Used in pharmaceutical and nutraceutical formulations.	Widely used in food, beverages, and dietary supplements.

pharmaceutical and nutraceutical applications and (4) Controlled release: Liposomal systems can be designed to release PUFAs in a controlled manner, ensuring sustained delivery over time.

35.3.3.2 Emulsions

Emulsions are another promising technology used to enhance the bioavailability of PUFAs (Vellido-Perez et al., 2021). An emulsion is a mixture of two immiscible liquids, typically oil and water, stabilized by surfactants (emulsifiers). In the context of PUFA delivery, emulsions are particularly useful for improving the solubility and absorption of hydrophobic compounds like omega-3 fatty acids, which are poorly soluble in water. In emulsions, PUFAs are dispersed within the oil phase, which is then stabilized by surfactants to form droplets. These droplets reduce the particle size of PUFAs, increasing their surface area and enhancing their absorption in the gastrointestinal tract. The emulsion system facilitates the breakdown of oil droplets by bile salts and digestive enzymes, promoting the release of PUFAs and enhancing their bioavailability. Benefits of emulsions in PUFA delivery: (1) Increased surface area: THE small droplet size in emulsions increases the surface area of PUFAs, leading to improved absorption in the intestines, (2) Improved stability: Emulsions protect PUFAs from oxidation by encapsulating them in oil droplets and preventing direct exposure to oxygen and light, (3) Enhanced solubility: By dispersing PUFAs in an aqueous phase, emulsions significantly improve the solubility of PUFAs, allowing for better absorption and (4) Sustained release: Emulsions can be formulated to release PUFAs slowly over time, providing sustained delivery and prolonged effects in the body.

Both liposomes and emulsions offer significant advantages for the enhanced bioavailability of PUFAs. Liposomes provide excellent protection against oxidative degradation and offer controlled release, making them ideal for pharmaceutical and nutraceutical applications. Emulsions, on the other hand, are particularly effective in improving the solubility and absorption of PUFAs, especially in food products and supplements. By employing these advanced delivery systems, the therapeutic and nutritional benefits of PUFAs can be maximized, offering enhanced efficacy in human health applications.

35.3.4 Smart delivery systems for targeted release of polyunsaturated fatty acids

Smart delivery systems have emerged as an innovative solution to enhance the bioavailability, stability, and targeted release of PUFAs, ensuring their controlled absorption and maximum efficacy. Smart delivery systems offer a powerful approach to enhancing the stability, bioavailability, and targeted release of PUFAs (Muthukrishnan, 2022). By leveraging nanotechnology, biopolymer engineering, and stimuli-responsive carriers, these systems can ensure efficient PUFA delivery for improved health benefits. The selection of the appropriate system depends on the intended application, whether in functional foods, pharmaceuticals, or nutraceutical formulations (Table 35.3).

35.4 Next-generation product formulations of functional foods and beverages enriched with polyunsaturated fatty acid

The PUFAs' susceptibility to oxidation, poor solubility, and low bioavailability have presented challenges in their incorporation into functional foods and beverages. Next-generation product formulations are addressing these issues by employing advanced delivery systems, innovative stabilization techniques, and novel food matrices to enhance the stability, sensory properties, and bioavailability of PUFAs. Next-generation PUFA-enriched functional foods and beverages are driven by cutting-edge food science and technology, ensuring enhanced stability, bioavailability, and consumer appeal. By integrating nanoencapsulation, emulsification, protein-binding, and smart hydrogel technologies, food manufacturers can develop highly effective and palatable PUFA-fortified products (Liu et al., 2024). Future innovations, including 3D-printed foods, personalized nutrition, and PUFA-enhanced fermented products, will further expand the reach and impact of functional PUFA formulations in the health and wellness industry (Table 35.4).

35.5 Personalized nutrition and tailored polyunsaturated fatty acid solutions

The paradigm of personalized nutrition, which tailors dietary guidance to an individual's genetic profile, lifestyle, and health objectives, is transforming approaches to health and wellness. Within this framework, PUFAs—encompassing omega-3 and omega-6 families—are recognized for their foundational contributions to cardiovascular and cognitive health, as well as inflammatory modulation. Determining the ideal PUFA intake, however, requires personalization, as requirements diverge significantly based on genetic predisposition, metabolic efficiency, dietary patterns, and specific health statuses. Tailored PUFA solutions leverage advancements in nutrigenomics, precision delivery systems, and smart food technologies to provide targeted and effective supplementation (Table 35.5). Moreover, personalized nutrition is

TABLE 35.3 Mechanism, advantages, and applications of smart delivery systems for targeted release of polyunsaturated fatty acids.

Delivery system	Mechanism	Advantages	Applications	References
Nanostructured lipid carriers	Encapsulates PUFAs in a hybrid solid-liquid lipid matrix for controlled release.	High oxidative stability, improved absorption, sustained release.	Nutraceuticals, pharmaceuticals, functional foods.	Fang et al. (2013)
Functionalized liposomes	Phospholipid bilayers modified with ligands for targeted PUFA delivery.	Enhanced bioavailability, site-specific release, PUFA protection.	Pharmaceutical formulations for cardiovascular and neurological health.	Sonju et al. (2021)
Nanoemulsions	PUFA-loaded nanosized droplets stabilized in an aqueous phase.	High surface area for absorption, oxidation protection, and easy food incorporation.	Functional foods, dietary supplements, and medical nutrition.	Dey et al. (2018)
Smart hydrogels	PUFAs encapsulated in biopolymer matrices that respond to pH or temperature.	Controlled and sustained release, high gastrointestinal stability.	Drug delivery systems, functional food coatings.	Wang et al. (2021)
Stimuli-responsive microcapsules	PUFA-loaded microcapsules break down under specific digestive conditions.	Enhanced PUFA stability, targeted intestinal release, sustained effect.	Fortified foods, pharmaceutical-grade supplements.	Cai et al. (2022)
Layer-by-layer encapsulation	Multiple alternating biopolymer layers for precise PUFA release control.	Customizable release profiles, superior PUFA protection, personalized nutrition.	Personalized nutrition, functional food packaging, therapeutic applications.	Shchukina and Shchukin (2012)

TABLE 35.4 Key innovations in polyunsaturated fatty acid -enriched functional foods and beverages.

Innovation	Description	Benefits	Example applications	References
Nanoencapsulation technologies	Encapsulating PUFAs in nanosized carriers (liposomes, NLCs, nanoemulsions).	Improved stability, enhanced bioavailability, and controlled release.	Omega-3-enriched dairy products, functional oils.	Jurić et al. (2022)
Microencapsulation techniques	PUFA protection within solid microcapsules (spray drying, coacervation, extrusion).	Increased oxidative stability, better taste masking, and prolonged shelf life.	Fortified cereals, powdered meal replacements.	Timilsena et al. (2017)
Emulsified PUFA systems	PUFA-loaded emulsions (nanoemulsions, Pickering emulsions) for water-based formulations.	Improved solubility in beverages, reduced oxidation, and better mouthfeel.	Omega-3-enriched juices, plant-based milks.	Shchukina and Shchukin (2012)
PUFA-enriched protein matrices	Binding PUFAs with proteins (whey, casein, soy) to enhance stability and delivery.	Improved dispersibility, oxidation protection, and sustained release.	Fortified yogurt, protein bars.	Jacobsen (2015)
PUFA-infused smart hydrogels	Hydrogels that encapsulate and release PUFAs under specific digestive conditions.	Controlled release, prolonged bioactivity, and enhanced absorption.	PUFA-fortified gummies, functional confectionery.	Wang et al. (2021)
PUFA-fortified fermented foodS	Incorporation of PUFAs into probiotic-rich products like yogurt, kefir, and kombucha.	Synergistic gut health benefits, increased bioavailability.	Probiotic omega-3 yogurts, PUFA-enhanced kombucha.	Augustin et al. (2024)
3D-printed functional foods	Customizable PUFA-enriched food structures created using 3D food printing technology.	Precision nutrition, tailored PUFA delivery, enhanced consumer engagement.	Personalized PUFA-fortified snacks, meal replacements.	Portanguen et al. (2019)

TABLE 35.5 Key approaches in personalized polyunsaturated fatty acid nutrition.

Approach	Description	Benefits	Example applications	References
Nutrigenomics-based PUFA optimization	Using genetic testing to determine an individual's ability to metabolize and utilize PUFAs.	Identifies personalized omega-3: omega-6 ratios and prevents deficiencies.	DNA-based nutrition plans, customized supplement formulations.	Hosseiniara and Hosseini Zijoud (2024)
AI-driven dietary assessments	Machine learning and AI analyze diet and lifestyle data to recommend optimal PUFA intake.	Precision-based nutrition guidance, real-time dietary adjustments.	AI-powered meal planning apps, smart nutrition trackers.	Prasad et al. (2025)
Microbiome-targeted PUFA delivery	Adjusting PUFA supplementation based on gut microbiota composition to enhance absorption.	Improved gut health synergy, enhanced PUFA bioavailability.	PUFA-enriched probiotics, microbiome-friendly omega-3 capsules.	Theofilis et al. (2024)
Customized PUFA supplements	Personalized PUFA blends are formulated based on individual health markers and goals.	Tailored dosing, reduced risk of over or under consumption.	Custom omega-3 softgels, liquid blends for cardiovascular health.	El-Bayoumy and Manni (2020)
3D-printed PUFA foods	Creating personalized foods with specific PUFA compositions using 3D food printing.	Precision PUFA delivery, enhanced consumer engagement.	Personalized omega-3 snacks, PUFA-fortified protein bars.	Portanguen et al. (2019)
Smart PUFA-infused beverages	Functional beverages with adjustable PUFA levels based on health monitoring data.	Real-time nutritional adjustments, improved absorption.	PUFA-enriched sports drinks, brain-boosting omega-3 smoothies.	Anna and Boris (2012)
Wearable nutrition trackers	Devices that track fatty acid levels and recommend personalized PUFA intake.	Continuous monitoring, proactive nutrition adjustments.	Smart PUFA supplement dispensers, biosensor-based recommendations.	de Toro-Martín et al. (2017)

transforming PUFA supplementation by moving away from one-size-fits-all approaches toward precision-based, customized solutions (Singar et al., 2024).

The integration of nutrigenomics, AI-driven dietary assessments, microbiome research, and smart food technologies ensures that individuals receive the right type, dosage, and delivery format of PUFAs tailored to their unique health needs. With the rise of wearable nutrition trackers, AI-powered dietary tools, and personalized 3D-printed foods, PUFA solutions will become increasingly adaptive, enhancing long-term health and well-being.

35.6 Technological advancements in polyunsaturated fatty acid processing

The subject of PUFA technology is constantly evolving, driven by rising global demand for these critical nutrients in a variety of industries, including medicines, nutraceuticals, food, and skincare. This evolution necessitates a shift toward innovative processing methodologies that not only improve extraction and purification efficiencies but also prioritize sustainability by reducing environmental impact through the use of green technologies like supercritical fluid extraction (SFE) and enzyme-assisted extraction. Future advancements in PUFA processing are focused on improving the quality of final products by implementing advanced stabilization techniques, such as microencapsulation and nanoemulsions, to prevent oxidation and ensure prolonged shelf-life, as well as exploring enzymatic modifications to create tailored PUFA structures with enhanced bioavailability and specific functional properties (Fig. 35.1) (Calder, 2017).

35.6.1 Green extraction technologies

The future of PUFA extraction is clearly leaning toward ecologically harmless methods, driven by increased concerns about sustainability and resource efficiency. SFE, notably employing carbon dioxide (scCO2), is fast gaining popularity as a demonstrably green approach for PUFA recovery from diverse sources, including valuable fish by-products and lipid-rich microalgae (Adeoti & Hawboldt, 2014; Tzima et al., 2023). This shift is crucial as traditional solvent-based extractions often rely on hazardous chemicals, contributing to environmental pollution. SFE, utilizing scCO2, offers significant advantages such as a substantial reduction in energy consumption compared to conventional techniques, the employment of nontoxic and readily recyclable solvents, and the critical ability to prevent thermal and chemical degradation of the sensitive PUFA extracts (Tzima et al., 2023). The preservation of PUFA integrity is critical to

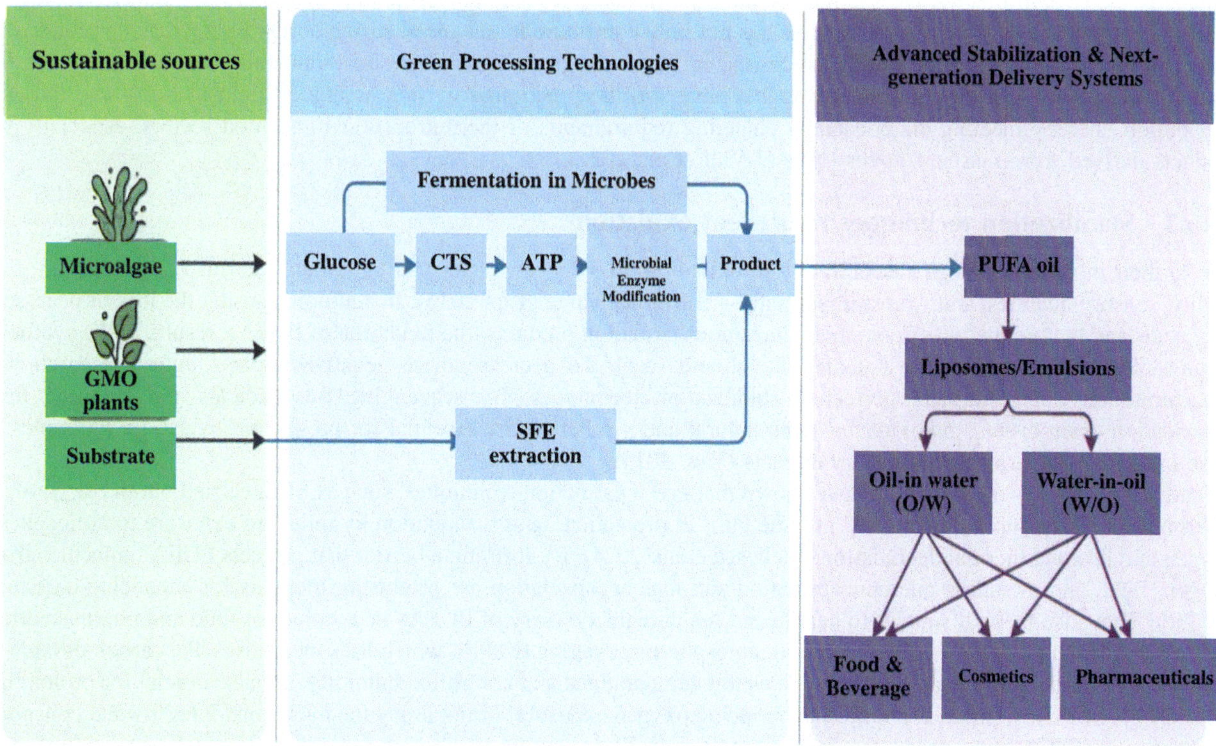

FIGURE 35.1 Schematic overview of major technological pathways for sustainable polyunsaturated fatty acid (PUFA) production and delivery.

preserving their nutritional and functional characteristics. The selectivity of SFE can be accurately controlled by methodically altering parameters such as pressure and temperature, taking use of the peculiar solvent characteristics of scCO2. Furthermore, the strategic use of cosolvents, such as ethanol, can effectively increase its efficacy for extracting polar PUFAs, widening the range of extractable molecules (Tzima et al., 2023). Recent advances in SFE technology include the optimization of extraction parameters through advanced experimental designs, such as response surface methods, and the use of thermodynamic models to acquire a deeper process understanding and anticipate extraction yields (Herrero et al., 2010). These simulations enable the modeling of solute-solvent interactions and the optimization of process settings. Beyond PUFA extraction, SFE is being actively investigated for the comprehensive recovery of additional useful compounds from biomass, including pigments and bioactive compounds from microalgae, connecting neatly with the concepts of the biorefinery concept and creating a circular economy (Tzima et al., 2023). This comprehensive strategy not only optimizes resource use but also reduces waste output, resulting in a more sustainable and ecologically responsible processing paradigm.

35.6.2 Enzymatic modification and structuring of polyunsaturated fatty acids

Enzymatic modification and structure of PUFAs are fast gaining attention as sustainable and effective ways for both the extraction and targeted modification of PUFAs, especially from aquatic sources (Marsol-Vall et al., 2022). Enzymes, including proteases and lipases, are effectively utilized in enzymatic-assisted extraction conducted under mild conditions, such as controlled temperature and pH, achieving comparable oil recovery and PUFA compositions to traditional solvent-based methods, while significantly minimizing oxidation levels and preserving the integrity of the delicate PUFAs, crucial for maintaining their nutritional value, as detailed in reviews on fish oil processing (Bonilla-Méndez et al., 2018). Lipase-catalyzed processes, such as ethanolysis, are being carefully researched and optimized for the precise concentration and enrichment of n-3 PUFAs, meeting the increasing need for highly purified omega-3 supplements and personalized lipid products (Marsol-Vall et al., 2022).

To improve the efficiency of enzymatic extraction, pre-treatment methods such as microwave and ultrasound irradiation are being used to effectively disrupt cell walls, thereby facilitating enzyme access and increasing PUFA release from raw materials, particularly from algal and fish by-product sources, aligning with the principles of sustainable resource utilization. (Marsol-Vall et al., 2022). Furthermore, enzymatic splitting, lipase utilization, and deacidification methods are actively investigated for the purification of PUFA-rich oils, effectively reducing free fatty acid concentration and enhancing the overall quality and stability of the final product, a vital step in refining fish oils (Bonilla-Méndez et al., 2018). These multifaceted enzymatic approaches not only contribute to enhanced sustainability by decreasing reliance on toxic substances and costly to operate processes, in line with green technology developments, but also allow for the accurate creation of specific lipid structures that have specific functionality, such as higher bioavailability and targeted distribution, thereby meeting the constantly changing requirements of the nutraceutical and food sectors, especially for products derived from marine sources (Marsol-Vall et al., 2022).

35.6.3 Stabilization techniques to prevent oxidation

Due to their intrinsic and high susceptibility to oxidation, PUFAs can suffer substantial and detrimental effects on their quality, sensory qualities, and—most importantly—nutritional value (Tao, 2015). In addition, causing the loss of necessary fatty acids and the production of potentially hazardous oxidation products, the oxidation of PUFAs, results in the synthesis of unwanted volatile chemicals that alter flavor and scent. To decrease these negative impacts, future research will concentrate on improving and perfecting stabilization techniques. By scavenging free radicals and stopping lipid peroxidation chain events, antioxidants—both natural and synthetic—are essential for preventing oxidation. Examples of these include tocopherols and rosemary extracts (Tao, 2015).

Studies on anchovy oil extraction have shown that green extraction techniques, such as SFE, carried out in oxygen-free environments using supercritical CO_2, provide built-in protection against oxidation by reducing exposure to atmospheric oxygen and limiting thermal degradation (Bichescu et al., 2024). By forming a barrier that protects PUFA molecules from oxygen, light, and moisture, microencapsulation and nanoencapsulation are promising methods for enhancing oxidative stability. They also make it simpler to handle and regulate the delivery of PUFAs in a variety of food and pharmaceutical applications (Bichescu et al., 2024). Modified atmosphere packaging (MAP), which uses inert gases like carbon dioxide or nitrogen, and proper storage conditions, such as low temperatures and controlled humidity, are also crucial for prolonging the shelf life of PUFA-enriched products by reducing oxygen exposure. Maintaining the nutritional integrity and consumer acceptance of PUFA-based products over the long term will depend on combining several stabilization approaches, such as using MAP and adding antioxidants to microcapsules (Bichescu et al., 2024).

35.7 Sustainability and ethical considerations

Due to growing customer demand for ethically sourced and produced products that support human health and well-being, as well as growing environmental awareness, sustainability, and ethical considerations are becoming more and more important in the PUFA business (Mititelu et al., 2025). As noted by Mititelu et al. (2025) in their review on the role of PUFAs in modern nutritional balance, this increased emphasis calls for a shift towards sustainable sourcing of PUFA-rich raw materials, such as microalgae and fish by-products, to minimize reliance on traditional fisheries and mitigate ecological impact. In order to lessen waste production and environmental impacts, ethical considerations also apply to the use of green processing methods, such as enzyme-assisted extraction and SFE. The industry's dedication to providing products that not only meet nutritional needs but also adhere to social responsibility and environmental stewardship principles is demonstrated by the responsible use of PUFAs, frequently in combination with polyphenolic compounds from food sources, promoting a comprehensive approach to human health (Mititelu et al., 2025).

35.7.1 Sustainable sourcing of polyunsaturated fatty acid-rich raw materials

Due to their numerous industrial uses and acknowledged health advantages, PUFAs are becoming more and more in demand worldwide, which calls for a change in perspective from conventional sourcing practices (Dyall et al., 2022; Ferreri et al., 2022). There is an urgent need for alternative, sustainable solutions because of the heavy reliance on conventional sources like fish oil, which is causing serious worries about overfishing, the disturbance of marine ecosystems, and the overall impact on the environment (Mandal & Ghosh, 2024; Thiagarajan & Devarajan, 2024). To reduce environmental stress and provide a steady supply, PUFA production in the future will have more of an emphasis on sustainable and varied sources.

Microalgae serve as a primary and efficient biological source for key long-chain PUFAs, notably EPA and DHA, thereby providing these nutrients without reliance on fish-derived intermediates (Ribeiro Carvalho, 2022; Venegas-Calerón & Napier, 2023). Another sustainable pathway is provided by fungi, especially Zygomycetes, which may produce omega-6 PUFAs and even DHA from inexpensive agro-industrial by-products, supporting a circular economy (Dufossé et al., 2021).

The foundational omega-3 compound ALA, which the body converts into longer-chain forms, is abundant in plant-derived foods like flaxseeds and chia seeds, providing essential vegan-friendly options (Coates, 2013). Furthermore, the valorization of underutilized fish processing residues offers a substantial PUFA source, aligning with circular economy principles by optimizing resources and promoting sustainable industry practices (Xia et al., 2024). Green methods such as supercritical CO_2 extraction can effectively recover fish oil from these by-products while reducing their negative effects on the environment (Fornaro et al., 2024).

Additionally, land-based sources of genetically engineered plants, such as omega-3 canola, are being created to provide scalability and less dependence on marine resources (Venegas-Calerón & Napier, 2023). Consumer demand for plant-based omega-3s and continued research into innovative production techniques are what are driving these developments (Saidaiah et al., 2024).

The market trends show a notable movement towards omega-3s derived from algae and other alternative sources, demonstrating the industry's growing recognition of the significance of sustainable practices (Van der Voort et al., 2017). Growing consumer understanding of environmental issues and PUFAs' health benefits is supporting this change (Yan et al., 2024). Industry-academia partnerships are essential to advancing sustainable PUFA production. These collaborations promote innovation, ease the transfer of technology, and guarantee the creation of solutions that are profitable (Qin et al., 2023). Research is concentrated on creating new uses for PUFAs in a variety of industries, such as industrial applications, medicines, cosmetics, and nutraceuticals, as well as on simplifying production procedures and enhancing extraction and purification methods (Barta et al., 2021). A diversified strategy that incorporates microalgae, fungi, plant-based sources, and fish by-products is the way of the future for PUFA sourcing. It also involves constant innovation through genetic modification and green technologies to guarantee a sustainable and morally sound supply of these vital nutrients (Siddiqui et al., 2024).

35.7.2 Reducing environmental impact in polyunsaturated fatty acid production

The synthesis of PUFAs has a significant negative influence on the environment, which motivates innovation in sustainable methods. Due to its heavy reliance on wild-caught fisheries, traditional fish oil production increases greenhouse gas emissions through fuel consumption and transportation, worsens overfishing, disturbs marine ecosystems, and destroys habitat through destructive fishing practices like bottom trawling (Keller et al., 2017). By providing a land-based substitute, algal-based PUFA production, on the other hand, has a substantially smaller carbon footprint because algae growth absorbs CO2 during photosynthesis and lessens the strain on marine resources (Van der Voort et al., 2017). Additionally, by keeping trash out of landfills and fostering a circular economy, using waste streams—such as industrial and agricultural by-products—as growth substrates for fungi, particularly Zygomycetes, can further reduce environmental impact. To identify areas for improvement and optimize processes to reduce environmental impacts, life cycle assessments (LCAs) are essential for assessing and measuring the environmental sustainability of various PUFA manufacturing methods (Togarcheti & Padamati, 2021). To develop a holistic view of the environmental footprint associated with producing PUFAs, such as LCAs, routinely scrutinize several key metrics: energy demand, greenhouse gas outputs, water utilization, and the generation of waste streams.

35.7.3 Ethical implications of genetic engineering and biotechnology

There are serious ethical questions raised by the use of genetic engineering and biotechnology to increase PUFA synthesis, especially in plants and microbes. Although these technologies have the potential to boost sustainability by decreasing dependency on marine resources, improving nutritional profiles, and increasing yields, there are worries about the possible effects on ecosystems and biodiversity (MacDonald et al., 2019). In particular, the introduction of genetically modified organisms into the environment may have unforeseen repercussions, like the transfer of genes to wild relatives or the upset of natural equilibrium. To address these ethical issues, foster trust, and guarantee the safe and long-term use of these technologies, responsible development and open communication with stakeholders and customers are crucial (MacDonald et al., 2019). To address concerns and develop consensus, this involves carrying out thorough risk assessments, putting strict containment measures in place, and having open discussions with the public.

35.8 Challenges and opportunities in polyunsaturated fatty acid innovation

Considering the notable developments in PUFA technology, the sector still faces a number of obstacles as well as numerous chances for innovation and expansion, spurred by rising customer demand and shifting market trends (Magoni et al., 2022; Tocher et al., 2001).

35.8.1 Regulatory hurdles and safety considerations

One of the biggest obstacles to PUFA innovation is navigating the complicated regulatory environment, especially when it comes to safety regulations, labeling, and health claims, which vary greatly between jurisdictions (Granato et al., 2023; Mittal et al., 2024). Ensuring product safety is crucial for both regulatory compliance and consumer trust, especially when it comes to oxidation, which can result in the development of harmful substances and potential pollutants like heavy metals or environmental toxins (Mosconi, 2024). For market access and acceptance, it is essential to adhere to changing rules, such as those pertaining to omega fatty acid labeling and permissible statements, and to give customers clear and accurate information regarding the advantages and safety of PUFA-enriched products (Granato et al., 2023).

35.8.2 Consumer acceptance and market trends

The market is expanding due in large part to consumer knowledge of the health advantages of PUFAs, especially omega-3 fatty acids, which raises demand for PUFA-enriched functional foods, dietary supplements, and nutraceuticals (Karageorgou et al., 2023). Due to concerns about sustainability, dietary preferences for vegan and vegetarian diets, and an increasing interest in clean-label products, plant-based omega-3 options—derived from sources like flaxseeds, chia seeds, and algae—are becoming more and more popular (Lane et al., 2022). To improve bioavailability and user convenience, the market is additionally experiencing a trend toward higher concentration PUFA products, such as highly purified EPA and DHA oils, and novel delivery systems, like nanoemulsions and microcapsules (Zhou & Wei, 2023). Successful product development and expansion into the market depend on an understanding of and ability to adapt to these changing consumer preferences and market trends, such as the growing need for tailored nutrition and focused health solutions (Karageorgou et al., 2023).

35.8.3 Bridging the gap between research and commercialization

It takes efficient methods to close the gap between academia and industry to translate promising PUFA research—including developments in extraction, purification, and modification techniques—into commercially profitable products (Elazzazy et al., 2025; Finco et al., 2017). By encouraging information sharing, exchanging resources, and carrying out market-driven research that takes into account customer demands and real-world problems, cooperation between academics and businesses can promote innovation. Building pilot facilities, increasing production, and introducing new technologies—like innovative systems for growing algae or enzymatic processing techniques—all depend on having access to capital and investment. Successful commercialization also requires an understanding of market prospects, consumer wants, and regulatory restrictions to make sure that cutting-edge PUFA goods satisfy consumers and comply with the relevant regulations (Banović Fuentes et al., 2024).

35.9 Future applications of polyunsaturated fatty acids beyond food

Given their many functional qualities, PUFAs' adaptability goes well beyond the food industry, with promising uses in the pharmaceutical, cosmetic, and other industrial sectors (Liu et al., 2022).

35.9.1 PUFAs in pharmaceuticals and nutraceuticals

The clinical and preventive benefits of omega-3 fatty acids, including EPA and DHA, for conditions ranging from neurological and inflammatory disorders to cardiovascular disease and certain cancers, are gaining broader recognition (Kapoor et al., 2021). Consequently, these PUFAs are heavily incorporated into dietary supplements and nutraceuticals aimed at modulating immune response, supporting heart and brain health, and promoting overall wellness (Saidaiah et al., 2024). Current investigations are exploring novel pharmaceutical and nutraceutical applications, such as personalized nutrition protocols, targeted drug delivery mechanisms, and advanced formulations designed to maximize bioavailability and therapeutic effectiveness.

35.9.2 Cosmetic and dermatological applications

By supporting the function of the skin barrier, providing moisture, and having antiinflammatory properties, PUFAs are essential for maintaining healthy skin and can help treat disorders including eczema, psoriasis, and acne (Balić et al., 2020). In an effort to promote skin health, minimize inflammation, and improve skin appearance, they are increasingly being added to a variety of dermatological and cosmetic products, including cleansers, moisturizers, and serums (Balić et al., 2020).

35.9.3 Industrial and nonfood uses of polyunsaturated fatty acid derivatives

Because of their distinct chemical characteristics, PUFAs and their derivatives have a wide range of industrial uses. They are employed in the manufacturing of alkyd resins, which give paints and coatings their flexibility, toughness, and resilience to weather (Ahmed, 2024). The drying and film-forming qualities of inks, putty, sealants, and mastics are facilitated by the use of polyunsaturated vegetable oils like linseed and soybean oil (Singh et al., 2011). Additionally, PUFAs can be utilized to create bioplastics and other polymers, providing environmentally friendly substitutes for materials derived from petrochemicals (Zubair et al., 2021). Additionally, its potential for producing ethanol is being investigated, which will aid in the development of renewable energy sources (Alhammad et al., 2023).

35.10 Conclusions and future directions

PUFAs are essential bioactive lipids with profound health benefits, playing critical roles in cardiovascular, neurological, and inflammatory health. The advancements in PUFA technology and product development, as explored in this chapter, highlight the transformative potential of biotechnological innovations, sustainable sourcing, and advanced delivery systems. From genetic engineering of microorganisms and algae to precision fermentation, nanoencapsulation, and personalized nutrition, these innovations are addressing key challenges such as oxidative instability, bioavailability, and environmental sustainability. The convergence of science, technology, and consumer demand will continue to propel PUFA research and commercialization, offering transformative solutions for global health and wellness.

Acknowledgement for artifical intelligence use

The authors acknowledge the use of Grok 3, an artificial intelligence tool developed by XAI, for assistance in paraphrasing sections of this manuscript to enhance clarity and reduce textual similarity. All AI-generated content was thoroughly reviewed and edited by the authors to ensure accuracy, originality, and alignment with the study's objectives.

References

Abozid, M. M., & Ayimba, E. (2014). Effect of omega 3 fatty acids family in human health. *Journal of Advanced Research, 2*(3), 202–211.

Adeoti, I. A., & Hawboldt, K. (2014). A review of lipid extraction from fish processing by-product for use as a biofuel. *Biomass and Bioenergy, 63*, 330–340. https://doi.org/10.1016/j.biombioe.2014.02.011.

Ahmed, S. (2024). Alkyds from vegetable oils for surface application. In *In* vegetable oil-based polymers and their surface applications. Elsevier, 33–50. https://www.sciencedirect.com/science/article/pii/B9780128221891000015.

Alhammad, B. A., Jamal, A., Carlucci, C., Saeed, M. F., Seleiman, M. F., & Pompelli, M. F. (2023). Non-conventional oilseeds: Unlocking the global potential for sustainable biofuel production. *Catalysts, 13*(9), 1263.

Anna, K., & Boris, M. (2012). Smart fats", healthy brain and function of lipid-sensing NMDA receptors. *Advances in Biological Chemistry, 2012*.

Augustin, M. A., Hartley, C. J., Maloney, G., & Tyndall, S. (2024). Innovation in precision fermentation for food ingredients. *Critical Reviews in Food Science and Nutrition, 64*(18), 6218–6238.

Balić, A., Vlašić, D., Žužul, K., Marinović, B., & Bukvić Mokos, Z. (2020). Omega-3 versus omega-6 polyunsaturated fatty acids in the prevention and treatment of inflammatory skin diseases. *International Journal of Molecular Sciences, 21*(3), 741.

Banović Fuentes, J., Beara, I., & Torović, L. (2024). Regulatory compliance of health claims on omega-3 fatty acid food supplements. *Foods, 14*(1), 67.

Barta, D. G., Coman, V., & Vodnar, D. C. (2021). Microalgae as sources of omega-3 polyunsaturated fatty acids: Biotechnological aspects. *Algal Research, 58*, 102410.

Bichescu, C. I., Mihalcea, L., Raimondo, R., Cotârleț, M., Păcularu-Burada, B., Barbu, V., Râpeanu, G., Bahrim, G. E., & Stănciuc, N. (2024). Supercritical CO_2 fluid extraction and microencapsulation of oil from anchovy (engraulis mordax) by-products. *Food Technology and Biotechnology, 62*(3), 302–313. https://doi.org/10.17113/ftb.62.03.24.8336.

Bonilla-Méndez, J. R., Hoyos-Concha, J. L., Bonilla-Méndez, J. R., & Hoyos-Concha, J. L. (2018). Methods of extraction refining and concentration of fish oil as a source of omega-3 fatty acids. *Ciencia y Tecnología Agropecuaria, 19*(3), 645–668. https://doi.org/10.21930/rcta.vol19_num2_art:684.

Cai, Y., Zhang, Y., Qu, Q., Xiong, R., Tang, H., & Huang, C. (2022). Encapsulated microstructures of beneficial functional lipids and their applications in foods and biomedicines. *Journal of Agricultural and Food Chemistry, 70*(27), 8165–8187.

Calder, P. C. (2017). Omega-3 fatty acids and inflammatory processes: From molecules to man. *Biochemical Society Transactions, 45*(5), 1105–1115. https://doi.org/10.1042/BST20160474.

Coates, W. (2013). ALA Sources—Plants, Seeds, and Nuts. In F. De Meester, R. R. Watson, & S. Zibadi (Eds.). *Omega-6/3 fatty acids* (pp. 309–316). Humana Press https://doi.org/10.1007/978-1-62703-215-5_16.

Deckelbaum, R. J., & Torrejon, C. (2012). The omega-3 fatty acid nutritional landscape: health benefits and sources. *The Journal of Nutrition, 142*(3), 587S–591S.

de Toro-Martín, J., Arsenault, B. J., Després, J. P., & Vohl, M. C. (2017). Precision nutrition: A review of personalized nutritional approaches for the prevention and management of metabolic syndrome. *Nutrients, 9*(8), 913.

Dey, T. K., Banerjee, P., Chatterjee, R., & Dhar, P. (2018). Designing of ω-3 PUFA enriched biocompatible nanoemulsion with sesame protein isolate as a natural surfactant: Focus on enhanced shelf-life stability and biocompatibility. *Colloids and Surfaces A: Physicochemical and Engineering Aspects, 538*, 36–44.

dos Reis, G. A., Rodrigues, C., Wiatek, A. M., de Melo Pereira, G. V., de Carvalho, J. C., Martinez-Burgos, W. J., & Soccol, C. R. (2024). Exploring the potential of Thraustochytrids and other microorganisms for sustainable omega-3 production: A comprehensive review of patents, perspectives, and scale-up strategies. *Systems Microbiology and Biomanufacturing, 4*(2), 448–462.

Dufossé, L., Fouillaud, M., & Caro, Y. (2021). Fungi and fungal metabolites for the improvement of human and animal nutrition and health. *Journal of Fungi, 7*(Issue 4), 274. MDPI https://www.mdpi.com/2309-608X/7/4/274.

Dyall, S. C., Balas, L., Bazan, N. G., Brenna, J. T., Chiang, N., da Costa Souza, F., Dalli, J., Durand, T., Galano, J.-M., & Lein, P. J. (2022). Polyunsaturated fatty acids and fatty acid-derived lipid mediators: Recent advances in the understanding of their biosynthesis, structures, and functions. *Progress in Lipid Research, 86*, 101165.

Elazzazy, A. M., Baeshen, M. N., Alasmi, K. M., Alqurashi, S. I., Desouky, S. E., & Khattab, S. M. (2025). Where biology meets engineering: scaling up microbial nutraceuticals to bridge nutrition, therapeutics, and global impact. *Microorganisms, 13*(3), 566.

Ebrahimi, M., Rajion, M. A., Jafari, S., Faseleh Jahromi, M., Oskoueian, E., Qurni Sazili, A., & Ghaffari, M. H. (2018). Effects of dietary n-6: n-3 polyunsaturated fatty acid ratios on meat quality, carcass characteristics, tissue fatty acid profiles, and expression of lipogenic genes in growing goats. *PLoS One, 13*(8), e0188369.

El-Bayoumy, K., & Manni, A. (2020). Customized prevention trials could resolve the controversy of the effects of omega-3 fatty acids on cancer. *Nutrition and Cancer, 72*(2), 183–186.

Fang, C. L. A., Al-Suwayeh, S., & Fang, J. Y. (2013). Nanostructured lipid carriers (NLCs) for drug delivery and targeting. *Recent Patents on Nanotechnology, 7*(1), 41–55.

Ferreri, C., Sansone, A., Chatgilialoglu, C., Ferreri, R., Amézaga, J., Burgos, M. C., Arranz, S., & Tueros, I. (2022). Critical review on fatty acid-based food and nutraceuticals as supporting therapy in cancer. *International Journal of Molecular Sciences, 23*(11), 6030.

Finco, A. M. D. O., Mamani, L. D. G., Carvalho, J. C. D., De Melo Pereira, G. V., Thomaz-Soccol, V., & Soccol, C. R. (2017). Technological trends and market perspectives for production of microbial oils rich in omega-3. *Critical Reviews in Biotechnology, 37*(5), 656–671. https://doi.org/10.1080/07388551.2016.1213221.

Fornaro, F. A., Zarli, A., Serangeli, C., Salladini, A., Piemonte, V., Iaquaniello, G., & Di Paola, L. (2024). Technological analysis of the sustainable production of ømega-3 from fish wastes in a biorefinery framework. *Waste and Biomass Valorization, 15*(7), 3953–3967.

Granato, D., Zabetakis, I., & Koidis, A. (2023). Sustainability, nutrition, and scientific advances of functional foods under the new EU and global legislation initiatives. *Journal of Functional Foods, 109*, 105793.

Giordano, D., Coppola, D., Russo, R., Denaro, R., Giuliano, L., Lauro, F. M., & Verde, C. (2015). Marine microbial secondary metabolites: Pathways, evolution and physiological roles. *Advances in Microbial Physiology, 66*, 357–428.

Gong, Y., Wan, X., Jiang, M., Hu, C., Hu, H., & Huang, F. (2014). Metabolic engineering of microorganisms to produce omega-3 very long-chain polyunsaturated fatty acids. *Progress in Lipid Research, 56*, 19–35.

Guo, D. S., Ji, X. J., Ren, L. J., Li, G. L., Sun, X. M., Chen, K. Q., & Huang, H. (2018). Development of a scale-up strategy for fermentative production of docosahexaenoic acid by Schizochytrium sp. *Chemical Engineering Science, 176*, 600–608.

Jacobsen, C. (2015). Some strategies for the stabilization of long chain n-3 PUFA-enriched foods: A review. *European Journal of Lipid Science and Technology, 117*(11), 1853–1866.

Jafari, S., Jafari, S. M., Ebrahimi, M., Kijpatanasilp, I., & Assatarakul, K. (2023). A decade overview and prospect of spray drying encapsulation of bioactives from fruit products: Characterization, food application and in vitro gastrointestinal digestion. *Food hydrocolloids, 134*, 108068.

Jafari, S., Ebrahimi, M., Assatarakul, K., & Jafari, S. M. (2022). Plant oils rich in essential fatty acids. *Handbook of Food Bioactive Ingredients: Properties and Applications*, 1–24.

Jagadevan, S., Banerjee, A., Banerjee, C., Guria, C., Tiwari, R., Baweja, M., & Shukla, P. (2018). Recent developments in synthetic biology and metabolic engineering in microalgae towards biofuel production. *Biotechnology for Biofuels, 11*, 1–21.

Jia, Y. L., Wang, L. R., Zhang, Z. X., Gu, Y., & Sun, X. M. (2022). Recent advances in biotechnological production of polyunsaturated fatty acids by Yarrowia lipolytica. *Critical Reviews in Food Science and Nutrition, 62*(32), 8920–8934.

Jurić, S., Jurić, M., Siddique, M. A. B., & Fathi, M. (2022). Vegetable oils rich in polyunsaturated fatty acids: Nanoencapsulation methods and stability enhancement. *Food Reviews International, 38*(1), 32–69.

Harwood, J. L. (2019). Algae: Critical sources of very long-chain polyunsaturated fatty acids. *Biomolecules, 9*(11), 708.

Herrero, M., Mendiola, J. A., Cifuentes, A., & Ibáñez, E. (2010). Supercritical fluid extraction: Recent advances and applications. *Journal of Chromatography. A, 1217*(16), 2495–2511. https://doi.org/10.1016/j.chroma.2009.12.019.

Hosseiniara, S. M., & Hosseini Zijoud, S. S. (2024). Nutrigenomics: A promising frontier in chronic disease prevention. *Journal of Preventive and Complementary Medicine, 3*(4), 195–200.

Kaka, A., Haron, W., Yimer, N., Channo, A., Jahejo, A. R., Ebrahimi, M., & Kalhoro, D. H. (2023). Enhancement of frozen-thawed quality of bull semen after enrichment of docosahexaenoic acid extended in tris-extender. Journal of Animal Health and Production, *11*(1), 7–13.

Kapoor, B., Kapoor, D., Gautam, S., Singh, R., & Bhardwaj, S. (2021). Dietary polyunsaturated fatty acids (PUFAs): Uses and potential health benefits. *Current Nutrition Reports, 10*, 232–242.

Karageorgou, D., Rova, U., Christakopoulos, P., Katapodis, P., Matsakas, L., & Patel, A. (2023). Benefits of supplementation with microbial omega-3 fatty acids on human health and the current market scenario for fish-free omega-3 fatty acid. *Trends in Food Science & Technology, 136*, 169–180.

Keller, H., Reinhardt, G., Rettenmaier, N., Schorb, A., Dittrich, M., de Wolf, P.L., van der Voort, M.P. J., Spruijt, J., Potters, J.I., & Elissen, H.J. H. (2017). Environmental assessment of algae-based PUFA production. PUFAChain. https://edepot.wur.nl/441803

Khoshnoudi-Nia, S., Forghani, Z., & Jafari, S. M. (2022). A systematic review and meta-analysis of fish oil encapsulation within different micro/nanocarriers. *Critical Reviews in Food Science and Nutrition, 62*(8), 2061–2082.

Lane, K. E., Wilson, M., Hellon, T. G., & Davies, I. G. (2022). Bioavailability and conversion of plant-based sources of omega-3 fatty acids – A scoping review to update supplementation options for vegetarians and vegans. *Critical Reviews in Food Science and Nutrition, 62*(18), 4982–4997. https://doi.org/10.1080/10408398.2021.1880364.

Liu, Y., Ren, X., Fan, C., Wu, W., Zhang, W., & Wang, Y. (2022). Health benefits, food applications, and sustainability of microalgae-derived N-3 PUFA. *Foods, 11*(13), 1883.

Liu, X., Song, Z., Tian, W., Abdullah, Huang, Q., Chen, M., & Xiao, J. (2024). Advancements in lipid-based delivery systems for functional foods: A comprehensive review of literature and patent trends. *Critical Reviews in Food Science and Nutrition*, 1–17.

Lopes, P. A., Bandarra, N. M., Martins, S. V., Martinho, J., Alfaia, C. M., Madeira, M. S., & Prates, J. A. (2017). Markers of neuroprotection of combined EPA and DHA provided by fish oil are higher than those of EPA (Nannochloropsis) and DHA (Schizochytrium) from microalgae oils in Wistar rats. *Nutrition & Metabolism, 14*, 1–17.

Lumanlan, J. C., Williams, M., & Jayasena, V. (2022). Edible insects: Environmentally friendly sustainable future food source. *International journal of food science & technology, 57*(10), 6317–6325. http://doi.org/10.1111/ijfs.16006.

MacDonald, C., Colombo, S., & Arts, M. T. (2019). Genetically engineered oil seed crops and novel terrestrial nutrients: Ethical considerations. *Science and Engineering Ethics, 25*(5), 1485–1497. https://doi.org/10.1007/s11948-018-0074-9.

Magoni, C., Bertacchi, S., Giustra, C. M., Guzzetti, L., Cozza, R., Ferrari, M., Torelli, A., Marieschi, M., Porro, D., & Branduardi, P. (2022). Could microalgae be a strategic choice for responding to the demand for omega-3 fatty acids? A European perspective. *Trends in Food Science & Technology, 121*, 142–155.

Mandal, A., & Ghosh, A. R. (2024). Role of artificial intelligence (AI) in fish growth and health status monitoring: A review on sustainable aquaculture. *Aquaculture International, 32*(3), 2791–2820.

Marsol-Vall, A., Aitta, E., Guo, Z., & Yang, B. (2022). Green technologies for production of oils rich in n-3 polyunsaturated fatty acids from aquatic sources. *Critical Reviews in Food Science and Nutrition, 62*(11), 2942–2962. https://doi.org/10.1080/10408398.2020.1861426.

Martinsson, H. (2016). Seaweed products on the Swedish market as a source of omega-3 fatty acids.

Mittal, R. K., Mishra, R., Sharma, V., & Purohit, P. (2024). Bioactive exploration in functional foods: Unlocking nature's treasures. *Current Pharmaceutical Biotechnology, 25*(11), 1419–1435. https://doi.org/10.2174/0113892010282580231120041659.

Mititelu, M., Lupuliasa, D., Neacşu, S. M., Olteanu, G., Busnatu, Ştefan S., Mihai, A., Popovici, V., Măru, N., Boroghină, S. C., Mihai, S., Ioniţă-Mîndrican, C.-B., & Scafa-Udrişte, A. (2025). Polyunsaturated fatty acids and human health: A key to modern nutritional balance in association with polyphenolic compounds from food sources. *Foods, 14*(1). https://doi.org/10.3390/foods14010046 Article 1.

Mosconi, G. (2024). Determination of contaminants in fishery products to support food safety. https://air.unimi.it/handle/2434/1118608

Mozafari, M. R., Flanagan, J., Matia-Merino, L., Awati, A., Omri, A., Suntres, Z. E., & Singh, H. (2006). Recent trends in the lipid-based nanoencapsulation of antioxidants and their role in foods. *Journal of the Science of Food and Agriculture, 86*(13), 2038–2045.

Muthukrishnan, L. (2022). Nanonutraceuticals—Challenges and novel nano-based carriers for effective delivery and enhanced bioavailability. *Food and Bioprocess Technology, 15*(10), 2155–2184.

Patel, A., Karageorgou, D., Rova, E., Katapodis, P., Rova, U., Christakopoulos, P., & Matsakas, L. (2020). An overview of potential oleaginous microorganisms and their role in biodiesel and omega-3 fatty acid-based industries. *Microorganisms, 8*(3), 434.

Prasad, G., Padhiary, M., Hoque, A., & Kumar, K. (2025). AI-driven personalized nutrition apps and platforms for enhanced diet and wellness. In *Food in the Metaverse and Web 3.0 era: Intersecting food, technology, and culture*. IGI Global Scientific Publishing, 125–158.

Portanguen, S., Tournayre, P., Sicard, J., Astruc, T., & Mirade, P. S. (2019). Toward the design of functional foods and biobased products by 3D printing: A review. *Trends in Food Science & Technology, 86*, 188–198.

Qin, J., Kurt, E., LBassi, T., Sa, L., & Xie, D. (2023). Biotechnological production of omega-3 fatty acids: current status and future perspectives. *Frontiers in Microbiology, 14*, 1280296.

Ribeiro Carvalho, M. (2022). Innovative feeds based on novel omega-3 sources to improve the production of mediterranean fish (PhD Thesis). https://accedacris.ulpgc.es/bitstream/10553/114856/1/Tesis%20doctoral%20Marta%20Carvalho.pdf

Riekkinen, K., Väkeväinen, K., & Korhonen, J. (2022). The effect of substrate on the nutrient content and fatty acid composition of edible insects. *Insects, 13*(7), 590.

Ruiz-Lopez, N., Usher, S., Sayanova, O. V., Napier, J. A., & Haslam, R. P. (2015). Modifying the lipid content and composition of plant seeds: Engineering the production of LC-PUFA. *Applied Microbiology and Biotechnology, 99*, 143–154.

Saidaiah, P., Banu, Z., Khan, A. A., Geetha, A., & Somraj, B. (2024). A comprehensive review of Omega-3 fatty acids: Sources, industrial applications, and health benefits. *Annals of Phytomedicine, 13*(1), 209–225.

Saini, R. K., & Keum, Y. S. (2018). Omega-3 and omega-6 polyunsaturated fatty acids: Dietary sources, metabolism, and significance—A review. *Life Sciences, 203*, 255–267.

Siddiqui, S. A., Ucak, İ., Afreen, M., Sasidharan, A., Yunusa, B. M., Bhowmik, S., Pandiselvam, R., Ambartsumov, T. G., & Shah, M. A. (2024). Microalgae as a potential raw material for plant-based seafood alternatives: A comprehensive review. *Food Science & Nutrition, 12*(11), 8559–8593. https://doi.org/10.1002/fsn3.4313.

Singh, K. K., Mridula, D., Rehal, J., & Barnwal, P. (2011). Flaxseed: A potential source of food, feed and fiber. *Critical Reviews in Food Science and Nutrition, 51*(3), 210–222. https://doi.org/10.1080/10408390903537241.

Shchukina, E. M., & Shchukin, D. G. (2012). Layer-by-layer coated emulsion microparticles as storage and delivery tool. *Current Opinion in Colloid & Interface Science, 17*(5), 281–289.

Singar, S., Nagpal, R., Arjmandi, B. H., & Akhavan, N. S. (2024). Personalized nutrition: Tailoring dietary recommendations through genetic insights. *Nutrients, 16*(16), 2673.

Soni, R., Suyal, D. C., & Morales-Oyervides, L. (2023). *Microbial bioactive compounds: Industrial and agricultural applications*. Springer Nature Eds.

Sonju, J. J., Dahal, A., Singh, S. S., & Jois, S. D. (2021). Peptide-functionalized liposomes as therapeutic and diagnostic tools for cancer treatment. *Journal of Controlled Release, 329*, 624–644.

Subedi, U., Jayawardhane, K. N., Pan, X., Ozga, J., Chen, G., Foroud, N. A., & Singer, S. D. (2020). The potential of genome editing for improving seed oil content and fatty acid composition in oilseed crops. *Lipids, 55*(5), 495–512.

Tao, L. (2015). Oxidation of polyunsaturated fatty acids and its impact on food quality and human health. Advances in Food Technology and Nutritional Sciences, *1*(6), 135–142.

Thiagarajan, C., & Devarajan, Y. (2024). The urgent challenge of ocean pollution: Impacts on marine biodiversity and human health. *Regional Studies in Marine Science*, 103995.

Theofilis, P., Vlachakis, P. K., Oikonomou, E., Tsioufis, K., & Tousoulis, D. (2024). Targeting the gut microbiome to treat cardiometabolic disease. *Current Atherosclerosis Reports, 26*(2), 25–34.

Timilsena, Y. P., Wang, B., Adhikari, R., & Adhikari, B. (2017). Advances in microencapsulation of polyunsaturated fatty acids (PUFAs)-rich plant oils using complex coacervation: A review. *Food hydrocolloids, 69*, 369–381.

Tocher, D. R., Agaba, M., Hastings, N., Bell, J. G., Dick, J. R., & Teale, A. J. (2001). Nutritional regulation of hepatocyte fatty acid desaturation and polyunsaturated fatty acid composition in zebrafish (*Danio rerio*) and tilapia (*Oreochromis niloticus*). *Fish Physiology and Biochemistry, 24*(4), 309–320.

Togarcheti, S. C., & Padamati, R. B. (2021). Comparative life cycle assessment of EPA and DHA production from microalgae and farmed fish. *Clean Technologies, 3*(4), 699–710.

Tzima, S., Georgiopoulou, I., Louli, V., & Magoulas, K. (2023). Recent advances in supercritical CO_2 extraction of pigments, lipids and bioactive compounds from microalgae. *Molecules (Basel, Switzerland), 28*(3). https://doi.org/10.3390/molecules28031410 Article 3.

Van der Voort, M.P., Spruijt, J., Potters, J.I., & Elissen, H.J. H. (2017). Socio-economic assessment of algae-based PUFA production: The value chain from microalgae to PUFA ('PUFACHAIN'). PUFAChain. https://edepot.wur.nl/441763

Vellido-Perez, J. A., Ochando-Pulido, J. M., Brito-de la Fuente, E., & Martinez-Ferez, A. (2021). Novel emulsions–based technological approaches for the protection of omega–3 polyunsaturated fatty acids against oxidation processes–a comprehensive review. *Food Structure, 27*, 100175.

Venegas-Calerón, M., & Napier, J. A. (2023). New alternative sources of omega-3 fish oil. In *Advances in food and nutrition research, 105*, Elsevier, 343–398. https://www.sciencedirect.com/science/article/pii/S1043452623000013.

Venkatraman, S., Rajendran, D. S., & Vaidyanathan, V. K. (2024). Development and scale-up of the bioreactor system in biorefinery: A significant step toward a green and bio-based economy. In *Biotechnological advances in biorefinery*. Singapore: Springer Nature Singapore, 207–230.

Visentini, F. F., Perez, A. A., & Santiago, L. G. (2019). Self-assembled nanoparticles from heat treated ovalbumin as nanocarriers for polyunsaturated fatty acids. *Food Hydrocolloids, 93*, 242–252.

Wang, J. Z., Wu, C. K., Yan, C. H., Chen, H., You, S., Sheng, S., & Wang, J. (2021). Nutritional targeting modification of silkworm pupae oil catalyzed by a smart hydrogel immobilized lipase. *Food & Function, 12*(14), 6240–6253.

Xia, F. L. W., Supri, S., Djamaludin, H., Nurdiani, R., Seng, L. L., Yin, K. W., & Rovina, K. (2024). Turning waste into value: Extraction and effective valorization strategies of seafood by-products. *Waste Management Bulletin, 2*(3), 84–100.

Xie, D., Jackson, E. N., & Zhu, Q. (2015). Sustainable source of omega-3 eicosapentaenoic acid from metabolically engineered *Yarrowia lipolytica*: From fundamental research to commercial production. *Applied Microbiology and Biotechnology, 99*, 1599–1610.

Xue, Y. F., Alain, I. T., Yin, N. W., Jiang, J. Y., Zhao, Y. P., Kun, L. U., & Chai, Y. R. (2023). Biotechnology of α-linolenic acid in oilseed rape (*Brassica napus*) using FAD2 and FAD3 from chia (*Salvia hispanica*). *Journal of Integrative Agriculture, 22*(12), 3810–3815.

Xu, P., Bhan, N., & Koffas, M. A. (2013). Engineering plant metabolism into microbes: From systems biology to synthetic biology. *Current Opinion in Biotechnology, 24*(2), 291–299.

Yan, K., Guo, F., Kainz, M. J., Li, F., Gao, W., Bunn, S. E., & Zhang, Y. (2024). The importance of omega-3 polyunsaturated fatty acids as high-quality food in freshwater ecosystems with implications of global change. *Biological Reviews, 99*(1), 200–218. https://doi.org/10.1111/brv.13017.

Zelikina, D., Chebotarev, S., Komarova, A., Balakina, E., Antipova, A., Martirosova, E., & Semenova, M. (2022). Efficiency of an oral delivery system based on a liposomal form of a combination of curcumin with a balanced amount of n-3 and n-6 PUFAs encapsulated in an electrostatic complex of WPI with chitosan. *Colloids and Surfaces A: Physicochemical and Engineering Aspects, 651*, 129630.

Zhao, W., Zhu, J., Yang, S., Liu, J., Sun, Z., & Sun, H. (2024). Microalgal metabolic engineering facilitates precision nutrition and dietary regulation. *Science of The Total Environment,* 175460.

Zhou, Q., & Wei, Z. (2023). Food-grade systems for delivery of DHA and EPA: Opportunities, fabrication, characterization and future perspectives. *Critical Reviews in Food Science and Nutrition, 63*(15), 2348–2365. https://doi.org/10.1080/10408398.2021.1974337.

Zhu, Q., & Jackson, E. N. (2015). Production of omega-3 and omega-6 polyunsaturated fatty acids by metabolic engineering of *Yarrowia lipolytica. ACOS Lipid Library.*

Zubair, M., Pradhan, R. A., Arshad, M., & Ullah, A. (2021). Recent advances in lipid derived bio-based materials for food packaging applications. *Macromolecular Materials and Engineering, 306*(7), 2000799. https://doi.org/10.1002/mame.202000799.

Chapter 36

Harnessing the potential of polyunsaturated fatty acids for health and sustainable food systems

Ravi Sanjana[1], Sureshkumar Sujithra[1], K.S. Krithiga[1], Safreena Kabeer[1], Kalaiselvi Krishnamoorthy[2], and Pothiyappan Karthik[1]

[1]*Department of Food Technology, Faculty of Engineering, Karpagam Academy of Higher Education, Coimbatore, Tamil Nadu, India,* [2]*Centre for Herbal Pharmacology and Environmental Sustainability, Chettinad Hospital and Research Institute, Chettinad Academy of Research and Education, Chennai, Tamil Nadu, India*

36.1 Introduction

In recent decades, the food and nutrition fields have received more attention due to consumer preferences and lifestyle changes. Modern technologies involve foods that also need to fulfill the required amount of nutrients and maintain well-being. Polyunsaturated fatty acids (PUFAs) play a vital part in human metabolism (Majhi et al., 2022). Omega-3 and omega-6 fatty acids are subgroups of the PUFA; both types are broadly analyzed for their role in neurological, cardiovascular disease (CVD) and anti-inflammatory activities (Mallick et al., 2024; Zárate et al., 2017). Apart from that, PUFAs are involved in numerous cellular actions such as cell signaling, fluidity of the cell membrane, structural integrity, blood pressure regulation, blood sugar levels, nerve system, and blood clotting (Mukerjee et al., 2021; Xu et al., 2025). Omega-3 types are "Alpha-linolenic acid (ALA), Eicosapentaenoic acid (EPA), and Docosahexaenoic acid (DHA)," where ALA is a plant-based fatty acid existing in vegetables, flaxseed, walnuts, and chia seeds. EPA is present in marine organisms such as fatty fish and algae. DHA is a crucial structural lipid in retinal membranes, vital for cognitive and visual development. While "Linoleic acid (LA), Arachidonic acid (AA), and Dihomo-gamma-Linolenic acid (DGLA)" are representatives of omega-6 PUFAs, LA is most abundantly present in vegetable oils, ALA is found in animal-based products, and DGLA is predominantly found in grains, meats, and dairy products (Geetha et al., 2025; Basak et al., 2021).

The 21st century has changed very rapidly in the food sector due to consumer cravings and food habits (Kumari et al., 2025). This led to the innovative techniques involved in functional food production (Seth et al., 2025). Specifically, the requirement of PUFA is fulfilled by food technologists, because PUFA-based agricultural products provide rich sources of oil-seed crops (Saini et al., 2021). Fortified dairy products and bakery items, to beverages and infant formulas are also products where PUFAs are widely used. In addition to boosting individual health, PUFAs are essential in supporting general health and nutrition security at the global level. From an aspect of public health, consuming PUFA reduces the threat of non-communicable diseases (NCDs). To commercialize the PUFA, consumer awareness plays a major role. Growing interest in the use of functional foods need to fulfill the nutritional benefit, as well as consumer needs (Mititelu et al., 2024). At present, PUFA is commercialized in various products like ready-to-eat meals and sports nutrition. This clearly reflects that PUFA-based products are gradually being accepted and reaching consumers at a global level (Attia et al., 2017). However, the next barrier is its availability everywhere in the world. While PUFA-enriched foods are often found in high-income countries, low- and middle-income communities frequently have limited access to them because of distribution and cost difficulties (Pérez-Palacios et al., 2019). In order to overcome this gap and ensure that the advantages of PUFAs are distributed internationally, public policy, international collaboration, and consumer education are vital and crucial.

Omega-3 and Omega-6 Polyunsaturated Fatty Acids in Food Systems. DOI: https://doi.org/10.1016/B978-0-443-43810-3.00022-1

The current chapter focuses on the differences between omega-3 and omega-6 families, their physiological properties, and the benefits of human health. Furthermore, PUFA involvement in the global transition toward functional and sustainable foods is also being elaborated. Overall, the chapter highlights both nutritional and ecological resources of PUFA.

36.2 Nutritional and therapeutic significance of polyunsaturated fatty acids

36.2.1 Biochemistry and physiology of polyunsaturated fatty acids

Lipids constitute one of the most significant biomolecules in nature as they act as the major source of energy to the human body. They provide the structural framework for cells and tissues. They also act as precursors to the hormones and other biologically active compounds (Frydrych et al., 2025). Fatty acids are considered the building blocks of most lipids. They are divided into saturated and unsaturated fatty acids based on the existence of the double bonds between the carbon atoms. A fatty acid is characterized by a long-chain hydrocarbon with a COOH group at one end and a methyl group at another (Hulbert et al., 2005). The saturated fatty acids contain only one single bond in their chain structure, and the carbon backbone is fully saturated by hydrogen atoms. Saturated fatty acids are referred to as solid, and they have higher melting points. Unsaturated fatty acids contain one or more double bonds and usually have a bend in the position of the double bond (Harayama & Antonny, 2023). If there are multiple double bonds in a fatty acid, it is known as a PUFA (De Carvalho & Caramujo, 2018).

The two principal PUFA families of fatty acids are omega-3 and omega-6, which differ in the position of the first double bond from the methyl end of the carbon chain. These are considered essential fatty acids, as humans do not have the desaturase enzymes required to synthesize them and are added to the daily diet, making dietary intake necessary (Calder, 2010). PUFAs mainly occur in the cis configuration, in which hydrogen atoms adjacent to the double bond occur on the same side. This type of configuration produces a bend in the fatty acid chain. But the trans configuration lies in a straighter structure, reducing membrane flexibility (Mozaffarian and Wu, 2011).

The enzymes such as desaturase and elongase convert the omega-3 (ALA) and omega-6 (LA) fatty acids into long-chain metabolites. Omega-3 fatty acid is converted into EPA. EPA is reported to help in heart health by decreasing triglyceride levels in blood vessels. They also support endothelial function and regulate inflammatory responses. It is further converted into DHA. DHA is present in the brain and retina, and it helps in supporting cognitive and visual function and neuron signaling. But excessive intake of EPA and DHA may increase bleeding in the blood vessels and interrupt the immune balance in the human body (Calder, 2010; Petermann et al., 2022). LA is further converted into gamma-linolenic acid (GLA), DGLA, and AA in order. The eicosanoids such as prostaglandin E_2 and leukotriene B_4 are derived from AA. These are essential for immunity and tissue healing. At the same time, DGLA-derived compounds may exhibit anti-inflammatory effects (Das, 2021).

36.2.2 Health benefits of polyunsaturated fatty acids

Omega-3 fatty acids, mostly EPA and DHA, play a vital role in regulating heart health. They help in maintaining blood triglyceride levels by enhancing lipoprotein lipase action. They can suppress lipogenic genes such as sterol regulatory element-binding protein-1c and fatty acid synthase. Apart from controlling lipid control, omega-3 fatty acids can generate anti-inflammatory mediators like resolvins and protectins, reducing cytokine levels including tumor necrosis factor-alpha (TNF-α) and interleukin-6 (IL-6), and they also reduce the activity of cyclooxygenase-2. They enhance endothelial function by promoting nitric oxide release, supporting better blood flow. When these actions are put together, it can be said that PUFAs can reduce cardiovascular risk (Howell et al., 2009; Michaeloudes et al., 2023).

Omega-3 fatty acids such as EPA and DHA are declared to support insulin sensitivity through coordinated mechanisms. They can activate peroxisome proliferator-activated receptor gamma, and this receptor enhances glucose uptake in muscles and adipose tissue from the food. They suppress nuclear factor kappa-light-chain-enhancer of activated B cells signaling and lower cytokines such as TNF-α and IL-6, and they protect insulin signaling pathways (Botta et al., 2018; Calder, 2010). These omega-3 fatty acids may help in regulating body weight by increasing lipid metabolism activities. They can also influence adipokine secretion and insulin sensitivity, and support a healthier metabolic balance if they are consumed in appropriate amounts (Kalupahana et al., 2011). Fig. 36.1 consolidates the health benefits of PUFA.

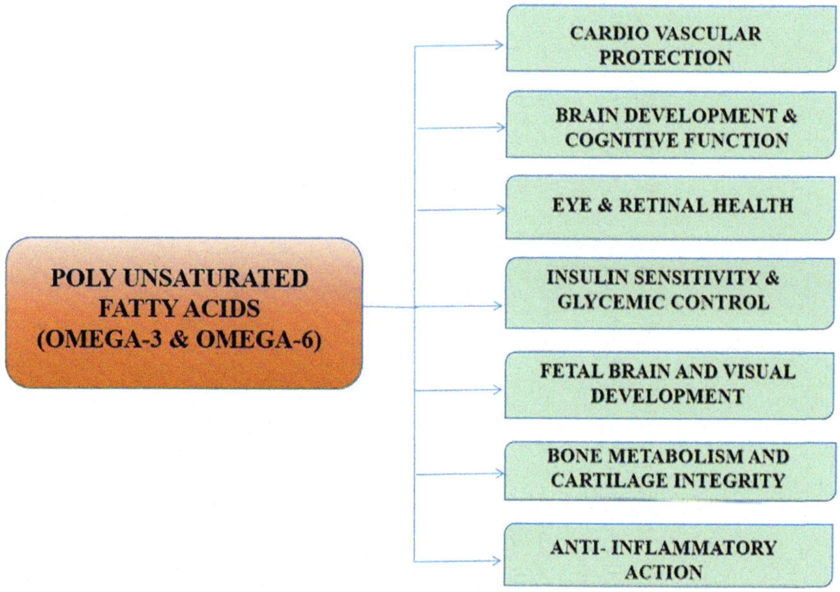

FIGURE 36.1 Health benefits of polyunsaturated fatty acids.

36.2.3 Clinical and epidemiological evidence

The scientific studies, in the past decades, have progressed immensely; from testing the total fat intake to measuring the concept of metabolism of fatty acids, the quantitative and qualitative measures have improved. A significant reduction in coronary heart diseases has been observed when the saturated fatty acids were substituted with PUFA (Mozaffarain et al., 2010). But results have not been identified as identical across all experiments. These variations are due to the dosage level, diet habits, and the use of medicine and treatment. Yurko-Mauro et al. (2010) conducted a 24-week clinical study to analyze the effect of DHA supplementation (900 mg/d) on improved cognitive and memory function which resulted in a positive outcome. Similarly, Li et al., 2025 showed that PUFA supplementation improved the lipid profile and glucose metabolism in diabetic patients. Alternatively, some studies show neutral to significant improvement on the required outcome. Singh et al. (2010) demonstrated that the PUFA supplementation did not show any effect on Sjögren's disorder in saliva production when compared to wheat germ oil. A similar neutral outcome was obtained by Theander et al. (2002), who used GLA from primrose oil to test the efficacy of saliva production for Sjögren's disorder. Table 36.1 consolidates multiple epidemiological studies and the clinical significance of PUFA.

36.2.4 Dietary recommendations, global intake patterns, and public health implications

PUFAs do not have global standard recommended dietary intake values like vitamins and minerals. But experts have provided adequate intake (AI) levels or guidelines based on heart and metabolic outcomes. The European Food Safety Authority (EFSA) recommends that the intake of approximately 250 mg/day and 500 mg/day of combined EPA and DHA for adults can support cardiovascular activity (EFSA Panel on Dietetic Products, Nutrition and Allergies (NDA), 2012). Similarly, the American Heart Association also advises that two servings of fatty fish per week containing 500 mg/day of long-chain omega-3 fatty acids can help in cardiovascular health (Siscovick et al., 2017). In the case of α-linolenic acid, it was recommended that intake can range from 1.1 to 1.6 g/day in North America for adults. Western dietary patterns often exhibit an omega-6 to omega-3 ratio exceeding 15:1, which is a distribution that is thought to promote the production of pro-inflammatory eicosanoids and reduce the efficiency of endogenous conversion of α-linolenic acid into longer chain metabolic compounds.

In spite of much research conducted, the intake level of omega-3 PUFAs has been uneven across the global populations. In the regions where marine foods are not consumed regularly, intake levels of EPA and DHA fall behind the recommended intake levels. These lower levels have induced public health strategies highlighting the dietary strategies, encouraging greater consumption of fatty fish, nuts, seeds, and plant-derived oils such as sunflower oil and olive oil, etc., rather than depending on dietary supplements. Whole diet patterns, including Mediterranean dietary style, consistently relate to improved metabolic results in research studies, suggesting that the fatty acids work synergistically within the dietary foods (Mozaffarian & Wu, 2011).

TABLE 36.1 Study of polyunsaturated fatty acids (PUFA) in clinical and epidemiological evidence.

Study/evidence type	Population/design	Intervention/exposure	Key numerical findings reported in text	References
Randomized placebo-controlled trial	>20,000 generally healthy U.S. adults	1 g/day marine-derived omega-3 fatty acids	No statistically significant reduction in major cardiovascular health	Manson et al. (2019)
Randomized, double-blind, placebo-controlled, clinical study	485 healthy subjects, aged ≥55	900 mg/d of DHA supplementation	Improved memory, learning, and cognitive function with aging	Yurko-Mauro et al. (2010)
Prospective, randomized, and placebo-controlled study	Double-blind clinical trial, 61 participants with Sjögren's	1.750 mg of omega-3 fatty acids (1 g of flaxseed, 450 and 300 mg of EPA and DHA, respectively)	No significant changes for Sjögren's due to PUFA supplementation	Singh et al. (2010)
Prospective, randomized, and placebo-controlled study	87 participants (Women: 79, men: 8)	GLA: 1600 mg/day	No significant changes in dryness and fatigue	Theander et al. (2002)
Meta analysis	Randomized controlled trials	-	Omega-3 fatty acids improved the lipid and glucose levels, although no significant changes were observed for blood pressure and inflammation	Li, Lin, et al. (2025)

36.3 Dietary sources of polyunsaturated fatty acid

36.3.1 Natural sources of polyunsaturated fatty acid

The PUFA is naturally sourced from vegetables, fruits, and marine sources such as soybean, sunflower, safflower, rapeseed oil, flaxseed, chia seed, fatty fish, etc. The major classes of PUFA are omega-3 fatty acids and omega-6 fatty acids, as illustrated in Fig. 36.2 (Duan et al., 2023). Since the body cannot synthesize PUFA, the natural dietary sources play a vital role in maintaining the required levels for important body functioning of the brain, reproduction, and neural development (Jovanovic et al., 2021). The plant oils contribute to the vegetarian sources of the PUFA with varying amounts of ALA, LA, etc. The soybean oil has 54.17% of LA, while the ALA is minimal. The canola oil has 25% of LA and 9.5% of ALA (Dorni et al., 2018). The α-linolenic acid is highest in the oil of *Ocimum basilicum* with 63.8%, followed by *Eucommia ulmoides* oliver with 61.36%. The chia seed and flaxseed follow the same trend with 54.5% and 53.4%, respectively. The chia seed is considered generally recognized as safe and also has good antioxidant properties along with valuable nutritional attributes, including protein and fiber content. Additionally, chia seeds have exceptional water-absorbing capacity, making them applicable in food industries as emulsifiers and directly in baked goods as flour, oil, etc (Zettel & Hitzmann, 2018). Stearidonic acid (18:4), an intermediate of ALA, offers direct health benefits in cardiovascular health and acts as a great alternative to fish oil. This type is rich in corn gromwell and purple viper's bugloss with 21% and 11%, respectively (Saini et al., 2021). Many evidences show the positive impact of the consumption of fish and its oil on heart health. In a study by Albert et al. (2002), men with low levels of DHA and EPA were more susceptible to cardiac arrest. Omega-3 from fish reduces the chance of blood clotting and improves antiinflammatory properties, thereby decreasing atherosclerosis and thrombosis (Calder, 2004). PUFA also imparts anticancer effects and improves the activity of cancer treatment drugs (Serini et al., 2011).

36.3.2 Microbial and synthetic sources of polyunsaturated fatty acid

The emergence of PUFA and its interests have grown among the population due to its huge health benefits. Ward and Singh (2005) suggested that the consumption of PUFA (1 g of DHA and EPA) through diet to impart the required functional benefit would be difficult. Intake of large quantities of fish and related products was associated with numerous health issues, including marine pollutants that accumulated in the food chain. Additionally, the fish products usually impart a bad odor, which poses a threat to consumer perception. Bio-synthesis of PUFA may risk overfishing and loss of biodiversity. To overcome these conditions and contamination, other sources of PUFA are widely preferred, including microbial and synthetic sources from biotechnological innovations (Martins et al., 2013).

Single-cell oil producers are "oleaginous microorganisms" that store lipid in them and are used as a major source of PUFA synthesis. Although the production cost could be high, they can be grown in huge quantities in bulk with pure

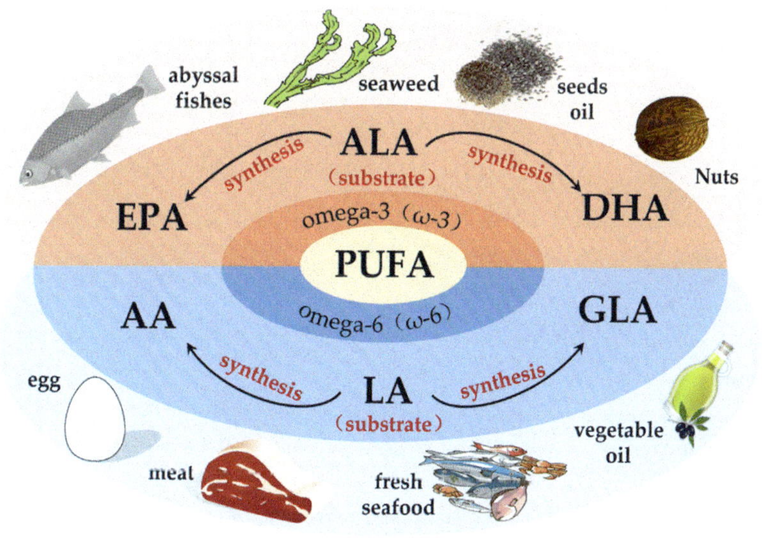

FIGURE 36.2 Classification of polyunsaturated fatty acid sources (Duan et al., 2023).
Source: From Duan, Hao, Song, Wei, Zhao, Jian & Yan, Wenjie. (2023). Polyunsaturated Fatty Acids (PUFAs): Sources, Digestion, Absorption, Application and Their Potential Adjunctive Effects on Visual Fatigue. Nutrients, 15(11). https://doi.org/10.3390/nu15112633.

standards. Whereas, the biotechnological treatments of PUFA synthesis use different agro-based waste materials as the raw material or substrate (Kothri et al., 2020). For microbial conversion of monounsaturated fatty acid to PUFA using the aerobic pathway, certain enzymes such as elongases and desaturases are required. These enzymes are present in the microbes, including microalgae, fungi, and bacteria (Khozin-Goldberg et al., 2011). In some prokaryotes and eukaryotes, the anaerobic pathway (polyketide synthase) is also used to synthesize PUFA, without the aid of these enzymes (Shah et al., 2022). Oleaginous fungi such as *Umbellopsis isabellina* and *Cunninghamella echinulata*, and yeast varieties such as *Candida*, *Cryptococcus*, *Schizochytrium*, etc., are used to synthesize PUFA. Genetically modified strains, including *Mortierella alpina* 1S-4, *M. alpina* ST1358, and *Yarrowia lipolytica*, are also employed for the same purpose (Kothri et al., 2020). Illustrate the production of EPA and DHA from the bio-engineered yeast *Y. lipolytica in* Fig. 36.3. According to the published review by Kothri et al. (2020), some of the highest DHA-yielding fungal species are *Aurantiochytrium sp*., *Schizochytrium sp*., and *Thraustochytrium sp*., with 48.5%, 44.3%, and 45.3%, respectively. Zygomycete fungi such as *Mucor circinelloides strains* produce 27.1% of GLA, followed by *C. echinulata* with 22% of GLA yield, and *Y. lipolytica* produces 56.6%–58% of EPA. In microalgal species, *Dunaliella salina* is reported to yield 33.8% of GLA. *Amphidinium sp.* and *Heterocapsa tricuetra* produce 26.3% and 25.4% of DHA, respectively. PUFAs extracted from bacterial sources are of high demand in the nutraceutical industries as they usually produce a single PUFA rather than a mix, making it easier to process and cost-efficient. Bacteria such as *Photobacterium, Shewanella*, and *Vibrio* are among the top PUFA (DHA and EPA) producing species (Shah et al., 2022).

PUFA synthesis can be improved using certain techniques, such as the usage of mutant strains of *M. alpina* 1S-4, which produce more AA and EPA. Another genetic engineering technique is to alter or manipulate the desaturase genes to produce more PUFA (EPA and GLA). Similarly, incorporation of the antioxidant superoxide dismutase enzyme-producing gene in *Schizochytrium sp.* reduces the damage caused by reactive oxygen species, reducing the strain in the cell, thereby improving the function and production of DHA (Sakuradani et al., 2013; Zhang et al., 2018). Change of the physicochemical conditions of the PUFA manufacturing can alter the efficiency of the production. Li et al. (2015) evaluated the effect of DHA yield by *Aurantiochytrium limacinum* SR21 in different substrates (glucose + glycerol and glucose) used in the production. The mixture substrate produced 15.24% more DHA than the glucose-only substrate. Different microorganisms require different pH and temperature in the fermentation stages for effective DHA production. Similarly, the aeration rate should be between 0.2-1.0 vvm (volumetric airflow/reactor volume) with the agitation rate

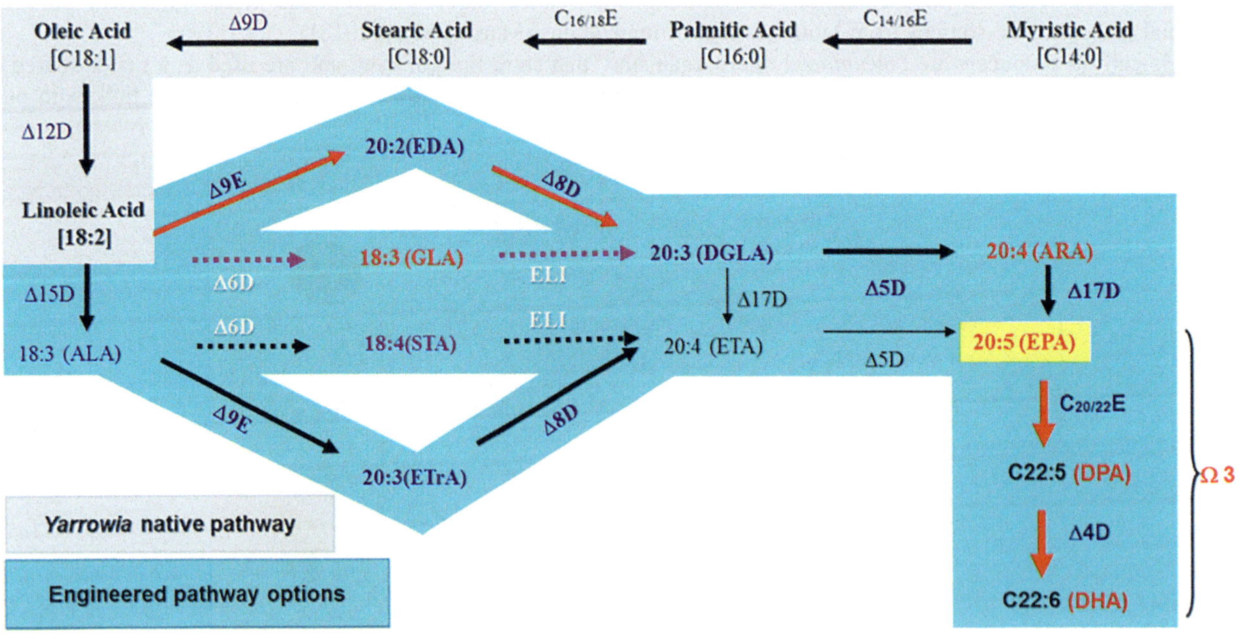

FIGURE 36.3 Polyunsaturated fatty acid synthesis using biotechnological engineering in *Yarrowia lipolytica* (Gray pathway is a conventional process, green pathway is a bio-engineered process) (Xie et al., 2015).
Source: From Xie, D., Jackson, E.N. & Zhu, Q. (2015). Sustainable source of omega-3 eicosapentaenoic acid from metabolically engineered Yarrowia lipolytica: from fundamental research to commercial production. Applied Microbiology and Biotechnology, 99(4), 1599–1610. https://doi.org/10.1007/s00253-014-6318-y.

between 50-400 rpm (Verma et al., 2019). Although different sources of PUFA are inspected for synthesis, extraction, and application in various industries, it is crucial to understand the safety and quality measures of the oil-producing organism to explore its complete potential for clinical and nutritional uses.

36.3.3 Barriers to adequate intake of polyunsaturated fatty acids

The knowledge on sources, health, and nutritional benefits of PUFA has been well studied and documented previously. However, the AI of PUFA is affected by various factors, including dietary preferences, bioavailability, sustainable choice, contaminants, etc. Recent studies indicate that people consuming a plant-based diet have a PUFA deficiency, especially EPA and DHA (Neufingerl & Eilander, 2022). Apart from dietary preferences, personal taste and flavor choices play an important component in the consumption of PUFA as a supplement. Derbyshire (2019) reported that PUFA levels were lower in females, children, and adolescent groups, establishing the influence of the type of diet and gender. 7.3% of kids consuming oily fish don't satisfy the recommended level of PUFA in their diet. A recent study informed that the decreasing levels of DHA in the pregnant woman's body over the gestation period, attributing to the fact that the requirement levels of EPA, DHA, and ALA are increasing due to pregnancy hormones like estrogen and progesterone (Lanier et al., 2023). Microplastics ingestion by the fish affects the gastrointestinal tract and gills, causing toxic effects to humans (Alberghini et al., 2023). Sensory barriers of smell and taste, and cooking knowledge and skills were also concluded as a barrier in PUFA consumption. In this study, the omega-3 intake of 35 elite female athletes was studied. The results revealed an inconsistent intake of fish and omega-3 supplements compared to the prescribed amount due to personal choice as a crucial sensory barrier (Hooks et al., 2023). Another study compared the socioeconomic status and education levels of the mother with the PUFA concentration. This revealed that highly educated college graduate mothers have higher levels of PUFA in plasma than those with lesser educational qualifications (Hergenrader et al., 2023). Overcoming these barriers requires proper awareness of nutrition, new products fortified with PUFA suitable for all dietary needs that suit the individual culture and personal preferences.

36.4 Sustainability dimensions of polyunsaturated fatty acid production

36.4.1 Environmental impact of traditional sources

As the demand for PUFA has increased worldwide and is continuing to rise steadily due to its numerous health benefits, difficulties in sourcing are also considered a serious threat. The traditional sourcing of PUFA from fish remains a challenge to the marine ecosystem and its biodiversity. The negative shift in the ocean resources and the depletion of the ecosystem due to overfishing impact the sustainability of the environment. Global warming and climatic changes that contribute to a high carbon footprint are some other effects of biomass shift and overfishing (Kang 2011). This includes expensive feed for the fish to maintain the required PUFA levels (Remize et al., 2021). The ocean sources are contaminated with heavy metals and other inorganic pollutants due to industrialization. This phenomenon affects the quality of the PUFA supplements, including fish oil. Other organic contaminants in the supplements, including biphenyls, cause toxicity if consumed by humans (Kang 2011). The "life cycle assessment" is used to study the environmental effects of various PUFA production techniques. This estimates the extent through raw material extraction, production of PUFA, and further synthesizing and purification processes (Togarcheti and Padamati, 2021). Studies show that microalgae used for PUFA synthesis release 30%–40% of global warming potential (GWP) compared to fish oil as substrate (Davis et al., 2021). Effective waste valorization of fish waste through proper process optimization to obtain multiple coproducts, can be used to improve the sustainability aspect. Governmental policies should implement strategies to produce low-impact PUFA production. Deville et al. (2025) studied the environmental impact of fish meal and fish oil in Peru, South America. Production of 1 tonne of fish oil and fish meal resulted in greenhouse gas emissions of 320 kg CO_2eq and 4430 kg CO_2eq. It was also estimated that 45% of greenhouse gases were emitted, contributing to the maximum impact on the sustainability front. Seves et al. (2015) studied the fish consumption pattern and the environmental sustainability aspects. The greenhouse gas emissions varied between wild fish and cultured fish, with cultured fish showing higher emissions than the wild fish. Similarly, the land usage was found to be more for cultured fish than for wild fish. Some studies show that temperature fluctuation due to global warming affects the enzymatic activity of elongases and desaturases that aid the production of PUFA. Similarly, high temperatures produce more saturated fatty acids than unsaturated fats (Morales-Sánchez et al., 2020). All these sustainable issues have instigated the research on other alternative sustainable sources, such as microalgal sources, precision fermentation in microbial engineering, and ecological practices for plant-based PUFA crops.

36.4.2 Alternative sustainable sources

Microalgal PUFA synthesis is considered the most viable option for sustainable PUFA synthesis. PUFA synthesis involving microalgae primarily involves the aerobic pathway with desaturases and elongases. In the initial step, Δ6- and Δ12-desaturases convert the saturated fats to unsaturated ones, followed by elongases that elongate the chain length. Δ6-desaturases are used in the production of omega-3, whereas the Δ12-desaturases are used in the production of omega-6 fatty acids (Sun et al., 2024). The efficiency of PUFA synthesis from the microalgae depends on the species, nutrient demands, growth conditions, environmental factors (physical and chemical), etc. Optimizing the factors such as temperature, salinity, CO_2, nutrients, and light intensity gives better growth conditions for microalgae to produce more PUFA (Zakaria et al., 2025). *Crypthecodinium cohnii* was recorded with 60.0% highest PUFA (DHA) accumulation, followed by *Aurantiochytrium sp.* with 46.70%. For EPA, *Phaeodactylum tricornutum* was recorded as highest PUFA accumulation with 35%. Similarly, for ALA, *Chlorella vulgaris* has 27% highest PUFA accumulation. Whereas *Chaetoceros muelleri* and *Rhodomonas baltica* were among the microalgae species that contained a wide variety of PUFA, making them an excellent source for nutraceutical application (Ulmann et al., 2017). The nutrient ratio of Nitrogen and phosphorus in the ratio 15:1 in the culture medium is considered ideal for microalgal growth. Increased temperature improves the photosynthesis and respiration rate, favoring cell growth. It was reported that the desaturase synthesizing gene in *Synechocystis* sp. encoded better in low temperatures and yielded more PUFA (Eungrasamee et al., 2020). Higher light intensity induced cell growth in PUFA-containing thylakoid membrane of the microalgae (Jimbo et al., 2021). Higher saline conditions influence the PUFA production in freshwater microalgae (*Scenedesmus* sp.) to maintain the membrane fluidity (Arora et al., 2017).

Microalgae have been used in various food products such as pasta and cookies to enhance the flavor and nutritional value. *Nannochloropsis oculata* can be incorporated upto 30% of the flour to give enough amount of EPA without altering the properties such as color, biomass, etc. The omega-3 was found to be 98 mg in 100 g of cookie when fortified with 1% of *N. oculata*. The green color incorporated was stable up to 2 months. A more compact and firm texture of the cookie was observed. When compared to control (wheat and maida flour) with 1.8 N, the microalgal pasta had better firmness of 2.9-4 N. These results correspond to other fortified pastas with spirulina and other legume flour (Fradique et al., 2010). The future aspects include metabolic engineering and genetic manipulation of the strains to improve productivity and application prospects in the nutraceutical and food industry.

36.5 Polyunsaturated fatty acid fortification and food system integration

A multidisciplinary challenge for improving public health nutrition is the fortification and integration of PUFA. Anti-inflammatory effects, cardiovascular protection, and neurological function are leveraged through fortification of foods with PUFA (Venugopalan et al., 2021). Stability in fortified products, bioavailability, consumer acceptance, and technological processing are the key issues involved in the integration and fortification of PUFA in food systems. Especially marine sources such as fish oils abundant in DHA and EPA counteract contamination and shelf-life issues (Moi et al., 2018). Marine bacteria, microalgae, and a variety of plant oils rich in omega-3 fatty acids like stearidonic acid and genetically modified plants are the alternate sources of PUFA (Chen et al., 2023; Rizzo et al., 2023). These sources are novel and offer pathways to meet increasing global demands while dealing with environmental and customer acceptability disputes. Technological improvement enables the fortification of omega-3 PUFA in different food systems and beverages through various approaches, such as fortification of PUFA-rich oil extracted from microalgae and incorporation into different food systems and enriching animal feeds with PUFA (Liue et al., 2022). Fig. 36.4 shows the proportion of PUFA-enriched product in the global market (Liu et al., 2022).

Chemical instability is the major technical challenge due to lipid oxidation in the fortification of PUFA, which can develop off-flavors, decrease stability, and minimize nutritional value and bioavailability (Jurić et al., 2020). To trounce these problems, technologies such as microencapsulation and nanoencapsulation use food-grade delivery systems, including liposomes, emulsions, and hydrogels, have been utilized to protect PUFAs from oxidation, mask undesirable taste and off-flavors, and maximize bioavailability (Venugopalan et al., 2021; Jurić et al., 2020). Solid forms produced by encapsulation techniques such as spray and freeze-drying aid in the incorporation of PUFA into various food systems (Jacobsen, 2010; Siddiqui et al., 2004). Sensory attribute is a major concern that is easily affected by the addition of PUFA in food systems, which may develop unacceptable taste and reduce product appeal (Jacobsen, 2010). Besides sustainability in PUFA-integrated foods, the safety and regulatory framework also play a major role. In addition to safety and regulatory aspects, fortification also addresses precise nutritional needs, which shows potential for enhancing immune and disease outcomes (Sartorio et al., 2022).

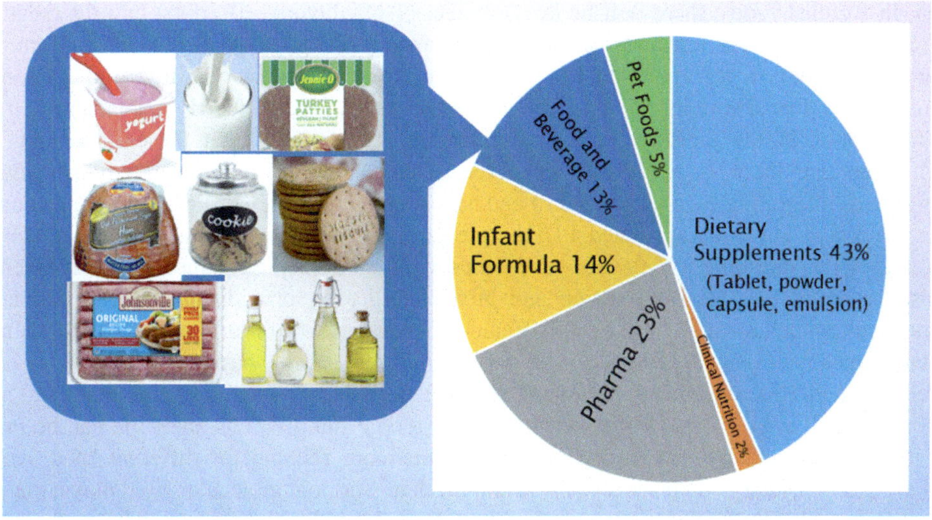

FIGURE 36.4 Proportion of polyunsaturated fatty acid-enriched product in the global market (Liu et al., 2022).
Source: From Liu, Yanjun, Ren, Xiang, Fan, Chao, Wu, Wenzhong, Zhang, Wei & Wang, Yanwen. (2022). Health Benefits, Food Applications, and Sustainability of Microalgae-Derived N-3 PUFA. Foods, 11(13). https://doi.org/10.3390/foods11131883.

36.5.1 Functional foods and fortification programs

Functional foods such as dairy, cereal products, and beverages are fortified with PUFA to improve bioavailability, nutritional value, and convey health benefits. PUFA fortified foods employ different techniques such as encapsulation, gel preparation, and emulsification to incorporate fish oil, which enable the effective delivery of omega-3 fatty acids and overcome issues related to oxidation and organoleptic qualities linked with PUFA integration (Jacobsen, 2010; Wallace et al., 2000). A major platform for PUFA fortification is dairy products, where omega-3 enrichment can be accomplished via alteration of animal feed or incorporation of plant or fish oils during processing. Reduced cardiovascular risk factor profiles have been achieved with omega-3-enriched dairy products (Savatinova & Ivanova, 2024). Likewise, an alternative source for essential fatty acids is omega-3 integrated eggs and chicken meat; omega-3 indices are raised by regular consumption of the enriched products, which also proved to have clinically relevant reductions in blood pressure (Stanton et al., 2020).

The fortification of snack foods, bakery, and beverages with omega-3 fatty acids and other PUFAs causes difficulties such as oxidation, stability, and acceptability issues. Consumer acceptance and nutritional quality are usually reduced by lipid oxidation, but the development of recent technologies, such as encapsulation techniques and antioxidant strategies, has effectively reduced these effects (Jacobsen, 2010; Ren et al., 2013). Remarkably, the stability of omega-3-enriched eggs with antioxidants has increased during cooking and storage, showing enhancement in technical solutions for fortification of PUFA (Ren et al., 2013). Global and national fortification programs largely encourage PUFA fortified foods to tackle omega-3 deficiency diseases such as developmental, cardiovascular, and inflammatory diseases. Due to ecological issues and fewer fish source stocks, alternative and sustainable PUFA sources, namely marine bacteria and fungi like *M. alpina*, have been discovered to hold up ongoing fortification programs (Moi et al., 2018; Sakuradani, 2010). Antiinflammatory effects, neuroprotection, and antibacterial properties are the major functional benefits of PUFA sources, which emphasize the significance of a fortification approach (Denis et al., 2015; Huang & Ebersole, 2010). Global and national efforts highlight the enhancement of dietary omega-3 intake via such fortified products to alleviate key public health concerns related to PUFA deficiencies (Metcalf et al., 2003).

36.5.2 Bioavailability and stability challenges

PUFA, particularly omega-3 PUFAs, are highly recommended for health benefits, including cardioprotective, neuroprotective, and metabolic advantages (Shahidi & Ambigaipalan, 2018). On the other hand, the integration of foods with PUFAs poses stability and bioavailability challenges mainly due to their chemical and structural integrity. The major challenge in PUFA fortification is that it is prone to oxidation as it contains many double bonds, building them highly susceptible to sudden oxidation on exposure to heat, light, and oxygen during processing, transportation, and storage.

Due to oxidation, in fortified foods, there will be development of off-flavors, off-odors, and degradation in nutritional quality, which may limit the shelf life and consumer acceptance (Venugopalan et al., 2021; Homroy et al., 2023). Furthermore, the complication in incorporating PUFAs, which have low water solubility, into aqueous food matrices, which in turn minimizes the absorption in the gastrointestinal tract. The reduced bioavailability results from low dissolution and absorption in the digestive system, constraining the benefits that these fatty acids can carry upon consumption. To overcome these issues, novel techniques such as encapsulation and emulsification can be used. Encapsulation engrosses integrating PUFAs into micro and nano-size binders such as liposomes, emulsions, and hydrogels from food-grade materials. These encapsulated PUFAs are protected from oxidative damage by developing barriers against oxygen and light, masking off-flavors, and improving solubility in aqueous environments. In addition, encapsulation also promotes enhanced absorption and bioavailability by providing improved contact and uptake of PUFAs at the intestinal epithelium (Gill et al., 2024; Venugopalan et al., 2021; Jurić et al., 2020; Homroy et al., 2023).

Nanoencapsulation techniques, such as the use of metal-organic frameworks, have better results for enhanced stability and controlled release of PUFAs, which can improve their beneficial effects related to therapeutics and minimize adverse effects from oxidation (Gill et al., 2024). Moreover, handling, storage stability, and shelf life can be increased by spray drying the oils into powder and by making PUFA fortification more reliable for different food system applications (Venugopalan et al., 2021). Dietary composition, absorption mechanisms, and molecular form play a major role in making the PUFAs enhance bioavailability in the gastrointestinal tract. Diets loaded with omega-3 PUFAs can transform fatty acid absorption patterns by tailoring the circulation and inhibitory effects on saturated fat absorption, which improve their bioavailability (Yang et al., 2017).

36.5.3 Innovations in food product development

EPA and DHA play an important role in the development of the neurological system, regulation of the immune system, and cardiovascular health (Kapoor et al., 2021). PUFA fortified foods provide potential benefits regarding school feeding programs and elderly nutrition. Requirements of PUFAs for the development of brain and cognitive function are essential in children. Various studies emphasize the significance of sufficient consumption of PUFA in childhood to maintain neuronal growth and minimize the risks of attention deficit hyperactivity disorder (ADHD). The children with ADHD have resulted in taking a lesser amount of PUFA sources (Fuentes-Albero et al., 2019; Lattka et al., 2012).

Certain studies have been verified to boost the consumption efficiency and enhance the blood and tissue PUFA levels in the general population due to the uptake of PUFA-fortified foods such as milk, margarine, sausages, and eggs (Metcalf et al., 2003). Age-associated declines in cognitive, cardiovascular, and inflammatory health associated with elderly people are combated with PUFA supplements. Cell membrane integrity, modulating inflammatory responses, and metabolic functions can be maintained with long-chain PUFA, which are essential in elderly nutrition to minimize the menace of chronic diseases and improve the quality of life (Kapoor et al., 2021). The challenge in the emergence of PUFA fortified foods affects the palatability mostly, as fish oil can bring undesirable fishy flavors, which in turn are minimized by advanced purification techniques, making them acceptable among all age groups, including children and the elderly (Ganesan et al., 2013).

36.6 Socioeconomic and policy implications of polyunsaturated fatty acid-enriched interventions

PUFA-enriched interventions have become a vital strategy to improve population health outcomes. This global rise will prevent NCDs and reduce the persistent burden of malnutrition (Ola et al., 2025; Rajeev et al., 2025). Beyond their physiological importance, PUFA-enriched interventions carry significant policy and socioeconomic relevance. The global nutrition has led to increased consumption of processed foods high in saturated and trans fats. Subsequently, improving the quality of dietary fat has become a major public health priority (Kotzaoglan, 2026).

Replacing unhealthy fat with omega-3 and omega-6 fatty acids provides an evidence-based approach to minimize diseases like CVD, type-2 diabetes, and other diet-related NCD (Tayebi-Khorrami et al., 2025). At the same time, providing appropriate consumption of PUFA among vulnerable populations like pregnant women, infants, and low-income communities can help to address the awareness of essential fatty acid deficiencies (Valle-Valdez et al., 2025). They can address the effects of the deficiency that can contribute to impaired growth, weakened immunity, and poor cognitive outcomes. Therefore, integrating PUFA-focused strategies into nutrition policies, food systems planning, and health promotion programs offers a dual benefit (Westheim et al., 2023). It can oppose both undernutrition and overnutrition while promoting long-term economic productivity and sustainable development. As shown in Table 36.2,

TABLE 36.2 Socioeconomic and policy implications of polyunsaturated fatty acid (PUFA)-enriched interventions.

Theme	Focus	Health impact	Economic and policy significance	References
Cost-effectiveness	Fortification, supplementation, and dietary diversification	Reduced cardiovascular disease risk and improved neurodevelopment	Lower healthcare costs; supports preventive health strategies	Al-Ewaidat et al. (2025)
Malnutrition and NCD prevention	Maternal-child programs: replacing saturated and trans fats	Reduced stunting; improved immunity; lower coronary heart disease risk	Long-term human capital gains; reduced NCD burden	Rajeev et al. (2025)
Global and national policies	Fat intake guidelines; food reformulation; labeling laws	Improved dietary fat quality	Alignment with WHO and Food and Agriculture Organization recommendations	Valle-Valdez et al. (2025)
Equity in access	Subsidies, social protection, and culturally appropriate diets	Reduced nutrition disparities	Promotes inclusive public health strategies	Westheim et al. (2023)
Sustainable production	Fisheries, aquaculture, oilseed diversification, and algae sources	Stable PUFA supply; environmental sustainability	Supports blue economy; agricultural subsidy reforms	Westheim et al. (2023)

PUFA-enriched interventions have substantial economic and health implications, ranging from reduced cardiovascular risk to sustainable production strategies.

36.6.1 Cost-effectiveness of polyunsaturated fatty acid-enriched interventions

PUFA-enriched interventions are widely regarded as cost-effective strategies in public health. They emphasize disease prevention rather than exclusive clinical treatment. By improving the quality of dietary fat, particularly through increasing the intake of omega-3 and omega-6, it helps to decrease the risk of CVD (Sadeghi et al., 2025). Nutrition-based preventive strategies offer a more viable and cost-efficient model for health systems. Food fortification and targeted supplementation programs further improve cost-effectiveness (Borpatra & Saikia, 2025). When integrating into the existing food production systems, the addition of PUFAs to commonly consumed foods such as cooking oils, dairy products, and infant formulas involves relatively low marginal cost (Trujillo-Cayado et al., 2025). Supplemental programs that enhance immunological functions, visual acuity, and cognitive development for pregnant women and young children provide substantial returns on investment. These benefits reduce future healthcare expenditures and help to improve educational performance and workforce productivity (Purkiewicz et al., 2025).

Based on the socioeconomic perspective, investing in PUFA-enriched interventions strengthens human capital development (Li, Wang, et al., 2025). The risk of mortality and disability can be reduced through these interventions. This enhances the neurodevelopment in early childhood and supports long-term economic participation. Governments are placing greater emphasis on preventive healthcare models. Incorporating PUFA-focused strategies into national nutrition and health policies represents a financially viable approach that yields substantial economic health benefits (Gutierres et al., 2025).

36.6.2 Role in addressing malnutrition and noncommunicable diseases NCDs

PUFAs play a critical twin role in opposing both undernutrition and NCDs (Leziak et al., 2025). In underdeveloped countries, diets are heavily reliant on staple carbohydrates and often lack dietary diversity. This is mainly due to the deficiencies in essential fatty acids, which can weaken our immune systems, impair growth, and hinder cognitive development in children (Candra & Handini, 2025). The implementation of PUFA-rich foods from fish, nuts, seeds, and fortified products into maternal and child nutrition programs establishes educational programs for people to learn about these nutritional deficiencies. The study shows that using this method will lead to better brain development results and increased health benefits for infants (Ahmad et al., 2025).

The primary global health threat stems from NCDs, which PUFAs can both prevent and treat. The replacement of saturated and trans fats with PUFAs brings multiple health advantages, which include better lipid profiles, decreased systemic inflammation, and reduced chances of developing CVD, hypertension, and type-2 diabetes (Nuriddinov et al., 2025). Omega-3 fatty acid consumption will lead to better heart health, reduced triglyceride levels, and improved endothelial function. Various programs have been established to educate pregnant women and parents of infants and children about the need to prevent fatty acid deficiencies. The process will help develop cardiovascular systems and metabolic functions throughout a person's entire life. The application of PUFA interventions produces actual health improvements because they serve as verified medical methods for enhancing public health (Ashraf, 2025).

36.6.3 Policies promoting polyunsaturated fatty acid-rich diets

Both global and national policies play a vital role in promoting the consumption of PUFA-rich diets to enhance population health outcomes. International organizations such as the WHO and the Food and Agriculture Organization provide evidence-based dietary guidelines (Vargas et al., 2025). These guidelines require the use of PUFA to replace saturated and trans fats. Foods rich in omega-3 and omega-6 fatty acids, such as fatty fish, nuts, seeds, and fortified oils, can be relatively expensive or limited in availability. There are several additional factors, such as socioeconomic disparities, geographic location, and cultural dietary practices, that can influence the consumption of these foods (Jayasinghe et al., 2025). Women, children, and marginalized groups are particularly vulnerable to inadequate intake of PUFA, which may cause health inequalities. To address these problems, awareness programs such as targeted policy interventions and social protection initiatives. For example, anganwadi centers or nongovernment organizations can help to distribute PUFA-rich foods (Hirani et al., 2025). They can include fortified products in school meals and provide awareness classes that integrate both maternal and child nutrition programs.

36.6.4 Incentives and subsidies for sustainable polyunsaturated fatty acid production

Sustainable production systems that achieve nutritional targets through their environmental and economic impacts will establish permanent PUFA-rich food sources, which require sustainable production systems to maintain their supply. Marine fish serve as the main source of EPA and DHA, which face permanent dangers because of overfishing and ecosystem destruction (Dhillon, 2025). The solution demands that governments create economic incentives that promote sustainable fisheries management alongside their efforts to develop aquaculture systems. The method guarantees ongoing access to PUFA-rich seafood products. The world needs sustainable methods to produce omega-3 through algae-based systems, which fulfill the increasing global demand. The agricultural sector requires that governments provide financial support to farmers who grow oilseed crops, which include flaxseed, canola, and soybean, because this subsidy will help increase domestic omega-3 and omega-6 fatty acid production (Mustafa et al., 2025). Biofortification represents this practice. The fatty acid content of essential crops will improve through these methods, which help create a permanent supply of PUFA. By encouraging sustainable production practices, governments can ensure long-term access to essential fatty acids while simultaneously promoting economic development and ecological resilience.

36.7 Future prospects and research directions

Many clinical and research studies collectively prove that PUFAs, mainly omega-3 fatty acids, support the nutritional significance and therapeutic potential. Genetic engineering and synthetic biology have emerged recently to reduce the variations that represent the next phase in PUFA science. Long-chain omega-3 fatty acids such as EPA and DHA are mainly obtained from marine fish. But marine ecosystems face issues such as overfishing, marine pollution, and loss of biodiversity. To address this issue, transgenic *Camelina sativa* has been reported to possess the ability to accumulate significant levels of EPA and DHA in seed oils. This plant offers a suitable alternative to fish-derived oils (Ruiz-Lopez et al., 2013; Napier et al., 2020). Synthetic biology approaches are emerging as new techniques in PUFA research. It has been shown that the optimization of PUFA yield can be enhanced through modifications in pathways and control in metabolism in modified microalgae and yeast strains. These strategies are reported to reduce the dependence on marine biodiversity and also make the industrial production under controlled environments possible (Xie et al., 2015).

Climatic conditions in various regions can remain a new challenge for PUFA supply chains. Modifications in ocean temperature and agricultural conditions can interrupt fatty acid composition in plants and marine sources. Thus, future research may focus on climate-resilient oilseeds and algae cultivation to regulate fatty acid composition. Algae cultivation in controlled photo-bioreactors helps to reduce the dependence on staple crops for PUFA composition (Borowitzka, 2013). PUFA production through microbial fermentation is emerging as a new technique in PUFA research. EPA and DHA can be produced on an industrial scale by microorganisms, which can result in good quality, traceability, and low contamination. Further, encapsulation technologies like nanoencapsulation improve PUFA stability, bioavailability, and shelf life in nutraceuticals (Jacobsen, 2010). Thus, the chances for oxidative degradation in PUFA can be reduced efficiently by these advanced methodologies. Also, the food systems should be designed by scientists and technologists to balance affordability, as an imbalance in omega-3 and omega-6 fatty acids at the population level can be related to chronic inflammatory issues (Simopoulos, 2016).

Next, personalized nutrition is a recent trend in the processing of PUFA-enriched foods. Glaser et al. (2011) state that genetic variations in fatty acid desaturase genes can influence an individual's ability to convert ALA into EPA and DHA. Understanding these issues can lead to formulating dietary recommendations based on metabolism. Many digital health technologies can support PUFA management individually. Advancements like wearing biosensors, diet tracking applications, and AI-driven nutritional platforms allow monitoring of the daily dietary intake of PUFA. These ways can help people regulate omega-3 intake for heart health, neural function, and inflammatory responses. Watson et al. (2018) report that research evidence suggests that there are interactions between gut microbes and the metabolism of fatty acids that can help in regulating PUFA recommendations.

36.8 Conclusion

PUFA has gained immense prevalence in research and industry sectors in the past decades due to health benefits, in enabling support for chronic diseases, physiological disorders, and adaptation to sustainable food systems. Various sources of PUFA, in terms of oils, including plants, oil seeds, algal and microbial origin, and other novel techniques, are vastly researched for PUFA enrichment. This will help overcome the excessive exploitation of natural marine resources.

Incorporation of PUFA in foods and beverages and other functional foods is improved by emulsion and encapsulation techniques. Consumer acceptance is a vital factor that influences the PUFA-enriched product's success in the food systems. Optimization of sensory analysis with a wide range of trials with varied composition of participants will be helpful to mitigate the challenges in the real-time industry. Shelf-life improvement, along with prevention against rancidity and off-flavor are also crucial to maintaining the product stability. Therefore, PUFA incorporation in the food systems is transitioning worldwide towards nutritional, healthier, and sustainable foods.

References

Ahmad, M. F., Alsayegh, A. A., Khanam, A., Ahmed, A., Raposo, A., Bantun, F., Zeyaullah, M., Babalghith, A. O., Aldairi, A. F., Mozaffar, B., Bajahzer, M. F., Abdelrahman, M. H., & Alam, M. I. (2025). Efficacy of omega-3 fatty acids as a functional food: A multifaceted approach to health reinforcement. *Journal of the Science of Food and Agriculture*. https://doi.org/10.1002/jsfa.70346, http://onlinelibrary.wiley.com/journal/10.1002/(ISSN)1097-0010.

Alberghini, L., Truant, A., Santonicola, S., Colavita, G., & Giaccone, V. (2023). Microplastics in fish and fishery products and risks for human health: A review. *International Journal of Environmental Research and Public Health, 20*(1), 789. https://doi.org/10.3390/ijerph20010789.

Al-Ewaidat, Ola A., Gogia, S., & Naffaa, M. M. (2025). Omega-3 PUFAs: a multifaceted approach to lifespan brain health, neurodevelopment, and precision therapeutics with implications for ASD, ADHD, and cognitive function. *Diseases & Research, 5*(2), 77–99. https://doi.org/10.54457/dr.202501005.

Albert, C. M., Campos, H., Stampfer, M. J., Ridker, P. M., Manson, J. E., Willett, W. C., Ma, J., et al. (2002). Blood levels of long-chain n–3 fatty acids and the risk of sudden death. *New England Journal of Medicine, 346*(15), 1113–1118. https://doi.org/10.1056/nejmoa012918.

Arora, N., Patel, A., Sharma, M., Mehtani, J., Pruthi, P. A., Pruthi, V., & Poluri, K. M. (2017). Insights into the enhanced lipid production characteristics of a fresh water microalga under high salinity conditions. *Industrial and Engineering Chemistry Research, 56*(25), 7413–7421. https://doi.org/10.1021/acs.iecr.7b00841, http://pubs.acs.org/journal/iecred.

Ashraf, S. A. (2025). Food fortification as a sustainable global strategy to mitigate micronutrient deficiencies and improve public health. *Discover Food, 5*(1). https://doi.org/10.1007/s44187-025-00512-5, https://www.springer.com/journal/44187.

Attia, Y. A., Al-Harthi, M. A., Korish, M. A., & Shiboob, M. M. (2017). Fatty acid and cholesterol profiles, hypocholesterolemic, atherogenic, and thrombogenic indices of broiler meat in the retail market. *Lipids in Health and Disease, 16*(1). https://doi.org/10.1186/s12944-017-0423-8, http://www.lipidworld.com/home/.

Borowitzka, M. A. (2013). High-value products from microalgae-their development and commercialisation. *Journal of Applied Phycology, 25*(3), 743–756. https://doi.org/10.1007/s10811-013-9983-9.

Basak, S., Mallick, R., Banerjee, A., Pathak, S., & Duttaroy, A. K. (2021). Maternal supply of both arachidonic and docosahexaenoic acids is required for optimal neurodevelopment. *Nutrients, 13*(6), 2061. https://doi.org/10.3390/nu13062061.

Borpatra, P. J., & Saikia, B. S. (2025). *Zinc supplementation as a preventive measure for zinc deficiency strategies to alleviate human zinc deficiency*. India: IGI Global, 159–192. https://www.igi-global.com/book/strategies-alleviate-human-zinc-deficiency/339898, https://doi.org/10.4018/979-8-3693-5355-4.ch007.

Botta, M., Audano, M., Sahebkar, A., Sirtori, C. R., Mitro, N., & Ruscica, M. (2018). PPAR agonists and metabolic syndrome: An established role? *International Journal of Molecular Sciences, 19*(4). https://doi.org/10.3390/ijms19041197, http://www.mdpi.com/1422-0067/19/4/1197/pdf.

Calder, P. C. (2004). n-3 Fatty acids and cardiovascular disease: Evidence explained and mechanisms explored. *Clinical Science, 107*(1), 1–11. https://doi.org/10.1042/CS20040119.

Calder, P. C. (2010). Omega-3 fatty acids and inflammatory processes. *Nutrients, 2*(3), 355–374. https://doi.org/10.3390/nu2030355, http://www.mdpi.com/2072-6643/2/3/355/pdf.

Candra, A., & Handini, L. S. (2025). The relationship between stunting and body resistance to infection in children. *Journal of Diverse Medical Research: Medicosphere, 2*(3), 110–117. https://doi.org/10.33005/jdiversemedres.v2i3.93.

Chen, W., Li, T., Du, S., Chen, H., Wang, Q., et al. (2023). Microalgal polyunsaturated fatty acids: Hotspots and production techniques. *Frontiers in Bioengineering and Biotechnology, 11*. https://doi.org/10.3389/fbioe.2023.1146881.

Davis, D., Morão, A., Johnson, J. K., & Shen, L. (2021). Life cycle assessment of heterotrophic algae omega-3. *Algal Research, 60*, 102494. https://doi.org/10.1016/j.algal.2021.102494.

Das, U. N. (2021). Essential fatty acids and their metabolites in the pathobiology of inflammation and its resolution. *Biomolecules, 11*(12), 1873. https://doi.org/10.3390/biom11121873.

De Carvalho, C. C. C. R., & Caramujo, M. J. (2018). The various roles of fatty acids. *Molecules (Basel, Switzerland), 23*(10). https://doi.org/10.3390/molecules23102583, https://www.mdpi.com/1420-3049/23/10/2584/pdf.

Denis, I., Potier, B., Heberden, C., & Vancassel, S. (2015). Omega-3 polyunsaturated fatty acids and brain aging. *Current Opinion in Clinical Nutrition and Metabolic Care, 18*(2), 139–146. https://doi.org/10.1097/mco.0000000000000141.

Derbyshire, E. (2019). Oily fish and omega-3s across the life stages: A focus on intakes and future directions. *Frontiers in Nutrition, 6*. https://doi.org/10.3389/fnut.2019.00165.

Deville, A., Vázquez-Rowe, I., Avadí, A., Miranda, F., & Kahhat, R. (2025). Identifying current trends in the environmental impacts linked to fishmeal and fish oil production in Peru. *Aquaculture, 600*, 742239. https://doi.org/10.1016/j.aquaculture.2025.742239.

Dhillon, O. (2025). *Role of omega-3-fatty acids in aquaculture feeds and their impact on human health aquaculture: Enhancing food security and nutrition*. India: Springer Science+Business Media, 245–272. https://doi.org/10.1007/978-3-031-92858-1_12.

Dorni, C., Sharma, P., Saikia, G., & Longvah, T. (2018). Fatty acid profile of edible oils and fats consumed in India. *Food Chemistry, 238*, 9–15. https://doi.org/10.1016/j.foodchem.2017.05.072.

Duan, H., Song, W., Zhao, J., & Yan, W. (2023). Polyunsaturated fatty acids (PUFAs): Sources, digestion, absorption, application and their potential adjunctive effects on visual fatigue. *Nutrients, 15*(11), 2633. https://doi.org/10.3390/nu15112633.

Eungrasamee, K., Incharoensakdi, A., Lindblad, P., & Jantaro, S. (2020). Synechocystis sp. PCC 6803 overexpressing genes involved in CBB cycle and free fatty acid cycling enhances the significant levels of intracellular lipids and secreted free fatty acids. *Scientific Reports, 10*(1). https://doi.org/10.1038/s41598-020-61100-4.

EFSA Panel on Dietetic Products, Nutrition and Allergies (NDA). (2012). Scientific opinion on dietary reference values for fats, including saturated fatty acids, polyunsaturated fatty acids, monounsaturated fatty acids, trans fatty acids, and cholesterol. *EFSA Journal, 10*(3), 2815.

Fradique, M., Batista, A. P., Nunes, M. C., Gouveia, L., Bandarra, N. M., & Raymundo, A. (2010). Incorporation of *Chlorella vulgaris* and *Spirulina maxima* biomass in pasta products. Part 1: Preparation and evaluation. *Journal of the Science of Food and Agriculture, 90*(10), 1656–1664. https://doi.org/10.1002/jsfa.3999Portugal, http://www3.interscience.wiley.com/cgi-bin/fulltext/123438086/PDFSTART.

Frydrych, A., Kulita, K., Jurowski, K., & Piekoszewski, W. (2025). Lipids in clinical nutrition and health: Narrative review and dietary recommendations. *Foods, 14*(3), 473. https://doi.org/10.3390/foods14030473.

Fuentes-Albero, M., Martínez-Martínez, M. I., & Cauli, O. (2019). Omega-3 long-chain polyunsaturated fatty acids intake in children with attention deficit and hyperactivity disorder. *Brain Sciences, 9*(5), 120. https://doi.org/10.3390/brainsci9050120.

Ganesan, B., Brothersen, C., McMahon, D. J., et al. (2013). Fortification of foods with omega-3 polyunsaturated fatty acids. *Critical Reviews in Food Science and Nutrition, 54*(1), 98–114. https://doi.org/10.1080/10408398.2011.578221.

Gill, R., Al-Badr, M., Alghouti, M., Mohamed, N. A., Abou-Saleh, H., & Rahman, M. M. (2024). Revolutionizing cardiovascular health with nano encapsulated omega-3 Fatty Acids: A nano-solution approach. *Marine Drugs, 22*(6). https://doi.org/10.3390/md22060256, http://www.mdpi.com/journal/marinedrugs.

Gutierres, D., Pacheco, R., Reis, C. P., et al. (2025). The role of omega-3 and omega-6 polyunsaturated fatty acid supplementation in human health. *Foods, 14*(19), 3299. https://doi.org/10.3390/foods14193299.

Glaser, C., Lattka, E., Rzehak, P., Steer, C., Koletzko, B., et al. (2011). Genetic variation in polyunsaturated fatty acid metabolism and its potential relevance for human development and health. *Maternal & Child Nutrition, 7*(s2), 27–40. https://doi.org/10.1111/j.1740-8709.2011.00319.x.

Geetha, P., Bharathi, D., Deepa, N., Gopi, G., Begum, S., & Devi, T. (2025). Effectiveness of alpha lipoic acid in type 2 diabetes mellitus patients with cardiac autonomic neuropathy. *Research Journal of Science and Technology*, 286–288. https://doi.org/10.52711/2231-5713.2025.00043.

Harayama, T., & Antonny, B. (2023). Beyond fluidity: The role of lipid unsaturation in membrane function. *Cold Spring Harbor Perspectives in Biology, 15*(7), a041409. https://doi.org/10.1101/cshperspect.a041409.

Hergenrader, A., VanOrmer, M., Slotkowski, R., Thompson, M., Freeman, A., Paetz, O., Sweeney, S., Wegner, L., Ali, K., Bender, N., Chaudhary, R., Thoene, M., Hanson, C., & Anderson-Berry, A. (2023). Omega-3 polyunsaturated fatty acid levels in maternal and cord plasma are associated with maternal socioeconomic status. *Nutrients, 15*(20), 4432. https://doi.org/10.3390/nu15204432.

Hirani, K., Sundheim, B., Blaschke, M., Lemos, J. R. N., & Mittal, R. (2025). A global call to action: Strengthening strategies to combat dysglycemia and improve public health outcomes. *Frontiers in Public Health, 13*. https://doi.org/10.3389/fpubh.2025.1597128.

Hooks, M. P., Madigan, S. M., Woodside, J. V., & Nugent, A. P. (2023). Dietary intake, biological status, and barriers towards omega-3 intake in elite level (Tier 4), female athletes: Pilot study. *Nutrients, 15*(13). https://doi.org/10.3390/nu15132821, http://www.mdpi.com/journal/nutrients/.

Howell, G., Deng, X., Yellaturu, C., Park, E. A., Wilcox, H. G., Raghow, R., & Elam, M. B. (2009). N-3 polyunsaturated fatty acids suppress insulin-induced SREBP-1c transcription via reduced trans-activating capacity of LXRα *Biochimica et Biophysica Acta - Molecular and Cell Biology of Lipids, 1791*(12), 1190–1196. https://doi.org/10.1016/j.bbalip.2009.08.008.

Homroy, S., Chopra, R., Singh, P. K., Dhiman, A., Chand, M., & Talwar, B. (2023). Role of encapsulation on the bioavailability of omega-3 fatty acids. *Comprehensive Reviews in Food Science and Food Safety, 23*(1). https://doi.org/10.1111/1541-4337.13272.

Huang, C. B., & Ebersole, J. L. (2010). A novel bioactivity of omega-3 polyunsaturated fatty acids and their ester derivatives. *Molecular Oral Microbiology, 25*(1), 75–80. https://doi.org/10.1111/j.2041-1014.2009.00553.x.

Hulbert, A. J., Turner, N., Storlien, L. H., & Else, P. L. (2005). Dietary fats and membrane function: Implications for metabolism and disease. *Biological Reviews of the Cambridge Philosophical Society, 80*(1), 155–169. https://doi.org/10.1017/S1464793104006578.

Jacobsen, C. (2010). Enrichment of foods with omega-3 fatty acids: A multidisciplinary challenge. *Annals of the New York Academy of Sciences, 1190*(1), 141–150. https://doi.org/10.1111/j.1749-6632.2009.05263.x.

Jayasinghe, S., Byrne, N. M., & Hills, A. P. (2025). Cultural influences on dietary choices. *Progress in Cardiovascular Diseases, 90*, 22–26. https://doi.org/10.1016/j.pcad.2025.02.003.

Jimbo, H., Yuasa, K., Takagi, K., Hirashima, T., Keta, S., Aichi, M., & Wada, H. (2021). Specific incorporation of polyunsaturated fatty acids into the sn-2 position of phosphatidylglycerol accelerates photodamage to photosystem II under strong light. *International Journal of Molecular Sciences, 22*(19), 10432. https://doi.org/10.3390/ijms221910432.

Jovanovic, S., Dietrich, D., Becker, J., Kohlstedt, M., & Wittmann, C. (2021). Microbial production of polyunsaturated fatty acids—high-value ingredients for aquafeed, superfoods, and pharmaceuticals. *Current Opinion in Biotechnology, 69*, 199–211. https://doi.org/10.1016/j.copbio.2021.01.009.

Jurić, S., Jurić, M., Siddique, M. A. B., Fathi, M., et al. (2020). Vegetable oils rich in polyunsaturated fatty acids: nanoencapsulation methods and stability enhancement. *Food Reviews International, 38*(1), 32–69. https://doi.org/10.1080/87559129.2020.1717524.

Kapoor, B., Kapoor, D., Gautam, S., Singh, R., & Bhardwaj, S. (2021). Dietary polyunsaturated fatty acids (pufas): uses and potential health benefits. *Current Nutrition Reports, 10*(3), 232–242. https://doi.org/10.1007/s13668-021-00363-3.

Kang, J. X. (2011). Omega-3: A link between global climate change and human health. *Biotechnology Advances, 29*(4), 388–390. https://doi.org/10.1016/j.biotechadv.2011.02.003.

Kalupahana, N. S., Claycombe, K. J., & Moustaid-Moussa, N. (2011). (n-3) fatty acids alleviate adipose tissue inflammation and insulin resistance: mechanistic insights. *Advances in Nutrition, 2*(4), 304–316. https://doi.org/10.3945/an.111.000505.

Kothri, M., Mavrommati, M., Elazzazy, A. M., Baeshen, M. N., Moussa, T. A. A., & Aggelis, G. (2020). Microbial sources of polyunsaturated fatty acids (PUFAs) and the prospect of organic residues and wastes as growth media for PUFA-producing microorganisms. *FEMS Microbiology Letters, 367*(5). https://doi.org/10.1093/femsle/fnaa028, http://femsle.oxfordjournals.org/.

Khozin-Goldberg, I., Iskandarov, U., Cohen, Z., et al. (2011). LC-PUFA from photosynthetic microalgae: occurrence, biosynthesis, and prospects in biotechnology. *Applied Microbiology and Biotechnology, 91*(4), 905–915. https://doi.org/10.1007/s00253-011-3441-x.

Kotzaoglan, R. (2026). Nutritional risk factors related to non-communicable diseases in the world. *Developments and Experiments in Health and Medicine, 40*(1), 1–14. https://doi.org/10.18614/dehm.1873505.

Kumari, P., Sharma, J., Khare, P., et al. (2025). Recent advancements and strategies for omega-3 fatty acid production in yeast. *Journal of Basic Microbiology, 65*(3). https://doi.org/10.1002/jobm.202400491.

Lanier, K., Wisseman, B., Strom, C., Johnston, C. A., Isler, C., DeVente, J., Newton, E., Pawlak, R., Allman-Tucker, B. R., McDonald, S., & May, L. E. (2023). Self-reported intake and circulating epa and dha concentrations in US pregnant women. *Nutrients, 15*(7). https://doi.org/10.3390/nu15071753, http://www.mdpi.com/journal/nutrients/.

Lattka, E., Klopp, N., Demmelmair, H., Klingler, M., Heinrich, J., Koletzko, B., et al. (2012). Genetic variations in polyunsaturated fatty acid metabolism – implications for child health? *Annals of Nutrition and Metabolism, 60*(Suppl. 3), 8–17. https://doi.org/10.1159/000337308.

Leziak, A., Lipina, J., Reclik, M., & Kocelak, P. (2025). Dietary modulation of metabolic health: From bioactive compounds to personalized nutrition. *Metabolites, 15*(9), 624. https://doi.org/10.3390/metabo15090624.

Li, J., Lin, Y. C. D., Zuo, H. L., Huang, H. Y., Zhang, T., Bai, J. W., & Huang, H. D. (2025). Dietary omega-3 PUFAs in metabolic disease research: A decade of omics-enabled insights (2014–2024). *Nutrients, 17*(11). https://doi.org/10.3390/nu17111836, http://www.mdpi.com/journal/nutrients/.

Li, R., Wang, Y., Xu, J., Yu, J., & Li, B. (2025). Effects of n-3 polyunsaturated fatty acid supplementation on cardiovascular indices in type 2 diabetes: A meta-analysis of randomized controlled trials. *Reviews in Cardiovascular Medicine, 26*(2). https://doi.org/10.31083/RCM25882, https://www.imrpress.com/journal/RCM/26/2.

Liu, Y., Ren, X., Fan, C., Wu, W., Zhang, W., & Wang, Y. (2022). Health benefits, food applications, and sustainability of microalgae-derived N-3 PUFA. *Foods, 11*(13), 1883. https://doi.org/10.3390/foods11131883.

Mallick, R., Basak, S., Das, R. K., Banerjee, A., Paul, S., Pathak, S., & Duttaroy, A. K. (2024). Fatty acids and their proteins in adipose tissue inflammation. *Cell Biochemistry and Biophysics, 82*(1), 35–51. https://doi.org/10.1007/s12013-023-01185-6, https://www.springer.com/journal/12013.

Majhi, P., Mohanty, M. K., & Samantaray, S. M. (2022). Biosynthesis of polyunsaturated fatty acids from microalgae for nutraceuticals. In *Advances in agricultural and industrial microbiology: Volume 1: Microbial Diversity and Application in Agroindustry*. Springer Nature Singapore, 205–216. https://doi.org/10.1007/978-981-16-8918-5_11.

Manson, J. A. E., Cook, N. R., Lee, I. M., Christen, W., Bassuk, S. S., Mora, S., Gibson, H., Gordon, D., Copeland, T., D'Agostino, D., Friedenberg, G., Ridge, C., Bubes, V., Giovannucci, E. L., Willett, W. C., & Buring, J. E. (2019). Vitamin D supplements and prevention of cancer and cardiovascular disease. *New England Journal of Medicine, 380*(1), 33–44. https://doi.org/10.1056/NEJMoa1809944, http://www.nejm.org/medical-index.

Martins, D., Custódio, L., Barreira, L., Pereira, H., Ben-Hamadou, R., Varela, J., & Abu-Salah, K. (2013). Alternative sources of n-3 long-chain polyunsaturated fatty acids in marine microalgae. *Marine Drugs, 11*(7), 2259–2281. https://doi.org/10.3390/md11072259.

Metcalf, R. G., James, M. J., Mantzioris, E., & Cleland, L. G. (2003). A practical approach to increasing intakes of n-3 polyunsaturated fatty acids: Use of novel foods enriched with n-3 fats. *European Journal of Clinical Nutrition, 57*(12), 1605–1612. https://doi.org/10.1038/sj.ejcn.1601731.

Michaeloudes, C., Christodoulides, S., Christodoulou, P., Kyriakou, T.-C., Patrikios, I., & Stephanou, A. (2023). Variability in the clinical effects of the omega-3 polyunsaturated fatty acids DHA and EPA in cardiovascular disease—possible causes and future considerations. *Nutrients, 15*(22), 4830. https://doi.org/10.3390/nu15224830.

Mititelu, M., Lupuliasa, D., Neacşu, S. M., Olteanu, G., Busnatu, S. S., Mihai, A., Popovici, V., Măru, N., Boroghină, S. C., Mihai, S., Ioniță-Mîndrican, C.-B., & Scafa-Udriște, A. (2024). Polyunsaturated fatty acids and human health: a key to modern nutritional balance in association with polyphenolic compounds from food sources. *Foods, 14*(1), 46. https://doi.org/10.3390/foods14010046.

Moi, I. M., Leow, A. T. C., Ali, M. S. M., Rahman, R. N. Z. R. A., Salleh, A. B., & Sabri, S. (2018). Polyunsaturated fatty acids in marine bacteria and strategies to enhance their production. *Applied Microbiology and Biotechnology, 102*(14), 5811–5826. https://doi.org/10.1007/s00253-018-9063-9, link.springer.de/link/service/journals/00253/index.htm.

Morales-Sánchez, D., Schulze, P. S. C., Kiron, V., & Wijffels, R. H. (2020). Temperature-dependent lipid accumulation in the polar marine microalga chlamydomonas malina RCC2488. *Frontiers in Plant Science, 11*. https://doi.org/10.3389/fpls.2020.619064.

Mozaffarian, D., & Wu, J. H. Y. (2011). Omega-3 fatty acids and cardiovascular disease. *Journal of the American College of Cardiology, 58*(20), 2047–2067. https://doi.org/10.1016/j.jacc.2011.06.063.

Mozaffarian, D., Micha, R., & Wallace, S. (2010). Effects on coronary heart disease of increasing polyunsaturated fat in place of saturated fat: a systematic review and meta-analysis of randomized controlled trials. *PLoS Medicine, 7*(3), e1000252. https://doi.org/10.1371/journal.pmed.1000252.

Mukerjee, S., Saeedan, A. S., Ansari, M. N., & Singh, M. (2021). Polyunsaturated fatty acids mediated regulation of membrane biochemistry and tumor cell membrane integrity. *Membranes, 11*(7). https://doi.org/10.3390/membranes11070479, https://www.mdpi.com/2077-0375/11/7/479/pdf.

Mustafa, H. S. B., Munir, H., Farah, U., Arshad, A. W., ul Hasan, E., Zahra, F., Waqar, M., Khan, B., Tahir, A., Athar, M. H., Gill, A. N., Qamar, R., Raza, M. M., & Laique, A. (2025). Enhancing global nutrition: Biofortifying oilseed crops for sustainable health. *Plant Bulletin, 4*(1), 72–87. https://doi.org/10.55627/pbulletin.004.01.927.

Napier, J. A., Haslam, R. P., Olsen, R.-E., Tocher, D. R., & Betancor, M. B. (2020). Agriculture can help aquaculture become greener. *Nature Food, 1*(11), 680–683. https://doi.org/10.1038/s43016-020-00182-9.

Neufingerl, N., & Eilander, A. (2022). Nutrient intake and status in adults consuming plant-based diets compared to meat-eaters: A systematic review. *Nutrients, 14*(1), 29. https://doi.org/10.3390/nu14010029.

Pérez-Palacios, T., Ruiz-Carrascal, J., Solomando, J. C., & Antequera, T. (2019). Strategies for enrichment in ω-3 fatty acids aiming for healthier meat products. *Food Reviews International, 35*(5), 485–503. https://doi.org/10.1080/87559129.2019.1584817, www.tandf.co.uk/journals/titles/87559129.asp.

Petermann, A. B., Reyna-Jeldes, M., Ortega, L., Coddou, C., & Yévenes, G. E. (2022). Roles of the unsaturated fatty acid docosahexaenoic acid in the central nervous system: Molecular and cellular insights. *International Journal of Molecular Sciences, 23*(10). https://doi.org/10.3390/ijms23105390, https://www.mdpi.com/1422-0067/23/10/5390/pdf?version=1652326413.

Purkiewicz, A., Regin, K. J., Mumtaz, W., & Pietrzak-Fiećko, R. (2025). Breastfeeding: The multifaceted impact on child development and maternal well-being. *Nutrients, 17*(8), 1326. https://doi.org/10.3390/nu17081326.

Rajeev, A. M., Malisetty, H., Baidya, O. P., Vamshy J, K., Siddhanta, S., & Dharan, B. G. (2025). Pediatric nutrition and its role in preventing non-communicable diseases: A review. *Cureus, 17*(7). https://doi.org/10.7759/cureus.87431.

Remize, M., Brunel, Y., Silva, J. L., Berthon, J.-Y., & Filaire, E. (2021). Microalgae n-3 PUFAs production and use in food and feed industries. *Marine Drugs, 19*(2), 113. https://doi.org/10.3390/md19020113.

Ren, Y., Perez, T. I., Zuidhof, M. J., Renema, R. A., & Wu, J. (2013). Oxidative stability of omega-3 polyunsaturated fatty acids enriched eggs. *Journal of Agricultural and Food Chemistry, 61*(47), 11595–11602. https://doi.org/10.1021/jf403039m.

Rizzo, G., Baroni, L., & Lombardo, M. (2023). Promising sources of plant-derived polyunsaturated fatty acids: a narrative review. *International Journal of Environmental Research and Public Health, 20*(3), 1683. https://doi.org/10.3390/ijerph20031683.

Ruiz-Lopez, N., Haslam, R. P., Usher, S. L., Napier, J. A., Sayanova, O., et al. (2013). Reconstitution of EPA and DHA biosynthesis in Arabidopsis: Iterative metabolic engineering for the synthesis of n–3 LC-PUFAs in transgenic plants. *Metabolic Engineering, 17*, 30–41. https://doi.org/10.1016/j.ymben.2013.03.001.

Sadeghi, R., Norouzzadeh, M., HasanRashedi, M., Jamshidi, S., Ahmadirad, H., Alemrajabi, M., Vafa, M., & Teymoori, F. (2025). Dietary and circulating omega-6 fatty acids and their impact on cardiovascular disease, cancer risk, and mortality: A global meta-analysis of 150 cohorts and meta-regression. *Journal of Translational Medicine, 23*(1). https://doi.org/10.1186/s12967-025-06336-2.

Saini, R. K., Prasad, P., Sreedhar, R. V., Naidu, K. A., Shang, X., & Keum, Y. S. (2021). Omega−3 polyunsaturated fatty acids (PUFAs): Emerging plant and microbial sources, oxidative stability, bioavailability, and health benefits—A review. *Antioxidants, 10*(10). https://doi.org/10.3390/antiox10101627, https://www.mdpi.com/2076-3921/10/10/1627/pdf.

Sakuradani, E. (2010). Advances in the production of various polyunsaturated fatty acids through oleaginous fungus *Mortierella alpina* breeding. *Bioscience, Biotechnology, and Biochemistry, 74*(5), 908–917. https://doi.org/10.1271/bbb.100001Japan, http://www.jstage.jst.go.jp/article/bbb/74/5/908/_pdf.

Sakuradani, E., Ando, A., Shimizu, S., & Ogawa, J. (2013). Metabolic engineering for the production of polyunsaturated fatty acids by oleaginous fungus *Mortierella alpina* 1S-4. *Journal of Bioscience and Bioengineering, 116*(4), 417–422. https://doi.org/10.1016/j.jbiosc.2013.04.008.

Sartorio, M. U. A., Pendezza, E., Coppola, S., Paparo, L., D'auria, E., Zuccotti, G. V., & Berni Canani, R. (2022). Potential role of omega-3 polyunsaturated fatty acids in pediatric food allergy. *Nutrients, 14*(1). https://doi.org/10.3390/nu14010152, https://www.mdpi.com/2072-6643/14/1/152/pdf.

Savatinova, M., & Ivanova, M. (2024). Functional dairy products enriched with omega-3 fatty acids. *Food Science and Applied Biotechnology, 7*(1), 1. https://doi.org/10.30721/fsab2024.v7.i1.301.

Serini, S., Fasano, E., Piccioni, E., Cittadini, A. R. M., & Calviello, G. (2011). Differential anti-cancer effects of purified epa and dha and possible mechanisms involved. *Current Medicinal Chemistry, 18*(26), 4065–4075. https://doi.org/10.2174/092986711796957310.

Seth, T., Mishra, G. P., Chattopadhyay, A., Deb Roy, P., Devi, M., Sahu, A., Sarangi, S. K., Mhatre, C. S., Lyngdoh, Y. A., Chandra, V., Dikshit, H. K., & Nair, R. M. (2025). Microgreens: Functional food for nutrition and dietary diversification. *Plants, 14*(4). https://doi.org/10.3390/plants14040526, www.mdpi.com/journal/plants.

Seves, S. M., Temme, E. H. M., Brosens, M. C. C., Zijp, M. C., Hoekstra, J., & Hollander, A. (2015). Sustainability aspects and nutritional composition of fish: evaluation of wild and cultivated fish species consumed in the Netherlands. *Climatic Change, 135*(3-4), 597–610. https://doi.org/10.1007/s10584-015-1581-1.

Shah, A. M., Yang, W., Mohamed, H., Zhang, Y., & Song, Y. (2022). Microbes: A hidden treasure of polyunsaturated fatty acids. *Frontiers in Nutrition, 9*. https://doi.org/10.3389/fnut.2022.827837, journal.frontiersin.org/journal/nutrition.

Nuriddinov, S., Bozorov, S., Abdukhalimova, S., Tsay, E., Yakubov, M., Dalimova, D., et al. (2025). Chemical transformations of vegetable oils during cooking: implications for cardiovascular diseases and type 2 diabetes. *Universum:Chemistry & biology, 128*(2). https://doi.org/10.32743/unichem.2025.128.2.19250.

Shahidi, F., & Ambigaipalan, P. (2018). Omega-3 polyunsaturated fatty acids and their health benefits. *Annual Review of Food Science and Technology, 9*, 345–381. https://doi.org/10.1146/annurev-food-111317-095850, http://www.annualreviews.org/journal/food.

Siddiqui, R., Shaikh, S., Sech, L., Yount, H., Stillwell, W., & Zaloga, G. (2004). Omega 3-fatty acids: Health benefits and cellular mechanisms of action. *Mini-Reviews in Medicinal Chemistry, 4*(8), 859–871. https://doi.org/10.2174/1389557043403431.

Simopoulos, A. (2016). An increase in the omega-6/omega-3 fatty acid ratio increases the risk for obesity. *Nutrients, 8*(3), 128. https://doi.org/10.3390/nu8030128.

Singh, M., Stark, P. C., Palmer, C. A., Gilbard, J. P., & Papas, A. S. (2010). Effect of omega-3 and vitamin e supplementation on dry mouth in patients with Sjögren's syndrome. *Special Care in Dentistry, 30*(6), 225–229. https://doi.org/10.1111/j.1754-4505.2010.00158.x.

Siscovick, D. S., Barringer, T. A., Fretts, A. M., Wu, J. H. Y., Lichtenstein, A. H., Costello, R. B., Kris-Etherton, P. M., Jacobson, T. A., Engler, M. B., Alger, H. M., Appel, L. J., & Mozaffarian, D. (2017). Omega-3 polyunsaturated fatty acid (fish oil) supplementation and the prevention of clinical cardiovascular disease. *Circulation, 135*(15). https://doi.org/10.1161/cir.0000000000000482.

Sun, K., Meesapyodsuk, D., & Qiu, X. (2024). Molecular cloning and functional analysis of a plastidial ω3 desaturase from Emiliania huxleyi. *Frontiers in Microbiology, 15*. https://doi.org/10.3389/fmicb.2024.1381097.

Stanton, A. V., James, K., Brennan, M. M., O'Donovan, F., Buskandar, F., Shortall, K., El-Sayed, T., Kennedy, J., Hayes, H., Fahey, A. G., Pender, N., Thom, S. A. M., Moran, N., Williams, D. J., & Dolan, E. (2020). Omega-3 index and blood pressure responses to eating foods naturally enriched with omega-3 polyunsaturated fatty acids: A randomized controlled trial. *Scientific Reports, 10*(1). https://doi.org/10.1038/s41598-020-71801-5, www.nature.com/srep/index.html.

Theander, E., Horrobin, D. F., Jacobsson, L. T. H., & Manthorpe, R. (2002). Gammalinolenic acid treatment of fatigue associated with primary sjögren's syndrome. *Scandinavian Journal of Rheumatology, 31*(2), 72–79. https://doi.org/10.1080/03009740252937577.

Tayebi-Khorrami, V., Fadaei, M. R., Rajabi, M. J., Askari, V. R., et al. (2025). *Handbook of public health nutrition*. Springer Nature Switzerland, 1–33. https://doi.org/10.1007/978-3-031-32047-7_61-1.

Trujillo-Cayado, L. A., Sánchez-García, R. M., García-Domínguez, I., Rodríguez-Luna, A., Hurtado-Fernández, E., & Santos, J. (2025). Emerging trends in sustainable biological resources and bioeconomy for food production. *Applied Sciences, 15*(12), 6555. https://doi.org/10.3390/app15126555.

Togarcheti, S. C., & Padamati, R. B. (2021). Comparative life cycle assessment of EPA and DHA production from microalgae and farmed fish. *Clean Technologies, 3*(4), 699–710. https://doi.org/10.3390/cleantechnol3040042.

Ulmann, L., Blanckaert, V., Mimouni, V., Andersson, M. X., Schoefs, B., & Chenais, B. (2017). Microalgal fatty acids and their implication in health and disease. *Mini-Reviews in Medicinal Chemistry, 17*(12). https://doi.org/10.2174/1389557516666160722132736.

Valle-Valdez, B., Terrazas-Lopez, X., Gonzalez-Rocha, A., Astiazaran-Garcia, H., & Armenta-Guirado, B. (2025). Dietary patterns of docosahexaenoic acid intake and supplementation from pregnancy through childhood with a focus on low- and middle-income countries: A narrative review of implications for child health. *Nutrients, 17*(24), 3931. https://doi.org/10.3390/nu17243931.

Vargas, M., Álvarez Sánchez, C., Tyler, V., & Hachem, F. (2025). Putting food at the centre of learning: An evidence-based and practice-informed model of holistic food education in schools. *The Lancet Planetary Health, 9*(11), 101219. https://doi.org/10.1016/s2542-5196(25)00033-6.

Venugopalan, V. K., Gopakumar, L. R., Kumaran, A. K., Chatterjee, N. S., Soman, V., Peeralil, S., Mathew, S., McClements, D. J., & Nagarajarao, R. C. (2021). Encapsulation and protection of omega-3-rich fish oils using food-grade delivery systems. *Foods, 10*(7). https://doi.org/10.3390/foods10071566, https://www.mdpi.com/2304-8158/10/7/1566/pdf.

Verma, M. L., Kishor, K., Sharma, D., Kumar, S., & Sharma, K. D. (2019). *Microbial production of omega-3 polyunsaturated fatty acids biotechnological production of bioactive compounds*. India: Elsevier, 293–326. http://www.sciencedirect.com/science/book/9780444643230, https://doi.org/10.1016/B978-0-444-64323-0.00010-2.

Wallace, J. M. W., McCabe, A. J., Robson, P. J., Keogh, M. K., Murray, C. A., Kelly, P. M., Márquez-Ruiz, G., McGlynn, H., Gilmore, W. S., & Strain, J. J. (2000). Bioavailability of n–3 polyunsaturated fatty acids (PUFA) in foods enriched with microencapsulated fish oil. *Annals of Nutrition and Metabolism, 44*(4), 157–162. https://doi.org/10.1159/000012839.

Watson, H., Mitra, S., Croden, F. C., Taylor, M., Wood, H. M., Perry, S. L., Spencer, J. A., Quirke, P., Toogood, G. J., Lawton, C. L., Dye, L., Loadman, P. M., & Hull, M. A. (2018). A randomised trial of the effect of omega-3 polyunsaturated fatty acid supplements on the human intestinal microbiota. *Gut, 67*(11), 1974–1983. https://doi.org/10.1136/gutjnl-2017-314968, http://gut.bmj.com/content/by/year.

Ward, O. P., & Singh, A. (2005). Omega-3/6 fatty acids: Alternative sources of production. *Process Biochemistry, 40*(12), 3627–3652. https://doi.org/10.1016/j.procbio.2005.02.020.

Westheim, A. J. F., Stoffels, L. M., Dubois, L. J., van Bergenhenegouwen, J., van Helvoort, A., Langen, R. C. J., Shiri-Sverdlov, R., & Theys, J. (2023). The modulatory effects of fatty acids on cancer progression. *Biomedicines, 11*(2). https://doi.org/10.3390/biomedicines11020280, www.mdpi.com/journal/biomedicines.

Xie, D., Jackson, E. N., & Zhu, Q. (2015). Sustainable source of omega-3 eicosapentaenoic acid from metabolically engineered Yarrowia lipolytica: from fundamental research to commercial production. *Applied Microbiology and Biotechnology, 99*(4), 1599–1610. https://doi.org/10.1007/s00253-014-6318-y.

Xu, R., Molenaar, A. J., Chen, Z., & Yuan, Y. (2025). Mode and mechanism of action of omega-3 and omega-6 unsaturated fatty acids in chronic diseases. *Nutrients, 17*(9). https://doi.org/10.3390/nu17091540, http://www.mdpi.com/journal/nutrients/.

Yang, Q., Wang, S., Ji, Y., Chen, H., Zhang, H., Chen, W., Gu, Z., & Chen, Y. Q. (2017). Dietary intake of n-3 PUFAs modifies the absorption, distribution and bioavailability of fatty acids in the mouse gastrointestinal tract. *Lipids in Health and Disease, 16*(1). https://doi.org/10.1186/s12944-016-0399-9, http://www.lipidworld.com/home/.

Yurko-Mauro, K., McCarthy, D., Rom, D., Nelson, E. B., Ryan, A. S., Blackwell, A., Salem, N., & Stedman, M. (2010). Beneficial effects of docosahexaenoic acid on cognition in age-related cognitive decline. *Alzheimer's & Dementia, 6*(6), 456–464. https://doi.org/10.1016/j.jalz.2010.01.013.

Zakaria, M. F., Mat Zaidi, F. N. A., Ahmad Kamal, A. H., Aleng, N. A., Abd Wahid, M. E., Katayama, T., & Jusoh, M. (2025). PUFA from microalgae: Challenges, factors affecting high production and industrial application. *Aquaculture and Fisheries, 10*(4), 545–555. https://doi.org/10.1016/j.aaf.2025.01.004, https://www.sciencedirect.com/science/journal/2468550X.

Zárate, R., el Jaber-Vazdekis, N., Tejera, N., Pérez, J. A., & Rodríguez, C. (2017). Significance of long chain polyunsaturated fatty acids in human health. *Clinical and Translational Medicine, 6*(1). https://doi.org/10.1186/s40169-017-0153-6.

Zettel, V., & Hitzmann, B. (2018). Applications of chia (*Salvia hispanica* L.) in food products. *Trends in Food Science & Technology, 80*, 43–50. https://doi.org/10.1016/j.tifs.2018.07.011.

Zhang, S., He, Y., Sen, B., Chen, X., Xie, Y., Keasling, J. D., & Wang, G. (2018). Alleviation of reactive oxygen species enhances PUFA accumulation in *Schizochytrium* sp. through regulating genes involved in lipid metabolism. *Metabolic Engineering Communications, 6*, 39–48. https://doi.org/10.1016/j.meteno.2018.03.002, http://www.journals.elsevier.com/metabolic-engineering-communications/.

Index

Note: Page numbers followed by "*f*" and "*t*" refer to figures and tables, respectively.

D

E

N

P

Q

R

S

T

U

V

W

Y

Z

Printed and bound by CPI Group (UK) Ltd, Croydon, CR0 4YY
14/09/2026
02216388-0017